PRECLINICAL SAFETY EVALUATION OF BIOPHARMACEUTICALS

PRECLINICAL SAFETY EVALUATION OF BIOPHARMACEUTICALS

A SCIENCE-BASED APPROACH TO FACILITATING CLINICAL TRIALS

Edited by

Joy A. Cavagnaro
Access BIO

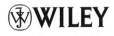

A JOHN WILEY & SONS, INC., PUBLICATION

Published by John Wiley & Sons, Inc., Hoboken, New Jersey
Published simultaneously in Canada

For general information on our other products and services or for technical support, please contact our Customer Care Department within the United States at (800) 762-2974, outside the United States at (317) 572-3993 or fax (317) 572-4002.

Wiley also publishes its books in a variety of electronic formats. Some content that appears in print may not be available in electronic formats. For more information about Wiley products, visit our web site at www.wiley.com.

Library of Congress Cataloging-in-Publication Data:

Preclinical safety evaluation of biopharmaceuticals : a science-based approach to facilitating clinical trials / [edited by] Joy A. Cavagnaro.
    p. ; cm.
  Includes bibliographical references and index.
  ISBN 978-0-470-10884-0 (cloth)
1. Pharmaceutical biotechnology—Safety measures. 2. Drugs—Testing.
I. Cavagnaro, Joy A.
  [DNLM: 1. Clinical Trials as Topic—methods. 2. Biological Products.
3. Clinical Trials as Topic—legislation & jurisprudence. 4. Drug Evaluation, Preclinical—methods. QV 771 P9228 2008]
  RS380.P74 2008
  615′.19–dc22

                                                    2007050275

Printed in the United States of America

10 9 8 7 6 5 4 3 2 1

CONTENTS

JOY A. CAVAGNARO, PhD, DABT, RAC, and ANTHONY D. DAYAN, LLB, MD, FRCP, FRCPath, FFOM, FFPM, FIBiol

Biopharmaceutical research represents the use of various biotechnology techniques to discover and manufacture potential new medicines, to test their safety, and to prove their value in treating or preventing disease in humans and animals. It employs the skills and hard work of discovery and development scientists, pharmacologists, immunologists, toxicologists, pharmacokineticists, pharmacists and manufacturers, clinical scientists, and clinical research organizations representing the public interest, healthy and patient volunteers, ethics committees, and regulatory agencies.

The public, venture capitalists, media, and even novelists have looked to biotechnology for health care solutions with high expectations. Bringing the safest possible new medicines into public use is critical for society as a whole, from human and veterinary medical and economic perspectives, and also to maintain public trust in the industry. However, no drug can ever be "100% safe." Drugs are developed and approved because they show benefits that outweigh foreseeable risks for specific indications in specific populations. Once marketed, a drug can be less safe if it is used in a way that decreases foreseeable benefits, or that increases risks if the actual risks are greater than or differ from the predicted risks. What then are the most appropriate and reasonable ways to answer the essential questions about possible risks versus benefits during the lengthy process of developing a new drug? What can be predicted from preclinical studies and of what value are the predictions?

Before testing new medicines in humans, various in vitro and in vivo preclinical studies are performed in selecting the lead candidate for clinical development. In particular, studies are designed to support a first in human (FIH) dose for phase 1 clinical trials. Phase 1 trials are principally designed to examine safety of single and sometimes several doses in about 20 to 80 study subjects, usually healthy volunteers. Phase 2 trials are designed to confirm safety, determine clinical activity, and help define an optimal dose, usually following one- to three-month dosing, for the subsequent phase 3 trials. Phase 2 are controlled studies of approximately 100 to 300 volunteer subjects with disease. Phase 3 trials are designed to prove efficacy and safety of the drug. These trials are double-blinded and placebo-controlled involving hundreds to thousands of research subjects with the intended disease in clinics and hospitals. The duration of dosing for drugs administered chronically can last six months or longer. Each phase is supported by in vivo animal studies based on consideration of the population being tested and the duration of the clinical trial. Following the completion of all three phases of clinical trials, the sponsor of the trial analyzes all the data and files a marketing application with one or more regulatory authorities. Once approved, the new medicines become available for physicians to prescribe. For some drugs the process from discovery to approval can take as long as 10 years or more. Sponsors are also required to submit periodic reports, including any cases of adverse reactions and appropriate quality control records even after a product is approved. The phase 4 or postmarketing study commitments, which may involve additional preclinical as well as clinical studies, are for evaluation of long-term effects as well as detection and definition of previously unknown or inadequately quantified adverse reactions and related risk factors.

A pre-approved capitalized cost estimate for development of a new bio-pharmaceutical has recently been estimated at over $1 billion (US dollars) with $615 million estimated for all R&D costs, including basic research and preclinical development prior to initiation of clinical testing and $626 million for clinical testing [1]. These estimates take into account the significant attrition rates over the course of clinical development.

In order to facilitate clinical development, it is important to define risk and benefit in the most reasonable and appropriate way. Preclinical studies are the foundation for the initial and ongoing assessment of potential risks and as such should be designed in order to realize their maximum value. The primary objective of preclinical safety evaluation studies is to provide data that clinical investigators can use to better predict adverse effects in study subjects and to help researchers design clinical studies that will minimize their occurrence. The same information will also help to guide research toward new, less toxic drugs and, if harmful effects cannot be entirely avoided, to suggest means to lessen or alleviate the adverse actions.

In this context the term "nonclinical" is often used interchangeably with "preclinical," particularly to define the preclinical studies performed after a product has advanced into the clinic (and thus is no longer in the preclinical development phase). Diverse studies are performed at different times to answer specific questions that only become relevant during particular phases of clinical development; for example, carcinogenicity studies are done to answer questions that ultimately arise at the end of lifetime administration to patients. Based on the explicit objective of safety studies to reveal or exclude potential adverse effects *before* they occur in healthy subjects or patients, the term "preclinical" will be used throughout this book to highlight the importance of the data to be derived *prior* to the specific clinical phase they are designed to support.

The expanding role of preclinical safety evaluation has changed the discovery/development interface for conventional small-molecule pharmaceuticals as well as large-molecule biopharmaceuticals. A larger proportion of scientific staff and resources are required to support research and screening efforts. There has been an increasing emphasis on mechanistic studies, exploratory research, and a systems biology approach to detect and investigate an expanding range of predictable and unexpected harmful effects, always with the intention of improving the predictive value of the positive and negative information obtained.

Major technological advances in platform technologies have had a major impact on the pathways and timelines of pharmaceutical development. These include high-throughput assays for profiling and probing new molecules: "omics" technologies, exposure technologies, delivery technologies, and "informatics" technologies. A number of strategies have evolved to improve the predictive value and increase the safety knowledge based including the validation and acceptance of alternative methods, in vitro cellular models, in silico techniques and animal-based simulation models, use of nontraditional animal models and animal models of disease including humanized transgenic mice, development of noninvasive and minimally invasive technologies, and increased efforts in computational toxicology and data mining have also evolved to improve predictive value and increase the safety knowledge base and provide feedback from failed and successful development programs. A practical challenge has been the prioritization and validation of these innovative technologies.

Integration and optimization of results from early evaluation models have been essential components in improving the predictive value of preclinical studies. Programs have been accelerated through innovative study designs that can incorporate efficacy, pharmacokinetics, and safety/toxicity endpoints in the same model, thus speeding the delivery of safer therapeutic and prophylactic medicines. Lead candidate selection has been advanced by the clinical exploration and acceptance of microdosing and exploratory investigational new drug application (IND) regulatory mechanisms that support early investigation of new drugs in humans based on the results of focused preclinical information sufficient to exclude unacceptable risks and obtained with limited but proportionate expenditure of time and resources. Such strategies meet the goal of hastening development without increasing risks to the subjects involved.

Conventional FIH studies designed to determine the maximum safe dosage while ensuring the greatest possible safety in healthy volunteers may not always suffice to meet clinical needs and development and financial timelines. For accelerated development plans, FIH studies should be designed not only to identify development-limiting adverse effects but to establish proof of concept or initial effectiveness, ideally this may mean studying in an index population (i.e., a disease population). Accordingly preclinical development strategies need to be designed to support early treatment of patients and seamless progress into full clinical development.

Sometimes a product will be shown not to be ready for the widespread use and must go back for refinement. It is, however, very difficult from preclinical studies or during the early stages of clinical trials to make the decision to stop or delay development because of findings that point to potentially unacceptable risks. When a product is delayed in meeting certain milestones or if it never reaches registration and marketing at all, the consequences can be devastating for the developer, particularly for small, one-product companies. The challenge of preclinical work is to be efficient and effective in order to be able to make the "no go" decision as early as possible in the process to conserve resources and gain insight for future products. This opportunity to discontinue a product's development early and to redirect research and development effort should ultimately lead to better products.

The history of drug development, especially its preclinical aspects, has been one of irregular advances, often based on ad hoc means intended to detect recent clinical problems and adverse effects and commonly based on national expertise and practices. The result was a patchwork of overlapping and even conflicting but commonly mutually exclusive data requirements in different countries. Additional barriers to facilitating clinical development have been the various multiple national and local standards and guidance that often resulted in duplication, inefficiency, and delays. By common consent this "internationally disharmonized state of drug development" slowed and inhibited the development of new treatments for rare and common diseases and led to much waste of scarce and precious resources.

It took many years but eventually careful discussions between regulatory agencies representing the public interest, drug industry, and academic experts led to a continuing international process to agree on guidelines for the different aspects of drug development. In the early 1990s the International Conference on Harmonization of Technical Requirements for Registration of Pharmaceuticals for Human Use (ICH) representing industry and regulators in the United States, Europe, and Japan was established to work on international guidelines in the areas of manufacturing (quality), preclinical evaluations (safety), and clinical evaluations (efficacy).

For small molecules, experience with conventional pharmaceuticals (new chemical entities, NCEs) has shown that relatively standardized approaches have generally been appropriate to support clinical development, but for biopharmaceuticals (novel biological entities, NBEs), scientific and clinical appreciation of their special properties has shown that it is unwise to provide detailed general guidelines applicable to every NBE because their nature, actions, and the reactions of the treated recipient differ so greatly between products and biological and clinical circumstances. Thus the broad nature of the information required to assess probable safety prior to obtaining clinical experience can be and has been defined but not the detailed procedures and investigative strategies required in providing it.

In 1997 the ICHS6 guidance on preclinical safety evaluation of biotechnology-derived products [2] introduced the concept of the "case-by-case" approach. This means that each new test article (product) or product class must have a science-based testing program custom prepared for that product based on its chemistry, pharmacology, kinetics and biological properties and effects, and its clinical indication. This strategic approach replaced naive reliance on what had been done for the last product tested. The testing program is expected to be iterative, as we should learn from and adapt testing to what has been discovered from all previous testing with the product and from advances in biological, physiological, immunological, and pathological understanding. "Science-based" means that the testing program is defendable in terms of the scientific understanding of the biological effects of the product and the testing is performed with an appropriate scientific rationale.

Preclinical safety evaluation of biopharmaceuticals has evolved through the application of scientific insight, historical and anecdotal experiences, and common sense. The scientific community has relied on the exchange of ideas among academia, industry, and regulatory scientists. However, despite the implementation of up-to-date, optimal preclinical testing strategies to assess safety and rigorous product surveillance programs in the clinic, novel biopharmaceuticals sometimes still cause unanticipated adverse clinical effects, contributing to skepticism by some as to the purpose and/or relevance of preclinical studies. It should be realized that unexpected effects may occur because of unknown changes in the product, because of unanticipated actions of the substance and individual or idiosyncratic responses by treated subjects. Tighter pharmaceutical control and better-focused preclinical studies, both guided by past experience of adverse actions, will minimize the first two risks, and cautious investigation of carefully increased doses will limit the potential harm of unusual individual responses. There can be no direct defense against idiosyncratic responses. Fortunately, they are rare, and cautious investigation of each novel substance in humans has protected us against this form of harm, as every clinical study has to balance risk to every subject against the possible benefit to the participant and to humankind in general. The value of prudently designed and conducted clinical studies is so great that they are justifiable provided that precautions are taken that reflect the nature and activities of the biopharmaceutical product and any special features of the subjects to be given it, all interpreted in the light of the basic and preclinical knowledge of the product's actions.

In a world of more fully informed patients, increased public scrutiny, and greater debate about ethics, manufacturers, developers, and regulators are demonstrating increased interest in patient welfare. Many small start-up biotech companies still enter the business to take on the challenges of producing safe and effective products to meet "unmet" medical need despite the high development costs and risk of failure. The expanded use of biotechnology in a broader range of diseases and conditions has opened a public debate about societal issues surrounding the expanded use of biotechnology, such as broadening the use of genetic testing to predict an individual's susceptibility to a particular disease, the use of stem cells for tissue regeneration, the implications of genomic and potentially transmissible changes produced by gene therapy, and the availability of allograft or xenograft organs and tissues for transplantation.

Heightened public awareness means industry must initiate interactions with regulators and their scientific and medical advisers and with public interest representatives early in development to select the most promising products, to ensure that the rationale for each project is acceptable, and to obtain agreement that the development and testing strategy will provide valid and appropriate information to justify approval of the product as a prescribable medicine. It is important for industry to understand not only the regulatory review process but also to prepare development plans that comply with the process and address particular requirements. It is equally important for regulators to provide guidance that is consistent to enable strategic planning and yet flexible enough to allow tailored development of individual therapies to meet regulatory expectations for individual companies. Industry as a whole will also have to meet their legal and other official expectations.

Creating a cooperative atmosphere and processes to maintain increased trust and easy communication between "regulators" and "industry," meaning scientists, clinicians, and industrialists, is becoming a key element in the growth and strength of the industry, which sees itself as the originator of life-saving, life-enhancing, and life-extending treatments and therapies. In the same way it is no less necessary to maintain trust and ready communication with academics and the public and their representatives and especially with regulators, whose mandate is to protect and enhance the public health.

The publication of the results of clinical trials and preclinical research has resulted in the general understanding that biopharmaceuticals can be toxic as well as beneficial in humans and animals and that many aspects of their toxicity can be studied with relevance in animals. Toxicology as a science has benefited from this experience in many ways by improved and widely applicable understanding of basic biological mechanisms of health and disease and the introduction of novel methods to detect and assess effects. Case-by-case assessment based on science encourages scientific advancement in toxicology and infuses excitement and quality research into safety assessment.

This book is intended to provide a comprehensive account of the past 20 years of biopharmaceutical preclinical development practices. Although the book was written from the viewpoint of biopharmaceutical research, development, and evaluation, the principles and concepts presented can be used for other stakeholders in the clinical research enterprise, including academic research scientists, clinical investigators, ethics committees, venture capitalists, and consultants to the pharmaceutical industry. The goal is to provide a comprehensive reference book for the preclinical discovery and development scientist whose responsibilities span target identification, lead candidate selection, pharmacokinetics, pharmacology, and toxicology and for the regulatory scientist whose responsibilities include the evaluation of novel therapies.

The scope of this book covers the entire clinical development continuum from selection of lead candidate to first-in-human studies to ultimate product approval. This book is devoted to the principles and practices of preclinical safety evaluation. It is divided into eight parts including (Part I) background, which provides definitions and methods of production of biopharmaceuticals; (Part II) discussion of the principles of ICHS6 and the global implementation of the principles; (Part III) current practices and comparisons to small molecule development; (Part IV) the importance and criteria for selection of relevant species; (Part V) a consideration of the various toxicity endpoints "icities" as they relate to biopharmaceuticals; (Part VI) specific considerations based on each product class; (Part VII) practical considerations in design, implementation, and analysis of biopharmaceuticals; and finally (Part VIII) the ultimate transition to clinical trials. The parts of the book are self-contained but may be interrelated or cross-referenced for more general or specific details.

Many new challenges in biopharmaceutical clinical development lie ahead. New technologies such as nanotechnology, microelectronics, tissue engineering, and regenerative medicine utilizing stem cells are progressing rapidly. These technologies and potential products not yet envisioned will continue to challenge toxicologists. Additional challenges and advances will come from efforts devoted to site-directed delivery or site-specific expression. Open dialogue among scientists who are regulators, academics, or who work in industry will be critical in ensuring that the new products that are safe and effective are made available without unnecessary delay. A regulatory environment that encourages innovation will make this possible. Society has a large role as a neutral facilitator of ongoing discussions and as the receiver of the benefits and risks of the new developments. The concepts, justified uses, and limitations of the new medicines must be explained and understood at all levels of the community. How toxicologists respond to the challenges ahead will influence whether we will continue to seize the opportunity to advance toxicology and enjoy medical and scientific progress or whether we will lose rigor and default to previous inefficiencies and weaknesses as it is often easier to maintain old habits than to develop and justify new approaches.

REFERENCES

1. DiMasi JA. Measuring trends in the development of new drugs: time, costs, risks and returns. SLA Pharmaceutical and Health Technology Division Spring Meeting, Boston, March 19, 2007. http://units.sla.org/division/dpht/meetings/spring2007/dimasi_2007s.ppt

2. Guidance for Industry S6 Preclinical Safety Evaluation of Biotechnology-Derived Pharmaceuticals. http://www.fda.gov/cder/guidance/index.htm

■■■■■ ACKNOWLEDGMENTS

In February of 2005 I received an invitation from Jonathan Rose, then assistant editor for sponsoring and acquisitions with Wiley's Scientific, Technical and Medical Division, to develop a book on the preclinical assessment for biopharmaceuticals. Since that time Jonathan Rose has been promoted to Editor of Wiley-Blackwell, and I have become a bit wiser in accepting such invitations in the future.

This book is a reality today because of the dedication of colleagues who accepted the invitation to participate in this comprehensive "bio-knowledge transfer mission." I thank each of them for their expert contributions and for not blocking my e-mails and phone calls during the editing process; I am much the wiser because of their efforts.

I am fortunate to have had personal experiences across the clinical development continuum. I am grateful to my academic mentors Dr. James Clegg (JC), Dr. David Holbrook, Dr. Chi-Bom Chae, and the late Dr. Michael Osband for introducing me to basic research (my first love); to my industry mentors Dr. Terry Hayes, the late Professor Gerhard Zbinden, and the late Dr. Raymond Cox for giving me an appreciation of applied research and testing in supporting the development of important new medicines; and to my regulatory mentors Dr. Carolyn Hardegree, Dr. Janet Woodcock, and Dr. Kathryn Zoon for showing me the importance of regulatory science in ensuring the availability of safe and effective new medicines.

To my "relevant" ICH S6 Expert Working Group colleagues: Professor Giuseppe Vicari, Dr. Marisa Papaluca-Amati, Dr. Jennifer Sims, Dr. Jorgen Carstensen, Dr. Wolfgang Neumann, Dr. Tohru Inoue, Dr. Mashiro Nakadate, Dr. Eliji Maki, Dr. Mutsufumi Kawai, and Dr. James Green: I do not think we would have predicted the impact or the scrutiny.

Most of all I thank my husband, Dr. Richard Lewis, and our daughters Sara, Adrianne, and Jacqueline for their unconditional love and support. I dedicate this work to them.

jc

CONTRIBUTORS

Laura Andrews, PhD, DABT, Vice President, Pharmacology and Toxicology, Genzyme, 1 Mountain Road, Framingham, MA 01701; laura.andrews@genzyme.com

Bruce Babbitt, PhD, Principal Consultant, PAREXEL Consulting, 200 West Street, Waltham, MA 02451; bruce.babbitt@parexel.com

Edward W. Bernton, MD, 3842 Garrison St. NW, Washington, DC 20016; ebernton@pathwaypharmacology.com

Timothy A. Bertram, DVM, PhD, Tengion, Inc., 3929 Westpoint Blvd., Suite G, Winston-Salem, NC 27103; tim.bertram@tengion.com

Curt W. Bradshaw, Vice President, Chemistry, 9381 Judicial Drive, Suite 200, San Diego, CA 92121; cbradshaw@covx.com

Jennifer G. Brown, PhD, Viventia Biotech Inc., 147 Hamelin Street, Winnipeg, Manitoba, Canada, R3T 3Z1; jbrown@viventia.com

Peter Bugelski, PhD, FRCPath, R-4-2, Centocor R&D, 145 King of Prussia Road, Radnor, PA 19807; pbugelsk@cntus.jnj.com

Jeanine L. Bussiere, PhD, DABT, Executive Director of Toxicology, Amgen, Inc., One Amgen Center Dr., MS 29-2-A, Thousand Oaks, CA 91320-1799; bussierj@amgen.com

Joy A. Cavagnaro, PhD, DABT, RAC, President, Access BIO, PO Box 240, Boyce, VA 22620; jcavagnaro@accessbio.com

Joel Cornacoff, DVM, PhD, DABT, Centocor R&D, 145 King of Prussia Road, Radnor, PA, 19807

Nathan Cortez, Assistant Professor of Law, Southern Methodist University, PO Box 750116, Dallas, TX 75205; ncortez@smu.edu

Mary Ellen Cosenza, PhD, MS, DABT, RAC, Executive Director, Regulatory Affairs, Amgen Inc., One Amgen Center Dr., Thousand Oaks, CA 91320; mcosenza@amgen.com

Anthony D. Dayan, LLB, MD, FRCP, FRCPath, FFOM, FFPM, FIBiol, Emeritus Professor of Toxicology, University of London, 21 Heathgate, London NW11 7AP, UK; a.dayan@toxic.u-net.com

Damon R. Demady, PhD, Director of Preclinical Development, Knopp Neurosciences Inc., and independent consultant, 2100 Wharton St. Suite 615, Pittsburgh, PA 15203; demadyd@yahoo.com

A. Marguerite Dempster, PhD, DABT, Director, Biopharmaceutical Projects, Non-clinical Safety Projects, GlaxoSmithKline Research and Development Ltd, Park Road, Ware, Herts SG12 0DP, UK; maggie.a.dempster@gsk.com

Jacques Descotes, MD, PharmD, PhD, Fellow ATS, Poison Center and Pharmacovigilance Department, Lyon University Hospitals, 162 avenue Lacassagne, 69424 Lyon cedex 03, France; jacques-georges.descotes@chu-lyon.fr

Joycelyn Entwistle, PhD, Viventia Biotech Inc., 147 Hamelin Street, Winnipeg, Manitoba, R3T 3Z1, Canada; jentwhistle@viventia.com

Werner Frings, PhD, Covance Laboratories GmbH, Kesselfeld 29, Muenster D-48163, Germany; werner.frings@covance.com

Antje Fuches, PhD, Covance Laboratories GmbH, Kesselfeld 29, Muenster D-48163, Germany; antje.fuchs@covance.com

Hanan Ghantous, PhD, DHHS/FDA/CDER/OND, Bldg. WO22, Rm 6488, Silver Spring, MD 20993

Nick Glover, PhD, Viventia Biotech Inc., 5060 Spectrum Way, Suite 405, Mississauga, ON, Canada, L4W 5N5; nglover@viventia.com

Martin D. Green, PhD, DHHS/FDA/CBER/OVRR/DVRPA, WOC 1, 2318 Rockville, MD 20852; martin.green@fda.hhs.gov

William C. Hall, VMD, PhD, DACVP, Hall Consulting, Inc., 12337 Sherwood Forest Drive, Mt. Airy, MD 21771; hallconsulting@earthlink.net

Melanie Hartsough, PhD, Senior Consultant, Biologics Consulting Group, Inc., 12526 Timber Hollow Place, Germantown, MD; mhartsough@bcg-usa.com

Richard Haworth, FRCPath, DPhil, Director, Discovery and Regulatory Pathology, GlaxoSmithKline Research and Development Ltd, Park Road, Ware, Herts SG12 0DP UK; richard.i.haworth@gsk.com

Shawn M. Heidel, DVM, PhD, Head, Nonclinical Safety Assessment, Eli Lilly and Company, Lilly Research Laboratories, PO Box 708, Greenfield, IN 46140; sheidel@lilly.com

Scott P. Henry, PhD, DABT, Isis Pharmaceuticals, Inc., 1896 Rutherford Road, Carlsbad, CA 92008; shenry@isisph.com

Christopher Horvath, DVM, MS, DACVP, Archemix Corp., 300 Third Street, Cambridge, MA 02142; chorvath@archemix.com

Ying Huang, PhD, Center for Biologics Evaluation and Research, U.S.-FDA, 1401 Rockville Pike, Suite 200N, Rockville, MD 20852-1448

David Hutto, PhD, DVM, Senior Director, Comparative Pathology, Biogen Idec, Inc., 14 Cambridge Ctr., Cambridge, MA 02142

Manuel Jayo, DVM, PhD, Tengion, Inc., 3929 Westpoint Blvd., Suite G Winston-Salem, NC 27103; manuel.jayo@tengion.com

Wim Jiskoot, PhD, Division of Drug Delivery Technology, Leiden/Amsterdam Center for Drug Research (LACDR), Leiden University, PO Box 9502, 2300 RA Leiden, The Netherlands; w.jiskoot@lacdr.leidenuniv.nl

Johan te Koppele, PhD, TNO Quality of Life, Utrechtseweg 48, Zeist, The Netherlands

David Jacobson-Kram, PhD, DABT, DHHS/FDA/CDER/OND, Bldg. WO22, Rm. 6488, Silver Spring, MD 20993; david.jacobsonkram@fda.hhs.gov

Arthur A. Levin, PhD, Biotech & Pharmaceutical Consulting, 15951 Avenida Calma, Rancho Sante Fe, CA 92091; art.levin@gmail.com

Richard M. Lewis, PhD, Chief Executive Officer, Access BIO L.C., PO Box 240, Boyce, VA 22620; rlewis@accessbio.com

Glen C. MacDonald, PhD, Viventia Biotech Inc., 147 Hamelin Street, Winnipeg, Manitoba, R3T 3Z1, Canada; gmacdonald@viventia.com

Pauline L. Martin, PhD, Centocor Research and Development, Inc., 145 King of Prussia Road, Radnor, PA 19087; pmarti27@cntus.jnj.com

Elisabeth Mertsching, PhD, Senior Scientist, Immuno Discovery Biology, Biogen Idec Inc., 14 Cambridge Ctr., Cambridge, MA 02142

Takahiro Nakazawa, PhD, Eli Lilly Japan, 7-1-5 Isogamidori, Chuo-ku, Kobe 651-0086 Japan; nakazawa@lilly.com

Michael Niehaus, PhD, Covance Laboratories GmbH, Kesselfeld 29, Muenster D-48163, Germany; michael.niehaus@covance.com

Michael O'Callaghan, DVM, PhD, MRCVS, Vice President, Preclinical Biology, Genzyme, 1 Mountain Road, Framingham, MA 01701; mike.ocallaghan@ genzyme.com

Anita Marie O'Connor, PhD, ANITA OCONNOR CONSULTING, LLC, PO Box 1750, Pinehurst, NC 28370; aoconnor728@yahoo.com

Ingrid Osterburg, PhD, Covance Laboratories GmbH, Kesselfeld 29, Muenster D-48163, Germany

Todd Page, PhD, Research Scientist, Eli Lilly and Company, Lilly Research Laboratories, PO BOX 780, Greenfield, IN 46140; pagetj@lilly.com

Rafael Ponce, PhD, DABT, Director, Safety Assessment, Preclinical Development, ZymoGenetics, Inc., 1201 Eastlake Ave. E., Seattle, WA 98102; poncer@ zgi.com, reap@zgi.com

Shari A. Price-Schiavi, PhD, DABT, Pathologist, Charles River Laboratories, Pathology Associates (PAI), Maryland, 15 Worman's Mill Court, Suite I, Frederick, MD 21701; shari.price-schiavi@us.crl.com

Theresa Reynolds, BA, DABT, Associate Director, Safety Assessment, Genentech, Inc., 1 DNA Way, South San Francisco, CA 94080; reynolds.theresa@gene. com

Nicola Rinaldi, PhD, Scientist, Biogen Idec, Inc., 14 Cambridge Ctr., Cambridge, MA 02142

Stanley A. Roberts, PhD, DABT, Vice President, Preclinical Development, 9381 Judicial Drive, Suite 200, San Diego, CA 92121; sroberts@covx.com

Jennifer L. Rojko, DVM, PhD, DACVP, Director, Molecular and Immunopathology Division, Charles River Laboratories, Pathology Associates (PAI), Maryland, 15 Worman's Mill Court, Suite I, Frederick, Maryland 21701; jennifer.rojko@us.crl.com

Peter Ryle, PhD, DipRCPath (Tox), FRCPath, PR BioServices Ltd., Ramsey St. Mary's, Huntingdon, CAMBS PE26 2SR, United Kingdom; pryle@prbio.co.uk

Clifford Sachs, PhD, DABT, Centocor R&D, 145 King of Prussia Road, Radnor, PA, 19807

Barry S. Sall, RAC, Principal Consultant, PAREXEL Consulting, 200 West Street, Waltham, MA 02451; barry.sall@parexel.com

Tanya Scharton-Kersten, Head, Regulatory Affairs, CMC and Compliance, Marburg D35041, Germany; tanya.scharton-kersten@novartis.com

Huub Schellekens, MD, PhD, Dept. of Pharmaceutical Sciences, Dept. of Innovation Studies, Utrecht University, PO Box 80.082, 3508 TB Utrecht, The Netherlands; h.schellekens@uu.nl

Mercedes A. Serabian, MS, DABT, Chief, Pharmacology/Toxicology Branch, FDA/CBER/OCTGT/DCEPT, 1401 Rockville Pike, Rockville, MD 20852-1448; Mercedes.serabian@fda.hhs.gov

David J. Snodin, PhD, FRSC, MChemA, MSc, Vice President, Nonclinical Consulting, Parexel Consulting, 101-105 Oxford Road, Uxbridge, Middlesex UB8 1LZ, United Kingdom; david.snodin@parexel.com

Meena Subramanyam, PhD, Senior Director, Clinical Science & Technology, Biogen Idec, Inc., 14 Cambridge Ctr., Cambridge, MA 02142; meena. subramanyam@biogenidec.com

George Treacy, MS, Vice President, Toxicology and Investigational Pharmacology, Centocor Research and Development, Inc., 145 King of Prussia Road, Radnor, PA 19087; gtreacy@cntus.jnj.com

Lincoln Tsang, PhD, FRSC, FIbiol, FRPharmS, Partner, Arnold & Porter LLP, Tower 42, 25 Old Broad Street, London EC2N 1HQ, England; Lincoln.Tsang@ aporter.com

Thierry Vial, MD, Poison Center and Pharmacovigilance Department, Lyon University Hospitals, 162 avenue Lacassagne, 69424 Lyon cedex 03, France

Jennifer Visich, PhD, Senior Scientist, LSPKPD Immunology Group Leader, Genentech, Inc., 1 DNA Way, MS 70, South San Francisco, CA 94080; jennievi@gene.com

Gerhard F. Weinbauer, Director Research and Safety Assessment, Covance Laboratories GmbH, Kesselfeld 29, Muenster D-48163, Germany; Gerhard. Weinbauer@covance.com

Joan Wicks, DVM, PhD, DACVP, Charles River Laboratories, Pathology Associates (PAI), 15 Worman's Mill Court, Suite I, Frederick, MD 21701

Patricia D. Williams, PhD, Summit Drug Development Services, LLC, 15204 Omega Drive, Suite 200, Rockville, MD 20850; pwilliams@summitdrug.com

Renger F. Witkamp, PhD, Professor in Nutritional Pharmacology, Department of Human Nutrition, Wageningen University, PO Box 8129, Wageningen 6700 EV, The Netherlands, and TNO Quality of Life, Zeist, The Netherlands; renger.witkamp@wur.nl

Gary W. Wolfe, PhD, DABT, Vice President, Preclinical Services, Summit Drug Development Services, LLC, 15204 Omega Drive, Suite 200, Rockville, MD 20850; gwolfe@summitdrug.com

Gary Woodnutt, PhD, Vice President, Biology, 9381 Judicial Drive, Suite 200, San Diego, CA 92121; gwoodnutt@covx.com

PART I

BACKGROUND

CHAPTER 1

Biopharmaceuticals: Definition and Regulation

LINCOLN TSANG, PhD, FRSC, FIBiol, FRPharmS, and NATHAN CORTEZ

Contents

1.1 INTRODUCTION

Compared with other types of pharmaceutical products, products derived from a biological source or a biotechnological process are structurally complex and involve manufacturing processes that require tight control to ensure their safety, quality, and efficacy. Biological products, because of their sheer size, are orders of magnitude more complicated than small-molecule drugs. This can be seen by a comparison of molecular weight, which can be used as a measure of the size of a given product. Moreover the product arising from the manufacturing process is often not a pure, homogeneous mixture. Rather, various forms of these molecules are usually present in the final product.

Preclinical Safety Evaluation of Biopharmaceuticals: A Science-Based Approach to Facilitating Clinical Trials, edited by Joy A. Cavagnaro
Copyright © 2008 by John Wiley & Sons, Inc.

In scientific terms, conventional biological products such as blood-derived clotting products, vaccines, and those derived from high technology such as those employing a recombinant DNA technology are characterized as biological products. Because of these differences in respect of the product characteristics and manufacturing process, the regulatory oversight of biological products is distinguishable from conventional pharmaceutical products based on small molecules. This chapter addresses legal framework governing biological products principally in the United States and in the European Union. The regulatory landscape in Japan is briefly described particularly in relation to the recent changes to Japan's Pharmaceutical Affairs Law.

1.2   UNITED STATES

The United States has one of the most active and sophisticated systems in the world for ensuring the safety and effectiveness of biopharmaceuticals. To understand this system, it is important to understand (1) how the United States defines biopharmaceuticals and biologics, (2) the legal foundations for regulating these products, and (3) the rules that apply during various stages, including research, development, approval, and marketing. This section also highlights how the United States regulates biologics in relation to drugs.

1.2.1   How the United States Defines Biologics and Biopharmaceuticals

US law does not have a single, simple definition for *biologics* or *biopharmaceuticals*. The Food and Drug Administration (FDA) recognizes that most biologic products "are complex mixtures that are not easily identified or characterized" [1]. Traditionally *biologics* are substances that are derived from living organisms, such as humans, animals, plants, and microorganisms [2]. Today *biologics* include these substances as well as those produced by biotechnology [2]. A federal statute defines *biological product* as a virus, therapeutic serum, toxin, antitoxin, vaccine, blood, blood component or derivative, allergenic product, or analogous product, or arsphenamine or derivative of arsphenamine (or any other trivalent organic arsenic compound) that is "applicable to the prevention, treatment, or cure of a disease or condition of human beings" [3]. The corresponding federal regulation uses similar language, but clarifies several key terms [4]:

1. A *virus* is interpreted to be a product containing the minute living cause of an infectious disease and includes filterable viruses, bacteria, rickettsia, fungi, and protozoa, among other things.
2. A *therapeutic serum* is a product obtained from blood by removing the clot or clot components and the blood cells.

3. A *toxin* is a product containing a soluble substance poisonous to laboratory animals or to human in doses of one milliliter or less (or equivalent in weight) of the product, and having the property, following the injection of nonfatal doses into an animal, of causing to be produced therein another soluble substance that specifically neutralizes the poisonous substance and that is demonstrable in the serum of the animal thus immunized.

4. An *antitoxin* is a product containing the soluble substance in serum or other body fluid of an immunized animal that specifically neutralizes the toxin against which the animal is immune.

The regulation also clarifies how additional products may be biologics if they are "analogous" to certain categories of products listed in the definition. A product is a biologic if it is analogous to the following [5]:

1. A *virus*, if prepared from or with a virus or agent actually or potentially infectious, without regard to the degree of virulence or toxicogenicity of the specific strain used.

2. A *therapeutic serum*, if composed of whole blood or plasma or containing some organic constituent or product other than a hormone or an amino acid, derived from whole blood, plasma, or a serum.

3. A *toxin* or *antitoxin*, if intended, regardless of its source of origin, to be applicable to the prevention, treatment, or cure of diseases or injuries of human through a specific immune process.

Although these definitions seem to be relatively concrete, biological products come in many forms, including drugs, devices, and "combination" products [6]. The FDA regulates biopharmaceuticals as both drugs and biologics because they meet both definitions. US law, as described above, defines *biological products* by referring to several categories of tangible products. In contrast, the law defines *drugs* by their functions [7]. The term *drug* means "articles intended for use in the diagnosis, cure, mitigation, treatment, or prevention of disease in man" and "articles (other than food) intended to affect the structure or any function of the body of man" [8]. Thus the definitions of *drugs* and *biologics* are not mutually exclusive, which allows the FDA to regulate some products as both.

1.2.2 Legal Foundations for Regulating US Biopharmaceuticals

To understand how biopharmaceuticals are regulated in the United States, it is helpful to understand the underlying legal bases for regulation, how these laws have evolved, and how regulatory responsibility for biologics has shifted. Currently the Public Health Service Act authorizes the FDA to ensure the safety, purity, and potency of biologics. The FDA approves biologics for marketing under section 351 of the Act [9]. The FDA also regulates biopharmaceuticals as drugs under the Federal Food, Drug, and Cosmetic Act. Thus the FDA now delegates responsibility for regulating biopharmaceuticals to two centers within the agency: the Center for Drug Evaluation and Research (CDER) and the Center for Biologics Evaluation and Research (CBER). Regulation under the Public Health Service Act precludes the manufacture of generic, or "follow-on" biologicals and "biosimilars."

The foundations for this regulatory system were set in 1902 with the Biologics Control Act, the first legislation to regulate a specific class of drugs [7]. The Biologics Control Act was a response to tragedies in St. Louis, Missouri, and Camden, New Jersey, in which several people died after taking diphtheria and small pox vaccines [10]. The purpose of the Act was to authorize the regulation of certain biologics, require manufacturers to obtain licensing, and authorize the government to inspect manufacturing facilities [7]. The Act prohibited companies from selling or transporting biologics that were either not manufactured at facilities licensed and inspected by the government or not labeled with the manufacturer's name and an expiration date [7].

Since the 1902 Act, the laws and regulations for biologics have steadily evolved, and responsibility for regulating biological products has shifted several times. In 1903, the federal government issued the first biologics regulations, administered by the Hygienic Laboratory in the Public Health and Marine Hospital Service. The regulations required manufacturers to annually renew their licenses and make their facilities available for unannounced inspections. In 1919, the regulations were amended to require manufacturers to report changes in manufacturing methods, equipment, and personnel. The regulations also required manufacturers to maintain manufacturing records and submit certain product samples for government inspection and approval [7].

These initial laws and regulations laid the foundation for the current biologics regulatory scheme. From the beginning the United States regulated biologics and drugs differently. The government did not regulate nonbiologic drugs until it passed the Pure Food and Drugs Act in 1906, which did not address biologics or the 1902 Biologics Control Act [7]. In fact Congress did not formally recognize the difference between drugs and biologics until after it passed the 1938 Federal Food, Drug, and Cosmetic Act (FDCA) [12]. In 1944, Congress reenacted the 1902 Biologics Control Act and recodified the Public Health Service Act. A major issue was the definitional overlap between drugs and biologics [12].

Between 1902 and 1972, regulatory responsibility for biologics transferred several times, ultimately settling with FDA, as shown by this brief timeline of the relevant transfers:

1930   The Hygienic Laboratory within the Public Health and Marine Hospital Service is redesignated as the National Institutes of Health (NIH).

1937	The NIH is reorganized, and responsibility for biologics is transferred to the Division of Biologics Control. In 1944 it is renamed the Laboratory of Biologics Control.
1948	The Laboratory of Biologics Control is integrated into the NIH's National Microbiological Institute, which later becomes the Institute of Allergy and Infectious Diseases.
1955	Responsibility for biologics is transferred to the new Division of Biologics Standards, a new independent entity within the NIH.
1972	The Division of Biologics Standards is transferred from the NIH to the FDA, becoming the Bureau of Biologics.
1982	The Bureau of Biologics is merged with the Bureau of Drugs to form the National Center for Drugs and Biologics (NCDB).
1983	The biologics component of the NCDB is renamed the Office of Biologics Research and Review, within the Center for Drugs and Biologics (CDB).
1988	CDB split into two centers, the Center for Biologics Evaluation and Research (CBER), and the Center for Drug Evaluation and Research (CDER).
2003	Transfer of therapeutic biological products from CBER to CDER.

The steady stream of reorganizations in many ways reflects the difficulty of both categorizing and regulating biologics. The FDA continues to struggle with these responsibilities. For instance, since the FDA created CBER in 1988, the agency has both overhauled the way it approves biologics, and once again shifted responsibility for certain biologics. First, the FDA established a single approval application, the Biological License Application (BLA) through the Food and Drug Modernization Act of 1997 (FDAMA), the most comprehensive rewrite of food and drug laws since 1938. Second, in 2003, the FDA shifted responsibility for therapeutic biologics from CBER to CDER, given CDER's role in regulating therapeutic drugs. CDER's new responsibilities include a wide array of biological products, including monoclonal antibodies for in vivo use, therapeutic proteins, and immunomodulators [10]. CBER retained authority over traditional biologic products such as vaccines, allergenic extracts, antitoxins, blood, and blood products, as well as products composed of human, bacterial, or animal cells [10].

1.2.3 Legal Requirements for US Biopharmaceuticals

The regulation of biologics continues to evolve. The transcendent growth of biotechnology research, spurred by the Human Genome Project, almost ensures that biologic regulations will require further tinkering to accommodate new products. The following is a brief synopsis of relevant US laws and regulations at various stages, including research, development, approval, and marketing. Where relevant, we highlight where the rules for biologics differ from drugs.

Research and Development   The United States heavily regulates the research and development of biologics. At the preclinical stage, FDA requires companies to comply with regulations on good laboratory practices (GLPs) at 21 CFR part 58. The GLP regulations seek to ensure the quality and integrity of preclinical safety data submitted to the FDA. GLPs apply to nonclinical (preclinical) laboratory studies intended to support research or marketing applications, and address a broad range of topics, including personnel, facilities, and equipment. Ideally preclinical studies to support safety are subject to GLPs and should be supported by a statement that the study was conducted in compliance with the good laboratory practice regulations in 21 CFR part 58, or if the study was not conducted in compliance with those regulations, a brief statement of the reason for the noncompliance (21 CFR 312.23 (8) (iii)).

At the clinical stage, FDA sets minimum standards for clinical trials through several regulations and guidance documents, collectively known as good clinical practices (GCPs). GCPs are designed to ensure the quality and integrity of data submitted to FDA and protect the rights of human subjects. GCPs govern key personnel involved in clinical trials—particularly sponsors, and investigators—and address several important areas, including informed consent, institutional review boards (IRBs), and investigational new drug (IND) requirements.

Informed consent is governed by both federal and state law [14]. These laws generally require that before participating in clinical trials, human research subjects state in writing that they understand the risks of the trial and are participating voluntarily. Each informed consent document must contain several elements required by FDA regulations [15].

IRBs are also governed by federal and state law. FDA regulations require IRBs to provide initial and continuing review of clinical trials [16]. IRBs must ensure that investigators and sponsors protect the study subjects, obtain adequate informed consent, and adhere to other safeguards and reporting requirements [16]. Moreover FDA regulations require IRBs members to meet specific membership criteria [17].

Investigational biologics are subject to the FDA's investigational new drug (IND) requirements [18]. The IND application is the first formal submission to FDA, and the application must be submitted before initiating any clinical studies [7]. It is not a request for commercial marketing approval; rather, it is a request to be exempt from the federal statute that prohibits shipping "unapproved" drugs across state lines. Thus an IND permit allows the product to be shipped during investigational studies. The purpose of the IND requirement is to assure the FDA that the safety and rights of subjects will be protected in all phases of the investigation, and that the quality of the studies are adequate to permit the FDA to evaluate the product's safety and effectiveness [13].

Approval The FDA approves biologics for marketing through the biological license application (BLA), which requires the applicant to show that the product is safe, pure, and potent [19]. The BLA submission is typically the culmination of years of research and development, through which the company submits preclinical and clinical data, physiochemical information, biological activity results, and manufacturing information [7]. Previously the FDA approved biologics through two license applications, the product license application (PLA) and the establishment license application (ELA). In 1996, CBER consolidated these applications into a single BLA for certain products, and in 1997, Congress extended the BLA to all biological products.

Although the BLA process differs in some ways from the new drug approval (NDA) application process for nonbiologic drugs, the required showing of safety and efficacy is similar, if not identical, between drugs and biologics [20]. While the FDA requires biologics to be "safe, pure, and potent," the agency interprets this language as requiring the same type of evidence in NDAs for nonbiologic drugs [20]. Nevertheless, there are differences between the BLA and NDA that reflect CBER's historical emphasis on manufacturing and process control. For instance, the FDA requires BLA applicants to submit detailed information on manufacturing processes so that the FDA can determine whether the manufacturer can produce a product consistent with current good manufacturing practices (cGMPs) and the manufacturing specifications listed in the BLA. The manufacturer's facility is also a major factor—its construction, design, layout, validation processes, and environmental monitoring must meet FDA standards.

After approval, biologics manufacturers must comply with the FDA's cGMP regulations [21]. These regulations govern the manufacturer's use of raw materials, buildings and facilities, production and process controls, packaging and labeling, laboratory controls, stability testing, expiration dates, production records, and the company's overall quality system. Although the same cGMP regulations apply to drugs and biologics, manufacturing biologics can be quite different. Physically and chemically, biologics act differently than drugs [11]. They are less defined, less pure, less stable, and degrade in more complex ways than most drugs [11]. Their potency also depends greatly on the underlying organisms from which they are produced [11]. Thus, if a manufacturer makes relatively minor changes to the manufacturing process of a biologic, the FDA may require the manufacture to demonstrate through new clinical studies that the process produces the same results as the original clinical studies [11].

Marketing and Postapproval Requirements Once the FDA approves a biopharmaceutical for marketing, the agency applies a different set of regulatory standards. The main postapproval requirements govern: (1) adverse event reporting, (2) manufacturing under cGMPs, (3) lot release testing, (4) general reporting, and (5) postmarketing studies.

- The FDA's adverse event reporting system does not differ significantly between drugs and biologics. However, the FDA did not have a comprehensive adverse event reporting system for biologics until 1994 [22]. Biologics manufacturers can use two reporting systems: MedWatch and the Vaccine Adverse Event Reporting System (VAERS). MedWatch is administered by the FDA and covers drugs, biologics, medical devices, and special nutritional products. VAERS is jointly administered by the FDA and the Centers for Disease Control and Prevention (CDC), and covers adverse events following immunizations. FDA regulations require manufacturers to report serious, unexpected adverse events within 15 days. Less serious reports can be submitted in periodic follow-up, or distribution reports.

- The FDA's cGMP regulations specify minimum standards for manufacturing facilities and their production controls. These regulations generally apply to both drugs and biologics, but the FDA has additional cGMP-related regulations that focus on biologics [23]. CBER has also tailored cGMP requirements for "specified biotechnology and synthetic biological products" to be as similar to drug requirements as possible.

- The FDA's lot release regulations allow the agency to require manufacturers to submit samples of any licensed biological products for testing [24]. Manufacturers must submit to CBER representative samples of each lot, a lot release protocol, and a summary of the test results. Lots may not be released until CBER authorizes an "official release." However, CBER does not require lot release in all circumstances.

- The FDA requires manufacturers to report certain changes in the product, production process, quality controls, equipment, facilities, personnel, or labeling that are established in the approved license application [25]. The manufacturer must demonstrate that the change does not adversely affect the identity, strength, quality, purity, or potency of the product that may affect the product's safety or effectiveness. FDA regulations and guidance categorize each change as "minor," "moderate," or "major" based on the risk to the product's quality, safety, and effectiveness. The FDA must give prior approval before the manufacturer can implement "major" changes. "Moderate" changes must be reported to the FDA within 30 days. Minor changes must be reported annually.

- The FDA may require, at the time of product approval, that the manufacture agree to conduct additional testing on its biological product, called phase 4 studies. These postmarketing studies may further evaluate the product's safety, efficacy, or manufacturing methods. Sponsors that agreed to conduct phase 4 studies as part of their BLA approval must update the FDA annually.

1.3 EUROPEAN UNION

1.3.1 How EU Law Defines a Biological Medicinal Product

In the European Union the regulation of biological products is subject to continuing review taking account of the evolving science and technology. Directive 87/22/EEC (now repealed) provided the first time in EU law the legal definition of a medicinal product developed by a biotechnological process. The following processes were considered as biotechnological: recombinant DNA technology, controlled expression of genes coding for biologically active proteins in prokaryotes and eukaryotes including transformed mammalian cells, hybridoma, and monoclonal antibody methods. This definition remains unchanged since 1987, and it is now used for defining a biotechnological medicinal product as set out in the Annex to Regulation (EC) 726/2004 [26], which repealed Regulation (EC) 2309/93 [27] governing the European centralized procedure.

The definition of a process based on biotechnology is sufficiently broad to capture a wide arrange of medicinal products, such as recombinant proteins and gene-based therapeutics, and prophylactics, such as gene transfer medicinal products and DNA vaccines. Medicinal products manufactured by biotechnological processes as defined in the Annex to Regulation (EC) 726/2004 must be authorized centrally pursuant to article 3 of the Regulation.

In June 2003 the European Commission adopted a new Annex I to Directive 2001/83/EC [28] on the EU code relating to medicinal products for human use. This new Annex was adopted in the form of Commission Directive 2003/63/EC [29]. The new Annex was adopted for implementation of the International Conference on Harmonization (ICH) Common Technical Document (CTD) format. Annex I sets out the particulars and documents accompanying an application for marketing authorization irrespective of the EU procedure used for obtaining a marketing authorization. Directive 2003/63/EC defines a biological medicinal product, and this definition consists of two essential elements. First, the active substance is a biological substance. A biological substance is a substance that is produced by or extracted from a biological source. Any one of the following source is considered as a biological source: microorganisms, organs and tissues of either plant or animal origin, cells or fluids (including blood or plasma) of human or animal origin, and biotechnological cell constructs utilizing cell substrates. If the product is produced from primary cells such as certain prophylactic vaccines, the product is considered a biological medicinal product. Second, the product requires for its characterization and the determination of its quality a combination of physicochemical-biological testing together with the production process and its control.

The Commission has indicated that the following are considered as biological medicinal products: immunological medicinal products and medicinal products derived from human blood and human plasma. EU law defines an immunological medicinal product as any medicinal product consisting of vaccines, toxins, serums, or allergen products. Vaccines, toxins, and serums cover, in particular, agents used to produce active or passive immunity, and to diagnose the state of immunity. An allergen product means any medicinal product that is intended to identify or induce a specific acquired alteration in the immunological response to an allergizing agent.

Medicinal products derived from human blood or human plasma means those based on blood constituents that are prepared industrially by public or private establishments, such as albumin, coagulation factors, and immunoglobulins of human origin. This definition reflects the way plasma derived medicinal products are manufactured in the European Union. This class of products may be produced by privately owned industry or by public organizations that are owned by the member state.

1.3.2   Legal Foundation for Regulation of Biological Medicinal Product

The regulatory framework governing biological medicinal products is based on the European Community Treaty, which aims at the free movement of goods within the European Union. Although the legal base is built on the principle of free trade of medicinal products within the European Union, the essential aim of any rules governing the production, distribution, and use of medicinal products must be firmly based on protection of public health. Recital 3 of Directive 2001/83/EC notes that the objective of public health protection must be attained by means that do not hinder the development of the pharmaceutical industry or trade in medicinal products within the European Union.

The EU regulatory system is based on cooperation among the competent authorities of the member states (including the member states of the European Economic Area, e.g., Norway, Liechtenstein, and Iceland) and various relevant European institutions such as the European Commission and the European Medicines Agency (formerly called the European Agency for the Evaluation of Medicinal Products). The European Medicines Agency (EMEA) was formally established in 1995 by virtue of Regulation (EC) 2309/93, which is now replaced by Regulation (EC) 726/2004. The EMEA's role is narrowly defined in the Regulation as a body responsible for coordinating the existing scientific resources put at its disposal by member states for the evaluation, supervision, and pharmacovigilance of medicinal products. In practice, the scientific work is carried out by the member states through the EMEA's advisory committees and working parties.

The Committee for Medicinal Products for Human Use (CHMP) is one of the main committees responsible for preparing the opinion of the EMEA on any question relating to the assessment of medicinal products for human use. Pursuant to Regulation (EC) 141/2000 [30] the Committee for Orphan Medicinal Products (COMP) was established to provide scientific opinion on whether a medicinal product meets the criteria under EU law for it to be designated as an orphan medicinal product.

The sector-specific rules governing medicinal products are set out in various legal instruments and administrative guidance which follow the following hierarchy [31].

- A Regulation is directly applicable and binding in its entirety on in all member states. Therefore it does not require a period of transposition into the domestic laws of the member states.
- A Directive is directly effective that requires it to be transposed into domestic laws in order to give effect to the Directive. Under EU law, member states are only required to implement the Directive with respect to its objectives and EU law does not control the manner and form of how a Directive is transposed into the national laws.
- A Decision is binding in its entirety upon persons to whom it is addressed.
- Opinion is not legally binding.

In addition the Commission has issued a number of technical and administrative guidelines such as those set out in various volumes of the Notice to Applicants in order to explain how EU law can workably put into practice. The EMEA has developed a body of scientific guidelines regarding the technical requirements for addressing issues relating to safety, quality and efficacy. Although guidelines are not legally binding, the European Courts have increasingly relied on such documents as an aid in interpretation of the legal requirements.

Research and Development   Clinical development in the European Union is regulated by Directive 2001/20/EC [32], which is commonly known as the Clinical Trials Directive. This Directive regulates all stages of clinical development in the European Union, including Phase I clinical studies involving healthy volunteers. The competent authorities of the member states are responsible for assessing the applications for clinical trial authorization. In assessing whether an approval should be granted, the competent authorities are required to ensure that conduct of the clinical trials comply with the principles of good clinical practice and the relevant ethical principles. Reference is made to the principles set out in the ICH E6 Guideline on Clinical Practice and the applicable version of the Declaration of Helsinki. Under the Clinical Trials Directive, competent authorities are required to make a determination of an application for clinical trial authorisation within 60 days from the date of submission. However, the Directive permits the member states to extend the statutory time limit for certain investigational medicinal products such as gene therapy, xeno-transplantation, and products that are derived from biological source.

Compliance with the requirements of Directive 2001/20/EC is important. This is because Annex I to Directive 2001/83/EC (as amended) expressly requires that for the purpose of obtaining a marketing authorization, all clinical trials conducted within the European Union to comply with Directive 2001/20/EC. For clinical trials conducted outside the European Union and the data of which are used in support of an application for a marketing authorization, such clinical trials must be designed, implemented, and reported on the basis of principles that are equivalent to the provisions of Directive 2001/20/EC and carried out in accordance with the ethical principles that are reflected in the Declaration of Helsinki.

EU law expressly requires nonclinical (pharmacotoxicological) studies to be carried out in conformity with the provisions related to good laboratory practice set out in Directive 2004/10/EC [33] and Directive 2004/9/EC [34] on the inspection and verification of laboratory practice.

Approval   Approval process for biological medicinal products is the same as other chemically synthesized small molecules. The legal test is firmly based upon an assessment of risk–benefit balance. However, in assessing risk–benefit balance of a biological medicinal product, EU law requires the applicant to provide certain additional information. If the medicinal product contains a new biological active substance, the applicant must comply with the requirements set out in article 8(3) of Directive 2001/83/EC by providing results of the pharmaceutical and nonclinical testing, and clinical trials.

Given the safety and efficacy of a biological medicinal product is determined largely by the starting material used and the process, EU law requires applicants to describe and document the origin and history of starting materials. Starting materials mean any substance of biological origin such as microorganism, organs, and tissues of either plant or animal origin; cells or fluids of human or animal origin; and biotechnological cell constructs, including the cell substrates whether or not they are recombinant. Moreover, for medicinal products that are manufactured based on a cell bank system, the cell characteristics must be shown to have remained unchanged at the passage level used for the production and beyond. It is also a requirement to test all materials used in the process for adventitious agents, including animal spongiform encephalopathy agents. If the presence of potentially pathogenic adventitious agents is inevitable, the corresponding material must only be used when further processing is demonstrated to be capable of eliminating and/or inactivating such adventitious agents. The capability of the process must be validated. In comparison with chemically synthesized products, greater emphasis is placed on the in-process controls to ensure batch to batch consistency.

With respect to preclinical testing, EU law expressly states the testing program must be adapted for individual products. It is for the applicant for a marketing authorization to justify the testing program to elucidate the preclinical safety and biological activity of the product. EU law states that in establishing the testing program, the following must be taken into account:

- All tests requiring repeated administration of the product must be designed to take account of the possible induction of, and interference by antibodies.
- Examination of reproductive function, of embryo-fetal and perinatal toxicity of mutagenic potential and of carcinogenic potential must be considered. However, constituents other than the active substance(s) are incriminated, validation of their removal may replace the study.
- The toxicology and pharmacokinetics of an excipient used for the first time in the pharmaceutical field must be investigated.
- Where there is a possibility of significant degradation during storage of the medicinal product, the toxicology of degradation products must be considered.

In general, according to EU law, applicants are expected to carry out controlled clinical trials, randomized and as appropriate against a placebo and an established medicinal product (an active comparator) of proved therapeutic value. However, applicants may justify use of other trial design. The treatment of the control groups will vary from case to case and also will depend on ethical consideration and therapeutic area. In some cases it may be more justified to compare the efficacy of a new medicinal product with that of an established medicinal product of proved therapeutic value rather than with a placebo.

In the new European pharmaceutical legislation, a new regulatory path has been created for approval of a similar biological medicinal product, which is commonly known as a biosimilar medicinal product. The definition of a similar biological medicinal product as set out in article 10(4) of Directive 2001/83 (as amended by Directive 2004/27/EC) [35] to mean a biological medicinal product that is similar to a reference product does not mean the conditions in the definition of generic medicinal products owing to, in particular, differences relating to raw materials or differences in manufacturing processes of the biological medicinal product and the reference biological medicinal product. In such cases the results of appropriate nonclinical tests and/or clinical trials relating to these conditions must be provided. The EMEA has developed has now developed a series of technical guidelines to address the type and quantity of supplementary data to be provided [36].

Marketing and Postapproval Requirements   Regardless of whether a medicinal product is considered a conventional pharmaceutical product or a biological product, after grant of an approval, the holder of the marketing authorization is required to monitor the continuing risk–benefit balance of the product. In relation to the method of manufacture, in addition to ensuring compliance with good manufacturing practice in accordance with Directive 2003/94/EC [37] the authorization holder must take account of scientific and technical progress and introduce any changes that may be required to enable the product to be manufactured and controlled by means of generally accepted scientific methods. Immunological products such as vaccines and products derived from human blood or plasma may be subject to official batch release testing at the request of a competent authority.

In the new pharmaceutical legislation, greater emphasis is placed on pharmacovigilance and risk management. Indeed, at pre-approval, applicants are required to submit to the competent authority a detailed description of the pharmacovigilance and of the risk amangement system that the applicant will introduce. In general, it is a requirement for the marketing authorization holder to record all suspected serious adverse reactions and to report them promptly to the competent authority within a defined time frame as set out in EU law. For new products, the marketing authorization holder is required to provide periodic, updated safety report at least every six months during the first two years following the initial placing on the market and once a year for the following two years. Thereafter the reports must be submitted at three yearly intervals or immediately on request by the competent authority. The Commission has developed a guidance document published in volume 9 of the Rules governing medicinal products in the European Union, which is currently being revised. This guidance takes account of various guidelines promulgated under the International Conference on Harmonization.

In order to establish and maintain a pharmacovigilance system, the holder of the marketing authorization is required to have permanently and continuously at his or her disposal an appropriately qualified person. This qualified person is personally responsible for ensuring that information about all adverse reactions that are reported to the personnel of the company and to medical representatives is collected and collated. This qualified person is also responsible for ensuring that all suspected serious adverse reactions are reported to the competent authority concerned.

1.4   JAPAN

On 25 July 2002, the Japanese House of Representatives passed the revised Pharmaceutical Affairs Law (PAL), which dates back to 1943. Although amendments have been made in the 1940s, 1960s, and 1970s, certain parts of the legislation required updating to take account of changes in science and technology, and the need for the liberalization of the Japanese market. Companies can now outsource the manufacturing process, allowing pharmaceutical companies to market their products in Japan without operating their own production facilities. Changes made to the PAL have also fueled growth in the clinical trial sector in Japan. Notwithstanding the revision of the PAL, the basic purpose of the law remains intact in that it is designed to protect public health by ensuring the safety, quality, and efficacy of medical products in Japan.

The revised PAL of 2002 aims at addressing the following challenges:

- The need to strengthen the safety measures related to medical devices
- The need to strengthen regulatory control over products based on biotechnology and genomic technology
- The need to strengthen the postmarketing safety monitoring and take account of the efforts in international harmonization for the technical assessment of pharmaceutical products

A new regulatory agency, the Pharmaceuticals and Medical Devices Agency (PMDA), has been created with the executive function of overseeing regulation of pharmaceutical products and medical devices. Similar to the system adopted by the United States and the European Union, the regulatory control of medicinal products in Japan is through a system of approval/licensing for certain regulated activities such as conduct of clinical trials, manufacture, marketing, distribution, sale, and supply of specific pharmaceutical products. The Japanese Pharmacopoeia is an integral part of the regulatory framework as it sets out the quality standards for certain pharmaceutical products or substances.

Japan is a party to the tripartite ICH process. Therefore all the adopted guidelines have been implemented as the basic technical standards for the evaluation of safety, quality, and efficacy for pharmaceutical and biotechnological products. In addition the requirements for good laboratory practices for conducting nonclinical safety testing of pharmaceutical products have been applied since the 1980s in the form of administrative instruction. The requirements for conducting clinical trials in accordance with good clinical practice have been implemented since 1990. Such standards have now been enforced through various ministerial ordinances.

The PAL sets out the broad legislative framework for regulating medical products. However, the Ministry for Health, Labor, and Welfare (MHLW) has the authority to issue ordinances and notifications setting out the details for regulating certain product types, such as pharmaceutical products, medical devices, in vitro diagnostic reagents, cosmetic and quasi-drugs. For example, Ministerial Ordinance No. 136, 2004 sets out standards for quality assurance for drugs, quasi-drugs, cosmetics, and medical devices. This Ordinance seemingly applies to drugs based on cells or tissues. The basic structure of this ordinance reflects the principles of good manufacturing practice where a focus is placed on the quality management system, quality control, personnel, training, documentation, and self-inspection.

Given that global trade and international harmonization are key to the development of a sustainable life sciences industry, closer international cooperation is key to tackling technical barriers to trade in medicines. In addition to the ICH process, increasingly regulatory authorities have entered into agreements to enable them to exchange confidential information about approval and safety of medicines.

In February 2007 the European Commission and the EMEA signed a confidentiality agreement with the MHLW and PMDA to enable both parties to exchange confidential information relating to all legislation and guidance documents, postapproval pharmacovigilance, scientific advice, orphan designation, good clinical practices inspections, and so forth [39]. The US FDA has established a similar confidentiality arrangement with the European Commission and the EMEA.

1.5 CONCLUSION

This chapter introduces the legal and regulatory aspects pertaining to biological products in the United States and in the European Union. The regulatory laws in these two jurisdictions distinguish between conventional pharmaceutical products based on small molecules and biological products. While the legal test for regulatory approval is firmly based on an assessment of risk–benefit balance, the approach to such an assessment is distinctly different with respect to biological products. This is exemplified by the publication of a recent scientific review commissioned by the health ministers following serious adverse reactions that occurred in a first-in-human clinical trial involving a monoclonal antibody TGN 1412 at Northwick Park Hospital in London (March 2006). Six healthy volunteers experienced severe systemic adverse reactions after administration with the biological product. The adverse reactions were characterized as associated with cytokine release. The report emphasizes the importance of performing appropriately conducted preclinical studies in identifying the safe starting dose in humans. The report appears to accept that the conventional approach based upon NOAEL (no observed adverse effect level), a concept that is generally applicable to chemically synthesized small molecules, may not be appropriate. Instead, the principle based on minimal anticipated biological effect level (MABEL) is a good model for defining the safe starting dose, taking account of the novelty of the agent, its biological potency, its mechanism of action, the degree of species-specificity of the agent, the dose–response curves in vitro and in vivo. This concept is also articulated in the FDA guidance in consideration of lowering the starting dose based on a variety of factors that include the pharmacologically active dose (PAD) [38].

REFERENCES

1. FDA, Center for Biologics Evaluation and Research (CBER). Frequently Asked Questions. http://www.fda.gov/cber/faq.htm
2. CBER. Science and the Regulation of Biological Products: From a Rich History to a Changing Future 6 (2001). http://www.fda.gov/cber/inside/centscireg.htm
3. Public Health Service Act §351(i), 42 USC §262(i).
4. 21 CFR §600.3(h).
5. Id. at §600.3(h)(5).

6. CBER. Frequently Asked Questions; FDA, Selected Guidance Documents Applicable to Combination Products. http://www.fda.gov/oc/combination/guidance.html

7. Mathieu M, ed. Biologics Development: A Regulatory Overview. 2004. See also Pub. L. No. 57-244, 32 Stat. 728, 1902. (An Act to Regulate the Sale of Viruses, Serums, Toxins, and Analogous Products in the District of Columbia, to Regulate Interstate Traffic in Said Articles, and for Other Purposes).

8. Federal Food, Drug, and Cosmetic Act §321(g)(1), 21 USC §201(g)(1).

9. Public Health Service Act §351, 42 USC §262.

10. Kracov DA. FDA's role in regulating biologics. In Pines WJ, ed. *FDA: A Century of Consumer Protection.* 2006, 195.

11. Buday PV. Fundamentals of United States biological product regulations. *Regul Affairs* 1991;3:223.

12. Korweck EL. Human biological drug regulation: Past, present, and beyond the year. *Food Drug LJ* 1995;50:123.

13. 21 CFR §312.22.

14. For example, 21 CFR part 50; 45 CFR part 46.

15. 21 CFR §50.25.

16. See 21 CFR part 56.

17. 21 CFR §56.107.

18. FDCA §505, 21 USC §355; 21 CFR part 312.

19. 21 CFR §601.2.

20. Beers DO. FDA regulation of biologic drugs. In *Generic and Innovator Drugs: A Guide to FDA Approval Requirements §13.02,* 6th ed. 2004.

21. 21 CFR parts 210, 211, and 600.

22. 21 CFR §600.80.

23. For example, 21 CFR parts 600, 601, 606, 607, 610, 630, 640, 660, 680.

24. 21 CFR §610.2(a).

25. 21 CFR §§610.12, 610.14.

26. Regulation (EC) No 726/2004 of the European Parliament and of the Council of 31 March 2004 laying down Community procedures for the authorization and supervision of medicinal products for human and veterinary use and establishing a European Medicines Agency. OJ L136, 31.03.2004, p1.

27. Council Regulation (EEC) No 2309/93 of 22 July 1993 laying down Community procedures for the authorization and supervision of medicinal products for human and veterinary use and establishing a European Agency for the Evaluation of Medicinal Products. OJ L214, 24.08.1993, p1.

28. Directive 2001/83/EC of the European Parliament and of the Council of 6 November 2001 on the Community code relating to medicinal products for human use. OJ L311, 28.11.2001, p67.

29. Commission Directive 2003/63/EC of 25 June 2003 amending Directive 2001/83/EC of the European Parliament and of the Council on the Community code relating to medicinal products for human use. OJ L159, 27.06.2003, p46.

30. Regulation (EC) No 141/2000 of the European Parliament and of the Council of 16 December 1999 on orphan medicinal products. OJ L18, 22.01.2000, p1.

31. Article 249 of the Treaty Establishing the European Community.

32. Directive 2001/20/EC of the European Parliament and of the Council of 4 April 2001 on the approximation of the laws, regulations and administrative provisions of the member states relating to the implementation of good clinical practice in the conduct of clinical trials on medicinal products for human use. OJ L121, 01.05.2001, p34.

33. Directive 2004/10/EC of the European Parliament and of the Council of 11 February 2004 on the harmonization of laws, regulations, and administrative provisions relating to the application of the principles of good laboratory practice and the verification of their applications for tests on chemical substances (codified version). OJ L50/44, 20.02.2004, p44.

34. Directive 2004/9/EC of the European Parliament and of the Council of 11 February 2004 on the inspection and verification of good laboratory practice (GLP) (codified version). OJ L50, 20.02.2004, p28.

35. Directive 2004/27/EC of the European Parliament and of the Council of 31 March 2004 amending Directive 2001/83/EC on the Community code relating to medicinal products for human use (text with EEA relevance). OJ L136, 30.04.2004, p34.

36. Tsang L, Beers D. Follow-on biological products: the regulatory minefield. In *Global Counsel Handbooks Life Sciences 2004/05*. Practical Law Company.

37. Commission Directive 2003/94/EC of 8 October 2003 laying down the principles and guidelines of good manufacturing practice in respect of medicinal products for human use and investigational medicinal products for human use (text with EEA relevance). OJ L262, 14.10.2003, p22.

38. FDA Guidance for Industry Estimating the Maximum Safe Starting Dose in Initial Clinical Trials for Therapeutics in Adult Healthy Volunteers (July 2005).

39. Press Release, Brussels 5 February 2007. Closer ties on medicines safety between EU and Japan (IP/07/135).

CHAPTER 2

Methods of Production of Biopharmaceutical Products and Assessment of Environmental Impact

PATRICIA D. WILLIAMS, PhD

Contents

2.1 INTRODUCTION

The genomics revolution over the past 20 years and subsequent sequencing of the human genome have provided opportunities for the pharmaceutical

Preclinical Safety Evaluation of Biopharmaceuticals: A Science-Based Approach to Facilitating Clinical Trials, edited by Joy A. Cavagnaro
Copyright © 2008 by John Wiley & Sons, Inc.

industry in terms of drug targeting and identification of novel therapeutics. Advances in molecular biology and genetics have also played significant roles in the pharmaceutical development of these novel products. Specifically, the biomanufacture of protein therapeutics has relied on genetically engineered production systems. Biomanufacturing has evolved out of heterologous gene expression technology of the 1980s and 1990s and continues to evolve. From bacterial hosts to yeast to mammalian cells to even transgenic plants and animals, novel approaches have been developed to increase the capacity, efficiency, and safety of biopharmaceuticals.

In parallel, protein purification and characterization techniques have also markedly improved, increasing the yields and speeding analysis time for biologically active proteins. With this developing technology, biopharmaceutical production has been able to diversify from bacterial cells to yeast to mammalian cells and now into transgenic "bioreactors" (e.g., goats, cattle). Through an understanding of these novel production systems, the advantages of this new technology in contributing to the successful production of novel biopharmaceutical products can be realized.

At present, over 20 therapeutics produced via recombinant technology are currently on the market [1]. These products range from monoclonal antibodies to interferons (IFNs) to growth factors to human insulin. While in many cases relatively small-scale production in bacterial, yeast, or cell culture systems are amenable for proteins required in microgram quantities, new products are being developed requiring significantly higher doses and long-term administration. Thus the need for higher capacity manufacturing systems has arisen. In particular, protein production in transgenic animals has become the method of scale-up or a necessary choice for some protein therapeutics. Production in milk of transgenic sheep, goats, or cattle may yield between 5 and 30 g/L of recombinant protein, which is far beyond the production capacity of mammalian culture systems [2].

In 1969 the National Environmental Policy Act (NEPA) was enacted. This act requires that all federal agencies assess the environmental impacts of their actions and ensure that the interested and affected public is informed of environmental analyses [3]. The Food and Drug Administration (FDA) is required under the NEPA to consider the environmental impact of approving drug and biologic applications as an integral part of its regulatory process. The FDA's regulations in 21 CFR part 25 specify that environmental assessments (EAs) must be submitted as part of certain new drug applications (NDAs), abbreviated applications, applications from marketing approval of a biological products (BLAs), supplements to such applications, investigational new drug applications (INDs), and for various other actions (see 21 CFR 25.20), unless the action qualifies for categorical exclusion [3].

The issue of product comparability when manufacturing processes or systems are changed, in particular, poses an important challenge to the pharmaceutical and biotechnology industry. For example, how should a sponsor demonstrate that proteins secreted into the milk of transgenic cattle or goats are comparable with those produced in *E. coli* or CHO cell systems? What methodologies should be employed to demonstrate product comparability? The need for analytical studies, in vitro testing, preclinical animal studies, or new clinical data will depend on the significance of the change in the system and the potential effect on the biologic product.

The systems available for production of biopharmaceuticals, and the approaches to introducing new technologies into the drug development process are discussed in the sections that follow.

2.2   HOST SYSTEMS FOR BIOPHARMACEUTICAL PRODUCTION

An overview of the manufacturing systems employed for the production of protein therapeutics is presented in Table 2.1. The advantages and disadvantages of the various manufacturing systems, as well as examples of therapeutic proteins currently marketed or under development utilizing these systems, are also presented.

One of the earliest and simplest expression systems for biopharmaceutical production is the eukaryotic bacteria, *E. coli*. The biology of *E. coli* is well understood, and bacteria are simple to grow and genetically stable. *E. coli* can accumulate extremely high concentrations of exogenous proteins in their cytoplasm (up to 20% of their total cellular protein), and can translocate proteins from the cytoplasm to the periplasm [4]. Although *E. coli* has proved to be a suitable host for a number of therapeutically useful proteins including IFNs, growth factors, and tissue plasminogen activator (tPA), *E. coli* cannot perform many of the same posttranslational modifications achievable in mammalian cells, and hence their utility is limited. Moreover many proteins expressed in *E. coli* will form insoluble inclusion bodies, and purification may be complicated [5].

Yeast strains such as *Saccharomyces cerevesia* and *Pichia pastoris* have also proved useful for expression of biotherapeutics. Yeast are rapidly growing eukaryotic cells, and they perform many of the same secondary protein modifications as mammalian cells. Yeast are inexpensive to grow and maintain, and can also secrete recombinant proteins directly into the culture media. This makes yeast very suitable for large-scale production of recombinant human proteins. *Pichia pastoris* are specifically capable of expressing correctly folded, secreted proteins, including those containing high levels of disulfide bonding. Secreted proteins can often be easily and efficiently purified from the fermentation media, often with only a single chromatographic step. For example, recombinant insulin was among the first proteins to be produced in large quantities in yeast [6]. While yeast do serve as excellent hosts for expression of recombinant proteins, they still do not perform all functions similar to mammalian cells, and can be extremely sensitive to temperature, aeration, and methanol concentration [7]. Marketed recombinant proteins produced in yeast include human insulin (Novolin®), granulocyte macrophage colony stimulating

TABLE 2.1 Expression systems for biopharmaceutical production

System	Advantages	Disadvantages	Examples
Bacterial (*E. coli*)	• High growth rate • Simple nutritional demands • Genetic consistency • Relative ease of purification • High protein yield • Well-defined biology • Approved products	• Inability to properly fold, glycosylate, phosphorylate, and acylate proteins • Difficulty in isolating proteins from inclusion bodies • Rapid doubling time potential for mutation	• **Betaseron®** (**interferon β-1b**) • **Trastuzumab®** (**monoclonal antibody**) • **Nutropin®** (**human growth hormone**) • **Numega®** (**interleukin-11**)
Saccharomyces Cerevisiae (yeast)	• Eukaryotic • Rapid growth, low cost • Ease of genetic manipulation • Protease-deficient strains • Secreted or intracellular protein products • Approved products	• Improper posttranslation modification • Temperature, O_2 sensitivity • Differences in codon usage from mammalian cells • Improper or excessive glycosylation	• **Engerix-B®** (**HBV vaccine**) • **Novolin-B®** (**insulin**) • **Humulin®** (**insulin**) • **Leukine®** (**granulocyte macrophage colony stimulating factor**)
Pichia pastoris (yeast)	• Rapid growth, low cost • Ease of genetic modification • Protein folding capabilities • Direct protein secretion into media • Relative ease of purification	• Potential codon bias • Posttranslation modification • Sensitivity to aeration, methanol concentration, and temperature	• Influenza neuraminidase • Botulinum neurotoxin A binding domain • CC49 single-chain variable fragments • Bovine tumor necrosis factor receptor I • Insulin
Mammalian cell	• Many cell types available • Posttranslational modification • Growth in selectable markers • Both suspension and adherent cultures • Inducible expression • Cytoplasmic, membrane, and secreted proteins produced • Proper RNA splicing • Approved products	• Requirement for adherent growth • Cost of scale-up • Time to develop well-characterized stable cell lines • Lower levels of expression • Limited passage number • Low yields relative to cost of production • Potential under sialylation of products	• **Retavase®** (**tPA**) • **Epogen®** (**Erythropoeitin**) • **Benefix™** (**coagulation factor IX**) • **Avonex™** (**interferon β-1a**) • **Pulmozyme®** (**DNAse I**) • **Reopro®** (**monoclonal antibody**)

System	Advantages	Disadvantages	Products
Baculovirus	• Eukaryotic—similar protein processing, modifications to mammalian cell culture • Ease of suspension culture • Soluble intracellular proteins • Large viral genome can accommodate large proteins • Noninfectious to mammalian cells	• Insect cell system—potentially different processing • Inefficient splicing of large products • Nonmammalian system • Requires characterization of both cells and virus stocks • Distinct glycosylation patterns	• HIV-1 gp160 IIIB • Carcinoembryonic antigen • Influenza vaccine • Hemagglutinin • Gp 160 (HIV protein)
Transgenic plant systems	• Low cost of raw materials • Able to assembly of multimeric proteins • Time to scale-up • Safety (plants are not hosts for human pathogens) • Efficient production of secretory IgAs (SIgAs) in tobacco	• Concerns with posttranslational modifications including acylation, glycosylation, phosphorylation, and plant proteases • Susceptibility to drought, elements • Incompatibility of mammalian proteins in plant cells • Presence and characterization of plant impurities in final products • Use of pesticides/herbicides	• CaroRx™ (antistreptococcus) • IgG (phase 1) • *E. coli* LT (phase 1)
Transgenic animal systems	• Substantially-increased yields • Decreased long-term costs • Ease of purification from milk • Variety of production species (goat, sheep, cattle) • Mammary specific expression • Ability to utilize both genomic and cDNA clones for effective expression	• Time to full scale-up • Animal to animal variation • Variations in feeding and milk production • Controlling for animal illness	• Alpha-1-antitrypsin (sheep) • Fibrinogen (sheep) • Protein C (porcine) • Antithrombin III (goat) • Monoclonal antibody (goat)

Note: **Products in bold are on the market [1]**

factor (Leukine®), and hepatitis B vaccine *(Engerix®)* [1]. Other products currently under study produced in yeast include influenza neuraminidase, botulinum neurotoxin A binding domain, and monoclonal antibody variable fragments [8].

Recombinant proteins can also be expressed in mammalian cell systems including Chinese hamster ovary (CHO) and baby hamster kidney (BHK) cells. While the initial bioreactor setup for these mammalian systems can be more costly than for either bacterial or yeast systems, mammalian cells can still produce large quantities of posttranslationally modified, viable recombinant product [2]. Indeed the majority of biopharmaceutical products marketed today are produced in mammalian cells, primarily CHO cells (Table 2.1). Mammalian cell approaches are often required when protein function is heavily dependent on posttranslational modifications, including glycosylation, phosphorylation, or acylation. Many protein biopharmaceutical products including DNAse I (Pulmozyme®), tissue plasminogen activator (Retavase®), erythropoietin (Epogen®), and FSH (Follistem®) can only be produced in their native structure in mammalian cells. Many mammalian cell systems are also highly inducible, meaning that expression of the desired product can be tightly controlled and highly stimulated. Methotrexate, for example, was used to select for high levels of dihydrofolate reductase (DHFR) expression in CHO cells producing recombinant tPA [2]. Among other advantages of mammalian cell systems are the numbers of distinct, specialized cell types available, growth of some cell types in suspension culture, and the ability of host cells to sequester proteins into specific cell compartments or secrete proteins directly into the culture media [9].

Despite these many advantages mammalian cells do not possess all the necessary enzymatic machinery to properly posttranslationally modify every recombinant protein. In many cases mammalian cell lines lack the enzymes necessary for proper sialylation of proteins [2]. While it is possible to stably introduce these sialyltransferases into the host cell, expression of these enzymes normally decreases with time and adds an extra variable to an already complicated cellular process. Another challenge with mammalian cells is that they often require a solid matrix for adherent growth. While many cells can be grown in suspension, others such as CHO must utilize large-scale spinner culture or microbead technology to achieve maximum yields. In many cases expression and growth of mammalian cells is not indefinite. Most cells exhibit a limited passage number, decrease their expression of recombinant protein, and cease to grow. Thus well-developed master cell banks and working cell banks must be constantly maintained in the event of contamination or loss of the culture [2]. Additionally mammalian cell culture is significantly more costly than bacterial culture with respect to growth media components such as serum and antibiotics.

Recombinant human proteins may also be expressed in baculovirus, such as *Spodoptera frugiperd*a (SF9) cells. These viruses possess large genomes capable of accommodating extremely large exogenous DNA sequences.

Numerous shuttle vectors are available that facilitate convenient transfer from bacteria or mammalian cells. Proteins such as HIV Gp 160, carcinoembryonic antigen, and a form of influenza vaccine have successfully been expressed in baculovirus systems [9]. Potential disadvantages of this system include inappropriate posttranslational modifications, use of insect rather than mammalian cells, and characterization of both the baculovirus and SF9 insect cells used.

In the future, neoplastic cells including spontaneous or virus-transformed cells, or other immortalized cell lines, may also serve as a preferred cell substrate for recombinant protein production. The use of malignant cells as host systems for recombinant proteins represents a natural extension of using neoplastic cells to produce purified biologicals, including interferons and monoclonal antibodies [10]. Obvious concerns with these agents as host systems for vaccine production include contamination with viable tumor cells or other adventitious agents. Contamination from residual DNA or biologically active proteins is also a possibility. Finally tumors are by nature heterogeneous, often consisting of numerous cell types exhibiting several distinct phenotypes and genotypes. Controlling for this heterogeneity represents an additional challenge for development of vaccines from neoplastic cell systems [10].

Transgenic plants might also be used for production of recombinant proteins. While many of these systems are still early in the development stage, plants offer very robust and high-capacity system for biopharmaceutical production. Since plants cannot always properly modify proteins as mammalian cells, their utility may be limited. However, early studies suggest that plants may serve as useful hosts for production of vaccines and antibodies. For example, HepB surface antigen has been successfully expressed in potatoes [11], and clinical trials are underway with secretory antibodies (SIgAs), such as CaroRx™, developed in plants [12].

Expression in transgenic animals, particularly dairy cattle, sheep, and goats, is a viable option for achieving large-scale recombinant protein production. Unlike bacterial, yeast, or mammalian cell systems, transgenic animal systems can express recombinant proteins in the milk at quantities up to 30 g/L. In addition to vastly increased capacity, milk provides a relatively simple matrix for purification [2]. Monoclonal antibodies, for instance, have successfully been expressed in transgenic mice and goats [13]. Furthermore transgenic animals are also capable of producing complex proteins folded with many of the posttranslational modifications such as glycosylation, amidation, and gamma-carboxylation [14].

As with any other biological system, transgenic animals are still susceptible to those adventitious agents capable of affecting bacterial, mammalian cell, or yeast systems. Moreover, unlike cells and bacteria, a somewhat greater degree of intraindividual genetic variation may be observed with a transgenic herd. Variability in food intake and/or milk production also represent points to consider in the development of transgenic animal populations. Characteristics of these various expression systems and examples of recombinant proteins produced using these technologies are described in Table 2.1.

2.3 GUIDELINES FOR THE PRODUCTION AND ACCEPTANCE OF RECOMBINANT PROTEINS IN BIOLOGIC SYSTEMS

As is the case for any new chemical entity, the FDA, the CPMP, and the International Conference on Harmonisation of Technical Requirements for Pharmaceuticals (ICH) have developed standards and guidelines for the production and characterization of recombinant biological products. In the subsequent section we will discuss some of the standards for manufacturing, release and finally, comparability of biologics produced in conventional versus transgenic systems. For reference, one may consult the ICH Tripartate Guidelines on Test Procedures and Acceptance Criteria for Biotechnological/Biological Products [15], and the FDA Points to Consider in the Manufacturing and Testing of Therapeutic Products for Human Use Derived from Transgenic Animals [16], the CPMP's Guideline on Comparability of Medicinal Products Containing Biotechnology-Derived Proteins as Active Substance [17], and the Points to Consider in the Characterization of Cell Lines Used to Produce Biologicals [18].

The FDA and ICH both convey messages that biologic manufacturers must thoroughly characterize all aspects of their manufacturing process, including the starting raw materials, strains of microbials or animals used, growth conditions, methods of introducing the novel genes into the host system, methods of isolation of the product, product characterizations including all analytical methods utilized, batch acceptance and rejection criteria, storage, expiration, and shipping. Regardless of the source of the recombinant protein, these elements must be addressed to ensure the safety and efficacy of the final product.

2.3.1 Manufacturing Criteria for Cellular Systems

For cellular systems (bacterial, mammalian cell-based, etc.) manufacturers must describe the origin of the cell lines used, the general characteristics, and genotype (if known) of the master and working cell lines, including any known genetic markers and the source tissue (if known). Growth conditions, including all components of the culture media, antibiotics, and/or growth factors should also be described. Production, characterization, and storage of both the master and working cell banks should be discussed. Master cell banks should be characterized for morphology, species of origin, split ratio, functionality, and identity. Working cell banks should be routinely characterized for contamination, sterility, and presence of viruses. Composition and source of the culture media and any other additional factors (serum, antibiotics) should be described.

Manufacturers should include reasonable detail about the source of the gene to be expressed, including, if known, the complete DNA sequence and any regulatory elements, the method of introduction of the recombinant gene into the host cell, and methods for identification of the transformed host.

Manufacturers should also describe all reagents utilized, selection criteria, methods for screening for recombinant protein and monitoring for stability or maintenance of gene expression (periodic testing). Production conditions should also be described, including the length of collection, the total batch size (cell number or volume), and frequency of recovery. Isolation procedures, including centrifugation techniques, chromatographic, or other biochemical techniques required for product purification, should also be described and validated for each biologically produced material. Finally, stability of the product should be determined, and storage conditions for the purified material and standards for acceptance or rejection should also be well defined [19].

2.3.2   Manufacturing Criteria for Transgenic Animals

The FDA and EU have also established specific guidelines for the manufacture and testing of therapeutic products derived from transgenic animals [16]. The FDA has specified its expectations on the use of transgenic animals for production of biopharmaceuticals, including relevant scientific points that should be addressed in any subsequent regulatory submission. Guidelines for biologic production in transgenic animals essentially follow those for cell-based systems.

Similar to cell-based systems, it is expected that sponsors provide detailed information on their genetic construct, including description of the native protein, the genetic structure of the transgene, any cloning and purification methods used, and any vectors such as yeast artificial chromosomes (YACs). The sponsor's strategy to create the final transgene construct should also be described. Specific DNA elements within the transgene, including enhancers, promoters, repressors, or other control regions, should be discussed, particularly if they are to have a planned effect on expression of the transgene.

The manufacturer should further describe production of the initial founder animals, including the history of the animals donating the gametes. Like master cell banks, transgenic production animals should have detailed veterinary records. The method of introduction of the transgene into the recipient animal(s) should be described, as well as characterization of methods used to assess transgene expression. Again, acceptance criteria should be established for presence of the transgene and to confirm expression of the transgene within desired limits in the transgenic animals. Also any deleterious effect of transgene expression on the animal's health should be duly noted.

Next, the transgenic animals must be monitored for stability of the transgene. This should continue through several rounds of germ-line passage using DNA analytical methods such as Southern blots. Then, stability of expression of the transgene must be established. While the transgene may be present in the transgenic animal, expression must be maintained. Unlike cell lines, transgenic animals cannot be stored indefinitely. Thus approaches must be developed to ensure that the transgenic product remains available for an extended period of time. This can be likened to the use of master cell banks (MCBs) and working cell banks (WCBs). These might be termed Master Transgenic Bank and Master Working Transgenic Bank, respectively.

Breeding techniques and animal husbandry methods should be described, including addition or elimination of animals from the production herd. Animal feed and housing should be thoroughly described. Standards for registered facilities may be found in the *NIH Guide for the Care and Use of Laboratory Animals* [20].

Last, purification and characterization of the transgenic product should be adequately described. Procedures such as milking, exsanguination or extirpation of tissues should be detailed so as to "maximize safety, sterility, potency, and purity of the product." Although collection of the biologic material may not occur under sterile conditions, the area should be as clean as possible. The actual production lot should be well defined, and those tests found to be sensitive to potential changes in the product should be incorporated into the lot release protocol. Naturally, products derived from transgenic animals (milk, blood urine, semen, etc.) will have a unique set of concerns compared to a product derived from asceptic cell culture. As is the case for the ICH guidelines, the FDA expects that any biopharmaceutical product derived from transgenic animals be thoroughly characterized with respect to safety, purity, and potency. "The manufacturer should describe all tests performed for in-process control and final product acceptability." This is particularly important in transgenics, since unlike a relatively homogeneous cell population, a transgenic herd may consist of numerous unique individuals with material harvested at different times of the year in different temperatures. However, it is not very different from using blood donations from unique human individuals for composition of the starting pool for purification of plasma products.

2.4 CRITERIA FOR RELEASE OF RECOMBINANT PROTEIN PRODUCTS

The ICH expectations are that "acceptance criteria" or limits of acceptability will be established prior to final product characterization, regardless of the host cell system. More important, with respect to system, the final product should be compared to appropriate reference standards (if available), and ideally, with the naturally occurring protein. Products should be thoroughly characterized with respect to five distinct criteria (ICH Guideline, Specification: Test Procedures and Acceptance Criteria for Biotechnological/Biological Products [15]):

- Physiochemical properties
- Characterization of biologic activity
- Immunochemical properties
- Characterization of purity and potential impurities
- Yield (quantity)

In 1999 the ICH recommended the adoption of a series of guidelines defining the test procedures and acceptance criteria for biotechnological and biological products. This document provides general principles for setting a uniform set of international specifications for biotechnology products. The principles apply to "all proteins and polypeptides, their derivatives, and products of which they are components." It is assumed that these proteins are produced from recombinant or nonrecombinant cell-culture expression systems or transgenic animal systems, and that they will be highly purified and characterized using appropriate analytical procedures.

2.4.1 Physiochemical Properties

Any protein product, regardless of the host cell system, must be extensively characterized. This involves describing not only the primary amino acid structure but also information regarding any higher order structure (if known), which may be acquired by various biochemical and analytical means including, but not limited to, a mass spectrum, amino acid analysis and SDS-polyacrylamide gel electrophoretic (SDS-PAGE) analysis. Other characterizations might include isoelectric focusing, anion exchange or gel filtration chromatography, HPLC analysis, fluorescence spectroscopy, tryptic mapping, or even circular dichroism spectra.

The manufacturer must also characterize the degree of heterogeneity in the product with respect to glycosylation or other posttranslational modifications using standard biochemical analyses: SDS-PAGE, Western blotting, and RP-HPLC. Again, standards should be developed for such secondary modifications and limits set for acceptance or rejection of a particular lot of material. If a consistent degree of heterogeneity is maintained and is deemed acceptable for biological activity, then extensive evaluations of efficacy and safety may not be required.

2.4.2 Biologic Activity

As for any new lot of material, assessments of biological activity should be performed to demonstrate the efficacy of the product. This may be achieved though the use of animal-based biological assays, cell-based assays that evaluate the material at the cellular level, and biochemical activity assays such as enzymatic action. Standards should be properly defined. Potency and efficacy for individual lots of material can therefore be defined.

2.4.3 Immunochemical Properties

The immunochemical properties of the biopharmaceutical should also be fully characterized. This may include binding assays of the antibody to purified antigens, using defined regions of the antigen. Additionally the target antigen, and if possible, the specific epitope should also be biochemically defined, particularly if immunochemical activity defines the primary biologic action.

2.4.4 Purity and Potential Impurities

Manufacturers should be able to demonstrate purity of the material. Posttranslational modifications do not necessarily represent impurities, provided that they can be shown to be consistent and without effect on the biological activity. Because of the complex nature of biological systems, it is understood that certain impurities may be present. In this case they should be characterized and shown to be without biological effect. Acceptance criteria should be equal to or exceed results obtained in preclinical studies. Contamination should be strictly controlled using well-defined in-process acceptance criteria. Product stability should be likewise characterized based on real time studies conducted with representative material [19].

2.4.5 Product Content

Protein or peptide content should be well defined by an appropriate physiochemical test. If the quantity of product can be well correlated to a specific biological activity (standard curve), then an elaborate physiochemical test does not need to be performed.

2.4.6 Products Made Transgenically

With respect to the final product, transgenic recombinant proteins are essentially no different from proteins produced in bacterial, yeast, or mammalian cell systems. Donor DNA must be entirely characterized, as well as the methods for introduction of the recombinant. Production conditions should be well defined as will be methods for product harvest, purification, and storage. The product must be characterized for its physical and biologic properties. Many of the primary concerns with the use of transgenic animals in fact have already been considered during the development of purified human proteins. A number of marketed biologics derived from human plasma or serum, such as IFN α-N3 (Alferon N®) or Coagulation Factor IX (Mononine®) are prepared from pooled donor plasma, representing diverse donors in distinct environments. The plasma or serum obtained must then be extensively tested for purity and viral contamination. In a similar manner, transgenic recombinant products will routinely be pooled from multiple individuals and examined for adventitious agents. Following sample collection, postharvest techniques should again be similar to those used for bacterial or mammalian cell systems. Table 2.2 highlights the various aspects of the manufacturing process and release criteria for biopharmaceutical products. It becomes apparent that transgenic animal products must meet the same criteria as those required for other host systems.

TABLE 2.2   Biologic manufacturing of recombinant proteins

Element of System	Cell Substrate		
	Bacterial	Mammalian Cell	Transgenic Animal
DNA expression construct	• Sequence • Expression vector • Regulatory Elements • Method of Production • Purification • Purity standards	Same	Same
Host cell/animal system • History of Cell Line • Master and Working Cell Banks • Environmental Growth Conditions	• Monitor contamination	• Monitor contamination	• Animal pedigree • Monitor for illness
Method of gene transfer	• Transformation	• Transfection	• Embryo manipulation
Methods of identifying or characterizing recombinant proteins	• Growth selection	• Antibiotic resistance	• Southern blots • PCR
Production conditions (environmental)	• Controlled	• Controlled	• Less controlled • Distinct individuals
Method of product recovery	• Batch fermentation	• Batch Fermentation	• Pool multiple individuals
Product stability	• Product specific	• Product specific	• Product specific
Product storage	• Product specific	• Product specific	• Product specific
Criteria for release/ acceptance	• Physiochemical • Biologic activity • Immunochemical • Purity/impurities • Yield	Same	Same

2.5   ENVIRONMENTAL ASSESSMENT AND CATEGORICAL EXCLUSIONS

Any submission requiring action by the FDA must include either an environmental assessment (EA) or a claim of categorical exclusion from the requirement for an EA (21 CFR 51.15(a)). When an EA is submitted, it is evaluated by the FDA and either an environmental impact statement (EIS) or a finding of no significant impact (FONSI) is filed by the Agency (21 CFR25.15(b)).

The following actions are generally categorically excluded from needing an EA or an EIS:

- If use of the active moiety does not increase
- If use of the active moiety increased, but the concentration of the substance at the point of entry into the aquatic environment (estimated introduction concentration; EIC) will be below 1 part per billion
- If the substance occurs naturally in the environment and the action does not alter significantly the concentration or distribution of the substance, its metabolites, or degradation products in the environment
- Action on an IND

The following assumptions are made in determining the EIC.

1. All of the drug product is used and enters the publicly owned treatment works,
2. Drug product usage occurs throughout the United States in a distribution that is proportional to the population, and amount of wastewater generated.
3. No metabolism occurs

A protein or nucleic acid comprised of naturally occurring amino acids or nucleosides, but having a sequence different form that of a naturally occurring substance, will normally qualify as a naturally occurring substance after considering metabolism.

The estimated introduction concentration (EIC) =

Kilogram (kg) of drug/biologic produced per year $\div$ 365 days $\times$ 10^9 micrograms per kg $\times$ liters of water per day entering the POTW (publicly owned treatment works; 1.2×10^{11} liters/day) (1996 Needs Survey, Report to Congress at www.epa.gov/own)

Refinements to the calculations can be made to correct for metabolism, pharmacological activity of metabolites, nonproportional distribution of release, and other factors.

The maximum expected environmental concentration (MEEC) is the concentration that organisms would be exposed to in the environment. It is derived from the EIC after taking into account any spatial or temporal accumulation or depletion factors, such as dilution, degradation, or bioaccumulation. If a drug is rapidly inactivated or degraded under environmental conditions, then it is generally not necessary to institute further testing. If not, then tiered environmental (ecotoxicity) testing is required.

INDs generally involve relatively small amounts of drug and treatment of a limited number of recipients, so the environmental exposure is usually low. INDs are evaluated on a case-by-case basis to determine if extraordinary circumstances exist. Extraordinary circumstances include situations where there is potential for serious harm to the environment at the expected level of exposure, lasting effects on ecological community dynamics, or an adverse effect on an endangered specie or habitat of an endangered specie. The determination of extraordinary circumstances can be based on information from the agency, the sponsor, published sources, and other sources. Most commonly INDs will be submitted with a request for categorical exclusion from EA.

An example of an EA for a typical IND is provided below:

[Company name] certifies that [drug or biologic name] is intended for use in clinical studies in which waste will be controlled and the amount of waste expected to enter the environment is expected to be nontoxic. Therefore, in accordance with 21 CFR 25.31, we request categorical exclusion from providing an environmental assessment.

2.6 DEMONSTRATION OF COMPARABILITY WHEN A MANUFACTURING SYSTEM IS CHANGED

In its Guidance on Demonstration of Comparability of Human Biologic Products, including Biotechnology Derived Products [18], the FDA formally elaborated its position on the steps manufacturers must take to demonstrate comparability following manufacturing changes (see Chapter 8). The FDA's position is for sponsors to discuss any potential changes with them prior to implementation to prevent unnecessary duplication of resources. These guidelines are applicable to any type of manufacturing change including changes from bacterial to mammalian cell to transgenic expression systems. While this list is not exhaustive, some of these potential changes include the following:

- Changes in DNA vector
- Changes in host cell system
- Changes in fermentation/culture process
- Equipment changes
- Changes in raw materials
- Changes in purification techniques
- Changes in storage conditions

Sponsors may make changes in manufacturing processes for a particular product for a number of reasons, including improvement of quality, yield, or simply manufacturing efficiency. Such changes may be frequent, and manufacturing changes have been successfully made during or even after the completion of clinical studies. In these situations comparability data have provided assurance that the product would continue to be safe, pure, and effective. For example, in the past such changes have included conversion from pilot plant to full-scale production, a move of the production facilities from one location to another, and implementation of changes in different stages of the process such as fermentation, purification, and formulation. For changes made prior to product approval, the sponsor must fully describe the changes in any license application or investigational new drug application (IND). The criteria for establishing product comparability include the following:

- Biochemical characterization
- In vitro and in vivo bioactivity
- Pharmacokinetics
- Safety

In terms of product identity and biochemical characterization, when manufacturers transition from one system of production to another, qualified product standards are used to judge product identity and purity. Biologic activity testing either in vitro or in vivo are also frequently standardized and can be consistently performed on protein products derived from any production system whether it be bacterial, mammalian, or intact organism. In most cases, however, mimicking the biological activity in the clinic following a change in the manufacturing process would not be required provided that cell or biochemical assays can be shown to correlate to clinical response.

Regardless of the cell substrate utilized for biologic production, consistency in both upstream and downstream production processes will also play an important role in validating any novel biological system. Detailed knowledge of the stepwise manufacturing paradigm and elaboration of these methodologies may compensate to a large extent for changes in starting materials. Nevertheless, manufacturers should make available to the FDA extensive chemical, physical, and biological comparisons with side-by-side analyses of the old and new lots of material. Most important, tests should include those routinely used for release of the bulk drug substance and final drug products in addition to those tests aimed at evaluating the impact of the change on the product. Basically the regulatory position suggests that sponsors follow their normal procedures when implementing a manufacturing change, namely demonstrating comparability. The tests should be sensitive to detect any alteration induced by the manufacturing change [21]:

> These tests should include tests routinely done on all production lots, those initially used to fully characterize product structure and identity and establish product consistency from one production lot to another . . .

An example of changes in manufacturing system and how comparability was assessed from a regulatory perspective involves interferon β-1a (IFNβ-1a).

Recombinant IFNβ-1a is produced in CHO cells, and the primary amino acid sequence of the recombinant protein produced by these cells was identical to the naturally occurring IFNβ. IFNβ-1a is a single, glycosylated polypeptide 166 amino acids in length. An initial batch of drug product, termed BG9015 was used in phase 3 clinical trials. The sponsor subsequently developed a new CHO cell line carrying the IFNβ-1a gene and designated the product isolated from these cells BG9216. These particular CHO cells harboring the IFNβ-1a gene were adapted for the suspension culture. Data supporting the use of this cell line were submitted to the FDA, and it was determined that the specific activity of BG9216 was greater than BG9015 and contained an additional peak in the peptide map. Pharmacokinetic studies also demonstrated that BG9216 was not equivalent to BG9015. With these data the FDA determined that BG9216 was not comparable to BG9015.

The sponsor then developed yet another IFNβ-1a cell line, and the product produced by these cells was designated BG9418. This product was extensively characterized and compared side by side with BG9015. Biological, biochemical, and biophysical analyses demonstrated that the two molecules were comparable. Biological activities of each molecule were similar using several different antiviral and antiproliferative assays. Chromatography of peptides derived by proteolysis of the two proteins was nearly identical. Carbohydrate analysis was also performed, and both forms exhibited similar patterns. In this case the sponsor further performed clinical pharmacokinetic studies and showed that the two forms behaved identically. Based on these data, the FDA determined that drugs BG9015 and BG9418 were comparable and that data obtained during the study of BG9015 would support the licensing of the BG9418 molecule [22].

Change to an entirely new host cell system can also have either minor or significant effects on recombinant protein production. In a comparison of five distinct eukaryotic cell expression systems, Geisse et al. [9] assessed the expression of human leukemia inhibitory factor (hu-LIF) in five of the most commonly used cell lines. The yields and quality of protein product were assessed in CHO, Sp2/0, MEL, COS, and baculovirus-infected insect cells. Although recombinant, biologically active product was produced in every case, yields and glycosylation patterns varied widely among the systems. To date, such significant changes have yet to be implemented into a biologic manufacturing paradigm.

2.7 APPLICATION OF COMPARABILITY CRITERIA TO A NEW MANUFACTURING TECHNOLOGY

The potential impact induced by changes in manufacturing systems cannot be assumed. Thus major changes in the host system may or may not impact a product's identity or activity. Applying sound scientific principles of safety and efficacy will permit manufacturers and regulators to objectively assess the impact of manufacturing changes.

Changes can occur in the manufacturing system at any point in the drug development cycle, and the extent of comparability testing may be related to the timing of such changes. Regardless of the stage of development, the FDA encourages sponsors to consult with them prior to instituting any major change in the manufacturing process. For biological products that the FDA has approved, the sponsor should submit information about manufacturing changes pursuant to 21 CFR 601.12 or 21 CFR 314.70(g) along with any FDA guidance on the changes described. The European Agency for the Evaluation of Medicinal Products (Committee for Proprietary Medicinal Products) has issued similar comparability statements in its year-end 2003 publication [17].

In general, the later in the development process a change takes place, the more studies may be expected to be conducted. Thus it is advantageous for biologic manufacturers to select an overall manufacturing approach as soon as possible. Similarly manufacturers will likely need to demonstrate some form of comparability each time major change takes place in the development process (see Figure 2.1.). Naturally, the best time to make significant changes to a biomanufacturing system is during the early development phase. If this is the case, few or potentially no comparability studies may be needed. When manufacturing changes are instituted during the preclinical (pre-IND) phase, limited batch comparison studies may be required to demonstrate comparability, but formal bioequivalence testing, including animal toxicology or pharma-

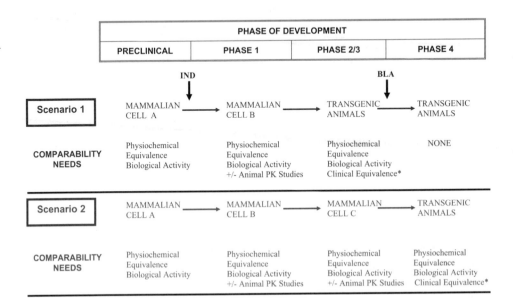

*Pharmacodynamic equivalence as demonstrated by validated surrogate markers or primary clinical endpoints.

Figure 2.1 Comparability needs in relationship to development stage.

cokinetic studies, may not be required. The sponsor, in its application, should provide a rationale for the types of comparability testing performed based on the nature of the change in the manufacturing system.

In most cases changes in a manufacturing paradigm are unlikely to impose drastic changes in product quality. However, even if purity and identity can be unequivocally established following a change in manufacturing system, animal pharmacokinetic or pharmacodynamic studies may be warranted. While a subtle change in product quality may have little or no impact on the toxicological profile of a biologic, changes in glycosylation, in protein folding, or in the tertiary structure could impact the pharmacodynamics of a biologic. Ultimately, if clinical studies are warranted, product innovators will frequently have at their disposal surrogate markers of efficacy and/or toxicity. These markers should allow more limited studies with defined surrogate endpoints in lieu of costly pivotal clinical trials. Identification and validation of these surrogate markers in Phase 2 and 3 studies, respectively, will be an increasingly important step in the development of any novel biologic.

When a manufacturing change occurs during the clinical phase (between the IND and BLA or NDA), the sponsor will need to demonstrate that batches used are chemically, biologically, and perhaps clinically equivalent. Again, pharmacodynamic equivalence should be verified using a validated animal model. Clinical pharmacokinetic studies might be warranted if chemical, biochemical, and animal pharmacodynamic studies cannot demonstrate comparability with the earlier product. This is demonstrated in scenario 1 in Figure 2.1. As was the case for IFN β-1a discussed above, the sponsor needed to demonstrate that the product produced in the new CHO cell line was biologically equivalent to the earlier version used in an initial clinical study.

Finally, manufacturing changes might also be introduced in the post-approval phase (Figure 2.1, scenario 2), namely after the initial, approved version of the product has already been on the market. Sponsors might pursue limited pharmacodynamic studies provided that chemical and biochemical equivalence can be established. In such a case that physiochemical or biologic comparability cannot be demonstrated following a manufacturing change during the postmarketing phase, clinical batch-to-batch comparability must be demonstrated.

2.8   SUMMARY AND CONCLUSIONS

Numerous manufacturing systems are presently available for large-scale expression of recombinant proteins. Bacteria, yeast, mammalian cells, and transgenic animals have all been successfully utilized for large-scale production of recombinant biologics. In most cases the recombinant product is a cloned version of a previously purified human or animal protein; thus reference standards are available for comparison. The FDA and the European Regulatory Agency have since developed standards for both the production and characterization of protein therapeutics produced using recombinant technology. These standards address the identity, purity, stability, and biological activity for recombinant proteins. Moreover, since it is expected that novel technology will facilitate conversion from one production method to another, both the FDA and the European CPMP have provided guidance on demonstrating comparability following changes to a manufacturing system. These guidances have provided a common pathway that can be followed for incorporating and evaluating changes within a biologic manufacturing system.

Any submission requiring action by the FDA must include either an environmental assessment (EA) or a claim of categorical exclusion from the requirement for an EA. INDs are frequently submitted with a request for categorical exclusion from EA, since they generally involve relatively small amounts of drug and treatment of a limited number of recipients such that the environmental exposure is usually low.

The criteria for demonstrating comparability are dependent on both the final product and its stage of development, rather than on perceived degree of change, especially as one may change host systems radically. While recombinant proteins in general are often more complex than small molecule drugs, the approach and standards for product comparability are similar. Structure, identity, purity, and biologic activity still remain the final endpoints of analysis, regardless of whether a novel drug is a small molecule or large, recombinant protein. While the process and its consistency and predictability are very important, the final drug product is the entity from which safety and efficacy will be evaluated. It is the responsibility of drug manufacturers to demonstrate product safety and efficacy of the final drug product throughout the development cycle where changes in process and manufacturing systems are common. With adherence to scientific principles and regulatory guidance, the development and commercialization of novel protein therapeutics utilizing manufacturing systems that meet the production needs of new lifesaving therapeutics should be realized.

REFERENCES

1. PDR, *Physician's Desk Reference.* 2006. Thomson PDR, Montvale, NJ, USA.
2. Werner RG, Noe W, Kopp K, Schluter M. Appropriate mammalian expression systems for biopharmaceuticals. *Arzneimittelforschung* 1998;48(8):870–80.
3. Guidance for Industry Environmental Assessment of Human Drugs and Biologics Applications (1998).
4. Pines O, Inouye M. Expression and secretion of proteins in *E. coli. Mol Biotechnol* 1999;12(1):25–34.
5. Janne J, Hyttinen J-M, Peura T, Tolvanen M, Alhonen L, Halmekyto M. Transgenic animals as bioproducers of therapeutic proteins. *Ann Med* 1992;24:273–80.
6. Ladisch MR, Kohlmann KL. Recombinant human insulin. *Biotechnol Prog* 1998; 8(6):79–81.

7. Eckart MR, Bussineau CM. Quality and authenticity of heterologous proteins synthesized in yeast. *Curr Opin Biotech* 1996;7:525–30.

8. Pennell CA, Eldin P. In vitro production of recombinant antibody fragments in Pichia pastoris. *Res Immunol* 1998;149(6):599–603.

9. Geisse S, Gram H, Kleuser B, Kocher HP. Eukaryotic expression systems: A comparison. *Protein Express Purific* 1996;8:271–82.

10. Lewis AM, Krause P, Peden K. A Defined Risks Approach to the Regulatory Assessment of the Use of Neoplastic Cells as Substrates for Viral Vaccine Manufacture. US FDA, 1999.

11. Mason HS, Lam DM, Arntzen CJ. Expression of hepatitis B surface antigen in transgenic plants. *Proc Natl Acad Sci USA* 1992;89(24):11745–9.

12. Larrick JW, Yu L, Chen J, Jaiswal S, Wycoff K. Production of antibodies in transgenic plants. *Res Immunol* 1998;149(6):603–8.

13. Bruggemann M, Neuberger MS. Strategies for expressing human antibody repertoires in transgenic mice. *Immunol Today* 1996;17(8):391–7.

14. Clark AJ. The mammary gland as a bioreactor: Expression, processing, and production of recombinant proteins. *J Mammary Gland Biol Neoplasia* 1998;3(3): 337–50.

15. Specifications: Test procedures and Acceptance Criteria for Biotechnological/Biological Products, ICH Harmonized Tripartite Guideline, 1999.

16. US FDA, CBER, Points to Consider in the Manufacture and Testing of Therapeutic Products for Human Use Derived from Transgenic Animals. 1995.

17. Committee for Proprietary Medicinal Products (CPMP). Guidance on Comparability of Medicinal Products Containing Biotechnology-Derived Proteins as Active Substance. EMEA, 2003.

18. US FDA. Points to Consider in the Characterization of Cell Lines Used to Produce Biologicals. 1993.

19. US FDA. ICH Q5C Quality of Biotechnological Products: Stability Testing of Biotechnological/Biological Products. 1996.

20. Office for the Protection from Research Risks. Guide for the Care and Use of Laboratory Animals. Washington: National Academy Press, 1996.

21. Cavagnaro JA. Establishment of criteria for determining comparability of "well-characterized" proteins. *Dev Biol Stand* 1998;96:79–81.

22. US FDA. Summary Basis of Approval for Interferon beta-1a. PLA#95-0979, 1995.

PART II

PRINCIPLES OF PRECLINICAL DEVELOPMENT

CHAPTER 3

The Principles of ICH S6 and the Case-by-Case Approach

JOY A. CAVAGNARO, PhD DABT, RAC

Contents

3.1   HISTORY OF PRECLINICAL SAFETY EVALUATION

The conduct of toxicology studies in laboratory animals has been driven by experience, historical precedence, and governmental requirements, and the results of these studies usually, and reasonably, have led to restrictions on the use, or method of use, of the chemicals concerned [1]. The primary objective of pharmaceutical preclinical safety evaluation is to provide information essential for the initiation of clinical trials. Scientific rationale and controlled reproducible data are used to show that the initial human risk is so low as to be ethically and practically acceptable in relation to the medical value of the information to be obtained from humans. Preclinical safety studies performed throughout the course of product development facilitate and may guide work

Preclinical Safety Evaluation of Biopharmaceuticals: A Science-Based Approach to Facilitating Clinical Trials, edited by Joy A. Cavagnaro
Copyright © 2008 by John Wiley & Sons, Inc.

TABLE 3.1   Objectives of preclinical safety evaluation

- To permit initiation of clinical trials and to support subsequent clinical investigations
- To recommend safe starting dose, dose escalation scheme, regimen, and route of administration
- To identify potential target organs of toxicity
- To identify parameters to monitor in the clinical trial (e.g., biomarkers of safety and activity)
- To discern the mechanism of activity/toxicity and reversibility or delay of effects
- To identify "at-risk" human populations by thorough definition of study subject inclusion/exclusion criteria
- To provide safety data to support product labeling claims
- To provide data to support potential product liability concerns
- To provide critical information to support termination of a potentially unsuccessful development program in a timely manner

in healthy volunteers and patients by confirming the acceptability of the risk–benefit ratio of the proposed clinical development and how to minimize any foreseeable risks (see Table 3.1). Efforts devoted to improving the predictive value of preclinical studies are critical to achieving these objectives.

In the early 1950s guidelines and standard approaches for general toxicity testing were introduced in the form of acute subchronic and chronic toxicity studies to help predict human risks. The increase in the number of new drugs, chemicals, and environmental pollutants led to the introduction of additional toxicological tests to screen for specific mutagenic, teratogenic, and other reproductive and/or carcinogenic activities to better determine toxicity to specific organ systems. This testing became standardized. During this time these approaches for toxicity testing were considered essential in ensuring adequate coverage of potential risks and in promoting consistency and improving the quality of data for review. They also provided guidance to industry on testing strategies that would generally be acceptable for evaluation by regulatory authorities.

In the late 1960s the FDA Goldenthal guidelines described, in general, the types of preclinical studies that could be used in support of the several phases of clinical investigation as well as the approval of a new drug application. Admittedly the guidelines were not intended to be used as protocols, but merely as guides [2]. The agency stated that it was in full agreement with the critics of current practices—and that the toxicology assessment of new drugs should keep pace with the more sophisticated technology, consistent with the objective of being as critical and comprehensive as possible. It was acknowledged that development of new methods in drug evaluation was proceeding at a rapid rate. The agency correctly cautioned that general acceptance of new procedures would be predicated on their applicability and predictive value [2].

When originally promulgated, the 1968 guidelines were intended to provide a framework of guidance on which a testing program for a specific compound could be built. In practical usage the term "guideline" has come to connote a list of necessary tests to meet minimum regulatory requirements. Although guideline connotes various meanings to different individuals, to the toxicologist it has traditionally meant a comprehensive set of rules to follow for the testing of new drugs for registration with regulatory authorities. In the extreme it is a "check box" approach to the toxicity testing of new compounds for safety assessment. Thus lists of specific tests have come to be seen as absolute requirements for product registration, and not doing a test would mean not following the guidelines. However, comprehensive guidelines can only be based on what is known or can be anticipated [3].

Similar approaches were adopted by major regulatory authorities in other countries, including the United Kingdom, France, Germany, Italy, and Scandinavia and subsequently the European Union. The official agencies and the pharmaceutical industries' own experts have published recommendations for a wide range of types of toxicity tests to provide comprehensive data in stardardized form for assessment.

3.2   ICH S6: A NEW APPROACH TO PRECLINICAL SAFETY EVALUATION

Biopharmaceuticals have brought new challenges to toxicologists. In the early 1980s neither industry toxicologists nor regulatory scientists were sure of what constituted an appropriate toxicological assessment program for biopharmaceuticals. It was fortuitous that interferon, an extremely species-specific protein was one of the first human biopharmaceutical products. Despite performing a "traditional" toxicity package, including assessment in multiple species, toxicologists found that the animal studies did not predict the common adverse events observed in humans [4].

In 1986 the Biotechnology Working Party was established in Europe to focus on specific issues related to the development of biotechnology-derived pharmaceuticals. In July 1986 a Satellite Symposium to the IV International Congress of Toxicology was held in Tokyo, Japan. Approximately 135 scientists representing virtually all major countries attended the symposium. Among the attendees were government regulatory scientists, university scientists, and industrial scientists and research managers, all with an interest in the development of new biotechnology products [5]. A few statements made during this meeting are worth noting as they introduced an approach to preclinical safety evaluation that would distinguish the practice of biopharmaceutical preclinical development for the ensuing two decades.

> The availability of modern biotechnology products opens a wide range of exciting therapeutic possibilities. ... For many areas of potential toxicity, no satisfactory safety tests are available, and most of the existing models are not yet properly validated. Nevertheless, since progress can only be made through

accumulation of experience, it appears reasonable to suggest that a considered effort be made to develop and to use scientifically sound experimental systems, and to refrain from following the beaten track of routine toxicity testing. [4]

There is no place for detailed programs of rigidly pre-defined tests to be applied automatically to all products. Instead, useful information will only be obtained if the need for any experimentation at all is decided according to the specific properties and planned uses of each compound. Then, the nature of the studies should be adapted to those individual circumstances. Toxicity testing in this area is most like a series of pharmacological explorations and should not be expected to follow conventional rigid guidelines. [6]

In part our [FDA] experience with the endocrine drug products (the peptides) has influenced our approach for other proteins. We recognize that we do not know enough about the pharmacology of many of the new immunomodifiers and many of the other protein products. I believe the case-by-case approach is the most sensible course at this time I'm sure that as we learn more about the pharmacology of a class of proteins, for example, that our approach will be modified for that class. [7]

Consistent with the case-by-case approach, some toxicological studies will follow a traditional approach, while others may deviate. Instead of focusing on procedures (length of studies, number of groups, number of animals, number of species, etc.) it would be best to focus on the goal behind such testing in order to identify and understand the potential toxicity of the agent. [8]

Based on experiences gained over the intervening decade, a concept paper was proposed by the FDA in 1995, under the auspices of the International Conference on Harmonization of Technical Requirements of Pharmaceuticals (ICH), for a new safety topic specifically relating to the preclinical safety evaluation of biotechnology-derived products. In February 1997 the Thirteenth CMR International Workshop provided an opportunity for international experts to discuss experiences and difficulties encountered in designing scientifically based preclinical safety evaluation programs for biopharmaceuticals. This two-day meeting brought together toxicologists and clinicians, from 32 pharmaceutical and biotechnology companies and regulators and regulatory advisors from the European Medicines Evaluation Agency and 9 countries: Denmark, France, Germany, Italy, Japan, the Netherlands, Sweden, the United Kingdom and the United States [9]. Recommendations arising from the CMR Workshop were taken into consideration by the Expert Working Group for the final drafting of ICH S6 guideline and agreement was reached at ICH 4 in Brussels in July 1997 [10].

At the ICH 4 meeting ICH M3 was also finalized, acknowledging that that there had been marked changes in the kinds of therapeutic products being developed (e.g., biotechnology-derived products) and that existing paradigms for safety evaluation might not always be appropriate or relevant. As such the safety evaluation of biotechnology-derived products should be considered on a case-by-case basis, as described in ICH S6 [11].

The principles of case-by-case assessment were also suggested in a 1998 paper by DeGeorge et al. entitled "Regulatory Considerations for Preclinical Development of Anticancer Drugs." The authors acknowledged that basic research continues to provide information about new cellular mechanisms central to malignancy and often leads to drugs that attempt to exploit those mechanisms. The optimal development of a new class of drug may differ from successful approaches used in the development of older well-established classes. The authors commented that new biological endpoints and new methods in toxicology may be discovered that cannot be anticipated. The recommendations in the manuscript emphasized the concerns to be addressed and the importance of avoiding excessively restrictive and specific guidelines so as not to impede the development of innovative therapies for clinical use [12].

3.3 PRINCIPLES VERSUS PRACTICES

The basic principles of toxicology are applicable across product classes. It is the specific attributes of the product that have the greatest influence on the successful practice of biopharmaceutical toxicology (see Table 3.2). This focus on product attributes has defined the case-by-case approach. Table 3.3 provides a further definition of the case-by-case approach (see Table 3.3).

Pharmaceuticals and biopharmaceuticals can be viewed as a product continuum based on size and complexity in molecular structure. However, as products have evolved, there has been a blurring of product attributes. Small molecules have become larger as the result of alternative scaffolding technologies (e.g., forming protein conjugates and fusion proteins) in order to improve exposure characteristics and dosing regimens. Large molecules have become smaller (e.g., antibody fragments and protein mimetics) in order to improve distribution and decrease potential immunogenicity. There are small molecules in development that exhibit unique species specificity making the traditional test species, rat and/or the dog, less relevant for safety assessment. Novel delivery technologies are also enabling alternative routes of delivery for biopharmaceuticals, such as by the oral and inhalation routes. Some products such as oligonucleotide drugs (ODNs) may have combined product attributes. For example, ODNs are synthetically derived but have complex chemical profiles and are catabolized in ways similar to those followed by certain biopharmaceuticals. Although toxicity assessments are designed to address hybridization-independent effects, some ODNs can also exhibit species specificity where analogous sequences may be needed to assess hybridization-dependent effects, namely toxicity related to exaggerated pharmacology.

3.4 IMPLEMENTATION OF ICH S6 GUIDANCE

The optimal preclinical development of a biopharmaceutical product has benefited from experience. This is because the strategy for designing programs is

TABLE 3.2 Comparative product attributes

Product Attribute	Pharmaceutical	Biopharmaceutical
Manufacture	Chemical synthesis	Biological synthesis (cell culture, transgenic plants, transgenic animals)
Composition	Commonly organic chemical	Protein, carbohydrate, DNA, virus, bacteria, cell
Structure	Well-defined, linear	Complex, tertiary structure
Size	Generally <1 kDa	Generally >30 kDa up to 800 kDa
Purity	Homogeneous single-entity high chemical purity (except racemic mixtures)	Heterogenous mixture (microheterogeneity, aggregates)
Impurities	Easy to qualify; toxicity testing may be required	Difficult to qualify; toxicity generally not an issue but may affect immunogenicity
Product characterization	Specifications defined early in development, generally little change; usually one bioanalytical method (mostly LC/MS-MS)	Broadly defined at initial stages of developed and refined; several bioanalytical assays (e.g., HPLC, SDS-PAGE, MALDI-TOF)
Potency	Not determined	Required; generally in vivo but for some products in vitro acceptable.
Stability	Stable and not heat sensitive	Less stable and sensitive to heat and shear
Route of administration	Oral, topical, inhalation	Parenteral or targeted (IV, SC, IM, intracardiac, intrathecal, intraarticular, etc.)
Pharmacokinetics	Half-life usually minutes to hours	Half-life usually days to weeks
ADME	Rapid entry through blood capillaries, distribution to many organs/tissues, metabolized to active and non-active metabolites	Distribution limited based on size to plasma a/o extracellular fluid, degraded (catabolized) to endogenous amino acids
Drug–drug interactions	Influenced by metabolism (enzyme induction or inhibition)—can be significant	Interactions related to additive or synergistic pharmacological activity not metabolism

TABLE 3.2 *Continued*

Product Attribute	Pharmaceutical	Biopharmaceutical
Dose response	Linear—establishment of maximum tolerated dose (MTD)	Can be bell-shaped—establishment of optimum biological dose (OBD)
Targets	Intracellular or ligand–receptor	Cell–matrix, cell–cell, or ligand–receptor
Pharmacological activity	Active in standard screening and functional assays	Not active in standard screening assays; novel models created to address activity (e.g., transgenic animals, homologous test material)
Species specificity	Species independent; preclinical assessments for generally toxicity generally performed in one rodent (generally rat) and one nonrodent (generally dog)	Species specific; nonhuman primates often the only relevant species or design of specific animal models
Toxicological effects	Unpredictable; can be related to metabolites or unrelated to mechanism of action	Predictable based on known mechanism of action "exaggerated pharmacology"; animal models of disease often used to assess safety in addition to activity
Immunogenicity	Rare; allergic or hypersensitivity reactions may occur	Common; may affect PK or result in immune-mediated adverse events other than allergic and/or hypersensitivity responses
Dosing interval	Daily	Intermittent
Dose formulation	Complex	Simple
Demonstration of equivalence	Bioequivalence (generic equivalents)	Comparability within a development program (more difficult to define biogeneric)

Source: Adapted from Cavagnaro (2002), Baumann (2006), and Horvath (personal communication).

influenced not only by the amount of existing knowledge concerning the pharmacology and toxicology for the specific product and product class but also by the expanding knowledge base of a number of product classes. A number of articles have been published over the years highlighting the challenges of

TABLE 3.3   Case-by-case approach to preclinical safety evaluation

Is Not …	Is …
• Consistent with the "traditional" practices for small molecules	• Consistent with the principles for safety evaluation of small molecules
• Standardized approach	• Product or product-class specific
• Unique to biopharmaceuticals	• Science-based
• A minimalist approach	• Questions-based
• An opportunity to "get a better label"	• Experiential-based
• Just what a sponsor wants to do	• Targeted
• Practiced by all developers of biopharmaceuticals	• Flexible
• Embraced by all regulators	• Fair
• Easy to predict "if acceptable" to regulatory authorities	• More difficult to predict "if acceptable" to regulatory authorities

preclinical development of biopharmaceuticals [13–20] as well as the valuable experiences in implementing the case-by-case approach [21–30]. The following is a discussion of a few key areas.

3.4.1   Use of Animal Models

A guiding principle in the design of preclinical safety studies is to parallel as closely as possible the clinical conditions of exposure. In accordance with the principle, much attention is paid to the dosing regimen with respect to the route of administration, duration of exposure, and dosing interval. With respect to mirroring the characteristics of the patient population to be exposed, normal animals appropriately parallel the typical phase 1 population in normal subjects (healthy volunteers). Where toxicologists deviate from the principle of correlation of clinical conditions of exposure is in the evaluation of potential toxicity in patients in the later safety and efficacy trials in phase 2 and beyond. The deviation from this principle relates primarily to the physiological state of the clinical populations involved as they are no longer healthy volunteers but rather individuals who have a specific disease and/or are very ill. Thus a relevant question for the toxicologist is to ask whether toxicology studies in normal animals adequately assess the risks in sick people. The answer to this question has even greater significance for biopharmaceuticals as first in human (FIH) phase 1 trials are often conducted in subjects with disease for ethical and practical reasons.

Animal models of disease play a critical role in the drug discovery process and are important in the lead candidate selection process as well. Categories of animal disease models include spontaneous disease, induced models (e.g., chemically, immunologically), xenograft models, infection models, and genetically modified models (e.g., transgenic knockouts (KOs) or knock-ins (KIs), humanized animals (e.g., expressing the human protein or receptor). The subsequent evaluation and demonstration of biological activity of test articles in these animal models is often pivotal for further progression of these agents in the clinic.

The principle of estimating a therapeutic index prior to clinical trials typically involves determining the no observable adverse effect level (NOAEL) and comparing that to the projected human dose. In providing the estimate, the efficacious dose is typically obtained from in vitro data with human cells or tissues and in vivo preclinical pharmacology studies that involve animal disease models. Not infrequently the species used to estimate the toxic level is different from the species used to estimate an efficacious level. Thus the therapeutic index is not a true ratio as the units (species and/or conditions) are often different. On the other hand, if one were to obtain information relating to toxicity as well as efficacy from studies employing animal models of disease, a direct estimate of therapeutic index could be made provided that appropriate models had been characterized or validated in the relevant species.

The decision on the use animal models of disease for assessing safety is based on a consideration of a number of factors, not the least of which is whether an animal model of disease is available for the intended disease. There are also ethical and welfare considerations as in any proposal to use animals in scientific work. Animal models of human disease may not mimic all aspects of disease or be more sensitive. However, as long as there is a good understanding of the human disease as well as acknowledgment of specific limitations of the model, studies should allow for better predictions of risk in the intended disease populations (see Table 3.4).

TABLE 3.4   Use of animal models of disease

Potential Advantages	Potential Disadvantages
• Ethical considerations in protection of humans	• Ethical considerations in use of animals
• May be useful to screen compounds for lead candidate	• Relative paucity of background data
• Potential for increased sensitivity	• Inherent variability
• Disease condition may parallel target population	• May only represent one aspect of the disease
• Early opportunity to define biomarkers of safety and activity more relevant to intended population	• Excess mortality may confound data interpretation
• Direct estimate of therapeutic index feasible	• Increased sensitivity may not be relevant
• Opportunity to understand the pathogenesis of treatment related findings	• May be limited in size of group
• Support human safety and efficacy when human clinical trial is not feasible or ethical ("animal rule")	• Potential limitations in study design
	• Potential interference of disease process with safety evaluation

A variety of transgenic animals have been used over the years to help characterize the activity and safety of biopharmaceuticals. Knockout animals have been used to assess a worst-case scenario for maximum inhibition (e.g., MAbs blocking a receptor and suppression of endogenous cytokines or proteins); knock-in animals have been used to describe a worst-case scenario for overexpression (e.g., consequences of growth factor induced proliferation) and humanized transgenic animals (e.g., expressing the human receptor). In the latter case the clinical material can be directly assessed rather than relying on the species specific homologue or on indirect extrapolation from the actions of the clinical (human) therapy acting on targets in another species. In all cases, however, the models lack historical control data. There may be additional concerns with respect to potential differences related to epitope density, localization/compartmentalization, signal transduction pathways, regulation, unknown compensatory mechanisms, host defense mechanisms, or natural life history. Thus as a caution, models may either overestimate or underestimate identification and the magnitude of of a hazard.

3.4.2   Selection of Relevant Species

Traditionally toxicologists have used at least one rodent and nonrodent species for multidose toxicity studies. The use of two species is important for assessing potential variability of metabolism, for products with extensive distribution, and in cases where a relevant species has not been defined. The rat and dog are selected in most cases, usually on an empirical basis [2] without an open-minded consideration of whether alternate species might be better in terms of biochemistry and metabolism [1].

In 1987 Zbinden identified three main areas of concern for biopharmaceuticals: (1) the toxicity per se (intrinsic toxicity), (2) the adverse effects related to the pharmacodynamic properties (exaggerated pharmacology), and (3) the undesirable responses mainly due to indirect biological responses not related to pharmacodynamic properties [4]. Since contaminants are usually present only in small amounts (e.g., host cell proteins, contamination with viruses, DNA, endotoxin, antibiotics), their intrinsic toxicity is considered of minor significance and best addressed through rigorous quality control. Intrinsic toxicity is defined as toxicity unrelated to a product's pharmacodynamic properties, such as the clinical syndrome, flu-like symptoms, fever, nausea, and malaise, observed in humans following interferon administration, or fluid retention and interstitial pulmonary edema following IL 2 administration. The information gained from clinical observations are used to guide toxicological experiments in animals to gain a better understanding of the intrinsic toxic potential and hopefully define more predictive animal models. However, standard toxicological test procedures are poorly suited to a priori identify intrinsic effects. Toxicity that occurs as a consequence of the desired pharmacodynamic effect can often be predicted especially when the biological characteristics are known. Biological toxicity due to indirect biological responses unrelated to pharmacodynamic properties includes toxicity related to structure such as the allergic and sensitizing potential of biopharmaceuticals [4]. See also immunogenicity discussed below.

ICH S6 states that safety evaluation programs should include relevant species demonstrating pharmacological activity. As such the mechanism of toxicity is defined by exaggerated pharmacology. Importantly, relevant pharmacological species can also be used to assess biological toxicity and in some cases intrinsic toxicity. In some cases it may be necessary to consider animal models of disease to evaluate intrinsic toxicity. For small molecules where toxicity may be the result of metabolites or due to extensive distribution to nontarget tissues, a species lacking the target may be relevant as the mechanism of toxicity may be unrelated to exaggerated pharmacology. In such cases the most sensitive species becomes the most relevant species with respect to dose extrapolation. A variety of techniques (e.g., immunochemical or functional tests) can be used to identify a relevant species.

There has been the misconception that only one species is expected for assessing general toxicity of biopharmaceuticals. However, the language in ICH S6 explicitly states that safety evaluation programs should normally include two relevant species, but in certain justifiable cases, one relevant species may suffice (e.g., when only one relevant species can be identified or where the biological activity of the biopharmaceutical is well understood). The guidance intentionally did not specify use of the "most relevant" in order to avoid the routine consideration of use of higher primate species (e.g., greatest homology of a protein or a receptor with chimpanzees or baboons). Demonstration of binding of the biopharmaceutical to a receptor or other target may not be sufficient to define a relevant species as not all molecules that bind actually induce activity. Therefore primary consideration should be given to receptor-mediated activity. Determining biological activity is based on an understanding of in vitro receptor occupancy, affinity, distribution, and in vitro and in vivo pharmacological effects. Importantly, toxicity studies in nonrelevant species are discouraged.

The ICH reproductive toxicology guidance considers the acceptability of a single species if it can be shown by means of pharmacological and toxicological data that the species selected is a relevant model for humans. ICH further states that there is little value in using a second species if it does not show the same similarities [31].

3.4.3 Cross-Reactivity

Tissue cross-reactivity studies for monoclonal antibody products were originally intended to explore off-target tissue binding. Studies have thus been used to screen candidates to avoid off-target binding. As stated in ICH S6, an animal species that does not express the desired epitope may be of some relevance for assessing toxicity if comparable unintentional tissue cross-reactivity to humans is demonstrated. For example, if cross-reactivity was observed in human tissues, assessments of potential binding to nonhuman primate tissue is recommended in order to determine if similar binding is observed in order to justify the use of a nonhuman primate. If similar binding is not observed, the data could be used to justify use of rodents especially in cases where the epitope is not present in normal animals (e.g., tumor antigens). Tissue cross reactivity, however, has inappropriately expanded to testing a variety of animal species in order to select a relevant species for assessing general toxicity. As discussed above, selection of a relevant species is more correctly justified by pharmacological-based receptor or other specific target studies. Similar off-target binding to nonhuman primate nonreproductive tissues justifying use in general toxicity studies does not justify use of the nonhuman primate in reproductive or developmental toxicity studies. The design and relevance of tissue cross-reactivity studies for bispecific and trispecific antibodies, conjugated antibodies, and fusion proteins may differ from monoclonal antibody applications.

Unintentional cross-reactivity may also be suggested by Basic Local Alignment Search Tool (BLAST) that are routinely performed electronically to identify potential binding to nontarget tissue or to determine if there is unintentional cross-reactivity with an endogenous molecule such as following administration of a monoclonal antibody or a vaccine [32]. CEREP assay platforms routinely performed for small molecules for determining off-target binding are not used for biopharmaceuticals.

3.4.4 Analogous Products

For biopharmaceuticals that are unique in their species specificity (i.e., reacting only with monkeys, chimpanzees, and/or humans) use of the homologous protein or more broadly defined analogous products that recognize the ortholog of the original human target, have been considered in order to assess general and/or specific toxicity. The term "surrogate molecule" has been used incorrectly especially if one considers the judicious use of the term when referring to surrogate endpoints in clinical development. The acceptability of a surrogate endpoint requires extensive validation.

While analogous products are often used in early discovery and development to provide data in support for proof of concept, there is concern regarding their use for assessing safety unless they have been shown to be comparable to the clinical material (see Table 3.5). The use of analogous products is most often considered for assessing reproductive/development toxicity based on the inherent limitations of nonhuman primate models for characterizing reproductive risks. Analogous products are also considered for assessing carcinogenic risk for products intended for chronic use. Interestingly both of these preclinical risks are communicated in product labels. Since the manufacturing process is different than that of the clinical material, the product may contain

TABLE 3.5 Considerations for use of analogous products

Potential Advantages	Potential Disadvantages
• Useful for understanding early pharmacological properties of the drug • Useful for developing early proof of concept • Provides the ability "to do" toxicology studies • Opportunity to use a lower order species (rodents vs. NHP) • May be only feasible approach if no usable species responding to the clinical biopharmaceutical is available (e.g., no terminable studies feasible in chimpanzees, carcinogenicity testing not feasible in NHPs)	• Could have different manufacturing process and thus difference in range of process related impurities/contaminants • Could have different PK • Could have different pharmacological activity and/or feedback control (toxicity profile may be different if based on exaggerated pharmacology) • May be different for monoclonal antibody isotype (with associated activity) • Could have different intrinsic toxicity unrelated to pharmacological activity • Inability to assess relative immunogenicity of the clinical product • May be of questionable relevance in following up mechanism of toxicity of adverse events in clinic

differences in impurity contaminant profiles as well as stability. More important, however, there can be significant differences in potency and pharmacological activity.

In cases where analogous products are not used to establish proof of concept for a development candidate, such information would need to be developed prior to the conduct of toxicology studies. If an analogous product is not sufficiently comparable to the clinical product but utilized in order to satisfy the assessment of general toxicity in two species, it is unclear how to interpret the relevance of any adverse findings with the analogous product especially in cases where similar findings are not observed with the clinical material in a relevant species. The cost, production capabilities, and the additional resources required for a parallel product development program of an analogous product may also be prohibitive.

3.4.5 Use of Relevant Test Systems

ADME Since metabolism and formation of active metabolites are not a concern for unmodified biopharmaceuticals, mass balance studies are uninformative. Tissue concentration of radioactivity using radioactive proteins is also difficult to interpret due to unstable radiolabel linkage, rapid in vivo catabolism, and recycling of radiolabeled amino acids into non–drug-related proteins/peptides.

PK-mediated interactions are unlikely except for the rare examples of certain hormones that may be displaced by various chemicals form the tight binding of specific transport proteins, and the depressant action of certain interferons and other cytokines on hepatic P450s.

In vitro Safety Pharmacology   Specific guidance on safety pharmacology, ICH S7B, was published after ICH S6. This guidance specifically excluded biopharmaceuticals, acknowledging that, since biopharmaceuticals achieve highly specific receptor targeting, it has usually been sufficient to evaluate safety pharmacology endpoints as a part of toxicology and /or pharmacodynamic studies [33]. Nevertheless, assessment of in vitro cardiotoxicity, such as in vitro IKr assays (human ether a-go-go related gene, hERG), has been performed for some biopharmaceuticals even though mechanistically biopharmaceuticals are not likely to enter cells and bind a site within the potassium channel due to their molecular size. With the exception of some highly selective peptide toxins, there are no data to support binding to proteins on the cell surface mediating subsequent effects on ion channels.

Genotoxicity   Biopharmaceuticals do not have the same distribution properties as small molecules, and they are therefore not expected to pass through cell and nuclear membranes to interact with DNA. Experience has confirmed that the standard battery of genotoxicity assays is not relevant for products that do not directly interfere with DNA or mitosis to induce gene mutations, chromosome aberrations, or DNA damage. While studies may be applicable for protein conjugates with a chemical organic linker, consideration is warranted if there is precedence of use with the linker or if there is no evidence of degradation of the protein conjugate. Additionally, unlike small molecules where there may be a cause for concern for testing for genotoxic impurities, process-related impurities associated with biopharmaceuticals include residual host cell proteins, fermentation components, column leachables, and detergents rather than organic chemicals.

Immunogenicity   The injection of human proteins in sufficient quantity into animals should be expected to elicit an immunological response. Interestingly some analogous products have also induced immune responses in the derivative species. The presence of neutralizing antibody can change the PK/PD profile and thus impact exposure margins and estimates of toxicity. In early studies with biopharmaceuticals the development of antibodies in a toxicology study was considered a reason to stop studies; however, we now know that we can "dose through" in animals similar to dosing practices in humans. While the presence of antibodies in animals is generally not predictive for humans, the information has helped in defining relative immunogenicity and identifying potential consequences of an immune response such as neoantigenicity, autoantigenicity, immune complex deposition, complement activation, and antibodies crossing the placenta.

Clinically relevant antibodies include clearing antibodies, sustaining anti-bodies, neutralizing antibodies, and antibodies that cross-react with endoge-nous proteins and other molecules.

A reliable antibody screening assay capable of detecting high- and low-affinity antibodies is recommended. The sampling time for antibody assess-ment is also important, in allowing long washout periods in some cases in order to ensure that components in the serum sample do not prevent the assay from detecting a true positive (e.g., interference by the biopharmaceutical due to a long half-life).

Although assays for cell-mediated immunity are more complex and demand-ing, the possible need for them should always be considered because they may represent the source of a "toxic" action while accompanying antibodies are only a signal that an immune response has occurred.

The possibility of induced autoimmune responses should also be considered as a cause of damage to nuclei, cytoplasm, and cells and tissues as well as the stimulus for antibody formation.

Dose: Selection, Schedule, Duration, and Response   According to ICH S6, dose levels should be selected to provide information on a dose response including a toxic dose and NOAEL [10]. While the NOAEL is generally con-sidered for purposes of recommending initial doses for first in human studies, it was recognized that for certain classes of drugs or biologics (e.g., vasodilator, anticoagulants, monoclonal antibodies, or growth factors) where toxicity may arise from exaggerated pharmacology that the pharmacologically active dose (PAD) in these cases may be a more sensitive indicator of potential toxic-ity than the NOAEL and might therefore warrant lowering the minimum recommended starting dose (MRSD) [34]. More recently it has been suggested that the starting dose for the FIH for certain classes of biopharmaceuticals should be below the MABEL (minimal anticipated biological effect level) as predicted from all the available preclinical data (in vitro in humans and in vivo in animals) [35,36]. Importantly a number of factors have to be con-sidered to optimize dose extrapolation (see Table 3.6). It is also important to consider if these initial trials are performed in normal subjects or subjects with disease.

Ideally the design of the toxicology studies should mimic the clinical trial. However, because of more rapid clearance in test animals, more frequent dosing than proposed for the clinical trial may be needed to model for the equivalent exposure. Importantly, when longer intervals are anticipated, such as once a month or once every six months, a more accelerated or contracted dosing scheme may be needed as longer intervals generally serve as immuniz-ing regimen (e.g., similar to the intervals used for vaccines intended to induce an immune response). It is also important to understand whether dosing strat-egies induce tolerance, as was the case for IL 12 [37].

While identifying a maximum tolerated dose is preferred when designing toxicity studies in some cases, such a dose has been difficult to achieve for

TABLE 3.6   Considerations for optimizing dose extrapolation across species

- Receptor binding affinity
- Receptor saturation
- Potency to the target
- Upregulation of soluble receptors
- Tissue expression
- Stimulation of biological cascades by agonists at immune cell receptors
- Knowledge of other downstream signaling
- Potential for biological amplification
- Delayed induction of secondary mediator release
- Temporal dissociation of pharmacological effects from plasma levels due to persistent activity in nonplasma compartments
- Redundancy
- Homeostasis

Note: Specific considerations based on product class.

biopharmaceuticals. The use of a limit dose has been acceptable as the high dose for pharmaceuticals if an MTD cannot be achieved (e.g., 1 g/kg/day [31] and 1.5 g/kg/day ICH S1CR [38]). For biopharmaceuticals a limit dose is often defined as a maximum feasible dose (MFD) based on the physiological properties of the test material or dosage form allied to route of administration that may impose practical limitations in the amount that can be administered. A maximum absorbed dose (MAD) or pharmacodynamic maximum response dose (PMRD) based on saturation of absorption has also generally been acceptable for pharmaceuticals. However, in cases where for biopharmaceuticals with inherently low toxicity a maximum sensible dose (MSD) (A. Pilaro, personal communication) may need to be considered, a good understanding of the mechanism of action of the product, as well as of the intended clinical subject (i.e., normal volunteer vs. patient), is needed to support the adequacy of proposed multiples (e.g., 10–20X) for the high dose. In cases where lower multiples are justified, a more conservative estimate of FIH dose could be considered. Ironically it can be more difficult to select a FIH dose for a "safe drug."

3.5   FUTURE OF PRECLINICAL SAFETY EVALUATION AND ICH S6

The speed at which clinical development is expected to take place to bring novel therapies to market is challenging not only for small start-up companies but also for large established global companies. The inability to better assess and predict product safety can lead to failures during clinical development and, occasionally, after marketing [39]. Emerging technologies and novel therapies created the need and also the opportunity for considering novel approaches to toxicological testing in efforts to improve the predictive value of the data from preclinical studies for clinical decision making.

Many novel therapies could be considered "high risk" if only based on their uniqueness and lack of precedence. The introduction of novel therapies into the clinic has been facilitated by the cooperation between industry and regulatory scientists, and an adherence to sound scientific principles, common sense, and an approach based on flexibility. The "case-by-case" approach is dependent on acceptance by both regulators and industry that the interpretation of the data has to reflect best scientific practice and that no study in experimental animals can predict with certainty the outcome when a drug is given to humans [40].

In 2007 ICH S6 was proposed for updating ("maintenance") under the auspices of the ICH. Since the optimal design of preclinical programs is experiential based, the revisions would reflect accumulated experiences as well as advancements in science over the past decade—"a knowledge transfer." There is a concern, however, that revising this document may result in formalizing the emerging increase in studies performed for biopharmceuticals. The recent increase in the number and types of studies over the last few years has been attributed in part to both industry practice and regulatory expectations at better "aligning" preclinical development programs of biopharmaceuticals with pharmaceutical without consideration of the specific product attributes. As previously mentioned, flexibility in program design may also be needed for novel pharmaceuticals that share product attributes similar to biopharmaceuticals such as species specificity. The revised guidance could reduce the current flexibility in programs if new programs are expected to follow the "case studies" discussed in the guidance. The specific examples may not be applicable to either current or future novel products.

On the other hand, a revision may be an opportunity to redirect the emerging trend of increasing studies and increasing regional guidance. It could discourage the application of ICH guidance documents where biopharmaceuticals are specifically excluded and provide a better understanding of current regulatory expectations. Specific sections could be clarified to ensure optimal interpretation, for example, of species selection, immunogenicity assessment, duration of chronic studies, the number of species needed to assess chronic toxicity, the use of analogous products including interpretation of findings when an analogous product is not sufficiently comparable especially when toxicity differs significantly from results obtained with the clinical product, reproductive toxicity assessment strategies, carcinogenicity assessment strategies including whether "enhanced" chronic studies could inform the carcinogenicity section of the label. Other sections could be added, for example, on dose selection to support the first in human dose based on pharmacological activity, developmental immunotoxicity testing for immunomodulatory products, and information regarding risk management and communication.

Alternatively, ICH S6 could serve as an umbrella document. More specific guidance regarding the types of studies and areas of concern could then be provided as addendums or annexes with respect to product class, for example, monoclonal antibodies, protein conjugates, growth factors, soluble receptors, oligonucleotide drugs.

3.6 CONCLUSION

Supported by advances in biotechnology and other enabling technologies, the practice of toxicology has shifted form a ritualistic standards-based approach to a rational science-based approach, which is best defined by studies designed to ask specific questions with an understanding of what need to be known and the ability to make acceptable assumptions. Studies are data driven and practical to obtain maximum information. Designs are modified, based on additional information. Identification of limitations and knowledge gaps are acknowledged and identified, and effort to develop new models to replace outdated models embracing novel technologies is an ongoing process.

Development principles for preclinical safety assessment have been and will continue to be a dynamic process that is strongly controlled by the expanding knowledge and improvements in product design. The full investigation of the potential usefulness of biopharmaceuticals requires the development of reliable animal model systems that allow assessment of toxicity and provide pharmacokinetic data that can be successfully scaled to humans in order to reduce risk factors before clinical testing. The design of relevant preclinical safety evaluation programs is consistent with global initiatives to facilitate and to improve clinical development programs. In the coming years stakeholders will be facing the issue of how to implement preclinical development programs for biopharmaceuticals and pharmaceuticals that better anticipate adverse effects, including development of new test systems that produce reliable results faster and at lower cost. Hopefully, preclinical evaluation programs will evolve and mature concurrently with more novel products and will focus on improving the predictive value of preclinical safety testing, targeting the toxicity testing to provide information to ensure that the correct data are collected from the most appropriate studies.

ACKNOWLEDGMENT

The author would like to thank Dr. Richard Lewis and Dr. Tony Dayan for critically reviewing the manuscript.

REFERENCES

1. Olson H, Betton G, Robinson D, Thomas K, Monro A, Kolaja G, Lilly P, Sanders J, Sipes G, Bracken W, Dorato M, Van Deun K, Smith P, Berger B, Heller A. Con-

cordance of the toxicity of pharmaceuticals in humans and animals. *Regul Toxicol Pharmacol* 2000;32:56–67.

2. Goldenthal EI. Current views on safety evaluation of drugs. FDA Papers May 1968.

3. Hayes TJ, Cavagnaro JA. Progress and challenges in the preclinical assessment of cytokines. *Toxicol Letts* 1992;64/65:291–7.

4. Zbinden G. Biotechnology Products Intended for Human Use, Toxicological Targets and Research Strategies. In CE Grahm (ed) *Preclinical Safety of Biotechnology Products Intended for Human Use: Clinical and Biological Research*, Vol. 235, Alan R. Liss, New York, 1987, pp 143–59.

5. Giss HE. Foreword. In CE Grahm (ed) *Preclinical Safety of Biotechnology Products Intended for Human Use: Clinical and Biological Research*, Vol. 235, Alan R. Liss, New York, 1987, pp xiii–xv.

6. Dayan AD. Rationality and regulatory requirements—A view from Britain. In CE Grahm (ed) *Preclinical Safety of Biotechnology Products Intended for Human Use: Clinical and Biological Research*, Vol. 235, Alan R. Liss, New York, 1987, pp 89–106.

7. Galbraith WM. Symposium discussion. In CE Grahm (ed) *Preclinical Safety of Biotechnology Products Intended for Human Use: Clinical and Biological Research*, Vol. 235, Alan R. Liss, New York, 1987, pp 189–206.

8. Finkle BS. Genetically engineered drugs: Toxicology with a difference. In CE Grahm (ed), *Preclinical Safety of Biotechnology Products Intended for Human Use: Clinical and Biological Research*, Vol. 235, Alan R. Liss, New York, 1987, pp 161–7.

9. Griffith SA, Lumley CE. Non-clinical safety studies for biotechnologically-derived pharmaceuticals: Conclusions for an International workshop. *Hum Exper Toxicol* 1998;17:63–83.

10. ICH S6 Preclinical Safety Evaluation of Biotechnology-Derived Pharmaceuticals. http://www.fda.gov/cder/guidance/index.htm.

11. ICH M3 Nonclinical Safety Studies for the Conduct of Human Clinical Trials for Pharmaceuticals. http://www.fda.gov/cder/guidance/index.htm.

12. DeGeorge JJ, Ahn C-H, Andrews PA, Brower ME, Giorgio DW, Goheer MA, Lee-ham DY, McGuinn WD, Schimdt W, Sun CJ, Tripathi SC. Regulatory considerations for preclinical development of anticancer drugs. *Cancer Chemother Pharmacol* 1998;41:173–85.

13. Dayan AD. Testing biotechnology recombinant DNA (rDNA) products. *BIRA J* 1990;9:7–10.

14. Zbinden G. Safety evaluation of biotechnology products. *Drug Safety* 1990;5(Suppl. 1):58–64.

15. Zbinden G. Predictive value of animal studies in toxicology. *Regul Toxicol Pharmacol* 1991;14:167–77.

16. Bass R, Kleeburg U, Schroder H, et al. Current Guidelines for the Preclinical Safety Assessment of Therapeutic Proteins. *Toxicol Letts* 1992;64/65:339–47.

17. Cavagnaro JA. Science-based approach to preclinical safety evaluation of biotechnology products. *Pharmaceutl Eng* 1992;12:32–3.

18. Claude JR. Difficulties in conceiving and applying guidelines for the safety evaluation of biotechnologically-produced drugs: Some examples. *Toxicol Letts* 1992; 64/65:349–55.

19. Terrell TG, Green JD. Issues with biotechnology products in toxicologic pathology. *Toxicol Pathol* 1994;22:187–93.

20. Cavagnaro JA. Preclinical safety assessment of biological products. In Mathieu M, ed. *Biologics Development: A Regulatory Overview*. Waltham, MA: Parexel International, 1993;23–40.

21. Sims J. Assessment of biotechnology products for therapeutic use. *Toxicol Letts* 2001;120:59–66.

22. Dayan AD. Safety evaluation of biological and biotechnology-derived medicines. *Toxicology* 1995;105:59–68.

23. Thomas JA. Recent developments and perspectives of biotechnology-derived products. *Toxicology* 1995;105:7–22.

24. Serabian MA, Pilaro AM. Safety assessment of biotechnology-derived pharmaceuticals: ICH and beyond. *Toxicol Pathol* 1999;27:27–31.

25. Ryan AM, Terrell TG. Biotechnology and its products. In *Handbook of Toxicologic Pathology*, 2nd ed. San Diego: Academic Press, 2002;479–500.

26. Verdier F. Preclinical safety assessment of vaccines in biotechnology and safety assessment. In Thomas JA, Fuchs RL, eds. *Biotechnology and Safety Assessment*. 3rd ed. Academic Press, San Diego, 2002;397–412.

27. Brennan FR, Shaw L, Wing MG, Robinson C. Preclinical safety testing of biotechnology-derived pharmaceuticals. *Mol Biotechnol* 2004;27:59–74.

28. Nakazawa T, Kai S, Kawai M, Maki E, Sagami F, Onodera H, Kitajima S, Inoue T. "Points to Consider" regarding safety assessment of biotechnology-derived pharmaceuticals in non-clinical studies (English Translation). *J Toxicol Sci* 2004;29: 497–504.

29. Cavagnaro JA. Predicting safety for novel therapies. *Regul Affairs J* 2006;(June): 1–4.

30. Snodin DJ, Ryle PR. Understanding and applying regulatory guidance on the non-clinical development of biotechnology-derived pharmaceuticals. *Biodrugs* 2006;1: 25–52.

31. ICH S5A Detection of Toxicity to Reproduction for Medicinal Products, September 1994.

32. BLAST. http://www.ncbi.nlm.nih.gov/Education/blasttutorial.html.

33. ICH S7B Nonclinical Evaluation of the Potential for Delayed Ventricular Repolarization (QT Interval Prolongation) by Human Pharmaceuticals, October 2005. http://www.fda.gov/cder/guidance/index.htm.

34. Estimating the Maximum Safe Starting Dose in Initial Clinical Trials for Therapeutics in Adult Healthy Volunteers, July 2005.

35. Early Stage Clinical Trial Taskforce, Joint ABPI/BIA Report, July 2, 2006. http://www.abpi.org.uk/information/pdfs/BIAABPI_taskforce2.pdf.

36. Expert Scientific Group on Phase One Clinical Trials, Final Report ("Duff Report"), November 30, 2006. http://www.dh.gov.uk/assetRoot/04/14/10/43/04141043.pdf.

37. Leonard JP, Sherman MT, Fisher GL, Buchanan LJ, Larsen G, Atkins MB, Sosman JA, Dutcher JP, Vogelzang NJ, Ryan JL. Effects of single dose interleukin-12 exposure on interleukin-12 associated toxicity and interleukin-γ production. *Blood* 1997;90:2541–8.

38. ICH S1C(R) Guidance on Dose Selection for Carcinogenicity Studies of Pharmaceuticals: Addendum on a Limited Dose and Related Notes, December 1997 http://www.fda.gov/cder/guidance/index.htm.

39. FDA Challenge and Opportunity on the Critical Path to New Medical Products, March 2004. http://www.fda.gov/oc/initiatives/criticalpath/whitepaper.html.

40. Academy of Medical Sciences Forum Safer Medicines Report. Pre-clinical Toxicology Working Group Report. November 2005.

CHAPTER 4

Implementation of ICH S6: EU Perspective

PETER R. RYLE, PhD, DipRCPath (Tox), FRCPath, and DAVID J. SNODIN, PhD, FRSC, MChemA, MSc

Contents

4.1 INTRODUCTION

The development and regulatory approval of biopharmaceuticals in the European Union (EU) has lagged slightly behind that in the United States. But

Preclinical Safety Evaluation of Biopharmaceuticals: A Science-Based Approach to Facilitating Clinical Trials, edited by Joy A. Cavagnaro
Copyright © 2008 by John Wiley & Sons, Inc.

over the last decade this class of drug has assumed increasing importance in the development pipelines of EU-based pharmaceutical companies. In addition, many US and Japanese companies conduct development of their products in Europe for the EU market. Some countries in the European Union have acquired a reputation for innovation in the biopharmaceutical field, with various clusters of start-up and small biotechnology companies becoming established, particularly in the United Kingdom (mainly around the university cities of Oxford and Cambridge) and Germany. More recently France, the Netherlands, the Scandinavian countries (Sweden, Denmark, Norway, Finland), and smaller countries such as Belgium and Ireland can claim to have flourishing biotechnology industries, producing potential biopharmaceutical development candidates. Although Switzerland is not a member of the European Union, its location and the presence of both long-established large multinational pharmaceutical, as well as some smaller biotechnology start-up companies, make it a major contributor to the biopharmaceutical sector in Europe.

Examples of biopharmaceutical products that have received approval in the European Union are shown in Table 4.1. In addition to the approval of novel biopharmaceutical products, the first EU approval of a "generic" or "biosimilar" biopharmaceutical product (Omnitrope®) was granted in 2006 [1]. In general, most major new biopharmaceutical products that are approved by the US regulatory authority (FDA) are approved in the European Union at about the same time, or shortly after FDA approval for marketing. There are relatively few biopharmaceutical products that undergo region-specific development and marketing, largely due to the high cost of development of these products, and reflecting the fact that the drugs are often for areas of unmet medical need. In addition the EU population (slightly under 500 million) makes it one of the most attractive potential markets for new pharmaceutical products. Therefore the trend of an increasing proportion of new drugs in development or receiving EU marketing approval that are biotechnology derived probably reflects the situation in the United States and other regions. In 2004, 8 of 19 new therapeutics approved for use in the United Kingdom were biopharmaceuticals.

In terms of the application and implementation of ICH guidelines in the European Union, the approach from a technical and scientific viewpoint can be regarded as similar to that in the other major ICH regions (the United States and Japan). The major difference relates to the regulatory administrative structure within the European Union, as will be discussed below. Sponsors developing biopharmaceuticals for the US and Japanese markets will deal with a single regulatory agency for those regions throughout the development cycle. The EU situation is rather more complex, such that early in the development cycle the sponsor may interact with one or two EU national authorities to enable phase 1 and 2 trials to be initiated. As the development cycle proceeds, interactions with more national authorities and the central European Medicines Agency (EMEA) are likely to take place, working toward approval of the product by the central agency, through the so-called centralized procedure.

TABLE 4.1 Examples of biopharmaceuticals approved in the European Union

Product Name	Action	Company	Therapeutic Use	Year Approved
Actrapid	Insulin analogue	Novo Nordisk	Diabetes mellitus	2002
Avastin	Anti-VEGF monoclonal Ab	Roche	Colo-rectal carcinoma	2005
Avonex	Interferon-α	Biogen IDEC	Multiple sclerosis	1997
Betaferon	Interferon-β	Schering	Multiple sclerosis	2000
Cerezyme	β-cerebrosidase	Genzyme	Gaucher's disease	1997
Dynepo	Epoetin	Shire	Anaemia	2002
Enbrel	Anti-TNFα fusion protein	Wyeth	Rheumatoid arthritis/psoriasis	2000
Erbitux	Anti-EGF monoclonal Ab	Merck	Colo-rectal carcinoma	2004
Herceptin	Anti-HER2 monoclonal Ab	Roche	Breast cancer	2000
Humalog	Lispro insulin analogue	Eli Lilly	Diabetes mellitus	1996
Humira	Anti-TNFα monoclonal Ab	Abbott	Rheumatoid arthritis	2003
Intron A	Interferon-α	Schering-Plough	Hepatitis/lymphoid tumors	2000
Kineret	IL-1 antagonist	Amgen	Rheumatoid arthritis	2002
Liprolog	Insulin analogue	Eli Lilly	Diabetes mellitus	2001
Mabcampath	Anti-CD52 monoclonal Ab	Genzyme	Chronic leukaemia	2001
Mabthera	Anti-CD20 monoclonal Ab	Roche	Rheumatoid arthritis/lymphoma	1998
Neulasta	PEG-G-CSF	Amgen	Neutropenia	2002
NovoSeven	Factor VIIa	Novo Nordisk	Haemophilia	1996
Osigraft	Osteogenic Protein-1	Howmedica	Bone non-union	2001
Pegasys	PEG-interferon alpha	Roche	Chronic hepatitis	2002
Raptiva	Anti-CD11a monoclonal Ab	Serono	Psoriasis	2004
Remicade	Anti-TNFα monoclonal Ab	Centocor BV	Rheumatoid arthritis/Crohn's	1999
Simulect	Anti-CD25 monoclonal Ab	Novartis	Immune suppression	1998
Tysabri	Anti-α4 integrin monoclonal Ab	Elan	Multiple sclerosis	2006
Xolair	Anti-IgE monoclonal Ab	Novartis	Asthma	2005

This chapter will therefore concentrate mostly on the major differences in regulatory structure between the European Union and other regions, which has bearing on obtaining regulatory guidance and scientific advice during the development of a biopharmaceutical for the European market. Such interactions with the regulatory agencies are crucial to the application of the case-by-case approach to preclinical development of biopharmaceuticals advocated by the ICH S6 guideline.

4.2 EUROPEAN UNION

The European Union per se was created in November 1993 when the Treaty on European Union came into effect. At that time 12 European countries had already joined the European Community (EC), formed in 1967 as a merger of the European Coal and Steel Community (ECSC, founded in 1952), the European Economic Community (EEC, founded in 1958), and the European Atomic Energy Community. The 12 countries that were part of the European Union in 1993 were Belgium, France, Italy, Luxembourg, the Netherlands, West Germany, Denmark, Ireland, the United Kingdom, Greece, Portugal, and Spain.

Since 1993 other countries have joined the European Union, with Austria, Finland, and Sweden joining in 1995, Cyprus, Czech Republic, Estonia, Hungary, Latvia, Lithuania, Malta, Poland, Slovakia, and Slovenia joining in 2004, and Bulgaria and Romania joining in January 2007. At the present time, there are 27 countries or "member states" in the European Union. At the time of writing, Turkey and Croatia are in "accession" negotiations to join the European Union, with several other countries, such as Macedonia, Albania, Montenegro, and Serbia, as potential future member states.

The European Union has a number of high-level institutions, the most important being as follows:

The Council of Ministers. The Council is the main decision-making body of the European Union. The ministers of the member states meet within the Council, and depending on the issue on the agenda, each country will be represented by the minister responsible for that subject (foreign affairs, finance, social affairs, transport, agriculture, etc.). The presidency of the Council is held for six months by each member state on a rotational basis.

The European Parliament. Following elections held in June 2004, the European Parliament had 732 members elected in the 25 member states of the European Union. Each member is elected for a five-year term. Most of the time Parliament and its members are based in Brussels where its specialist committees meet to scrutinize proposals for new EU laws.

The European Commission. Based in Brussels, the Commission consists of 27 commissioners, one from each member state, appointed for a five-year term by member states' governments. The Commission, which acts as the

European Union's civil service, and comprises approximately 14,000 officials, has the right of initiative, that is, to draw up proposals for Union
legislation. The Commission negotiates on behalf of the member states
in multilateral and bilateral trade matters and in the drawing up of association and membership agreements with nonmember countries.

The European Court of Justice. The European Court of Justice, consisting
of 15 judges (appointed by the Member States) and 9 Advocates-General,
is based in Luxembourg. It is responsible for arbitrating in disputes relating to the interpretation and application of EU legislation.

4.3 EU DRUG REGULATORY FRAMEWORK

4.3.1 Pharmaceutical Legislation and Regulation

Pharmaceutical regulation in the European Union is applied centrally and
nationally in individual member states. In general, after joining the European
Union, a member state is required to harmonize or revoke its existing legislation and to incorporate any new provisions agreed centrally into its national
legislation. European Union pharmaceutical legislation dates back to the
1960s; Directive 65/65/EEC remained the basis of European Union rules
for many years. This has been superseded by Directive 2001/83/EC (e.g., as
amended by 2004/27/EC) relating to medicinal products for human use, which
essentially consolidated previous relevant directives into one text. As
explained in the preamble to Directive 2001/83/EC, the key aim of EU pharmaceutical legislation is the protection of public health, provided that this is
achieved by means that will not hinder drug development. A committee
system ("comitology") is often used in the European Union as a vital part of
the adoption and implementation of legal statutes. Most EU legislation is
passed by the Commission under powers delegated by the Council of Ministers, and in such cases there is no formal involvement of the general public,
national parliaments, or the European Parliament. One example in drug regulation is Annex I to Directive 2001/83/EC, an annex containing a variety of
definitions and concepts that forms the basis of technical requirements
involved in drug regulation. An updated Annex 1 (Directive 2003/63) is now
in operation [2].

Other important legal documents are as follows:

- Directive 2001/20/EC, which mainly concerns approval of clinical trials in
  the European Union.
- Council Regulation 726/2004/EC (updates and expands the previous regulation 239/1993/EC), which mainly concerns the duties of the European
  Medicines Agency (EMEA), establishment of the Committee for Medicinal Products for Human Use (CHMP), and the scope and mechanisms of
  the centralized procedure for marketing authorization applications
  (MAAs) and pharmacovigilance issues.

All the above-mentioned legal treatises apply to the European Economic Area (EEA; this comprises the 27 EU member states plus Liechtenstein, Iceland, and Norway—Switzerland chose by referendum not to join the EEA, but has certain Swiss–EU bilateral agreements). Switzerland acts as the representative of the European Free Trade Association, which is an observer in the ICH (International Conference on Harmonization) process, accepts ICH guidelines, but is not part of the European Economic Area. There is a legal obligation for the Swiss competent authority, Swiss Agency for Therapeutic Products (Swissmedic), to take account of decisions/authorizations in other territories that have equivalent medicinal product control.

4.3.2 European Medicines Agency and National Competent Authorities

Each member state has a national medicines agency, which is usually located in the capital city (but not, e.g., in Germany, the Netherlands, and Sweden). These agencies are listed in Table 4.2. Some national agencies combine the

TABLE 4.2 Regulatory bodies (competent authorities) for human medicines in Europe

Country	Agency	Web Site
Austria	Bundesamt für Sicherheit im Gesundheitswesen	www.ages.at
Belgium	Directoraat generaal Geneesmiddelen Direction générale Médicaments	www.afigp.fgov.be
Denmark	Lægemiddelstyrelsen	www.dkma.dk
Europe	European Medicines Agency (EMEA)	www.emea.europa.eu
Finland	Lääkelaitos	www.nam.fi
France	Agence Française de Sécurité Sanitaire des Produits de Santé	www.afssaps.sante.fr
Germany	Bundesministerium für Gesundheit und Soziale Sicherung	www.bmgs.bund.de www.bfarm.de/de/index.php
	Bundesinstitut für Arzneimittel und Medizinprodukte Paul-Ehrlich-Institut	www.pei.de
Germany	Zentralstelle der Länder für Gesundheitsschutz bei Arzneimitteln und Medizinprodukten	www.zlg.nrw.de
Greece	National Organization for Medicines	www.eof.gr
Iceland	Lyfjastofnun	www.lyfjastofnun.is
Ireland	Irish Medicines Board	www.imb.ie
Italy	Ministero della Salute	www.ministerosalute.it
Liechtenstein	Liechtensteinische Landesverwaltung Amt für Lebensmittelkontrolle und Veterinärwesen Kontrollstelle für Arzneimittel	www.llv.li

TABLE 4.2 *Continued*

Country	Agency	Web Site
Luxembourg	Ministère de la Santé Division de la Pharmacie et des Médicaments	www.etat.lu/MS
Netherlands	Staatstoezicht op de volksgezondheid Inspectie voor de Gezondheidszorg	www.igz.nl
Netherlands	College ter Beoordeling van Geneesmiddelen (CBG)	http://www.cbg-meb.nl
Norway	Statens Legemiddelverk	www.legemiddelverket.no
Portugal	Instituto Nacional da Farmácia e do Medicamento	www.infarmed.pt
Spain	Agencia española del medicamento	www.agemed.es
Sweden	Läkemedelsverket	www.mpa.se
United Kingdom	Medicines and Healthcare products Regulatory Agency	www.mhra.gov.uk
Bulgaria	Bulgarian Drug Agency	www.bda.bg
Cyprus	Ministry of Health	www.pio.gov.cy
Czech Repbulic	State Institut for Drug Control	www.sukl.cz www.uskvbl.cz
Estonia	State Agency of Medicines	www.sam.ee
Hungary	National Institute of Pharmacy	www.ogyi.hu
Latvia	Food and Veterinary Service	zaale.vza.gov.lv
Lithuania	State Medicines Control Agency	www.vvkt.lt
Malta	Medicines Authority	www.medicinesauthority.gov.mt
Poland	Office for Medicinal Products	http://www.urpl.gov.pl
Romania	National Medicines Agency	www.anm.ro/home.html
Slovak Republic	State Institute for Drug Control	www.sukl.sk
Slovenia	Agency of the Republic of Slovenia for Medicinal Products and Medical Devices	http://www2.gov.si/mz/ mz-splet.nsf
Switzerland	Swissmedic, Schweizerisches Heilmittelinstitut	www.swissmedic.ch

regulation of medicines and medical devices (e.g., Medicines and Healthcare products Regulatory Agency, called MHRA, in the United Kingdom) while others regulate both human and veterinary medicines. The European Medicines Agency (EMEA) is a pan-European regulatory agency, responsible for both human and veterinary medicines, located in Canary Wharf on the east side of London. It was established on February 1, 1995, and its staff numbers have grown year by year; the EMEA budget for 2007 makes provision for up to 441 staff. The EMEA functions in a different manner to the US Food and Drug Administration. Its role is mainly in policy and coordination while technical expertise is provided by staff from the national agencies [3]. There is a network of approximately 3500 European experts that are drawn mainly from the national agencies and academia [4] whose main roles relate to undertaking assessment of application dossiers, providing scientific advice, developing new guidelines, and sitting on various committees, working groups, and advisory groups. The mission statement and main tasks and responsibilities of the EMEA are shown in Table 4.3. More details on committees, working groups, and scientific advisory groups are shown in Table 4.4.

TABLE 4.3 EMEA: Mission statement and main responsibilities

Mission statement

In the context of a continuing globalization, to protect and promote public and animal health:
- By developing efficient and transparent procedures to allow rapid access by users to safe and effective innovative medicines and to generic and nonprescription medicines through a single European marketing authorization
- By controlling the safety of medicines for humans and animals, in particular, through a pharmacovigilance network and the establishment of safe limits for residues in food-producing animals
- By facilitating innovation and stimulating research, hence contributing to the competitiveness of EU based pharmaceutical industry
- By mobilizing and coordinating scientific resources from throughout the European Union to provide high-quality evaluation of medicinal products, to advise on research and development programs, to perform inspections for ensuring fundamental GXP provisions are consistently achieved, and to provide useful and clear information to users and health-care professionals

Main tasks and responsibilities

- Scientific advice to member states and Community institutions on quality, safety, and efficacy of human and veterinary medicinal products
- Centralized (and to a lesser extent decentralized) authorization procedures: administration of these procedures to achieve a single evaluation and marketing authorization for medicinal products
- Pharmacovigilance and inspection: organization of procedures for effective surveillance (and possibly withdrawal) of medicinal products in the European Union, and to reinforce national inspection activities
- Advice to companies on drug development (scientific advice and protocol assistance)
- Committees, working parties, and scientific advisory groups
- Guidance documents
- EPARs (European Public Assessment Reports) and Withdrawal Public Assessment Reports
- List of European experts

Note: GXP means "good clinical practice" (GCP), "good manufacturing practice" (GMP), and "good laboratory practice" (GLP) collectively.

TABLE 4.4   EMEA: Committees, working groups, and scientific advisory groups on human medicines

Committees

* Management Board
* Committee on Human Medicinal Products (CHMP)
* Committee on Orphan Medicinal Products (COMP)
* Committee on Herbal Medicinal Products (HMPC)

Working parties (WPs)

* Safety Working Party (SWP)
* Quality Working Party (QWP)
* Efficacy Working Party (EWP)
* Other WPs: Pharmacogenetics (PgWP), Pharmacovigilance (PhVWP), Biologics (BWP), Gene Therapy (GTWP), Vaccines (VWP), Blood Products (BPWP), Cell-Based Products (CPWP), Scientific Advice (SAWP)
* Temporary WPs: Pediatric (PEG), Similar Biological (Biosimilar) Medicinal Products (BMWP)

Scientific advisory groups (SAGs)

* The role of the SAGs is to provide, on request from the committee concerned, an independent recommendation on scientific and technical matters relating to products under evaluation or any other scientific issues relevant to the work of the respective committees. While views expressed by SAGs are taken into account, the ultimate responsibility for the final opinions rests with the respective scientific committee.
* SAGs created to date: Oncology, Diagnostics, Anti-Infectives, Diabetes/ Endocrinology, Cardiovascular Issues, Central Nervous System, HIV/Viral Diseases

4.3.3   Marketing Authorization Applications (MAAs)

Four routes are available for obtaining a marketing authorization (MA) for a human medicinal product in the European Economic Area: independent national procedure, mutual recognition procedure (MRP), decentralized procedure (DCP), and centralized procedure (CP) [5–7].

Independent National Procedure   If a company wishes to market a product in one country only and there are no legal obligations to use a route other than the national one (which would apply if the type of drug or therapeutic area were within the scope of the centralized procedure), then an application can be made to one health authority, leading to a marketing authorization in that country alone.

Mutual Recognition Procedure (MRP)   This procedure begins with a national application to one member state (MS), and when a marketing authorization has been obtained the applicant applies for "mutual recognition" of this initial authorization by the reference member state (RMS) in some or all of the other European economic area countries, called concerned member states (CMSs).

Decentralized Procedure (DCP) The decentralized procedure was established as an application route in late 2005. This procedure is essentially a combination of the national and the mutual recognition procedures. The applicant chooses a reference member state to undertake the initial assessment. On completion of the RMS assessment, the concerned member states can put forward additional questions to those raised by the reference member state. If the questions are answered by the applicant to the satisfaction of the reference member state and concerned member states, the drug can be authorized. The benefit of the decentralized procedure is that all concerned member states are provided with the application dossier from the start of the procedure.

Centralized Procedure (CP) This is the procedure of most interest for biopharmaceuticals, as this is the mandatory route for review and approval of such drugs in the European Union. In the centralized procedure a single application is submitted to the European Medicines Agency (EMEA). A variety of presubmission activities, starting six months before the intended start date of the centralized procedure, are required [8]. Two initial assessments by a "Rapporteur" and "Co-rapporteur" national authorities (one from each of two member states chosen by the EMEA) are made, leading to Day 80 Critical Assessment Reports. A consolidated list of questions (LoQ) is provided to the applicant at Day 120 when there is a clock stop, normally of three months, to allow the preparation and submission of responses. Following satisfactory negotiation of other steps in the procedure, the Committee on Human Medicinal Products will recommend authorization at Day 210, with authorization by the Commission at Day 277.

The centralized procedure is mandatory for the following cases:

- Medicinal products developed by means of one of the following biotechnological processes: recombinant DNA technology, controlled expression of genes coding for biologically active proteins in prokaryotes and eukaryotes including transformed mammalian cells, hybridoma and monoclonal antibody methods.
- New chemical entities for the following indications: acquired immunodeficiency syndrome (AIDS), cancer, neurodegenerative diseases, diabetes. Two more categories (autoimmune diseases and other immune dysfunctions, and viral diseases), will be included with effect beginning May 20, 2008.
- Orphan medicinal products.
- Biosimilar products.

The current CP application fee is 232,000 Euros for a single strength associated with one pharmaceutical form. Although the fees are high and the Committee on Human Medicinal Products review is extremely thorough, if successful the centralized procedure leads to an authorization that is valid in all European Economic Area countries, and for this reason is attractive to companies that have a presence in only one or a few European countries.

4.3.4   Clinical Trial Authorizations (CTAs)

Clinical trials are regulated by individual member states in the European Union. An applicant (or sponsor) submits data on the investigational medicinal product (IMP), and details of the proposed clinical trial, to the competent authority in the country in which the trial is to be carried out. The ethics committee responsible for the site where the trial is to take place also needs to give approval.

Clinical trials and clinical trial authorizations in the European Union are controlled under the Clinical Trial Directive, 2001/20/EC [9], and all member states are bound by its requirements. Under the provisions of the Directive, a clinical trial is an investigation in human subjects that is intended to discover or verify the clinical, pharmacological, and/or other pharmacodynamic effects of one or more medicinal products, identify any adverse reactions or study the absorption, distribution, metabolism, and excretion, with the object of ascertaining the safety and/or efficacy of those products. This definition includes pharmacokinetic studies.

All submissions need to include a completed application form and, prior to submitting the application, a reference number (EudraCT number) must be obtained [10]. In addition the applicant needs to supply additional documents (depending on the type of trial and investigational medicinal product), but normally including:

- Investigator's brochure (IB)
- Clinical trial protocol
- Investigational medicinal product dossier (IMPD)
- Subject information leaflet
- Informed consent

Detailed guidance on the preparation of the Investigational Medicinal Product Dossier is available [11]. In terms of preclinical aspects, the key considerations are:

- The investigational medicinal product dossier can be stand-alone or be constructed by cross-reference to relevant sections of the IB (applies to preclinical and clinical data only).
- Summaries of preclinical data should be provided, preferably using tabular formats. The headings for the preclinical part should follow those for

written summaries in the Common Technical Document (CTD) module 2.6. In contrast to the situation with the US FDA, full study reports and individual data (line listings) for the nonclinical studies are not required.

- An overall risk assessment should be included. This is intended to be a brief integrated summary that analyzes the preclinical and clinical data in relation to the potential risks and benefits of the proposed trial. Safety margins should be expressed on the basis of relative systemic exposure rather than applied dose.

The CTA approval process should take no longer than 60 days. Approval times are often shorter (e.g., 14–21 days for a healthy volunteer trial in the United Kingdom) and vary among member states.

4.3.5 Scientific Advice

The case-by-case approach that is needed for the effective preclinical development of biopharmaceuticals requires close collaboration and agreement between the sponsor and the regulatory agency at all stages of development. In the United States, such collaboration and scientific advice is often achieved through interaction with the FDA at pre-IND, end of phase 2, or pre-NDA meetings with the Agency.

In the European Union, scientific advice can be sought from national agencies at any stage of drug development [12,13]. Details are provided on agency Web sites (e.g., MHRA) [14], and fees are charged depending on the nature of the advice requested (one or more of quality, preclinical, clinical, regulatory, pharmacovigilance plans). Scientific advice (called "protocol assistance" in the case of orphan drugs) can also be obtained centrally from the EMEA. The concepts are similar to those for national scientific advice, but the procedures are considerably more complex (sometimes involving joint sessions with FDA), of longer duration, and more costly in terms of applicant fees [15]. EU guidance emphasizes that it is not the role of the Committee on Human Medicinal Products (CHMP) to substitute the industry's responsibility in the development of their products, and that any advice given is not legally binding with respect to any future marketing authorization application for the product concerned, although in the Notice to Applicants it is a requirement to include a copy of any formal scientific advice in the application dossier.

In terms of the particular questions asked as part of EMEA scientific advice, questions that can be answered by consulting a particular guideline are discouraged, although a question based on interpretation of a guideline would probably be acceptable. There is no direct equivalent of the US FDA pre-IND or end-of-phase-2 meeting in Europe. Since clinical trials are regulated on a national basis, and the review times for clinical trial submissions are quite short, most companies would submit an application for a CTA without holding a meeting beforehand, unless the treatment in question was potentially controversial (e.g., involving a monoclonal antibody, gene therapy, or cell therapy). Once a program has negotiated phase 1, obtaining scientific advice either nationally and/or centrally would be strongly considered by most companies.

4.4 THE EUROPEAN UNION AND ICH

The European Union was and still is a major contributor to ICH, through the input of the European Commission (which represents the 27 member states) and the European pharmaceutical industry (European Federation of Pharmaceutical Industries and Associations, EFPIA) to the process. European technical and scientific support for the ICH process was provided by the Committee for Medicinal Products for Human Use (CHMP, formerly CPMP) of the European Medicines Agency (EMEA), on behalf of the European Commission. Therefore EU-based regulatory and industry professionals were actively involved in the development of the ICH guidelines, including the S6 guideline that covers preclinical testing of biotechnology-derived pharmaceuticals. The content and principles of the ICH S6 guideline have been covered in detail in other chapters, so it will not be addressed further here. Obviously the key message from the ICH S6 guidance was the need for a case-by-case approach to the preclinical testing of biopharmaceuticals, taking into account factors such as species specificity and immunogenicity of the products.

Prior to the implementation of the ICH S6 [16] guideline, an EU guideline covering the preclinical testing of biotechnology-derived drugs [17] was adopted in 1988. The ICH S6 guideline was approved by the CPMP of the EU regulatory agency (EMEA) in September 1997 and came into operation in member states in March 1998. The implementation of the ICH S6 guideline effectively replaced the previous 1988 guidance document. At the time of adoption of the ICH S6 guideline, there was only one other document in place that provided some preclinical guidance on biopharmaceuticals, a guideline covering the production and quality control of monoclonal antibodies [18]. This guidance recommended the use of tissue cross reactivity studies that are usually performed on monoclonal antibody products. A more recent initiative to update the EU monoclonal antibody guidance indicated that the update should concentrate on quality aspects only, since preclinical testing of these products was adequately addressed by adoption of the ICH S6 guidance [19].

4.5 EU-SPECIFIC REGULATORY GUIDANCE

Since the adoption of the ICH S6 guideline, and with the growing number of biopharmaceuticals entering development, the EMEA have developed a number of specific guidelines in relation to the preclincial testing of biopharmaceuticals. The current draft and approved EU-specific preclinical guidance documents that apply to biopharmaceuticals are listed in Table 4.5. In addition

TABLE 4.5 **EU-specific preclinical guidelines on biopharmaceuticals**

Relevant Product Type	Guideline	Date
Vaccines (excluding DNA or viral vector vaccines)	CPMP/SWP/465/95: Preclinical pharmacological and toxicological testing of vaccines [31]	1997
Gene therapy, DNA vaccines, genetically modified tissue or cell-based products	CPMP/BWP/3088/99: Quality, preclinical, and clinical aspects of gene transfer products [32]	2001
Insulin analogues	CPMP/SWP/372/01: Nonclinical assessment of carcinogenic potential of insulin analogues [33]	2001
Insulin analogues	CPMP/SWP/2600/01: Need for assessment of reproductive toxicity of insulin analogues [34]	2002
Biotechnology-derived proteins	CPMP/3097/02: Comparability of medicinal products containing biotechnology-derived proteins as drug substance—preclinical and clinical issues [35]	2003
Gene therapy, DNA vaccines, genetically modified tissue or cell-based products.	EMEA/273974/05: Draft Annex on nonclinical testing for inadvertent germ-line transmission of gene transfer vectors [36]	2005
Vaccine adjuvants	CHMP/VEG/134716/2004: Guideline on adjuvants in vaccines for human use [37]	2005
Biotechnology-derived proteins	EMEA/CHMP/BMWP/101695/2006: Guideline on comparability of biotechnology-derived medicinal products after a change in the manufacturing process [38] (will replace CPMP/3097/02)	2007

Note: The term guideline is used here to refer to testing guidelines, "Notes for guidance," as well as "Points to consider" documents.

to use of the guiding principles laid out in ICH, there are EU-specific preclinical guidelines relating to gene transfer medicinal products, vaccines, vaccine adjuvants, and insulin analogues. There has also been much recent activity with respect to evolution of guidelines for addressing comparability of biotechnology products after production process changes, and the development of biosimilar products, that contain some guidance on the preclinical data requirements. EU-specific guidelines relating to "biosimilar" products are listed in Table 4.6, and these include some guidance directed toward some specific "generic" forms of biopharmaceutical product that are likely to be coming off-patent in the coming years. Such products include recombinant forms of human insulin, growth hormone, and erythropoeitein.

TABLE 4.6   EU preclinical guidelines on biosimilar medicinal products

Guideline	Type	Start Date
CHMP/437/04: Similar biological medicinal products [39]	Regulatory guideline	2005
EMEA/CHMP/42832/05: Similar biological medicinal products containing biotechnology-derived proteins as active substance—preclinical and clinical issues [40]	Testing guideline	2006
EMEA/CHMP/94526/05: Annex guideline—preclinical and clinical issues on similar medicinal products containing recombinant erythropoietins [41]	Testing guideline	2006
EMEA/CHMP/94528/05: Annex guideline—preclinical and clinical issues on similar medicinal products containing somatropin [42]	Testing guideline	2006
EMEA/CHMP/94529/05: Annex guideline—preclinical and clinical issues on similar medicinal products containing recombinant granulocyte-colony stimulating factor [43]	Testing guideline	2006
EMEA/CHMP/32775/05: Annex guideline—preclinical and clinical issues on similar medicinal products containing recombinant human insulin [44]	Testing guideline	2006

In addition to the EU guidance documents that relate specifically to biopharmaceuticals, there are also a few other EU general preclinical guidelines that may need to be referred to in the planning of toxicity studies on biopharmaceuticals. For example, there is a guidance relating to toxicokinetic sampling of control animals in toxicity studies, in order to check for cross contamination with test substance [20]. An indication of potential evolution of new or modified guidance on nonclinical issues in the European Union can be gained from reference to the "work plan" for the Safety Working Party (SWP) on the EMEA Web site [21].

4.6   APPLICATION OF THE ICH S6 GUIDELINE IN THE EUROPEAN UNION

In addition to the unique regulatory structure in the European Union and the specific guidelines referred to above, there are a few other comments and issues relating to the interpretation and application of the ICH guidance.

4.6.1   General Comments on Application of the Guidance

All the national regulatory agencies, and the central agency (EMEA) in the European Union recognize and are generally familiar with the principles laid out in the ICH S6 guideline. In view of the considerable expertise that has been gained in the various agencies through review of preclinical programs on the large number of approved biopharmaceuticals in the EU region, the level of scientific expertise and quality of advice given to applicants can be regarded as equivalent to that in the other major territories covered by ICH (the United States and Japan). In general, there is a good understanding of the need for a case-by-case approach to preclinical testing of biopharmaceutical products, and most EU preclinical assessors are anxious to avoid unnecessary animal studies that will add little to the human risk assessment. The strategies employed for preclinical testing of biopharmaceuticals have been generally similar to the flexible approaches that have been a hallmark of the Center for Biologics Evaluation and Research (CBER) at the US FDA. While some observers have commented that since the recent switch of assessment of many biotechnology-derived drugs from CBER to the drugs division of FDA (CDER—Center for Drugs Evaluation and Research), a more rigid small-molecule approach has been applied by the US agency, not strictly in the spirit of the ICH S6 guideline [22], a similar trend is not evident among the EU agencies. The EU approach is generally harmonized across all types of biopharmaceutical products, and it seems to be firmly anchored around the principles laid out in the ICH S6 guideline, as evidenced by recent publications on safety assessment of these products by regulators in Germany [26], as well as comments in the report from UK industry bodies (Association of British Pharmaceutical Industry, ABPI and BioIndustry Association, BIA) issued following the TGN1412 incident in 2006 [23] (see later). These publications reinforce the concept that preclinical studies on biopharmaceuticals should only be performed in species that show target homology with humans, and where the relevant human pharmacology/pharmacodynamics can be demonstrated. This approach is reinforced by the fact that human toxicity caused by biologicals normally results from "on-target" effects (i.e., exaggerated pharmacology), while the opposite tends to be the case for small-molecule drugs. There does not appear to be any drift toward a more conventional two-species (rodent/nonrodent) approach to toxicity testing for biopharmaceuticals in the European Union, regardless of species relevance, that has become evident recently in the United States, since CDER took over assessment of many of these products from CBER [21].

In Germany, where potentially two different agencies (PEI and BfArM) may review biopharmaceutical products (predominantly PEI, which has responsibility for review of blood/tissue products, vaccines, gene/cellular therapies and antibody products, although some biopharmaceuticals are reviewed by BfArM), the between-agency approach is consistent and ICH S6 compliant.

The major difference between application of the ICH S6 guideline in the European Union, compared to the United States and Japan, is the rather more complex interaction with the regulatory agencies in relation to agreeing on the preclinical testing strategy for biopharmaceuticals. While sponsor companies in the United States and Japan will work with a single agency (FDA or MOHW) during the development cycle, in the European Union several national agencies, and then the EMEA, may be consulted for scientific advice. Prior to initiation of the first human study on a biopharmaceutical in the European Union, the sponsor company will file a CTA with the relevant national authority for the country where the trial will be conducted, and may seek scientific advice from that authority prior to filing. For novel biopharmaceuticals, some sponsor companies also adopt a strategy of approaching a selection of national authorities in the EU countries that have had the opportunity to amass significant experience in the assessment of biopharmaceutical products (e.g., United Kingdom, Germany, France, the Netherlands, and Sweden) for scientific advice, fairly early in the development cycle, to obtain a general impression of likely EU data requirements. This process may then be further supported by a request for scientific advice from the EMEA, before submission of the MAA. Prior to and following MAA submission, further interaction between the sponsor and the appointed Rapporteur authority may take place to resolve any outstanding issues in the data submission. It may be a point of concern that due to the rather flexible case-by-case approach to preclinical studies advocated by ICH S6, there could be differences of opinion about data requirements between national authorities, but it is the role of the EMEA and the Rapporteur authorities to act as "moderators" in this regard. There is ample opportunity, particularly in the preclinical overview (section 2.4 of the Common Technical Document or CTD), for sponsor companies to defend their preclinical program and to justify any apparent data gaps. Major disputes during late development, or at the MAA, regarding the adequacy of the preclinical programme for a biopharmaceutical in the European Union appear to occur rarely, which seems to indicate that the scientific advice process and sponsor/agency relationships work quite well.

4.6.2 "High-Risk" Compounds and Clinical Trials

The severe, unexpected toxicity, not predicted by a 28-day toxicity study in the monkey, observed in a phase 1 study with a CD28 agonist monoclonal antibody (TGN1412) in healthy volunteers conducted in London in March 2006, has had repercussions regarding the extrapolation from preclinical data to starting doses in human phase 1 studies for some biopharmaceuticals, as well as some so-called high-risk small-molecule drugs. Following the TGN1412 phase 1 study incident, an Expert Scientific Group (ESG) was established in the United Kingdom to investigate why the adverse events seen in the volunteers had not been predicted by the preclinical safety studies in animals and to make recommendations about the future conduct of phase 1 clinical trials in the United Kingdom. The ESG, led by Professor Gordon Duff, published its final report in November 2006 [24]. As a result of the review process following the TGN1412 trial, the ESG made 22 recommendations regarding the preclinical and early clinical development of compounds that might pose a "high risk" to volunteers or patients in early clinical studies. In the subsequent CHMP guideline that has been issued, relating to mitigation of risk for such studies [25], it is stated that all compounds entering the clinic should be assessed for certain "factors of risk," namely:

- Novelty of the mode of action, including possibility of pleiotropic effects or triggering of biological cascades (e.g., cytokine release).
- Nature of the target in humans, and level of available knowledge of the target.
- Relevance of animal species and models used for preclinical studies.

For drugs that might be identified to pose a "high risk" based on assessment of these criteria, prior to conduct of a phase 1 study (or possibly other types of trial) in the United Kingdom, a data package (basically the CTA package, supplemented by specific responses to some standard questions; see Table 4.7), is submitted to the UK authority (MHRA) for consideration by an Expert Advisory Group (EAG). Prior to submission of the CTA package, it is possible to request an opinion from MHRA as to whether the trial might be regarded as "high-risk," thereby warranting referral of the CTA package to the EAG

TABLE 4.7 Standard questions requiring response prior to conduct of phase 1 trials with "high-risk" pharmaceuticals in the United Kingdom

Question	Information/Data Requested
1	A discussion of the function of the target in human.
2	A discussion of the ability of the subject to maintain a normal physiological response to challenge in the presence of the investigational product.
3	A rationale for the transition from preclinical to human testing, particularly with regard to highly species-specific molecules.
4	A discussion of the potential for on-target and off-target effects and how these will be handled in the clinic.
5	A discussion of the doses used in the relevant animal species (particularly with regard to the use in the animal model of the starting dose to be used in human).
6	A rationale for the starting dose in human (e.g., including receptor occupancy).
7	A rationale for the study population (particularly for the use of healthy volunteers).
8	A rationale for the administration schedule for the initial and subsequence cohorts. This should include the time interval between dose administered to individual subjects.
9	A rationale for the dose escalation particularly with regard to potential adverse effects.
10	The proposed trial site, including the facilities available.

for review. The scope and remit of assessments performed by the EAG is as follows:

- First Time in Man (FTIM) studies with new compounds acting (directly or indirectly) via the immune system with a novel target or a novel mechanism of action or having a secondary potential effect on the immune system via a mechanism of action which currently is not well characterized.
- FTIM studies with novel compounds acting via a possible or likely species specific mechanism.
- Any FTIM studies which are otherwise seen as requiring expert advice.
- Other clinical trials involving classes of compound where MHRA may wish to seek external expert advice.
- Provide expert advice on whether a product's mechanism of action is novel and comes within the scope of the EAG.
- Provide MHRA with expert advice on pre-meeting scientific advice documentation for within scope compounds.
- Other clinical trials where MHRA may wish to seek advice or where there is a difficult risk/benefit balance.
- Other clinical trials involving products where a new class safety issue has been identified.

EAG review of a CTA package referred to the EAG by MHRA takes 40–45 days, after which time the CTA can be submitted to MHRA provided the EAG gives a positive opinion. This new process for assessment of CTAs for drugs that might pose a "high risk" in early human trials has already been implemented by the UK regulatory authority (MHRA). As mentioned above, following the TGN1412 event, and due to political pressure, the Safety Working Party (SWP) of EMEA has issued an EU guidance document with regard to the identification and mitigation of risk for first-in-man human clinical trials for investigational medicinal products [25].

At a practical level, the TGN1412 incident is likely to have an influence on the preclinical testing of certain biopharmaceutical products (particularly monoclonal antibodies and other immunomodulatory products), in the following respects:

- There will need to be clearer understanding of the relevance of the species used in preclinical studies to humans. This is likely to involve generation of relative receptor expression/density data between animals/humans and relative potency between animals/humans using suitable cell/tissue preparations, to be taken into account in interspecies dose scaling. Although the ICH S6 guideline makes reference to these issues, they will now assume greater importance and a more thorough examination as a result of the TGN1412 incident.

- Additional preclinical data to address potential for specific adverse events, such as cytokine release syndrome, may be required in some cases.
- The approach to setting the starting dose for "high-risk" human clinical trials may no longer be based on extrapolation from the no-observable-adverse-effect-level (NOAEL) in the animal toxicity studies, but rather on the "minimal anticipated biological effect level" (MABEL), derived from in vitro potency data, combined with predictive modeling of the kinetic behavior of the drug in man and/or estimates of potential receptor occupancy at the human starting dose. Examples of various approaches to calculation of MABEL values are given in the Final Report of the ESG on Phase One Clinical Trials [24], as well as in the ABPI/BIA report on early stage clinical trials [23]. An overview of the TGN1412 incident and the implications for conduct of phase 1 trials in Germany has been published by assessors from one of the German authorities, the Paul-Ehrlich Institute (PEI) [26]. Some other EU countries have also modified their assessments and procedures for approval of first-in-man clinical trials following the TGN1412 incident (e.g., the French agency, AFSSAPS, issued guidance on conduct of human phase 1 studies in July 2006, including recommendations for starting dose selection and dose escalation, although this guidance no longer seems to be available in English on their website).

4.6.3   Primate Supply and Use

Due to the high degree of species specificity of action of many biopharmaceuticals, and potential immunogenicity in lower species, primates are quite extensively used in preclinical safety testing of these products. There is a slight misconception in some regions outside the European Union that there are tight controls and some difficulties regarding the conduct of preclinical studies in primates in Europe. The reality of the situation is as follows:

- Breeding facilities for primates for laboratory use are limited within the European Union, with the exception of marmosets.
- There are well-established supply channels for import of purpose-bred monkeys (mainly cynomolgus monkeys, and some rhesus monkeys) into the European Union from breeding colonies in Eastern Asia or Mauritius.
- Monkeys used for drug development are almost exclusively "purpose bred," the use of wild-caught animals actually not being allowed in many member states.
- The use of primates in research has to be fully justified, and is subject to special review in some member states. However, provided that scientific justification can be provided, preclinical studies on primates are permitted, and there are a number of major contract research organizations

(CROs) throughout the EU that perform primate toxicity studies on a routine basis.

- Studies using great apes (e.g., chimpanzees) are generally not permitted in many member states, and there are no readily available colonies of great apes for research use in the European Union.

The protection of experimental animals in the European Union is covered by Directive 86/609/EEC [27]. This Directive is currently undergoing a process of review and update, a public consultation exercise on the proposed revisions having recently been undertaken. There are some proposed changes to the Directive that could impact on primate use, and potentially on biopharmaceutical development in the European Union:

- A proposal to restrict primate use to F2 animals (and subsequent generations) of wild-caught breeding stock. At present, many EU laboratories still use F1 generation animals, and a switch to F2 animals would lead to supply problems in the coming years, while breeders set aside a significant number of the F1 animals normally supplied to the European Union, for breeding purposes.
- An EU-wide ban on the use of great apes, with very limited exceptions. In reality this change may have little impact, since statistics show that virtually no great apes have been used for research purposes in the European Union in recent years (only six animals in 1999, and zero in 2002). However, for monoclonal antibodies that only show cross reactivity in humans and chimpanzees, it is still fairly common for a limited safety study in chimpanzees to be conducted to support the phase 1 human studies. Such studies would have to be conducted outside of the European Union, although it should be pointed out that it is unlikely that an EU national regulatory authority would expect chimpanzee data to be submitted as part of a CTA for a human-specific monoclonal antibody product. Data from literature sources, in vitro data, as well as data from any relevant transgenic mouse or rodent homologue antibody models would probably be used in the risk assessment in these circumstances.

There are efforts to reduce primate use in the European Union, which could impact on the use of monkeys for biopharmaceutical development programs in the future. For example, the National Centre for Replacement, Refinement and Reduction of Animals in Research (NC3Rs, based in the Union Kingdom) has recently hosted a workshop and published proposals in relation to the reduction in primate use in monoclonal antibody development [28]. They are advocating that so-called alternative approaches to safety testing of monoclonal antibodies, using transgenic rodents that express the human receptor for the antibody, or using rodent homologue versions of the human antibody, should be employed more routinely so as to reduce the numbers of primates used. This initiative, while well-intentioned, possibly fails to understand the technical difficulties and interpretative challenges associated with the alternative approaches, and it remains to be seen whether such approaches would be accepted in place of primate toxicity studies by regulatory agencies in all ICH regions. In addition, while such approaches have been used in a few instances where human antibodies show no cross reactivity with conventional laboratory animal species (e.g., the anti-CD11a antibody, Efalizumab [29]), there has been no validation of the alternative approaches for an antibody that does cross react with monkeys, to assess whether the transgenic or rodent homologue models provide equivalent, relevant safety data compared to those obtained from a standard primate toxicity study. This debate will probably continue for some time, but for the present, sponsors based outside the European Union probably just need to be aware that there are groups working to reduce primate use in Europe.

4.6.4 Duration of Chronic Toxicity Studies

There has been some confusion regarding the required duration of chronic toxicity studies on biopharmaceutical products. The ICH S6 guideline states that studies of six months duration are usually adequate for biotechnology-derived drugs. In contrast, some regulators (including some assessors at CDER in the US agency) have referred to the ICH M3 guidance [30] on this topic, and suggested that 9 or 12 month toxicity studies may be necessary for chronic use biopharmaceuticals, using a small-molecule drug approach to the preclinical studies. In the European Union such confusion does not seem to exist, such that all agencies accept the ICH S6 guidance that a six-month animal study is generally adequate to address chronic toxicity of biopharmaceutical products.

4.6.5 Comparability Testing of Biopharmaceutical Products

It is reasonable to comment that the state of the art of comparability testing, as well as approaches used for assessment of biosimilar or follow-on biologics may actually be slightly more advanced in the European Union than in some other regions, due the effort that has been expended in the development of a number of guidelines in this area. These guidelines include specific documents on particular product types (e.g., insulins, growth hormone) that are likely to be developed as biosimilars in the coming years.

4.7 CONCLUDING REMARKS

ICH S6 has been uniformly implemented across the EU member states, and considerable experience of the application of the guiding principles in this document has been gained both locally (in many of the national authorities) as well as centrally (within the EMEA). There is no evidence that there are major differences in the interpretation of the guideline within the European Union, compared to the other major ICH territories (the United States and Japan). The major difference in application of the guidance stems from the rather more complex regulatory structure and process for obtaining scientific advice, compared to the single-agency model that applies in the United States and Japan. Therefore much attention has been paid in this chapter to an explanation of the unique regulatory structure and the options for obtaining drug approvals within the European Union.

Safety evaluation of novel biopharmaceuticals has come into the spotlight in the European Union over the last year, as a result of the serious adverse events observed in the TGN1412 phase 1 clinical trial. This has already led to new initiatives with regard to extrapolation from preclinical animal data to early human trials, which will place more emphasis on a full understanding of species differences in pharmacology of biotechnology-derived drugs, as well as novel approaches to deriving starting doses for first-in-human studies for some of these molecules. In the short term there is likely to be a more cautious approach to setting of starting dosages for phase 1 studies on immunomodulatory biopharmaceuticals in the European Union, although there is no evidence that the TGN1412 incident has led to increased requirements for preclinical animal studies. In contrast, there has probably been an increased interest in additional in vitro studies to assist in pharmacokinetic/pharmacodynamic correlations between animals and humans so as to better understand the relevance of the animal safety data to humans. These activities are basically an extension of some of the principles originally laid out in the ICH S6 guideline, and should serve to further enhance the relevance and value of preclinical studies on biopharmaceuticals.

REFERENCES

1. European Medicines Agency Press Release: European Medicines Agency adopts first positive opinion for a similar biological medicinal product. 27 January 2006. http://www.emea.europa.eu/pdfs/human/press/pr/3179706en.pdf

2. Commission Directive 2003/63/EC. Official Journal of the European Union. 27 June 2003. http://ec.europa.eu/enterprise/pharmaceuticals/eudralex/vol-1/dir_2003_63/dir_2003_63_en.pdf

3. Harman RJ. The EMEA–Drug regulation at a supranational level. *Pharm J* 2002;269:752–6.

4. European Experts. European Medicines Agency Web site. http://www.emea.europa.eu/htms/aboutus/experts.htm

5. Pignatti F, Boone H, Moulon I. Overview of the European regulatory system. *J Ambul Care Manage* 2004;27:89–97.

6. Bertele' V, Li Bassi L. A critique to the European regulatory system. *J Ambul Care Manage* 2004;27:98–104.

7. Ainsworth MA. New drugs and European procedures of approval. The European Agency for Evaluation of Medicinal Products' role. *Ugeskr Laeger* 2003;165: 1648–9.

8. EMEA pre-submission flowchart. European Medicines Agency Web site. http://www.emea.europa.eu/htms/human/presub/q31.htm

9. Directive 2001/20/EC of the European Parliament and of the Council of 4 April 2001 on the approximation of the laws, regulations and administrative provisions of the member states relating to the implementation of good clinical practice in the conduct of clinical trials on medicinal products for human use. http://europa.eu.int/eur-lex/lex/LexUriServ/LexUriServ.do?uri=CELEX: 32001L0020:EN:HTML

10. European Clinical Trials Database. EudraCT supporting documentation. http://eudract.emea.eu.int/document.html

11. Detailed guidance for the request of authorization of a clinical trial on a medicinal product for human use to the competent authorities, notification of substantial amendments and declaration of the end of the trial. October 2005. http://ec.europa.eu/enterprise/pharmaceuticals/eudralex/vol-10/11_ca_14-2005.pdf

12. Kock M, Thomsen MK. Contact and dialogue between drug companies and the global regulatory authorities throughout research and development phase. *Ugeskr Laeger* 2003;165:1649–52.

13. Dejas-Eckertz P, Shaffner G. Scientific advice by the nationally competent authority and the EMEA on the conduct of clinical trials. *Bundesgesundheitsblatt Gesundheitsforschung Gesundheitsschutz* 2005;48:423–8.

14. MHRA Web site. Scientific advice for license applicants. http://www.mhra.gov.uk/home/idcplg?IdcService=SS_GET_PAGE&nodeId=121

15. European Medicines Agency. New framework for scientific advice and protocol assistance. EMEA/267/187/2005 Rev. 1, 26 April 2006. http://www.emea.europa.eu/pdfs/human/sciadvice/26718705en.pdf

16. ICH Harmonized Tripartite Guideline S6: Preclinical Safety Evaluation of Biotechnology-Derived Pharmaceuticals. July 1997. http://www.ich.org/LOB/media/MEDIA503.pdf

17. Pre-clinical biological safety testing on medicinal products derived from biotechnology (3BS13a). European Commission. http://pharmacos.eudra.org/F2/eudralex/vol-3/pdfs-en/3bs13aen.pdf

18. Guideline on Production and Quality Control of Monoclonal Antibodies. Document III/5271/94 in Volume 3AB4a of the Rules Governing Medicinal products in the European Union. http://www.tga.gov.au/docs/pdf/euguide/vol3a/3ab4aen.pdf

19. Concept paper on the need to revise the guideline on production and quality control of monoclonal antibodies. CHMP/BWP/64/04, 21 October 2004. http://www.emea.eu.int/pdfs/human/bwp/006404en.pdf

20. European Medicines Agency—Committee for Proprietary Medicinal Products. Guideline on the Evaluation of Control Samples In Nonclincial Safety Studies: Checking for Contamination with the Test Substance. CPMP/SWP/1094/04. 17 March 2005. http://www.emea.europa.eu/pdfs/human/swp/109404en.pdf

21. European Medicines Agency. Work plan for the Safety Working Party. EMEA/154420/2006 corr. January 2007. http://www.emea.europa.eu/pdfs/human/swp/15242006en.pdf

22. Schwieterman WD. Regulating biopharmaceuticals under CDER versus CBER: an insider's perspective. *Drug Disc Today* 2006;11:945–51.

23. Joint ABPI/BIA Report: Early stage clinical trial taskforce. 24 July 2006. http://www.abpi.org.uk/information/pdfs/BIAABPI_taskforce2.pdf

24. Expert Scientific Group on Phase One Clinical Trials. Final report. 30 November 2006. http://www.dh.gov.uk/en/Publicationsandstatistics/PublicationsPublicationsPolicyAndGuidance/DH_063117

25 European Medicines Agency—Committee for Medicinal Products for Human Use (CHMP). Guideline on Strategies to Identify and Mitigate Risks for First-in-Man Human Clinical Trials with Investigational Medicinal Products. EMEA/CHMP/SWP/2836707/2007. 19 July 2007. http://www.emea.europa.eu/pdfs/human/swp/2836707enfin.pdf

26. Liedert B, Bassus S, Schneider C, Kalinke U, Löwer J. Safety of phase 1 clinical trials with monoclonal antibodies in Germany—The regulatory requirements viewed in the aftermath of the TGN1412 disaster. *Int J Clin Pharmacol Ther* 2007;45:1–9.

27. Council Directive of 24 November 1986 on the approximation of laws, regulations and administrative provisions of the member states regarding the protection of animals used for experimental and other scientific procedures (86/609/EEC). http://ec.europa.eu/food/fs/aw/aw_legislation/scientific/86-609-eec_en.pdf

28. Chapman K, Pullen N, Graham M, Ragan I. Preclinical safety testing of monoclonal antibodies: the significance of species relevance. *Nature Drug Disc* 2004;6:120–6.

29. Clarke J, Leach W, Pippig S, et al. Evaluation of a surrogate antibody for preclinical safety testing of an anti-CD11a monoclonal antibody. *Reg Toxicol Pharmacol* 2004;40:219–26.

30. ICH Harmonized Tripartite Guideline M3: Nonclinical Safety Studies for the Conduct of Human Clinical Trials for Pharmaceuticals. November 2000. http://www.ich.org/LOB/media/MEDIA506.pdf

31. European Medicines Agency—Committee for Proprietary Medicinal Products. Preclinical pharmacological and toxicological testing of vaccines. CPMP/SWP/465/95. London, 17 December 1997. http://www.emea.eu.int/pdfs/human/swp/046595en.pdf

32. European Medicines Agency—Committee for Proprietary Medicinal Products. Note for Guidance on the Quality, Preclinical and Clinical Aspects of Gene Transfer Medicinal Products. CPMP/BWP/3088/99. London, 24 April 2001. http://www.emea.eu.int/pdfs/human/bwp/308899en.pdf

33. European Medicines Agency—Committee for Proprietary Medicinal Products. Points to Consider on the Non-clinical Assessment of the Carcinogenic Potential of Insulin Analogues. CPMP/SWP/372/01. London, 15 November 2001. http://www.emea.eu.int/pdfs/human/swp/037201en.pdf

34. European Medicines Agency—Committee for Proprietary Medicinal Products. Points to Consider on the Need for Assessment of Reproductive Toxicity of Human Insulin Analogues. CPMP/SWP/2600/01 final. London, 1 March 2002. http://www.emea.eu.int/pdfs/human/swp/260001en.pdf

35. European Medicines Agency—Committee for Proprietary Medicinal Products. Guideline on the Comparability of Medicinal Products Containing Biotechnology-

Derived Proteins as Active Substance. Nonclinical and Clinical Issues. 17 December 2003. http://www.emea.europa.eu/pdfs/human/ewp/309702en.pdf

36. European Medicines Agency—Committee for Proprietary Medicinal Products. Note for Guidance on the Quality, Preclinical and Clinical Aspects of Gene Tansfer Medicinal Products. Draft annex on the non-clinical testing for inadvertent germline transmission of gene transfer vectors. 17 November 2005. http://www.emea.europa.eu/pdfs/human/genetherapy/27397405en.pdf

37. European Medicines Agency—Committee for Proprietary MedicInal Products. GuidelIne on Adjuvants in Vaccines for Human Use. EMEA/CHMP/VEG/134716/2004. London, 20 January 2005. http://www.emea.eu.int/pdfs/human/vwp/13471604en.pdf

38. European Medicines Agency—Committee for Proprietary Medicinal Products. Guideline on Comparability of Biotechnology-Derived Medicinal Products after a Change in the Manufacturing Process. EMEA/CHMP/BMWP/101695/2006. 24 January 2007. http://www.emea.europa.eu/pdfs/human/biosimilar/10169506en.pdf

39. European Medicines Agency—Committee for Medicinal Products for human use. Guideline on Similar Biological Medicinal Products. CHMP/437/04, 30 October 2005. http://www.emea.europa.eu/pdfs/human/biosimilar/043704en.pdf

40. European Medicines Agency—Committee for Medicinal Products for Human Use. Similar Biological Medicinal Products Containing Biotechnology-Derived Proteins as Active Substance: Nonclinical and Clinical Issues. EMEA/CHMP/42832/05. 22 February 2006. http://www.emea.europa.eu/pdfs/human/biosimilar/4283205en.pdf

41. European Medicines Agency—Committee for Medicinal Products for Human Use. Annex Guideline: Nonclinical and Clinical Issues on Similar Medicinal Products Containing Recombinant Erythropoietins. EMEA/CHMP/94526/05. 22 March 2006. http://www.emea.europa.eu/pdfs/human/biosimilar/9452605en.pdf

42. European Medicines Agency—Committee for Medicinal Products for Human Use. Annex Guideline: Nonclinical and Clinical Issues on Similar Medicinal Products Containing Somatropin. EMEA/CHMP/94528/05. 22 February 2006. http://www.emea.europa.eu/pdfs/human/biosimilar/9452805en.pdf

43. European Medicines Agency—Committee for Medicinal Products for Human Use. Annex Guideline: Nonclinical and Clinical Issues on Similar Medicinal Products Containing Recombinant Granulocyte-Colony Stimulating Factor. EMEA/CHMP/94529/05. 22 February 2006. http://www.emea.europa.eu/pdfs/human/biosimilar/3132905en.pdf

44. European Medicines Agency—Committee for Medicinal Products for Human Use. Annex Guideline: Preclinical and Clinical Issues on Similar Medicinal Products Containing Recombinant Human Insulin. EMEA/CHMP/32775/05. 22 February 2006. http://www.emea.europa.eu/pdfs/human/biosimilar/3277505en.pdf

■■■■■ CHAPTER 5

Implementation of ICH S6: Japanese Perspective

TAKAHIRO NAKAZAWA, PhD

Contents

5.1 INTRODUCTION

Biotechnology-derived pharmaceuticals (biopharmaceuticals) appeared for the first time in the 1980s for medical treatment of diseases, such as diabetes mellitus and hypophysical dwarfism. Since then the number and types of biopharmaceuticals have climbed and continue to dramatically increase. One reason for the increase is the evolution of recombinant manufacturing of biopharmaceuticals. This has provided sufficient amounts of proteins for development and clinical use, whereas, for example, the amount of insulin or growth hormones extracted from animal or human tissues had been limited. Another

Preclinical Safety Evaluation of Biopharmaceuticals: A Science-Based Approach to Facilitating Clinical Trials, edited by Joy A. Cavagnaro
Copyright © 2008 by John Wiley & Sons, Inc.

benefit of recombinant technology is the production of proteins with primary amino acid sequences that are identical to those of endogenous human proteins. This reduces immunogenicity, which was a problem with the use of animal proteins in humans. Long-term use of bovine or porcine insulin induces the production of an antibovine insulin or antiporcine insulin antibody that can sometimes decrease its efficacy, change the pharmacokinetics, and cause immunological adverse effects. Human proteins are expected to have sufficiently low or no immunogenicity to be used for the long term in humans. Human insulin produced by recombinant DNA technology was shown to induce the production of the antibody at much lower level in humans than bovine or pork insulin. Although immunogenicity is reduced, long-term administration of human insulin also induces the production of antibody in humans in some patients. Similarly to human insulin, the immunogenicity of biopharmaceuticals in humans remains an issue.

From a preclinical point of view, human protein biopharmaceuticals may be immunogenic in animals. In the case where a human protein is highly immunogenic in animals, the safety evaluation may have technical limitations. Over a decade ago the following concerns/questions were raised about the scientific justifications on the safety assessment of biopharmaceuticals in preclinical studies: If low or no toxicity is observed at high doses of a biopharmaceutical in an animal that does not respond to the biological activity of the biopharmaceutical, can it simply be concluded that the failure of demonstrating toxicity in animals would mean low or absence of toxicity in humans? How is the potential toxicity of a biopharmaceutical interpreted if toxicity decreases after repeated administration due to the production of neutralizing immunogenicity? Should developers conduct a battery of genotoxicity studies for a biopharmaceutical? A human protein biopharmaceutical is positive in an antigenicity study [1], but is this meaningful? Should ADME studies be conducted with radiolabeled biopharmaceuticals?

To answer these questions, guidelines and/or Points-to-Consider documents were issued in the European Union, the United States, and Japan. However, differences in approaches for safety evaluation of biopharmaceuticals among those regions were identified, indicating the need for harmonizing these approaches among the three regions. In 1997 the three regions reached an agreement concerning preclinical safety evaluation of biotechnology-derived pharmaceuticals (ICH S6). On the basis of this ICH S6 guideline, Notification 326 was issued as ICH Step 5 by the Ministry of Health and Welfare (MHW) in 2000 [2]. Subsequently scientists from the National Institute of Health Sciences (NIHS), the Pharmaceuticals and Medical Devices Evaluation Center (currently, Pharmaceuticals and Medical Devices Agency, called PMDA), and Japan Pharmaceutical Manufacturers Association (JPMA) collaborated to publish a Japanese Points-to-Consider document regarding the safety assessment of biopharmaceuticals in preclinical studies in 2002 [3]. An English translation was published in 2004 [4].

5.2 ANALYSIS OF DATA FROM THE JPMA QUESTIONNAIRE SURVEY REGARDING ICH S6 IMPLEMENTATION IN JAPANESE PHARMACEUTICAL COMPANIES

A JPMA working group conducted a survey in 2001 to examine how the ICH S6 guideline was being implemented by the 83 pharmaceutical companies that belonged to JPMA at that time [5]. Responses to general principles were obtained from 54 out of 83 pharmaceutical companies. Moreover 34 biopharmaceuticals from 25 pharmaceutical companies were examined with respect to each company's specific points of considerations in their preclinical studies. In this section the key survey results are summarized along with the interpretation of the JPMA working group.

5.2.1 Understanding the General Principles

Animal Species Selection Almost all pharmaceutical companies select animal species for preclinical studies on the basis of the results of the responsiveness of a test animal to the biological activity of a biopharmaceutical and its production of neutralizing antibodies. Such considerations are specifically applicable to biopharmaceuticals but not to new chemical entities (NCEs). This survey finding suggests that most pharmaceutical companies in Japan understand and implement the animal species selection in good accordance with ICH S6.

ICH S6 allows the use of only one species for subsequent long-term studies when the toxicity profiles of two species are comparable in a short-term study. JPMA's questionnaire included a question on whether the toxicity profiles are concluded to be similar when no toxicity is observed in the two species that are responsive to the biological activity of a biopharmaceutical. The most common response was that this decision is made on a case-by-case basis considering pharmacological and pharmacokinetic data. The second most common was that the toxicity profiles are considered similar when the highest dose for testing is scientifically justified (as discussed in the next section), closely followed by the third most common answer that profiles are not concluded to be similar since the comparison of toxicological changes cannot be done. There may not be a correct single answer. Because in many cases only the biological changes due to exaggerated pharmacological effects are observed, the JPMA working team concluded that it may be practical to consider these toxicity profiles as similar and to use only one species in the subsequent long-term studies as long as the pharmacologically responsive animal and the dose selection are appropriate.

Highest Dose Selection It is sometimes difficult to set the highest dose for safety programs of a biopharmaceutical when low or no toxicity is observed in animals. The JPMA questionnaire survey revealed that most pharmaceutical companies set the highest dose of a biopharmaceutical using the maximum feasible dose, which is the highest concentration that can be prepared based on the solubility of the biopharmaceutical, and the largest administration volume that can be administered to animals. The second most common response was a dose that is 10 to 100 times higher than the expected clinical dose, and the third was to use a dose several to 10 times higher than the clinical dose. However, the JPMA working team did not agree that the maximum feasible dose or a large multiple of the clinical dose is scientifically appropriate. More important is to determine the adverse biological changes induced by any exaggerated pharmacological effects at doses relevant to the expected clinical dose rather than toxicological changes induced by unrealistic doses. Moreover animal data gathered at maximum feasible doses or at doses that are 100 times higher than the clinical dose cannot ensure the safety of biopharmaceuticals in humans without the consideration of the difference in responsiveness to the biological activity between the test animals and humans and the intended clinical indication. Therefore the JPMA working team concluded that the test doses should be determined on the basis of the responsiveness of animal species to the biological activity of a biopharmaceutical and the clinical usage conditions.

5.2.2 Japanese Practices in Preclinical Studies

Types of Biopharmaceuticals Survey data on preclinical safety assessment programs were analyzed for 34 biopharmaceuticals cases. The numbers of antibodies, human proteins, and human protein analogues either in the development or marketed as of 2001 in Japan were 13, 12, and 6, respectively. The remainder were bioconjugates, DNA-derived vaccines, and human T cell epitopes. Thus antibodies and human proteins are the two major biopharmaceuticals.

In vivo Studies The in vivo preclinical studies conducted for 34 biopharmaceuticals are shown in Table 5.1. Single-dose and repeated-dose toxicity studies up to three months were conducted in most cases using rodents and nonrodents. Repeated-dose toxicity studies longer than three months were conducted for a third of the 34 cases. Nonrodents were used more often than rodents in considering the biological responsiveness of test animals to the biopharmaceuticals. Levels of antibodies were measured in most repeated-dose toxicity studies (31 out of 34 cases). The alteration of pharmacokinetics or pharmacodynamics by antibodies was observed in 13 out of 31 cases, which did not result in the discontinuation of the studies nor required significant changes in the study design. The JPMA working group agreed with the continuation of such studies, since neutralizing antibodies do not always interfere with the outcome of a toxicological response. However, the production of neutralizing antibodies precludes long-term studies, such as carcinogenicity studies. Reproductive toxicity studies were conducted for 11 out of 34 cases.

TABLE 5.1   In vivo preclinical studies conducted for 34 biopharmaceuticals

In vivo Preclinical Studies	Cases
Rodent single-dose toxicity study	24
Nonrodent single-dose toxicity study	21
Rodent repeat-dose toxicity study (not longer than 3 months)	24
Nonrodent repeat-dose toxicity study (not longer than 3 months)	29
Rodent repeat-dose toxicity study (longer than 3 months)	8
Nonrodent repeated dose toxicity study (longer than 3 months)	13
Antigenicity studies	12
Immunogenicity studies (excepting antigenicity studies)	11
Reproductive toxicity study (segment 1)	13
Rodent reproductive/developmental toxicity study (segment 2)	14
Nonrodent reproductive/developmental toxicity study (segment 2)	17
Reproductive/developmental toxicity study (segment 3)	11
Genotoxicity studies	16
Carcinogenicity study (long-term)	2
Carcinogenicity study (short- to mid-term)	1
Local irritation studies	24
General pharmacology studies (category A)	9
General pharmacology studies (category B)	3
Safety pharmacology studies (core battery)	9
Safety pharmacology studies (follow-up or additional studies)	5
Other	6

Antigenicity studies (active sensitization test in guinea pigs, PCA in rabbits or guinea pigs, passive hemagglutination reaction using sensitized rabbit serum, investigation of IgE-type antibody production capacity, degree of covalent bonding with proteins, polymerization of the drug or cross-antigenicity) defined by a book entitled *Drug Approval and Licensing Procedures in Japan* [1] were conducted for 11 out of 34 cases. The antigenicity studies were conducted in most cases before the ICH S6 notification. It was concluded by the ICH S6 expert working group that antigenicity studies conducted with biopharmaceuticals are not scientifically justified. A description of antigenicity studies was taken out of the 2006 edition of the book. The in vivo genotoxicity studies were done for 16 biopharmaceuticals; almost all the cases were prior to the ICH S6 notification. A few carcinogenicity studies were conducted for 34 biopharmaceuticals examined (e.g., recombinant hormones).

On the questionnaire was also a question asking what in vivo preclinical studies commonly conducted for NCEs were intentionally omitted for the 34 biopharmaceuticals (Table 5.2). Rodent repeated-dose toxicity, antigenicity, reproductive toxicity, in vivo genotoxicity, and carcinogenicity studies were in this category for a third to half of the 34 cases. The main reason for not conducting rodent repeated-dose toxicity studies was the lack of rodent responsiveness to the biological activities of the biopharmaceuticals. The reasons for not conducting reproductive toxicity studies were related to the

TABLE 5.2   In vivo preclinical studies intentionally not conducted for 34 biopharmaceuticals

In vivo Preclinical Studies	Cases
Rodent single-dose toxicity study	9
Nonrodent single-dose toxicity study	8
Rodent repeat-dose toxicity study (not longer than 3 months)	11
Nonrodent repeat-dose toxicity study (not longer than 3 months)	5
Rodent repeat-dose toxicity study (longer than 3 months)	10
Nonrodent repeat-dose toxicity study (longer than 3 months)	6
Antigenicity studies	15
Immunogenicity studies (excepting antigenicity studies)	4
Reproductive/developmental toxicity study (segment 1)	11
Rodent reproductivedevelopmental toxicity study (segment 2)	11
Nonrodent reproductive/developmental toxicity study (segment 2)	8
Reproductive/developmental toxicity study (segment 3)	11
In vivo genotoxicity studies	11
Carcinogenicity study (long-term)	15
Carcinogenicity study (short- or mid-term)	6
Local irritation studies	3
General pharmacology studies (category A)	5
General pharmacology studies (category B)	4
Safety pharmacology studies (core battery)	6
Safety pharmacology studies (follow-up or additional studies)	5
Other	0

administration period in a clinical setting, the patient population, nonresponsiveness of animal species to biological activity, and the existence of extensive safety data for humans on natural proteins. The main reason for not conducting antigenicity and in vivo genotoxicity studies was that those studies are not required by ICH S6. The main reasons for carcinogenicity studies were the lack of biological responsiveness and the production of neutralizing antibodies.

In vitro Studies   Table 5.3 shows the in vitro preclinical studies conducted for the 34 biopharmaceuticals. Most were in vitro genotoxicity studies that are not required by the ICH S6 guideline. This is not the case of poor understanding of the ICH S6. In vitro genotoxicity studies are usually conducted at the early stage of development. Almost all the in vitro genotoxicity studies examined by the JPMA survey in 2001 were conducted before the ICH S6 notification. The cross-reactivity studies were used to understand interspecies reactivity to a biopharmaceutical, especially in case of antibodies.

ADME Studies   Absorption, distribution, metabolism, and excretion studies were conducted for 24, 21, 17, and 19 out of the 34 biopharmaceuticals, respectively. No radiolabeled proteins were used for 20, 2, 1, and 13 out of the 34

TABLE 5.3   In vitro preclinical studies conducted for 34 human proteins

In vitro Preclinical Studies	Cases
Ames tests	14
Chromosomal aberration test	10
Mouse lymphoma TK test	3
Cross reactivity study	9
In vitro general pharmacology studies (category A)	4
In vitro general pharmacology studies (category B)	3
In vitro safety pharmacology studies	3
Other	3

biopharmaceuticals, respectively. The types of radiolabeled proteins in the remaining studies included conjugates of ^{125}I-, ^{14}C-, and ^{3}H-. When using radiolabeled proteins, it is important to demonstrate that a radiolabeled test material maintains its activity and biological properties equivalent to those of the unlabeled material. In most cases this was done before using the radiolabeled protein. Other concerns are stoichiometric radiolabeling, the loss of radiolabel, recycling of a radiolabeled amino acid into non–drug-related protein, and disruption of stability. It is well known that there are technical limitations to the use of radiolabeled proteins for ADME studies. For example, when using ^{125}I-radiolabeled proteins in distribution studies, the formation of inorganic iodine by deiodinization in vivo should be considered. Free ^{125}I thus produced is accumulated in the thyroid gland: therefore a ^{125}I-radiolabeled biopharmaceutical seems to distribute mainly in the thyroid gland. However, the JPMA working group agreed that with a good understanding of the technical limitations, ADME studies using radiolabeled proteins may provide some useful information for the planning of human study.

5.3   POINTS-TO-CONSIDER DOCUMENT IN JAPAN

Scientists from NIHS, PMDA, and JPMA collaborated to publish a Points-to-Consider document regarding the safety assessment of biopharmaceuticals in preclinical studies in 2002 [3]. The collaboration team intended to clarify their interpretation of the ICH S6 guideline and share recent Japanese practices on this matter. However, it was written in Japanese. Thus the collaboration team made an English translation of the document and also collected comments on the contents from experts in the United States and the European. The experts agreed to most ideas presented in the Japanese Points-to-Consider document. They also suggested more clarification of some other ideas. In light of these comments, the collaboration team revised and published the English translation of the document, such that the nonnative Japanese could correctly understand the contents [4]. In this section, I summarize the key points of the document, as they may be of some help to scientists in the pharmaceutical industries and regulatory reviewers in countries other than Japan. However, it is important to note that the Points-to-Consider document is not a regulatory requirement in Japan. There may even be a gap between the contents of the document and some individual cases. Therefore the application of the contents to individual cases should be made on a scientifically justified case-by-case manner.

5.3.1 Classification of Biopharmaceuticals

A significant contribution of the Japanese Points-to-Consider document is the classification of biopharmaceuticals. When ICH S6 was written, the types of biopharmaceuticals whose information was available for discussion were mainly human proteins/peptides and diagnostic antibodies. Several new types of bio-pharmaceutical have been developed since the notification of the ICH S6. However, the knowledge on and experiences in the development of the new types of biopharmaceutical have not been shared. Thus the classification and considerations for many of the newer types is proposed in the Japanese Points-to-Consider document. Discussed next are the key points of the document [4].

   Biopharmaceuticals covered by the ICH S6 guideline include protein and peptide products consisting of natural amino acids. The top portion of Table 5.4 shows the subcategories of biopharmaceuticals. Antibodies were initially considered to be included under the protein subcategory classification, as they consist of amino acids, but ended up being a separate category because the biological activities of antibodies differs substantially from those of other protein products. In recent years the development of human protein analogues has sporadically been observed with the intent of improving efficacy. Therefore approaches to the development of these analogues are also described. The ICH S6 covers the safety evaluation of biopharmaceuticals by taking into account the type and clinical applications. The considerations for each type of biopharmaceutical are described below. The safety of impurities and degradation products in biopharmaceuticals needs to be comprehensively assessed with respect to their quality and bioactivity.

Proteins   When a human protein is used at a concentration in blood exceeding the physiological level, studies for safety evaluation should be designed with reference to many of the considerations mentioned in the ICH S6 guideline. Moreover an entirely different physiological secretion pattern in humans should be considered. Changes in concentration in blood are considered more significant than the concentration itself for some classes of proteins. Biopharmaceuticals intended for use in sustained-release formulation show changes in blood concentration that diverge much from the physiological secretion pattern. Therefore, when the changes in the blood concentration of an exogenous human protein in blood differ from the physiological secretion patterns of an endogenous protein, attention should be paid to the potential changes in the physiological action.

TABLE 5.4 Type of biopharmaceuticals/related biological medicines and scope of the ICH S6 guideline

PROTEINS *(covered by ICH S6)*
  Human-type protein
  Nonhuman protein
  Human-type protein analog consisting of natural amino acid
  Human-type protein analog containing nonnatural amino acid
  Bioconjugate of human-type protein and other protein
  Bioconjugate of human-type protein and organic linker

PEPTIDES *(covered by ICH S6)*
  Human-type peptide
  Nonhuman-type peptide
  Human-type peptide analogue consisting of natural amino acid
  Human-type peptide analogue containing nonnatural amino acid

ANTIBODIES *(covered by ICH S6)*
  Monoclonal antibodies/chimera antibodies
  Immunoconjugates

PEPTIDE MIMICS *(not covered by ICH S6 but its basic principles can be used as reference)*
  NCEs having a selective affinity to human peptide receptors

OLIGONUCLEOTIDE MEDICINES *(not covered by ICH S6 but its basic principles can be used as reference)*
  Anti-sense compounds
  RNAi
  Aptamer

OTHER BIOLOGICAL MEDICINES *(not covered by ICH S6 and safety evaluation conforms to other standards)*
  Antibiotics
  Allergen extracts
  Vitamins
  Viral vaccines, etc.

For animal proteins or human-type protein analogues consisting of natural amino acids (i.e., human-type protein analogues with the original human protein amino acids substituted with other natural amino acids, added natural amino acids, or deleted amino acids) potential differences in the potency and quality of biological activity between these pharmaceuticals and the original human proteins should be considered. For example, in the case of a human-type protein analogue in which the substituted site is in receptor recognition sites, its biological activity may be enhanced or diminished, and even a new biological activity may occur. Moreover, depending on the type and site of the amino acid replaced, a new antigen determinant (epitope) may be expressed that results in changes of immunogenicity.

For human-type protein analogues with nonnatural amino acids, in addition to the considerations above, attention should be paid to the potential biological activity and pharmacokinetic behavior in the fragment containing the site in which this protein has been metabolized. For example, no genotoxicity studies are required for proteins that cannot pass through cell membranes, whereas the applicability of these studies should be discussed on a case-by-case basis for fragments containing nonnatural amino acids. No metabolism studies are required for proteins that are degraded into only amino acids, whereas metabolism studies may provide useful information on proteins containing nonnatural amino acids.

Two types of bioconjugates may exist. A bioconjugate of a human-type protein and another protein may have the combined biological activity of both proteins, and their effects on the body may be altered due to their interaction. Therefore conducting safety evaluation in pharmacological studies should be considered. On the other hand, a bioconjugate of a human-type protein and an organic linker can be studied similarly to human-type protein analogues containing nonnatural amino acids.

Peptides   Peptides, similar to proteins, consist of amino acids, although their molecular weights are lower than those of proteins. Therefore the considerations above for proteins are also applicable to peptides. Antibody formation, which is a key issue in animal experiments on human-type proteins, generally depends on molecular weight (i.e., the probability of antibody formation is low if the molecular weight is low). The guideline covers not only biotechnologically produced peptides but also chemically synthesized peptides.

Antibodies   Antibodies are usually targeted to specific receptors, particularly monoclonal antibodies. Many of these antibodies are inherently species-specific. It is important for the developer to verify species specificity in order to justify the use (or non-use) of a particular animal species in safety studies. In the cases where an appropriate animal model is not available, the use of homologous antibodies for animals or the use of relevant transgenic animals expressing human antigens should be considered. In addition, when an IgG antibody is used in possibly pregnant or lactating women, and on the basis of the intended indication, reproductive toxicity should be investigated because of the potential of the antibody to be transferred to the placenta or milk. Immunoconjugates of antibodies, conjugated with either other proteins or organic linkers, should be handled the same way as for the bioconjugates described above.

Peptide Mimics and Oligonucleotide Medicines   The middle section of Table 5.4 shows new types of pharmaceuticals not classified as biopharmaceuticals, although they may have a selective pharmacological action similar to that of biopharmaceuticals. Their safety evaluation in animals is sometimes difficult to conduct. The ICH S6 guideline does not cover these pharmaceuticals, but its basic principles can be used as reference. Peptide mimics, antisense compounds, RNAi, and aptamer fall in this category. (Refer to the Points-to-Consider paper [4] for references.)

Other Biological Medicines   The conventional biologics shown in the bottom section of Table 5.4 are not covered by the ICH S6 guideline. Preclinical safety evaluation based on relevant standards is necessary for this group of pharmaceuticals. (Refer to the Points-to-Consider paper [4] for references.)

5.3.2   Individual Considerations

Additional useful ideas included in the Japanese Points-to-Consider document are summarized that require further clarification.

Highest Dose Selection   The highest dose for safety assessment programs in the preclinical studies should be selected by considering the intended maximum clinical exposure of a biopharmaceutical on the basis of its AUC. There is generally no need to investigate biopharmaceuticals at exposures much higher than the intended clinical exposure, unlike the case of NCEs. Another consideration is that the highest dose is as the dose at which the pharmacodynamic response has reached the plateau (pharmacodynamic maximum dose).

Toxicological Effects and Pharmacological Action   In some cases only exaggerated pharmacological effects may be observed in the toxicological studies of the biopharmaceuticals. Sometimes these effects are difficult to distinguish from a compound-related toxicity. However, if the effect is related to the mechanism (predictable) and is reversible, it should not be considered as an adverse effect.

In the event of lethality observed in a toxicity study it is prudent to determine whether the death is due to toxicity or an exaggerated pharmacological effect considering the clinical application. For example, death due to hemorrhage is sometimes observed in healthy animals after administration of biopharmaceuticals with an anticoagulation activity. Likewise death due to hypoglycemia can occur in healthy animals after administration of insulin. To attribute these death cases to toxicity has little value for determining human safety in clinical practice. Because these changes are observed only in healthy animals, and because biopharmaceuticals are prescribed for the normalization of abnormal functions in patients (e.g., hypercoagulopathy or hyperglycemia) through their pharmacological activity, one can easily assume that hemorrhage or hypoglycemia due to excessive expression of the pharmacological actions may occur.

Metabolism Study   The degradation of a protein to peptides and an amino acid moiety is commonly expected as a representative metabolic pattern. Therefore conventional biotransformation studies are not needed for biopharmaceuticals consisting of natural amino acids. However, metabolism studies of biopharmaceuticals containing nonnatural amino acid may provide useful information. In such cases radiolabeled proteins should be prepared to trace the pharmacokinetic behavior of the nonnatural amino acid fragments.

In vitro Electrophysiological Study   In vitro electrophysiological studies are generally not applicable to biopharmaceuticals. This is because NCEs act on each cellular channel after passing through the cell membrane, whereas biopharmaceuticals are not expected to act similarly because they cannot pass through the cell membrane.

Single-Dose Toxicity Study   An objective of single-dose studies is to define the relationship of dose with systemic and/or local toxicity. For biopharmaceuticals repeatedly administered clinically, the data from single-dose toxicity studies can be used to select doses for repeated-dose toxicity studies. Repeated-dose toxicity studies of biopharmaceuticals that have minimal toxicity can be performed without conducting single-dose toxicity studies under GLP conditions. Therefore single-dose toxicity studies in two animal species are not considered to be as necessary for these biopharmaceuticals as they are for NCEs. When a single-dose toxicity study is necessary, single-dose toxicity can be evaluated as a component of safety pharmacology or primary pharmacodynamic studies using animal models. When the doses set for the repeated-dose toxicity study are reasonable, the initial administration data obtained from the repeated-dose toxicity study can be used as data for single-dose toxicity studies. Since biopharmaceuticals need not be examined at high doses such as the approximate lethal dose, conducting single-dose toxicity studies merely to obtain information on the potential of toxic substances among others would be meaningless. Single-dose toxicity studies in nonrodents only should be considered in cases where rodents are not considered a relevant species.

Repeat-Dose Toxicity Studies   Typically toxicity studies are performed in two animal species. However, for toxicity studies for which there is only one relevant animal species, these studies may be performed using one animal species. When two animal species show the same toxicity profile in short-term studies, only one animal species may be used in long-term studies. Comparison of toxicity profiles means comparing the type and severity of any toxicity observed. However, biopharmaceuticals with a low toxicity may display no toxicity at high doses in some cases. It such cases it may still be important to select one species for assessment of chronic toxicity. More important, in cases where toxicity has not been clearly demonstrated justification of human safe human doses would be based on an understanding of the therapeutic index (i.e., minimum effective biological dose and the maximum feasible dose).

Reproductive and Developmental Toxicity Studies The requirement for reproductive and developmental toxicity studies depends on the clinical indication and intended patient population. For example, when (1) no relevant animal species exists, (2) a biopharmaceutical is not used for pregnant women or women of child-bearing potential (3) there is a structurally comparable natural biopharmaceutical for which there is much experience in clinical practice, or (4) a biopharmaceutical is indicated for patients with minimal child-bearing potential and indicated for those with serious diseases, reproductive, and developmental toxicity studies could be obviated.

When standard reproductive and developmental toxicity studies are not feasible due to problems of neutralizing antibody formation, although it is deemed necessary, the study design and dosing schedule may be modified on the basis of factors related to species specificity, immunogenicity, biological activity, and/or elimination half-life. For example, a reproductive and developmental toxicity study with a shorter periodic dosing than the whole-period dosing shown in the toxicology guideline for NCE can be meaningful. In addition alternative studies using relevant transgenic animals, or homologous proteins, should be considered. However, as reproductive performance in transgenic animals has not yet been clarified, careful selection of a study system is required.

The points to consider on the need for assessment of reproduction toxicity of human insulin analogues have been published [6].

Carcinogenicity Studies When the following points are confirmed, generally, carcinogenicity studies are not necessary even when a biopharmaceutical is used for a long period:

1. It is used for substitution therapies at the physiological level.
2. It has no physiological activity that differs from that of endogenous substances.
3. Its biological action is not significantly stronger than that of endogenous substances.
4. It has no potential to induce tumor cell division (in the case of growth promoters).
5. It neither locally retains nor accumulates at a high concentration for a long period of time.
6. It does not have a sustained pharmacological action.
7. In repeated-dose toxicity studies when a dosing duration adequate for evaluation is attained, no preneoplastic lesions are observed.

8. The results of genotoxicity studies are negative in the case that the studies are relevant and have been conducted (e.g., bioconjugate with organic chemical linker).

Assessment of the carcinogenic/tumorigenic potential should be considered for some biopharmaceuticals because of the dosing duration, the relationship of target diseases with cancer, the biological activity of a product, the presence or absence of immunosuppressive action, in vitro data, and so forth. In the cases where a product is biologically active and nonimmunogenic in rodents and other studies have not provided sufficient information to allow an assessment of carcinogenic potential, then the use of one rodent species should be considered. Careful consideration should be given to the selection of dose. The use of a combination of pharmacokinetic and pharmacodynamic endpoints, with consideration of comparative receptor characteristics and intended human exposures, represents the most scientific approach to defining the appropriate dose. The rationale for the selection of dose should be provided. Points-to-consider on the preclinical assessment of the carcinogenic potential of insulin analogues have been published [7].

Genotoxicity Studies   It is generally not applicable to routinely implement the genotoxicity studies of biopharmaceuticals as required for NCEs. Proteins and peptides are not expected to interact directly with DNA or other chromosomal materials by passing through the cell membrane. On the other hand, ICH S6 describes "With some biopharmaceuticals, there is a potential concern about accumulation of spontaneously mutated cells (e.g., via selectively facilitating a predominating factor of proliferation) leading to carcinogenicity, alternative in vivo or in vitro models to address such concerns may have to be developed and evaluated." When in vitro or in vivo data suggest a potential biopharmaceuticals' ability to strongly stimulate cell proliferation, carcinogenicity studies should be considered. In the case of human-type proteins or peptides, it would be helpful to assess the necessity of conducting further studies to compare the physiological concentration of a biopharmaceutical in blood or tissue with that at which an enhanced activity of the biopharmaceutical on cell proliferation is observed. Human protein analogues should be evaluated for potential difference in activity from natural human-type proteins.

Genotoxicity studies should be considered for bioconjugates having an organic chemical linker molecule or proteins with nonnatural amino acids. The requirement for genotoxicity studies depends on whether a biopharmaceutical is a natural protein or an analogue such as a bioconjugate. Genotoxicity studies are not required for natural proteins, because they are not expected to interact directly with DNA or other chromosomal materials after passing through the cell membrane and because natural proteins are degraded into only natural amino acids. In the case of protein analogues containing nonnatural amino acids, it may be necessary to assess their genotoxicity under metabolic activation conditions, since there might be a possibility that chemical compounds having unknown activity can be formed by metabolic degradation. However, genotoxicity studies can be obviated even by demonstrating the inability of such a protein analogue and the fragments into cells using radiolabeled biopharmaceuticals or by other scientific evidence for their lack of genotoxicity.

5.3.3 Items for Future Update of Japanese Points-to-Consider Document

New Types of Biopharmaceuticals There is accumulated knowledge and experience on new types of biopharmaceuticals since the issuance of the Japanese Points-to-Consider document in 2002 [3]. One of new types of biopharmaceuticals are the bioconjugates, namely PEGylated proteins. PEGylation is a useful method of improving the therapeutic potential of proteins by changing pharmacokinetics and in vivo pharmacodynamics. The preclinical information from a number of PEGylated proteins is helpful for the further clarification of safety assessment programs (particularly, metabolism, in vitro electrophysiological and genotoxicity studies) for bioconjugates. Another new category of biopharmaceuticals is therapeutic antibodies. The section on antibodies in the Japanese Points-to-Consider document should be revised because there are examples of therapeutic antibodies that have much more potent biological activity than those developed in the 1990s. These antibodies act strongly on biological systems of the body and sometimes induce marked biological changes. Furthermore some of the therapeutic antibodies acting on the immune system may induce cytokine release that results in a "cytokine release syndrome" in humans. This syndrome is one of the most serious adverse events caused by biopharmaceuticals in humans. Therefore intensive investigations on the mechanism underlying this syndrome and preclinical studies of the prediction of cytokine release syndrome are needed for those biopharmaceuticals with potent pharmacology toward activation of the immune system.

New Technologies and Assays The use of transgenic animals for the safety assessment of biopharmaceuticals has become easier and less costly over the years. Transgenic animals can provide useful information when no relevant animal species are available, although there are limitations in terms of the historical background and how data will be used in the evaluation of the margin of safety. The use of homologous proteins is also a useful alternative when the biological activity of a biopharmaceutical is not properly studied in animals. Homologous proteins should be designed to produce similar biological activities in animals used for the safety assessment to those of biopharmaceuticals that will be used in humans.

In vitro electrophysiological studies have been introduced in ICH S7B [8] for the evaluation of the potential of QT prolongation of ECG for NCEs. Those studies are usually not applicable for biopharmaceuticals. This is because NCEs act on each type of cellular channel after passing through the cell membranes, whereas biopharmaceuticals consisting of natural amino acids are not expected to act similarly because they cannot pass through the cell membrane. However, we may need to confirm whether this argument is relevant for bioconjugates and proteins containing nonnatural amino acids, since there might be a possibility that unknown chemical compounds can be formed by metabolic degradation. Likewise we should revisit the justification for not conducting genotoxicity studies for bioconjugates and proteins containing nonnatural amino acids. Preclinical studies of prediction of cytokine release syndrome are required for some categories of therapeutic antibodies acting on the immune system, as described in the previous section. There would be a species difference in responsiveness in terms of cytokine release induced by humanized antibodies. Therefore an in vitro cytokine release assay using human blood may also need to be considered.

Timing of Preclinical Studies   Neither ICH S6 [2] nor ICH M3 [9] defines the timing of preclinical studies to support biopharmaceutical clinical development. Considering limitations in the prediction of adverse effects in humans using preclinical models, it may be most important to clarify what preclinical information is useful for the first trial in humans. One should note that no toxicity is often observed even at a high dose of a biopharmaceutical in animals that are not biologically responsive to the biopharmaceutical. Preclinical programs that support the first dosing in humans may need to be optimized on a case-by-case basis. In particular, the necessity for in vitro electrophysiology, genotoxicity, and cytokine release studies should be justified by taking into consideration the types of biopharmaceutical and available information on the class of biopharmaceutical tested. There are some differences in preclinical studies required for phases 2 and 3 of clinical trials and registration between biopharmaceuticals and NCEs. For example, the durations of nonrodent repeat dosing studies are six and nine months for biopharmaceuticals and NCEs, respectively. ICH S6 allows the use of only one species for subsequent long-term studies if the toxicity profiles of a biopharmaceutical in two species are comparable in a short-term study. Moreover only one animal species may be used for a carcinogenicity study for a biopharmaceutical when the study is required. These different approaches described in ICH S6 are useful for most biopharmaceuticals. Therefore the preclinical programs after conducting the first trial in humans should be optimized on a case-by-case basis rather than determined by a common study package.

5.4   CONCLUSION

The safety assessment of biopharmaceuticals in preclinical studies has been improved in Japan with the implementation of the ICH S6. The analysis of data from a questionnaire survey conducted by JPMA suggests that the ICH S6 was well understood and adequately implemented in Japan. The Japanese

Points-to-Consider document helps industry scientists and regulatory reviewers understand the ICH S6 guideline. In particular, it is helpful for the clarification of case-by-case approaches to preclinical programs depending on the biopharmaceutical type. However, further updates of the Japanese Points-to-Consider document may be needed as newer types of biopharmaceuticals, technologies, and assays have developed.

ACKNOWLEDGMENT

I deeply appreciate valuable comments from Drs. T. Inoue and S. Kitajima from NIHS, H. Onodera from PMDA, F. Sagami from JPMA, and M. Kawai and S. H. Heidel from Eli Lilly.

REFERENCES

1. Antigenicity tests. *Drug Approval and Licensing Procedures in Japan 1992.* Yakugyo Jiho, Tokyo, 1992, pp. 128.
2. Ministry of Health and Welfare. Preclinical Safety Evaluation of Biotechnology-Derived Pharmaceuticals, 2000. Notification No. 326.
3. Pharmaceutical Non-clinical Investigation Group. "Points-to-consider" regarding safety assessment of biotechnology-derived pharmaceuticals in non-clinical studies. In *Handbook on Non-clinical Guidelines for Pharmaceuticals 2002.* Tokyo: Yakujinipposya, 2002, pp 83–94.
4. Nakazawa T, Kai S, Kawai M, Maki E, Sagami F, Onodera H, Kitajima S, Inoue T. "Points-to-consider" regarding safety assessment of biotechnology-derived pharmaceuticals in non-clinical studies (English translation). *J Toxicol Sci* 2004; 29:497–504.
5. Kamita Y, Shiga T, Koga T, Nomura A, Shibata M, Maeda Y, Horigome H, Kurokawa M, Suzuki I, Niwano Y, Nakazawa T, Matsuzawa T. Points-to-consider on non-clinical safety studies on biotechnology-derived pharmaceuticals—Analysis of questionnaire survey data by JPMA. *Iyakuhin kenkyu* 2003;34:358–67.
6. CPMP/SWP/2600/01. Points-to-Consider on the need for Assessment of Reproduction Toxicity of Human Insulin Analogues, 2002. www.emea.eu.int
7. CPMP/372/01. Points-to-Consider on the Non-clinical Assessment of the Carcinogenic Potential of Insulin Analogues, 2001. www.emea.eu.int
8. ICH S7B Step 4. Non-clinical Evaluation of the Potential for Delayed Ventricular Depolarization (QT Interval Prolongation) by Human Pharmaceuticals, 2005.
9. Ministry of Health and Welfare. Non-clinical Safety Studies for the Conduct of Human Clinical Trials for Pharmaceuticals (revision), 2000. Notification No. 1831.

CHAPTER 6

Implementation of ICH S6: US Perspective

MARY ELLEN COSENZA, PhD, MS, DABT, RAC

Contents

6.1 INTRODUCTION

Several years ago an ICH guidance (ICH S6 Preclinical Safety Evaluation of Biotechnology-Derived Pharmaceuticals) was written to address the preclinical development and safety issues of products derived from biotechnology. ICH S6 defined biotechnology-derived pharmaceuticals as "products derived

Preclinical Safety Evaluation of Biopharmaceuticals: A Science-Based Approach to Facilitating Clinical Trials, edited by Joy A. Cavagnaro
Copyright © 2008 by John Wiley & Sons, Inc.

from characterized cells through the use of a variety of expression systems including bacteria, yeast, insect, plant, and mammalian cells" [1]. The scope of the guidance included proteins, peptides, derivatives of these or products of which they are components. It also states that these principles may apply to "recombinant DNA protein vaccines, chemically synthesized peptides, plasma derived products, endogenous proteins extracted from human tissues, and oligonucleotide drugs," but does not cover "antibiotics, allergenic extracts, heparin, vitamins, cellular blood components, conventional bacterial or viral vaccines, DNA vaccines, or cellular and gene therapies."

Regulatory agencies throughout the world define biopharmaceuticals differently, and in part this has affected how they are regulated. In the United States most, but not all, biopharmaceutical products have been developed in accordance with ICH S6 since its publication in 1997. However, some product classes specified in the guidance at that time fell under the FDA definition of hormones and chemically synthesized products (e.g., oligonucleotides) and were thus considered "drugs." These "drugs" were reviewed by regulatory scientists in the Center for Drug Evaluation and Research (CDER) and approved as new drug applications (NDAs). Therapeutic proteins, including antibodies, were regulated as "biologics" and were reviewed by regulatory scientists in the Center for Biologics Evaluation and Research (CBER) and approved as biologics license applications (BLAs). In 2003, the divisions of CBER responsible for review of ICH S6-specified, biotechnology-derived pharmaceuticals merged with CDER. This merger changed the FDA center responsible for primary review of these products. The products, however, were, and continue to be, approved as BLAs [2]. The "traditional biologicals" (i.e., vaccines and blood products and the novel cellular, tissue, and gene therapy products including tissue engineered products) remained in CBER (see Table 6.1). In June 2003 the CBER staff (pharm/tox experts and medical officers) in the Office of Therapeutics were transferred to CDER, and resided in a new Office of Drug Evaluation, ODE VI. More recently this office was eliminated, and the various "biologics" reviewers were reassigned by therapeutic or disease area to be consistent with how pharmaceutical products are reviewed. Thus the review of biopharmaceuticals now takes place in the same review division as traditional drug therapeutics for similar indications.

Even before final approval there was a rapid adoption of the principles outlined by in the ICH S6 guideline both by industry and by the FDA. The main tenet of the ICH S6 guidance is to create a case-by-case, science-driven approach to biotechnology preclinical product development. That is to say, each molecule should be evaluated for both its physical and pharmacological properties. Therefore a product's pharmacological attributes needs to be understood in addition to its clinical use before embarking on a preclinical safety assessment development plan. The overarching goal of a preclinical development plan is to provide information for designing and conducting clinical trials ("the principles"). A case-by-case rational, science-based approach ("the practice") was defined, and has proved to be, the most appropriate way to develop biotechnology-derived products [3]. The approach

TABLE 6.1 Regulation of biotechnology products

Products formally regulated by CBER, now by CDER

- Proteins and modified proteins
- Cytokines
- Growth factors
- Ligands and receptors
- Antibodies

Products regulated by CDER

- Hormones
- Chemically synthesized peptides
- Oligonucleotides

Products still regulated by CBER

- Gene therapies
- Cellular therapies
- Engineered tissue products
- Vaccines
- Blood and blood products
- Antitoxins

defined in S6 is appropriate for any pharmaceutical, regardless of its chemical or biological nature, that demonstrates species specificity, has an extended half-life, or requires a novel route of delivery.

6.2 HISTORICAL PERSPECTIVE

Over the past two decades many biotechnology-derived products have been approved in the United States. A selected list of these products is provided in Table 6.2. The products include recombinant endogenous-replacement proteins, cytokines, monoclonal antibodies, and fusion molecules. Other chapters in this book give more detailed "product-class-specific" descriptions of the preclinical development programs for many of these molecules.

In the early days of biotechnology product development, the focus was on "quality" issues [4] or process-related impurities. The concerns at that time were for carryover of other cellular proteins and DNA and for contamination with endotoxins, chemicals, and viruses. Of course, these concerns still exist, but methods for purification and assays for evaluation of clearance have alleviated the need for the safety assessment scientist to focus on contaminants; instead they are now asked to focus on the pharmacological activity of the molecules. An ICH guidance (Q6B Specifications: Test Procedures and Acceptance Criteria for Biotechnological/Biological Products) addresses the specific issues related to the manufacturing process [6]. Other product-related issues such as impurities do need to be considered by the safety assessment scientist, for

TABLE 6.2 Examples of marketed biotechnology products

Year of Approval	Approved Biologics	Trade Name
1982	Insulin	Humulin®
1985	Growth Hormone	Protropin®
1986	Interferon-alpha	Roferon®, Intron A®
1986	Muromonab CD3	Orthoclone OKT3®
1987	TPA (Alteplase)	Activase®
1989	Epoetin-alfa	Epogen®
1990	Interferon-gamma	Actimmune®
1991	Filgrastim (G-CSF)	Neupogen®
	Sargramostim (GM-CSF)	Leukine®
1992	Interleukin-2	Proleukin®
	Antihemophilic factor	Recombinate®rAHF
1993	Interferon-beta	Betaseron®
	Dornase Alfa	Pulmozyme®
1994	Imiglucerase	Cerezyme®
	Abciximab	ReoPro®
1997	Rituximab	Rituxan®
	Daclizumab	Zenpax®
	Oprelvekin	Neumega®
	Becaplermin gel	Regranex®
1998	Traztuzumab	Herceptin®
	Infliximab	Remicade®
	Basiliximab	Simulect®
	Palivizumab	Synagis®
2000	Tenecteplase	TNKase®
2001	Pegfilgrastim	Neulasta®
	Darbepoetin	Aranesp®
	Alemtuzumab	Campath®
	Drotecogin alpha	Xigris®
2002	Interferon beta 1-a	Rebif®
	Ibritumomab tiuxetan	Zevalin®
2003	Alefacept	Amevive®
	Tositumomab	Bexxar®
	Efalizumab	Raptiva®
	Omalizumab	Xolair®
2004	Bevacizumab	Avastin®
	Natalizumab	Tysabi®
	Palifermin	Kepivance®
	Technetium 99m Tc fanolesomab	NeutroSpec®
2005	Abatacept	Orencia®

Sources: www.fda.gov; and www.bio.org.

example, genetic variants, aggregate forms, chemical linkers, and differences in glycosylation patterns.

In 1997 the FDA issued an addendum to the original Points-to-Consider Document for Developing Monoclonal Antibodies. This document addressed issues covering all aspects of drug development for these molecules. Items specific to safety assessment included the requirement for tissue cross-reactivity studies. These studies allow for evaluation of binding in tissues from different species with the idea that this could help justify species selection. Over the years other more specific methods have generally been used to select appropriate species for safety assessment studies. Binding is no longer considered sufficient to justify the selection of a species. Other proof of biological activity is generally desired as well. The next section reviews specific sections of the ICH S6 document and discuss how this guidance has been implemented in the United States.

6.3 ICH S6 GUIDANCE

6.3.1 General Principles

The General Principles section acknowledges that "conventional approaches to toxicity testing of pharmaceuticals may not be appropriate for biopharmaceuticals." This has led to the proposal for case-by-case, science-driven drug development. Some of the unique challenges that the biopharmaceutical molecules face include species specificity, immunogenicity, unique routes of administration, and intermittent dosing schedules. The addition of pharmacological parameters to standard GLP toxicology studies, or the addition of toxicology parameters to pharmacology studies, allows for the judicious use of animals. The challenge of conducting some of these assays under GLPs was recognized in this guidance and by the FDA. Over the years more and more of these specialty assays (e.g., immunotoxicity assessment in primates using flow cytometry) have been validated and are being conducted in compliance with GLPs.

6.3.2 Animal Species Selection

One of the greatest challenges in the preclinical development of biotechnology-derived molecules is that of species specificity. Unlike traditional "small molecules," such a molecule cannot be assumed to be active in the standard species used for toxicity testing. The lack of pharmacological activity in a species can then lead to "no effects" in that species. With a few exceptions, where there were potential effects of contaminants, these studies had little purpose and a questionable use of animals. Justification for using only one species can be based on the lack of a second species with biological activity or when the biological activity of the molecule or target toxicity can be adequately defined in just one species.

An example where the original species was not relevant is that of the early work performed on the interferons. The studies were performed in nonrelevant species and generated misleading information [7]. Several studies were conducted in rodents with recombinant human interferons with little evidence of toxicity. This did not predict what was to occur in humans. Activity in monkey studies was more predictive, but there was the additional challenge of relative differences in the activity level between humans and nonhuman primates.

The Animal Species Selection section of the ICH document also refers to the use of homologous proteins and transgenic animals that express the human receptor. One example of a development program that relied on surrogates for safety assessment is that of infliximab [8]. Many of the challenges of these models are acknowledged in this section. Animal models of disease are also discussed and can be used with strong scientific rationale.

6.3.3 Administration/Dose Selection

Unlike most traditional pharmaceutical small molecules, biologics are not given once or twice a day, orally, in a pill or capsule. They are almost all dosed via a parenteral route and are not given (or "taken") daily. Some of these therapeutics are given in hospital settings or in clinicians' offices. Several are now self-administered on an approximately weekly basis. The dose regimen for the safety assessment studies should reflect the dosing regimen plan for the human studies. The dosing interval in the toxicology studies may be different depending on the half-life of the molecule in animals versus humans. Also the development of antibodies in the animals may alter the pharmacokinetics, and modifying the dosing interval has been shown to reduce the incidence of antibodies.

Dose selection can be a challenge with biopharmaceuticals. Often the dose-limiting toxicity is related to the pharmacology (often referred to as exaggerated pharmacology), and it can be difficult to establish a margin of safety. The slope of the dose–response curve between the intended level of effect and an effect that leads to toxicity (even if it is the same effect, e.g., an increase in hematocrit with erythropoietin-like molecules) may be very steep. The ability to produce formulations of proteins that allow for "high" doses can be difficult, especially if the protein formulation is viscous. Doses can be limited by practicality as well (dosing volume limits, maximal stable concentrations, etc.). There is always the desire to study a dose without effect, but this can be an additional challenge for molecules that are active at doses in the μg/kg level.

Other factors that need to be considered in dose selection are related to pharmacokinetics and drug metabolism. One area generally not deemed relevant for biologics is metabolism studies. Mass balance studies have not proved useful when performed with proteins. Radiolabeled studies have limited usefulness as these labeled molecules undergo rapid metabolism and the label is often unstable. Protein biologics undergo proteolytic degradation into smaller peptides and then into individual amino acids. Distribution is viewed more from the perspective of target distribution, except for gene and cell therapies and viral or bacterial vectors.

Recovery periods are very important considerations for studies with biopharmaceuticals. For many biopharmaceuticals, the pharmacodynamic effects are prolonged either pharmacologically, through secondary "cascading" effects through various pathways, and/or as a consequence of a long half-life. It is important to have a recovery/washout period of the test agent in order to properly test for antibody levels. The longer recovery can greatly increase the ability of the assays to detect antibodies to the drug. Active test article levels in blood samples can interfere with the ability to measure true antibody levels.

6.3.4 Immunogenicity

It is generally well accepted that immunogenicity is not well predicted across species. It has also been well documented that many biological compounds intended for human use are immunogenic in animals [9]. ICH S6 states: "Most biotechnology-derived pharmaceuticals intended for humans are immunogenic in animals." Traditional antigenicity studies or guinea pig anaphylaxis studies are not useful for predicting immunogenicity in humans and are now generally recognized as not being appropriate studies for biologics. When these studies were conducted years ago, at the request of some regulators, they were generally positive and led to adverse effects in animals. Since there is little to no predictive value in these studies, and they were not considered appropriate, such studies have not been conducted since publication of ICH S6.

All preclinical (and clinical) studies with biopharmaceuticals should include measurements of total incidence of antibodies and a further characterization as to whether these antibodies are neutralizing. Assays to determine antibodies have become more sophisticated over the years, and the newest technologies allow detection at lower levels than was achievable with traditional ELISAs. Clinically relevant antibodies include those that are clearing, sustaining, neutralizing, and/or cross-react with endogenous proteins [10]. It is important to screen for the presence and development of antibodies to the test article throughout development. Since the consequence of these antibodies may range from no clinically significant effects to serious safety effects, assays need to be developed to determine if antibodies that appear are able to block the biological activity of the test compound. This may occur either by direct binding to an epitope with activity or by binding to a site in close proximity, resulting in steric hindrance to the active site.

Immunogenicity is a substantial complication for preclinical safety assessment studies. Antibodies can invalidate the animal model species. Antibody production alone, however, should not necessarily prohibit the conduct of these studies. The effect on pharmacokinetics and pharmcodynamics needs to be measured and evaluated. The potential consequences of the antibodies on endogenous molecules also needs to be evaluated. Secondary effects, such as antibody deposition, should be measured. The lack of ability to predict absolute human immunogenicity does not preclude the use of animals to assess the relative potential for an immune response.

6.4 ICH S6 SPECIFIC CONSIDERATIONS

6.4.1 Safety Pharmacology/Single-Dose Studies

Safety pharmacology parameters (e.g., cardiovascular) can be incorporated into standard toxicology studies, including single-dose studies if that is most appropriate. Molecules that cross-react in traditional species (rodents and dogs) allow for more flexibility in designing these studies. Molecules that only have activity in nonhuman primates can be more challenging. Knowledge of the intended molecular target and its presence on these target organs can aid in the decision as to whether specific studies will need to be conducted. Primates can be telemeterized for cardiovascular assessments. In recent years many CNS parameters have been validated in primates as well. In vitro assessments are generally not relevant for biologics for many of the same technical reasons well recognized with in vitro genotoxicity assays.

6.4.2 Exposure

Toxicokinetics must be assessed in preclinical toxicology studies, as with traditional pharmaceuticals. These data are necessary to prove exposure (which may differ with route) and to monitor the potential effects of antibodies on the exposure levels over time. Perhaps the greatest difference between small-molecule pharmaceuticals and large-molecule biopharmaceuticals is the potential for immunogenicity, which can greatly affect pharmacokinetics as previously discussed.

6.4.3 Repeat-Dose Studies

The ICH S6 document states: "This duration of animal dosing has generally been 1–3 months for most biotechnology derived pharmaceuticals." And then: "for chronic indications, studies of 6 months duration have generally been appropriate, although in some cases shorter or long durations have supported marketing authorizations." Most important, it states: "the duration of long-term toxicity studies should be scientifically justified." The six-month paradigm was based on the idea that all or most toxicity would be elicited during this time frame for molecules that are highly targeted and for which their toxicity is mainly based on exaggerated pharmacology. Although it may not always be as straightforward as this, six months has proved to be sufficient for the elucidation of chronic toxicity for almost all biologics that have been developed. Requests for longer term toxicity studies (9 or 12 months) have rarely added useful information to the safety assessment of these molecules [11]. This does not mean that six months should be a default without rigorous scientific evaluation. If there are indications of unexpected toxicities, or other scientific reasons to expect delayed effects, then longer term studies should be considered. Without these concerns six months should continue to be sufficient. If there are indications of carcinogenic potential, then those questions should be dealt with via more specific studies. The issues of species specificity or the use of homologous proteins makes these questions more complicated and are another reason to consider the need to conduct longer term studies carefully. Longer term dosing may also increase the possibility of immunogenicity.

6.4.4   Immunotoxicity Studies

Since many biotechnology products are designed to modulate the immune system, basic immunotoxicity parameters have traditionally been evaluated as part of standard toxicity studies. Over time more and more immunotoxicity specific parameters have been validated in toxicology species, including primates. These parameters (humoral and cell-mediated) should be measured as appropriate. Other specific issues for biopharmaceuticals include immunogenicity, as previously discussed.

6.4.5   Reproductive/Developmental Studies

When a biopharmaceutical product cross-reacts with traditional reproductive toxicology species, these studies should be conducted as appropriate for the intended clinical population. When conducting these studies in rodents and rabbits, care should be taken to select the dosing regimen and to consider the impact of immunogenicity. The timing of dosing in these studies might need to be more frequent to ensure that there is adequate exposure during the pivotal stages of gestation. The exposure period for the segment 2 studies in rodents and rabbits is usually short enough to avoid a strong immunogenic response, but samples should be taken to measure test article levels and antibodies in the dose–range-finding studies.

When a molecule does not cross-react with rodents or rabbits, then a decision must be made as to whether to conduct these studies in primates or to make a rodent surrogate. There are several factors that need to be considered. For example, human IgGs are known to cross the placental barrier, and their response to teratogens has been shown to be similar to humans. Compared to rodents, nonhuman primates have a small number of offspring (usually just one offspring per mother), they are very expensive, and their gestation period is 150 days. In addition nonhuman primates have a low conception rate and a high spontaneous abortion rate, and the historical database for primate reproductive studies is not that large. The FDA has been more accepting of primate studies than agencies in other geographic regions. (See Chapters 17 and 18 for discussions of reproductive toxicity studies for biopharmaceuticals.) The considerations above must also be balanced against the challenges of developing and validating a surrogate to use in rodents or rabbits.

6.4.6   Genotoxicity Studies

It is generally accepted now that genotoxicity studies are not applicable for biopharmaceuticals, unless there is a "chemical" linker or toxic conjugate to the molecule. This is also clearly stated in the FDA Points-to-Consider Document for Monoclonal Antibodies [5].

6.4.7 Carcinogenicity

Carcinogenicity studies are generally considered inappropriate for biopharmaceuticals. Both the ICH S6 document and the ICH S1A (The Need for Long-term Rodent Carcinogenicity Studies of Pharmaceuticals) support this position [12]. ICH S6 states that need for evaluation of carcinogenic potential of these molecules depends on "duration of clinical dosing, patient population, and/or biological activity." Most of the early biotechnology molecules developed were for severe clinical indications and/or addressed unmet medical needs.

Currently (December 2007) there are no published traditional carcinogenicity studies for ICH S6 specified biotechnology-derived pharmaceuticals. Conducting a traditional two-year bioassay with these molecules is extremely challenging due to species specificity, immunogenicity, and the challenges of using homologous molecules. When there are reasons to be concerned about related issues such as potentially enhancing the growth of existing tumors through the intended pharmacological activity, then more specific studies have been considered. These studies have included (among others) assessments of the presence or absence of the drug's receptor on relevant tumor cells, effects of the drug on in vitro tumor cell growth rate, and effects of the drug on the growth rate of tumor cell xenografts in mice. Measurements of cell proliferation have also been added in some cases to repeat-dose animal studies as per ICH S6 when there is cause for concern.

6.4.8 Local Tolerance

Local tolerance assessments are usually incorporated into repeat-dose toxicity studies. Specific assessments include clinical observations (e.g., Draize scoring) and macroscopic and microscopic evaluations of the injection site. These types of studies may also be used to test formulation changes during the course of clinical development.

6.5 SUMMARY

The safety evaluation of biotechnology products has been an evolving process over the past two decades. ICH S6 did much to help give guidance to preclinical scientists (both in industry and government) on how to approach these development plans. In the future the basic questions for these products will remain the same, but the challenges will be greater. Global strategies for development of biopharmaceuticals should be more science driven and problem focused. If we (industry scientists) want the reviewers (regulatory scientists) at the FDA (and at all agencies worldwide) to stick to the scientific principles addressed in ICH S6, then the safety assessment industry scientist must be able to use science (e.g., target liability) to justify development plans as well. Defaulting to ICH S6 without scientific justification is as imprudent as conducting traditional small-molecule pharmaceutical studies on biopharmaceuticals inappropriately.

With the changes in the global regulatory environment there are likely to be additional challenges. The overarching goal should still be to evaluate preclinically the potential effects of these molecules and to provide guidance to the clinicians. Safety assessments approaches should have a strong scientific rationale and use the appropriate animal species judiciously.

REFERENCES

1. ICH S61. Preclinical Safety Evaluation of Biotechnology-Derived Pharmaceuticals. July 1997.

2. Schwieterman WD. Regulating biopharmaceuticals under CDER versus CBER: An Insider's perspective. *Drug Discov Today* 2006;11:19–20.

3. Cavagnaro JA. Preclinical safety evaluation of biotechnology-derived pharmaceuticals. *Nat Rev* 2002;1:469.

4. Dayan AD. Safety Evaluation of biological and biotechnology-derived medicines. *Toxicology* 1995;105:59.

5. FDA, CBER. Points to Consider in the Manufacture and Testing of Monoclonal Antibody Products for Human Use, 1997.

6. ICH Q6B. Specifications: Test Procedures and Acceptance Criteria for Biotechnological/Biological Products, August 1999.

7. Serabian MA, Pilaro AM. Safety assessment of biotechnology-derived pharmaceuticals: ICH and beyond. *Toxicol Pathol* 1999;27:2.

8. Treacy G. Using an analogous monoclonal antibody to evaluate the reproductive and chronic toxicity potential for a humanized anti-TNFα monoclonal antibody. *Hum Exper Toxicol* 2000;19:226.

9. Shankar G, Shores E, Wagner C, Mire-Sluis A. Scientific and regulatory considerations on the immunogenicity of biologics. *TRENDS Biotech* 2006;24:274–80.

10. Koren E, Zuckerman LA, Mire-Sluis AR. Immune responses to therapeutic proteins in humans—clinical significance, assessment and prediction. *Curr Pharmaceut Biotech* 2002;3:349.

11 Clarke J, Hurst C, Martin P, et al. Duration of chronic toxicity studies for biotechnology-derived pharmaceuticals: is 6 months still appropriate? *Regul Toxicol Pharmacol* 2008;50:2–22.

12. ICH S1A. The Need for Long-term Rodent Carcinogenicity Studies of Pharmaceuticals, March 1996.

PART III

CURRENT PRACTICES IN PRECLINICAL DEVELOPMENT

Comparison of Preclinical Development Programs for Small Molecules (Drugs/Pharmaceuticals) and Large Molecules (Biologics/Biopharmaceuticals): Studies, Timing, Materials, and Costs

CHRISTOPHER HORVATH, DVM, MS, DACVP

Contents

Preclinical Safety Evaluation of Biopharmaceuticals: A Science-Based Approach to Facilitating Clinical Trials, edited by Joy A. Cavagnaro
Copyright © 2008 by John Wiley & Sons, Inc.

7.1   INTRODUCTION

Successful and efficient development of a new pharmaceutical requires the planning of an integrated development program that coordinates the trilogy of product manufacture—chemistry, manufacturing, and controls (CMC), preclinical studies (distribution, metabolism, and pharmacokinetic [DMPK], pharmacology and toxicology), and clinical trials—within the framework of the regulatory development strategy. Preclinical (often referred to as nonclinical) safety studies must support each successive phase of clinical development, as well as any significant changes to the method(s) of manufacturing, formulating, or administering the pharmaceutical. A desirable goal for the preclinical portion of the integrated development program should be to enable each phase of clinical development and each significant change in CMC methodology without ever becoming rate-limiting to the pharmaceutical development time line. At face value, this would seem to be a relatively simple task if one adheres to available guidance documents: International Conference on Harmonization (ICH) M3 [1] outlines the necessary types of studies and their timing relative to phase 1, 2, or 3 clinical trials, additional ICH guidelines (S1A through S8) [2–13] discuss selected types of safety studies in detail, ICH S6 [14] discusses special considerations for biopharmaceuticals (biotechnology-derived pharmaceuticals), and ICH Q5E [15] addresses comparability testing for biopharmaceuticals. However, the preclinical program must also evaluate potential changes in pharmacology, DMPK, immunogenicity, and/or safety properties as evolutionary changes are made to the process or scale of manufacture, the formulation, and the route or method of administration of the pharmaceutical.

This chapter had its origins in a discussion that occurred during a June 2004 meeting between Food and Drug Administration (FDA) pharmacology and toxicology reviewers and BioSafe, a committee of experts experienced in preclinical development of biotechnology-derived products organized under the auspices of the Biotechnology Industry Organization (BIO). The intent of that meeting was to review and discuss some of the inherent differences among preclinical development programs for biologics and drugs, particularly the complexities of reproductive toxicology testing of biologics. It was agreed that, consistent with ICH S6, preclinical programs for biopharmaceuticals should be designed on a case-by-case basis to address *relevant* safety issues, and that novel approaches might be necessary to accomplish this. For example, the preclinical program might require the use of nontraditional study designs, species, or endpoints or even the invention and use of a homologous (surrogate) test article. In these discussions it was difficult to reach agreement on what constitutes a *relevant* preclinical program, as the relevance of each preclinical program might depend on both the results of the component studies and their acceptance by the assigned FDA reviewers. Thus a conundrum was recognized: How does one design a program that might of necessity be unlike any other yet be reasonably likely to provide relevant and acceptable answers regarding safety?

For members of the pharmaceutical industry engaged in the biologics development this question raises practical concerns as well. While the resources and time needed for a traditional drug development program are well known, those for a nontraditional biologics development program are less well known, but might reasonably be expected to be greater. In addition, while the acceptability of a traditional drug development program is well established, the acceptability of each nontraditional biologics development program must be established. The degree of acceptability will be dependent on the degree of relevance, which can only be "known" retrospectively, or after completion of the program. Attempts to gain the a priori approval from FDA reviewers for nontraditional preclinical development programs are not always successful. Therefore nontraditional preclinical development programs may be run at risk of not attaining the necessary relevance and acceptability. For members of a pharmaceutical company's management this dilemma signals greater risk and a lower probability of success, and thus creates pressures to "de-risk" the preclinical development program for biologics.

From a purely pragmatic point of view, most pharmaceutical companies are interested in trying to determine the costs, resources, and time required to complete various different possible development programs for a product. For drugs or biologics, if multiple development pathways are possible and scientifically sound, it may be appropriate to pursue the path that is least costly or most rapid. For most drugs, the development path is relatively straightforward and well-trodden. For most biologics, finding an appropriate development path is often an exercise in trailblazing. The uncertainty of this process, as well as the inherent difference in some of the issues to be addressed for biologics, has the potential to result in more risky, costly, and time-consuming development programs.

To attempt to investigate some of the issues described above, I volunteered to try to assemble a comparative evaluation of the studies, timing, materials, and costs associated with preclinical development of a drug instead of a biologic. I based the comparison on experiences I have had with the preclinical programs for both a drug and a biologic (a monoclonal antibody) being developed for very closely related therapeutic targets in the same clinical indications. The resulting comparison was first presented at a February 2005 BioSafe/FDA reviewer workshop[1] and subsequently at the June 2005 BIO convention.[2]

7.2 OBJECTIVE AND METHODS

The objective of this chapter is to compare to the studies, materials, and costs associated with hypothetical preclinical development programs intended to

---

[1]Preclinical development of biologics and biotech derived pharmaceuticals: Principles and practices. University of Maryland Conference Center, Rockville, February 1, 2005.

[2]Key considerations in designing preclinical safety evaluation programs for biopharmaceuticals. Program designs and material needs: Investing for success. BIO 2005, Philadelphia, June 20, 2005.

support the clinical development of a small molecule (drug) and a large molecule (biologic).

To accomplish this objective, a detailed clinical development program was designed, from investigational new drug application (IND) through new drug or biologic licensing application (NDA or BLA). The respective preclinical development programs to support each filing were planned for a drug and biologic. Individual GLP- and ICH-compliant studies for both preclinical programs were then designed and submitted to different preclinical contract research organizations (CROs) for price estimates, to allow determination of the average price for each study. Although this comparison was conducted in 2004 and the study prices are likely no longer accurate, the relative prices of these study should remain comparable over time (see Chapter 37 updated listing of cost estimate for preclinical study designs). For an estimation of the amount of each test article needed for each study, the study designs included the doses to be evaluated, based on information available on each product at that time, and on common industry practices for setting doses.

7.3 DISTINGUISHING BIOLOGICS FROM DRUGS

For the purposes of this discussion, drugs are chemically synthesized pharmaceuticals, often described as "small molecules" or "new chemical entities"; biologics are "large molecules" or "biopharmaceuticals."

7.3.1 Properties of Drugs and Biologics

In addition to great differences in biophysical characteristics, the properties of biologics are vastly different than those of drugs. Key differences in the properties of drugs and biologics are summarized in Chapter 3. It should be noted that some drugs have properties of biologics, and vice versa.

7.3.2 Influence of Drug and Biologic Properties on Development Program Design

The inherent differences in the properties of drugs and biologics strongly influence the design of their respective development programs. Some key considerations for the design of preclinical development programs for drugs and biologics are summarized in Table 7.1. Detailed discussion of each of these considerations is beyond the scope of this chapter. However, the magnitude of these differences can be illustrated by discussing one of the key considerations: selection of relevant specie(s) for preclinical testing.

As specified in ICH M3, general toxicology testing (e.g., single- and repeated-dose studies) should be conducted in two species: a rodent and a nonrodent. For drugs, the "default" choices are rats and dogs. The selection of these species (or occasionally other species) as the relevant species for preclinical studies is generally justified on the basis of comparative in vitro metabolism testing and demonstration of the extent to which the species-specific metabolism of the

TABLE 7.1 Considerations in the design of preclinical safety evaluation programs for drugs and biologics

	Drugs	Biologics
Species specificity and activity	Often have pharmacologic activity in multiple species	Generally have pharmacologic activity restricted to a limited number of species
Selection of relevant rodent and nonrodent species for preclinical testing	Generally based on shared in vitro metabolite profile with humans. Pharmacologic activity is a secondary consideration. Rodent and nonrodent species are easily identified.	Generally based on shared pharmacologic activity. Identification of rodent species is generally difficult, if not impossible. Identification of nonrodent species is occasionally difficult.
Route of administration	Seldom changed during development	Often changed during development (e.g., IV to SC)
Manufacturing process and scale	May change manufacturing scale but seldom change process	Often change cell clone (e.g., higher producing), process, and/or scale (e.g., 500 to 2000 L)
Formulation	Seldom change formulation	Often change formulation (e.g., liquid to lyophilized)
Support to product changes during development	Generally established via biochemical specifications, occasionally with in vivo bioequivalence (PK or PK/PD) studies	Generally established via in vivo comparability testing. Often need to assess pharmacologic activity (PD) and immunogenicity in addition to PK.
Rate-limiting portion of development	Generally rate-limited by time needed for toxicology studies	Generally rate-limited by time needed for manufacturing material
Preclinical studies	Generally follow traditional, resource-defined designs	Often follow nontraditional (alternative), resource-intensive designs
Unique preclinical issues	Uncommon, though changing as drugs with properties of biologics are being developed (e.g, species-restricted pharmacologic activity)	Lack of relevant species compromises toxicity testing (e.g., limit to 1 species, unable to evaluate reproductive toxicity). Exposure-limiting immunogenicity compromises chronic studies
Availability of competent testing facilities	Readily available	Can be difficult to identify testing facilities with experience with nontraditional species, end points, study designs, routes of administration, assays, etc.
Acceptability of preclinical program to FDA reviewers	Predictable; often no need to get feedback from FDA reviewers prior to conduct or submission	Unpredictable. Generally a compelling need to get feedback from FDA reviewers prior to submission, and prior to conduct if possible.

parent compound and the resulting metabolite profile is similar to that for humans. The intent is to identify any *active* metabolite(s) that might contribute to pharmacologic responses and to study in animals any *inactive* metabolite(s) that might contribute to toxicologic effects in humans. Pharmacologic activity in the chosen species, though desirable and often present, is not essential for toxicology testing. Because the focus of traditional toxicology testing is to discover and characterize unexpected and/or "off-target" toxicity, this approach to selection of relevant species is considered scientifically sound, even if the drug is not the pharmacologic activity in the chosen species. Thus the selection of relevant species for toxicity testing of drugs is generally based on metabolism and not on the pharmacologic mechanism of action.

In contrast, as specified in ICH S6, the primary consideration for the selection of a relevant species for toxicity testing of biologics is pharmacologic activity. This is because biologics are generally catabolized (degraded) rather than metabolized (chemically altered), and therefore generation of active metabolites with pharmacologic effects or inactive metabolites with toxicologic effects is uncommon. Thus off-target (nonpharmacologically mediated) toxicity is unlikely for biologics. This fundamental difference in the disposition of drugs and biologics means that the observed toxicity of biologics often represents "superpharmacology." It also means that an animal species in which there is no pharmacologic activity is generally not relevant for studying the safety of biologics. In recognition of this point, ICH S6 made allowances for use of only a single, relevant species in toxicity testing when such a decision could be scientifically justified.

7.3.3   Applicable Regulatory Guidelines for Drugs and Biologics

The ICH guidances pertaining to preclinical development [1–13] are generally applicable to both drugs and biologics, except as noted, with additional guidances specific to biotechnology-derived products [14, 15]. Careful reading and interpretation of all guidances is necessary to facilitate planning of the preclinical programs.

In addition to the ICH guidances discussed above, additional specific guidances related to pharmacology/toxicology evaluations to support clinical development should be considered based upon product class and/or indication (specific considerations for medical imaging agents, therapeutic radiopharmaceuticals, and pediatric drug products, as wells as for photo-safety testing, safety testing of drug metabolites, etc.).

7.4   COMPARATIVE PRECLINICAL DEVELOPMENT PROGRAMS FOR A HYPOTHETICAL DRUG AND BIOLOGIC

For this hypothetical comparison of the preclinical development programs for a drug and a biologic it was necessary to make some general assumptions about the preclinical development programs, to define the therapeutic target, mechanism of action and clinical indication, to define the clinical development program, and then to make some specific assumptions for the drug and biologic.

7.4.1 General Assumptions

The general assumptions about the preclinical development programs were as follows:

- The comparison would begin at the point of nomination of the compound for clinical development; that is, the first series of studies would be IND-enabling.
- The respective preclinical development programs would represent typical, but idealized programs, with the focus being on safety only (e.g., no consideration of pharmacology or DMPK studies).
- All studies would be outsourced to contract research organizations (CROs) for study conduct, including any bioanalytical or other assays.
- All studies would comply with GLP regulations, as well as other appropriate guidelines (ICH M3, S6, etc.).
- All animals would be observed until test article had cleared (estimated to be five half-lives).
- All regulatory filings would be on final study reports.
- The manufacture of the respective test articles used in the studies would be outsourced to contract manufacturing organizations (CMOs) and sequential use of research-grade/non-GMP and GMP material would be allowed, if appropriate.
- The clinical development plan to be supported would be idealized, with minimal delays between phases and without substantive changes to the test article (e.g., no changes to manufacturing process or formulation) or the route of administration.
- No "run-at-risk" strategies would be allowed, such as concurrently validating the PK assay while collecting the samples to be assayed.

These assumptions were made to try to keep the number of variables to a minimum to allow this comparison, although hypothetical, to be as realistic as possible. Last, the key metrics to be compared would include the numbers and types of studies and their durations and costs, the quantity of material (test article) needed, the time required for manufacture and its costs, and the timing of the studies relative to clinical development.

7.4.2 Therapeutic Target, Mechanism of Action, and Clinical Indication

Designing an appropriate preclinical development program requires a complete understanding of the therapeutic target, mechanism of action, clinical indication, and disease biology. This information is essential in choosing the relevant specie(s) and endpoints to be assessed. In addition it is necessary to have an understanding of the intended clinical route of administration, projected therapeutic concentration, projected therapeutic dose, projected dosing regimen, and the intended duration of dosing and exposure. These attributes are often summarized in the target product profile (TPP) that is generated by a project team during the development candidate nomination process. Detailed discussion of the methods for establishing this information is beyond the scope of this discussion.

For this hypothetical comparison, however, most of this information was known. The therapeutic targets were G protein-coupled receptors that were expressed on the cell surface of T cells, monocytes, and tissue macrophages. Through ligand-binding interactions these receptors were implicated in leukocyte trafficking, particularly to sites of active inflammation in autoimmune disease settings such as might be present in rheumatoid arthritis or multiple sclerosis. The intended mechanism of action was blockade of the receptor and thus prevention of ligand binding and subsequent leukocyte trafficking. The intended pharmacologic effect was downregulation of inflammation, or immune modulation. Data from animal models of disease induced in homozygous receptor knockout mice supported the targets, clinical indications, mechanism of action, and immunomodulatory effects of target knockout.

7.4.3   Clinical Development Plan to Be Supported

The proposed clinical development plan is summarized in Table 7.2 and illustrated in Figure 7.1. Based on the therapeutic target(s) and mechanism(s)

TABLE 7.2   Proposed clinical development program

Phase	1a	1b	2a	2b	3
Subjects	NHV	NHV	Patients	Patients	Patients
Women enrolled?	No	No	Post-menopausal	WCBP, DBP	WCBP
Regimen	SAD	MAD	MAD	MD	MD
Duration of dosing	Once	2 weeks	1 month	3 months	≥6 months
Phase duration (enrollment to report)	6 months	8 months	18 months	2 years	3 years

Note: DBP = double-barrier protection, MAD = multiple (repeated) ascending dose, WCBP = women of child-bearing potential, MD = multiple (repeated) dose, NHV = normal human volunteers, SAD = single ascending dose.

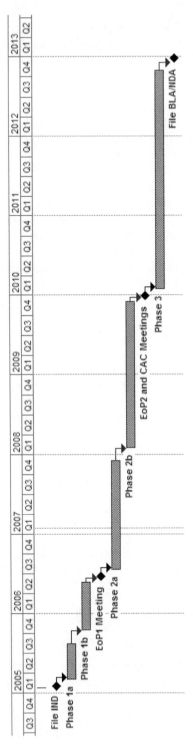

Figure 7.1 Proposed clinical development program.

Starting date was assumed to be 18 January 2005.

of action, the clinical indication to be supported is chronic administration in a non–life-threatening autoimmune and/or inflammatory disease. The plan calls for sequential conduct of phase 1a, 1b, 2a, 2b, and 3 clinical trials that enroll normal human volunteers (NVH) in phase 1 and patients in phases 2 and 3.

Dosing progresses from single ascending doses (SAD), to multiple ascending doses (MAD), to multiple doses (MD), as the duration of dosing increases from a single administration to dosing over 2-week, 1-month, 3-month, and ≥6-month periods. The duration of each clinical trial (from first patient in to clinical report) increases successively from 6 months to 3 years, with the duration of the entire clinical program, from IND through BLA filing, being 8 years. Milestones are incorporated to allow end of phase 1 (EoP1), end of phase 2 (EoP2), and the Carcinogenicity Assessment Committee (CAC) meetings. This clinical development program is idealized, as minimal time is allowed for the transition from completion of one phase to initiation of the next phase. As such, this clinical plan will put considerable pressure on the preclinical program to deliver the required support in advance of the need for it.

7.4.4 Specific Assumptions

The specific assumptions about the drug were as follows:

- The doses to be tested in humans in various studies would be 1, 3, 10, 30, and 100 mg/kg, administered orally once daily. The top viable dose would be 100 mg/kg.
- The relevant species were monkeys (in which the drug was pharmacologically active and metabolism was comparable to humans), rabbits, and rats (in which there was no pharmacologic activity but comparable metabolism).
- The route of administration would be oral, with daily dosing at doses of 3, 10, 30, 100, 300, and 1000 mg/kg utilized in various studies.
- The no observable adverse effect (dose) level (NOAEL) would be 100 mg/kg, with a maximum tolerated dose (MTD) of 1000 mg/kg.
- The cost of manufacturing test article for preclinical use would range from $10,000 to $70,000 per kilogram, with a cost of $25,000 per kilogram at the commercial scale.

The specific assumptions for the biologic, a monoclonal antibody (mAb), were as follows:

- The doses to be tested in humans in various studies would be 0.1, 0.3, 1, 3, and 10 mg/kg, administered intravenously once monthly. The top viable dose would be 10 mg/kg.
- The relevant species was the monkey, in which the biologic was pharmacologically active, with comparable affinity and activity to human test

systems in vitro. The mAb was not active in any other species, including mice, rats, guinea pigs, rabbits, dogs, and pigs.

- The route of administration would be intravenous, with weekly dosing at doses of 10, 30, and 100 mg/kg utilized in various studies.
- The NOAEL would be 100 mg/kg, without an MTD being established.
- The mAb would be immunogenic in monkeys, with approximately 50% of the animals developing anti-mAb antibodies, and approximately 25% of the animals developing neutralizing and/or clearing antibodies.
- The cost of manufacturing test article for preclinical use would range from $3000 to $30,000 per gram, with a cost of $1000 per gram at the commercial scale.

Obviously some of these specific assumptions could be questioned, and the associated costs might be very different for different products or within different companies. At the time, however, these were reasonable assumptions for the two products being compared, and these specific assumptions allowed calculation of the amount, time, and cost associated with manufacture of the test articles.

7.4.5 "Traditional" Preclinical Development Plans to Support Clinical Development by Phase

The first comparison to be made evaluates "traditional" preclinical development plans to support each phase of clinical development. While the term "traditional" might be thought to apply only to drugs, it is also true that certain preclinical programs for biologics have been established as well as accepted, and therefore could be regarded as traditional. This initial comparison assumes direct, uninterrupted progression of the product along a relatively simple development pathway. For the biologic this means that a relevant species has been identified and there are no planned changes to the cell line, manufacturing process, formulation, or route of administration during development. The need for "nontraditional" or "alternative" development pathways to address these issues will be discussed later.

Essential Components Required for Starting Preclinical Development Prior to the design and initiation of a preclinical development program, there are a number of essential components that should be in place, as outlined in Table 7.3. These components include important information on the manufacture and characterization of the product, as well as the reagents and assays necessary for evaluation of the PK and PD properties and, for biologics, the immunogenicity and tissue cross-reactivity. In addition, most preclinical development programs would not be started without identification of the relevant species and some preliminary non–GLP-compliant studies to establish some general parameters, such as those associated with "discovery toxicology." These preliminary studies, generally conducted to facilitate nomination of a

TABLE 7.3 Essential components required for starting preclinical development

	Criteria	Drug	Biologic (mAb)
Product information	Material selected	Compound and salt form	Initial cell line, growth conditions
	Production process known	Yes	Yes
	Initial material characterization	Impurities, solvents	LPS, viral, host cell proteins
	Pilot scale material produced in-house	≤1 kg	≤20 g
	Other criteria	NA	Potency (activity) assay
Assays and reagents	Dose retain analysis	HPLC	ELISA
	PK	LC/MS/MS	ELISA
	PD (receptor-ligand binding inhibition)	FACS	FACS
	Immunogenicity (PAHA)	NA	ELISA
	Tissue cross-reactivity	NA	IHC
Preclinical studies	Relevant species selected	Based on shared in vitro metabolite profile with humans. Rodent and nonrodent species identified.	Based on shared pharmacologic activity. Identification of rodent species is generally difficult, if not impossible. Identification of nonrodent specie(s) is occasionally difficult.
	Genetic toxicology screened	Mini-Ames In vitro micronucleus	NA
	Discovery toxicology has set doses	Non-GLP 14-day rodent, non-GLP 14-day nonrodent	Non-GLP single-dose PK/PD/toxicity in relevant species
	Other criteria	Non-GLP receptor screening	Non-GLP tissue cross-reactivity

Note: ELISA = enzyme-linked immunosorbent assay, FACS = fluorescence-activated cell sorting, HPLC = high-performance liquid chromatography, IHC = immunohistochemistry, LC/MS = liquid chromatography/MS = mass spectrometry, LPS = lipopolysaccharide (endotoxin), NA = not applicable, PAHA = (nonhuman) primate anti-human antibodies.

candidate for development, are intended to ensure that preclinical development has the appropriate preliminary information and/or tools to assess safety and that there are few surprises during development.

Preclinical Support to Phase 1   The studies, time, materials, and costs associated with preclinical support to phase 1 are summarized in Table 7.4 and illustrated in Figure 7.2. For the drug, the studies necessary to support phase 1 would typically consist of in vitro and in vivo genetic toxicity studies, dedicated safety pharmacology studies evaluating cardiovascular, central nervous system (CNS) and respiratory function,[3] and general toxicology studies of 1-month (28-day) dosing duration (with a 2-week recovery period) in a rodent and nonrodent species.[4] For this particular drug, a receptor antagonist, a study would also be conducted to assess species cross-reactivity in vitro by screening receptor binding on target cells from different species.[5]

Except for the general toxicology studies, phase 1-supporting studies are independent in nature and can be conduct in parallel. The general toxicology studies ideally would not be initiated until after the PK and PD assays are validated, by which time there may be some useful toxicity information from the safety pharmacology studies. This IND-enabling preclinical program for a drug requires approximately 10 months and costs around \$1.2 M, including the roughly \$40 K cost and 2 months required for manufacturing approximately 1.3 kg of non–GMP-compliant material. For a drug, most sponsors would elect to use GMP-compliant material, with the attendant delay in the ability to start.

For the mAb, the studies necessary to support phase 1 include tissue cross-reactivity and general toxicology studies; in accordance with ICH S6, dedicated safety pharmacology and genetic toxicology studies are not required. The general toxicology studies can be conducted in a single, pharmacologically relevant species and include both a single-dose[6] and 1-month repeated-dose study, with longer recovery periods (one and three months, respectively) to allow for the slower clearance of the mAb. Relative to those for a drug, these studies can be much more complicated and expensive, as they would routinely incorporate assay for immunogenicity (in addition to PK and PD) and assessment of safety pharmacology (cardiovascular, respiratory and CNS)

---

[3]Prior to beginning development, many sponsors would also have conducted in vitro safety pharmacology studies (e.g., hERG inhibition) to assess cardiovascular concerns, as well as single-dose and 5- to 7-day repeated-dose non–GLP-compliant studies to assess toxicity and help set doses for the GLP-compliant studies (see Table 7.3).

[4]A 14-day dosing duration would also be acceptable to support phase 1 single-dose to 2-week studies, although many sponsors are electing to conduct 28-day studies to support up to 1-month trials.

[5]Some sponsors would also screen related targets, if available, for recognition by the drug, which might be associated with secondary pharmacologic activity.

[6]A single-dose study is generally useful to fully characterize the clearance of a compound, such as this mAb, with a long half-life.

TABLE 7.4 Preclinical support to phase 1

Phase 1	Drug				Biologic			
		Time (Mo)	Material (g)	Cost ($K)		Time (Mo)	Material (g)	Cost ($K)
Assay validation	PK (LC/MS/MS)	4	1	15	PK (ELISA)	10	1	30
	PD (LBI; FACS)	6	1	50	PD (LBI; FACS)	6		50
					Immunogenicity (ELISA)	10		30
					Tissue cross-reactivity (IHC)	2		20
Cross-reactivity	Receptor screening	2	1	15	Tissue cross-reactivity	2	1	80
Genetic toxicology	Mutagenicity (Ames)	2.5	2	6				
	Chromosomal aberration in vitro (CHO)	2.5	2	22				
	Chromosomal aberration in vivo (RMN)	2.5	2	30				
Safety pharmacology	Cardiovascular, monkey	2.5	25	150				
	Respiratory, rat	2.5	5	38				
	CNS, rat	2.5	5	20				
General toxicology	1 mo (+2 wk rec) rat	4	250	200	Single-dose (+1 mo rec) monkey	4	3	150
	1 mo (+2 wk rec) monkey	4	1000	600	1 mo (+2 mo rec) monkey	7	30	600
Studies		10	—	1146		17	—	960
Material		2	1293	40		6	35	1600
Total		**10**	**1293**	**1186**		**17**	**35**	**2560**

Note: CHO = Chinese hamster ovary cells, ELISA = enzyme-linked immunosorbent assay, FACS = fluorescent-activated cell sorting or flow cytometry; IHC = immunohistochemistry, LBI = ligand-binding inhibition, rec = recovery, RMN = rat micronucleus.

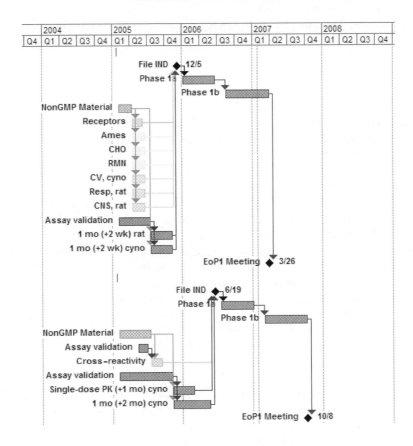

Preclinical programs to support a drug (top) or biologic (bottom). For comparison purposes, the starting date was assumed to be 18 January 2005.

Figure 7.2 Preclinical support to phase 1.

parameters. This preclinical IND-enabling program for a mAb requires approximately 17 months and costs $2.6 M, including the $1.6 M cost and 6 months required to manufacture approximately 35 g of non–GMP-compliant material. Thus, relative to the program for the drug, the program for the mAb requires fewer studies and less material, but will take approximately 7 months longer and require $1.4 M more in total costs. Both the added cost and time are primarily related to the manufacture of material, although the longer time required for validation of the biological assays and clearance of the test article in the recovery periods also contribute to this.

Both of these IND-enabling preclinical programs could reasonably be expected to be acceptable to regulatory agencies, so there may be little need to try to obtain a preliminary agreement as to their acceptability from regulatory reviewers. That is, it would not be essential to arrange a pre-IND meeting (to present preliminary results) or even an earlier (pre-pre-IND) meeting (to discuss planned studies) to assess whether the appropriate studies were done to support the phase 1 trial.[7]

Preclinical Support to Phase 2   The studies, time, materials, and costs associated with preclinical support to phase 2 are summarized in Table 7.5 and illustrated in Figure 7.3. For the drug, the studies necessary to support phase 2 would consist of rodent and nonrodent 3-month repeated-dose general toxicology studies and reproductive and developmental toxicology studies. The latter would include embryo/fetal (segment 2) studies in pregnant female rats and rabbits, and fertility (segment 1) studies in males and female rats. Range-finding (pilot) studies to establish maternal toxicity prior to segment 2 studies would be necessary as well. The use of rabbits and rats, in which pharmacologic activity is absent, for developmental toxicology can be justified on the basis of metabolic profiles comparable to humans in vitro. Such a decision is not unusual for drugs, where toxicology unrelated to the mechanism of action is a primary concern. A significant advantage to the use of rats and rabbits is the short gestation periods and less expensive animal costs. This preclinical program to support phase 2 for the drug takes approximately 9 months and costs $1.8 M, including the nearly $125 K cost and 2 months required for manufacturing approximately 5 kg of GMP-compliant material.

For the mAb, the studies necessary to support phase 2 would consist of a monkey 3-month repeated-dose general toxicology study (with a 2-month recovery period), segment 2 studies in pregnant female monkeys and segment 1 studies in male and female monkeys.[8] Although the duration of dosing in the latter studies is relatively short (1 to 3 months), these studies can be very difficult and time-consuming to conduct as they typically last at least 12 months. This time is required to identify females in estrus and to breed and enroll pregnant female monkeys into the studies. This preclinical program to support phase 2 for the mAb requires approximately 17 months and costs $4.3 M, including the $1.2 M cost and 5 months required for manufacturing approximately 400 g of GMP-compliant material. Thus, the program for the mAb is approximately 8 months longer, and $2.5 M more expensive than the program for the drug, primarily due to the use of monkeys (with long gestation periods) for reproductive and developmental toxicology.

As was the case for support for phase 1, these development programs to support phase 2 follow ICH guidelines and are therefore not controversial. They are unlikely to require advanced indication of their acceptability to regulatory agencies.

---

[7]This discussion understandably cannot address whether the *results* of the preclinical studies that were conducted would support the proposed clinical trials (e.g., the proposed first-in-human dose). For that reason, or for other reasons, a development project team might choose to request a pre-IND meeting or an earlier meeting.

[8]It should be noted that there are very few CROs that offer reproductive toxicity testing in nonhuman primates. To date, most of the reproductive toxicology studies in monkeys have been segment 2 (teratology) studies. Segment 1 (fertility) studies would be difficult to conduct.

TABLE 7.5 Preclinical support to phase 2

Phase 2		Drug			Biologic		
		Time (Mo)	Material (g)	Cost ($K)		Time (Mo)	Material (g)	Cost ($K)
General toxicology	3 mo (+1 mo rec) rat	7	700	253				
	3 mo (+1 mo rec) monkey	7	3000	650	3 mo (+2 mo rec) monkey	9	100	650
Reproductive and developmental toxicology	Segment 2 RF, rat	2.5	40	43				
	Segment 2 RF, rabbit	2.5	500	57				
	Segment 2, rat	3.5	100	128				
	Segment 2, rabbit	3.5	500	185	Segment 2, monkey (1 mo)	12	50	950
	Segment 1, rat, male	6	50	193	Segment 1, monkey, male (3 mo)	12	120	710
	Segment 1, rat, female	6	50	119	Segment 1, monkey, female (3 mo)	12	120	742
Studies		7	—	1628		12	—	3052
Material		2	4940	125		5	390	1200
Total		**9**	—	**1753**		**17**	—	**4252**

Note: Rec = recovery, RF = range-finder.

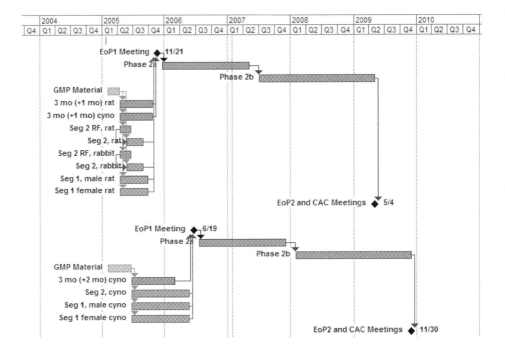

Preclinical programs to support a drug (top) or biologic (bottom). For comparison purposes, starting date was assumed to be 18 January 2005.

Figure 7.3 Preclinical support to phase 2.

Preclinical Support to Phase 3 and Registration The studies, time, materials, and costs associated with preclinical support to phase 3 and registration are summarized in Table 7.6 and illustrated in Figure 7.4.

For the drug, the studies necessary to support phase 3 include chronic toxicology in rats and monkeys (6 and 12 months, respectively) and perinatal/postnatal (segment 3) toxicology studies in pregnant female rats. These studies take approximately 22.5 months and $1.6M, including the 2.5 months and $125K to manufacture 5 kg of material. To support registration of the drug, carcinogenicity studies must be conducted in two rodent species. This example uses a 2-year bioassay in rats and a 6-month study in transgenic mice. The cost to support registration is approximately 38 months and $2.9 M, including 2 months to manufacture 3 kg of material for $75 K.

For the mAb, the studies necessary to support phase 3 include a 9-month chronic toxicology study[9] and a segment 3 reproductive toxicology

---

[9]Although ICH S6 indicates that chronic toxicology studies of 6 months duration may be sufficient, many Sponsors have been recently requested to conduct nine-month studies.

TABLE 7.6 Preclinical support to phase 3 and registration

Phase 3	Study (Drug)	Study (Biologic)	Drug Time (Mo)	Drug Material (g)	Drug Cost ($K)	Biologic Time (Mo)	Biologic Material (g)	Biologic Cost ($K)
Reproductive and developmental toxicology	Segment 3, rat	Segment 3, monkey (3 mo rec + 3 mo)	9	250	350	18	120	1500
Chronic toxicology	6 mo (+2 mo rec) rat		11	1250	355			
	12 mo (+2 mo rec) monkey	9 mo (+3 mo rec) monkey	20	3600	770	16	400	750
Studies			20	—	1475	18	—	2250
material			2.5	5100	125	5	520	1800
Total			22.5	—	**1600**	**23**	—	**4050**
Registration								
Carcinogenicity	2 yr rat		36	3000	1700			
	5 d/1 mo RF, Tg mouse		4	10	225			
	6 mo Tg mouse		18	15	900			
Studies			36	—	2825	18	—	2250
Material			2	**3025**	75	5	**520**	1800
Total			38	—	**2900**	**23**	—	**4050**

Note: Rec = recovery, RF = range-finder, Tg = transgenic.

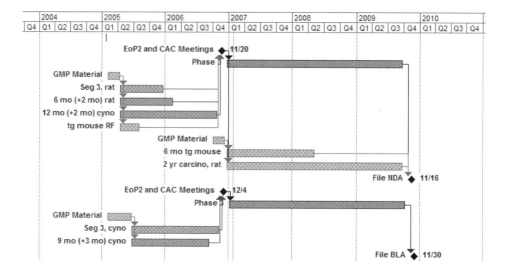

Preclinical programs to support a drug (top) or biologic (bottom). For comparison purposes, starting date was assumed to be 18 January 2005.

Figure 7.4   Preclinical support to phase 3 and registration.

study[10] in monkeys. These studies take approximately 23 months and $4.1 M, including 5 months and $1.8 M to manufacture approximately 500 g of material. In accordance with ICH S6, carcinogenicity studies would not be conducted for a biologic if no relevant and appropriate species can be identified. While monkeys are a relevant species for this mAb, they are not an appropriate species for carcinogenicity testing. Therefore, after chronic toxicity testing, no additional studies are necessary to support registration. Once again, relative to the drug, the cost of this preclinical support is greater for the mAb, primarily due to the cost of its manufacture. However, the time needed is about 15 months shorter due to the lack of carcinogenicity testing for this biologic.

Again, these preclinical safety evaluation programs to support Phase 3 are designed to follow ICH guidelines and are relatively likely to be acceptable to regulatory agencies.

The Integrated Preclinical Development Plans   The total time, materials and costs associated with preclinical support for phase 1 through registration are summarized in Table 7.7 and the integrated preclinical support to clinical development is illustrated in Figure 7.5.

[10]It should be noted that conducting true segment 3 studies in monkeys are not feasible, as this would require several years to follow the first filial (F1) generation to reproductive maturity. However, some sponsors developing immunomodulatory biologics have been evaluating the immune system function in F1 monkeys to address the most relevant portion of segment 3 concerns for their product. To do this, some sponsors elect to combine immune function assessment of the offspring from a segment 2 study when using monkeys for reproductive toxicology testing.

TABLE 7.7   Total time, materials, and costs for preclinical support for phase 1 through registration

	Drug			Biologic		
	Time (Mo)	Material (kg)	Cost ($M)	Time (Mo)	Material (kg)	Cost ($M)
Phase 1	10	1.293	1.186	17	0.035	2.560
Phase 2	9	4.940	1.700	17	0.390	4.252
Phase 3	22.5	5.100	1.600	23	0.520	4.050
Registration	38	3.025	2.900	—	—	—
Material	8.5	15	0.4	16	1	4.6
Studies	73	—	7.0	47	—	6.3
Total	105	~15	7.4	112	~1	10.9

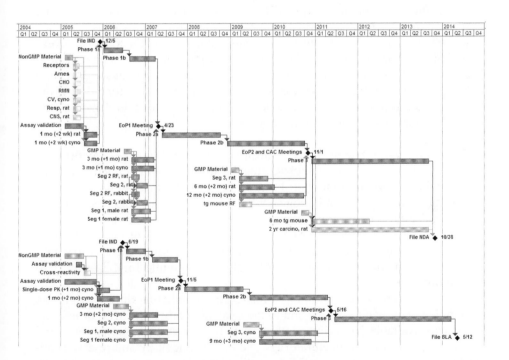

Preclinical programs to support a drug (top) or biologic (bottom). For comparison purposes, starting date was assumed to be 18 January 2005.

Figure 7.5   Integrated preclinical support to clinical development.

For the drug, the studies conducted require 73 months in total, at a cost of around $7.0 M. The amount of material required is 15 kg, manufactured over 8.5 months at a cost of $0.4 M. Of the $7.4 M total cost, manufacturing represents only 5.4%. In contrast, the studies for the mAb required only 47 months and $6.3 M. Only around 1 kg of material is required for the mAb, with about 16 months required to manufacture it, at a cost of around $4.6 M. Manufacturing represents 42% of the $10.9 M total costs. Thus, relative to the drug, material supply for preclinical development of the mAb takes twice as long and is 10 times as expensive, even though only 1/15th as much material is required. The studies for the mAb can be completed in almost half the time, but cost approximately the same. Overall, this comparison demonstrates that it is more expensive to provide comparable preclinical support to clinical development for the mAb than the drug.

If both programs were started at the same time and progressed as scheduled, it would take 105 months (8 years, 9 months) until filing the NDA for the drug and 112 months (9 years, 4 months) until filing the BLA for the mAb. The additional 7 months required to bring the mAb to registration can be traced directly to the additional 7 months required to enable phase 1, which was related primarily to a longer time to manufacture and the longer recovery period necessary to observe clearance of the mAb in the one-month repeated-dose study. This illustration reveals an important difference between drugs and biologics: the rate-limiting portion of preclinical development for a drug is the time required to conduct the toxicology studies, while for a biologic it is the time required to manufacture the material.

Critical Decisions to Be Made   The preceding examples have demonstrated that the time required for manufacturing the appropriate material for preclinical testing is an important contributor to the overall time line for preclinical development; more so for biologics. When planning these programs, there are critical decisions to be made related to reserving the necessary manufacturing capacity. Whether manufacturing is to be done internally or outsourced to a contract manufacturing organization (CMO), the lead time necessary to secure manufacturing time via contract is generally 3 to 6 months for a drug and 6 to 12 months for a biologic.[11]

The differences in lead time are related to the inherent differences in the complexity of manufacturing and to the relative number of CMOs or internal capacity available for each type of product. It is generally easier, quicker, and less expensive to manufacture drugs, and easier to identify and reserve available manufacturing capacity for drugs. Similar lead times for advanced reservation of CRO capacity are often needed for certain types of preclinical

---

[11]For a drug, the lead time necessary for reserving manufacturing capacity remains 3 to 6 months throughout development, while over time it declines from 6 to 12 months to 6 to 9 months for a biologic.

studies, such as those using monkeys or requiring complicated technical procedures.

A careful review of Figure 7.5 reveals that, because of the 3- to 6-month or 6- to 9-month lead time required for a drug or biologic, respectively, these critical decisions must generally be made prior to knowing whether the contractual commitment is justified. They therefore involve an element of risk. For example, a development project team must commit to manufacturing a drug or biologic for preclinical support to phase 1 as much as 5 or 18 months, respectively, ahead of the time when the material is actually needed for dosing. In many companies this would mean that a commitment to manufacture development material to facilitate preclinical support to phase 1 must be made before the product is officially accepted into development. This requirement for making critical decisions in advance of supportive results recurs in each phase of clinical development.

Some sponsors elect to pursue a minimal risk development strategy, with success of each phase of clinical development being demonstrated before preclinical or manufacturing support for the next phase is initiated. Sometimes such a strategy is dictated by financial constraints. This stage-gated approach imposes significant delays to the clinical development time line and ensures that the time until registration will be prolonged. The only way to prevent delays in clinical development that might arise from the preclinical program would be to manufacture the preclinical material and conduct the preclinical studies at risk. That is, complete all preclinical support to the next phase prior to knowing whether the current phase of clinical development will be successful, thereby rewarding the risk taken.

It is important to recognize that the magnitude of the resources, time, and money at stake for the manufacture of biologics is greater than for drugs, and that the manufacturing capacity is more limited. Sponsors may elect to accept certain risks to decrease the likelihood that there will be later delays. For example, sufficient quantities of a drug could be manufactured to enable multiple phases of preclinical and clinical development with minimal financial risk because manufacturing a drug is relatively inexpensive and quick. Furthermore, because of the inherent physicochemical properties of drugs, which lend themselves to early definition of the manufacturing specifications, there is also minimal risk that the material will not be representative of ("noncomparable" to) the "final" material, which is used in phase 3 trials. Relatively simple bioequivalence (comparative PK/PD) studies can be conducted in animals or humans to document this. This strategy is generally not viable for a biologic.

The most risk-filled phase of preclinical development, especially for a biologic, is that associated with the support to phase 3, which should be completed prior to the end of phase 2. Support to phase 3 is the most critical portion of preclinical development, as these are the pivotal studies that, with the carcinogenicity studies run concurrently with phase 3, will support registration. It is therefore essential that the material used to support phase 3 is representative of final product intended for use in humans.

When possible, GMP-compliant material from the clinical trial lots might be used, but waiting for this material may delay the start of the chronic toxicology studies. A drug manufactured by the final process and/or representative of the final process material is generally available for phase 3 support. A biologic manufactured by the final process (final cell line, scale, process, etc.) is seldom available when it is time to initiate the studies required for phase 3 support. Thus for a biologic, simple bioequivalence studies may be replaced by more complicated comparability studies that assess PK/PD parameters and immunogenicity at a minimum, and perhaps safety and efficacy if warranted by observed differences (see Chapter 8). The point is that each project team must consider many different critical decisions in designing the integrated development plans. Each of these decisions will carry with it an element of risk with regard to financial, scientific or regulatory aspects and to the development time line.

7.4.6 "Alternative" or Novel Preclinical Development Plans for Biologics

So far this exercise has focused on a "traditional" and uncomplicated development program for a biologic. To facilitate this, some assumptions were made, such as that a relevant species was identified and there were no planned changes to the cell line, manufacturing process, formulation, or route of administration during development. These assumptions, however, are not typical for most biologics. In reality the nature of many biologics is that they often require "nontraditional" or "alternative" development pathways. This is the essence of the "case-by-case" or science-driven program design espoused by ICH S6.

For example, it may be difficult to identify a relevant species, such as when a mAb does not cross-react with any species other than humans or cross-reactivity is limited to chimpanzees, a protected species that is difficult to access and has significant limitations in their use. Or the biologic may recognize the target in species other humans, but the target is expressed in different tissues or on different cells or has different functions than in humans. In these cases one may choose to develop a homologous (or surrogate) biologic for which a pharmacologically relevant (generally rodent) species can be identified.

Biologics are also different than drugs in that the product characteristics may differ as changes are made to the cell line or manufacturing process. These changes could affect PK, PD, immunogenicity, efficacy, and/or safety and typically require comparability studies to assess the potential differences. Likewise it is not uncommon for biologics to be tested initially in their simplest forms, such as an aqueous solution administered intravenously (IV), to attempt to get an indication of the viability of the product for the intended clinical indication. Later in development it might be prefered that the biologic be formulated for delayed release after subcutaneous (SC) administration. These changes could also affect the in vivo properties of the product and typically require "bridging" studies to assess potential differences.

Thus the second set of comparisons to be made evaluates "alternative" preclinical development plans to support the lack of a relevant species and planned changes to the cell line, manufacturing process, formulation, or route of administration during development.

Supporting Development without a Relevant Species
The simplest definition of a relevant species might be "one that is biologically comparable to humans and in which the test article has comparable pharmacologic and toxicologic properties." It is, however, sometimes much easier to describe a relevant species than to identify one. For the GPCRs that were the targets in this example, demonstrating biological comparability might involve comparison of the amino acid sequences, cellular and tissue expression in normal and disease states, and in vitro biological functions for humans and several other species, with the intent being to identify the most comparable species (see Chapters 9–13).

A robust preclinical safety program may devote as much or more effort to demonstrating biological comparability of the chosen species as to evaluating the toxicity of the product in that species. Prior to undertaking this effort, most project teams would evaluate the extent to which the product recognized or was active against the target in candidate species. Simple receptor binding affinity or ligand binding inhibition studies are often used for this purpose (see Chapter 9). If an acceptable level of cross-recognition or "cross-reactivity" is present in the tested species, then additional efforts would be justified to determine the relative activity and potency of the product in that species in vitro, or to evaluate pharmacologic activity of the product in vivo, such as in an animal model of disease (see Chapter 13). Despite these efforts to demonstrate comparable biology and pharmacology as the key components for identification of a relevant species for safety testing, it will only be after testing in humans that the degree of relevance of the selected species will become known.

Perhaps all biologics would be pharmacologically active in chimpanzees, our closest nonhuman primate relative. Most biologics would also be active in one or more monkey species, particularly of the *Macaca* genus (e.g., *M. mulatta* or *M. fascicularis*, the rhesus and cynomolgus monkeys, respectively). However, some biologics, particularly mAbs, have such restricted, species-specific cross-reactivity that they recognize the target only in humans and chimpanzees and thus are active only in these species. Although chimpanzees have been used for preclinical testing programs, their protected status, relatively limited numbers, lack of suitability for invasive measurements (e.g., histopathology) or chronic, reproductive or developmental toxicology studies, and past use for testing a variety of biologic agents (which can be associated with interfering immunogenic responses) makes chimpanzees not practical for most programs. Furthermore in some countries there is a ban on the use of chimpanzees to support clinical development. For these reasons, some biotechnology companies will no longer nominate as a development candidate any biologic that has cross-reactivity restricted to chimpanzees only.

While most biologics companies will first evaluate cynomolgus monkeys as a potential relevant species (because of their relative availability), that is not to say that monkeys are always the most relevant species or that other species are not relevant. The degree of relevance of the selected species must be demonstrated for each program.

When a relevant species cannot be identified for preclinical testing of a biologic, ICH S6 supports the use of (1) transgenic animals expressing the human target (in which the biologic might be tested, provided that the target was appropriately functional), (2) knockout or transgenic animals to evaluate the potential effects of target inhibition or replacement therapy, respectively, or (3) the use of "homologous proteins," which are often referred to as "surrogate" biologics. Any of these choices requires a commitment to thoroughly characterize the surrogate product and (surrogate) testing system. That is, the choice of testing system (species, strain, genotype, etc.) must be demonstrated to be relevant. For transgenic or knockout animals, this might mean genotyping individual animals, as well as fully describing the resulting phenotype. For a surrogate product, this might mean characterizing the pharmacologic activity of the surrogate in the test species, as well as the biological function of the target in this species. For example, for a non–cross-reactive mAb directed against a human target, a relevant surrogate mAb might be one directed against the same target in a rodent species, provided that the target functions comparably in the rodent species. Any of these alternative choices, if intended to support preclinical safety testing, must also comply with appropriate regulatory guidelines. For example, the material used might best be manufactured in compliance with GMP guidelines and the studies might best be GLP compliant. In these surrogate studies all of the usual endpoints should be assessed, such as PK, PD, and immunogenicity. In essence this means that the decision to adopt a surrogate program to address safety issues in a pharmacologically relevant species is a decision to double the amount of preclinical (and CMC) work to be done. However, adoption of a surrogate may allow testing of all aspects of toxicology, potentially even through carcinogenicity testing. Some would argue that, because these alternative methods do not directly evaluate the development product, some degree of relevance is lost. The counterargument to this point of view might be that if the biologic is not active in an animal species, there is no choice but to develop an alternative preclinical development program.

Figure 7.6 illustrated the hypothetical studies and time lines associated with preclinical support for a mAb that has cross-reactivity (pharmacologic activity) restricted to humans and chimpanzees. In this example, the strategy to support clinical development consists of conducting single-dose and 1- and 3-month repeated-dose studies in chimpanzees with the development mAb and use of a surrogate rat–anti-mouse mAb in a complete toxicology program in mice. Note that the portions of the program conducted in chimpanzees or mice would be essentially identical to what would be done in monkeys or rats if either were a relevant species. Once adopted, the surrogate mAb program

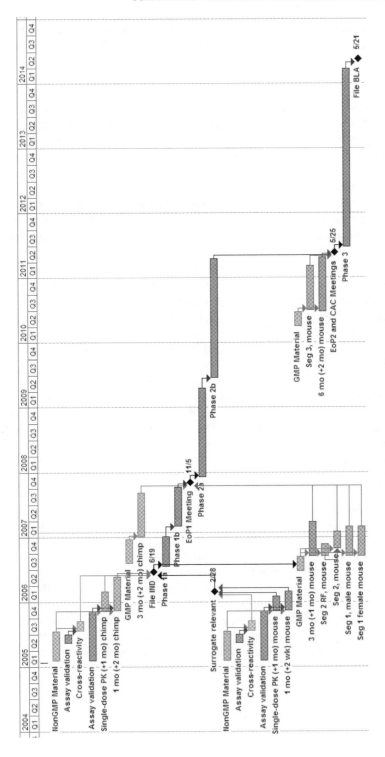

For comparison purposes, starting date was assumed to be 18 January 2005.

Figure 7.6 Supporting development without a relevant species.

cannot be abbreviated; to the extent possible, appropriate studies must be conducted to demonstrate that the surrogate is relevant. In this case the results of the chimpanzee studies with the development mAb and the mouse studies with the surrogate mAb could be compared.

As an aside, many biologics companies would choose one or the other of these alternative strategies, not both. In some cases it might not be logistically or technically feasible to conduct chimp studies. In some cases it might not be technically possible or pharmacologically appropriate to use a surrogate. In no case does ICH S6 recommend that a surrogate be developed for the purpose of allowing testing in a second (rodent) species if a single relevant species is identified.

This example of an integrated development plan assumes that the surrogate mAb cell line was already established, so that no time was required for establishing it. In this case the time until BLA filing is essentially unchanged from the previous example in which monkeys were used, but the total cost of the program is about $8.1 M, which is $2.8 M less expensive. This savings is primarily related to the use of mice rather than monkeys. However, the lower cost does not include the internal costs associated with the concurrent (parallel) development of both the surrogate and development mAb cell lines. If the surrogate mAb cell line was not yet established at the time it was decided to pursue this strategy, an additional roughly 9 to 12 months would be necessary, with the BLA then filed about 1 year later.

As with a traditional approach there are numerous critical decisions to be made during development. One of the most important considerations is the extent to which the data generated by use of a surrogate is likely to be viewed as acceptable to regulatory authorities. From the project team's point of view, it is unwise to commit resources to the conduct of studies that would not be acceptable.[12] From a regulator's point of view, acceptability will be assessed both on the quality of the studies (appropriateness, design, and compliance) and their eventual results (demonstration of apparent relevance). While a given study may be understood to be irrelevant a priori (e.g., one that uses a species in which there is no pharmacologic activity), it is not true that all studies that appear to be relevant will prove to be so. That is, the true relevance of any study can only be known *after* human data are available for comparison. It becomes therefore important for an alternative preclinical program to attempt to establish the degree of *apparent* relevance of a study. But it is equally important to try to establish the degree of apparent regulatory *acceptability* of alternative development programs. That means that there are several times during development, generally prior to large resource commitments, when discussions should be held with regulatory authorities as to the acceptability of the proposed alternative development programs.

---

[12]In this context, acceptability refers to the scientific rationale and the study designs, rather than to the results, which can only be assessed for acceptability retrospectively.

If one reviews Figure 7.6, it is apparent that discussions with regulatory authorities might be held at two critical times. The first is around 12 months prior to beginning manufacture of the surrogate, when the commitment to reserve manufacturing capacity is needed, and when the acceptability of the alternative strategy should be discussed. This discussion might address whether GMP-compliant material, GLP-compliant studies and validated assays would be expected. Without an agreement as to the apparent acceptability of the proposed program, the program may be run at risk of failure (nonacceptability) from a regulatory point of view. The second discussion should be held several months prior to the time of IND submission, when the apparent relevance of the surrogate should be demonstrable based on the results of the studies conducted to date. At this time, if the cumulative data from the surrogate studies suggest that the surrogate approach is not relevant, then this alternative approach is not viable. For example, if our hypothetical mAb binds to a cell surface receptor and inhibits activation of human T cells in vitro and chimpanzee T cells in vivo, but the rodent surrogate mAb binds to mouse T cells and inhibits T cell activation in vitro, yet induces T cell depletion in vivo, the surrogate would not be relevant because it does not share the pharmacologic properties of the development mAb. Perhaps numerous efforts to re-engineer the surrogate mAb to a nondepleting mAb would be unsuccessful also. Or a nondepleting surrogate might be discovered, but the cell line might not reach necessary productivity levels, leading to failure for technical reasons. Thus, even with a preliminary agreement that an alternative approach might be relevant and acceptable, there is still considerable risk that the alternative approach will eventually not be successful in supporting the clinical development program.

Supporting Changes to Cell Line, Manufacturing Process, Formulation, or Route of Administration

Biologics generally evolve over the lifespan of product development, with changes along the way to cell line, manufacturing process, formulation, and/or the method or route of administration. Many programs in fact undergo changes in each of these categories. Because each of these changes has the potential to affect one or more properties of a biologic, which may in turn affect the PK, PD, immunogenicity, safety, or efficacy, it has been said for biologics that "the process defines the product." Therefore the preclinical development program must also support all significant changes made to the product or its manner of use.

For the mAb in this comparison, the initial product is from an early cell line that is formulated as a liquid, stored frozen, and administered by IV injection. This is sufficient for initial safety, PK/PD, and pharmacologic activity assessments in phase 1 but is not an acceptable product profile for commercialization. To be competitive in the intended clinical indication, the product needs to be stored as a lyophilized powder (to increase shelf life and concentration), to be reconstituted and injected SC as needed. The acceptable volume for SC injection dictates a much more concentrated formulation.

Commercialization also dictates a highly productive cell line is in place prior to phase 3. Each of the significant evolutionary changes to be made during development may require some degree of "bridging" or comparability testing, to demonstrate that the most recent version of the product maintains the qualities of the previous version (see Chapter 8). The challenge to the project team will be to decide when it is most efficient to test the effects of which changes.

Figure 7.7 illustrates the hypothetical studies and time lines associated with preclinical support for a mAb that undergoes changes to the route of administration (IV to SC) prior to phase 2, formulation (frozen liquid to lyophilized powder) midway through phase 2, and cell line (high-producing new clone) prior to phase 3. The initial studies included IV single-dose and 1-month repeated-dose studies in monkeys. To support the planned change from IV to SC administration for phase 2, one might conduct: a single-dose SC PK/PD study for comparison to the single-dose IV results and, if they are acceptable, then conduct the 3-month repeated-dose safety study with SC dosing. These studies should demonstrate that the SC route is tolerated and provides comparable PK/PD properties to the IV route. Likewise, to support switching from frozen liquid to lyophilized material during phase 2, one might conduct a single-dose PK/PD comparability study of the frozen and lyophilized materials. Last, one would ideally like to defer evaluating chronic and reproductive toxicity testing until after establishment of the final, high-producing cell line intended for commercialization and manufacture of the pivotal phase 3 clinical trial material. If the material intended to be used in the pivotal 9-month chronic toxicity testing study is derived from a new cell line and has not previously been tested in monkeys, one might consider first conducting a 1-month repeated-dose study to assess safety and comparability. Although not discussed here, one might also conduct clinical comparability studies in humans to support the change from IV to SC prior to phase 1 and any changes occurring between phases 2 and 3.

As was true for the alternative program to support the lack of a relevant species, the additional support required for changes to the route of administration, formulation, and cell line adds time and money to the preclinical program. In this case about 12 more months and an additional $2.7 M are required to enable BLA filing.

From Figure 7.7 it becomes apparent that discussions with regulatory authorities should be held at several critical times. While meetings to discuss clinical comparability protocols are an accepted practice, it is less common, but potentially just as important, to do the same for preclinical programs. The first meeting(s) would be to present the proposed changes and to assess the acceptability of the planned comparability testing.[13] Subsequent meetings might occur soon after completion of the animal comparability/safety testing

---

[13]In vivo comparability testing may not be required if the in vitro or biochemical characterization of the biologic is sufficient to support comparability of the pre- and post-change products.

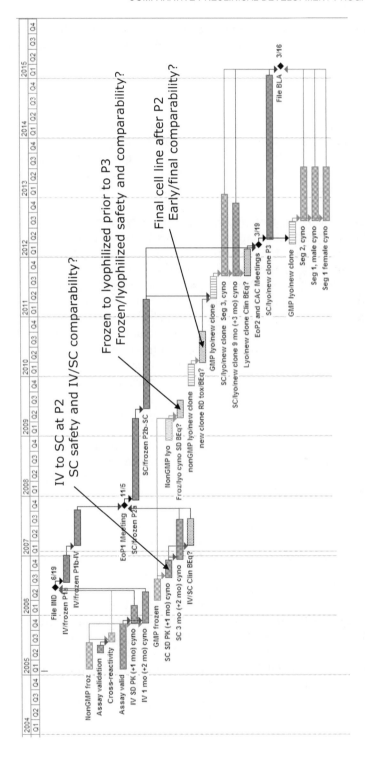

Figure 7.7   Supporting changes to route of administration, formulation, and cell line.

For comparison purposes, starting date was assumed to be 18 January 2005.

(to determine whether comparability was established) and prior to human comparability testing. The point to be made is that an understanding of the acceptability of the proposed changes and the effect of those changes on the product profile is needed prior to continuing to the next phase of development. Without regulatory agreement to the plan, there will be a risk that the method of comparability testing will not be acceptable, and therefore not useful. Even with an agreement, there remains a risk that comparability will not be demonstrated, in which case a significant portion of the supportive data derived from the earlier material will not be appropriate for support of the later material. Failure to demonstrate comparability means that some studies may need to be repeated with the new material.

The Challenge of Biologics Preclinical Development   The examples above demonstrated that alternative approaches to preclinical development, intended to address lack of a relevant species or to support changes to the product or its manner of use, are associated with significantly more time required for development and often with greater expense. The delays and costs are related to the need to dually develop the surrogate and the product, or to perform comparability assessments of earlier and later versions of the product. In reality, many biologics programs must address issues with both appropriate safety testing and support of product changes. In this example, if it was necessary to develop a surrogate mAb and to support changes to the product and its use, the total time until BLA filing might be as long as 10 years, 10 months, and require around $11 M.

These "nontraditional" concerns are generally not encountered with drugs. For this reason it is often feasible for a drug program to design, conduct, and submit a complete preclinical development program that has a defined budget and time line and is of relatively certain regulatory acceptability. Consultations with regulatory authorities are therefore not as essential for a drug (with the exception of dose-setting for carcinogenicity testing). In contrast, the challenge with biologics is in designing preclinical development programs that address the relevant safety issues but, if nontraditional, are acceptable to regulatory authorities. Gaining some assurance of this acceptability for a biologic requires more frequent and earlier discussions with regulatory authorities.

7.5   MESSAGES FOR PRECLINICAL DEVELOPMENT PROGRAMS FOR BIOLOGICS

The fundamental responsibility of preclinical development is to enable clinical development by consistently providing the relevant target biology, pharmacology, PK/PD, immunogenicity, efficacy, or safety information, as well the required regulatory support, in advance of when it is needed. The goal is for preclinical development to never be rate-limiting for clinical development. The hypothetical comparisons and examples that are presented here serve to illustrate what a challenge this can be for some programs. From this exercise, several key messages for preclinical development programs for biologics emerge:

- *Plan strategically.* The entire integrated development program should be planned early, to identify when each clinical phase will require the supportive preclinical information. Critical decision points must be identified and these decisions made in a timely fashion. A strategy must be planned to address potential issues, such as lack of a relevant species or changes to the product or manner of use.
- *Design relevant studies to answer relevant questions.* The preclinical development program should consist of relevant studies designed to answer relevant concerns about pharmacology, PK/PD, efficacy, and safety, as well as comparability. No study should be conducted if it is not potentially capable of adding useful information to the knowledge of the product.
- *De-risk high-risk plans.* Whenever possible, discussions should be had with regulatory authorities to determine the acceptability of the preclinical program or studies for support of clinical development. Conducting alternative programs without some assurance as to their potential acceptability is a run-at-risk proposition. While gaining preliminary approval of the development program will not guarantee that it will eventually be acceptable, it will at least determine that it is not unacceptable. Only the program results will determine the eventual acceptability of the program.
- *Add value to clinical development.* The greatest value that preclinical development can offer is to enlighten or inform upon clinical development. This is more than just meeting regulatory requirements without becoming rate limiting. It includes, through careful selection of relevant species and incorporation of relevant endpoints, the ability to inform upon the likely PK/PD, pharmacology, efficacy and safety results to be seen in human clinical trials.

7.6 SUMMARY

The objective of this chapter was to compare to the studies, materials, and costs associated with hypothetical preclinical development programs intended to support the clinical development of a drug and a biologic. To accomplish this objective, an integrated development program was planned, from IND through NDA or BLA, and the respective preclinical development programs to support each filing were then designed and compared. This exercise demonstrated that relative to preclinical programs for drugs, there are some important differences in preclinical programs for biologics:

- Biologics often require nontraditional or alternative testing strategies due to limited species cross-reactivity (pharmacologic activity).
- Biologics often require additional studies to support changes to the product or its manner of use and to demonstrate comparability.
- Biologics often require investment of additional time, effort, and money to support a given phase of clinical development.
- Biologics often have greater risks of failing for technical, scientific, and/or regulatory reasons.
- Biologics often require significantly different timing for key development decisions to facilitate clinical development and manage risk.

Success for biologics will be achieved by de-risking the integrated development program with early, detailed, long-range strategic planning, frequent review of progress against plan, and early and frequent interactions with regulatory reviewers to assess acceptability of the plan and the results.

ACKNOWLEDGMENTS

Learning the trade of preclinical development for biologics is a long and challenging, but fortunately shared, process. There seem to be no training programs that address the many nuances and differences from traditional drug development paradigms, the latter of which can be accessed in numerous texts. The results of development programs for biologics are generally not published, with the exception of summary information available after approval. However, the most valuable lessons to be learned often reside in the programs that do not reach approval. Thus much of what we can learn of biologics development comes from our colleagues. While I have had the opportunity to work on programs for a wide variety of biologics, I have been especially fortunate to have had the benefit of the council of others who have had more and different experiences than me. I am particularly grateful for the contributions of Lauren Black, Page Bouchard, Joy Cavagnaro, Mary Ellen Cosenza, James Green, Marie Green, Mark Milton, and George Treacy to my ongoing education.

REFERENCES

1. ICH M3(R1). Maintenance of the ICH Guideline on Non-clinical Safety Studies for the Conduct of Human Clinical Trials for Pharmaceuticals. International Conference on Harmonization of Technical Requirements for Registration of Pharmaceuticals for Human Use, 9 November 2000.
2. ICH S1A. Guideline on the Need for Carcinogenicity Studies of Pharmaceuticals. International Conference on Harmonization of Technical Requirements for Registration of Pharmaceuticals for Human Use, 29 November 1995.

3. ICH S1B. Testing for Carcinogenicity of Pharmaceuticals. International Conference on Harmonization of Technical Requirements for Registration of Pharmaceuticals for Human Use, 16 July 1997.

4. ICH S1C(R1). Dose Selection for Carcinogenicity Studies of Pharmaceuticals and Limit Dose. International Conference on Harmonization of Technical Requirements for Registration of Pharmaceuticals for Human Use, 17 July 1997, November 2005.

5. ICH S2A. Guidance on Specific Aspects of Regulatory Genotoxicity Tests for Pharmaceuticals. International Conference on Harmonization of Technical Requirements for Registration of Pharmaceuticals for Human Use, 19 July 1995.

6. ICH S2B. Genotoxicity: A Standard Battery for Genotoxicity Testing of Pharmaceuticals. International Conference on Harmonization of Technical Requirements for Registration of Pharmaceuticals for Human Use, 16 July 1997.

7. ICH S3A. Note for Guidance on Toxicokinetics: The Assessment of Systemic Exposure in Toxicity Studies. International Conference on Harmonization of Technical Requirements for Registration of Pharmaceuticals for Human Use, 27 October 1994.

8. ICH S3B. Pharmacokinetics: Guidance for Repeated Dose Tissue Distribution Studies. International Conference on Harmonization of Technical Requirements for Registration of Pharmaceuticals for Human Use, 27 October 1994.

9. ICH S4. Duration of Chronic Toxicity Testing in Animals (Rodent and Nonrodent Toxicity Testing). International Conference on Harmonization of Technical Requirements for Registration of Pharmaceuticals for Human Use, 2 September 1998.

10. ICH S5(R2). Detection of Toxicity to Reproduction for Medicinal Products and Toxicity to Male Fertility. International Conference on Harmonization of Technical Requirements for Registration of Pharmaceuticals for Human Use, November 2005.

11. ICH S7A. Safety Pharmacology Studies for Human Pharmaceuticals. International Conference on Harmonization of Technical Requirements for Registration of Pharmaceuticals for Human Use, 8 November 2000.

12. ICH S7B. The Non-clinical Evaluation of the Potential for Delayed Ventricular Repolarization (QT Interval Prolongation) by Human Pharmaceuticals. International Conference on Harmonization of Technical Requirements for Registration of Pharmaceuticals for Human Use, 12 May 2005.

13. ICH S8. Immunotoxicity Studies for Human Pharmaceuticals. International Conference on Harmonization of Technical Requirements for Registration of Pharmaceuticals for Human Use, 15 September 2005.

14. ICH S6. Preclinical Safety Evaluation of Biotechnology-derived Pharmaceuticals. International Conference on Harmonization of Technical Requirements for Registration of Pharmaceuticals for Human Use, 16 July 1997.

15. ICH Q5E. Comparability of Biotechnological/Biological Products Subject to Changes in Their Manufacturing Process. International Conference on Harmonization of Technical Requirements for Registration of Pharmaceuticals for Human Use, 18 November 2004.

■■■■■ CHAPTER 8

Demonstration of Comparability of a Licensed Product after a Manufacturing Change

RICHARD M. LEWIS, PhD

Contents

Preclinical Safety Evaluation of Biopharmaceuticals: A Science-Based Approach to Facilitating Clinical Trials, edited by Joy A. Cavagnaro
Copyright © 2008 by John Wiley & Sons, Inc.

8.1   INTRODUCTION

Biopharmaceuticals have traditionally been defined by their manufacturing processes. Over the course of a product's life cycle a biopharmaceutical manufacturer often faces the question of whether to make changes to the manufacturing process and when to implement such changes. The need to make a change may be driven by a variety of reasons, including contractual obligations, manufacturing capacity, improving purity, improving safety, increasing product yield, or optimizing the ultimate cost of goods of manufacture. There is also regulatory pressure to maintain current good manufacturing practices (cGMPs). The FDA has recently focused on maintaining cGMPs in their "GMPs for the twenty-first century" initiative [1]. Central to this proposal are the concepts of quality systems [2] and the process analytical technologies (PAT) initiative [3]. The PAT guidance is intended to describe a regulatory framework that will ensure the voluntary development and implementation of innovative pharmaceutical manufacturing and quality assurance [4]. The framework is intended to assist manufacturers in developing and validating new efficient tools to maintain product quality while controlling the manufacturing process. These concepts will need to be considered, among other decisions, when process changes are implemented. Since quality concepts need to be considered prior to implementing a process change, the most difficult decision for a product developer is when to implement manufacturing changes. Some of the issues to consider will be addressed in this chapter.

The initial goal in making a change is the demonstration that the original product has not changed in "identity, strength, quality, purity, and potency" and that previously developed safety and efficacy data will apply to the product processed using the new method. If any differences are observed, they must then be evaluated for their impact on the current product and relevance to the previously obtained data. Importantly, even minor changes must be considered as potentially altering the above-mentioned product attributes. This chapter will provide an overview of the key issues and considerations for implementing a manufacturing change. The process that a manufacturer will go through to determine these characteristics has been referred to as "comparability."

8.2   DEFINITION OF TERMS

8.2.1   Comparability

The concept of comparability was first introduced by the FDA in 1996 in its guidance, FDA Guidance Concerning Demonstration of Comparability of Human Biological Products, Including Therapeutic Biotechnology-derived Products [5]. The term *comparability* was specifically chosen (1) to recognize the possible lack of identity after a manufacturing change and (2) to distinguish the concept from other specific pharmaceutical regulatory terms: equivalence or bioequivalence. A successful demonstration of comparability between two biopharmaceutical materials does not mean that the products are identical in every way. Minor differences in the product may be identified, but the products can still be viewed as comparable. Similarly each batch or lot may not be exact but meet the boundaries or specifications that have been established for the process [6]. The challenge for developers, manufacturers, and regulators is to identify those characteristics that define the identity, strength, quality, purity, and potency. Although the term comparability is used in the FDA guidance, it is applied primarily to the changes in manufacturing; the FDA has also used comparability principles in other ways.

8.2.2 Equivalence

Equivalence is meant to be a demonstration of a specified statistical confidence that two compounds can achieve the same characteristics. It often has been used to describe the same outcome or endpoint frequency in clinical trials. Equivalence is not a comparative evaluation of similarity between different manufacturing methods of the same product or necessarily a comparison of extremely similar products. Equivalence also is a difficult statistical assurance to reach in a clinical trial, and therefore it is an extreme standard for comparison of manufacturing processes.

8.2.3 Generic Drugs and Bioequivalence

Bioequivalence is distinct from both equivalence and comparability and it is defined in the regulations for generic drugs. Generic drugs are approved on the basis of identity of strength, dosage form, safety, quality, performance characteristics, and route of administration. They must have the same indication for use and demonstrate bioequivalence. A generic drug is considered bioequivalent to an innovator if it exhibits the same rate and extent of absorption of the active or therapeutic ingredient, although inactive ingredients may vary, and becomes available at the site of drug action. Acceptable absorption parameters are those between 80% and 125% of those obtained with the proprietary agent under the same testing conditions. These mechanisms for approval are meant to address products that are identical to drugs, distinct from biologics, and have an innovator that has been approved as a drug. Generics are regulated under the Food Drug and Cosmetic (FD&C) Act, sections 505(b)(2) and 505(j). Under section 505(b)(2) of the FD&C Act, the FDA may rely on data for approval of a new drug application that is not developed by the applicant. Some or all of the clinical information can be provided by the literature or by references to a past FDA finding of safety and effectiveness for approved drugs. Generic drugs in the United States can be approved based on a demonstration of bioequivalence of pharmacokinetic data. Those products can be substituted (are interchangeable). The conditions which are accepted for bioequivalence are defined in the regulation but those for comparability are generally negotiated with the FDA and based on the best scientific information that is available. The decision about comparability is determined on a case-by-case basis initially using multiple analytical tests to characterize the chemical and physical attributes of the process materials together with considerations of the complexity of the product and the scope of the manufacturing change.

8.2.4 Biogenerics

Biological products that provide for generic medications were not part of the Hatch–Waxman amendments to the FD&C Act. In part due to historical precedence and in part due to scientific concerns of the FDA, biologics do not have regulatory mechanisms to provide for the approval of "generic" compounds for a previously approved biological drug. As a result of the large degree of interest globally in providing the same advantages to biologic drug development as the Hatch–Waxman Act provided to pharmaceuticals, the concept of biogenerics is being discussed widely in industry and regulatory venues as well as congressional and public settings.

European health authorities have developed regulations that allow a form of generic biologics for recombinant proteins and monoclonal antibodies. The Committee for Medicinal Products for Human Use (CHMP), of the European Medicines Agency (EMEA), issued a series of guidelines that address their expectations for applications as Marketing Authorization for Similar Biological Medicinal Products [7]. To support this new approach CHMP has issued additional guidelines: (1) regarding the demonstration of quality, Similar Biological Medicinal Products Containing Biotechnology-Derived Proteins as Active Substance: Quality Issues [8], and (2) for assessment of applications containing clinical and nonclinical data, Similar Biological Medicinal Products containing Biotechnology-Derived Proteins as Active Substance: Non-clinical and Clinical Issues [9]. The development of so-called biosimilars is dependent on the principles of comparability and thus the above-mentioned guidelines refer to the EMEA's previously issued Guideline on Comparability of Medicinal Products Containing Biotechnology-Derived Proteins as Active Substance: Quality Issues [10] and also Guideline on Comparability of Medicinal Products Containing Biotechnology-Derived Proteins as Active Substance: Non-clinical and Clinical Issues [11]. These guidelines, the concept of biosimilars, and the use of comparability principles add to the importance of, and confusion over, the term comparability. In the described CHMP comparability guidelines, comparability can be applied to either a manufacturing change by a single manufacturer or to the regulatory application of a biologic claiming similarity to a previously approved product after patent protection has ended. Thus the principle of comparability is central to the development of the so-called biosimilars. In fact, the first two biosimilar products, both for human DNA-recombinant growth hormone, were approved under these guidelines in 2006 [12].

It is beyond the scope of this chapter to discuss biogenerics and biosimilars, also referred to as follow-on biologics (in the United States), subsequent entry biologics (in Canada), and multisource biological products. The fate of a regulatory mechanism for approval of follow-on biologics in the United States is still undetermined, and the debate will likely continue as biopharmaceuticals take on an increasing share of the drug market and thus an increasing importance to the health care market [13].

8.3 REGULATORY GUIDANCE FOR DETERMINING COMPARABILITY

8.3.1 The FDA

The FDA guidance describes the possible evaluations that may be needed to demonstrate comparability to the US regulatory authorities. The document is broad enough to address changes in manufacturing at premarketing or after licensing, although it primarily addresses changes during development after some clinical studies have been completed. The comparability exercise may include a combination of analytical testing, biological assays (in vitro or in vivo), assessment of pharmacokinetics and/or pharmacodynamics and toxicity in animals, and clinical testing (clinical pharmacology, safety, or efficacy). The usual progression of complexity is from analytical to animal studies to human pharmacokinetics and/or pharmacodynamics to clinical safety and efficacy studies. Analytical testing is regarded as the most precise measure of a molecule's attributes and thus serves as the first tier for comparability determination. If product differences are observed in analytical testing, then additional preclinical studies or a clinical pharmacokinetic or limited pharmacodynamic study may be warranted. If differences are observed after additional limited clinical testing, or if there is insufficient product knowledge of the impact of differences on safety, purity, or potency, then data from larger clinical studies may be needed.

As previously mentioned, product manufacturing changes are made for many reasons: to increase product supply through process optimization such as to increase yield, to increase manufacturing capacity by scale-up or duplication and addition of viral reduction methods, or to increase compliance with cGMPs. The precise manufacturing process of all drug products must be described to regulatory agencies. In the United States, changes in manufacturing must be reported in either an active IND or to the BLA depending on stage of product life cycle. (See Section 8.6 for various types of license supplements that can be used to report changes.)

The ultimate goal of an investigational product is the demonstration of safety and efficacy and in the case of a licensed product that it has suitably provided that demonstration. Thus the primary concern after a manufacturing change is if that change will affect the safety or efficacy (safety, identity, purity, or potency) that has been demonstrated previously. The guidance points out that changes that appear minor may have major effects and major changes may exert minor effects. For this reason it is important to select those assays that can identify the characteristics that contribute to safety and efficacy.

8.3.2 The EMEA

The EMEA has also issued guidance on Comparability, as mentioned above, on quality issues [10] and for nonclinical and clinical issues [11]. In these guidelines the concept of comparability can be applied to either a manufacturing change by one manufacturer or to the application of a biologic claiming similarity to a previously approved product after patent protection has ended. This guidance offers more detail than either the ICH document or the FDA guidance. A complete section of the EMEA guideline addresses aspects of immunogenicity testing. It discusses factors that can contribute to changes in immunogenicity: measurement of antibody responses, antibody testing strategies, validation of antibody assays, and timing of sampling. The document insists that immunogenicity "be considered when a claim of comparability is made, especially when repeated administration is proposed."

8.3.3 The ICH

The International Conference on Harmonization has noted the importance of comparability and itself has issued guidance [14]. The FDA has accepted the ICH guidance, and it is a part of the material that offers advice in developing comparability data. In many respects it follows the previously published FDA guidance; however, with the benefit of an additional decade of experience with biopharmaceutical manufacturing processes and clinical validation, this document provides greater details for determining comparability.

The ICH published The Comparability of Biotechnological/Biological Products Subject to Changes in Their Manufacturing Process [14] in 2005. In comparison to the initial 1996 FDA guidance, this guidance addresses similar concerns with less emphasis on the preclinical and clinical aspects but it is similarly intended to address manufacturing changes for a product by a single manufacturer. It addresses changes that are made either during product development or manufacturing changes that are meant to improve the production of a marketed product. One principle, that is common to both documents and should be applied in all parts of the comparability exercise is that material before and after the manufacturing change should be compared in every analytical, biological, and stability evaluation as well as in nonclinical and clinical methods if deemed necessary.

By comparison to the EMEA document, the ICH guideline does not address immunogenicity in the same detail. It does suggest that immunochemical properties be a component of the characterization and considerations for immunogenicity should be a part of the planning of nonclinical and clinical

TABLE 8.1 Comparability guidance documents

Agency	Guidance	Purpose	Reference
EMEA	Guideline on similar biological medicinal products	Information requirements for the marketing authorization applications	5
EMEA	Similar biological medicinal products containing biotechnology-derived proteins as active substance: quality issues	Quality issues in demonstrating comparability of similar biological medicinal products containing recombinant DNA-derived proteins (proteins and peptides, their derivatives and products)	6
EMEA	Similar biological medicinal products containing biotechnology-derived proteins as active substance: nonclinical and clinical issues	Nonclinical and clinical requirements for demonstrating comparability of similar biological medicinal products	7
EMEA	Guideline on comparability of medicinal products containing biotechnology-derived proteins as active substance: quality issues	Quality of the comparability exercise for either change in a manufacturing process or to demonstrate similarity in a marketed product	8
EMEA	Guideline on comparability of medicinal products containing biotechnology-derived proteins as active substance: nonclinical and clinical issues	Quality of the comparability exercise for either change in a manufacturing process or to demonstrate similarity in a marketed product	9
ICH/U.S.FDA	Comparability of biotechnology-derived, ICH Q5E	Comparability of biotechnological/biological products for changes made in the manufacturing process	10
U.S. FDA	FDA guidance concerning demonstration of comparability of human biological products, including therapeutic biotechnology-derived products	Comparability testing for manufacturing changes made prior to product and after product approval for a single manufacturer	4

studies, in particular, when considering various aspects of the knowledge of the product use.

8.4   GENERAL PRINCIPLES AND PRACTICES

The scope of a comparability program should usually be established in relation to the significance of the change that is being evaluated, the stage of development, and the clinical indication. Each program should take into consideration how the change may affect the finished product as well as attempt to answer other questions: How much of a "difference" is acceptable? Is lack of "sameness" an issue for the particular stage of development? Are the pivotal safety and efficacy trials in progress? Do blood concentrations correlate with toxicity and/or efficacy [15]?

With a marketed product it is more important to provide assurance of comparability prior to committing to making the change. Even more than with a product in development, it is important to have confidence that the current manufacturing method produces a product on which there is confidence that there can be a reliance on previous data, including in vitro, preclinical, and clinical information, for the safety and efficacy of the current methods. Without complete confidence in the comparability, it will be difficult to evaluate trends in safety reporting.

In carrying out all aspects of the comparability exercise, it is important to consider previous knowledge of the product and, in particular, the relationship between the characteristics of the product and the effects documented by available preclinical and clinical experience. Other important considerations include recognizing the contribution of the particular production step that is changed, the potential impact of the change, and the ability to measure any predicted change. In evaluating the change, knowledge of the key physiological characteristics of the active product is central to selecting the proper traits to be tested and which manufacturing stages are relevant. In any case, the drug substance and drug product should both be included as part of the comparison. Also it is important to demonstrate a consistency of manufacturing, which is usually done with a limited number of manufacturing batches. The effect on stability should be measured and compared with the previous material [16].

Determining the potency of the final product and comparing the characteristics of drug substance and drug product are generally expected. However, in some cases the most sensitive step in the process to detect changes may be in intermediate fractions. In such cases key intermediate materials should be compared.

The effects that changes will have on the product at critical control points, in-process controls, and downstream steps must be considered and evaluated whenever possible. Samples from intermediate process steps may provide material that can be better evaluated for possible impurities or, in some cases, infectious agents. The milieu in which material is applied to purification matrices may affect separation parameters. As such, it is not only the degree of purity, specific activity, or concentration but also the consistency of the material in which it is isolated. The presence or absence of proteolytic enzymes or carriers may affect the chemical nature of the product. The FDA has recently emphasized process analytical technologies (PAT), and it should be recognized that upstream manufacturing changes can have important effects on in-process measurements [3]. A change in the purity profile, as well as the impurity profile, of one step has the potential to change the effectiveness of a subsequent manufacturing step. It is always important to note that the resulting material from one manufacturing step is the starting material for the following part of the process.

While it is likely that minor changes will result in a comparable product, a series of small changes over time can amount to a significant change in the product. For this reason manufacturers should evaluate the potential for gradual "drift" of the product or, taken together, there may be an interaction that is unforeseen and may be a reason for doing comparability studies. Also the changes may have some interactive function that cannot be predicted and will prompt the need for comparability studies.

It is very important that a side-by-side comparison be performed using the product from the previous process with the product from the new process. Sufficient "old" product and intermediates must therefore be available (retained) to allow for the comparability studies. During the initial characterization of the product, numerous assays are selected to ensure in-process consistency, including essential characteristics of key intermediates. It is assumed that these assays describe the important characteristics of the product. For this reason most of these assays will be employed in demonstrating comparability.

Biological assays, in particular potency assays, are meant to demonstrate a relationship between the product and the desired biological effect. The correlation between the activity measured by the potency assay and the resulting clinical effect is an important criterion in both dosing and the determination of efficacy. International or other accepted reference standards, when available, should be incorporated in the assay.

In theory, comparability is the provision of data so that there is sufficient confidence in product made by a new manufacturing method that one can rely on the data previously developed using the former manufacturing method. Although it is not necessarily a stepwise process, in practice comparison data are generated first in vitro, then in preclinical studies and finally in clinical trials. The need for a step up in each case generally is based on the data obtained in the current tier.

8.4.1 Comparability May Not Be Required

If the manufacturing change is carried out prior to any preclinical or clinical testing, there is little need to compare the products made by the two methods except for development purposes. The primary reason for determining comparability is to have a basis for reliance on previous data. The bar for establishing comparability will therefore likely be higher for changes made during or after phase 3 clinical studies.

8.4.2 Manufacturing Changes

The types of changes that a manufacturer might face are varied and diverse, from minor to major; to list some: transition from in vivo to in vitro production for a monoclonal antibody, changes in DNA vector, a new master cell bank, use of a different cell substrate (host cell system), changes in raw materials, different culture media and culturing conditions, different serum to serum-free tissue culture, changes in a purification step, changes in storage conditions, and changes in equipment and facilities including pilot versus full-scale product or a new production line. There may also be changes in the purity and impurity profiles, deliberate molecular modifications to the protein, or changes in the final formulation including changes in excipients, container closure, as well as a change from liquid to lyophilized product.

Some of the manufacturing changes that can alter biochemical structure include changes in cell substrate, raw materials, bioreactor conditions and purity [17]. These changes may lead to posttranslational modfications in glycosylation, may increase process- or product-related impurities that might be immunopotentiating, or may include degradation products that lead to aggregation. It is for this last reason that the FDA insists on evaluating the monomer pattern of the final product. A number of manufacturing changes have been shown to lead to aggregation. In one instance, merely the change in the container-closure system provided an increase in leached materials which induced aggregation [18]. Because aggregation can induce immunogenicity, alter pharmacokinetic (PK) characteristics, and induce hypersensitivity (e.g., intravenous immunoglobulin, IGIV), the evaluation of monomer patterns is usually a required evaluation in any comparability exercise.

There is a close relationship between the comparability of product made in different processes and in the applied current good manufacturing practices (cGMPs). The FDA has recognized that degree of GMP does not have to be as stringent for products in early phases of development [19,20]. It should also be noted that the better a product is characterized, the easier it is to demonstrate that a new process produces a comparable product.

8.4.3 Physicochemical Characterization

The availability of sensitive analytical tests to adequately characterize a product and to measure the predicted possible changes is central to a comparability assessment. Obviously tests should be chosen that will be the most likely to detect important changes. ICH Q6B offers advice on physicochemical, biological activity, and immunochemical properties, purity (impurity), contaminants and quantity [21]. The assay standards and statistical assurance of assay validity are also addressed as well as the application of testing to in-process material, drug substance, and drug product.

The importance of determining biological activity should be emphasized. The association of this activity with clinical effect is an important component of product characterization, in particular, potency and stability testing. Before embarking on animal or human trials to evaluate comparability, it is important to evaluate the data gathered in the quality testing and determine the need for additional studies. If any differences are observed, the nature of those differences will determine the need for animal or clinical studies. The association of the changes with known safety and therapeutic potential will help to contribute to the decision. In addition the dosing regimen, the therapeutic window, and the previous experience with the product will determine the need for in-life trials.

Often analytical testing and biological characterization are sufficient to provide evidence of comparability. One estimate of frequency of the use of clinical data for comparability demonstrations was 1% [22]. However, more recently the FDA has begun to request more clinical PK data for defining comparability of products in clinical development.

8.4.4 Preclinical Considerations

Changes in three-dimensional structure can ultimately affect pharmacokinetic profile, receptor affinity, and immunogenicity. Thus comparability programs often focus on those measures that can best be used to determine the retention of a molecular identity. While in most cases analytical testing and biological characterization are sufficient to provide evidence of comparability, various in vitro studies or in vivo animal studies may need to be considered. Animal pharmacokinetics may also be needed even in the absence of demonstrated differences in analytical testing of the functional assays for the product. This is because analytical testing may be insensitive to changes affecting pharmacokinetics and in vitro functional tests may not reflect the time-dependent aspects of distribution [5].

Assay performance criteria for biopharmaceuticals are often highly variable; therefore strict statistical criteria that attempt to rigorously establish traditional in vivo bioequivalence may not always be appropriate. In some cases an assessment of rate and extent of absorption as indicated by the maximum concentration (C_{max}), time of maximum concentration (T_{max}) and area under the curve (AUC) may be needed. In other cases complicating factors related to binding proteins, endogenous concentration, and unusual concentration-time profiles may need to be considered [15]. In cases where complications may arise from immune response to heterologous proteins, cross-over designs are inappropriate.

The extent of additional toxicology studies depends on where in the phase of clinical development or the life cycle of product the change is made, the previously developed safety profile and on the magnitude of the manufacturing change [15]. Additional animal studies or "bridging studies" may be needed where the product has a narrow therapeutic index or where specific safety concerns are present, such as when the process change raises concerns about possible toxic impurities or adventitious agents that cannot be assessed with analytical testing. Bridging studies may also be indicated if there is a significant change in the final formulation or route of administration.

8.4.5 Clinical Considerations

ICH Q5E is emphatic in stating that both preclinical and clinical data may not be necessary if the manufacturer can provide assurance of comparability through the previously described analytical program. However, when these data are insufficient, additional evidence may be required, and this is determined on a case-by-case basis. Various studies may be recommended based on the results of the analytical studies, knowledge of the product, and clinical information, in particular, regarding dosing indication, therapeutic index, and previous clinical experience. The studies may be PK, pharacodynamics (PD), efficacy, safety, immunogenicity, or phase 4 studies. Like all other parts of the program, these studies should be based on a direct comparison [15]. Similarly the 1996 FDA guidance states that usually the reason for the analytical studies is to avoid additional clinical trials. When needed, the additional human studies will be to evaluate changes that may affect pharmacodynamics and pharmacokinetics [5].

The EMEA, CHMP, offers more detail in their advice; however, the specific need for clinical data, like the ICH and FDA guidances, will depend on the degree of comparability measured in analytical methods. A wide variety of conditions for drug use and the availability of a surrogate marker may affect how the clinical comparison is performed. If a surrogate marker is available, PK/PD studies may be sufficient, and the degree of knowledge of the product along with the degree of difference will dictate the need for additional clinical data. It will be important, especially for marketed products, to follow closely the safety profile of the product using well-designed pharmacovigiliance methods to be assured that no additional safety concerns were introduced with the change.

When manufacturing changes are made prior to approval, comparability usually is demonstrated through analytical and sometimes animal studies before proceeding to the next phase of development. If late in development (e.g., during phase 3), it might be necessary or valuable to demonstrate comparability as part of the trial(s).

It is important to note that in order to be able to adequately compare product made from two different manufacturing schemes, material must be available from both. There has been more than one manufacturer who changed process without retaining sufficient material of the former method to do adequate comparisons. As discussed above, it should be noted that the final product is not always the best or only material to use for comparative studies. The concentration and nature of the impurities may be important in manufacturing steps further downstream.

8.4.6   Specific Considerations Regarding Immunogenicity

How does immunogenicity figure into comparability? Changes in manufacturing can undoubtedly give rise to changes in immunogenicity. The known association of particular molecular changes with changes in immunogenicity, such as secondary and tertiary conformational changes, may indicate the need for some assessment of the potential for an immune reaction to the new material if these changes are identified. Other considerations include the nature of the product itself, the dose schedule and route, the duration of therapy, and the immune status of the intended patient population. Given the nature of biological products, it is often difficult to determine the immunogenic potential of a particular product much less to be able to compare between similar products.

Immunogenicity concerns are based on a number of potential safety concerns. Adverse reactions can be based on the formation of immune complexes that can give rise to renal toxicity, complement activation, and, as recently reported, the induction of autologous antibodies that cross-react with the patient's own endogenous protein [23–28].

One example of a plasma-derived coagulation factor VIII showed a marked increase in inhibitor formation (antibodies to factor VIII that block activity) [29,30]. The question of immunogenicity is one of the most difficult questions to answer without clinical data. However, relative immunogenicity as measured by frequency of the development of antibodies or the relative magnitude of a reaction can be determined in animals, even though it is understood that treating animals with human proteins usually will result in the development of an immune reaction. The FDA has accepted one approach to demonstrate a lack of neo-antigenicity. This is the adsorption of antibodies against the novel material with the previous material. If all antibody activity can be adsorbed by the previous version, it suggests a lack of neo-antigenicity. The use of transgenic and knockout mice may also provide a means to evaluate neo-antigenicity. All evaluations of immunogenicity are dependent on the reliability, sensitivity, and specificity of the assays used.

Other chapters in this volume specifically address immunogenicity and preclinical models and may also be relevant in the context of comparability (Chapters 16 and 20). The FDA has allowed changes in production without a clinical evaluation of immunogenicity.

8.5   ADDITIONAL APPLICATIONS OF COMPARABILITY

The FDA has applied the concept of comparability in other unique ways in order to address specific regulatory needs. It has recently discussed the concept of comparability in its draft "Guidance for Industry: Minimally Manipulated, Unrelated, Allogeneic Placental/Umbilical Cord Blood Intended for Hematopoietic Reconstitution in Patients with Hematological Malignancies" [31]. Generally, comparability is used to demonstrate that there can be reliance that a novel process produces a safe and effective product based on data gathered from a previous method. (The "new product" relies on data gathered using the "old product.") In the umbilical cord blood guidance, the FDA has shown a willingness to use current data for licensure (i.e., as a demonstration of safety and efficacy) and to apply comparability principles to ensure safety and efficacy of product made under a previous method. In other words, rather than use comparability to make products available from a newer process, the FDA suggests using it to make products available from previous, unlicensed methods. (Data on the "new product" is used for confidence in the "old product.") This approach is important to ensure the availability of products for transplantation to individuals with very limited possibilities for matching donors. Because of the rapid changes in the field of umbilical cord blood transplantation, it is likely that many tests used today are not the same as those in a past decade nor validated in the same ways when these important products were first being collected and stored. Although much of the testing may not be identical, the cellular products may be the same or at least "comparable." With the assurance of comparability older products can be considered licensed.

In this guidance the FDA offers some direction for the demonstration of comparability. They request that the manufacturer provide evidence that the methods, facilities, and controls that were used to manufacture previous products conformed to cGMPs and to other applicable regulatory requirements. In addition they request the submission of validation summaries, as well as product characteristics such as total nucleated cell count, viable CD34 cell count, and number of colony-forming units. Stability data and information from the scientific literature can also be used. Clinical outcomes can be part of the comparability demonstration.

Upon approval of the application and the comparability data, all products could be made available under the license. Some of the concepts addressed for umbilical cord hematopoietic stem cells may be important in future comparability demonstrations in hematopoietic and other cell therapies.

8.6 REGULATORY SUBMISSIONS AFTER US MARKETING APPROVAL

For manufacturing changes that are made after marketing approval, the manufacturer must submit data demonstrating that the change does not affect the product. For licensed biologics, the submission will be as a biologics license supplement (BLS) and will fall in one of a few categories [32]. A prior approval supplement describes changes that have a substantial potential to have an adverse effect on the identity, strength, quality, purity, or potency of the product. The changes should not be implemented until the supplement has been reviewed and approval given. In changes that are thought to have a moderate impact on the product, a changes being effected in 30 days (CBE30) supplement, or a changes being effected (CBE) is submitted, which enables implementation within 30 days or immediately, respectively. Data documenting the change must be submitted and will be reviewed by the FDA. Other changes are reported in an annual report. A decreased time to distribution of product after the change in CMC can be facilitated if the manufacturer has the foresight to identify those changes that may be made in the future and/or a series of changes that may be implemented. It is also possible to decrease the reporting burden. This can be accomplished with the approval of a "comparability protocol."

> A comparability protocol is a well-defined, detailed, written plan for assessing the effect of specific CMC changes in the identity, strength, quality, purity, and potency of a specific drug product as these factors relate to the safety and effectiveness of the product. A comparability protocol describes the changes that are covered under the protocol and specifies the tests and studies that will be performed, including the analytical procedures that will be used, and acceptance criteria that will be achieved to demonstrate that specified CMC changes do not adversely affect the product [32].

It is important to note that the submission of a comparability protocol is a prospective approach. That is, the protocol with tests and acceptance criteria, including specifications, must be submitted even before the testing has begun. It is a protocol alone. It is more important in this effort to select the most appropriate analytical methods to be used. There are a number of advantages of this approach. Once the protocol is approved by the FDA, as a prior approval supplement, it can lower the type of biologics license supplement category. For example if the manufacturing change would need to be reported as a prior approval supplement, the approval of a comparability protocol could reduce that category to a changes being effected in 30 days (CBE30). Similarly a CBE30 could be reduced to reporting through an annual report. In addition the FDA, having approved a specific protocol, is less likely to ask questions that might delay final implementation.

The FDA has provided two separate guidances for submitting comparability protocols. One guidance is provided for therapeutic recombinant DNA-derived protein products, naturally derived protein products, plasma derivatives, vaccines, allergenics, and therapeutic DNA plasmids. This guidance also applies to new drug applications (NDAs), abbreviated new drug applications (ANDAs), or supplements to these applications for protein drug products, and peptide products that cannot be fully characterized (e.g., complex mixture of small peptides) [33]. Guidance is also available that addresses changes for comparability protocols that would be submitted in NDAs, ANDAs, or supplements to these applications, except for applications for protein products [34].

8.7   CONCLUSION

The demonstration of comparability has been addressed nationally and internationally by several published regulatory guidance documents. It should be noted that the better a product is characterized, the easier it is to demonstrate that a new process produces a comparable product. Importantly, the most relevant knowledge base for the physicochemical and biological characteristics of the product rests with the manufacturer. It is this specific knowledge that is paramount in developing the essential tests to use in the comparability exercise. As changes in manufacturing are inevitable, it is critical to retain material from certain product batches in order to be able to compare materials from the process before and after manufacturing changes, using in-process materials at critical control points and at manufacturing steps that will be the most sensitive for molecular changes that could offer the most risk. A manufacturer considering a process change should evaluate the overall process and determine the need and reason for making the change. The change should be viewed as part of research and development until there are satisfactory results from the comparability exercise. Once the tests are identified, samples collected from both processes, analysis performed and conclusions drawn, it will be possible to implement a well-documented manufacturing improvement.

REFERENCES

1. Pharmaceutical cGMPs for the 21st Century—A Risk-Based Approach Final Report, 2004. www.fda.gov/cder/gmp/gmp2004/GMP_finalreport2004.htm
2. Guidance for Industry, Quality Systems Approach to Pharmaceutical CGMP Regulations, 2006. http://www.fda.gov/cder/guidance/7260fnl.htm
3. Process Analytical Technologies Initiative, 2008. http://www.fda.gov/cder/OPS/PAT. htm
4. Guidance for Industry PAT—A Framework for Innovative Pharmaceutical Development, Manufacturing, and Quality Assurance, 2004. http://www.fda.gov/cder/guidance/6419fnl.pdf
5. FDA Guidance Concerning Demonstration of Comparability of Human Biological Products, Including Therapeutic Biotechnology-derived Products, 1996. http://www.fda.gov/cder/Guidance/compare.htm
6. Gerrard T. Statement to the Committee on Oversight and Government Reform, Safe and Affordable Biotech Drugs—The Need for a Generic Pathway, 2007.
7. Guideline on Similar Biological Medicinal Products, 2005. http://www.emea.europa.eu/pdfs/human/biosimilar/043704en.pdf
8. Similar Biological Medicinal Products Containing Biotechnology-Derived Proteins as Active Substance: Quality Issues, 2006. http://www.emea.europa.eu/pdfs/human/biosimilar/4934805en.pdf

9. Similar Biological Medicinal Products Containing Biotechnology-Derived Proteins as Active Substance: Non-clinical and Clinical Issues, 2006. http://www.emea.europa.eu/pdfs/human/biosimilar/4283205en.pdf

10. Guideline on Comparability of Medicinal Products Containing Biotechnology-Derived Proteins as Active Substance: Quality Issues, 2003. http://www.emea.europa.eu/pdfs/human/bwp/320700en.pdf

11. Guideline on Comparability of Medicinal Products Containing Biotechnology-Derived Proteins as Active Substance: Non-clinical and Clinical Issues, 2004. http://www.emea.eu.int/pdfs/human/ewp/309702en.pdf

12. Annual report of the European Medicines Agency, 2006. http://www.emea.europa.eu/pdfs/general/direct/emeaar/EMEA_Annual_Report_2006_full.pdf

13. Tsang L, Beers D. Follow-on Biological Products: The Regulatory Minefield. *Life Sciences, Global Counsel Handbooks* 2004;105.

14. Comparability of Biotechnological/Biological Products Subject to Changes in Their Manufacturing Process, Q5E 2005. http://www.fda.gov/cder/guidance/6677fnl.htm

15. Mordenti J, Cavagnaro J, Green J. Design of biological equivalence programs for therapeutic biotechnology products in clinical development: A perspective. *Phar Res* 1996;13:1427.

16. Guidance for Industry Q1A(R2). Stability Testing of New Drug Substances and Products, 2003. http://www.fda.gov/cder/guidance/5635fnl.htm

17. Swit M. Reg Aff. Focus, Hurdles on the Scientific Path to a Biogeneric Approval, 2005;10:43.

18. Rosenberg A, Worobec A. Risk-based approach to immunogenicity concerns of therapeutic protein products. Part 3: Effects of manufacturing changes in immunogenicity and the utility of animal immunogenicity studies. *BioPharm Int* 2005; 17:34–42.

19. Guidance for Industry INDs—Approaches to Complying with CGMP during Phase 1, 2006. http://www.fda.gov/CDER/guidance/6164dft.htm

20. Guidance for Industry, Investigators, and Reviewers Exploratory IND Studies, 2006. http://www.fda.gov/cder/guidance/7086fnl.htm

21. Specifications: Test Procedures and Acceptance criteria for Biotechnological/Biological Products, Q6B, 1999. http://www.ich.org/LOB/media/MEDIA432.pdf

22. Comparability Studies for Human Plasma-Derived Therapeutics, Workshop transcript, 2002. http://www.emea.europa.eu/pdfs/general/direct/emeaar/EMEA_Annual_Report_2006_full.pdfhttp://www.fda.gov/cber/minutes/plasma053002.htm

23. Bunn HF. Drug-induced autoimmune red-cell aplasia. *N Engl J Med* 2002;346: 522–3.

24. Casadevall N, Nataf J, Viron B, Kolta A, Kiladjian JJ, Martin-Dupont P, Michaud P, Papo T, Ugo V, Teyssandier I, Varet B, Mayeux P. Pure red-cell aplasia and antierythropoietin antibodies in patients treated with recombinant erythropoietin. *N Engl J Med* 2002;346:469–75.

25. Gershon SK, Luksenburg H, Cote TR, Braun MM. Pure red-cell aplasia and recombinant erythropoietin. *N Engl J Med* 2002;346:1584–6.

26. Zehnder JL, Leung LL. Development of antibodies to thrombin and factor V with recurrent bleeding in a patient exposed to topical bovine thrombin 1990;76: 2011–6.

27. Rapaport SI, Zivelin A, Minow RA, et al. Clinical significance of antibodies to bovine and human thrombin and factor V after surgical use of bovine thrombin. *Am J Clin Pathol* 1992;97:84–91.

28. Lawson JH, Lynn KA, Vanmatre RM, et al. Antihuman factor V antibodies after use of relatively pure bovine thrombin. *Ann Thorac Surg* 2005;79:1037–8.

29. Josic D, Buchacher A, Kannicht C, et al. Degradation products of factor VIII which can lead to increased immunogenicity. *Vox Sang* 1995;77:90.

30. Rosendaial F, Nieuwenhuis H, van den Berg H, et al. A sudden increase in factor VIII inhibiter development in multitransfused hemophilia A patients in the Netherlands. Dutch Hemophilia study group. *Blood* 1993;81:2180–6.

31. Draft Guidance for Industry: Minimally Manipulated, Unrelated, Allogeneic Placental/Umbilical Cord Blood Intended for Hematopoietic Reconstitution in Patients with Hematological Malignancies, 2006. http://www.fda.gov/cber/gdlns/cordbld.pdf

32. Changes to an Approved Application for Specified Biotechnology and Specified Synthetic Biological Products, 1997. http://www.fda.gov/cber/gdlns/chbiosyn.pdf

33. Guidance for Industry Comparability Protocols—Protein Drug Products and Biological Products–Chemistry, Manufacturing, and Controls Information, 2003. http://www.fda.gov/cber/gdlns/protcmc.pdf.

34. Guidance for Industry Comparability Protocols—Chemistry, Manufacturing, and Controls Information, 2003. http://www.fda.gov/cber/gdlns/cmprprot.pdf

PART IV

SELECTION OF RELEVANT SPECIES

CHAPTER 9

Selection of Relevant Species

MEENA SUBRAMANYAM, PhD, NICOLA RINALDI, PhD,
ELISABETH MERTSCHING, PhD, and DAVID HUTTO, PhD, DVM

Contents

9.1 INTRODUCTION

The goal of biopharmaceutical development is to maximize therapeutic benefit while minimizing the risk of treatment-related toxicity. To mimic putative interpatient treatment differences in test article responsiveness, it is important

Preclinical Safety Evaluation of Biopharmaceuticals: A Science-Based Approach to Facilitating Clinical Trials, edited by Joy A. Cavagnaro
Copyright © 2008 by John Wiley & Sons, Inc.

not only to select a relevant species for conducting safety assessment studies but also to understand the rank order pharmacologic sensitivity of the relevant common laboratory animal species. The ICH S6 guidance defines a relevant species as "one in which the test material is pharmacologically active due to the expression of the receptor or an epitope (in the case of monoclonal antibodies)." The guidance discourages conduct of studies in nonrelevant species because of concerns about generation of misleading information. Animal studies are critical to demonstrate cross-reactivity of the biopharmaceutical not only with target tissues but with nontarget tissues as well, which in turn facilitates risk assessment in humans. Appropriate selection of a pharmacologically relevant species that is sensitive to administration of the biopharmaceutical in question will enable identification of factors that most reproducibly affect the therapeutic index. A thorough evidence-based evaluation of the species selection criteria must therefore be performed prior to conducting toxicity studies. The feasibility of conducting such studies in two relevant species as per current regulatory requirement should also be evaluated.

This chapter will discuss various experimental approaches used to select the relevant species for conduct of toxicology studies for biopharmaceuticals, as well as highlight advances made in scientific approaches and technologies to facilitate this process. Methods discussed include the traditional immunohistochemistry and tissue cross-reactivity studies, flow cytometry, protein sequencing, and functional in vitro assays, as well as newer approaches such as utilization of microarray databases for genomic mRNA expression data and use of transcript profiling studies as an adjunct to functional assays, to understand similarity in pharmacological responsiveness between animals and humans.

9.1.1   Species Selection: Biologics versus Small Molecule Therapies

The rationale and experimental means by which relevant and appropriate species are selected for preclinical safety evaluations are different when comparing biopharmaceuticals with small molecular, chemically synthesized therapeutics. Unlike protein therapeutics that remain in the extracellular space, small molecular entities may be widely distributed within the biophase, may accumulate intracellularly, and may be associated with "off-target" toxicities, that is, toxicities not associated with or attributable to the targeted receptor or biochemical pathway. Moreover these molecules are frequently subject to metabolic biotransformation to other chemical entities either through enzymatically mediated chemical reactions (phase 1 metabolism) or conjugation with other biomolecules (phase 2 metabolism) that may alter the distribution, excretion and, importantly, toxicity of the metabolite. Biodistributive and metabolic effects on a given small molecule may vary widely among animal species, including humans. Therefore the relevance of candidate animal species for preclinical safety evaluation of small molecular therapeutics is based primarily on comparisons of the so-called metabolite profile of a particular chemical drug in a range of the common rodent and nonrodent laboratory animals. The question being asked in that instance is, which species most closely resembles humans with regard to the identity, number, and quantity of metabolites produced when the chemical therapeutic is added to an ex vivo or in vivo system containing the necessary metabolic components? In contrast, protein-based therapeutics remain in the extracellular space and are not metabolized, and generally induce toxicities via their known mechanism of action, so-called exaggerated pharmacology. Thus selection of species for preclinical safety evaluation of biopharmaceuticals is based on demonstration of the pharmacologic effect in that animal species. This can be done in a variety of ways, as discussed in detail below.

Even if a species is considered relevant based on pharmacological activity of the test article, the many limitations of using animals to predict toxicity of biopharmaceuticals in humans should be recognized. These limitations include variability in the expression pattern of the target, inherent differences in protein processing and clearing mechanisms in animals, differences in immune system development and phenotypes of immune cells, as well as the potential immunogenicity of biopharmaceuticals. By designing appropriate studies and experiments to identify the relevant species for conduct of toxicology studies, the risk of missing a major safety signal can be mitigated. The approaches and examples described in this chapter to illustrate the use of specific methodologies in the selection of a relevant species were selected from a diverse pool of experiments performed during the nonclinical development of either immunoglobulin fusion protein therapeutics or humanized monoclonal antibody therapeutics.

9.1.2 General Considerations for Relevant Species Selection

Numerous experimental approaches can be employed to test the hypothesis that a given laboratory animal species is relevant to humans with respect to a biopharmaceutical and its known target and mechanism of action. While the number of available evaluation methods can be expected to increase with the discovery and deployment of new technologies, the current commonly used methods comprise a relatively short list that can be rank ordered based on the ability of these methods to generate scientifically compelling data. Figure 9.1 depicts a proposed impact-based rank ordering of common methods. Many of these methods will be discussed in greater detail in subsequent sections of this chapter.

In general, it is reasonable to conclude that the data sets considered to be most compelling are those derived from relatively intact biological systems (whole animal- or cellular-based systems) while less compelling data could be expected to be produced through the analysis of isolated molecules (in vitro assays or in silico analyses). Further, even though a particular method may provide superior and desired data regarding species relevance, all therapeutics may not be amenable for evaluation using a given method. For example, not all biopharmaceuticals elicit measurable changes in a qualified pharmacodynamic marker, nor can a given biopharmaceutical be expected to have the inherent biochemical properties needed to perform as a useful assay reagent.

In vivo pharmacodynamic effect (Figures 9.2–9.4, Table 9.1):
Detectable test article exposure results in expected changes in a cellular or molecular marker known to be affected by the pharmacologic action of the drug, preferably proximate to the therapeutic mechanism. Pharmacologic sensitivity relative to humans is estimated.

In vivo interaction with known target:
Radio- or fluorophore-labeled test article is shown to bind to or impact expected target tissues / cells in vivo in the test species (whole body imaging).

Ex vivo biologic effect (Figures 9.5, 9.6):
Primary cells from the test species are shown to be altered by test article exposure in a manner known to be effected by the impacted signaling pathway (alteration of qualified gene products of affected pathway)

Presence and distribution of receptor in predicted tissues (Table 9.2):
Complete tissue sets are interrogated by molecular methods (IHC, ISH, northerns) to demonstrate the presence of putative biopharmaceutical target or ligand–receptor pairs. Tissue distribution patterns are compared between proposed test species and humans.

Ex vivo / in vitro interaction with known target (Figures 9.7, 9.8):
Labeled test article is shown to bind to or impact expected target tissue/cell ex vivo in tissues or cells of the test species (flow cytometry, tissue binding, etc.)

In vitro binding (Figure 9.9):
Immunoassays or other receptor binding assay formats demonstrate binding of test article to test species target. Quantitative binding data (affinity) is compared to human.

Transcript profiling (Figure 9.10):
Ex vivo (selected tissues from animals) or in vitro (using primary or transformed cells) analysis of mRNA changes effected by test article administration.

In silico analysis (Figure 9.11, Tables 9.3, 9.4):
Computational analysis of sequence homology of target between species, or electronic Northern blot examining target expression across tissues.

Figure 9.1 Proposed rank ordering of methods informing species selection for safety assessment of biopharmaceuticals. Various methods used for selecting pharmacologically relevant species for toxicological studies of biopharmaceuticals are presented, ordered (*top to bottom*) by the extent to which the data might impact the decision on which species to use. In cases where the methods are further discussed in this chapter, the relevant figure/table numbers are provided. These types of analyses may also be used for creating data packages for small molecules, although not typically for species selection.

As in all other areas of scientific inquiry, if one can interpret collected data, there is often value added in the collection of relevant data beyond that considered sufficiently compelling. It is also within the realm of possibility that the described methods for assessing species relevance may provide conflicting data. In such an instance, preference would be given to data derived from the higher order, intact biopharmaceutical systems.

The remainder of this chapter discusses the various methods in the order presented in Figure 9.1. However, this may not necessarily be the order in which the experiments are performed, as in silico and in vitro assays for an initial examination of species relevance may be easier and less costly to perform, and therefore worth completing prior to the more time-consuming and expensive in vivo assessments.

9.2 IN VIVO PHARMACODYNAMIC EFFECTS

The strongest line of evidence for selecting a pharmacologically responsive species will be the demonstration of similar pharmacodynamic effect across species, utilizing molecular markers reflective of the test article response. In cases where there is a known molecular marker of the test article effect in humans, illustration of a similar change in that marker in nonclinical species under consideration lends confidence to the selection of that species. This is particularly true if the marker is related to the mechanism of action (MOA). For novel molecules, markers of effect on the pathway could serve to demonstrate the desired effect (or lack thereof) of the novel molecule in species under evaluation for relevance. Apart from serving as reporters of the biopharmaceutical's activity to aid in species selection, pharmacodynamic markers also may assist in optimizing dose and frequency of administration, and in the understanding of the relationship between exposure (pharmacokinetics) and efficacy or safety.

One example in which clinical markers of exposure to a specific cytokine have been well studied is the upregulation of interferon-responsive genes and proteins upon administration of interferon-β (IFNβ). Clinical studies have demonstrated that serum neopterin levels (among others) are induced three- to fivefold by administration of interferon-β preparations, with a peak level reached at 24 to 48 hours after treatment [1,2,3]. A similar upregulation, in terms of both fold induction and timing of the induction, has also been observed in rhesus macaques (Figure 9.2). Neopterin, a catabolic product of guanosine triphosphate, is synthesized by macrophages upon stimulation by interferons, and is a marker of activation of cellular immunity. Based on the in vivo pharmacodynamic activity data, the rhesus monkey is considered an appropriate pharmacologically responsive species for toxicological evaluation of IFNβ.

Another molecular marker reflective of the pharmacological mode of the biopharmaceutical's action, and one that translated from rodent models to nonhuman primates and humans, was the reduction in the level of circulating

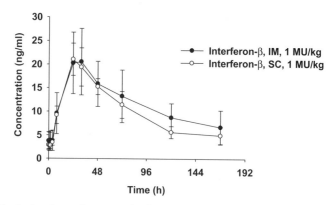

Figure 9.2 Induction of neopterin by administration of interferon-β to rhesus macaques. Mean neopterin concentration after a single dose administration of interferon-β in rhesus monkeys. Concentration over time profile plotted from animals treated IM (*closed circles*) or SC (*open circles*). MU = megaunits (=5 mcg/kg)

peripheral blood lymphocytes after administration of an immunoglobulin fusion protein. The fusion protein was designed to bind to a cell surface receptor expressed on lymphocytes and co-engage Fc_γ receptors expressed on antigen-presenting cells. The proposed mode of action of the therapeutic was the lysis of test article-bound target cells through the mediation of antibody-dependent cellular cytotoxicity like reaction by Fc_γ receptor-expressing cells.

In a chronic toxicity study conducted in 36 naive cynomolgus monkeys, the test article was administered weekly via intravenous injection for 12 months. The study comprised one control group and two test article-treated groups. Peripheral blood from the study animals was subject to flow cytometry analysis to determine the lymphocyte levels (counts/μl) in dosed animals compared to baseline. The percent change from pre-dose baseline and range for absolute lymphocytes and T cell subsets at week 52 are shown in Table 9.1. The absolute lymphocyte counts as well as counts of T cell subsets including $CD2^+$, $CD3^+$, $CD4^+$, and $CD8^+$ T cells were reduced in a dose-dependent manner following the administration of the test article, confirming test article exposure as well as pharmacologic activity.

The effect of a single course of weekly test article or placebo treatment was then studied in the patient population for a period of 12 weeks. The data on circulating lymphocyte levels were aggregated for the treatment group and compared to the placebo. Both groups had comparable total lymphocyte counts at baseline. There was approximately 39% reduction in total lymphocyte counts in the test article treated group over the course of treatment, although total lymphocyte count remained above the lower limit of normal throughout this time. The placebo group showed a stable profile over time (Figure 9.3).

TABLE 9.1   Mean reductions (range) in lymphocytes and T cell subsets in cynomolgus monkeys

Dose Group	Total Lymphs (%)	CD2$^+$ T Cells (%)	CD3$^+$ T Cells (%)	CD4$^+$ T Cells (%)	CD8$^+$ T Cells (%)
Saline	+34 (−6 to +187)	+38 (−3 to +163)	+43 (−12 to +176)	+42 (−15 to +175)	+48 (−8 to +171)
Test article dose level-1	−21 (−69 to +35)	−27 (−80 to +69)	−35 (−82 to +66)	−40 (−85 to +52)	−28 (−80 to +88)
Test article dose level-2	−46 (−66 to −15)	−63 (−79 to −41)	−75 (−94 to −31)	−85 (−98 to −34)	−64 (−89 to −27)

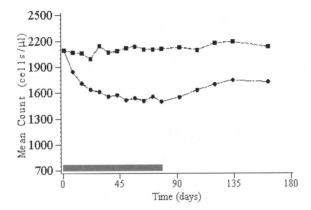

Figure 9.3   Mean total lymphocyte count after one course of treatment. Peripheral blood was collected from individuals administered test article (circles) or placebo (squares) on a weekly basis, and subject to flow cytometry analysis to determine mean lymphocyte counts. A standard panel of fluorochrome-conjugated antibodies was used to identify the various lymphocyte sub populations. The solid bar indicates the dosing interval.

Figure 9.4*a* and 9.4*b* provides a detailed analysis of the test article's effect on the CD4 and CD8 T lymphocyte populations, respectively. The CD4 counts showed a 47% reduction from baseline in the treatment group (circles, Figure 9.4*a*) and the CD8 counts showed a 53% reduction from baseline in the treatment group (circles, Figure 9.4*b*). The placebo group (squares, Figure 9.4*a* and 9.4*b*) showed a stable profile over time.

Overall, the pharmacodynamic effects of the test article exposure were qualitatively consistent between the cynomolgus monkeys and humans, confirming the similarity in the pharmacological activity of the test article.

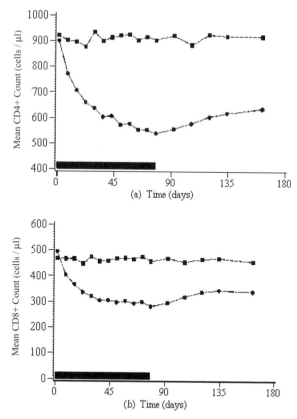

Figure 9.4 Mean T cell count after one course of treatment. Peripheral blood was collected from individuals administered test article (*circles*) or placebo (*squares*) on a weekly basis and stained for the presence of CD4 (*a*) or CD8 (*b*) lymphocytes using specific antibodies conjugated to fluorochromes. Samples were then analyzed on the flow cytometer to determine mean relative counts of each subpopulation of cells. The solid bar indicates the dosing interval.

9.3   EX VIVO BIOLOGICAL EFFECT

The practice of demonstrating functional activity of the therapeutic in the selected species is critical, as binding to the desired target does not always translate to functional receptor activation. Since the toxicity observed with biopharmaceuticals is most likely due to exaggerated pharmacology, it is necessary to confirm that the downstream effects observed upon binding of the test article to the target proteins are similar between humans and the selected species. For example, if the test article stimulates activation of subsets of T lymphocytes in humans with a specific activation profile, it is important that this function is conserved in the species selected for performing toxicology studies. Similarly a test article such as an immunoglobulin fusion protein may mediate antibody-dependent cellular cytotoxicity (ADCC) or complement-dependent cytotoxicity (CDC). Such activities can impact the overall toxicology assessments as they may be integrally linked to the MOA of the therapeutic. For well-characterized targets, information on their function in different species may be readily available in the literature. If the target protein is novel, however, its function will have to be characterized in pharmacology studies to determine the key biochemical drivers for test article activity.

9.3.1 Fixed Endpoint Assays

Endpoint assays such as proliferation or cytotoxicity assays are routinely used for functional assessments. For these assessments, primary cells, transformed cells, or cells transfected with the target receptor are exposed to range of concentrations of the test article. Proliferation or cytoxicity is then measured using a variety of methods such as crystal violet vital dye staining, MTT/MTS incorporation, or a luminescence readout like ATP lite. In addition, assays that analyze phosphorylation of specific transcription factors, or release of specific cytokines and chemokines, are also common. Figure 9.5 illustrates the measure of functional consequences of receptor–test article interaction by quantifying cytokine release. Cells from the species under evaluation were cultured in the presence of serial dilutions of the test article or control reagents, and supernatants harvested for determination of cytokine levels by ELISA (i.e.,

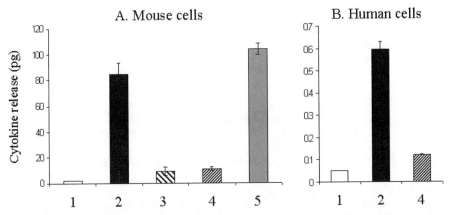

Figure 9.5 Inhibition of cytokine release in mouse and human cells. Mouse cells (*a*) and human cells (*b*) were stimulated in vitro with an antireceptor antibody and cytokine release was measured in the supernatant (in pg per million cells). Cytokine release was quantified in the supernatants of unactivated cells (bar 1), activated cells without biopharmaceutical Y (bar 2), and activated cells incubated with biopharmaceutical Y at 5 μg/ml (bar 3) or 10 μg/ml (bar 4). As a negative control, cells were exposed to an irrelevant fusion protein (bar 5).

enzyme-linked immunosorbent assay). Human and mouse cells were activated by cross-linking the receptor of interest using a specific antibody in the presence or absence of the test article, biopharmaceutical Y. Spontaneous cytokine release from unactivated cells was very low (Figure 9.5a and 9.5b, bar 1). In the absence of biopharmaceutical Y, stimulation of mouse and human cells resulted in the release of an expected cytokine (Figure 9.5a and 9.5b, bar 2). In the presence of biopharmaceutical Y, the production of the cytokine was strongly inhibited in both human and mouse cells (Figure 9.5a, bar 3 and 4; Figure 9.5b, bar 4). Release of the cytokine, however, was not inhibited when an irrelevant protein was used (Figure 9.5a, bar 5). Although the amounts of cytokine released by the human and mouse cells were substantially different, the inhibitory effect of biopharmaceutical Y was similar between the cell types. These results indicated that the test article was equally effective in blocking cytokine release mediated by target receptor activation in vitro in mouse and human cells.

9.3.2 Signaling Assays

Another approach to studying the similarities and differences in the pharmacology of the test article in species of interest involves the characterization of the signaling cascade downstream of the protein of interest. Signaling experiments, albeit more challenging, have the advantage of providing more clarity on the putative MOA of the test article. Binding of the test article to the target receptor may result in activation of kinases or other key transcription factors. In the example shown in Figure 9.6, the ability of biopharmaceutical Y to block signaling mediated through the target receptor was studied. Activation of the

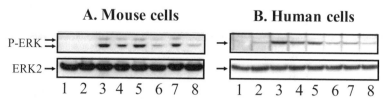

Figure 9.6 Effect of a fusion protein on ERK phosphorylation in activated mouse and human cells. Mouse bone marrow cells (*a*) and human cord blood cells (*b*) were activated with antireceptor Ab for 5, 10, and 15 minutes, lysed, and the total proteins loaded on a SDS-Page gel. After transfer to a membrane, ERK phosphorylation was detected using antibodies specific for the phosphorylated (active, P-ERK) form of ERK (upper blots). As a control for the amount of ERK in the samples, antibodies specific for total ERK (activated and nonactivated forms) were used (lower blots). Unstimulated cells untreated (lane 1) and treated with biopharmaceutical Y (lane 2) were used as controls. Cells were activated for 5 minutes (lanes 3, 4), 10 minutes (lanes 5, 6), or 15 minutes (lanes 7, 8) in the absence (lanes 3, 5, 7) or presence (lanes 4, 6, 8) of biopharmaceutical Y.

kinase protein ERK by phosphorylation was determined after stimulation of mouse and human cells. Presence of phosphorylated ERK and total ERK (phosphorylated and unphosphorylated) was detected using specific antibodies. As shown below, ERK phosphorylation was low in unstimulated mouse and human cells (Figure 9.6a and 9.6b, lane 1). Upon activation with antireceptor antibodies in the absence of biopharmaceutical Y, ERK phosphorylation was induced (Figure 9.6a and 9.6b, lanes 3, 5, 7). Pre-incubation of cells with the test article decreased activation-mediated phosphorylation of ERK at all time points in mouse and human cells (Figure 9.6a and 9.6b, lanes 4, 6, 8 compared to lanes 3, 5, 7 respectively).

Collectively, the results from the functional experiments illustrated in Figures 9.5 and 9.6 suggested that from a pharmacological perspective, the mouse was a relevant species for evaluating the toxicity of the test article.

9.4   PRESENCE AND DISTRIBUTION OF RECEPTOR IN PREDICTED TISSUES

In the area of relevant species identification, the objectives of immuno-histochemistry and tissue-binding studies (often referred to as tissue cross-reactivity studies) are to evaluate the relevance of a given species for use in toxicity studies with a biopharmaceutical and to identify expected and unexpected tissue binding of therapeutics in human and animal tissues.

Immunohistochemical methods can be used to evaluate the tissue distribution of the biopharmaceutical's target(s) or the tissue distribution of other relevant molecular components of a targeted biochemical pathway. A comparison of the distribution of these molecules between possible test species and humans often provides valuable information on the similarities or differences of tissue expression of molecules targeted by the test article between the queried species. The general expectation is to perform tissue cross-reactivity studies prior to human exposure to the new therapeutic. The purpose of these studies is to demonstrate, to the extent possible, what tissues and cells the intact biopharmaceutical binds to. Since monoclonal antibodies and other molecules containing an Fc region or additional binding sites may bind to more than one target, these experiments report localization of the test article to a tissue or cell irrespective of the known or expected binding mechanism. For therapeutic antibodies, the FDA recommends a comprehensive tissue cross-reactivity evaluation as defined in Points to Consider in the Manufacture and Testing of Monoclonal Antibody Products for Human Use (Docket No. 94D-0259). This document recommends conducting immunohistochemistry analysis at two antibody dilutions across triplicate specimens of approximately 32 frozen human tissue types (collected from three unrelated donors) for the therapeutic antibody and its isotype control. An analogous study is conducted in parallel in tissues from various animal species (two or three unrelated donors) for additional justification of the relevance of the toxicity species.

While this has been standard practice for a number of years, product developers have recently started questioning the relevance and utility of these types of studies for predicting human safety.

When test articles are chimeric, humanized, or fully human antibodies, three different staining methods can be used. These include avidin-biotin complex (when the test article is biotinylated), direct labeling of test article with fluorochromes such as fluorescein isothiocyanate (FITC) or rhodamine, or precomplexing the unlabeled test article with a labeled antihuman IgG. The latter method is most often used, as it allows secondary signal amplification by a variety of methods and, by precomplexing, avoids nonspecific binding of the secondary antihuman antibody to human antibodies that are present in the evaluated human tissue sections. It is also performed in instances where conjugation of biotin or a fluorochrome onto the test article could alter its affinity for the protein of interest. Even though this additional step often increases the backgound staining, the indirect approach has the advantage of amplifying the signal, and is therefore valuable when expression of the target protein is expected to be relatively low in tissues of interest.

For all test articles an isotype control antibody labeled in a similar fashion must be included to demonstrate specificity of staining observed with the test article. As with any assay procedure, both positive (containing cell types that express the target at high levels) and negative control tissues should be stained to assess extent of nonspecific binding under standardized immunohistochemical conditions. In general, the positive control may be a tissue element or cell line transfected with or known to express the target antigen, sepharose or agarose beads coated with the target antigen, or the target antigen spotted and cross-linked onto UV-resin slides. During optimization of the staining procedure the reactions of the test article with the positive control but not the negative control, as well as the lack of reactivity of the isotype control antibody, should be confirmed, to demonstrate the sensitivity, specificity, and reproducibility of the assay. A board-certified anatomical pathologist usually performs analysis of the immunolabeled tissues using a scoring system that assesses the identity and relative proportion of cells staining within a given immunopositive tissue, the relative intensity of staining, and the location (cytoplasm vs. cell surface) of staining. The slides are evaluated for integrity of the tissue sample as well as for specificity of the staining seen in the tissues based on knowledge of expression of the target antigen in question. For the reasons mentioned above, a biopharmaceutical known to have acceptable potency and binding affinity to its target may not perform well in a tissue-binding study. There are numerous examples of highly potent monoclonal antibodies that have been completely negative in tissue-binding studies, due to their poor performance as immunohistochemical reagents.

An example of results from a tissue cross-reactivity study comparing binding of a monoclonal antibody therapeutic to human, cynomolgus monkey, and mouse tissues is shown in Table 9.2. A cell line that did not express the target was used as negative control tissue; the same cell line transfected with the

TABLE 9.2   Cross-species tissue cross-reactivity study of a monoclonal antibody

Tissue	Cell Type	Human	Cynomolgus Monkey	Mouse
Urinary bladder	Urothelium	2 (3–4)	3 (3)	NS
Ureter	Urothelium	2 (3–4)	3 (2–4)	NA
Tonsil	Mucosal epithelium	3 (2–3)	3 (2–3)	NA
Uterus-cervix	Mucosa	3 (1–3)	1 (2)	NA
Eye	Corneal epithelium	1 (1)	NS	1 (1)[a]
Breast	Glandular epithelium	3 (1–3)	3 (1–3)	NS
Fallopian tube	Tubular epithelium	2 (1–2)	1 (3)	NS
Kidney	Tubular epithelium–cortex	3 (3)	1 (3)[b]	3 (1–2)
Lung	Alveolar epithelium	3 (2–3)	2 (3)	NS
Pancreas	Ductular epithelium	3 (2)	2 (1–2)	2 (1)
Prostate	Glandular epithelium	2 (1–2)	1 (2)	3 (2)[c]
Thyroid	Follicular epithelium	3 (2–3)	2 (2)	NS
Uterus-endometrium	Endometrial mucosa	2 (2)	NS	3 (1–3)[d]
Adrenal	Cortical epithelium	3 (1–2)	2 (1)	NS
Pituitary	Adenohypophysis epithelium	3 (2)	NS	NS
Liver	Sinusoidal mesenchymal cells	3 (2–4)	3 (2–3)	NS

Note: Cryosections of normal human, cynomolgus monkey, and mouse tissues listed (in addition to others) were obtained and stained with biotinylated test article. Data are shown for the optimal antibody concentration; the second concentration used was 5× higher (data not shown). The cell types that demonstrated staining are listed, along with the number (out of three) of sections that showed staining, with the staining intensity range in parentheses. 1 = Light staining or occasional cells stained—minimal. 2 = Light-medium staining and/or small numbers of cells/types of cells labeled—mild. 3 = Moderate staining and/or medium numbers of cells/types of cells labeled—moderate. 4 = Dark staining and/or large numbers of cells/types of cells labeled—marked. NS: No staining seen. NA: Tissue section not obtained.
[a]Lens fiber stained, not corneal epithelium.
[b]Tubular epithelium staining in papilla, not cortex.
[c]Tubular epithelium and intertubal stroma showed staining.
[d]Smooth muscle cells were also stained.

target was used as a positive tissue. Tissues were sectioned, frozen, and treated with avidin, biotin, and nonspecific IgG to block endogenous binding sites. Two concentrations of biotinylated test article (or control antibody) were applied to the tissue sections, followed by streptavidin HRP and substrate. After drying, the slides were read by a pathologist. Adequacy of tissues for staining was validated using an anti-CD31 (platelet endothelial cell adhesion molecule) antibody as positive control, and an isotype matched irrelevant antibody as a negative control. Semiquantitative results are shown in Table 9.2. Qualitatively, the pathologist determined that based on the staining intensity and localization of staining, the cynomolgus monkey, and human tissue samples showed a high degree of similarity in binding the test article, whereas only a few of the murine tissues were stained. Therefore a murine version of the antibody was used for mouse efficacy and toxicity studies, but the humanized antibody was used in the toxicology studies in the cynomolgus monkey.

9.5 EX VIVO / IN VITRO INTERACTION OF THE BIOPHARMACEUTICAL WITH KNOWN TARGET

To demonstrate functional pharmacological similarities between humans and the animal species under evaluation, biological assay systems are routinely utilized. In some instances primary cells expressing the target are utilized in these functional experiments. In most cases, however, cell lines containing the appropriate signaling machinery are transfected with the related cell-surface receptor from the test species. Specificity of interaction of test article to target is demonstrated initially through binding assays and then extended to other qualified endpoints such as phosphorylation or nuclear translocation of relevant proteins in the signaling cascade.

9.5.1 Binding Assays: Flow Cytometry Based Methods

Flow cytometry based assays are routinely utilized to measure binding of bio-therapeutics to various target cells (peripheral blood lymphocytes, bone marrow derived cells) from multiple species. This analysis can provide insight into the types of cells that the biopharmaceutical can bind, as well as the relative number of receptors on the cells. In instances where the target acts by dimerizing or trimerizing with signaling partners, it is important to determine whether the affinity of binding and the binding partners are similar between species. Flow-based methods require appropriate positive and negative controls, as well as an isotype control or irrelevant protein control to rule out nonspecific binding. Besides primary cells, binding assays can also be performed with cells transfected with proteins of interest or with cultured commercially available cells from various species, provided that the target receptor is expressed on the cell types.

The flow cytometry experiments described below outline a series of experiments conducted with primary cells collected from various species to determine the ability of a human biopharmaceutical (X) to bind in vitro to the target protein in these species. Figure 9.7 illustrates a flow cytometry assay conducted using murine bone marrow derived cells expressing the murine homologue of the biopharmaceutical's target receptor. The ligand for the target human receptor was used as a positive control in the assay, as an antibody to directly stain the murine homologue was not available. Fluorochrome conjugated secondary antibodies specific for the test article were used as detection agents. As shown in Figure 9.7a, biopharmaceutical X did not bind to the receptor expressed on mouse bone marrow derived cells. The human ligand also did not bind to the mouse receptor. Figure 9.7b illustrates an independent experiment performed using the murine version of biopharmaceuti-

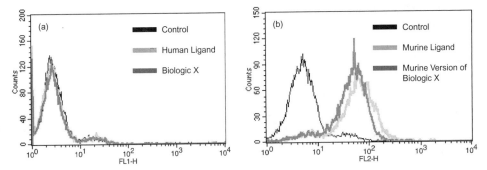

Figure 9.7   Evaluation of biopharmaceutical X binding to mouse bone marrow derived cells. (*a*) Biopharmaceutical X binding to mouse bone marrow-derived cells was evaluated using flow cytometry. Mouse cells were incubated with biopharmaceutical X or the human ligand. Secondary antibodies that cross-reacted with both biopharmaceutical X and the natural human ligand were used to detect binding. Cells were stained with the secondary antibodies only, to detect non-specific binding (control). (*b*) Bone marrow derived mouse cells were stained as described above with a murine version of biopharmaceutical X and the murine ligand for the receptor. Secondary antibodies that cross-reacted with the murine version of biopharmaceutical X and the murine ligand were used to detect binding. See color insert.

cal X and the natural ligand for the mouse receptor as the positive control. As expected, the murine version of biopharmaceutical X and the murine ligand bound to mouse cells, thereby confirming the expression of the target receptor. These results indicated that biopharmaceutical X did not cross-react with murine receptors and therefore the mouse was not a suitable species for conduct of toxicology studies.

Receptor-ligand binding assays with biopharmaceutical X were then performed on cynomolgus monkey peripheral blood cells. Cells were incubated first with the test article, and then with antibodies specific for the target receptor. Binding of biopharmaceutical X did not interfere with binding of the antibody, as the two molecules interacted with distinct epitopes on the target protein. As shown in Figure 9.8 (left panel), presence of cells in the upper-right quadrant in the plot demonstrated that all the cynomolgus cells that stained with the antireceptor antibody (*X*-axis) had also bound the human ligand (*Y*-axis). Figure 9.8 (right panel) shows the binding pattern of biopharmaceutical X to the cynomolgus cells. Presence of a large population of cells in the upper-right quadrant indicated that the test article bound to the same subset of cells that stained positively with the antireceptor antibody. The test article, however, also exhibited nonspecific binding to cells that did not show reactivity with the ligand or the antireceptor antibody.

The in vitro binding data shown in Figures 9.7 and 9.8 supported the selection of the cynomolgus monkey over mice as a relevant species for conduct of toxicology studies for biopharmaceutical X.

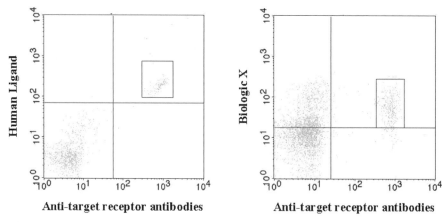

Figure 9.8 Evaluation of binding of biopharmaceutical X to cynomolgus monkey peripheral blood cells. Cynomolgus monkey cells were stained with fluorochrome-labeled biopharmaceutical X or the natural ligand for the human receptor. Expression of the target receptor on the cynomolgus cells was detected using antibodies specific for the target receptor.

9.5.2 In vitro Binding Affinity Determination

Besides qualitative determination of binding to the target receptor, more specific dose–response studies and binding affinity measurements can be performed to confirm selection of appropriate species. This determination may be necessary for agonist therapeutics for which the affinity and avidity of binding determine the strength of the signal induced. In the example illustrated in Figure 9.9, the affinity of binding of a humanized monoclonal antibody (MAb) therapeutic to cultured fibroblasts from humans and cynomolgus monkeys was compared. Various concentrations of the humanized MAb were added to the cells. Background binding was determined using an isotype control antibody.

The functional affinities of the humanized antibody for the target protein on human and cynomolgous cells were computed to be 0.05 and 0.03 nM, respectively. These results indicated that the humanized MAb bound with similar affinity to the target receptor on human and cynomolgus cells.

9.6 TRANSCRIPT PROFILING

Another approach, taking advantage of recent technological developments, is to determine the similarity of the pharmacological responsiveness between species through the conduct of a transcript-profiling study. This will typically be performed using either primary cells or transformed cell lines, with primary cells being preferable due to the greater relevance to the in vivo scenario. Cells

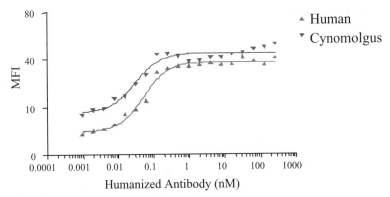

Figure 9.9 Affinity of binding of a humanized antibody to cultured human and cyno-molgus fibroblast cells. Cultured human (triangles) and cynomolgus fibroblast (upside-down triangles) cells were removed from the flasks by trypsin and washed with PBS. One million cells were incubated with various concentrations of humanized Ab, at 4°C for 2 hours. The cells were washed, and binding was detected with PE-conjugated goat antihuman IgG using a FACSCalibur flow cytometer. The binding of another human-ized Ab of the same isotype as the test article, but with irrelevant specificity, was used as an isotype control (data not shown). The mean fluorescence intensities (MFI) for each sample were plotted against the antibody concentration.

from the likely target organ(s) from different species can be exposed to the test article, then mRNA purified from the cells, and gene expression studies performed using microarrays. Commercially available microarrays exist for many of the species commonly used for toxicological studies, including mice, rats, dogs, and rhesus and cynomolgus monkeys. If pharmacological markers are already known from prior research, up- or downregulation of those markers can be confirmed in the additional species being assessed. In addition the overall overlap in gene expression response can be compared between species (taking into account the overlap between genes assayed on the microarray). Ideally the most relevant species would show similarly high up- or downregu-lation of prior known pharmacological markers, and of additional biologically relevant genes that are significantly changed. Further a high overall gene expression response similarity indicating that analogous pathways are affected across species is desirable. A gene ontology analysis can be performed for each species, where the functions of up- or downregulated genes are evaluated to determine whether, in general, the same biological functions are affected. The changed genes can also be classified as belonging to known biological path-ways, to determine whether there are any pathways that are affected in one species and not others.

In the preclinical development of biopharmaceuticals, restricted species cross-reactivity may limit the species in which toxicology evaluations can be performed. In higher order species such as chimpanzees, very limited safety data can be derived as organ and tissue collection is not feasible for detailed analysis and sufficient numbers of animals may not be available for chronic toxicity testing. In order to support extended clinical dosing, and to provide a more comprehensive safety assessment, a surrogate (or homolog) approach can be used. A surrogate of the therapeutic that interacts with rodent or other nonhuman primate species can be utilized in the conduct of toxicology studies, as long as similarity in in vitro and in vivo pharmacology is demonstrated. In the example described below, a surrogate of a humanized MAb therapeutic was evaluated for pharmacological similarity, due to restricted species cross-reactivity of the therapeutic. A transcript profiling experiment, besides additional studies, was performed, to demonstrate the similarity in the in vitro pharmacological effect of the biopharmaceutical and the surrogate antibody.

Transcript profiling was used to determine whether similar transcripts were induced or repressed when three cell lines (colon carcinoma cell line, primary endothelial cells, and primary fibroblasts) were treated with the MAb (biopharmaceutical Z) or the surrogate antibody. Cells were grown to confluence, and treated with a fixed dose of cytokine plus vehicle, or cytokine plus biopharmaceutical Z, surrogate antibody, nonspecific antibody control, or positive control. The cytokine was used in order to amplify the activation response through the target receptor. Cells were lysed after two hours of treatment, and transcript profiling was performed using the human HG-U133 Plus 2.0 Affymetrix® GeneChips®.

Initial analysis confirmed that the cell lines were responsive to treatment, as the positive control caused up- or downregulation of genes to approximately the same extent across all three cell lines. Biopharmaceutical Z and the surrogate antibody caused specific changes (after the effect of the nonspecific control was removed) to the same extent in the three cell lines, although the effects were not nearly as significant as with the positive control. In addition biopharmaceutical Z was known to upregulate expression of several cytokines; this upregulation was confirmed in the three cell lines examined, and a similar magnitude of upregulation was seen using the surrogate antibody. Next genes that were selected as meeting statistical cutoffs in the biopharmaceutical Z treated samples, and in the surrogate treated samples, were compared between the two treatments (Figure 9.10). These graphs illustrate that the overall magnitude of intensity and ratios were highly similar between the two treatments. In addition treatment with biopharmaceutical Z (and the surrogate antibody, data not shown) showed similar up- or downregulation as treatment with the positive control, although selected transcripts were upregulated to a greater degree by the positive control. Finally, gene ontology analysis found very similar biological functions affected by biopharmaceutical Z and the surrogate antibody, and differences were overwhelmingly due to transcripts in one treatment or the other barely failing to meet statistical cutoffs.

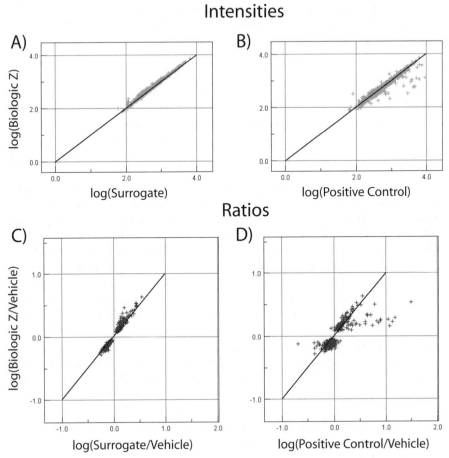

Figure 9.10 Comparison of signal intensities and ratios between treatments. Signal intensities (*a, b*) and ratios (*c, d*), comparing transcripts meeting significance cutoffs for biopharmaceutical Z with the surrogate antibody (*a, c*) and the positive control (*b, d*). Identical intensities or ratios will fall on the 1 : 1 diagonal line. The overall pattern of signal intensities and ratios was highly similar between biopharmaceutical Z and the surrogate antibody, with marginally higher intensities/ratios following treatment with biopharmaceutical Z. The positive control upregulated a set of transcripts to a higher degree than biopharmaceutical Z; these fall to the right of the 1:1 diagonal line.

9.7 IN SILICO ANALYSIS

9.7.1 Sequence Homology of Target Protein in Various Species

Another question to address is the likelihood of the biopharmaceutical candidate binding to the target protein in the animal species being examined for relevance. A convenient and commonly used approach to investigate this is to determine the sequence homology of the target protein between humans and the selected species. When a protein shares a high degree of homology across species, the probability of the test article binding to the protein across species is high. The implicit assumption when sequences are highly similar across species is that there is a shared commonality of function such as similar pharmacological function. Reciprocally, protein sequences in other species that share little or low homology to their human counterpart are less likely to bind a biopharmaceutical candidate targeted to the human protein. However, like all experimental methods, demonstration of sequence identity or similarity between species has limitations, as the relative importance of each amino acid in the sequence is not equivalent and is complicated to assess. For example, amino acids directly involved in the binding of the test article must be conserved across species, as well as those involved in the maintenance of the secondary and tertiary structure of the protein. This method will therefore provide a definitive answer only for proteins with sequences that are totally homologous to the human sequence, and only for those proteins that function as monomers. In all other cases determination of percent sequence homology will facilitate identification of those species that have the highest probability of binding the test article. Follow on in vitro binding assays will be needed to confirm these results. Figure 9.11 illustrates the protein sequence homology of $Fc_\varepsilon RI$-alpha chain across a range of species and Table 9.3 summarizes the percent sequence homology across species.

The homology of the macaque's (cynomolgus and rhesus) protein sequences to the human sequence was over 90%. In contrast, dog, rat, and mouse sequences shared low homology with the human $Fc_\varepsilon RI$-alpha protein. Based on these results, the receptor of nonhuman primates would be more likely to bind a biopharmaceutical designed to interact with the human $Fc_\varepsilon RI$-alpha chain. This conclusion, however, would have to be confirmed in additional in vitro binding assays.

9.7.2 Utilization of Microarray Data

In addition to the standard methods for determining the pattern of target expression, the availability of genomic mRNA expression data allows for in silico experiments. Since the advent of microarray technology in the mid-1990s [4,5,6], hundreds of thousands of mRNA samples have been tested on microarrays. Data have been generated from normal and diseased tissues of many species. Many of the datasets associated with published literature are publicly available; in addition private companies provide such data for a fee. The relative level of expression of genes in the targeted pathway, or of the gene targeted by a monoclonal antibody, can then be assessed across multiple tissue types, in diseased tissues, or in disease models. The expression pattern in potential species for preclinical studies can be compared with the expression pattern in human tissues. A metric to select the most relevant species might be difficult to construct; however, species that are clearly not relevant based on lack of

```
             1        10        20        30        40        50        60        70        80        90       100
             |--------+---------+---------+---------+---------+---------+---------+---------+---------+---------+
Human     MAPAMESPTLLCVALLFFAPDGVLAVPQKPKVSLNPPWNRIFKGENVTLCNGNHFEVSST-KWFHNGSLSEETNSSLNIVNAKFEDSGEYKCQHQQVN
Cyno      MAPAMESPTLLCVALLFFAPDGVLAVPQKPTVSLNPPWNRIFKGENVTLCNGSNFFEVSSH-KWFHNGSLSEVNSSWNIVNADFEDSGEYKCQHQQFD
Rhesus    MAPAMESPTLLCVALLFFAPDGVLAVPQKPTVSLNPPWNRIFKGENVTLCNGSNFFEVSSH-KWFHNGSLSEVANSSLNIVNADFEDSGEYKCQHQQFD
Dog       MPASMGGPALLALALLLSSPGVMSSDTLKPTVSHNPPWNTILKDSVTLTCTGNNSLEVDSA-VALHNNTHQETTSRLDINKAQIQDSGEYRCRENRSI
Rat       MDTGGSARLCLALVLISLGVMLTATQKSVVSLDPPWIRILTGDKVTLICNGNNSSQMNST-KAIHNDSISNVKSSHWVIVSATIQDSGKYICQKQGFY
Mouse     MVTGRSAQLCLALLFMSLDVILTATEKSVLTLDPPWIRIFTGEKVLSCYGNNHLQMNSTTKAIHNGTVSEVNSSHLVIVSATVQDSGKYICQKQGLF
Consensus m...mg.pallclALif.spdv.l..tqKp.vs$#PPWnrIfkg#.VTLCnGnW..#v.St.kW.HNgs.s#v..S.l.Iv.A..#DSGeY.Cq.#...

            101      110       120       130       140       150       160       170       180       190       200
             |--------+---------+---------+---------+---------+---------+---------+---------+---------+---------+
Human     ESEPVYLEVFSDWLLLQASAEVYWEGQPLFLRCHGWRWDVYKVIYYKDGEALKYWAYENHNISLTNATVEDSGTYYCTGKVWQLDYESEPLNITVIKAP-
Cyno      DSEPVHLEVFSDWLLLQASAEVYWEGQPLFLRCHSWRWDVYKVIYYKDGEALKYWAYENHNISLTNATVEDSGTYYCTGKLWQLDCESEPLNITVIKAQ-
Rhesus    DSEPVHLEVFSDWLLLQASAEVYWEGQPLFLRCHSWRWDVYKVIYYKDGEALKYWAYENHNISLTNATVEDSGTYYCTGKLWQLDCESEPLNITVIKAQ-
Dog       LSDPVYLTVFTEWLLQASANVYWEGESFLIRCHSWKWLRLTKVTVYKDGIPIRYWAYENFNISLSNVTKNSGNYSCSGIQQQKGYTSKVLNIIVKKEPT
Rat       KSKPVYINVMQEWLLLQVSDWGSFDIRCRSHKKWKVYHKVIYYKDIWFKYSYDSNNISIRKAIFNDSGSYHCIGTYLNKVECKSDKFSIAVVKDY-
Mouse     KSKPVYLNVTQDWLLLQTSADHILVHGSFDIRCHGWKWAHVRKVIYYRNDHAFNYSYESP-VSIREATLNDSGTYHCKGYLRQVEYESDKFRIAVVKAY-
Consensus .S.PVyL.VF.#WLlLQaSA#v!$eg.sf.iRChsWkkw.v.KVIYYK#g.a.kYwY#n.n!SI.naT..#SGtY.CtG.l.q..yeS..lnI.V.Ka..

            201      210       220       230       240       250       261
             |--------+---------+---------+---------+---------+---------+-|
Human     -REKY-WLQFFIPLLVVILFAVDTGLFISTQQQVTFLLKIKRTRKGFRLLNPHPKPNPKNN
Cyno      -HDKY-WLQFLIPLLVAILFAVDTGLFISTQQQVTFLLKIKRTRKGFKLLNPHPKPNPKSN
Rhesus    -HDKY-WLQFLIPLLVAILFAVDTGLFISTQQQVTFLLKIKRTRKGFKLLNPHPKPNPKSN
Dog       KQNKYSGLQFLIPL-VVILFAVDTGLFISTKQQLTVLQLKRTRKNKK---PEPGKN
Rat       -TIEYRWLQLIFPSLAVILFAVDTGLWFSTHKQFESILKIQKTGKGKKKG
Mouse     -KCKYYWLQLIFPLLVAILFAVDTGLLLSTEEQFKSVLEIQKTGKYKKVETELLT
Consensus ...kY.wLQf.iPllvvILFAVDTGLfiST.qQ.t.llkIkrTrKgkk...p.P..n.....
```

Figure 9.11 Alignment FcεRI-alpha chain protein sequences across species. Human, mouse, rat, dog, cynomolgus macaque, and rhesus macaque protein sequences coding for the alpha chain of the IgE receptor (FcεRI) were aligned and compared. Residues that are identical in all six species are highlighted in red. Residues common to more than half the sequences are listed in blue, and residues found to be identical in half the sequences or less are shown in black. See color insert.

TABLE 9.3   FcεRI-alpha protein sequence homology across species

Species	FcεRI-alpha Chain Percent Sequence Homology
Mouse	51
Rat	49
Dog	55
Cynomolgus macaque	91
Rhesus macaque	92

expression of a target or pathway in the appropriate organs can be excluded from further consideration.

This technology is well established, but caveats to its use remain. One drawback to overcome is the lack of data on most species. Currently databases of human, mouse, and rat tissues are extensive, but data from additional species are sparse. In addition only selected strains of mice and rats have been profiled. This might require use of those strains for toxicology studies or confirmation of results in the desired strains through additional transcript profiling or quantitative PCR experiments. Another caveat is that microarray results are not quantitative, and cannot be reliably compared in terms of absolute amounts across species because of differences in the sequences printed on the microarray, and differences in hybridization kinetics, among others. Also quantitation at the RNA level does not always correlate with quantification at the protein level. For a truly quantitative comparison, additional experiments would need to be performed. Finally, the computational methods for determining the most similar patterns of expression require further exploration as there is considerable debate on the optimal statistical analysis methods that can be utilized to identify meaningful differences in expression patterns. Moreover reliability of results generated with this approach are dependent on the purity of the tissue sample and quality of the RNA extracted, as well as the probes selected for analysis. Contamination with blood or other cell types is sometimes difficult to avoid and may alter the conclusions. For all the reasons mentioned above, information derived from such databases needs to be confirmed with other techniques.

For example, the expression of EGF was assessed using the Gene Logic® Ascenta® database. The "eNorthern" (electronic Northern blot, to examine mRNA expression across tissue types) function was used to find which tissues expressed EGF, and at approximately what level. The data were collected by Gene Logic® using the Affymetrix® GeneChip® platform, where oligonucleotides spotted on a microarray probe the expression of tens of thousands of mRNAs. Two metrics result from these experiments: a present (absent) call indicating whether the mRNA was detected in the sample, and a signal measurement suggestive of the number of copies of that mRNA present. The results of the assessment of EGF expression are shown in Table 9.4. EGF was

TABLE 9.4 Assessment of expression of EGF across species and strains

Organ	Human		Mouse (129S3)		Mouse (C57BL6)		Mouse (DBA)		Rat (Wistar)		Rat (Sprague–Daweley)	
	Present	Median Signal	Present	Median Signal	Present	Median Signal	Present	Median Signal	Present	Median Signal	Present	Median Signal
Bladder	0%	18	14%	5	0%	4	14%	8	0%	12	0%	10
Bones	50%	23	0%	37	0%	28	13%	29	NA	NA	NA	NA
Brain	15%[c]	19[c]	0%	7	0%	10	0%	4	6%	5	NA	NA
Breast	79%	54	40%	68	14%	47	63%	80	NA	NA	NA	NA
Colon	15%	14	0%	5	0%	32	0%	32	83%	23	NA	NA
Esophagus	14%	8	100%	236	100%	286	100%	173	0%	12	NA	NA
Heart	39%	36	17%	33	0%	24	0%	10	0%	10	0%	9
Kidney	94%	368	100%[a]	2623[a]	100%[a]	3616[a]	100%[a]	4071[a]	100%[b]	474[b]	100%[a]	540[a]
Liver	50%	18	13%	5	0%	6	0%	3	22%	13	NA	NA
Lung	22%	14	0%	8	0%	6	0%	5	0%	11	NA	NA
Lymph node	20%	12	0%	151	NA	21	67%	114	NA	NA	NA	NA
Ovary	5%	10	0%	9	NA	NA	0%	3	0%	12	NA	NA
Pancreas	96%	179	100%	488	33%	343	100%	464	NA	NA	NA	NA
Prostate	47%	22	80%	326	100%	741	100%	924	NA	NA	NA	NA
Spleen	12%	15	0%	11	0%	5	0%	11	NA	NA	NA	NA
Stomach	4%	12	0%	25	29%	51	86%	35	13%	11	NA	NA
Testis	0%	7	0%	23	0%	12	0%	127	0%	17	NA	NA
Thymus	3%	8	0%	5	0%	5	0%	11	NA	NA	NA	NA
Uterus	14%	12	0%	5	0%	5	0%	3	NA	NA	NA	NA

Note: Results from eNortherns of EGF in the Gene Logic® Ascenta® database are shown. The probe sets selected were 206254_at (human), 102774_at (mouse), and U04842_at (rat). The data were exported, and tissues with data across multiple species selected. NA indicates that the given tissue was not profiled in that species/strain. Shown are the percentages of tissues expressing EGF (% present) and the median of the signal for each tissue type (arbitrary units).

[a] Average of left and right kidney samples.
[b] Left kidney only.
[c] Average over multiple brain sections.

consistently present across 94% of kidney samples and 96% of pancreas in the human samples tested, with relatively high signal intensities in both. It was also present in 100% of kidney samples across both mice and rats. EGF was present in only 33% of pancreas samples from the mouse C57BL6 strain, suggesting a difference from humans and possibly that this strain would be less appropriate for use in testing an anti-EGF therapy. The pancreas was not assessed in the rats. Another significant difference across species was that EGF was expressed in the esophagus in the mouse strains but not in the human samples. This may suggest a potential difference in toxicity between the two species.

9.8 CONCLUSIONS

Biopharmaceuticals pose unique challenges to clinical development, wherein exaggerated pharmacology becomes the main driver for toxicities observed. This increases the importance of defining a pharmacologically relevant species for preclinical safety assessment. A variety of experimental approaches and technologies are available to assist in the selection of the relevant species for conduct of toxicology studies or, as stated previously, to test the proposed null hypothesis that a given laboratory animal species is not relevant to humans with respect to a biopharmaceutical and its known target and mechanism of action. These methods for analysis, however, should be selected prudently based on the test article and its pharmacology. An evidence-based approach is needed to rule in or rule out species with the understanding that experimental data from various methods may not always be aligned to rule in the species as biologically and pharmacologically relevant. Appropriate design of these experiments, with adequate controls, will ultimately aid in proper interpretation of the data that will form the basis for the selection of the species for conduct of toxicology studies. The diligence paid during the species selection exercise will facilitate the minimization of risks and, more important, create better awareness of risks, during clinical development of biopharmaceuticals.

ACKNOWLEDGMENTS

Experimental data discussed in this chapter were derived from Biogen Idec sponsored studies. The authors wish to acknowledge the contributions of many scientists in the Research and Development organization at Biogen Idec in the design and execution of these studies.

Study protocols involving use of animals were approved by the Institutional Animal Care and Use Committee at the institution where the study was performed. Further information is available upon request.

REFERENCES

1. Williams GJ, Witt PL. Comparative study of the pharmacodynamic and pharmacologic effects of Betaseron and AVONEX. *J Interferon Cytokine Res* 1998;18(11): 967–75.

2. Sturzebecher S, Maibauer R, Heuner A, Beckmann K, Aufdembrinke B. Pharmacodynamic comparison of single doses of IFN-beta1a and IFN-beta1b in healthy volunteers. *J Interferon Cytokine Res* 1999;19(11):1257–64.

3. Bagnato F, Pozzilli C, Scagnolari C, Bellomi F, Pasqualetti P, Gasperini C, Millefiorini E, Galgani S, Spadaro M, Antonelli G. A one-year study on the pharmacodynamic profile of interferon-beta1a in MS. *Neurology* 2002;58(9):1409–11.

4. Pease AC, Solas D, Sullivan EJ, Cronin MT, Holmes CP, Fodor SP. Light-generated oligonucleotide arrays for rapid DNA sequence analysis. *Proc Natl Acad Sci USA* 1994;91(11):5022–6.

5. Lipshutz RJ, Morris D, Chee M, Hubbell E, Kozal MJ, Shah N, Shen N, Yang R, Fodor SP. Using oligonucleotide probe arrays to access genetic diversity. *Biotechniques* 1995;19(3):442–7. Review.

6. Schena M, Shalon D, Davis RW, Brown PO. Quantitative monitoring of gene expression patterns with a complementary DNA microarray. *Science* 1995;270(5235): 467–70.

Tissue Cross-Reactivity Studies for Monoclonal Antibodies: Predictive Value and Use for Selection of Relevant Animal Species for Toxicity Testing

WILLIAM C. HALL, VMD, PhD, DACVP, SHARI A. PRICE-SCHIAVI, PhD, DABT, JOAN WICKS, DVM, PhD, DACVP, and JENNIFER L. ROJKO, DVM, PhD, DACVP

Contents

Preclinical Safety Evaluation of Biopharmaceuticals: A Science-Based Approach to Facilitating Clinical Trials, edited by Joy A. Cavagnaro
Copyright © 2008 by John Wiley & Sons, Inc.

10.1   INTRODUCTION

With the advent of hybridoma technology where murine myeloma cells could be programmed to produce antibody targeted to a specific epitope [1], a new era was ushered in for biomedical research that resulted in a legion of applications for these novel molecules. The first monoclonal antibody approved for human use was OKT3, which was initially used for rescue therapy for acute renal graft rejection by suppressing CD3+ T cells [2], and later expanded to prevent acute graft rejection for multiple organs in early postoperative periods [3–5]. Prior to the development of OKT3 murine monoclonal antibody, anti-thymocyte globulin of equine or lagomorph origin was similarly used to accomplish immunosuppression [6]. Both worked well, but the specificity of the monoclonal antibody proved more potent as an immunosuppressive agent than did the more variable polyclonal anti-bodies used previously. The serum half-life of OKT3 murine monoclonal antibody was only about 50 hours, so activity was short-lived. Part of the reason for the shortened half-life was the development of antibodies (human anti-mouse antibody [HAMA]) against the foreign OKT3 mouse IgG [6]. Subsequently, technologies were developed to provide antibodies that would not be immunogenic in an effort to prolong the circulation time (i.e., duration of treatment) of the molecule, improve efficacy, and reduce unwanted side effects. This was begun by the substitution of human Ig molecule sequences in the murine moiety to reduce antigenicity, followed by humanization of the Ig by site directed mutagenesis to further reduce antigenicity. Finally, fully human antibodies were developed using transgenic mice that expressed human immunoglobulins.

Because of the wave of technology, the regulatory agencies needed to ensure the safety of these novel molecules in some manner that differed from traditional drug safety. Hence, the FDA composed a Draft Points to Consider in the Manufacture and Testing of Monoclonal Antibody Products for Human Use in 1994, which was modified in 1997. The purpose of the Points to Consider and the subsequent International Conference on Harmonization Guidelines for Preclinical Safety Evaluation of Biotechnology-Derived Pharmaceuticals (ICH guidelines, S6) was to establish guidelines for industry to ensure the safety of these novel molecules. Nothing was clad in stone when these documents were put into place, and each molecule was and still is considered unique, both in the target of the antibody as well as in the antibody structure and biologic characteristics themselves.

Among other things, regulatory guidance addresses determination of the structural integrity, specificity (quantifying affinity, avidity, and immunoreactivity), and potency of the antibody. Once these data are obtained for an antibody, a tissue cross-reactivity study on normal human tissues should be conducted in order to determine if binding of the molecule to intended and unintended targets is observed by immunohistochemistry.

Monoclonal antibodies generally bind to an epitope consisting of 5 or 6 amino acids, and characterization of the complementarity determining region

(CDR) of the molecule is very important to identify the amino acids recognized. Since there are 20 amino acids, the theoretical probability of the antibody having full cross-reactivity with a linear epitope identical to that recognized by the CDR region is 1 in 20^6 or 1 in 64,000,000. At first glance there appears to be a low probability of cross-reactivity with the proteins in human tissues, but considering the large number of proteins throughout the cells of the body, there is actually a high probability of a cross-reactivity occurring with any given monoclonal antibody. The number indicated above does not include partial binding of an epitope with the CDR, nor conformational epitopes, both of which could greatly increase that probability. For example, roughly 5% of over 800 murine monoclonal antibodies directed against viral antigens from herpes simplex, cytomegalovirus, Epstein–Barr, vaccinia virus, myxoviruses, paramyxoviruses, arenaviruses, flaviviruses, orthoviruses, rhabdoviruses, coronaviruses, and human retroviruses cross-reacted with normal mouse tissues [7]. These represent viral antigens, but monoclonal antibodies directed against bacterial antigens react similarly. Moreover, almost all monoclonal antibodies directed against tumor antigens cross-react with the counterpart antigen found on the normal cell of origin of that tumor. If one accesses the human genome database with a BLAST search (http://www.ncbi.nlm.nih.gov/BLAST), and searches for the occurrence of 6 arginines in sequence in a protein, approximately 384 "hits" are generated (at least today), indicating that this sequence is present in a number of various human proteins. Thus, the probability of exposing a cross-reactivity in human tissues with a monoclonal antibody is high.

What does a tissue cross-reactivity study actually measure and why is it useful? Cross-reactivity assays measure what cells or noncellular tissue elements express the target epitope recognized by the CDR region of the monoclonal antibody and the location of that antigen on, within, or around various cells. Cross-reactivity assays also recognize off-target (cross-reactive) epitopes in tissue. Under optimized conditions cross-reactivity assays should not measure Fc binding of the monoclonal antibody, which is hopefully blocked by the addition of serum-containing immunoglobulins that bind to the Fc receptors in the tissues. Immunohistochemical cross-reactivity assays are useful because they provide information regarding target epitope distribution, off-target epitope distribution, and in vitro species comparisons (e.g., human versus monkey or rodent profiles) that assist in species selection for in vivo (preclinical) safety studies.

Let us digress a bit to discuss in general (specifics will follow) the tissue cross-reactivity study. Human tissues are obtained from autopsy or surgical specimens and snap frozen. Cryosections are prepared and fixed in a manner wherein antigens are not lost or altered. The samples are then blocked with serum, treated to block endogenous reaction enzymes (peroxidases, alkaline phosphatases, etc.) and other substances (endogenous biotin) that may interfere with interpretation of the reaction, run through a series of approximately a dozen more wash and reagent steps, desiccated, counterstained, and coverslipped for interpretation. Tissue binding (target or off-target) is then evaluated microscopically. The procedures are lengthy and must be highly controlled to ensure accuracy of all tissue elements stained. These conditions definitely are not exactly what a monoclonal antibody would experience following injection into a human. The goal is to ensure the accuracy of the staining and minimize background. In other words, the goal is to provide an assay and not replicate the conditions obtained in vivo.

Since most of the monoclonal antibodies currently under development are human or humanized, the goal of the assay is to detect the bound monoclonal antibody and not the background endogenous immunoglobulins in the tissues. This means labeling the antibody or utilizing a secondary antibody that recognizes only the monoclonal antibody that is labeled (or unlabeled) so that it can be differentiated from the endogenous Ig.

As a preclinical tool, the tissue cross-reactivity assay is one of the first assays that should be performed to provide guidance to the investigator for the applicability of the particular monoclonal antibody clone for in vivo use. Careful scrutiny at this stage could save years of additional preclinical investigation of an unwanted cross-reactivity. In addition, the immunohistochemistry procedures are of great assistance in finding a relevant animal model for the in vivo preclinical studies. Thus, the purpose of this chapter is not to detail the immunohistochemical methods used in a tissue cross-reactivity study, but rather to outline important considerations in the conduct of the tissue cross-reactivity study and provide best practices guidelines for interpreting the information gained from this assay relative to human safety. In addition, the use of this assay along with others can be used to determine a relevant species (one that expresses the target or off-target cross-reactive epitopes) for preclinical safety studies.

10.2 ANTIBODY TYPES AND THEIR EVOLUTION

In humans, there are five isotypes of antibodies, IgG, IgA, IgD, IgE, and IgM, which are defined by the structures of their heavy chains and their abilities to form multimers (Figure 10.1) [8]. IgG is the most abundant isotype present in serum with average serum concentrations ranging from 0.5 to 9 mg/ml depending on the IgG subtype. This is followed by IgA (3 mg/ml), IgM (1.5 mg/ml), IgE (0.05 mg/ml), and IgD (trace). Each antibody isotype has unique functions. Critical functions of IgG include opsonization, complement activation, antibody-dependent cell-mediated cytotoxicity (ADCC), passive immunity, and regulation of B cells. Both IgM and IgD act as antigen receptors on naive B cells, and soluble, multimeric forms of IgM are involved in complement activation. IgA is involved in mucosal and passive neonatal immunity, while IgE is involved in immediate hypersensitivity [8].

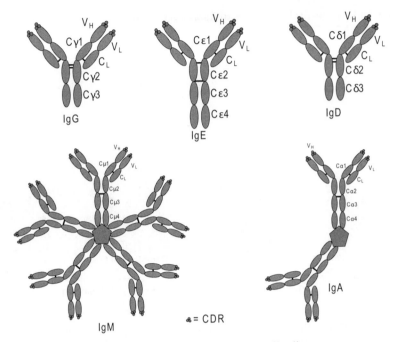

Figure 10.1   Isotypes of human antibodies.

Because of their relatively large size and other physicochemical character-istics, antibodies generally have prolonged serum half-lives compared to smaller circulating proteins with averages as follows: IgG—23 days; IgA—6 days; IgM—5 days; IgD—3 days; and IgE—2 days [8]. Antibody fragments such as Fabs and $F(ab')_2$ have significantly shorter half-lives that range from minutes to hours [9]. In general, the smaller the antibody fragment, the shorter the serum half-life, as the smaller antibody fragments are cleared through the kidneys more quickly than larger fragments or whole antibodies (discussed in more detail in Chapter 11). In addition, the ability of the antibody to reach its target antigen is affected by size and affinity or avidity (discussed in more detail in Chapter 11). The choice of whole antibody or antibody fragment for a therapeutic candidate thus depends on several factors including the location of the target antigen, the desired activity of the antibody or fragment, affin-ity/avidity of antigen binding, and desired serum concentrations of the thera-peutic candidate.

Most therapeutic antibodies on the market or in development are IgG or some fragment or derivative thereof. IgG is divided into four subtypes: IgG1, IgG2, IgG3, and IgG4, with IgG1 being the most abundant and IgG4 being least abundant in serum (Table 10.1). As with the main isotype groups, each subtype of IgG has unique properties and functions (Figure 10.2). The choice

TABLE 10.1   Biological properties of human IgG isotypes

	IgG$_1$	IgG$_2$	IgG$_3$	IgG$_4$
Serum concentration (%)	65	23	8	4
Fc binding	+++	+	+++	±
Placental passage	++	±	++	++
ADCC	+++	+	+++	±
CF	+++	++	++++	±

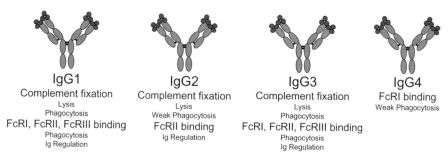

IgG1
Complement fixation
Lysis
Phagocytosis
FcRI, FcRII, FcRIII binding
Phagocytosis
Ig Regulation

IgG2
Complement fixation
Lysis
Weak Phagocytosis
FcRII binding
Ig Regulation

IgG3
Complement fixation
Lysis
Phagocytosis
FcRI, FcRII, FcRIII binding
Phagocytosis
Ig Regulation

IgG4
FcRI binding
Weak Phagocytosis

Figure 10.2   Isotype subgroups of human IgG molecules.

of isotype subgroup is dependent upon the desired activities for a given therapeutic candidate. There are several ways to generate these antibody-based
therapeutics. Briefly, mouse monoclonal antibodies can be generated by standard methods after immunization of mice (Figure 10.3a). When the clone of
choice has been selected, the variable regions can be cloned using routine
molecular biology strategies. The resulting variable region fragments can then
be cloned into an expression vector encoding human antibody light and heavy
chain regions to generate a mouse/human chimeric antibody (approximately
30% mouse and 70% human). These chimeric antibodies can be expressed by
and purified from stably transfected cell lines such as CHO or NSO cells. To
generate humanized antibodies, the chimeric versions can be mutagenized in
the variable regions to make the variable framework more similar to human
antibody sequences, which may be selected from human antibody sequences
found in antibody databases such as Kabat and others. The resulting humanized antibody (approximately 3% mouse and 97% human) can then be
expressed and purified.

There are two main methods for generating fully human antibodies (Figure
10.3b). In the first, transgenic mice that express fully human IgG can be immunized with target antigen and the resulting antibody of choice can be cloned
and expressed as described above. In the second, phage display libraries
expressing fully human antibody Fabs can be screened or "panned" using the
antigen of interest and the clone of choice can be cloned into and expressed

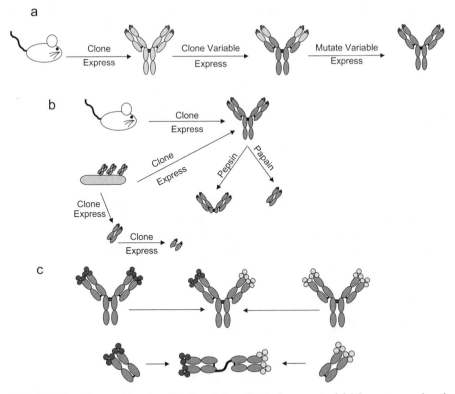

Figure 10.3 Generation of antibodies and antibody fragments. (*a*) Mouse monoclonal antibodies are produced after immunization and production of hybridomas. Chimeric antibodies are produced by cloning the variable regions of a mouse antibody onto a human antibody framework. Humanized antibodies are produced by site directed mutagenesis of chimeric antibodies to make the variable regions of the mouse antibody more closely resemble a human antibody. (*b*) Fully human antibodies are produced by immunization of transgenic mice that express fully human antibodies or by screening human antibody phage display libraries. (*c*) Antibody fragments are produced by enzymatic cleavage of human antibodies or screening phage display libraries. Bispecific or multivalent antibody fragments can be made using standard molecular biology techniques.

from a human antibody expression vector. Bispecific antibodies, which recognize two different antigens, can be generated in a similar way from two different "parental" antibodies (Figure 10.3*c*).

Antibody fragments can be generated by papain digestion of full antibodies to yield Fab fragments (V_H, CH1, V_L, C_L) or pepsin to yield $F(ab')_2$ fragments (Figure 10.3*b*). In these cases the resulting antibody fragment must be purified from the byproduct Fc region or fragments. As this extra purification step can complicate (and add additional cost) the development of antibody fragments, it is more common to screen phage display libraries that display antibody Fabs or other antigen binding fragments and then to clone the candidate of interest into a desired format and expression vector. This way it is easy to produce other types of antibody fragments such as Fv's or scFv's or bispecific and multivalent fragments.

Regardless of the type of resulting product (whole antibody or fragment, monospecific or bispecific), tissue cross-reactivity testing should be performed prior to toxicity studies to establish patterns of on- and off-target tissue binding and to confirm the relevance of the selected species for toxicity testing. For tissue cross-reactivity testing of any type of antibody-based therapeutic candidate, a similar irrelevant negative control antibody or fragment should be produced. In the case of whole antibodies, a human IgG of the same isotype (IgG1, IgG2, etc.) should be used, and for antibody fragments (which do not contain Fc or heavy chain regions) a similar fragment directed against an irrelevant epitope or the same non–cross-reactive epitope from a different species should be used. Ideally the negative control whole antibody would be identical to the test article except for an inactive or different CDR region.

10.3 BIOLOGICAL EFFECTS OF ANTIBODIES

As mentioned briefly above, antibodies have multiple, complex functions. In the body, the main effector functions of antibodies include pathogen/toxin neutralization, activation of phagocytosis and antibody-dependent cellular cytotoxicity (ADCC), and complement activation. Therapeutic approaches using antibodies or antibody fragments take advantage of these natural activities.

Pathogen or toxin neutralization occurs when an antibody CDR region binds to a pathogen or toxin and sterically hinders or blocks binding of the pathogen or toxin to its respective cellular receptor. As neutralizing activity can be mediated by the antibody CDR regions, it can be performed by antibodies of any isotype or even antibody fragments, if one ignores the role that the Fc or other non-CDR regions may play in the antibody activity. This neutralizing activity is utilized in passive vaccination and in therapeutic antibodies directed against specific pathogens or toxins such as Synagis®, which prevents respiratory syncytial virus binding to its cellular receptor by binding to and blocking RSV F protein (reviewed in [10]). In addition, this neutralization strategy is commonly used for other therapeutic strategies such as those for inflammatory and cardiovascular disease where the antibody or antibody fragment is used to block binding of an inflammatory cytokine or pro-thrombotic protein to its receptor either by binding to the ligand or its receptor. For example, Infliximab®, a chimeric anti–TNFα antibody, is used to neutralize TNFα activity in various inflammatory diseases [11]. In cardiovascular conditions, ReoPro®, an anti-IIb/IIIa Fab, blocks the platelet glycoprotein IIb/IIIa receptors, thus inhibiting fibrinogen binding, platelet cross-linking and thrombus formation [12].

Antibodies also can mediate phagocytosis and ADCC via their Fc receptor binding regions. Antibody bound to target antigen may bind through the Fc region of the antibody to Fc receptors expressed on phagocytic cells such as macrophages and neutrophils (Fc receptors are discussed in more detail in Chapter 11). Upon Fc receptor binding, signal transduction pathways are activated that result in engulfment and degradation of the bound particle as well as release of inflammatory mediators. Likewise, for ADCC, binding of antigen-bound antibody to Fc receptors on effector cells such as NK cells results in activation of the cells to release cytokines and cytolytic granules. In general, both phagocytic and cytotoxic functions are more efficient when multiple antibodies are bound to cell surface antigens resulting in higher avidity binding to the Fc receptors on the effector cells. If the desired effect of a therapeutic antibody is phagocytic or cytolytic activity, the isotype subgroup chosen should be one that binds to Fc receptors expressed on phagocytic or cytolytic cells (IgG1 or IgG3). Herceptin® and Rituximab®, therapeutic antibodies directed against ErbB-2 and CD20, respectively, have been reported to produce antitumor effects through Fc-receptor mediated mechanisms (reviewed in [13]).

For complement-dependent cytotoxicity, a complex cascade of protein binding and cleavage occurs that culminates in final complement mediated effector functions of phagocytosis, recruitment and activation of leukocytes, and osmotic lysis. It has been reported that Rituximab® (anti-CD20) utilizes a complement-dependent mechanism for tumor cell destruction [14]. If the desired effect of a therapeutic antibody is complement-dependent activity, the isotype subgroup chosen should be one that binds to complement proteins (IgG1 or IgG3).

Besides these classical effector mechanisms, other antibody-based mechanisms of action may be utilized, including targeted delivery of drugs, inflammatory mediators, or toxins; induction of apoptosis by modulation of critical signaling pathways; and direct linkage of target and effector cells by bispecific or multivalent antibody fragments.

10.4 TISSUE CROSS-REACTIVITY PROCEDURES

As mentioned earlier, the purpose of this review is not to detail the actual methods used for tissue cross-reactivity studies but rather to highlight the many important factors that must be taken under consideration during the conduct, evaluation, and regulatory review and of the study. Specific details for tissue collection, generation of control materials, and staining procedures themselves are readily available in the literature.

10.4.1 The Tissues

Human Tissues   According to the Points-to-Consider and other regulatory documents, tissues from at least three unrelated human donors should be evaluated in a tissue cross-reactivity study in order to screen for individual variation. In a 3-donor, 37-tissue cross-reactivity study, up to 111 different donors could theoretically be represented. To the extent possible, both males and females should be equally represented.

Tissue banks are the most common source of human tissues. While surgical biopsy accessions are preferred, they are limited in availability and often unavailable for many tissues (e.g., brain and other vital organs). Therefore the majority of tissue samples used in cross-reactivity studies are those acquired at autopsy. For autopsy accessions all efforts must be made to minimize the time interval between death and tissue collection. Information provided with specimens generally includes age, gender, and usually race and some clinical history and/or cause of death. As suggested in the Points-to-Consider document, the tissues used in a standard tissue cross-reactivity study are acquired from adults (>18 years of age). Pediatric tissues are often very difficult to obtain and are usually not used in a standard tissue cross-reactivity study unless there is a clear pediatric indication for the test article.

Animal Tissues   The ICH S6 guidelines and the FDA's Points to Consider in the Manufacture and Testing of Monoclonal Antibody Products for Human Use (US FDA [CBER], 28 February, 1997) state that for biological products, preclinical testing must be accomplished in a relevant species. A relevant species can be determined by immunohistochemistry, flow cytometry, or pharmacologic procedures. For tissue cross-reactivity (immunohistochemistry) studies in animals, at least two donors are recommended, with equal gender representation as appropriate. Since animals such as inbred rodent strains have relatively limited heterogeneity, staining of more than two donors is not considered as important as in humans, nonhuman primates, or other outbred strains, where the amount of genetic variability is much more extensive. The degree of individual variability in nonhuman primates still is not considered to be as great as in humans, but there is a growing trend toward staining three donors for animal tissues.

Animal tissues are collected at necropsy of humanely euthanized, purpose-bred laboratory animals immediately following death. Some nonhuman primates used for tissue acquisition may be wild caught. The animals used are preferably matched as closely as possible to that of the strain or origin of the animals to be used for preclinical toxicity testing.

Considerations in Comparing Cross-Reactivity Results between Humans and Animals   Several factors must be taken under consideration when comparing tissue cross-reactivity results between humans and animals. First, conditions surrounding acquisition of animal tissues are clearly different from those of human tissues. Thus, the quality of the animal tissues is much easier to control because the tissues are taken at necropsy and are frozen within a short time following death. For human tissues the relative age of the donors used is likely to be greater than that of the animal donors, and therefore normal aging changes may not be as prominent in the animal tissues. Further the cause of death of animals used as tissue donors is euthanasia, in contrast to humans where the cause of death is due to a variety of causes including trauma, myocardial infarction, or stroke (any of which may have overt or subtle systemic effects). Combined with the relatively young ages of the animal donors, it can be assumed that underlying disease processes such as diabetes, high blood pressure, or cardiovascular disease are not present in animal tissues. Finally, the physiological processes that occur during natural death of human tissue donors might influence antigen expression and the resulting observed staining pattern of a particular test article. These are considerations that will be addressed further in the interpretation of the relevance of the species for the tissue cross-reactivity study.

Tissue Microarrays   Tissue microarrays containing tissue core samples of all the required tissue types in the FDA Points-to-Consider document are available. While tissue microarrays can be useful for preliminary investigation of reactivity of a test article, they have several disadvantages for optimal evaluation of antibody cross-reactivity in tissues. The tissue cores (usually ≤2 mm each) represent only a very small sample of the tissue and generally do not present a wide panorama of the variety of tissue elements present in a larger sample (epithelium, vascular and/or intrinsic smooth muscle, mesothelium, etc.). For example, a 2 mm core sample collected from the medulla of the kidney might not contain glomeruli or proximal tubular epithelium. In the kidney there are indeed multiple types of tubules, all with a variety of antigen expression patterns depending on their functional roles and location in the kidney. Even for a particular cell type (e.g., epithelium in the internal os versus external os of the cervix), there may be heterogeneity in antigen expression patterns, and unless expression is widespread or diffuse in distribution, reactivity is more easily missed than it would be in a larger section of tissue. Finally, a key part of the evaluation of tissue cross-reactivity is examining the relationship between the cells of an organ and the stromal tissues. This is enhanced by size of the specimen.

Preparation of Tissues   Tissues are quick-frozen in OCT embedding media, and 4 to 6 μm cryosections are placed on slides and allowed to dry, or stored at 4 °C for a few days or at −80 °C for longer terms prior to fixation. Prolonged retention of tissue sections is usually to be avoided even at −80 °C as antigen deterioration can occur even under these conditions. Blood smears are prepared fresh and allowed to dry prior to fixation. Tissue preparation (sectioning, drying, fixation) is governed by the requirements needed to preserve the epitope on the positive control samples in preliminary studies to establish the correct conditions for the assay.

10.4.2   The Controls

Isotype Control Antibody   The isotype (or negative) control antibody should be an antibody of the same isotype subclass as the test material (IgG1, IgG2, etc.). The isotype control stained slide controls for staining due to binding to Fc receptors or similar non–CDR-mediated events. However, even with an isotype-matched control, nonspecific staining (non–CDR-mediated) can be observed with the test material but not with the negative control. Ideally the ideal negative control antibody is identical to the test antibody with a different CDR region. This type of control helps normalize or minimize variables such as glycosylation differences and allotypic variation of the antibody backbone that might contribute to non–CDR-mediated staining.

Assay Control   The assay control involves omission of the primary antibody (test article or negative control antibody) during the staining reaction and permits determination of staining by the secondary or tertiary antibodies or other components of the reaction process. This control slide may or may not be included based on the immunohistochemical method chosen.

Tissue Staining Control   Along with morphology, a tissue's ability to be stained for a common antigen provides evidence that the tissue is stainable and thus of sufficient quality to be used in a tissue cross-reactivity study. In the case of human tissues where the time between death and collection of tissues may be more prolonged compared to that for animal tissues, this control helps verify that proteins within the tissue have maintained their integrity. Depending on the lab, various staining control antibodies may be used including CD31, transferrin receptor, or β_2-microglobulin. The objective is to choose an antibody that recognizes an epitope that is expressed in all or most tissues. This indicates suitability of the tissues used in the cross-reactivity study but does not guarantee that the epitope recognized by the test article survived tissue collection, storage, and processing.

Positive and Negative Tissue Controls   In order to control the staining run and to determine if the method that has been chosen is adequately working, a positive tissue control is used. In addition a negative control tissue is used to ensure the specificity of the test article. A tissue with well-documented expression of the target antigen is the ideal positive tissue control because it is treated identically to the other tissues of the study. However, often a target antigen is not normally expressed by tissues, or on occasion may be washed from the tissues during the immunohistochemistry procedures. In these cases a neoplastic or other type of diseased tissue is used (e.g., rheumatoid arthritis or inflammatory bowel disease) or another type of positive control must be used as outlined below. A suitable negative tissue control consists of a tissue or tissue element that does not express the target antigen.

If acceptable positive control tissues are not available, target antigen-expressing cell lines may be used. In some cases there may be cell lines that normally express the target antigen. If such cell lines are not available, cell lines transfected with the target antigen may be used. Target antigen expression and the ability to detect expression of that antigen by immunohistochemistry may be verified through the use of a commercial antibody known to react with the target antigen. When using cell lines, an appropriate negative control cell line should also be evaluated. This cell line should be as similar to that of the positive control cell line as possible and should be grown under similar conditions (e.g., suspension versus monolayer, serum versus serum-free). If transfected cells are chosen as the positive control cell line, then nontransfected or mock transfected cells should be used as the negative control cell line. Often epitope density cannot be established for the cell line, but if available, high-density and low-density cell lines should be chosen to provide an internal sensitivity control for the assay.

When neither tissue nor cell lines are available, another alternative is purified target antigen. This type of control might be necessary when the test article is directed against a bacterial toxin and there is no cell line available that expresses the whole toxin or the targeted subunit. In these cases the negative "tissue" control would consist of a protein that is known to be nonreactive with the antibody being tested.

10.4.3 The Staining Method

In 1942 Coons et al. described an immunofluorescence technique for detecting cellular antigens in tissue sections [15]. This method utilized a fluorescent label bound to the primary antibody to localize the target antigen. In this case the fluorescent label was the detection method. The use of an "immunoenzyme" approach to detect binding of the primary antibody was introduced a quarter of a century later [16] with the introduction of peroxidase-labeled antibodies.

Immunohistochemical staining can be direct or indirect. Direct immunohistochemical staining methods utilize only a primary antibody, which may be conjugated to horseradish peroxidase, biotin, alkaline phosphatase, or other chromogens. In the case of biotin-labeled primary antibodies, avidin or streptavidin linked to peroxidase binds to the biotin allowing detection of reactivity of the test antibody with the tissue. Indirect immunohistochemical staining methods utilize secondary, tertiary, or even quaternary antibodies, any of which may be linked either to biotin or enzyme (e.g., peroxidase).

The ultimate choice of the method to be used in a tissue cross-reactivity study hinges on the fine balance between giving the best signal with the least amount of background or nonspecific staining. Background staining is associated with the detection methods used and endogenous or exogenous tissue pigments. While little can be done to affect the presence of tissue pigments, various blocks can be used to reduce staining associated with the detection methods. Detection enzymes such as horseradish peroxidase or alkaline phosphatase have counterparts endogenous to various tissues. For example, myeloperoxidase is present in mast cell and neutrophil granules. Myeloperoxidase utilizes the same substrate that is used during the chromogen development phase of the immunohistochemistry staining procedure. Several blocks are available that can be applied to the tissues prior to application of the horseradish peroxidase-labeled streptavidin or antibody that will substantially reduce the activity of the endogenous peroxidase enzyme. Other blocks are available for endogenous biotin present in tissue, thus preventing detection of endogenous biotin.

Protein blocks are applied to the tissues prior to application of the primary antibody to reduce nonspecific staining. Nonspecific staining is non–CDR-mediated staining. Protein blocks often contain serum, which contain immunoglobulins that bind to the Fc receptors in the tissues, blocking Fc attachment to those tissue receptors. Other proteins such as casein or BSA may be added to block nonspecific protein–protein interactions.

The following factors should be considered when choosing a staining method for a tissue cross-reactivity study: (1) test article forms that are available, (2) test article affinity, (3) proposed plasma level for clinical studies, (4) epitope stability, and (5) ability to scale up the method to stain a large number of tissues. These various issues are addressed below.

Test Article Forms   For preclinical testing (including tissue cross-reactivity) of antibody-based therapeutics, it is best to use the actual therapeutic candidate (or the closest derivative) to obtain the most accurate preclinical data about that therapeutic candidate. Most monoclonal antibody-based therapeutic candidates are fully human, humanized, or chimeric antibodies or fragments. This poses some challenge to tissue cross-reactivity studies on human and nonhuman primate tissues, as standard indirect immunohistochemical staining using an antihuman IgG secondary antibody yields excessive background staining of endogenous human IgG present in the tissue sections. For this reason antibodies or antibody fragments can be labeled in various ways to facilitate detection of binding to human or animal tissues. Labeling is particularly useful for facilitating detection of tissue binding of antibody fragments that do not contain an Fc region. However, any time an antibody or antibody fragment is labeled, it is critical to ensure that the label itself does not interfere with CDR-mediated binding to target epitope. At a minimum, characterization of the labeled antibody using techniques such as BiaCore, ELISA, and/or flow cytometry should be performed to evaluate the labeled antibody's ability to bind to target epitope and to determine any effect on epitope binding affinity and/or specificity. Although there are many different ways to label antibodies, one of the most common labels used for antibodies in tissue cross-reactivity studies is biotin.

Biotin is a member of the B vitamin family that is normally involved in various processes including biosynthesis of fatty acids, metabolism of branched amino acids, and gluconeogenesis. It binds with high affinity to avidin and streptavidin ($KD = 10^{-15}$ M). This small, bicyclic compound can be easily conjugated to macromolecules without disrupting their function. Biotin esters are most often used for antibody labeling. These compounds react with primary amino groups ($-NH_2$) present on lysines and at the N-terminus of the protein to form stable amide bonds. Other types of biotin reagents are available if biotinylation of groups other than primary amines is desired. After the labeling reaction, excess biotin and any other reaction by-products should be removed by column chromatography, dialysis, or desalting columns. Usually antibodies are labeled with three to six biotins per molecule, although this number can be different depending on how the reaction is set up and on how many available lysines are present for labeling. Excess biotin molecules can interfere with the CDR binding to the antigen. When an antibody or antibody fragment is labeled with biotin for cross-reactivity testing, a similarly labeled negative control antibody or antibody fragment should also be prepared.

Using biotinylated antibodies for immunohistochemical staining takes advantage of the high-affinity binding of biotin to avidin or streptavidin. For this reason biotinylated antibodies (either the primary antibody or secondary antibody) are easily detected using enzyme-conjugated (horseradish peroxidase or alkaline phosphatase) avidin or streptavidin. This type of procedure is useful when staining human or nonhuman primate tissues with chimeric, humanized, or human antibodies as it eliminates the need for an antihuman IgG secondary antibody. In addition this type of labeling facilitates staining with antibody fragments that do not contain an Fc region. Two important considerations when using biotinylated reagents for immunohistochemistry are use of a similarly labeled negative control antibody and adequate blocking of endogenous biotin in the tissue sections. Blocking of endogenous biotin is achieved by sequential incubation of the sections with avidin and biotin. In addition an assay control in which the primary antibody is omitted from the staining reaction should be performed to evaluate the level of endogenous biotin (to ensure adequate blocking) and other pigments as well as any nonspecific staining by secondary or detection reagents. A word of caution about the use of biotin is that its presence on some antibody molecules can result in non–CDR-mediated interactions forming between the tissues and the biotin resulting in nonspecific staining of the tissues. Depending on where the biotin molecules attach, biotinylation also can directly alter the test article CDR or trigger conformational changes in the test article antibody molecule that affects CDR-mediated binding. A concern is that the biotinylated negative control antibody may not behave in the same manner as the biotinylated test article.

As mentioned earlier, there are other ways to label antibodies for use in tissue cross-reactivity studies. Detailed discussion of various labels and staining methods associated with them are beyond the scope of this review. However, whatever the label chosen, careful consideration should be given to its effect on the test article and to the specifics of the staining method (controls, buffers, etc.) that must be used with that type of label.

In cases where the test article is derived from the same species as the tissue being stained and labeling is not feasible due to interference with the CDR, a precomplexing method may be attempted. This method involves precomplexing of the primary antibody and the anti-IgG secondary antibody prior to application to the tissue and has been described for both mouse and human antibodies [17–19]. Alternatively, if available, anti-idiotypic antibodies (antibodies that are directed specifically against the hypervariable region of the test article) can be used to detect test article binding to the tissues. Care should be taken to ensure that the anti-idiotypic antibodies do not recognize endogenous IgG or modulate test article binding directly.

Test Article Affinity   Different immunohistochemical staining methods have different levels of theoretical amplification (Table 10.2). For antibodies with relatively low affinities, it may be desirable or necessary to use a method with a high level of amplification, such as a tertiary indirect in order to see reactivity with the target antigen. For antibodies with relatively high affinity for the target antigen or for highly expressed antigens, the level of signal amplification may not be as critical for detection of staining.

Proposed Plasma Level for Clinical Studies   The tissue cross-reactivity study is an immunohistochemistry assay, which, because of its nature, does not replicate the conditions obtained in vivo. Moreover, one is looking at tissue sections where the cells are cleaved and all portions of the tissues and cells (membrane, cytoplasm, and nucleus) and surrounding milieu are exposed to the same concentration of the antibody, which is different from the intravascular and perivascular concentrations observed in vivo (see below). Since buffers, protein types, and electrolytes also differ in vivo compared to the immunohistochemistry conditions, one cannot expect to attain high concentra-

TABLE 10.2   Theoretical amplification and maximum test article concentration for various immunohistochemical procedures

Test Article Form	Method	Theoretical Amplification	Theoretical Maximum Test Article Concentration
Unconjugated	Secondary indirect	++ to +++	10–50 µg/ml
Unconjugated	Precomplex	+ to +++	10–20 µg/ml
Biotinylated	Direct	+ to +++	10–300 µg/ml
HRP-conjugated	Direct	+ to ++	10–300 µg/ml
Other labels	Indirect	++ to ++++	10–100 µg/ml
Anti-Id	Indirect	++ to +++	10–100 µg/ml

tions of the monoclonal antibodies in the in vitro assay compared to in vivo because of the background staining associated with high concentrations. It is good to attempt these concentrations, but for all practical purposes it is unrealistic for many, if not most, test articles. A less sensitive procedure providing less background could be chosen, but that would defeat the goal of the tissue cross-reactivity study to determine the possible cellular and tissue location of the antigen recognized by the antibody. The tissue cross-reactivity study is an in vitro experiment utilized to determine the location and density of an antigen. That said, an attempt should be made at least in preliminary studies to use the proposed clinical concentrations, but if excess background results, the higher concentrations would do little to assist in interpretation and should not be utilized. The data from the preliminary studies can be used to support the concentrations used.

Epitope Stability   How and whether to fix tissues to preserve morphology and maintain the reactive epitope is always a question. The secondary and tertiary structures of an epitope are modified by excessive fixation and sometimes drying, which can alter staining of the fixed tissues. Further, since protein structure is based on a number of factors, including hydrogen bonding between amino acid side chains, factors such as pH and salt will play a role in the protein structure and, in turn, in the antigen–antibody reaction if that reaction is dependent on a secondary, tertiary, or quaternary structure. While tissue collected and placed into formalin is not a consideration for tissue cross-reactivity studies, minor fixation of cryosections with standard fixatives aid in maintaining tissue morphology. Further, some antigens are preserved better with such minor fixation. Thus, different fixatives such as acetone, methanol, neutral buffered formalin, or paraformaldehyde may be considered. Each fixative has a different mechanism of action. Acetone is an organic solvent, methanol is dehydrating, and aldehydes cross-link amino acids. The effect of these fixatives on target and off-target antigen preservation should be considered during the method development.

Concentration Selection   During method development the primary antibody is titrated across a range of concentrations in order to determine both an ideal concentration (the lowest test article concentration that produces maximum binding to the target antigen) and a higher concentration of antibody that allows detection of reactivity that is of relatively lower affinity. The choice of this higher concentration is usually a multiple of the ideal concentration that approaches the proposed clinical concentration as determined by the levels of background staining. These two concentrations are commonly within a concentration range of 10 to 20-fold. If a study is conducted using lower-fold difference in high and low staining concentrations (e.g., threefold), appropriate justification should be provided. Rarely, three concentrations of antibody may be chosen if the range between the ideal concentration and the proposed plasma concentration is large (>50 to 100-fold).

10.5 INTERPRETATION OF TISSUE CROSS-REACTIVITY FINDINGS

10.5.1 CDR-Mediated "Specific" Staining

To interpret potential cross-reactivity findings correctly, the pathologist must consider the nature of the epitope-test article CDR interaction, the type of test article and staining method as well as the histologic characteristics of the tissue being stained. First, staining of a tissue component could indicate binding to the target epitope (e.g., a leukocyte CD marker) mediated by the test article CDR, or it could indicate CDR-independent binding (nonspecific sticking or Fc receptor mediated binding). Just because a test article binds to an unexpected tissue component does not mean the binding is nonspecific. It could mean that the target CD marker is expressed at that site. For example, CD4 was originally recognized as specific for helper T cells but was later found to be present on parathyroid epithelium [20,21] as well as monocytes and macrophages. Thus, finding CD4 on helper T cells was judged an expected, on-target, CDR-mediated staining, while finding CD4 on parathyroid epithelium was initially judged an unexpected, off-target, CDR-mediated staining. In contrast, the T10B9 anti-CD3 monoclonal antibody reacts with a monomorphic membrane CD3/T cell receptor complex epitope but does not react with cytoplasmic CD3 in human T lymphocytes and does not recognize membrane CD3/T cell receptor complex or cytoplasmic CD3 in rhesus monkey or cotton-top tamarin T lymphocytes [22]. However, T10B9 also reacts with cytoplasmic filaments in human, rhesus monkey, and cotton-top tamarin epithelial cells that do not express CD3/T cell receptor complex.[1] Thus finding T10B9 cross-reactive, non–CD3/non–T cell receptor complex-epitopes on human and non-human primate epithelial cells was judged an off-target, CDR-mediated staining.

10.5.2 Non–CDR-Mediated "Nonspecific" Staining

Whether expected or unexpected and on- or off-target, CDR-mediated binding is very different from non–CDR-mediated binding. Non–CDR-mediated binding can be due to binding of the Fc portion of the test article to Fc receptors on monocyte/macrophages or other cell types (Figure 10.4; reviewed in Chapter 11). Non–CDR-mediated binding can also be due to nonspecific stickiness, mediated by protein–protein, protein–nucleoprotein interactions, carbohydrate–carbohydrate (lectin-like) interactions, or van der Waals interactions. Thus, except for epitope : CDR matching, the types of physicochemical interactions that contribute to specific CDR binding are often similar to the types of physicochemical interactions that mediate nonspecific (non–CDR-mediated) binding. Additionally certain tissues or tissue components appear to be stickier than others. For example, vascular and intrinsic smooth muscle

---

[1]Interestingly this epithelial cytoplasmic filament cross-reactivity did not appear to lead to any toxic effects in clinical trials [23,24], reviewed in [25].

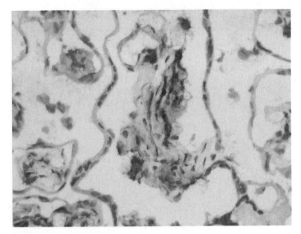

Figure 10.4 FcγR1 in human placenta. CD64 staining of Hofbauer cells and perivascular monocyte/macrophages and dendritic cells. No staining of placental trophoblast epithelium or endothelium. See color insert.

cells are often stickier than endothelial cells and/or perivascular collagen, as is mucin in the gastrointestinal tract and cervix. The stickiness of a tissue (and the propensity to bind antibody or protein reagents nonspecifically) also generally increases as the time between death and tissue collection increases. Additionally, as patients die, their peripheral tissues become poorly perfused and increasingly depleted of oxygen (anoxia). Anoxic endothelial cells contract and the spaces between adjacent endothelial cells widen, leading to protein leakage into the tissues. These serum proteins might coat (protect) the sticky sites on vascular smooth muscle cells. Alternatively, if the test article is directed against a serum protein (e.g., complement), the cross-reactivity staining patterns might appear greater than they really are due to reactivity with serum leaked into perivascular or more distal tissues.

10.5.3 Tissue Adequacy and Staining Adequacy

Interpretation of cryosections depends on tissue adequacy and staining adequacy. Tissue adequacy depends on the overall size and quality of each piece as well as whether the essential tissue components are adequately represented. For example, a piece of human uterus should have surface and glandular endometrium with endometrial stromal cells, muscular tunics, and, if possible, serosa (mesothelium). To ensure tissue adequacy, individual tissue cryosections should be used. Slides with multiple tissues (especially those with multiple small pieces—multitissue arrays) generally should not be used.[2] These

---

[2]Once a target or off-target reactivity is identified, a multitissue array might be useful in screening. For example, multitissue arrays might be used to identify how many livers are positive for a particular hepatocyte epitope.

small pieces often do not include all representative tissue components. Moreover in many cross-reactivity studies the key test article-stained cells might be evident in low numbers or in specialized portions of the tissue. For example, a tumor angiogenesis epitope might be present on normal endothelial cells in ovary that undergoes angiogenesis as part of postovulation corpus luteum formation during regular menstrual cycling. These test article-stained cells might only represent 1% of the endothelial cells of an ovary but are critical to identify as potential targets for that test article.

Staining adequacy is addressed by staining replicate cryosections from each tissue for an antigen known to be expressed on components common to all tissues (e.g., CD31, β_2-microglobulin, transferrin receptor), as discussed previously. This ensures that the tissue can be stained using immunohistochemical methods and thus is a suitable sample for the tissue cross-reactivity study.

10.5.4 Background Staining

Interpretation of cryosections depends on the level and type of background staining. Background staining can result from the staining procedure chosen for that test article or from endogenous or exogenous tissue pigments. Most immunohistochemical procedures used for tissue cross-reactivity are ultimately based on peroxidase cleavage of substrate–chromogen complexes to allow deposition of chromogen on tissue. If the staining procedure is avidin–biotin complex (ABC) based (e.g., biotinylated primary antibody), the tissue cryosections must be treated with specialty blocks to reduce endogenous biotin staining. These blocks generally are not required in staining of paraffin tissues unless antigen retrieval procedures are used. Certain tissue components (e.g., salivary gland duct epithelium) have higher endogenous biotin, which may compromise interpretation of that tissue component. Depending on the chromogen used in tissue cross-reactivity procedure, the background tissue pigments might have the same color or quality of staining as the chromogen. For example, the brown of diaminobenzidine is similar to the brown of melanin seen frequently in skin and eye sections. Other commonly encountered pigments include endogenous erythrocyte-derived pigments (reddish-yellow hemoglobin, yellowish-brown hemosiderin or hematoidin) or exogenous pigments (e.g., carbon pigments in macrophages in lungs from smokers or donors from polluted environments, india ink used to mark surgically obtained specimens).

10.5.5 Scoring

Scoring of test article staining in a tissue cross-reactivity study is a judgment call best made by a pathologist with broadly based experience in interpretation of frozen sections and comprehensive understanding of histology and immunohistochemistry. The actual scoring should include information regarding the cell or tissue component type, histologic location and pattern, subcellular location, and number or frequency of stained tissue components as well as the staining intensity. As a typical cross-reactivity study contains three donors per tissue, statistical analysis of the findings is generally not appropriate.

10.5.6 Types of Tissue Cross-Reactivity Staining Patterns

We have reviewed information from 161 typical cross-reactivity studies conducted by PAI-CRL.[3] These studies were selected from more than approximately 800 studies conducted between 1990 and 2006. The information is presented as percentages of total, but it is important to note that the percentages may exceed 100% as not all the studies had identical study design. For example, several studies included more than one test article, but the calculations were based on a per study basis. The specific data are proprietary, and only generalities are presented in the summary tables. The types and forms of the test articles and their epitopes are listed in Table 10.3, and the frequency of unexpected cross-reactivity is listed in Table 10.4.

The types and frequencies of cross-reactivity findings are listed by general category in Table 10.5. The most frequent unexpected cross-reactivities were recognized in neural, epithelial, or contractile filament components. Narrow-

TABLE 10.3 Test articles examined in 161 PAI-CRL tissue cross-reactivity studies

Types of test article	33% Human IgG1, 16% humanized IgG1
	7% Human IgG2, ≤1% human IgG3, 6% human IgG4
	2% Human Fab
	10% Chimeric, 10% mouse IgG1, 2% mouse IgG2a
	6% Fusion molecules or conjugates
Forms of test article	47% Unconjugated
	15% Biotinylated
	34% Fluoresceinated
	1% HRP-conjugated
	≤1% Other
Epitopes	29% CD markers
	25% Cytokine/chemokine receptors
	7% Integrins
	7% Infectious or toxic agents
	9% Other

TABLE 10.4 Frequency of unexpected cross-reactivity in 161 PAI-CRL tissue cross-reactivity studies

% Unexpected cross-reactivity	None (69%)
	Broad spectrum (6%)[a]
	Narrow spectrum (21%)[b]

[a]Multiple elements in multiple tissues.
[b]One to two elements in a few tissues, or one element in multiple tissues.

[3]Charles River Pathology Assoicates.

TABLE 10.5   **Types and frequencies of unexpected tissue cross-reactivity findings in 161 PAI-CRL studies**

Unexpected Cross-Reactivity	Broad Narrow-Spectrum?	% of Total Studies
Neural tissue components	Broad	4%
	Narrow	8%
		Axons, nerve endings—2%
		Neuropil—3%
		Schwann cells—2%
		Glial cells—1%
Endocrine tissue components	Broad	2%
	Narrow	4%
		Pituitary epithelium—2%
		Parathyroid epithelium—2%
Gonadal tissue components	Broad	1%
	Narrow	4%
		Seminiferous tubule cells—2%
		Gonadal fibroblasts—1%
		Oocytes—1%
Kidney tissue components	Broad	Not observed
	Narrow	Glomerular tuft cells—1%
Mucosal epithelium	Broad	4%
	Narrow	8%
		Stratified squamous epithelium—5%
		Basal lamina—1%
		Transitional cell epithelium (urinary)—1%
		Fallopian tube epithelium—1%
Gland or duct epithelium	Broad	2%
	Narrow	7%
		Apocrine gland epithelium—4%
		Salivary duct or acinar epithelium—2%
		Sebaceous duct epithelium—1%
		Pancreatic duct or acinar epithelium—1%
Cytoplasmic (contractile) filaments	Broad	7%
	Narrow	2%
		Myoepithelium—1%
		Cardiac myocytes—1%
		Skeletal myocytes—1%
		Myofibroblasts—1%
Endothelium	Broad	1%
	Narrow	1%
Other	Broad and/or narrow	Adipose (fat) cells—1%
		Mesothelium—1%
		Nuclei—1%
		Dendritic cells—1%

spectrum cross-reactivity (1–3 elements in a few tissues or 1 element in multiple tissues) was recognized more frequently than broad-spectrum cross-reactivity, except for contractile filaments in which broad-spectrum (multiple elements in multiple tissues) staining was recognized more often.

Examples of broad-spectrum and narrow-spectrum cross-reactivities are illustrated in Figures 10.5 and 10.6. Examples of unexpected staining of neural tissue elements are illustrated in Figures 10.7 and 10.8. Figure 10.8 also illustrates the very important point that large tissue sections are necessary for adequate evaluation of potential cross-reactivity. This particular cross-reactivity was seen in glial cells, primarily in dorsal but not ventral white

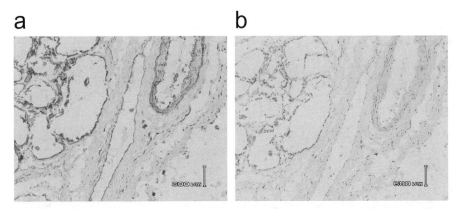

Figure 10.5   (*a*) Unexpected broad-spectrum cross-reactivity with epithelium, endothelium and selected vascular smooth myocytes. No staining of interstitial (stromal) cells, collagen, or nuclei. (*b*) No staining in replicate sections stained by negative control antibody at similar staining concentration. See color insert.

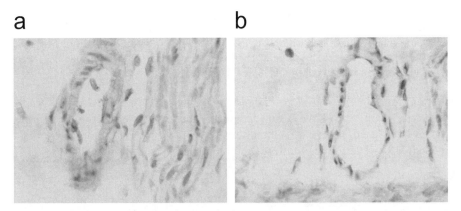

Figure 10.6   (*a*) Unexpected narrow-spectrum cross-reactivity with contractile filaments in vascular smooth myocytes. No staining of interstitial (stromal) cells, collagen, nuclei, or adjacent peripheral nerve. (*b*) No staining in replicate sections stained by negative control antibody at similar staining concentration. See color insert.

a   b

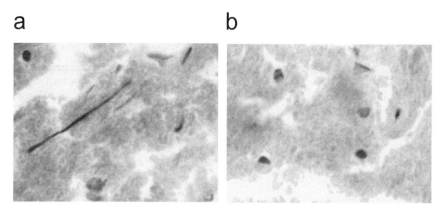

Figure 10.7   (*a*) Unexpected narrow-spectrum cross-reactivity with axons in human brain. No staining of neural tissue components. (*b*) No staining in replicate sections stained by negative control antibody at similar staining concentration. See color insert.

a   b

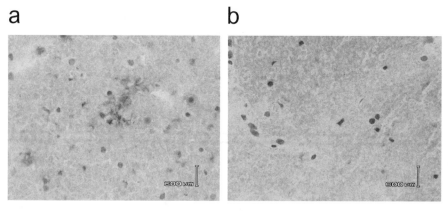

Figure 10.8   (*a*) Unexpected narrow-spectrum cross-reactivity with glial cells in dorsal tracts of human spinal cord. Clustering of glial cells might indicate a very small glial scar. No staining of neural tissue components. (*b*) Greatly reduced cross-reactivity with glial cells in ventral tracts of human spinal cord. See color insert.

matter tracts in the spinal cord. This difference (and potentially this cross-reactivity) would not have been recognized had smaller or incomplete tissue pieces been used. Figure 10.9 illustrates cross-reactivity with contractile filaments (cross-striations and intercalated discs) in heart muscle cells.

10.5.7   Context

Interpretation of test article staining should always be done in context of the published literature, knowledge of histology and physiologic processes, and common sense. We have previously seen staining of variably sized cytoplasmic inclusions in liver Kupffer cells when staining with antibodies directed against leukocyte markers. The staining did not represent true cross-reactivity with

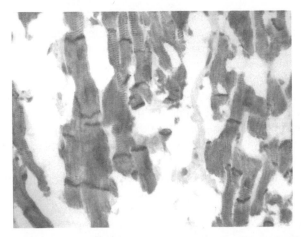

Figure 10.9   Unexpected cross-reactivity with contractile filaments (cross-striations, intercalated discs) in cardiac myocytes. No staining of sarcolemmal cells, interstitial cells or endothelium. See color insert.

Kupffer cell components but rather represented reactivity with leukocyte fragments that had been phagocytized by the Kupffer cells. Similar staining might be expected at other sites of leukocyte fragment clearance such as monocyte/ macrophages lining the cords of Billroth in spleen or subcapsular or medullary sinusoids in lymph node. Likewise, in staining human tissues for the presence of an integrin highly expressed on platelets, distinct particles in Kupffer cells that resembled platelets also stained. The initial thought was that Kupffer cells themselves were staining. To unravel this, a commercial antibody against glycoprotein 1b, an antigen expressed only on platelets, was purchased and applied to the tissues. The stained antigens were thus identified as platelets within the Kupffer cells, indicating that either platelets were phagocytized by the Kupffer cells before death or phagocytosis of platelets occurred as a postmortem event during the interval between death and autopsy.

10.5.8   Significance of Tissue Cross-Reactivity Findings

As discussed above, the FDA and other international regulatory authorities strongly recommend tissue cross-reactivity studies as part of any monoclonal antibody test article approval/registration package. Additionally, tissue cross-reactivity studies provide an immunohistochemical window through which to examine patterns of CDR-mediated and non–CDR-mediated staining. This window can reveal potential efficacy or toxicity targets as well as novel information regarding potential sites of expression of target epitope or related but off-target cross-reactive epitopes. However, the presence of tissue cross-reactivity does not equate to toxicity. Likewise, the absence of tissue cross-reactivity does not necessarily ensure safe administration of monoclonal antibody test articles. Rather, tissue cross-reactivity just reveals potential sites to monitor for test article binding. When the actual monoclonal antibody drug is administered to humans or animals, it becomes incorporated into the circulating immunoglobulin pool and is distributed, cleared, and/or salvaged by physiologic (and in heterologous species, immunologic) processes (Chapter 11). Whether monoclonal antibody test articles will bind to these or other (FcR, nonspecific, or non–CDR-mediated) sites will depend on the route of test article administration, extent of tissue distribution following administration, test article binding affinity, and the nature of, and potential access to, the cross-reactive subcellular sites and/or extracellular components.

The potential hierarchy of cross-reactivity findings according to site of test article staining is presented in Table 10.6. Test article cross-reactivity with membrane targets generally has been considered to be of greatest potential biological relevance or toxicity because access to this compartment is theoretically greater. Membrane binding to high-density epitopes also has been considered more likely to trigger events such as complement fixation and cell destruction, alterations in cell signaling, or ADCC than antibody binding to other cellular locations (see above).

The information in Table 10.6 is in fact oversimplified. Access to target and potential off-target epitopes is first and foremost affected by antibody distribution. The physiologic distribution of monoclonal antibody test articles (Chapter 11) suggests that the drug will be presented sequentially to intravascular components (blood cells, plasma components), endothelium, vessel wall, perivascular interstitial fluid and extracellular fibrils, cell membrane, cell cytoplasm (if receptor-mediated or nonspecific uptake occurs), nuclei (if nuclear uptake occurs). Additionally some of the administered antibody will be cleared, compartmentalized intracellularly, and/or salvaged by physiologic processes conducted by endothelium, monocytes/macrophages, and epithelium. Last, normal cell turnover might provide nuclear, membrane, or cytoplasmic fragments that could be present as possible binding targets in blood or tissue.

10.5.9   Animal Tissue Cross-Reactivity Testing

Animal tissue cross-reactivity studies can provide information regarding whether the animal species under consideration might provide relevant models for safety/toxicity testing. Cross-reactivity is one of a number of methods for determining a relevant species; others include flow cytometry and assessing expected pharmacologic events to a monoclonal antibody. However, the animal tissue cross-reactivity staining patterns alone are not sufficient to ensure or deny the relevance of toxicity testing in that species. The example cited earlier in this chapter of the differences in T10B9 staining of membrane CD3/TCR complex molecules on human T lymphocytes and cytoplasmic filaments in human and primate epithelial cells is useful [22]. While toxicity testing in the primate might not reveal anything about the potential for toxicity following T10B9 binding to T lymphocyte membranes, it might reveal information regarding access and/or toxicity to subcellular epithelial compartments. Finally, the appropriate use of a relevant species to identify any adverse events or to

TABLE 10.6   Potential for toxicity for cross-reactivity by cytologic or histologic location

Cytologic Location	Homologue(s)	Example(s) of Homologues	Potential for Toxicity for Unexpected Cross-Reactivity
Membrane	CD markers, receptors	CD3 in medullary thymocytes	Probably highest regulatory concern
Cytoplasm	Cytokines, chemokines, rare CD markers	CD3 in cortical thymoctyes	Probably limited in vivo access
Cytoplasmic filaments	Cytoskeleton, functional internal borders	Intermediate or contractile filaments	Probably limited in vivo access
Cytoplasmic granules	Organized subcellular sites (e.g., endosomes, lysosomes, ER/Golgi)	Pituitary hormones	Probably limited in vivo access
Nucleus	Nucleus, nucleolus	Steroid hormone receptors	Immune-mediated disease?
Soluble	Serum, interstitial fluid, urine, CSF, other body fluids	Cytokines, chemokines, complement factors, shed tumor antigens	Little to unknown
Extracellular structures	Basal lamina, basement membrane, interstitial fibers	Laminin, elastin, collagen, intercellular substance	Unknown? Immune-mediated disease?

make a final determination as to whether antibody binding actually occurs in vivo is important. Many of the cross-reacting antigens are cytoplasmic, and appropriately designed toxicity studies can help unravel their biological significance. Reviewing the animal tissues subsequent to injection of the monoclonal antibody into them for changes related to the antigens, and also demonstration of the injected monoclonal antibody binding to suspect tissues in vivo, can add a great measure to the safety of the product.

10.6   BIOLOGICAL RELEVANCE OF HUMAN TISSUE CROSS-REACTIVITY STUDIES

Several types of hypersensitivity reactions can occur in the host receiving mono-clonal antibody therapy, and the tissue cross-reactivity study might be predic-tive of some of these hypersensitivity reactions. Theoretically, adverse reactions result in tissue destruction because of the activation of complement or release of perforin and/or other inflammatory mediators by effector cells (K cells, neutrophils, macrophages) bound to the antibody by Fc receptors [26]. One example of a possible type II hypersensitivity reaction is described in Sections 10.6.2. In practice, type II hypersensitivity reactions are more likely elicited by anti-idiotypic responses to monoclonal antibody infusion than to the infusion itself. However, the anti-CD20 monoclonal antibody rituximab has been linked to cytokine release. This adverse reaction is speculated to be mediated by cross-linking of the antibody to target cell receptors, Fc engagement, and complement activation [27]. Other reactions, such as type I (IgE mediated hypersensitivity), types III (immune complex) and IV (cell mediated hypersensitivity), might also play a role in host disease. For example, administration of infliximab has been associated with type I, II, and III hypersensitivity reactions due to development of anti-idiotype antibodies [28]. Local injection site reactions to monoclonal antitumor necrosis factor-α antibodies (e.g., adalimumab) are reported to elicit type IV hypersensitivity reactions [29]. There are other considerations that assist in this evaluation of the biological relevance of human tissue cross-reactivity studies, such as the valence of the antibody, the subclass affecting Fc binding and cytokine release from effector cells, concentration and distribution of the antibody molecule in the tissues, and location of the stained cross-reacting antigen to determine its accessibility by the antibody.

In the tissue cross-reactivity studies, the antibody has equal access to all tissues and all cell components (membrane, cytosol, nucleus) of the tissues on the section. This is not true in vivo where access to the tissues is governed by passive diffusion of the antibody to the tissue. Moreover, unless uptake by tissues is receptor-mediated, cell membranes preclude entrance of an antibody into the cells. In addition there are blood–brain, blood–nerve, blood–eye, and blood–testis barriers characterized by specialized endothelium that reduce movement of immunoglobulin into these protected spaces. Thus, some tissues have relatively little access by antibodies compared to others. Likewise, antigens within cells have little chance of access to the antibody compared to cell membrane or transmembrane antigens.

Antibodies injected intravenously are more accessible to tissues associated with the vasculature (endothelium, blood leukocytes, platelets, and erythrocytes) compared with deeper, more complex tissues that are poorly perfused. Thus, the location of the cells in the body relative to vascular perfusion and diffusion of antibodies are important aspects of interpretation of the cross-reactivity studies. For example, ReoPro® (abciximab, c7E3 Fab) is an antibody Fab directed against glycoprotein IIb/IIIa on the platelet surface. This receptor is responsible for interacting with fibrinogen and von Willebrand factor that result in platelet aggregation and thrombosis. Blockage of these receptors prevents platelet aggregation and thrombosis [30].

10.6.1 Valence

ReoPro® a Fab monovalent, and this precludes cross-linking of platelets that would occur if the antibody were bivalent. The half-life of ReoPro® is approximately 10 minutes with a secondary half-life of 30 minutes in humans, in part because of the size of the molecule but, more important, because of the intravascular location of the platelets as well as the high affinity of the antibody for the platelet receptor. In clinical trials ReoPro® has proved to be an effective agent in preventing platelet aggregation and thrombosis. Additionally, a portion of the gpIIb/IIIa molecule is a β_3-integrin receptor (e.g., vitronectin receptor, $\alpha_v\beta_3$) expressed by different cell types, including neovascular endothelium and smooth muscle. The binding of ReoPro® to neovascular endothelium reportedly reduces attachment of the endothelial cells to the basal lamina, which is an important aspect of its usefulness as a therapeutic for coronary angioplasty [30–31]. A bivalent antibody produced against the same antigen in mice resulted in platelet loss [32].

10.6.2 ADCC

ADCC is a reaction that can occur with IgG1 and IgG3 antibodies where the antibody binds to the antigen in question and killer cells (K cells and CD8+ K cells, NK-cells) then bind to the Fc portion of the antibody by the FcγRIII or other receptors on the effector cells [26].

An IgG1 chimeric (mouse/human) antibody was developed against an antigen expressed on a large number of human colon carcinomas [33] and a cross-reactivity study was performed. The antibody bound to endothelial cells of the gray matter of the cerebrum (Figure 10.10). The same reactivity occurred in the cynomolgus monkey, and a toxicity study was conducted in this relevant species. In order to eliminate the possibility of cell repair and resolution of any lesions that might develop with this antibody, a small number of the

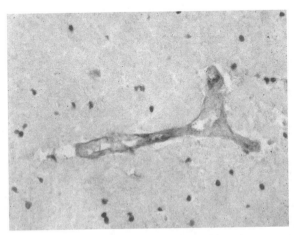

Figure 10.10 Staining of endothelium of human cerebral gray matter with chimeric antibody to a colon carcinoma antigen. The same endothelial staining pattern occurred in cynomolgus monkey cerebral gray matter. ABC Immunoperoxidase. See color insert.

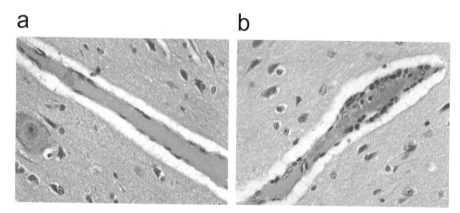

Figure 10.11   Vessels in the cerebral gray matter of control (*a*) and dosed (*b*) cynomolgus monkey 72 hours following IV injection of an antibody directed against colon carcinoma. Note the leukocytes adherent to the endothelium characteristic of ADCC. See color insert.

animals were sacrificed 72 hours following IV injection of the antibody. The pathology report was negative for any effects and a phase 1 trial was initiated. Of the six persons injected with the antibody, three developed dizziness and short-term memory loss, which subsided upon withdrawal of the drug. Additional review of the monkey brain tissues revealed the presence of mononuclear cells along the endothelial surface of small blood vessels in the cerebral cortical gray matter (Figure 10.11*a* and 10.11*b*). The cell infiltrates were not further characterized by staining for CD16 or any of the CD markers. The reaction nevertheless was consistent with ADCC, indicating the value of an appropriate model and careful interpretation of both the pathology and the cross-reactivity study.

10.6.3 Immune Complex Disease

In order to induce immune complex disease following immunization with a foreign protein (bovine gamma globulin), one generally needs to inject high levels of the foreign protein to produce the disease [32]. For symptoms and lesions of immune complex disease to occur, many immune complexes are needed. This usually means that the amount of protein injected must exceed the levels of antibodies produced in order to attain a level of antigen excess. For a nonhuman primate immunized against bovine gamma globulin, approximately 4.9 mg/kg is necessary to produce antibody equivalence for development of chronic immune complex disease [32–34]. For immune complex disease to occur, two conditions must be met: (1) the protein must be recognized by the host as foreign and (2) the levels of foreign protein must be high enough to exceed the level of antibody generated against them. The majority of monoclonal antibodies are human or humanized and therefore less likely than rodent antibodies to elicit anti-antibody responses, unless these are anti-idiotypic responses directed against the therapeutic antibody CDR. Moreover therapeutic levels of most monoclonal antibodies are much lower, resulting in a dose of less than 100 μg/ml of plasma or approximately 3 mg/kg body weight. Effective monoclonal antibody concentrations usually are much less than 100 μg/ml, on the order of 1 to 20 μg/ml.

The story is different for an antigen targeted by the monoclonal antibody (site-directed immune complex disease). Immune complex disease can result by reactivity of the host against the bound antibody. Again, little reactivity is observed against the monoclonal antibody having host specific characteristics (human, humanized, and in most cases, chimeric antibodies), but this differs with a xenogenic immunoglobulin. In a number of studies we have assessed where the toxicity model was other than the homologous antibody host species, site-directed immune complex disease has been observed. Generally, serum complement levels are reduced during the toxicity portion of the study, and there is the deposition of host Ig and C3 at the sites of antibody localization accompanied by infiltrates of various inflammatory cells.

Sometimes, development of immune disease that targets the antigen is a welcomed event. Some anti-tumor monoclonal antibodies (e.g., monoclonal antibody 17-1A directed against the colon carcinoma antigen) are expected to elicit an anti-idiotypic host response. The anti-idiotypic antibody structure mimics the tumor antigen and can act as a vaccine resulting in an anti-anti-idiotypic response against the antigen [38–40]. Response can be either antibody mediated or T cell mediated.

10.7 CONCLUSIONS

Tissue cross-reactivity studies, although burdensome, provide a rational in vitro assay to determine the range and intensity of distribution of potential epitopes reactive with a monoclonal antibody test article prior to its administration to humans. In addition, cross-reactivity studies provide a useful tool to identify animal species for safety assessment. The cross-reactivity profiles of different species can be compared to the profiles obtained in human tissues. The predictive value of the assay lies in incorporating the characteristics of the monoclonal antibody (isotype, subtype, and other molecular modifications) with the biological activity of the molecule itself, and the potential in vivo distribution of it.

REFERENCES

1. Kohler G, Milstein C. Continuous cultures of fused cells secreting antibody of predefined specificity. *Nature* 1975;256:495–7.
2. Cosimi AB, Colvin RB, Burton RC, Rubin RH, Goldstein G, Kung PC, Hansen WP, Delmonico FL, Russell PS. Use of monoclonal antibodies to T-cell subsets for

immunologic monitoring and treatment in recipients of renal allografts. *N Engl J Med* 1981;305:308–14.

3. Bristow MR, Gilbert EM, O'Connell JB, Renlund DG, Watson FS, Hammond E, Lee RG, Menlove R. OKT3 monoclonal antibody in heart transplantation. *Am J Kidney Dis* 1988;11:135–40.

4. Gay WA, Jr., O'Connell JG, Burton NA, Karwande SV, Renlund DG, Bristow MR. OKT3 monoclonal antibody in cardiac transplantation. Experience with 102 patients. *Ann Surg* 1988;208:287–90.

5. Norman DJ, Shield CF 3rd , Barry J, Bennett WM, Henell K, Kimball J, Funnell B, Hubert B. Early use of OKT3 monoclonal antibody in renal transplantation to prevent rejection. *Am J Kidney Dis* 1988;11:107–10.

6. Smith SL. Immunosuppressive therapies in organ transplantation. *Medscape* 2002. (http://www.medscape.com/viewarticle/437182).

7. Oldstone MB. Molecular mimicry and immune-mediated diseases. *Faseb J* 1998; 12:1255–65.

8. Abbas AK, Lichtman AH, Polischuk J. *Cellular and Molecular Immunology*, 4th ed. Philadelphia: WB Saunders.

9. Reff ME, Hariharan K, Braslawsky G. Future of monoclonal antibodies in the treatment of hematologic malignancies. *Cancer Control* 2002;9(2):152–66.

10. Le Calvez H, Yu M, Fang F. Biochemical prevention and treatment of viral infections—a new paradigm in medicine for infectious diseases. *Virol J* 2004;1:12.

11. Kirman I, Whelan RL, Nielsen OH. Infliximab: mechanism of action beyond TNF-alpha neutralization in inflammatory bowel disease. *Eur J Gastroenterol Hepatol* 2004;16:639–41.

12. Tcheng JE, Kereiakes DJ, Lincoff AM, George BS, Kleiman NS, Sane DC, Cines DB, Jordan RE, Mascelli MA, Langrall MA, Damaraju L, Schantz A, Effron MB, Braden GA. Abciximab readministration: results of the ReoPro Readministration Registry. *Circulation* 2001;104:870–5.

13. Brekke OH, Sandlie I. Therapeutic antibodies for human diseases at the dawn of the twenty-first century. *Nat Rev Drug Discov* 2003;2:52–62.

14. Harjunpaa A, Junnikkala S, Meri S. Rituximab (anti-CD20) therapy of B-cell lymphomas: direct complement killing is superior to cellular effector mechanisms. *Scand J Immunol* 2000;51:634–41.

15. Coons AH, Creech HJ, Jones RN, Berliner E. The demonstration of pneumococcal antigen in tissues by the use of fluorescent antibody. *J Immunol* 1942;45:159–63.

16. Avremeas S. Coupling of enzymes to proteins with glutaraldehyde: use of the conjugates for the detection of antigens and antibodies. *Immunohistochemistry* 1971;6:394.

17. Fung K, Messing A, Lee VM-Y, Trojanowski JQ. A novel modification of the avidin-biotin-complex method for immuniohistochemical studies of transgenic mice with murine monoclonal antibodies. *J Histochem Cytochem* 1992;40:1319–28.

18. Hierck BP, Iperen LV, Groot ACG-D, Poelmann RE. Modified indirect immunodetection allows study of murine tissue with mouse monoclonal antibodies. *J Histochem Cytochem* 1994;42:1499–1502.

19. Tuson JR, Pascoe EW, Jacob D. A novel immunohistochemical technique for demonstration of specific binding of human monoclonal antibodies to human cryostat sections. *J Histochem Cytochem* 1990;38:923.

20. Faure GC, Tang JQ, Mathieu P, Bene MC. A CD4-like molecule can be expressed in vivo in human parathyroid. *J Clin Endocrinol Metab* 1990;71:656–60.

21. Hellman P, Karlsson-Parra A, Klareskog L, Ridefelt P, Bjerneroth G, Rastad J, Akerstrom G, Juhlin C. Expression and function of a CD4-like molecule in parathyroid tissue. *Surgery* 1996;120:985–92.

22. Campana D, Thompson JS, Amlot P, Brown S, Janossy G. The cytoplasmic expression of CD3 antigens in normal and malignant cells of the T lymphoid lineage. *J Immunol* 1987;138:648–55.

23. Waid TH, Lucas BA, Amlot P, Janossy G, Yacoub M, Cammisuli S, Jezek D, Rhoades J, Brown S, Thompson JS. T10B9.1A-31 anti-T-cell monoclonal antibody: preclinical studies and clinical treatment of solid organ allograft rejection. *Am J Kidney Dis* 1989;14:61–70.

24. Waid TH, Thompson JS, McKeown JW, Brown SA, Sekela ME. Induction immunotherapy in heart transplantation with T10B9.1A-31: a phase I study. *J Heart Lung Transplant* 1997;16:913–16.

25. Bunin N, Aplenc R, Leahey A, Magira E, Grupp S, Pierson G, Monos D. Outcomes of transplantation with partial T-cell depletion of matched or mismatched unrelated or partially matched related donor bone marrow in children and adolescents with leukemias. *Bone Marrow Transplant* 2005;35:151–8.

26. Male D. Hypersensitivity type II. In Roitt I, Brostoff J, Male D (eds), *Immunology*. Mosby International, London, 1998, pp 319–28.

27. Winkler U, Jensen M, Manzke O, Schulz H, Diehl V, Engert A. Cytokine-release syndrome in patients with B-cell chronic lymphocytic leukemia and high lymphocyte counts after treatment with an anti-CD20 monoclonal antibody (rituximab, IDEC-C2B8). *Blood* 1999;94(7):2217–24.

28. Lee SJ, Kavanaugh A. Adverse reactions to biologic agents: focus on autoimmune disease therapies. *J Allergy Clin Immunol* 2005;116(4):900–5.

29. Zeltser R, Valle L, Tanck C, Holyst MM, Ritchlin C, Gaspari AA. Clinical, histological, and immunophenotypic characteristics of injection site reactions associated with etanercept: a recombinant tumor necrosis factor alpha receptor: Fc fusion protein. *Arch Dermatol* 2001;137(7):893–9.

30. Lefkovits J, Plow EF, Topol EJ. Platelet glycoprotein IIb/IIIa receptors in cardiovascular medicine. *N Engl J Med* 1995;332:1553–9.

31. Romagnoli E, Burzotta F, Trani C, Biondi-Zoccai GG, Giannico F, Crea F. Rationale for intracoronary administration of abciximab. *J Thromb Thrombolysis* 2007; 23(1):57–63.

32. Teeling JL, Jansen-Hendriks T, Kuijpers TW, de Haas M, van De Winkel JG, Hack CE, Bleeker WK. Therapeutic efficacy of intravenous immunoglobulin preparations depends on the immunoglobulin G dimers: studies in experimental immune thrombocytopenia. *Blood* 2001;98:1095–9.

33. Hurwitz E, Adler R, Shouval D, Takahashi H, Wands JR, Sela M. Immunotargeting of daunomycin to localized and metastatic human colon adenocarcinoma in athymic mice. *Cancer Immunol Immunother* 1992;35:186–92.

34. Noble B, Brentjens JR. Experimental serum sickness. *Meth Enzymol* 1988;162: 484–501.

35. Birmingham DJ, Hebert LA, Cosio FG, VanAman ME. Immune complex erythrocyte complement receptor interactions in vivo during induction of glomerulonephritis in nonhuman primates. *J Lab Clin Med* 1990;116:242–52.

36. Hebert LA, Birmingham DJ, Shen XP, Cosio FG, Fryczkowski A. Rate of antigen entry into the circulation in experimental versus naturally occurring immune complex glomerulonephritis. *J Am Soc Nephrol* 1994;5:S70–5.

37. Hebert LA, Cosio FG, Birmingham DJ, Mahan JD, Sharma HM, Smead WL, Goel R. Experimental immune complex-mediated glomerulonephritis in the nonhuman primate. *Kidney Int* 1991;39:44–56.

38. Fagerberg J, Frodin JE, Ragnhammar P, Steinitz M, Wigzell H, Mellstedt H. Induction of an immune network cascade in cancer patients treated with monoclonal antibodies (ab1). II. Is induction of anti-idiotype reactive T cells (T3) of importance for tumor response to mAb therapy? *Cancer Immunol Immunother* 1994;38: 149–59.

39. Fagerberg J, Frodin JE, Wigzell H, Mellstedt H. Induction of an immune network cascade in cancer patients treated with monoclonal antibodies (ab1). I. May induction of ab1-reactive T cells and anti-anti-idiotypic antibodies (ab3) lead to tumor regression after mAb therapy? *Cancer Immunol Immunother* 1993;37:264–70.

40. Mellstedt H, Frodin JE, Biberfeld P, Fagerberg J, Giscombe R, Hernandez A, Masucci G, Li SL, Steinitz M. Patients treated with a monoclonal antibody (ab1) to the colorectal carcinoma antigen 17–1A develop a cellular response (DTH) to the internal image of the antigen (ab2). *Int J Cancer* 1991;48:344–9.

CHAPTER 11

Physiologic IgG Biodistribution, Transport, and Clearance: Implications for Monoclonal Antibody Products

JENNIFER L. ROJKO, DVM, PhD, DACVP, and SHARI PRICE-SCHIAVI, PhD, DABT

Contents

Preclinical Safety Evaluation of Biopharmaceuticals: A Science-Based Approach to Facilitating Clinical Trials, edited by Joy A. Cavagnaro
Copyright © 2008 by John Wiley & Sons, Inc.

11.1 INTRODUCTION

Following administration, monoclonal antibodies become part of the endogenous IgG pool for distribution, transport and clearance unless these physiologic processes are altered by antibody CDR–epitope interactions or host anti-mononclonal antibody immune responses. This review focuses on physiologic (endogenous) IgG biodistribution, clearance and transport processes. Most of the information on these processes was derived from human clinical or laboratory studies. When available, information on exogenously administered monoclonal antibody test articles (data obtained from experimental studies in mice, monkeys or other species or clinical studies in humans) is included. The information is assumed to apply generally to humans and nonhuman primates (particularly cynomolgus monkeys), unless otherwise noted. Monoclonal antibody pharmacokinetics and pharmacodynamics were reviewed by Lobo and colleagues [1].

This review is intended to provide helpful information regarding potential monoclonal antibody IgG test article (non–CDR-mediated) binding to specific tissues, cell types or other tissue elements, and subcellular locations following exogenous intravenous administration in animal model test systems. Particulars specific to other routes of administration were reviewed by Lobo et al. [1].

Concerning plasma IgG characteristics in humans, endogenous human IgG (150 kd) has a plasma half-life greater than 21 days in humans [2]. The plasma level ranges from 8 to 16 mg/ml in healthy volunteers. Eighty percent of the total Ig in plasma is IgG with 65% of total IgG being IgG1 (Figure 11.1) [2]. With these levels of total IgG, administration of a therapeutic antibody, even at relatively high doses, is not expected to change the total level of plasma IgG or specifically IgG1 significantly. Therefore, it is safe to assume that exogenously administered antibodies will be distributed, transported, and cleared through normal physiologic processes [1].

Similar to that of endogenous IgG, the plasma half-life for human IgG1, IgG2, and IgG4 therapeutic antibodies can be up to three to four weeks in humans. This long plasma half-life has been ascribed to the protection from catabolism conferred by the neonatal Fc receptor (FcRn) as part of its role in regulating IgG homeostasis [3–5] (see below). In beta-2-microglobulin-

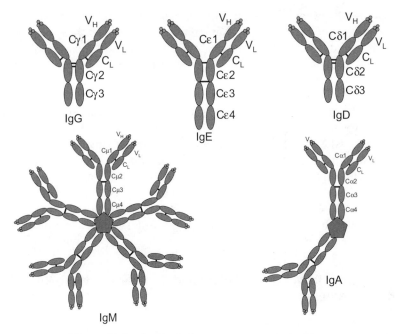

Figure 11.1   Antibody isotypes present in humans.

deficient mice, marked reductions in plasma IgG half-life (beta-phase [4]) are concomitant with reduced FcRn expression. On the other hand, the plasma half-life of human IgG3 is shorter due to a single amino acid difference (arginine substitution for histidine at position 435) in the FcRn binding domain [6] (see discussions of FcRn and isotype below) that results in less FcRn binding.

Fab (50 kd) and scFv (27 kd) antibody fragments have shorter plasma half-lives (0.5 to 21 hours) because of more rapid glomerular filtration and clearance [7]. Plasma clearance, particularly of the xenogenic (usually mouse) portions of humanized and/or chimeric monoclonal antibodies, might be accelerated by development of anti-mouse (or other species), anti-isotypic, anti-idiotypic, or anti-allotypic antibodies that foster immune complex formation or reticuloendothelial clearance via several different FcR forms or elicit allergic or anaphylactic responses [7,8].

11.2   BIODISTRIBUTION OF ENDOGENOUS IgG

Among the benefits of intravascular administration of antibody-based therapies are the rapid intravascular biodistribution and high-level bioavailability. Several factors influence the biodistribution of immunoglobulins within the vascular and tissue compartments. Intravascular fluid biodistribution of endogenous (or exogenous) IgG to any human tissue depends on the cardiac output (liver 28%, kidney 23%, brain 14%, skin 9%, skeletal muscle 16%, heart muscle 5%, rest of body 6% [9]) and vascularity of that tissue.[1] Within each tissue, IgG biodistribution is affected by the locations of capillary beds and postcapillary venules. Tissue compartment IgG levels are increased by processes promoting egress from vessels into tissue (convection, transcellular transport, receptor-mediated transport, and diffusion) and decreased when IgG is removed by catabolism or lymphatic drainage (convection, diffusion of fluid-phase antibodies, and migration of IgG or immune complexes associated with mononuclear or dendritic cells [1]). Further details of pharmacokinetic characteristics of exogenously administered monoclonal antibodies including CDR-mediated, epitope interaction-dependent influences on biodistribution and epitope-independent, plasma concentration-dependent clearance mechanisms were reviewed by Lobo et al. [1].

11.2.1 Egress from Intravascular Fluid Compartment into Interstitial Fluid Compartment

In liver, lung, kidney glomeruli, and spleen, the high vascularity and high cardiac output (first-pass effect) increases the potential for high uptake of antibody by that tissue. In less vascularized tissues (e.g., lymph node, remainder of kidney[2]), higher plasma concentrations are needed to generate higher concentration gradients to facilitate diffusion to more distant targets [13,14]. The rate of diffusion into interstitium is regulated by plasma concentration, plasma–interstitium concentration gradient, and outward diffusion into lymphatics, and this has been estimated as 5% to 10% of the rate of diffusion in aqueous solutions [1,15,16].

To reach the perivascular interstitium, immunoglobulins and other molecules must breach the endothelial cell barrier. Simionescu and Anthohe [17] note that an adult human contains more than 10^{13} endothelial cells which cover 7000 square meters and mass approximately 1 kg.[3] Egress to interstitium is affected by type of endothelium (continuous, fenestrated, or sinusoidal), endothelial uptake and transport processes (receptor-dependent or receptor-independent uptake, endocytosis and transcytosis[4]), paracellular (between or

---

[1]Cardiac output to rhesus monkey tissues was described by Forsyth et al. [10].

[2]The capillaries of the nonglomerular renal cortex (e.g., peritubular capillaries) represent a second capillary bed that derives from ramifications of the efferent glomerular arteriole. The vascular sequence is renal artery—arcuate arteries/arcuate arterioles—cortical arterioles—afferent (glomerular) arteriole—glomerular capillaries—efferent (glomerular) arteriole—peritubular capillaries [11,12].

[3]Pries and Kuebler [18] indicated a total surface area of 350 square meters and a mass of 100 g.

4Simionescu et al. [19] defined transcytosis as the polarized transport of plasma proteins across cells via caveolae or endosomal transport vesicles to the subjacent tissue or bidirectionally across other polarized cells such as epithelial cells.

alongside cells) transport, and tissue-specific barriers to macromolecule transport (e.g., blood–brain, blood–eye, or blood–nerve barriers; see below). Leakage of plasma proteins is greater from postcapillary venules than from capillaries as interendothelial pores are generally larger (50–60 angstroms compared with 18–20 angstroms [20]).

In addition molecules have been identified on continuous endothelium that facilitate binding of albumin to endothelium, increase capillary permeability, and theoretically can increase paracellular transport or transcytosis of albumin-bound molecules. An example of this is the gp60 albumin-binding glycoprotein molecule identified on continuous endothelium in multiple tissues (heart, lung, skeletal muscle, adipose, peritoneum, and intestinal smooth muscle) but absent from continuous endothelium in cerebral cortex, and sinusoidal or fenestrated endothelium in liver, adrenal, pancreas, and intestinal lamina propria [21,22].

Antibody fragments (either administered directly or generated by catabolism in the test species) distribute differently than whole IgG molecules. Monoclonal antibody fragments diffuse into interstitial fluid compartments faster and/or more completely than whole monoclonal IgG molecules in tissues with fenestrated or continuous vascular endothelium. However, antibody fragments and whole IgG molecules have comparable rates of diffusion in tissues with sinusoidal vascular endothelium (e.g., liver and spleen) in tumor-bearing mice [23]. The faster transfer across fenestrated or continuous capillary endothelium has been ascribed to the lower molecular weight (and increased capacity for diffusion) of the antibody fragments [23]. Antibody size-independent processes also limit IgG transfer from vessels to interstitium and include interstitial fluid/matrix pressure and cellular macromolecular exclusion [15]. Once within a tissue, exposure of potential target tissue elements to exogenously administered monoclonal antibodies can be affected by distance from blood vessels. Highly sticky monoclonal antibodies might associate with the first targets they encounter and will not distribute well to more distant targets. This might also rapidly decrease apparent plasma concentration and reduce concentration gradient across interstitium or parenchyma, further reducing distribution to more distant tissue elements.

Leukocyte-associated IgG egress from plasma is potentially mediated by binding of endogenous IgG or exogenously administered monoclonal antibodies to $Fc_\gamma RI$ or $Fc_\gamma RIII$ on circulating neutrophils and monocytes [2] or $Fc_\gamma RIIa$ on platelets [24,25]. Human peripheral blood monocytes also bear MHC class I-related FcRn that can transport IgG from plasma to tissue fluids, dendritic cells, or intestinal macrophages [26].

Transendothelial IgG transport may be mediated by binding of endogenous IgG or exogenously administered monoclonal antibodies to $Fc_\gamma RIIa,b$ on endothelium (e.g., $Fc_\gamma RIIa$ on skin microvessels [27]); $Fc_\gamma RIIb$ on placenta villous (fetal) endothelium [28,29]; or FcRn on placental syncytiotrophoblasts and fetal endothelium [28]. Transcellular transport is further described below under FcRn-mediated transport, $Fc_\gamma RIIa$-mediated transport, and specialized skin microvessel transport mechanisms.

Interendothelial (paracellular sieving) IgG transport is generally not efficient across continuous endothelium during homeostasis, but it can show increased efficiency in normally fenestrated, incomplete (kidney glomerulus) or sinusoidal endothelium (liver, spleen) or in inflamed vessels. Interendothelial paracellular sieving is generally restricted to the transport of water, ions, and other small molecules that can traverse the 6 nm gap found in about 30% of postcapillary venules [19]. Interepithelial paracellular IgG sieving may also occur. Paracellular sieving can increase early in inflammation when adjacent endothelial cells or epithelial cells retract and increase the paracellular space available [30].

Last, monoclonal antibodies or antibody fragments with specificity for endothelial transport systems (e.g., endosomal pathways) have been proposed as targeting devices to enhance therapeutic drug delivery or overcome tissue barriers [31].

11.2.2   Tissue-specific Barriers to IgG Transport/Uptake

In health, the blood–brain barrier is formed by tightly joined, nonfenestrated capillary endothelium with contributions by supporting perivascular astrocytic end-feet [32–34] and generally is thought to limit brain entry of endogenous IgG (or exogenously administered monoclonal antibody IgG test article) from plasma. However, endogenous IgG and other large hydrophilic molecules (including amyloid-$\beta_{1\text{-}40/42}$) can undergo brain–blood efflux [35]. This efflux is thought to be regulated by the adenosine triphosphate (ATP)-binding cassette transporter P-glycoprotein (P-gp) located within endothelial caveolae along with membrane and transport-related moieties cholesterol, caveolin-1, and caveolin-2 [36]. Additionally brain capillary endothelium expresses transferrin receptors; specific anti-transferrin receptor antibody-linked liposomes can be transferred into capillary endothelium but apparently do not enter brain parenchyma [37]. Whether the blood–brain movement of endogenous IgG or exogenously administered monoclonal antibodies is affected by $Fc_\gamma RI$-positive perivascular cells (macrophages, microglia) is not completely understood [38–44].

The blood–brain barrier can be overcome in certain circumstances. For example, in rats, uptake of mouse anti-*Cryptococcus neoformans* monoclonal antibodies into brain or cerebrospinal fluid is very limited after intravenous administration, but good uptake occurs after intrathecal administration [45]. Additionally, the blood–brain barrier can be overcome when molecules that are highly expressed by brain capillary endothelial cell membranes (e.g., transferrin) are targeted by specific antibodies as reported by Pardridge et al. [46] using a monoclonal anti-transferrin antibody in rats. In that study, the anti-transferrin antibody was cleared biexponentially, first by rapid, saturatable, transient hepatic extraction and later by slow continuous brain endothelial removal compared to the monoexponential clearance of isotype-matched negative control antibody by the liver [46].[5] Further non–CDR-mediated binding can theoretically occur to FcRn or other receptors on brain endothelium. In rats, confocal microscopy experiments demonstrated FcRn expressed by Glut1 transporter-coexpressing capillary endothelium at the blood–brain barrier as well as by choroid plexus epithelium [47].

The blood–brain barrier generally protects the retina of the eye, but the barrier is interrupted at the prelaminar optic nerve head [48]. The aqueous humor of the eye is accessible to plasma macromolecules and contains albumin, with lesser amounts of transferrin, IgA, and IgG [49]. Although avascular, the cornea receives nutrients via percolation from the limbal vasculature (i.e., scleral venous plexus and associated arterioles). Repeated intravenous infusion of rabbit polyclonal anti-HSA IgG into nonimmunized rabbits indicated slowly increasing centripetal diffusion into rabbit cornea (approximately 1% per day), with corneal anti-HSA IgG reaching the avascular central portions of the cornea and equilibrating at approximately 70% of serum anti-HSA IgG at approximately 70 days; diffusion and equilibration were independent of electrostatic charge [50]. Last, while the blood–brain barrier can protect the brain parenchyma, it cannot protect the meningeal tissue. Intravascular polyclonal immunoglobulin therapy has been associated with a single case of aseptic meningitis, but the pathogenesis was not detailed [51].

Peripheral nerves and spinal nerve roots (including endoneurium) are not protected by the blood–brain barrier but are afforded some protection by a blood–nerve barrier consisting of continuous endothelium with tight junctions and surrounding pericytes [52]. Experiments using Ig-coated erythrocytes have suggested that Schwann cells have $Fc_\gamma RIII$ (and perhaps low-affinity $Fc_\gamma RII$) but not $Fc_\gamma RI$, both of which readily bind IgG1 and IgG3 but bind only small amounts of IgG4 and fail to bind IgG2 [53,54].

Other blood–tissue barriers (e.g., blood–thymus, blood–testis) are less well defined [55,56]. An air–blood barrier also has been described that affects the systemic uptake of aerosolized molecules [57]. Therapeutants that target glycoprotein adhesion molecules on endothelium might surmount the blood–brain or other tissue barriers [58].

11.2.3 IgG within the Interstitial Fluid Compartment

Once egress from plasma is accomplished, IgG is the most abundant immunoglobulin in tissue and is particularly prominent in the interstitial fluid compartment [2]. In healthy adult human volunteers, dermal interstitial fluid endogenous IgG levels were demonstrated to be 30% of plasma IgG levels [59]. In mice, IgG transport from capillary beds into interstitium is most frequent in skin and muscle with equivalent or less transport in adipose tissue and liver and much less transport in other tissues [60–62] consistent with the

---

[5]Minor amounts were cleared by kidney, but virtually no clearance was achieved in heart or lung [46].

major sites of IgG catabolism originally reported by Waldmann and Strober [63]. Information regarding potential differences in catabolism between monkeys, humans, and rodents has been reported [62,64].

11.3 IMMUNOGLOBULIN CLEARANCE

Clearance of endogenous and exogenous immunoglobulin takes place via a number of mechanisms. Among these are phagocytosis by mononuclear phagocytic cells (reticuloendothelial clearance), lymphatic clearance, and other tissue-specific and/or specialized mechanisms (discussed in more detail below).

11.3.1 Lymphatic Clearance

Drainage of interstitial fluid IgG into lymphatics depends on the concentration gradient and occurs passively via convection [1]. The leg lymph fluid of humans contains less than 25% of the amount of IgG found in plasma [65]. Other specialized lymphatic channels drain peritoneal, pleural, or pericardial cavities. Lymphatic drainage enters lymph nodes via the subcapsular sinus, and the lymph fluid IgG is available for reticuloendothelial clearance of IgG (subcapsular sinus, perivascular or parenchymal macrophages, perivascular or parenchymal dendritic cells, sinusoidal endothelium) as detailed next.

11.3.2 Mononuclear Phagocyte System and Endothelial Cell Clearance of IgG–Fc$_\gamma$ Receptors

Mononuclear phagocytes (macrophages, Kupffer cells, spleen or lymph node) and sinusoidal or other specialized endothelium remove IgG from plasma, most frequently as IgG-containing immune complexes, IgG aggregates, or IgG bound to cell-associated epitopes [66–69]. The initial binding event often occurs between the Fc portion of the IgG molecule and specific Fc receptors (Fc$_\gamma$R) on reticuloendothelial cells (Figure 11.2).

Fc Receptors

Fc$_\gamma$RI High-affinity Fc$_\gamma$RI (CD64) are found constitutively on monocytes, macrophages, dendritic cells, mast cells, platelets, and microglia and mediate internalization of antigen–antibody complexes into antigen-presenting cells for processing, antigen presentation and/or clearance [2,38,42,67,68,70]. In addition binding of antibody to Fc$_\gamma$R through the Fc receptor binding domain of IgG heavy chains can elicit several cell-mediated effector functions. In monocyte-macrophages, Fc$_\gamma$RI binding can trigger phagocytosis, antibody-dependent, cell-mediated cytotoxicity or other functions, including respiratory burst and cytokine/chemokine release. γ-interferon and β-interferon have

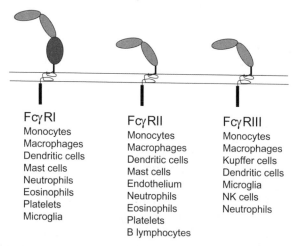

Fcγ RI	Fcγ RII	Fcγ RIII
Monocytes	Monocytes	Monocytes
Macrophages	Macrophages	Macrophages
Dendritic cells	Dendritic cells	Kupffer cells
Mast cells	Mast cells	Dendritic cells
Neutrophils	Endothelium	Microglia
Eosinophils	Neutrophils	NK cells
Platelets	Eosinophils	Neutrophils
Microglia	Platelets	
	B lymphocytes	

Figure 11.2 Fc receptors and the cell types upon which they are expressed.

opposing actions on monocyte-macrophage Fc$_\gamma$RI and function in vivo [71]. Immune complexes (e.g., monoclonal antibody–*Cryptococcus* neoformans) engage human and murine microglial Fc$_\gamma$RI (and Fc$_\gamma$RIII) to initiate microglial activation and chemokine release [42]. In vitro, Fc$_\gamma$RI are induced on human glomerular mesangial cells following treatment with IL-10 or γ-interferon but not IL-3, transforming growth factor-beta1 and granulocyte-macrophage colony-stimulating factor [72].

Fc$_\gamma$RII Low-affinity Fc$_\gamma$RII (CD32) exists as two isoforms: Fc$_\gamma$RIIa (CD32a) and Fc$_\gamma$RIIb (CD32b) on B lymphocytes, monocytes, macrophages, dendritic cells, and mast cells. Fc$_\gamma$RII (CD32) is also evident on endothelium with Fc$_\gamma$RIIb (CD32b) described on placental chorionic villous endothelium where FcRI (CD64) and Fc$_\gamma$RIIa (CD32a) are absent and where CD32b likely functions to transport IgG and/or scavenge immune complexes [29,67,68]. CD32a co-localizes with, and is negatively regulated by, CD31 (PECAM-1) in platelet plasma membranes [25]. Fc$_\gamma$RIIa (CD32a) also has been implicated in clearance of antibody-coated erythrocytes in vivo as treatment of Fc$_\gamma$RIIa-transgenic mice with antihuman CD32a monoclonal antibody. MDE-8 downregulates Fc$_\gamma$RIIa (and partially downregulates Fc$_\gamma$RI) and MDE-8 prevents immune-mediated hemolytic anemia [73]. Notably, Fc$_\gamma$RIIa-mediated phagocytosis of anti-RhD antibody-coated erythrocytes is favored by human IgG3 [74].

Fc$_\gamma$RIIa (CD32a) also has been demonstrated on natural killer cells [75], primary human brain microglial cells [42], and on small vessel endothelium in the papillary (superficial and periadnexal) dermis of the skin which do not express CD64 (Fc$_\gamma$RI) or CD16 (Fc$_\gamma$RIII) and in which Fc$_\gamma$RIIa engagement triggers Ca influxes and endosomal uptake of IgG [27]. Furthermore, although isolated human vein endothelial cells are normally negative for Fc$_\gamma$RIIa

(CD32a), they can express the molecules following activation by proteolytic enzymes (e.g., thrombin) or cytokines (e.g., tumor necrosis factor, γ-interferon [76]). Coggleshall has also proposed a role for Fc_γRIIb (CD32b) and associated phosphatases in the regulation of inhibitory responses of myeloid (particularly neutrophil and macrophage lineage) cells [77]. Binding of IgG1 and IgG2b but not IgM or IgG2a to the surface of monocyte precursors (e.g., HL60 cells) might influence monocyte differentiation at the expense of neutrophil differentiation [78].

Fc_γRIII Fc_γRIII (CD16) is observed on human monocytes, macrophages, Kupffer cells, dendritic cells, and microglia, and its presence likely is important in the clearance of circulating immune complexes [42]. Two isoforms have been identified: transmembrane Fc_γRIIIa (natural killer cells, macrophages, subset of T cells) and glycosylphosphatidylinositol-anchored Fc_γRIIIb (neutrophils, eosinophils [69,79]). In mice, the receptors for CD32, CD16, and CD14 are often closely associated on the membranes of monocyte cell lines [80]. Notably, CD16 and CD32 are closely associated in immature B lymphocytes, whereas mature B lymphocyes lose CD16 and only express CD32 [81].

Reticuloendothelial clearance of exogenously administered monoclonal IgG antibodies assumes binding to FcR on the reticuloendothelial (mononuclear phagocyte system) cells. High-dose intravenous IgGs might add themselves to circulating immune complexes to foster clearance of the complexes via macrophage Fc_γRIII receptors [82]. The rate of reticuloendothelial clearance of anti-RLD antibody-erythrocyte immune complexes in healthy human controls has been estimated by experimental half-life calculations ($t_{1/2} = 100 \pm$ 7.5 min [83]).

In monkeys, human(ized) test article administration can elicit primate antihuman antibodies (PAHA). PAHA binding to the human(ized) IgG test articles leads to formation of circulating immune complexes and subsequent clearance by reticuloendothelial cells or trapping by dendritic cells (e.g., follicular dendritic cells in spleen, lymph node, or mucosal-associated lymphoid tissues [67,68]). Alternatively, the test article might bind to its epitope (or a cross-reactive epitope) on circulating cells or intravascular protein, generating soluble or cell-associated immune complexes for reticuloendothelial clearance (e.g., depletion of CD45-positive leukocytes in monkeys following administration of monoclonal antihuman CD45 [13]).

Molecular Determinants of Binding of Human, Mouse, and Rabbit IgG Isotype/Subclass to FcR Plasma levels, biodistribution, and clearance of endogenous IgG and exogenously administered IgG are affected by species, isotype, and subclass. FcR binding is conferred by the hinge region of the heavy chain (C_H2) of human IgG. Amino acids at both ends of the hinge region determine affinity of isotype-specific hierarchical binding of monomeric human and mouse IgGs to high-affinity human Fc_γRI with preference for HuIgG1, HuIgG3, and MsIgG2a > HuIgG4 >> HuIgG2 [84–88]. MsIgG1 and MsIgG2b do not bind human Fc_γRI [85]. Each HuIgG and MsIgG2a molecule has two binding sites for Fc$_\gamma$RI with one within each heavy chain C$_H$2 domain. In HuIgG3, a unique first exon and replacement of a long flexible spacer for the more rigid spacer encoded by repetitive exons 2–4 in HuIgG1 confer segmental flexibility but reduce Fc$_\gamma$RI binding [89]. In HuIgG4, which retains a relatively rigid hinge, critical changes in the hinge-link region that decrease Fc$_\gamma$RI binding likely include leucine to phenylalanine at position 234 and serine to proline at position 331 [86]. In HuIgG2, the reduced affinity is mediated by changes in leucine (positions 234, 235), glycine (position 237), and threonine (position 337 [87,88]). Proteolysis shows the binding of rabbit IgGs to human Fc$_\gamma$RI to be mediated by rabbit IgG C$_H$3 domain with little role for the C$_H$2 domain (but molecular analysis was not done) [85]. Binding of human IgGs to Fc$_\gamma$RIII is also determined by the C$_H$2 domain [90].

Differences in Fc receptor γ-chain transmembrane domains (particularly polar or charged residues among the C-terminal 11 amino acids) influence cell membrane receptor expression and function [91]. The charged residues might protect Fc$_\gamma$RI and Fc$_\gamma$RIIIa receptors during membrane-associated receptor recycling in proteasomes associated with the endoplasmic reticulum or other intracellular structures [91].

FcRn binding is affected by amino acid changes in the C$_H$2 and C$_H$3 domains of IgG molecules, including the arginine substitution for histidine at position 435 characteristic of HuIgG3 but not HuIgG1 or HuIgG2 [6]. Determinants of MsIgG1 FcRn binding include C$_H$2 : C$_H$3 residues isoleucine 253, histidine 310, glutamine 311, histidine 433, and asparagine 434 [4]. While determinants of HuIgG1 FcRn binding include isoleucine 253, histidine 310, and histidine 435, histidine 433 is not involved [92]. Fc$_\gamma$RI stoichiometry allows binding of two IgGs (one per C$_H$2 domain); FcRn stoichiometry allows binding of only one IgG. Once FcRn binds to the C$_H$2 : C$_H$3 interface of the first IgG molecule, binding of the second IgG is prohibited as has been demonstrated for mouse antibodies [4,93,94].

Fc$_\gamma$R Polymorphisms   FcR polymorphisms are correlated with susceptibility to some infectious and immune-mediated diseases, and they also might influence monoclonal antibody transport, clearance, function, and beneficial (antitumor) or adverse (cytokine-eliciting) responses [95–99]. In rats, genetic influences such as allotype have been shown to affect the function of fibroblast-expressed Fc$_\gamma$RIIa [100]. In humans, eight genes on the long arm of chromosome 1 code for Fc$_\gamma$RI, Fc$_\gamma$RII, and Fc$_\gamma$RIII genes. Genetic polymorphisms in Fc$_\gamma$RIIa and Fc$_\gamma$RIIIa appear to influence IgG binding to FcR, and they might influence therapeutic responses. For example, the clinical response of human patients to the humanized anti-CD20 monoclonal antibody rituximab correlates with natural killer cell Fc$_\gamma$RIIIa polymorphisms and potentially with rituximab-armed NK antibody-dependent, cell-mediated cytotoxic responses [97,98]. Patients homozygous for valine at position 158 of the FCGR3A gene have better clinical responses than patients homozygous for phenylalanine at position 158 or heterozygotes [98]. Interestingly genetic polymorphisms in human monocyte $Fc_\gamma RIIa$ affect in vitro T cell proliferation induced by chimeric mouse-human IgG2 anti-CD3 monoclonal antibodies [95], and they might also influence cytokine release following monoclonal antibody administration.

11.3.3 Effect of IgG Structure on Plasma IgG Clearance and Tissue Catabolism

The rate of IgG clearance is proportional to the plasma IgG concentration, with faster clearance rates for higher plasma IgG concentrations [1,3]. Isotype, subclass, and amino acid changes in FcR-binding regions affect clearance [93,101] as does overall carbohydrate structure and composition [102–104]. Although less than 3% of endogenous IgG consists of carbohydrate, the carbohydrate structure and composition influences rapid liver clearance and/or catabolism but does not affect the slower IgG catabolism typical of skin and muscle [104]. Some of these effects are thought to be mediated by hepatic removal of IgG with galactosyl moieties by hepatocyte asialoglycoprotein receptors [102,104]. Hepatic and/or splenic removal of mannose-containing IgGs is mediated by mannose receptors on hepatic Kupffer cells and hepatic and/or splenic sinusoidal endothelium, macrophages, and/or dendritic cells [105–107]. Other tissues with the potential for IgG catabolism and relatively rapid IgG loss across mucosal surfaces include kidney and lung [104]. The effect of IgG isotype and subclass on FcR-mediated transport and the effect of carbohydrate moieties on IgG binding to Fc receptors (FcR) on brain microglia and other cells are discussed further below.

The carbohydrate content of IgG might affect IgG binding to FcR as deglycosylated IgG antibodies bind brain microglial FcR with reduced affinity [44], although an earlier study was unable to demonstrate differences between intact and aglycosylated antibody with regard to FcR binding and signal transport [108]. Certainly different methods of production result in different glycosylation patterns (e.g., mammalian cell lines—CHO, NSO, etc.—yeast, transgenic animals), but it remains unclear what effect differences in glycosylation patterns (i.e., what carbohydrate moieties are present, degree of glycosylation, and order of carbohydrate moieties) have on antibody binding.

11.4 SPECIALIZED TISSUE-SPECIFIC, IgG TRANSPORT OR CLEARANCE MECHANISMS

Once an antibody has egressed into the interstitial space, its movement is somewhat more complicated than simple diffusion around the interstitial space (until it binds to epitope) or flow into lymphatics for mononuclear phagocytic clearance. There are a number of mechanisms by which antibodies (that are not bound via CDR to target or a cross-reactive epitope) are transported across and to a variety of cell types. Below are discussed several specialized and/or tissue-specific mechanisms of IgG transport and/or clearance.

11.4.1 FcRn

Endogenous IgG is present in luminal secretions of human and monkey gastrointestinal, oral, respiratory, and urogenital mucosal epithelium (e.g., intestine, pharynx, lung, kidney, uterus), which is normally very resistant to passive diffusion of macromolecules as part of innate barrier function. These mucosal epithelia have developed specialized mechanisms, including transport organelles (vesicles, endosomes, etc.), that mediate transcytosis of macromolecules, including immunoglobulins [109,110]. The most important route probably is MHC class I related Fc receptor (FcRn) mediated IgG transport across and within multiple epithelia, including human (adult and neonatal) small intestine [26,111–115]. FcRn consists of a 3-domain α-subunit noncovalently bound to β_2-microglobulin [26,110,113]. IgG salvage, sorting and/or recycling occurs when cystosolic endosomes take up IgG at the plasma membrane. Polarized bidirectional transport has been described for human intestinal epithelium with FcRn and its associated endosomes localized in the apical cytoplasm in a punctate pattern (just below the apical membrane or zonula occludens tight junctions) with the apical pathway of transcytosis more efficient than the basolateral pathway [109]. Similarly FcRn is located apically in human (and mouse) placental syncytiotrophoblasts, where it mediates IgG uptake from the maternal circulation [28], and in human renal proximal tubule cells, where it mediates IgG salvage from the urinary filtrate [116]. The pH dependence of FcRn binding [26,109,117] is attributed to FcRn presence/function within acidic recycling and/or sorting endosomes [118–120], some of which become multivesicular bodies or are degraded in lysosomes and others of which release IgG to the environment either by dispersal into the plasma membrane or by sustained release from endosomes as they approach the plasma membrane from the peripheral cytoplasm [119,120]. Binding to the FcRn within the acidic endosomes presumably protects the sorted IgG from catabolism, allowing release of the salvaged IgG to plasma, interstitium, dendritic, and/or target cells at neutral pH. The process of FcRn-mediated transcytosis or transcellular transport thus consists of three phases: endocytosis, intracellular transport, and exocytosis, all of which might be pertinent to therapeutic monoclonal antibody development and administration [8].

The Fc portion (Fc_γ) of IgG is essential for FcRn-mediated transcytosis. Monoclonal antibodies have been designed with Fc_γ modifications that affect the affinity or pH of binding to FcRn and that can reduce FcRn-mediated salvage, and hasten clearance of other (endogenous or exogenously administered) IgG antibodies [121]. Such antibodies might be developed as therapeutic candidates to avert autoantibody-mediated damage.

FcRn was originally known as the Brambell receptor, based on multiple studies conducted by F. W. Brambell involving maternal transmission of antibodies across placenta and neonatal intestine in rabbits [3,5,122,123]. Transport was saturable with increases in plasma IgG leading to reductions in plasma half-life ($t_{1/2}$) according to the formula

$$t_{1/2} = \frac{C \ln 2}{a(C-b)},$$

where $a = +0.34$, $b = 2.5$, and C = total IgG concentration (mg/ml).

In adult mice, FcRn is expressed on endothelium in many tissues as well as on hepatocytes, where it serves a protective, anticatabolic, function by compartmentalizing, salvaging, and recycling IgG, but it does not mediate biliary clearance [4,62,124]. In mice, FcRn is preferentially expressed in cytoplasmic vesicles in small vessel endothelium (e.g., small arterioles, venules, and capillaries, liver sinusoids) skin, muscle, and liver, but it is not expressed by larger vessel endothelium (e.g., liver central veins or portal vessels in liver [62]) consistent with primary sites of IgG transport and catabolism in rodents [64]. FcRn is expressed on human placental endothelium [125] and also assumed to be expressed on widespread endothelium in adult humans but only secondary and not primary sources were reviewed herein [1,126]. FcRn is also expressed by monocytes, macrophages (including about one-fourth of intestinal macrophages), and dendritic cells; binds immune complexes; and is postulated to function in the acidic pH that characterizes inflammation or the tumor interstitium [26,127]. FcRn is preferentially expressed intracellularly by the majority of peripheral blood monocytes, with lower levels associated with the cell membrane [26]. The heavy chain of FcRn in humans is noncovalently associated with membrane molecules such as MHC class I molecule β_2-microglobulin expressed on endothelium, epithelium, leukocytes, placental syncytiotrophoblasts, dendritic cells, and macrophages as well as CD68 (macrosialin) and Nel-Macro on intestinal macrophages [26,110,128].

FcRn-mediated protection for endogenous IgG and exogenously administered human monoclonal antibodies is plasma concentration-dependent and epitope-independent, as has been reviewed recently [1]. However, Junghans et al. [129] suggest that human FcRn (in its Brambell receptor protective role) may differentially transport and catabolize antigen–antibody complexes formed between immune endogenous IgG and exogenously administered human and chimeric monoclonal antibodies via differential catabolism of antigen–antibody complexes.

FcRn binding is not affected by carbohydrate residues on IgG [130]. Last, at the time of this review there is no information regarding FcRn expression on surface lining cells (e.g., mesothelial cells, meningeal cells, or synoviocytes) available in the literature. Passive (nontranscytotic) mesothelial cell transport of IgG is discussed further below.

11.4.2   pIgR on Epithelium and Other Cell Types

The polymeric IgA receptor/secretory component (pIgA-R/SC, also designated pIgR) mediated transport represents another, less common and less utilized, form of specialized endosomal epithelial transcytosis. pIgR are found primarily on mucosal epithelium, including biliary epithelium, and hepatocytes in humans and rodents [131]. Immunofluorescence has demonstrated the secretory component (SC) on human intestinal and respiratory goblet cells, other mucosal epithelia (gall bladder, renal tubules), and gland and/or duct epithelia (pancreas, sweat glands [132,133]). In rodents, hepatocytes produce a secretory component, allowing dimeric IgA to attach to hepatocyte sinusoidal membrane pIgR and be translocated via cytoplasmic vesicles to the biliary canalicular membrane for excretion into bile [134,135].

Unlike FcRn-mediated transcytosis of IgG, pIgR is unidirectional and transports dimeric IgA (approximately 3 g per day in an adult human) more frequently than pentameric IgM. IgG transport occurs when monomeric IgG is complexed with polymeric IgA [136]. Information is not available as to whether pentameric IgM or IgM fragments can complex with monomeric IgG and facilitate transport IgG-IgM complex transport via pIgR. However, following monoclonal IgG antibody administration, heterologous (or less often homologous) IgM antimonoclonal IgG antibody responses can be detected. Thus, while pIgR-mediated transport of monoclonal IgG antibodies is likely to be infrequent in the homologous species (e.g., human antibodies in humans), it appears to occur more often as immune complexes in heterologous species used for efficacy or toxicity testing. The presence of pIgR on hepatocytes as well as mucosal surfaces might foster rapid liver clearance of exogenously administered IgG antibodies if antihuman IgM antibodies were present prior to, or as a result of, monoclonal IgG antibody administration in the heterologous species. Alternatively, both homologous and heterologous immunoglobulins can be taken up by hepatocyte asialoglycoprotein receptors (discussed with liver) and enter lysosomes for degradation [135].

Unlike FcRn-mediated transcytosis, the initial pIgR-Ig binding occurs at the cell surface rather than within endosomes, and usually leads to receptor degradation or loss to the apical environment rather than recycling [61,109]. Internalization occurs via a nocodozole-sensitive, microtubule-associated process [137,138].

pIgR is thought to be most prevalent in embryogenesis with less utilization in perinatal or adult human tissues. Immunoglobulins, secretory component, and the associated J chain are described in multiple embryonic tissues, including gastrointestinal, respiratory and urogenital tracts, gonads, endocrine tissues, mesothelial-lined surfaces, and functional blood–tissue barriers. As gestation progresses, the tissues remodel, and the distances between many mucosal and glandular epithelium increase while the distribution and function of pIgR/SC-mediated transport decrease [139]. pIgR is absent from adult human glomerular mesangial cells [140] but has been demonstrated on cultured human endometrial cells [141]. In adult mice, pIgR mediates Ig transport, principally of IgA and IgM, from the basolateral surface to the apical surface and lumen of intestine and bile canaliculi and ducts where it contributes to mucosal defense [142]. High concentrations of IgA and IgG are found in human and rat bile [143,144] and have been attributed to Ig transport by pIgR and FcRn, respectively [142,145], although nonspecific macromolecular transport (paracellular sieving [145]) might contribute when the liver is inflamed and IgG is produced locally.

Most of the mechanistic work on pIgR has focused on IgA transport rather than IgG transport. In polarized epithelial cells, receptors that mediate transcytosis (e.g., pIgR) are separated from other basolateral receptors (e.g., transferrin receptor) following delivery to recycling endosomes, although nearly 65% are re-transported rapidly to the basolateral surface via early endosomes [146]. About 35% of transferrin–transferrin receptor complexes and dimeric IgA–pIgR complexes enter into submembranous early endosomes and later co-localize into perinuclear recycling endosomes for a slower separatory phase [146]. The net transport of IgA is affected by four overlapping processes: surface clearance, endocytosis, basolateral recycling, and transcytosis [146].

pIgRs also are involved in disease pathogenesis. Pneumococci directly interact with pIgR to gain access to, or traverse, human respiratory epithelial cells [147,148]. Binding of Epstein–Barr virus (EBV) to EBV-specific IgA triggers internalization of the EBV–IgA complex by nasal epithelial cells and might initiate persistent nasal infection [149,150] cytomegalovirus (CMV) to CMV-specific IgA triggers internalization of the CMV–IgA complex.

11.4.3 Kidney

The glomerular capillary endothelial bed receives 23% of the cardiac output and serves as the primary blood filter. The glomerular capillary endothelium is fenestrated with discontinuous tight junctions and/or gap junctions (Kuhn et al., 1975) and glomerular endothelial cells express low affinity FcR distinct from $Fc_\gamma RI$, $Fc_\gamma RII$, and $Fc_\gamma RIII$ [151] now recognized as FcRn (reviewed in Lobo et al. [1]). This engenders direct contact between the underlying or intervening mesangial cells and the intravascular fluid within the glomerular capillary lumens, particularly at the glomerular angles [11,12,152,153], and both endothelium and mesangial cells probably participate in Ig recycling. The gap junctions of the mesangial cells [152] might facilitate this transport. Furthermore IgG molecules or their fragments can cross via the large pores in the glomerular basement membrane in healthy individuals [154]. Therefore the passage of exogenously administered monoclonal IgG test articles across the glomerular capillary endothelium into the mesangium might be expected, independent of antibody CDR specificity. Fab and scFv fragments have shorter plasma half-lives (0.5 to 21 hours) due to quicker glomerular filtration and clearance [7].

The mesangium also participates in removal of Ig (IgM, IgA > IgG) or immune complexes from blood via FcR (including $Fc_\gamma RI$ and $Fc_\gamma RIIIa$ on activated mesangium [72,155]) in humans and likely mediates nonspecific transport of macromolecules including Ig, possibly via integrin-mediated association with FcR-positive migrating leukocytes [153,156–158]. Glomerular epithelial cells (which also are in contact with mesangial cells as well as with the urinary filtrate in the urinary space) might complete the cycle of IgG transport and recycling by neonatal Fc receptor (FcRn)-mediated transcytosis [116] (see FcRn above). Alternatively, subepithelial deposition of immune complexes might occur subsequent to removal of immune complexes by attachment to FcRn on glomerular visceral epithelial cells (podocytes [116]). Last, exogenously administered monoclonal antibodies have been shown to delay the renal clearance of soluble epitopes from plasma (e.g., anti-Tac delays clearance of shed Tac [IL-2 receptor-alpha {IL-2Rα}] in mice [159]). Differential renal catabolism of the Tac–anti-Tac immune complex and the uncomplexed anti-Tac monoclonal antibody might be influenced by FcRn-mediated sorting/recycling in intracellular vesicles [129,159] (see FcRn below). There apparently is no contribution by pIgR or the asialoglycoprotein receptor as these structures are absent from adult human glomerular mesangial cells [140].

Renal proximal tubular epithelium (e.g., convoluted tubules) reclaim protein, including immunoglobulin, from the urinary filtrate via sorting/recycling mechanisms in intracellular vesicles. The apical (lumen-facing) surface of these cells features a specialized brush border which expresses FcRn closely associated with β_2-microglobulin [110,116]. Studies with cultured human renal proximal tubular epithelial cells have demonstrated bidirectional IgG transport and salvage by fully functional FcRn [110] as discussed further in the next section.

11.4.4 Breast (Mammary Gland)

Breast epithelium is responsible for the physiologic secretion of IgG into milk and, to a lesser extent, into nonlactating breast secretions. Although the biodistribution of exogenously administered monoclonal antibodies into breast milk or nonlactating breast secretion is not well understood, bovine IgG (and/or fragments thereof) is found in breast milk after dietary exposure [160]. This indicates the potential for transport of exogenously administered monoclonal antibodies (and/or antibody fragments) into breast milk or nonlactating breast secretion by physiologic mechanisms. FcRn have also been demonstrated on neoplastic human breast epithelial cells in tumors and lymph node metastases as well as morphologically normal adjacent epithelium but not tumor or adjacent endothelium [161].

11.4.5 Ovary

IgG is found in ovarian (intra)follicular fluid or corpus lutea secondary to ovarian (ovulation) hemorrhage or macrophage-mediated transport. Macrophages have been localized to ovarian stroma, to thecal layers of ovarian follicles, and within early, mid-, late, and regressing corpora lutea [162].

11.4.6 Placenta and Uterus

Different FcRs have different roles to play in maternal IgG transport across placental barriers in humans. $Fc_\gamma RI$, $Fc_\gamma RIIa$, $Fc_\gamma RIIb$, and $Fc_\gamma RIII$ are expressed at the surface of Hofbauer cells (placental macrophages), $Fc_\gamma RIIb$ and FcRn are expressed by chorionic (fetal) endothelium, and $Fc_\gamma RIII$ and FcRn are expressed by trophoblasts (fetal chorionic epithelium [28,29]). FcRn expression by syncytiotrophoblasts likely mediates a significant portion of maternal IgG transport in humans and IgG; β_2-microglobulin, and FcRn co-localize in plasma membrane granules or vesicles [28,29,128,163,164]. IgA and IgM do not cross placental barriers and are absent from fetal circulation. In contrast, fetal accumulation of maternal IgG (particularly IgG1) begins by human gestation week 16. Steady transplacental IgG increases lead to equivalent levels of maternally derived IgG1 in maternal and fetal circulation by gestation week 26, and greater IgG1 levels in fetal compared to maternal circulation at delivery. IgG3 and IgG4 levels are usually equivalent in maternal and fetal circulation at term while IgG2 levels remain greater in maternal circulation compared to fetal circulation [28,165]. The preference for IgG1 transport has also been shown using in vitro models of placental transport [166,167] and is reflected in the preference of high-affinity $Fc_\gamma RI$ for HuIgG1, HuIgG3 > HuIgG4 >> HuIgG2 [84–88]. The volume of IgG transported is consistent with in vitro calculations of placental binding site capacity (10^{15} sites/mg) and affinity (10^6 M) using paired fetal side-oriented and maternal side-oriented placental membrane vesicles [168]. Last, the discovery of FcRn by Brambell was based on rabbit studies in which whole IgG and Fc fragments easily crossed from mother to fetus, whereas F(ab')2 fragments failed to cross [3,5,122,123].

Functional pIgR has been described on a human endometrial cell line [141], but its role in maternal–fetal IgG transport or transcytosis in the nonpregnant uterus has not been described.

Immunoglobulin profiles of human cervical mucus indicate approximately twice as much IgG (30 mg/dl) as IgA (15 mg/dl) overall; however, there are both biphasic and menstrual cycle influences on Ig levels [169]. Different from blood plasma, the IgA2 subclass predominates in female genital tract secretions with lesser amounts of IgGA1 [170].

11.4.7 Seminal Fluid

IgG is more concentrated in seminal fluid than IgA, and only low levels of IgM are evident. As in blood plasma, more IgA1 than IgA2 is evident in seminal fluid.

11.4.8 Lung

Normal pulmonary (bronchoalveolar) lavage fluid contains IgG at lower concentrations (approximately 1%) than plasma. IgA is selectively concentrated relative to plasma proteins in bronchoalveolar lavage fluid, as is indicative of epithelial transcytosis rather than just leakage from vessels [171].

By immunoelectron microscopy, endogenous IgG has been localized to epithelial membranes, tubular myelin, and granular material within alveoli [172,173]. The major barrier to bidirectional air : blood exchange is composed of type I and type II alveolar epithelial cells (distal airways) that form zonulae occludens (tight junctions). Paracellular (between cells) diffusion of macro-molecules is considered very slight and probably insignificant in healthy (unin-flamed) lung regardless of direction (uptake or egress). Endothelium and interstitium contribute little to the blood–air–blood barrier. Alveolar protein (including IgG) transport is reduced by increasing molecular size and may be affected by protein catabolism (apical surface peptidases on alveolar lining epithelium [173]).

The rate of protein clearance has been estimated as 10% of the rate of fluid clearance from alveoli [173]. IgG clearance is probably mediated by FcRn transcytosis in distal type I alveolar epithelium and more proximal bronchial epithelium. Type I alveolar epithelium and bronchial epithelium contain the necessary subcellular structures for FcRn-mediated transcytosis: vesicles, membrane invaginations, caveolae, and clathrin-coated pits [173,174]. FcRn mRNA is expressed in lung although the cell types and locations have not yet been determined [112]. Moreover, primary alveolar epithelial monolayer cell cultures express functional FcRn [173]. pIgA–R/SC transcytosis is thought to contribute little to distal (alveolar) airway IgG transport but might mediate more proximal (bronchial or bronchiolar) IgA transport [173]. Uptake of an aerosolized IgG Fc-erythropoietin fusion molecule and subsequent erythro-poietin-induced reticulocytosis has been demonstrated in human and nonhu-man primates [175].

11.4.9 Skin

FcγRIIa (CD32a) is expressed in small-vessel endothelium in the papillary (superficial and periadnexal) dermis [27]. Binding of IgG or immune com-plexes to isolated human dermal microvessel endothelial cells initiates rapid receptor cross-linking, intracellular Ca fluxes, and endosomal internalization of the IgG–Fc$_\gamma$RIIa complexes [27]. FcRn is expressed principally in basal and suprabasal human keratinocytes in normal epidermis [176] and is also expressed in mouse skin [62]. In healthy adult human volunteers, dermal inter-stitial fluid endogenous IgG levels were demonstrated to be 30% of plasma IgG levels [59].

11.4.10 Liver

FcRn protein is expressed by rat hepatocytes, particularly at the canalicular surface [145] and might facilitate serum-to-bile IgG transport or prevent catabolism by hepatocytes [124,145]. The liver also has other specialized mechanisms for clearance and/or transport of glycoproteins and immunoglobulins–secretory component and the asialoglycoprotein receptor (ASGP-R). In the rat, asialoglycoproteins are taken up by liver hepatocytes for lysosomal degradation via the asialoglycoprotein receptor, while IgA, which is the predomiant immunoglobulin involved in immunological protection at mucous membrane surfaces, is cleared from plasma and transported through hepatocytes and into the bile via secretory component [135,177,178]. In humans, there is less hepatic transport of IgA because secretory component is expressed by biliary epithelium and there is more local synthesis of IgA within hepatobiliary tissues [177,178]. Humans are therefore unable to clear IgA–antigen complexes via the hepatic transport pathway, and this might contribute to development of IgA–mediated immune complex diseases [178]. For example, alcoholic liver disease is associated with deposition of IgA along the liver sinusoids in the majority of alcoholics [178]. Although there is considered to be minimal uptake of asialoglycoproteins by secretory component or IgA by ASGP-R, there is some evidence that heterologous immunoglobulin, specifically human IgA administered to rats, can bind to both receptors [135]. Many therapeutic glycoproteins including antibodies may further contain terminal GlcNAc and/ or Gal residues, which facilitate rapid clearance as a result of binding to mannose receptor and/or ASGP-R in the liver [179]. As described above, the liver is involved in the first-pass effect because of to its high vascularity and high cardiac output, so, it is probable that ASGP-R and/or secretory component plays a role in therapeutic (or exogenous) antibody transport or clearance.

11.4.11 Salivary Gland

Saliva contains IgA (0.6–49.2 mg/dL), IgG (0.03–4.86 mg/dl), small amounts of IgM (0.04–2.6 mg/dl), and secretory component [180]. pIgR expression has been described for human parotid salivary gland and is responsible for epithelial cell transport of IgA and secretory component into saliva [180,181]. The overwhelming majority (92–99%) of transported IgA is synthesized locally, while approximately half of transported IgG derives from serum with consistent accumulations in salivary interstitium [182]. IgA transport into saliva is increased by chewing [181]. The means of IgG transport into saliva has not been described; however, several authors have proposed local IgG production and nonspecific (transudative or paracellular sieving) of mucosal or serum IgG leaked from inflamed vessels into saliva or other oral fluids in reponse to viral or bacterial infections [180,183–185]. IgA, IgM, and IgG transport into saliva is reduced by some types of stimulation [180]. Increases in salivary IgG and IgM are also seen in patients with immunoglobulin-producing plasmacytomas or paraproteinemias [180,186].

The timing of IgG appearance in saliva (and nasal secretions) is delayed compared to its appearance in serum. Following subcutaneous administration of tetanus toxoid, peak anti-toxin IgG serum levels preceded peak anti-toxin IgG salivary and nasal secretion levels by two weeks. The levels of interstitial anti-toxin IgG were not measured [187].

11.4.12 Colon

In normal healthy volunteers, immunoglobulins are secreted into the colon lumen at the following rates: IgG (48 mg/day), polymeric IgA (220 mg/day), monomeric IgA (12 mg/day), and IgM (24 mg/day). For comparison, values for nonimmunoglobulin proteins were also calculated (e.g., albumin at 150 mg/day) by Prigent-Delecourt and colleagues [188].

11.4.13 Thyroid

Zimmer and colleagues [189,190] have reported that IgG is transported via epithelial transcytosis from the pericapillary basolateral aspect to the apical membrane of the follicular epithelium. Within the thyroid follicular epithelium, IgG has been localized to endoplasmic reticulum and Golgi by way of immunogold electron microscopy. IgGs also have been localized to the thyroid follicular lumen and at the apical membrane of the thyroid follicular epithelial cells [189,190]. Moreover normal thyroid follicular epithelium expresses FcRn while Graves's disease thyroid follicular epithelium expresses $Fc_\gamma RIIb$ as well as FcRn [191]. These molecules are thought to mediate IgG transport from the pericapillary basolateral aspect of the follicular cells to the apical membrane, although direct basal to apical movement has not been clearly demonstrated [191]. IgG transport is accelerated in the immune-mediated thyroid disease (e.g., Graves's disease), particularly in more susceptible females. The gender-dependence of susceptibility may be affected by androgen-mediated inhibition of $Fc_\gamma RIIb$ epithelial expression and transcytosis [191]. These associations might be particularly important in light of the localization of HLA-restricted class I and class II molecules and processed thyroglobulin to the same subcellular sites. This might facilitate antigen presentation or antigen–antibody complex formation leading to thyroid follicular epithelial cell damage [191]. In humans, pIgA-R/SC is also expressed by fetal thyroid, but it has not been described in adult thyroid [139] and has not been accorded a role in immune-mediated thyroid disease.

Thyroid clearance of exogenously administered monoclonal antibodies is reported to be affected by the concentration and injection volume of the administered drug. Following intraperitoneal administration of irrelevant CDR-containing mouse IgG2a monoclonal antibody to rats, thyroid uptake of radiolabeled mouse IgG2a monoclonal antibody has been demonstrated for higher doses and more concentrated solutions while lower doses or less concentrated solutions remain within blood vessels and do not penetrate the thyroid parenchyma [192].

11.4.14 Cytosolic Transport in Epithelium, Mesothelium, and Other Tissues

In epithelium, cytosolic or non–receptor-mediated transport is inefficient and often leads to lysosomal degradation of the macromolecule [109]. However, macromolecules, including IgG, are readily transported across the mesothelial surface of the peritoneum. The mesothelial lining cells are flat cells with pinocytotic vesicles but no caveolae comparable to endothelial cells [193]. Gap junctions separate interdigitated peritoneal mesothelial cells. IgG transport is known to be bi-directional and passive in rats [194–198] and also occurs in chronic peritoneal dialysis in humans [199].

There was no information regarding FcRn expression on mesothelial cells, meningeal cells, or synoviocytes available in the literature.

11.4.15 Erythrocyte CR1 (CD35) Clearance of IgG-Containing Immune Complexes

In primates, additional mechanisms exist for clearance of immune complexes. Erythrocyte CR1 (CD35) bind immune complexes via C3b and C4b ligand sites. Once bound to erythrocyte CR1, the immune complexes are transported to the liver where they are cleared by liver macrophages (Kupffer cells). Mouse antibody (MsIgG1-, MsIgG2a-, MsIgG2b-, and MsIgA-) containing immune complexes bind rapidly to erythrocyte CR1 and peak magnitude binding is high. MsIgG3- and MsIgM-containing immune complexes bind slowly to erythrocyte CR1, and the peak magnitude binding is low. Release rates are rapid for MsIgG2a- and MsIgG2b-containing immune complexes, intermediate for MsIgG1-containing immune complexes, relatively slow for MsIgA- and MsIgM-containing immune complexes, and very slow for MsIgG3-containing immune complexes [200]. Similarly, Kavai and colleagues [201] demonstrated reduced incorporation of C3b-iC3b into IgM-containing immune complexes compared to IgG-containing immume complexes. In general, high-affinity mouse antibodies activate complement better than, but bind to erythrocyte CR1 less well than, low-affinity mouse antibodies [202].

11.5 CONCLUSION

The movement of IgG through tissue is more complex than its circulation through the vasculature, its binding (or not binding) to target or off-target epitope, and its clearance. As described above, antibodies can move out of the vasculature and be carried through various cell types through interactions with a number of different molecules that are expressed in many different tissue types. As such, many tissue and/or cellular compartments are available to therapeutic antibodies—vascular, interstitial, cell membrane, and cytoplasmic. During the course of therapeutic antibody development, tissue cross-reactivity testing is required (see Chapter 10). In many cases the test article (therapeutic candidate) stains only expected tissue elements (cell types and subcellular locations). However, some test articles display tissue cross-reactivity with unexpected cell types and/or subcellular locations. Although tissue cross-reactivity results are not necessarily considered to be predictive of toxicity, they do yield information as to potential tissue sites that warrant closer scrutiny and/or additional evaluation during preclinical toxicity studies or early phase clinical trials. As a follow-up to tissue cross-reactivity testing, tissues submitted for histopathological evaluation during the toxicity studies can be stained using specialized techniques for detection of the test article (therapeutic candidate) to take a snapshot of its biodistribution at any given time point during the toxicity study. We have conducted approximately 20 of these studies in cynomolgus monkeys, rhesus monkeys, and marmosets. However, because of the proprietary nature of the work, specific details cannot be provided. In general, the test article (therapeutic candidate) was localized either at sites of expected or tissue cross-reactive staining as predicted by the tissue cross-reactivity study or at sites consistent with physiological IgG biodistribution, transport, and clearance. For most studies of this kind, the test article (therapeutic candidate) was localized at a variable subset of sites consistent with both the tissue cross-reactivity study results and the normal physiologic processes described above. Similar distribution patterns were recognized for exogenously administered antibody fragments in mice [62]. Specifically, $F(ab')_2$ fragments prepared from preimmune serum were cleared by renal filtration, whereas $F(ab')_2$ fragments prepared from anti-FcRn serum tended to localize in skin and muscle (and to a lesser extent, adipose tissue and liver) consistent with the distribution of FcRn [62]. These types of studies highlight the complexity of biodistribution, transport, and clearance of exogenous IgG. How these factors affect potential toxic effects of any therapeutic antibody is still unclear for many marketed antibody-based therapeutics and therapeutic candidates. However, greater understanding of IgG biodistribution, transport, and clearance will facilitate more efficient development of safer, more effective antibody-based therapeutics.

REFERENCES

1. Lobo ED, Hansen RJ, Balthasar JP. Antibody pharmacokinetics and pharmacodynamics. *J Pharm Sci* 2004;93(11):2645–68.
2. Roitt I. *Essential Immunology*. Oxford: Blackwell Scientific, 1994.
3. Brambell FW, Hemmings WA, Morris IG. A theoretical model of gamma-globulin catabolism. *Nature* 1964;203:1352–4.
4. Ghetie V, Hubbard JG, Kim JK, Tsen MF, Lee Y, Ward ES. Abnormally short serum half-lives of IgG in beta 2-microglobulin-deficient mice. *Eur J Immunol* 1996;26(3):690–6.

5. Junghans RP. Finally! The Brambell receptor (FcRB). Mediator of transmission of immunity and protection from catabolism for IgG. *Immunol Res* 1997;16(1): 29–57.

6. Ghetie V, Ward ES. Transcytosis and catabolism of antibody. *Immunol Res* 2002; 25(2):97–113.

7. Roskos LK, Davis CG, Schwab GM. The clinical pharmacology of therapeutic monoclonal antibodies. *Drug Dev Res* 2004;61:108–20.

8. Peterson E, Owens SM, Henry RL. Monoclonal antibody form and function: manufacturing the right antibodies for treating drug abuse. *AAPS J* 2006;8(2): E383–90.

9. Bard P. *Medical Physiology*, 11th ed. St. Louis: Mosby, 1961.

10. Forsyth RP, Nies AS, Wyler F, Neutze J, Melmon KL. Normal distribution of cardiac output in the unanesthetized, restrined rhesus monkey. *J Appl Physiol* 1968;25(6):736–41.

11. Venkatachalam MA, Kriz W. Anatomy. In Heppinstall RH, ed. *Pathology of the Kidney*, 4th ed. Boston: Little, Brown, 1992;1–92.

12. Tisher CC, Madsen KM. Anatomy of the kidney. In Brenner MD, ed. *Brenner and Rector's The Kidney*, 5th ed. Philadephia: WB Saunders, 1996;3–71.

13. Matthews DC, Appelbaum FR, Eary JF, et al. Radiolabeled anti-CD45 monoclonal antibodies target lymphohematopoietic tissue in the macaque. *Blood* 1991;78(7):1864–74.

14. Matthews DC, Appelbaum FR, Eary JF, et al. Phase I study of (131)I-anti-CD45 antibody plus cyclophosphamide and total body irradiation for advanced acute leukemia and myelodysplastic syndrome. *Blood* 1999;94(4):1237–47.

15. el-Kareh AW, Braunstein SL, Secomb TW. Effect of cell arrangement and interstitial volume fraction on the diffusivity of monoclonal antibodies in tissue. *Biophys J* 1993;64(5):1638–46.

16. Rippe B, Haraldsson B. Transport of macromolecules across microvascular walls: the two-pore theory. *Physiol Rev* 1994;74(1):163–219.

17. Simionescu M, Antohe F. Functional ultrastructure of the vascular endothelium: changes in various pathologies. *Handb Exp Pharmacol* 2006;(176 Pt 1):41–69.

18. Pries AR, Kuebler WM. Normal endothelium. *Handb Exp Pharmacol* 2006; 176(Pt 1):1–40.

19. Simionescu M, Gafencu A, Antohe F. Transcytosis of plasma macromolecules in endothelial cells: a cell biological survey. *Microsc Res Tech* 2002;57(5):269–88.

20. Palade GE, Simionescu M, Simionescu N. Structural aspects of the permeability of the microvascular endothelium. *Acta Physiol Scand Suppl* 1979;463:11–32.

21. Schnitzer JE. gp60 is an albumin-binding glycoprotein expressed by continuous endothelium involved in albumin transcytosis. *Am J Physiol* 1992;262(1 Pt 2): H246–54.

22. Tiruppathi C, Song W, Bergenfeldt M, Sass P, Malik AB. Gp60 activation mediates albumin transcytosis in endothelial cells by tyrosine kinase-dependent pathway. *J Biol Chem* 1997;272(41):25968–75.

23. Demignot S, Pimm MV, Baldwin RW. Comparison of biodistribution of 791T/36 monoclonal antibody and its Fab/c fragment in BALB/c mice and nude mice bearing human tumor xenografts. *Cancer Res* 1990;50(10):2936–42.

24. Tomiyama Y, Kunicki TJ, Zipf TF, Ford SB, Aster RH. Response of human platelets to activating monoclonal antibodies: importance of Fc gamma RII (CD32) phenotype and level of expression. *Blood* 1992;80(9):2261–8.

25. Thai IM, Ashman LK, Harbour SN, Hogarth PM, Jackson DE. Physical proximity and functional interplay of PECAM-1 with the Fc receptor Fc gamma RIIa on the platelet plasma membrane. *Blood* 2003;102(10):3637–45.

26. Zhu X, Meng G, Dickinson BL, et al. MHC class I-related neonatal Fc receptor for IgG is functionally expressed in monocytes, intestinal macrophages, and dendritic cells. *J Immunol* 2001;166(5):3266–76.

27. Groger M, Fischer GF, Wolff K, Petzelbauer P. Immune complexes from vasculitis patients bind to endothelial Fc receptors independent of the allelic polymorphism of FcgammaRIIa. *J Invest Dermatol* 1999;113(1):56–60.

28. Saji F, Samejima Y, Kamiura S, Koyama M. Dynamics of immunoglobulins at the feto-maternal interface. *Rev Reprod* 1999;4(2):81–9.

29. Lyden TW, Robinson JM, Tridandapani S, et al. The Fc receptor for IgG expressed in the villus endothelium of human placenta is Fc gamma RIIb2. *J Immunol* 2001;166(6):3882–9.

30. Minshall RD, Malik AB. Transport across the endothelium: regulation of endothelial permeability. *Handb Exp Pharmacol* 2006;176(Pt 1):107–44.

31. Ding BS, Dziubla T, Shuvaev VV, Muro S, Muzykantov VR. Advanced drug delivery systems that target the vascular endothelium. *Mol Interv* 2006;6(2):98–112.

32. Benarroch EE. Neuron-astrocyte interactions: partnership for normal function and disease in the central nervous system. *Mayo Clin Proc* 2005;80(10):1326–38.

33. Abbott NJ, Ronnback L, Hansson E. Astrocyte-endothelial interactions at the blood-brain barrier. *Nat Rev Neurosci* 2006;7(1):41–53.

34. Kim JH, Kim JH, Park JA, et al. Blood-neural barrier: intercellular communication at glio-vascular interface. *J Biochem Mol Biol* 2006;39(4):339–45.

35. Terasaki T, Ohtsuki S. Brain-to-blood transporters for endogenous substrates and xenobiotics at the blood-brain barrier: an overview of biology and methodology. *NeuroRx* 2005;2(1):63–72.

36. Jodoin J, Demeule M, Fenart L, et al. P-glycoprotein in blood-brain barrier endothelial cells: interaction and oligomerization with caveolins. *J Neurochem* 2003;87(4):1010–23.

37. Gosk S, Vermehren C, Storm G, Moos T. Targeting anti-transferrin receptor antibody (OX26) and OX26-conjugated liposomes to brain capillary endothelial cells using in situ perfusion. *J Cereb Blood Flow Metab* 2004;24(11):1193–204.

38. Ulvestad E, Williams K, Bjerkvig R, Tiekotter K, Antel J, Matre R. Human microglial cells have phenotypic and functional characteristics in common with both macrophages and dendritic antigen-presenting cells. *J Leukoc Biol* 1994;56(6):732–40.

39. Carson MJ, Reilly CR, Sutcliffe JG, Lo D. Mature microglia resemble immature antigen-presenting cells. *Glia* 1998;22(1):72–85.

40. Webster SD, Park M, Fonseca MI, Tenner AJ. Structural and functional evidence for microglial expression of C1qR(P), the C1q receptor that enhances phagocytosis. *J Leukoc Biol* 2000;67(1):109–16.

41. Webster SD, Galvan MD, Ferran E, Garzon-Rodriguez W, Glabe CG, Tenner AJ. Antibody-mediated phagocytosis of the amyloid beta-peptide in microglia is differentially modulated by C1q. *J Immunol* 2001;166(12):7496–503.

42. Song X, Shapiro S, Goldman DL, Casadevall A, Scharff M, Lee SC. Fcgamma receptor I- and III-mediated macrophage inflammatory protein 1alpha induction in primary human and murine microglia. *Infect Immun* 2002;70(9):5177–84.

43. Koenigsknecht-Talboo J, Landreth GE. Microglial phagocytosis induced by fibrillar beta-amyloid and IgGs are differentially regulated by proinflammatory cytokines. *J Neurosci* 2005;25(36):8240–9.

44. Rebe S, Solomon B. Deglycosylation of anti-beta amyloid antibodies inhibits microglia activation in BV-2 cellular model. *Am J Alzheimers Dis Other Demen* 2005;20(5):303–13.

45. Goldman DL, Casadevall A, Zuckier LS. Pharmacokinetics and biodistribution of a monoclonal antibody to Cryptococcus neoformans capsular polysaccharide antigen in a rat model of cryptococcal meningitis: implications for passive immunotherapy. *J Med Vet Mycol* 1997;35(4):271–8.

46. Pardridge WM, Buciak JL, Friden PM. Selective transport of an anti-transferrin receptor antibody through the blood–brain barrier in vivo. *J Pharmacol Exp Ther* 1991;259(1):66–70.

47. Schlachetzki F, Zhu C, Pardridge WM. Expression of the neonatal Fc receptor (FcRn) at the blood-brain barrier. *J Neurochem* 2002;81(1):203–6.

48. Hofman P, Hoyng P, vanderWerf F, Vrensen GF, Schlingemann RO. Lack of blood-brain barrier properties in microvessels of the prelaminar optic nerve head. *Invest Ophthalmol Vis Sci* 2001;42(5):895–901.

49. Bours J. The protein distribution of bovine, human and rabbit aqueous humour and the difference in composition before and after disruption of the blood/aqueous humour barrier. *Lens Eye Toxic Res* 1990;7(3–4):491–503.

50. Verhagen C, Breeboart AC, Kijlstra A. Diffusion of immunoglobulin G from the vascular compartment into the normal rabbit cornea. *Invest Ophthalmol Vis Sci* 1990;31(8):1519–25.

51. Marie I, Herve F, Lahaxe L, Robaday S, Gerardin E, Levesque H. Intravenous immunoglobulin-associated cranial pachymeningitis. *J Intern Med* 2006;260(2):164–7.

52. Hadden RD, Gregson NA, Gold R, Smith KJ, Hughes RA. Accumulation of immunoglobulin across the "blood-nerve barrier" in spinal roots in adoptive transfer experimental autoimmune neuritis. *Neuropathol Appl Neurobiol* 2002;28(6):489–97.

53. Vedeler CA. Demonstration of Fc gamma receptors on human peripheral nerve fibres. *J Neuroimmunol* 1987;15(2):207–16.

54. Vedeler CA, Matre R, Kristoffersen EK, Ulvestad E. IgG Fc receptor heterogeneity in human peripheral nerves. *Acta Neurol Scand* 1991;84(3):177–80.

55. Houston LL, Nowinski RC, Bernstein ID. Specific in vivo localization of monoclonal antibodies directed against the Thy 1.1 antigen. *J Immunol* 1980;125(2):837–43.

56. Badger CC, Krohn KA, Shulman H, Flournoy N, Bernstein ID. Experimental radioimmunotherapy of murine lymphoma with 131I-labeled anti-T-cell antibodies. *Cancer Res* 1986;46(12 Pt 1):6223–8.

57. Simionescu D, Simionescu M. Differentiated distribution of the cell surface charge on the alveolar-capillary unit. Characteristic paucity of anionic sites on the air-blood barrier. *Microvasc Res* 1983;25(1):85–100.

58. Lossinsky AS, Shivers RR. Structural pathways for macromolecular and cellular transport across the blood–brain barrier during inflammatory conditions. Review. *Histol Histopathol* 2004;19(2):535–64.

59. Svedman C, Yu BB, Ryan TJ, Svensson H. Plasma proteins in a standardised skin mini-erosion (I): permeability changes as a function of time. *BMC Dermatol* 2002;2:3.

60. Moldoveanu Z, Epps JM, Thorpe SR, Mestecky J. The sites of catabolism of murine monomeric IgA. *J Immunol* 1988;141(1):208–13.

61. Mestecky J, Moro I, Underdown BJ. Mucosal Immunology. Ogra PL, Mestecky J, Lamm ME, Strober W, Bienenstock J, McGhee JR, eds. *Mucosal Immunoglobulins*, 2nd ed. 1998. London: Academic Press, 1998;133–52.

62. Borvak J, Richardson J, Medesan C, et al. Functional expression of the MHC class I-related receptor, FcRn, in endothelial cells of mice. *Int Immunol* 1998; 10(9):1289–98.

63. Waldmann TA, Strober W. Metabolism of immunoglobulins. *Prog Allergy* 1969; 13:1–110.

64. Henderson LA, Baynes JW, Thorpe SR. Identification of the sites of IgG catabolism in the rat. *Arch Biochem Biophys* 1982;215(1):1–11.

65. Olszewski WL, Engeset A. Capillary transport of immunoglobulins and complement proteins to the interstitial fluid and lymph. *Arch Immunol Ther Exp (Warsz)* 1978;26(1–6):57–65.

66. Roccatello D, Picciotto G, Ropolo R, et al. Kinetics and fate of IgA-IgG aggregates as a model of naturally occurring immune complexes in IgA nephropathy. *Lab Invest* 1992;66(1):86–95.

67. Fanger NA, Wardwell K, Shen L, Tedder TF, Guyre PM. Type I (CD64) and type II (CD32) Fc gamma receptor-mediated phagocytosis by human blood dendritic cells. *J Immunol* 1996;157(2):541–8.

68. Fanger NA, Voigtlaender D, Liu C, et al. Characterization of expression, cytokine regulation, and effector function of the high affinity IgG receptor Fc gamma RI (CD64) expressed on human blood dendritic cells. *J Immunol* 1997;158(7): 3090–8.

69. Ravetch JV. Fc receptors. *Curr Opin Immunol* 1997;9(1):121–5.

70. Guyre CA, Keler T, Swink SL, Vitale LA, Graziano RF, Fanger MW. Receptor modulation by Fc gamma RI-specific fusion proteins is dependent on receptor number and modified by IgG. *J Immunol* 2001;167(11):6303–11.

71. Van WJ, Lipinski P, Abadie A, et al. Antagonistic action of IFN-beta and IFN-gamma on high affinity Fc gamma receptor expression in healthy controls and multiple sclerosis patients. *J Immunol* 1998;161(3):1568–74.

72. Uciechowski P, Schwarz M, Gessner JE, Schmidt RE, Resch K, Radeke HH. IFN-gamma induces the high-affinity Fc receptor I for IgG (CD64) on human glomerular mesangial cells. *Eur J Immunol* 1998;28(9):2928–35.

73. van Royen-Kerkhof A, Sanders EA, Walraven V, et al. A novel human CD32 mAb blocks experimental immune haemolytic anaemia in FcgammaRIIA transgenic mice. *Br J Haematol* 2005;130(1):130–7.

74. Wiener E, Dellow RA, Mawas F, Rodeck CH. Role of Fc gamma RIIa (CD32) in IgG anti-RhD-mediated red cell phagocytosis in vitro. *Transfus Med* 1996;6(3): 235–41.

75. Metes D, Ernst LK, Chambers WH, Sulica A, Herberman RB, Morel PA. Expression of functional CD32 molecules on human NK cells is determined by an allelic polymorphism of the FcgammaRIIC gene. *Blood* 1998;91(7):2369–80.

76. Favaloro EJ. Differential expression of surface antigens on activated endothelium. *Immunol Cell Biol* 1993;71(Pt 6):571–81.

77. Coggeshall KM. Regulation of signal transduction by the Fc gamma receptor family members and their involvement in autoimmunity. *Curr Dir Autoimmun* 2002;5:1–29.

78. Micouin A, Rouillard D, Bauvois B. Induction of macrophagic differentiation and cytokine secretion by IgG1 molecules in human normal monocytes and myelogenous leukemia cells. *Leukemia* 1997;11(4):552–60.

79. Ravetch JV, Perussia B. Alternative membrane forms of Fc gamma RIII(CD16) on human natural killer cells and neutrophils. Cell type-specific expression of two genes that differ in single nucleotide substitutions. *J Exp Med* 1989;170(2): 481–97.

80. Hisaka H, Kataoka M, Higuchi Y, Matsuura K, Yamamoto S. Close localization of mouse CD14 and CD32/16 in the cell surface of monocytic cell lines. *Pathobiology* 1999;67(2):92–8.

81. de AB, Mueller AL, Verbeek S, Sandor M, Lynch RG. A regulatory role for Fcgamma receptors CD16 and CD32 in the development of murine B cells. *Blood* 1998;92(8):2823–9.

82. Delire M. Different modes of action of high-dose immunoglobulins in rheumatoid arthritis. *Acta Univ Carol [Med] (Praha)* 1994;40(1–4):95–9.

83. Muller C, Traindl O, Schwarz M, et al. Increased Fc-receptor-mediated clearance via reticuloendothelial system in patients with nephrotic syndrome. *Nephron* 1991;58(2):150–4.

84. Anderson CL, Abraham GN. Characterization of the Fc receptor for IgG on a human macrophage cell line, U937. *J Immunol* 1980;125(6):2735–41.

85. McCool D, Birshtein BK, Painter RH. Structural requirements of immunoglobulin G for binding to the Fc gamma receptors of the human tumor cell lines U937, HL-60, ML-1, and K562. *J Immunol* 1985;135(3):1975–80.

86. Canfield SM, Morrison SL. The binding affinity of human IgG for its high affinity Fc receptor is determined by multiple amino acids in the CH2 domain and is modulated by the hinge region. *J Exp Med* 1991;173(6):1483–91.

87. Chappel MS, Isenman DE, Everett M, Xu YY, Dorrington KJ, Klein MH. Identification of the Fc gamma receptor class I binding site in human IgG through the use of recombinant IgG1/IgG2 hybrid and point-mutated antibodies. *Proc Natl Acad Sci USA* 1991;88(20):9036–40.

88. Chappel MS, Isenman DE, Oomen R, Xu YY, Klein MH. Identification of a secondary Fc gamma RI binding site within a genetically engineered human IgG antibody. *J Biol Chem* 1993;268(33):25124–31.

89. Tan LK, Shopes RJ, Oi VT, Morrison SL. Influence of the hinge region on complement activation, C1q binding, and segmental flexibility in chimeric human immunoglobulins. *Proc Natl Acad Sci USA* 1990;87(1):162–6.

90. Morgan A, Jones ND, Nesbitt AM, Chaplin L, Bodmer MW, Emtage JS. The N-terminal end of the CH2 domain of chimeric human IgG1 anti-HLA-DR is necessary for C1q, Fc gamma RI and Fc gamma RIII binding. *Immunology* 1995; 86(2):319–24.

91. Kim MK, Huang ZY, Hwang PH, et al. Fcgamma receptor transmembrane domains: role in cell surface expression, gamma chain interaction, and phagocytosis. *Blood* 2003;101(11):4479–84.

92. Kim JK, Firan M, Radu CG, Kim CH, Ghetie V, Ward ES. Mapping the site on human IgG for binding of the MHC class I-related receptor, FcRn. *Eur J Immunol* 1999;29(9):2819–25.

93. Kim JK, Tsen MF, Ghetie V, Ward ES. Identifying amino acid residues that influence plasma clearance of murine IgG1 fragments by site-directed mutagenesis. *Eur J Immunol* 1994;24(3):542–8.

94. Popov S, Hubbard JG, Kim J, Ober B, Ghetie V, Ward ES. The stoichiometry and affinity of the interaction of murine Fc fragments with the MHC class I-related receptor, FcRn. *Mol Immunol* 1996;33(6):521–30.

95. Parren PW, Warmerdam PA, Boeije LC, Capel PJ, van de Winkel JG, Aarden LA. Characterization of IgG FcR-mediated proliferation Of human T cells induced by mouse and Human anti-CD3 monoclonal antibodies. Identification of a functional polymorphism to human IgG2 anti-CD3. *J Immunol* 1992;148(3):695–701.

96. Wu J, Edberg JC, Redecha PB, et al. A novel polymorphism of FcgammaRIIIa (CD16) alters receptor function and predisposes to autoimmune disease. *J Clin Invest* 1997;100(5):1059–70.

97. Koene HR, Kleijer M, Algra J, Roos D, von dem Borne AE, De HM. Fc gammaRIIIa-158V/F polymorphism influences the binding of IgG by natural killer cell Fc gammaRIIIa, independently of the Fc gammaRIIIa-48L/R/H phenotype. *Blood* 1997;90(3):1109–14.

98. Cartron G, Dacheux L, Salles G, et al. Therapeutic activity of humanized anti-CD20 monoclonal antibody and polymorphism in IgG Fc receptor Fc gamma RIIIa gene. *Blood* 2002;99(3):754–8.

99. Su K, Wu J, Edberg JC, McKenzie SE, Kimberly RP. Genomic organization of classical human low-affinity Fc gamma receptor genes. *Genes Immun* 2002;3 Suppl 1:S51–6.

100. Haagen IA, Geerars AJ, Clark MR, van de Winkel JG. Interaction of human monocyte Fc gamma receptors with rat IgG2b: a new indicator for the Fc gamma RIIa (R-H131) polymorphism. *J Immunol* 1995;154(4):1852–60.

101. Medesan C, Matesoi D, Radu C, Ghetie V, Ward ES. Delineation of the amino acid residues involved in transcytosis and catabolism of mouse IgG1. *J Immunol* 1997;158(5):2211–7.

102. Mattes MJ. Biodistribution of antibodies after intraperitoneal or intravenous injection and effect of carbohydrate modifications. *J Natl Cancer Inst* 1987; 79(4):855–63.

103. Wright A, Morrison SL. Effect of altered CH2–associated carbohydrate structure on the functional properties and in vivo fate of chimeric mouse-human immunoglobulin G1. *J Exp Med* 1994;180(3):1087–96.

104. Wright A, Sato Y, Okada T, Chang K, Endo T, Morrison S. In vivo trafficking and catabolism of IgG1 antibodies with Fc associated carbohydrates of differing structure. *Glycobiology* 2000;10(12):1347–55.

105. Lennartz MR, Cole FS, Shepherd VL, Wileman TE, Stahl PD. Isolation and characterization of a mannose-specific endocytosis receptor from human placenta. *J Biol Chem* 1987;262(21):9942–4.

106. Stahl PD. The mannose receptor and other macrophage lectins. *Curr Opin Immunol* 1992;4(1):49–52.

107. Dong X, Storkus WJ, Salter RD. Binding and uptake of agalactosyl IgG by mannose receptor on macrophages and dendritic cells. *J Immunol* 1999;163(10):5427–34.

108. Groenink J, Spijker J, van den Herik-Oudijk IE, et al. On the interaction between agalactosyl IgG and Fc gamma receptors. *Eur J Immunol* 1996;26(6):1404–7.

109. Dickinson BL, Badizadegan K, Wu Z, et al. Bidirectional FcRn-dependent IgG transport in a polarized human intestinal epithelial cell line. *J Clin Invest* 1999; 104(7):903–11.

110. Kobayashi N, Suzuki Y, Tsuge T, Okumura K, Ra C, Tomino Y. FcRn-mediated transcytosis of immunoglobulin G in human renal proximal tubular epithelial cells. *Am J Physiol Renal Physiol* 2002;282(2):F358–65.

111. Simister NE, Mostov KE. Cloning and expression of the neonatal rat intestinal Fc receptor, a major histocompatibility complex class I antigen homolog. *Cold Spring Harb Symp Quant Biol* 1989;54(Pt 1):571–80.

112. Simister NE, Mostov KE. An Fc receptor structurally related to MHC class I antigens. *Nature* 1989;337(6203):184–7.

113. Junghans RP, Anderson CL. The protection receptor for IgG catabolism is the beta2-microglobulin-containing neonatal intestinal transport receptor. *Proc Natl Acad Sci USA* 1996;93(11):5512–6.

114. Story CM, Mikulska JE, Simister NE. A major histocompatibility complex class I-like Fc receptor cloned from human placenta: possible role in transfer of immunoglobulin G from mother to fetus. *J Exp Med* 1994;180(6):2377–81.

115. Mikulska JE, Pablo L, Canel J, Simister NE. Cloning and analysis of the gene encoding the human neonatal Fc receptor. *Eur J Immunogenet* 2000;27(4): 231–40.

116. Haymann JP, Levraud JP, Bouet S, et al. Characterization and localization of the neonatal Fc receptor in adult human kidney. *J Am Soc Nephrol* 2000; 11(4):632–9.

117. Zhu X, Peng J, Raychowdhury R, Nakajima A, Lencer WI, Blumberg RS. The heavy chain of neonatal Fc receptor for IgG is sequestered in endoplasmic reticulum by forming oligomers in the absence of beta2-microglobulin association. *Biochem J* 2002;367(Pt 3):703–14.

118. Teter K, Chandy G, Quinones B, Pereyra K, Machen T, Moore HP. Cellubrevin-targeted fluorescence uncovers heterogeneity in the recycling endosomes. *J Biol Chem* 1998;273(31):19625–33.

119. Ober RJ, Martinez C, Lai X, Zhou J, Ward ES. Exocytosis of IgG as mediated by the receptor, FcRn: an analysis at the single-molecule level. *Proc Natl Acad Sci USA* 2004;101(30):11076–81.

120. Ober RJ, Martinez C, Vaccaro C, Zhou J, Ward ES. Visualizing the site and dynamics of IgG salvage by the MHC class I-related receptor, FcRn. *J Immunol* 2004;172(4):2021–9.

121. Vaccaro C, Zhou J, Ober RJ, Ward ES. Engineering the Fc region of immunoglobulin G to modulate in vivo antibody levels. *Nat Biotechnol* 2005;23(10):1283–8.

122. Brambell FW, Hemmings WA, Oakley CL, Porter RR. The relative transmission of the fractions of papain hydrolyzed homologous gamma-globulin from the uterine cavity to the foetal circulation in the rabbit. *Proc R Soc Lond B Biol Sci* 1960;151:478–82.

123. Brambell FW. The transmission of immune globulins from the mother to the foetal and newborn young. *Proc Nutr Soc* 1969;28(1):35–41.

124. Telleman P, Junghans RP. The role of the Brambell receptor (FcRB) in liver: protection of endocytosed immunoglobulin G (IgG) from catabolism in hepatocytes rather than transport of IgG to bile. *Immunology* 2000;100(2):245–51.

125. Antohe F, Radulescu L, Gafencu A, Ghetie V, Simionescu M. Expression of functionally active FcRn and the differentiated bidirectional transport of IgG in human placental endothelial cells. *Hum Immunol* 2001;62(2):93–105.

126. Stevenson GT, Anderson VA, Leong WS. Engineered antibody for treating lymphoma. *Recent Results Cancer Res* 2002;159:104–12.

127. Tannock IF, Rotin D. Acid pH in tumors and its potential for therapeutic exploitation. *Cancer Res* 1989;49(16):4373–84.

128. Kristoffersen EK, Matre R. Co-localization of beta 2-microglobulin and IgG in human placental syncytiotrophoblasts. *Eur J Immunol* 1996;26(2):505–7.

129. Junghans RP, Carrasquillo JA, Waldmann TA. Impact of antigenemia on the bioactivity of infused anti-Tac antibody: implications for dose selection in antibody immunotherapies. *Proc Natl Acad Sci USA* 1998;95(4):1752–7.

130. Hobbs SM, Jackson LE, Hoadley J. Interaction of aglycosyl immunoglobulins with the IgG Fc transport receptor from neonatal rat gut: comparison of deglycosylation by tunicamycin treatment and genetic engineering. *Mol Immunol* 1992; 29(7–8):949–56.

131. Perez JH, Wight DG, Wyatt JI, Van SM, Mullock BM, Luzio JP. The polymeric immunoglobulin A receptor is present on hepatocytes in human liver. *Immunology* 1989;68(4):474–8.

132. Tourville DR, Adler RH, Bienenstock J, Tomasi TB, Jr. The human secretory immunoglobulin system: immunohistoligical localization of gamma A, secretory "piece," and lactoferrin in normal human tissues. *J Exp Med* 1969;129(2):411–29.

133. Tourville DR, Tomasi TB, Jr. Selective transport of gamma A. *Proc Soc Exp Biol Med* 1969;132(2):473–7.

134. Takahashi I, Nakane PK, Brown WR. Ultrastructural events in the translocation of polymeric IgA by rat hepatocytes. *J Immunol* 1982;128(3):1181–7.

135. Schiff JM, Fisher MM, Jones AL, Underdown BJ. Human IgA as a heterovalent ligand: switching from the asialoglycoprotein receptor to secretory component during transport across the rat hepatocyte. *J Cell Biol* 1986;102(3):920–31.

136. Kaetzel CS, Robinson JK, Lamm ME. Epithelial transcytosis of monomeric IgA and IgG cross-linked through antigen to polymeric IgA. A role for monomeric antibodies in the mucosal immune system. *J Immunol* 1994;152(1):72–6.

137. Hunziker W, Mellman I. Expression of macrophage-lymphocyte Fc receptors in Madin-Darby canine kidney cells: polarity and transcytosis differ for isoforms with or without coated pit localization domains. *J Cell Biol* 1989;109(6 Pt 2): 3291–302.

138. Hunziker W, Male P, Mellman I. Differential microtubule requirements for transcytosis in MDCK cells. *EMBO J* 1990;9(11):3515–25.

139. Gurevich P, Zusman I, Moldavsky M, et al. Secretory immune system in human intrauterine development: immunopathomorphological analysis of the role of secretory component (pIgR/SC) in immunoglobulin transport (review). *Int J Mol Med* 2003;12(3):289–97.

140. Leung JC, Tsang AW, Chan DT, Lai KN. Absence of CD89, polymeric immunoglobulin receptor, and asialoglycoprotein receptor on human mesangial cells. *J Am Soc Nephrol* 2000;11(2):241–9.

141. Ball JM, Moldoveanu Z, Melsen LR, et al. A polarized human endometrial cell line that binds and transports polymeric IgA. *In Vitro Cell Dev Biol Anim* 1995; 31(3):196–206.

142. Underdown BJ, Schiff JM. Immunoglobulin A: strategic defense initiative at the mucosal surface. *Annu Rev Immunol* 1986;4:389–417.

143. Manning RJ, Walker PG, Carter L, Barrington PJ, Jackson GD. Studies on the origins of biliary immunoglobulins in rats. *Gastroenterology* 1984;87(1):173–9.

144. Mullock BM, Shaw LJ, Fitzharris B, et al. Sources of proteins in human bile. *Gut* 1985;26(5):500–9.

145. Blumberg RS, Koss T, Story CM, et al. A major histocompatibility complex class I-related Fc receptor for IgG on rat hepatocytes. *J Clin Invest* 1995;95(5): 2397–402.

146. Sheff DR, Daro EA, Hull M, Mellman I. The receptor recycling pathway contains two distinct populations of early endosomes with different sorting functions. *J Cell Biol* 1999;145(1):123–39.

147. Zhang JR, Mostov KE, Lamm ME, et al. The polymeric immunoglobulin receptor translocates pneumococci across human nasopharyngeal epithelial cells. *Cell* 2000; 102(6):827–37.

148. Elm C, Braathen R, Bergmann S, et al. Ectodomains 3 and 4 of human polymeric Immunoglobulin receptor (hpIgR) mediate invasion of *Streptococcus pneumoniae* into the epithelium. *J Biol Chem* 2004;279(8):6296–304.

149. Sixbey JW, Yao QY. Immunoglobulin A-induced shift of Epstein-Barr virus tissue tropism. *Science* 1992;255(5051):1578–80.

150. Gan YJ, Chodosh J, Morgan A, Sixbey JW. Epithelial cell polarization is a determinant in the infectious outcome of immunoglobulin A-mediated entry by Epstein-Barr virus. *J Virol* 1997;71(1):519–26.

151. Aarli A, Matre R, Thunold S. IgG Fc receptors on epithelial cells of distal tubuli and on endothelial cells in human kidney. *Int Arch Allergy Appl Immunol* 1991; 95(1):64–9.

152. Kuhn K, Stolte H, Reale E. The fine structure of the kidney of the hagfish (*Myxine glutinosa L.*): A thin section and freeze-fracture study. *Cell Tissue Res* 1975; 164(2):201–13.

153. Latta H. An approach to the structure and function of the glomerular mesangium. *J Am Soc Nephrol* 1992;2(10 Suppl):S65–73.

154. Tencer J, Frick IM, Oquist BW, Alm P, Rippe B. Size-selectivity of the glomerular barrier to high molecular weight proteins: upper size limitations of shunt pathways. *Kidney Int* 1998;53(3):709–15.

155. Radeke HH, Gessner JE, Uciechowski P, Magert HJ, Schmidt RE, Resch K. Intrinsic human glomerular mesangial cells can express receptors for IgG complexes (hFc gamma RIII-A) and the associated Fc epsilon RI gamma-chain. *J Immunol* 1994;153(3):1281–92.

156. Gomez-Guerrero C, Hernandez-Vargas P, Lopez-Franco O, Ortiz-Munoz G, Egido J. Mesangial cells and glomerular inflammation: from the pathogenesis to novel therapeutic approaches. *Curr Drug Targets Inflamm Allergy* 2005;4(3):341–51.

157. Mauer SM, Fish AJ, Blau EB, Michael AF. The glomerular mesangium. I. Kinetic studies of macromolecular uptake in normal and nephrotic rats. *J Clin Invest* 1972; 51(5):1092–101.

158. Thompson EM, Evans DJ. Association of mesangial IgM with IgM deposits in the macula densa: an indication of non-specific macromolecule transport rather than immune reactant? *Nephrol Dial Transplant* 2001;16(9):1910–3.

159. Junghans RP, Waldmann TA. Metabolism of Tac (IL2Ralpha): physiology of cell surface shedding and renal catabolism, and suppression of catabolism by antibody binding. *J Exp Med* 1996;183(4):1587–602.

160. Clyne PS, Kulczycki A, Jr. Human breast milk contains bovine IgG. Relationship to infant colic? *Pediatrics* 1991;87(4):439–44.

161. Cianga P, Cianga C, Cozma L, Ward ES, Carasevici E. The MHC class I related Fc receptor, FcRn, is expressed in the epithelial cells of the human mammary gland. *Hum Immunol* 2003;64(12):1152–9.

162. Takaya R, Fukaya T, Sasano H, Suzuki T, Tamura M, Yajima A. Macrophages in normal cycling human ovaries; immunohistochemical localization and characterization. *Hum Reprod* 1997;12(7):1508–12.

163. Leach JL, Sedmak DD, Osborne JM, Rahill B, Lairmore MD, Anderson CL. Isolation from human placenta of the IgG transporter, FcRn, and localization to the syncytiotrophoblast: implications for maternal-fetal antibody transport. *J Immunol* 1996;157(8):3317–22.

164. Kristoffersen EK. Human placental Fc gamma-binding proteins in the maternofetal transfer of IgG. *APMIS* Suppl 1996;64:5–36.

165. Einhorn MS, Granoff DM, Nahm MH, Quinn A, Shackelford PG. Concentrations of antibodies in paired maternal and infant sera: relationship to IgG subclass. *J Pediatr* 1987;111(5):783–8.

166. Malek A, Sager R, Schneider H. Transport of proteins across the human placenta. *Am J Reprod Immunol* 1998;40(5):347–51.

167. Malek A. Ex vivo human placenta models: transport of immunoglobulin G and its subclasses. *Vaccine* 2003;21(24):3362–4.

168. Eaton BM, Oakey MP. Image analysis of protein profiles from paired microvillous and basal syncytiotrophoblast plasma membranes from term human placenta and characterization of IgG binding to membrane vesicles. *Placenta* 1997;18(7): 569–76.

169. Kutteh WH, Moldoveanu Z, Mestecky J. Mucosal immunity in the female reproductive tract: correlation of immunoglobulins, cytokines, and reproductive hormones in human cervical mucus around the time of ovulation. *AIDS Res Hum Retroviruses* 1998;14 Suppl 1:S51–5.

170. Moldoveanu Z, Huang WQ, Kulhavy R, Pate MS, Mestecky J. Human male genital tract secretions: both mucosal and systemic immune compartments contribute to the humoral immunity. *J Immunol* 2005;175(6):4127–36.

171. Delacroix DL, Marchandise FX, Francis C, Sibille Y. Alpha-2-macroglobulin, monomeric and polymeric immunoglobulin A, and immunoglobulin M in bronchoalveolar lavage. *Am Rev Respir Dis* 1985;132(4):829–35.

172. Bignon J, Jaurand MC, Pinchon MC, Sapin C, Warnet JM. Immunoelectron microscopic and immunochemical demonstrations of serum proteins in the alveolar lining material of the rat lung. *Am Rev Respir Dis* 1976;113(2):109–20.

173. Kim KJ, Malik AB. Protein transport across the lung epithelial barrier. *Am J Physiol Lung Cell Mol Physiol* 2003;284(2):L247–59.

174. Spiekermann GM, Finn PW, Ward ES, et al. Receptor-mediated immunoglobulin G transport across mucosal barriers in adult life: functional expression of FcRn in the mammalian lung. *J Exp Med* 2002;196(3):303–10.

175. Dumont JA, Bitonti AJ, Clark D, Evans S, Pickford M, Newman SP. Delivery of an erythropoietin-Fc fusion protein by inhalation in humans through an immunoglobulin transport pathway. *J Aerosol Med* 2005;18(3):294–303.

176. Cauza K, Hinterhuber G, Dingelmaier-Hovorka R, et al. Expression of FcRn, the MHC class I-related receptor for IgG, in human keratinocytes. *J Invest Dermatol* 2005;124(1):132–9.

177. Brown WR, Kloppel TM. The role of the liver in translocation of IgA into the gastrointestinal tract. *Immunol Invest* 1989;18(1–4):269–85.

178. Brown WR, Kloppel TM. The liver and IgA: immunological, cell biological and clinical implications. *Hepatology* 1989;9(5):763–84.

179. Raju TS, Briggs JB, Chamow SM, Winkler ME, Jones AJ. Glycoengineering of therapeutic glycoproteins: in vitro galactosylation and sialylation of glycoproteins with terminal N-acetylglucosamine and galactose residues. *Biochemistry* 2001; 40(30):8868–76.

180. Hurlimann J. Immunoglobulin synthesis and transport by human salivary glands. Immunological mechanisms of the mucous membranes. *Curr Top Pathol* 1971; 55:69–108.

181. Proctor GB, Carpenter GH. Chewing stimulates secretion of human salivary secretory immunoglobulin A. *J Dent Res* 2001;80(3):909–13.

182. Strober W, Blaese RM, Waldmann TA. The origin of salivary IgA. *J Lab Clin Med* 1970;75(5):856–62.

183. Malamud D. Oral diagnostic testing for detecting human immunodeficiency virus-1 antibodies: a technology whose time has come. *Am J Med* 1997;102(4A):9–14.

184. Takahashi K, Mooney J, Frandsen EV, Kinane DF. IgG and IgA subclass mRNA-bearing plasma cells in periodontitis gingival tissue and immunoglobulin levels in the gingival crevicular fluid. *Clin Exp Immunol* 1997;107(1):158–65.

185. Hochman N, Zakay-Rones Z, Shohat H, et al. Antibodies to cytomegalo and Epstein-Barr viruses in human saliva and gingival fluid. *New Microbiol* 1998; 21(2):131–9.

186. Brandtzaeg P. Human secretory immunoglobulins. II. Salivary secretions from individuals with selectively excessive or defective synthesis of serum immuno-globulins. *Clin Exp Immunol* 1971;8(1):69–85.

187. Newcomb RW, Ishizaka K, DeVald BL. Human IgG and IgA diphtheria antitoxins in serum, nasal fluids and saliva. *J Immunol* 1969;103(2):215–24.

188. Prigent-Delecourt L, Coffin B, Colombel JF, Dehennin JP, Vaerman JP, Rambaud JC. Secretion of immunoglobulins and plasma proteins from the colonic mucosa: an in vivo study in man. *Clin Exp Immunol* 1995;99(2):221–5.

189. Zimmer KP, Scheumann GF, Bramswig J, Bocker W, Harms E, Schmid KW. Ultra-structural localization of IgG and TPO in autoimmune thyrocytes referring to the transcytosis of IgG and the antigen presentation of TPO. *Histochem Cell Biol* 1997;107(2):115–20.

190. Zimmer KP, Schmid KW, Bocker W, et al. Transcytosis of IgG from the basolateral to the apical membrane of human thyrocytes in autoimmune thyroid disease. *Curr Top Pathol* 1997;91:117–28.

191. Estienne V, Duthoit C, Reichert M, et al. Androgen-dependent expression of FcgammaRIIB2 by thyrocytes from patients with autoimmune Graves' disease: a possible molecular clue for sex dependence of autoimmune disease. *FASEB J* 2002;16(9):1087–92.

192. Barrett JS, Wagner JG, Fisher SJ, Wahl RL. Effect of intraperitoneal injection volume and antibody protein dose on the pharmacokinetics of intraperitoneally administered IgG2a kappa murine monoclonal antibody in the rat. *Cancer Res* 1991;51(13):3434–44.

193. Feriani M, Biasioli S, Chiaramonte S, et al. Anatomical bases of peritoneal perme-ability: a reappraisal. Anatomy of peritoneum. *Int J Artif Organs* 1982;5(6): 345–8.

194. Flessner MF, Dedrick RL, Reynolds JC. Bidirectional peritoneal transport of immunoglobulin in rats: tissue concentration profiles. *Am J Physiol* 1992;263 (1 Pt 2):F15–23.

195. Flessner MF, Dedrick RL, Reynolds JC. Bidirectional peritoneal transport of immunoglobulin in rats: compartmental kinetics. *Am J Physiol* 1992;262 (2 Pt 2):F275–87.

196. Flessner MF, Dedrick RL. Monoclonal antibody delivery to intraperitoneal tumors in rats: effects of route of administration and intraperitoneal solution osmolality. *Cancer Res* 1994;54(16):4376–84.

197. Flessner MF. The role of extracellular matrix in transperitoneal transport of water and solutes. *Perit Dial Int* 2001;21 Suppl 3:S24–9.

198. Rosengren BI, Carlsson O, Venturoli D, al RO, Rippe B. Transvascular passage of macromolecules into the peritoneal cavity of normo- and hypothermic rats in vivo: active or passive transport? *J Vasc Res* 2004;41(2):123–30.

199. Krediet RT, Koomen GC, Vlug A, et al. IgG subclasses in CAPD patients. *Perit Dial Int* 1996;16(3):288–94.

200. Yokoyama I, Waxman F. Isotypic and clonal variations in the interactions between model monoclonal immune complexes and the human erythrocyte CR1 receptor. *Mol Immunol* 1992;29(7–8):935–47.

201. Kavai M, Rasmussen JM, Baatrup G, Zsindely A, Svehag SE. Inefficient binding of IgM immune complexes to erythrocyte C3b-C4b receptors (CR1) and weak incorporation of C3b-iC3b into the complexes. *Scand J Immunol* 1988;28(1): 123–8.

202. Marzocchi-Machado CM, Polizello AC, Azzolini AE, Lucisano-Valim YM. The influence of antibody functional affinity on the effector functions involved in the clearance of circulating immune complexes anti-BSA IgG/BSA. *Immunol Invest* 1999;28(2–3):89–101.

CHAPTER 12

The Role of Pharmacokinetics and Pharmacodynamics in Selecting a Relevant Species

MARTIN D. GREEN, PhD, and MELANIE HARTSOUGH, PhD

Contents

12.1   INTRODUCTION

A relevant animal species is one in which the biopharmaceutical product, as a function of orthologous receptors or antigens, causes a similar biological response and mediates similar effector pathways to that occurring in humans [1]. The appropriate selection and use of a relevant animal species in preclinical toxicity testing is dependent on pharmacokinetic (PK) and pharmacodynamic (PD) measures, and these measures are fundamental for the extrapolation of the preclinical toxicity data to the clinical situation. PD properties, starting with receptors, form the scientific basis for the selection of an animal species for preclinical safety assessment of a biopharmaceutical. Translating the PD findings from laboratory animals to humans is often accomplished through an

Preclinical Safety Evaluation of Biopharmaceuticals: A Science-Based Approach to Facilitating Clinical Trials, edited by Joy A. Cavagnaro
Copyright © 2008 by John Wiley & Sons, Inc.

understanding and extrapolation of PK relationships between these models and the clinical setting. In particular, PD responsiveness typically yields evidence of the intensity and dynamic range of a response, whereas PK parameters serve as the means to convert the PD relationships gained from the preclinical models, such as those relating to plasma levels, dose, and dosing regimens, into the practical issues involved in a clinical study (e.g., selection of an initial dose, dose escalation scheme, and patient monitoring scheme).

Although the selection of a relevant species is clearly recognized as a defining principle for the safety assessment of biopharmaceuticals, this concept is not generally instrumental in the safety assessment of drugs that are typically of significantly lower molecular weight.[1] However, a limited application of this concept may be applied to drugs of smaller molecular weight. In this approach animal models for use in preclinical toxicity evaluations [2] and carcinogenicity studies [3,4] are selected for toxicity assessment that possess clinically meaningful metabolites due to similarities in the pathways for cytochrome 450 enzymes (P_{450}). In general, evaluating the data for a drug given to animals that produces metabolites that are common to humans allows for a more accurate interpretation of the toxicity profile and a more representative risk–benefit assessment. As biopharmaceuticals do not undergo metabolism by P_{450}, this concept is not applicable to large molecular weight products. Nevertheless, a common perspective between biopharmaceuticals and drugs is the need to establish a predictive preclinical model for the evaluation of human safety and identification of clinically relevant outcomes.

12.2 PHARMACODYNAMIC PROPERTIES

For most biopharmaceuticals, exaggerated pharmacological responses are a major contributor to the profile of adverse clinical events. Thus, the use of a relevant animal species to determine the toxicity profile of a biopharmaceutical is essential to the process of assessing overall safety. In some cases, the frequency of potential adverse events is relatively common and readily predictable from the pharmacodynamics of a product. For example, tissue plasminogen activator (tPA) has a restricted pharmacological activity, which is the ability to lyse clots and induce fibrinolysis. These effects apply across a number of species, albeit with different relative potency, and they subsequently lead to an expected increased incidence of bleeding. In other instances, the exact nature of predicting a specific adverse event from the PD properties of a product is significantly less reliable. Such is the case for biopharmaceuticals that inhibit TNF function. Although a general immune suppression may be anticipated with these products, the immune suppression unexpectedly leads

---

[1]Drugs are defined as products made by synthetic chemical processes and have lower molecular weights than biopharmaceutical products, which are made by cells and have molecular weights often greater than 1000 daltons.

to an increased incidence of tuberculosis in humans. Thus, the utility of the toxicology findings in animals depends on the selection of an appropriate animal model, with an understanding of its limitations, the frequency of the adverse occurrence, and the degree of impact on safety, and all these are dependent on the ability to extrapolate preclinical findings in a comprehensive manner. Although many important clinically adverse events may often be linked to information related to exaggerated pharmacological responses and are logical extrapolations from the preclinical safety data, not all important adverse events lend themselves to be assessed in preclinical models. For example, traztuzumab, which is used to treat breast cancer, causes a cardiomyopathy that resembles the effects of anthracyclines. This adverse event is not linked to its pharmacological actions mediated by its binding to the HER2 receptor, its only known site of action.

Without a proper understanding of the PK and PD responsiveness of an animal model elected for preclinical safety evaluation, it is difficult to distinguish between true positive or negative findings and outcomes. In the early 1990s with FIAU (fialuridine) and more recently with TGN 1412, an agonist monoclonal antibody (mAb) acting on CD28, preclinical studies yielded a false sense of anticipated clinical safety, due to a lack of corresponding PD responsiveness between animal models used for preclinical safety assessment and subjects of the clinical investigations. For FIAU, an antiviral nucleoside, commonly used animal models such as the mice or dogs failed to demonstrate the liver toxicity that was later observed in patients with viral hepatitis [5]. Rats did reveal some evidence of potential liver toxicity but at doses approximately 2000-fold greater than those demonstrated to be toxic to patients. Although unusual as an animal model, the woodchuck was later identified as a relevant model of human hepatitis B infections that was similarly responsive in terms of liver toxicity and sensitivity to doses of FIAU [6]. Similarly, TGN 1412 was investigated in nonhuman primates that were relatively unresponsive in terms of symptoms exhibited and thus yielded a false sense of understanding in terms of potential toxicities to humans [7]. The simple realization that the animal models used were not pharmacodynamically responsive should have led to a more conservative approach to the design of the clinical study with respect to the number of patients put at risk in a given cohort, clinical monitoring, dose escalation scheme and duration of treatment.

12.2.1 Species Specificity

Sometimes PD properties are common across species, thus allowing for pertinent toxicity data to be collected from a variety of species. An example of this is granulocyte colony stimulating factor (G-CSF), a cytokine produced by various cells including monocytes, fibroblasts, and endothelial cells that regulates the production of neutrophils within the bone marrow, influences neutrophil proliferation and differentiation, and contributes to increased phagocytic function, respiratory burst, and antibody-dependent killing. Keller et al. [8] reported that recombinant, human G-CSF administered to mice, rats, hamsters, dogs, and nonhuman primates produced the expected neutrophil effects at doses ≥1 µg/kg/day in all of the species. In other instances the PD properties restrict the applicability of animal species commonly used for safety testing. For example, in contrast to G-CSF, recombinant human granulocyte-macrophage colony stimulating factor (rhGM-CSF) exerts strong effects in nonhuman primates (including cynomolgus and rhesus monkeys) but is pharmacologically inactive in rodents. In the rhesus monkey, rhGM-CSF increased the proliferation and differentiation of myeloid precursors, resulting in a 20-fold increase in mature granulocytes counts in blood and in an activation of granulocytes and monocytes. At high doses it caused inflammation of the serosal surfaces of the heart and liver and at the site of injection [9]. Moreover secondary to a significant increase in granulocyte count, cardiovascular adverse events such as thrombosis also occurred. These effects are similar to that observed in humans. Given the PD agreement in responsiveness to humans, it was found that the rhesus monkey, rather than rodents, was predictive of clinical outcomes.

Yet a potentially more complicated problem is one of properly interpreting and extrapolating the effects of some biopharmaceuticals across closely related animal species that are pharmacologically responsive, in order to determine the species most clinically predictive. This problem is exemplified by interleukin-2 (IL-2), a cytokine used clinically to treat metastatic, renal cell carcinoma. IL-2 is produced by activated T cells and mediates a variety of effects, such as stimulation of lymphocyte activation and proliferation, enhancement of lymphocyte-directed cytotoxicity, and induction of interferon-γ secretion. It is pharmacologically active in rodents, rabbits, sheep, and humans [10]. Similar PD effects to those in humans are observed in mice, but in rats a related, but different, set of consequences occurs, even though the same underlying causative mechanisms exist. Moreover, the relative potency of human, recombinant IL-2 is approximately 20-fold less in mice and 70-fold less in rats when compared to humans. These differences are also reflected in the relevancy of the toxicity profiles of the two rodent species to that observed in humans. For example, the most prominent clinical toxicity of IL-2 results from an increased vascular permeability, producing extravasation of fluid and subsequent pulmonary edema and pleural effusions. Ultimately, a condition collectively referred to as vascular or capillary leak syndrome, characterized by the loss of fluid and proteins out of the circulating blood volume and into surrounding tissues, is produced. This set of conditions leads to extremely low blood pressure, multiple organ failure, and shock. In the setting of oncology, the clinical use of IL-2 is characterized by weight gain due to retained fluid, pulmonary edema, pleural effusion, and ascites. Other clinically significant side effects include fever, nausea, eosinophilia, and thrombocytopenia. In rats given an intraperitoneal injection of IL-2, pleural effusion was inconsistently observed and minor in intensity. In addition, while lung weights were increased due to cellular infiltration, primarily eosinophilic in nature, frank evidence of pulmonary edema was not observed. Intravenous administration of IL-2 to rats also failed to yield similar effects as that in humans, perhaps due to a decreased systemic persistence. In contrast, mice given IL-2 presented with similar toxicities as humans, severe pulmonary edema and pleural effusion and lymphocytic cell infiltration [11,12,13].

Some biopharmaceuticals exhibit a high degree of species selectivity that may restrict their biological activity to nonhuman primates (e.g., cynomolgus and rhesus monkeys) for preclinical safety. Hart et al. [14] reported the use of an in vitro IL-4-dependent, T cell proliferation assay to identify relevant species for testing the toxicity of an anti-IL-4 mAb (a humanized version of the murine parent mAb 3B9). The findings of the assay revealed that the antihuman IL-4 antibody inhibited the T cell response to recombinant cynomolgus monkey IL-4, an orthologous molecule with an amino acid sequence identity of 93% to the clinical version. No reactivity was found with mouse, rat, cow, goat, or horse IL-4.

Among the most highly selective cytokine biopharmaceuticals are the interferons. Interferons are members of a large family of related proteins that may be divided into two categories: type I and type II interferons. Type I interferons (i.e., α- and β-interferon) possess antiviral and anti-proliferative properties, whereas type II interferons (i.e., γ-interferon) have immunostimulatory activity. Several animal species were examined for their responsiveness to interferons, and with the exception of nonhuman primates, all tested animal species were found to be unresponsive [15].

Increasingly, the selectivity and specificity of biopharmaceuticals for human receptors often limit the range of responsive animal models (as described above for interferons and IL-4 mAb) or require the creation and use of different strategies. Alternate approaches to the problem of obtaining useful information include the use of homologous (also referred to as analogous or surrogate) proteins for the biopharmaceutical, the creation of transformed animal models such as transgenic animals, and the use of models of disease. Preclinical studies based on these alternative approaches should display a parallel and hopefully correct relative PD relationship in order to yield predictive information.

In rare instances the number of pharmacologically responsive preclinical species is very narrow, and only a single species such as the chimpanzee may be available to appropriately assess preclinical PD and PK endpoints. Since toxicology testing cannot be performed in chimpanzees due to their protective status, alternative methods are usually considered for standard safety assessments. An example of this is described by Clarke et al. [16] for efalizumab, a humanized mAb directed against the α-chain component of lymphocyte function associated antigen1 (LFA-1), also known as CD11a, that binds only to chimpanzee and human forms of the molecule. Efalizumab is used clinically for the treatment of psoriasis, and the PD basis for treating psoriasis is the antagonization of T lymphocyte infiltration into psoriatic lesions by blocking the T cell surface molecule LFA-1, thereby preventing interaction with the endothelial cell surface protein ICAM-1. To provide an adequate safety assessment, muM17, a chimeric rat anti-mouse CD11a mAb, was created and evaluated. This analogous molecule bound with similar specificity and affinity as efalizumab to the human CD11a and was found to have similar pharmacological activities in mice as efalizumab in humans. In order to bridge the preclinical safety information obtained from muM17 to the human setting, a PK/PD model was developed in mice [17]. This model was useful in selecting a clinically relevant dose based on the PD rather than the PK profile because of differing capacities of the CD11a binding between mice and humans and its influence on pharmacokinetics.

In some cases animal models of disease that mimic the anticipated clinical situation are needed to provide a set of relevant safety data, since the pathophysiological background is essential in providing the appropriate receptor or effecter mechanism. For example, erythropoietin, a glycoprotein with a molecular weight of 30 kDa, stimulates division and differentiation of committed erythroid progenitor cells and is not species restricted in terms of its primary biological activity. It induces the release of reticulocytes from the bone marrow into the bloodstream where they mature into erythrocytes and increase hematocrit. Too rapid a response to this growth factor will increase the viscosity of blood, thereby increasing vascular resistance and likelihood of a stroke. Erythropoietin did not demonstrate any cardiovascular toxicities in the general toxicity studies or in the extensive cardiovascular safety pharmacology studies performed in healthy animals [18], perhaps due to inherent compensating mechanisms. In contrast to a lack of findings in normal animals, a difference in cardiovascular regulatory response was observed in either spontaneously hypertensive rats or in isolated tissues obtained from these animals [19,20]. When erythropoietin was used in patients with chronic renal failure, hypertension was observed as a major clinical toxicity.

12.2.2 Binding Properties

Binding properties of a biopharmaceutical are important determinants in establishing the relevance of a species for safety assessment. An empirical assessment of binding is often necessary to establish the extent and location of binding across species. For example, in vitro studies of adalimumab, a fully human recombinant mAb directed against human TNFα, have revealed it to be a potent inhibitor of TNFα-related actions for humans, cynomolgus monkeys, and dogs, whereas no binding to the rat TNFα and only weak inhibition of the murine TNFα were observed [21]. Another example is humanized mAb alemtuzumab. This antibody recognizes CD52 and cross-reacts with epitopes from cynomolgus monkeys, rhesus monkeys, and baboons. However, in rhesus monkey and baboons as well as some individual cynomolgus monkeys, CD52 expression is found on erythrocytes, in contrast to humans in which it is absent [22]. Moreover, the binding affinity of alemtuzumab to cynomolgus CD52 is approximately 16-fold less than that to the human epitope. Hence, the binding to erythrocytes in these preclinical models could yield a false positive signal of hemolytic anemia, relative to humans.

The role of the various subcomponents of a receptor or epitope may contribute to the overall complexity of biopharmaceutical binding, pharmacokinetics, and pharmacological responsiveness and, in fact, is often an unknown factor in PK and PD differences between species. For example, the IL-2 receptor is a trimeric receptor composed of α, β, and γ chains, and the assembly of different groupings of these subcomponents determines the pharmacological relationship to pharmacokinetics. The trimeric complex binds IL-2 with very high affinity (Kd = 10^{-11}M), when compared to IL-2's affinity for the IL-2R$\beta\gamma$ complex (Kd = 10^{-9}M) or IL-2Rα subunit (Kd = 10^{-8}M). Moreover, the IL-2Rα chain is not involved with intracellular signaling, whereas the IL-2Rβ and IL-2Rγ subunits are critically important for pharmacological activity. Thus the therapeutic activity of IL-2 is actually more complex than just cytokine receptor binding. It also requires the recruitment of antigen-activated T cells and CD56 bright NK cells, an event dependent on the expression of all three receptors subunits as a trimeric complex with high affinity. In contrast, the IL-2-induced toxicity is associated with the lower affinity complexes, in particular, the binding of IL-2 to the IL-2R$\beta\gamma$ complexes located on CD56 dim NK cells. Hence the relative affinity dictates the range of IL-2-dependent effects, as picomolar concentrations are associated with the therapeutic aspects of the pharmacological activity of IL-2 and nanomolar levels with toxicity [23,24].

In rare cases intra-species variation may be important when assessing overall clinical predictability. Similar to the differences in P_{450s} that may be observed within humans and animals, the binding properties may vary within a species (even within a relevant species), which may confound the overall interpretation of the toxicology study. A good example of this is provided by Klingbeil and Hsu [25]. The authors describe the safety testing of Hu1D10, a humanized mAb directed against the posttranslational form of HLA-DR expressed on normal B cells as well as B cell leukemias and lymphomas. Klingbeil and Hsu reported that Hu1D10 administration to some monkeys resulted in severe acute adverse effects (e.g., respiratory suppression, increased heart rate, and urticaria) that in some cases required life-sustaining intervention, while no such adverse effects were observed in other Hu1D10-treated monkeys or the control monkeys. The extreme differences in effect were associated with the variation of HLA-DR expression, in that those animals that were antigen-positive exhibited toxicities while those that were antigen-negative did not.

12.3 PHARMACOKINETICS

Pharmacokinetic studies are often used to establish the extent of exposure to a biopharmaceutical in a preclinical study. This information not only validates dosing but also provides a means of extrapolating exposure across species. It therefore can be used as the basis for selecting an initial, safe starting dose for clinical use, determining therapeutic targets based on plasma levels associated with pharmacological effects, and providing an upper limit to clinical dosing based on PK exposure.

In general, extrapolation of PK data across species is dependent on the molecular weight of the biopharmaceutical, the involvement of receptor-mediated uptake, and the disposition and the route of administration [26]. A clinical dose may be extrapolated from preclinical data on either a body weight or surface area basis [27]. The appropriate method of extrapolations depends on the underlying factors governing disposition. Surface area based extrapolations assume a proportionate first-order dependent process, which may have active components such as receptor-mediated uptake mechanisms or more passive ones such as glomerular filtration. Generally, larger molecular weight biopharmaceuticals of greater than 70 kDa will scale by body weight, and lower molecular weight products will more often be applicable to scaling based on body surface area conversion. It is not uncommon for the saturation of various active processes to result in a nonlinearity in PK between plasma levels and dose, thus complicating extrapolation and interpretation when a wide range of doses are studied. This range of doses often includes and extends beyond a range with clinical utility. Thus, it is important to consider doses that are clinically relevant to ensure that clearance across species is highly predictive, whether it is a function of body weight or surface area.

12.3.1 Disposition

The PK of biopharmaceuticals are governed by factors such as absorption, distribution, catabolism, and excretion (similar principles to drugs) as well as other factors such as binding proteins and antibodies directed against the biopharmaceutical. Unlike drugs that readily diffuse, biopharmaceuticals, due to their molecular weight and shape, do not diffuse but are initially confined to the circulating vasculature; however, with time they distribute to the extravascular space by various factors, including bulk flow and convection. Catabolism of biopharmaceuticals is achieved by the same proteolytic processes that break down endogenous proteins, occurs in many sites in vivo, and usually involves receptor-mediated endocytosis followed by proteolysis in lysosomes. In addition to the intracellular mechanisms, catabolism may also occur at extravascular sites, such as the mediation of degradation by local proteolytic activity after subcutaneous injection, a process that influences overall bioavailability [28,29]. The route of absorption from these extravascular sites is influenced by molecular size and is partitioned between direct absorption into the blood stream and lymphatic system. Similarly, the mechanisms of elimination of a biopharmaceutical from blood are also dictated by molecular size. For instance, biopharmaceuticals of greater than 70 kDa do not undergo renal glomerular filtration and degradation; instead, the liver plays a predominant role in their catabolism and PK behavior. In contrast, the smaller the biopharmaceutical the more likely the kidney, not the liver, will play a major role in elimination. Those biopharmaceuticals that undergo renal filtration are often readsorbed and/or degraded by various renal structures, including the brush border and tubules. While these disposition mechanisms are similar across species, it is important to understand that the certain aspects will vary across species due to physical differences. For example, upon administration of a biopharmaceutical into a tissue site, the ratio of the volume injected to the total volume of the organ may vary across species and result in different proportions of anatomical structures and cellular populations being exposed. Thus, it is important to understand what mechanisms are expected to influence absorption, distribution, catabolism, and excretion in humans to help elucidate the relevancy of the species with regard to extrapolation of PK endpoints.

Besides the influence of physical anatomical features such as the glomerular filtration, the PK behavior of biopharmaceuticals may be significantly affected by receptor-mediated processes and other uptake processes that outweigh more passive aspects of disposition. An example is the glycosylation patterns of a biopharmaceutical. The terminal glycoforms such as sialic acid and mannose residues play a significant role in regulating catabolism and influence several PK parameters, including systemic exposure, as measured by AUC and half-life. Glycosylation profiles may vary across species, which may result in different product clearance rates due to the disparate rates of uptake by, for example, the asialoglycoprotein or mannose/GlcNAc receptor-mediated pathways [30]. It is therefore important to consider these PK-related mechanisms when selecting a relevant species for preclinical testing.

In contrast to PD, in which the validity of the study for the assessment of safety often depends on specific receptors or antigens, the validity of PK studies are not as highly dependent on the presence of specific receptors or other mechanisms that are clinically homologous. For example, the disposition of tPA is strongly dependent on blood flow patterns to various organs, such as the liver, as well as on the presence of various receptors involved in uptake. It has a molecular weight of 65 kDa and is composed of a serine protease domain at the carboxyl terminal end joined to other domains typical of plasma proteases. Also contained in tPA is a fibronectin-type finger region, a growth factor domain and two kringle domains. About 8% of the total molecular mass consists of glycoforms, which play a significant role in the in vivo disposition. Included in the glycoforms is a high mannose type moiety. tPA circulates as both an unbound moiety and a complex consisting of plasminogen inhibitor (PAI-1) and other protease inhibitors such as plasminogen inhibitors 1 and 2, C1-esterase inhibitor, α2-macroglobulin and α- antiplasmin [31–34]. The PK of tPA have been studied in several different species, including mice, rats, rabbits, dogs, and monkeys [35–40]. A generally applicable and consistent linear PK pattern has emerged from these studies across varies species that is a good approximation of that found clinically. After infusion of tPA, plasma levels decrease in a rapid initial pattern that is characterized by a half-life of 1 to 3 minutes (α-phase). The initial phase is dominant with respect to exposure and includes approximately 70% of the total AUC. A second phase of disposition follows with a half-life of 10 to 40 minutes (β-phase) and finally a third phase with a half-life of 1 to 2 hours (γ-phase). The degree of compartmentalization is dependent on the quantitative ability and reliability of the assay used to measure tPA. The final phase of disposition only accounts for approximately 7% to 10% of the total AUC. Total plasma clearance of tPA closely approximates hepatic plasma flow in all species and ranges from 16 to 23 ml/min/kg; the initial volume of distribution corresponds to plasma volume of 46 to 91 ml/kg. A highly significant correlation was observed between tPA clearance and body weight in animal species and humans, and this provides the basis for predicting human PKs from animal data [41].

In the liver, tPA is taken up in various cellular populations and illustrates the varied nature of the distribution of a biopharmaceutical within an organ. A saturable, receptor-mediated endocytosis of tPA fundamentally occurs followed by lysosomal degradation when tPA is taken up by parenchymal, endothelial, and Kupffer cells in the liver [42]. In the rat, endothelial cells, as compared to parenchymal cells, accounted for a 20-fold higher amount of radioactive activity on a per milligram of protein basis [43,44]. Also Kupffer cells exhibited a 4-fold higher level of uptake, as compared to parenchymal cells. When the cellular mass of cells comprising the liver was considered, endothelial cells accounted for 55%, parenchymal cells 40%, and Kupffer cells 6% of the total uptake of tPA in the liver. The hepatic receptor-mediated uptake by these cells is regulated by two distinct systems. A receptor on endothelial cells that recognizes high-mannose glycoform is responsible for approximately one-half of the total [45]. Additionally a receptor that recognizes protein structure rather than glycoforms seems to be operant and attributes to the remaining disposition of the biopharmaceutical [46–48].

Other pathways exist for the interactions of biopharmaceuticals with receptors on cell surfaces, including receptor binding and shedding of the resulting complex into the circulation and receptor binding that is neither shed nor internalized but stable on the cell surface. Monoclonal antibodies undergo a recycling process via the FcRn receptor [49], as well as nonspecific uptake and the Fcγ receptor's binding. These mechanisms are generally found in various species, but their specificity and relative activity may vary and may need to be considered when selecting an appropriate animal model.

12.3.2 Immunogenicity

A major factor in extrapolating pharmacokinetics across species is the development of antiproduct antibodies, which, if this occurs, may confound interpretation of the PK data. Thus, the clinical relevance of PK and PD information based on preclinical data can only be understood to the extent that the nature, magnitude, and timing within the course of dosing is relative to the development of antiproduct antibodies. Furthermore, characteristics (e.g., precision, accuracy, and specificity) of the assays necessary to quantitate and characterize the antiproduct antibodies and the time of collecting samples in the preclinical study are important. Due to the potential assay interference from the presence of high blood concentrations of the biopharmaceutical, sufficient time must elapse between the last administration of dose and the collection of plasma samples to obtain accurate data. Conversely, with too much time allowed to pass after the last dose of the biopharmaceutic, the immune response may be undetectable. Nevertheless, a comparison of early and late levels at comparable points of time after dosing of the biopharmaceutic may provide a robust signal of immunogenicity. In preclinical studies, immunogenicity will vary among species and additionally among the strains of animals that may be used in safety studies, as the immune response to the biopharmaceutical may differ as the expression of major histocompatibility complexes varies among strains.

Although immunogenicity may arise in the course of exposure of biopharmaceuticals, preclinical PK studies may be successfully conducted by monitoring the development of antiproduct antibodies when this factor is considered in the analysis of the data. For example, preclinical studies conducted using lenercept provided useful PK information for extrapolation to humans [50]. Lenercept is a fusion protein that combines the extracellular domain of two human p55 tumor necrosis factor receptors with the hinge and constant domain C2 and C3 sequences of the human immunoglobulin G1 heavy chain. The biopharmaceutical has a molecular weight of 120 kDa and possesses eight potential sites of glycosylation. Lenercept was investigated for its potential application to various clinical conditions including rheumatoid arthritis. In the manuscript by Richter et al., the pharmacokinetics of lenercept were studied in RoRo rats, Himalayan rabbits, beagle dogs, and cynomolgus monkeys [50]. Several doses of lenercept was administered intravenous by bolus or short infusion; rats were given 0.2 or 5 mg/kg, rabbits 5 mg/kg, monkeys 4.0 or 5.0 mg/kg, and dogs 0.11 and 0.14 mg/kg. Groups sizes were relatively small and ranged from eight to two subjects per species, and blood samples were analyzed for lenercept levels with an ELISA. Neutralizing antibodies to the biopharmaceutical were also measured during the course of the investigation. Various PK endpoints were collected from the different species studied and examined for their fit in an allometric scaling procedure. Sample collection times for PK assessment extended into the period that the development of antiproduct antibodies were observed. The minimal sampling time was 192 hours for rats and a maximum of 437 hours for dogs after injection. A triphasic PK profile was observed, in monkeys, dogs, and rabbits, but not rats, given a dose of 5 mg/kg intravenously. Following an initial, rapid decrease in levels, a second, slower disposition phase occurred, followed by a third phase of rapidly decreasing levels between days 6 to 10. The third phase reflected an immune response directed toward lenercept that showed intra-subject variability. When the effect of antibodies to lenercept in the third phase are subtracted from the data set, the plasma levels were found to be superimposable and linear to dose across species, thus allowing for the allometric scaling of the PK parameters to the clinical situation. In fact, predicted human clearance and the volume of distribution at steady state based on the preclinical data were found to be in agreement with the clinical studies performed [51]. More likely the clearance of lenercept is a result of the uptake mediated by glycosylation and Fc binding and is not reflective of glomerular filtration as the molecular size exceeds 70 kDa.

12.4 CONCLUSION

Biopharmaceuticals represent a broad but discrete class of large molecular weight therapeutic entities that are characterized by their specific pharmacological activities and distinctive pharmacokinetics. The selection of an appropriate animal model is dependent on a combination of PD and PK factors. As described in this chapter, it is essential to understand the relationship of the basic pharmacology of a biopharmaceutical (signaling, receptor presence, binding properties, etc.) and the associated PK properties to that expected in humans, in order to select animal species that will have the most predictive value in safety assessments.

REFERENCES

1. ICH S6: Preclinical Safety Evaluation of Biotechnology-Derived Pharmaceuticals. http://www.fda.gov/cder/guidance/1859fnl.pdf
2. Obach RS, Baxter JG, Liston TE, Silber BM, Jones BC, Macintyre F, Rance DJ, Wastall P. The prediction of human pharmacokinetic parameters from preclinical and in vitro metabolism data. *J Pharmacol Exp Therapeut* 1977;283:46–58.
3. Hengstler JG, Van Der Burg B, Steinberg P, Oesch F. Interspecies differences in cancer susceptibility and toxicity. *Drug Metab Rev* 1999;31:917–70.
4. Morton DM. Importance of species selection in drug toxicity testing. *Toxicol Letts* 1998;102–3, 545–50.
5. McKenzie R, Freed MW, Sallie R, Conjeevaram H, Bisceglie AM, Yoon P, Savarese B, Kleiner D, Tsokos M, Luciano C, Pruett T, Stotka J, Straus SE, Hoofnagle JH. Hepatic failure and lactic acidosis due to Fialuridine (FIAU), an investigational nucleoside analogue for chronic hepatitis B. *N Eng J Med* 1995;333:1099–105.
6. Tennant BC, Baldwin BH, Graham LA, Ascenzi MA, Hornbuckle WE, Rowland PH, Tochkov IA, Yeager AE, Erb HN, Colacino JM, Lopez C, Engelhardt JA, Bowsher RR, Richardson FC, Lewis W, Cote PJ, Korba BE, Gerin JL. Antiviral activity and toxicity of fialuridine in the woodchuck model of hepatitis B virus infection. *Hepatology* 1998;28:179–91.
7. Expert Scientific Group on Phase One Clinical Studies. Final Report. The Stationery Office. Her Majesty's Stationery Office, St. Clements House, 2–16 Colegate, Norwich NR3 1BQ.
8. Keller P, Smalling R. Granulocyte colony stimulating factor: animal studies for risk assessment. *Int Rev Exp Pathol* 1993;34(pt A):173–88.

9. Robison RL, Myers LA. Preclinical safety assessment of recombinant human GM-CSF in rhesus monkeys. *Int Rev Exp Pathol* 1993;34A:149, 172.

10. Anderson TD, Hayes TJ. Toxicity of human recombinant interleukin-2 in rats. *Lab Invest* 1989;60:331–46.

11. Anderson TD, Hayes TJ, Gately MK, Bontempo JM, Stern LL, Truit GA. Toxicity of human recombinant interleukin-2 in the mouse is mediated by interleukin-activated lymphocytes: separation of efficacy and toxicity by selective lymphocyte subset depletion. *Lab Invest* 1988;59:598–612.

12. Gately MK, Anderson TD, Hayes TJ. Roles of asialo GM1-positive lymphoid cells in mediating the toxic effects of recombinant interleukin-2 in mice. *J Immunol* 1988;141:189–200.

13. Rosenstein M, Ettinghausen SE, Rosenberg SA. Extravasation of intravascular fluid mediated by the systemic administration of recombinant interleukin-2. *J Immunol* 1986;137:1735–42.

14. Hart TK, Blackburn MN, Brigham-Burke M, Dede K, Al-Mahdi P, Zia-Amirhoseine P, Cook RM. Preclinical efficacy and safety of pascolizumab (SB 240683): a humanized anti-interleukin-4 antibody with therapeutic potential in asthma. *Clin Exp Immunol* 2002;130:93–100.

15. Terrell TG, Green JD. Comparative pathology of recombinant murine interferon-γ in mice and recombinant human interferon-γ in cynomolgus monkeys. *Exp Pathol* 1993;34B: 73, 101.

16. Clarke J, Leach W, Pippig S, Joshi A, Wu BM, House R, Beyer J. Evaluation of a Surrogate Antibody for Preclinical Safety Testing of an AntiCD11a mAb. *Regul Toxicol Pharmacol* 2004;40:219–26.

17. Wu B, Joshi A, Ren S, Ng C. The application of mechanism-based PK/PD modeling in pharmacodynamic-based dose selection of muM17: a surrogate monoclonal antibody for Efalizumab. *J Pharmaceut Sci* 2006;95:1258–68.

18. Dempster AM. Pharmacological testing of recombinant human erythropoietin: implications for other biotechnology products. *Drug Dev Res* 1995;35:173–8.

19. Muntzel M, Hannedouche T, Lacour B, Drueke TB. Effect of erythropoietin on hematocrit and blood pressure in normotensive and hypertensive rats. *J Am Soc Nephrol* 1992;3:182–7.

20. Tsukade H, Ishimitsu T, Ogawa Y, Sugimoto T, Yagi S. Direct vassopressor effects of erythropoietin in genetically hypertensive rats. *Life Sci* 1992;52:1425–34.

21. Humira. Scientific Discussion. European Public Assessment Report. European Medicines Agency. http://www.emea.europa.eu/humandocs/Humans/EPAR/humira/humira.htm

22. MabCampath. Scientific Discussion. European Public Assessment Report. European Medicines Agency. http://www.emea.europa.eu/humandocs/Humans/EPAR/mabcampath/mabcampath.htm

23. Rao BM, Driver I, Lauffenburger DA, Wittrup KD. Interleukin 2 (IL-2) variants engineered for increased IL-2 receptor alpha-subunit affinity exhibit increased potency arising from a cell surface ligand reservoir effect. *Mol Pharmacol* 2004;66:864–9.

24. Rao BM, Girvin AT, Ciardelli T, Lauffenburger DA, Wittrup KD. Interleukin-2 mutants with enhanced alpha-receptor subunit binding affinity. *Protein Eng* 2003; 16:1081–7.

25. Kingbeil C, Hsu DH. Pharmacology and safety assessment of humanized monoclonal antibodies for therapeutic use. *Toxicol Pathol* 1999;27:1–3.

26. Mordenti J, Chen S, Moore J, Ferraiolo B. Interspecies scaling of clearance data for five recombinant proteins. *Pharmaceut Res* 1991;8:1351–9.

27. Mordenti J, Green JD. The role of PKs and PDs in the development of therapeutic proteins. In Rescigno A, Thakur A (eds), *New Trends in Pharmacokinetics*. New York: Plenum Press, 1991, pp 411, 424.

28. Supersaxo A, Hein WR, Steffen H. Effect of molecular weight on the lymphatic absorption of water-soluble compounds following subcutaneous administration. *Pharmaceut Res* 1990;7:167–9.

29. Supersaxo A, Hein WR, Gallanti H, Steffen H. Recombinant human interferon alpha-2a: delivery to lymphoid tissue by selected modes of application. *Pharmaceut Res* 1988;5:472–6.

30. Park EI, Yiling M, Unverzagt C, Gabius H-J, Baenziger JU. The asialoglycoprotein receptor clears glycoconjugates terminating with sialic acida2,6GalNAc. *Proc Nal Acad Sci USA* 2005;102:17125–9.

31. Higgins DL, Bennett WF. Tissue plasminogen activator: the biochemistry and pharmacology of variants produced by mutagenesis. *Ann Rev Pharmacol Toxicol* 1990; 30:91–121.

32. Lucore CL, Sobel BE. Interactions of tissue-type plasminogen activator with plasma inhibitors and their pharmacologic implications. *Circulation* 1988; 77:660–9.

33. Sprengers ED, Kluft C. Plasminogen activator inhibitors. *Blood* 1987;69:381–7.

34. Haggroth L, Mattsson C, Friberg J. Inhibition of the human tissue plasminogen activator in plasma from different species. *Thromb Res* 1984;33:583–94.

35. Tanswell P, Heinzel G, Greischel A, Krause J. Nonlinear pharmacokinetics of tissue-type plasminogen activator in three animal species and isolated perfused rat liver. *J Pharmacol Exp Ther* 1990;255:318–24.

36. Mohler MA, Refino CJ, Chen SA, Chen AB, Hotchkiss AJ. D-phe-pro-arg-chloromethylketone: its potential use in inhibiting the formation of in vitro artifacts in blood collected during tissue-type plasminogen activator thrombolytic therapy. *Thromb Hemostasis* 1986;56:160–4.

37. Krause J, Seydel W, Heinzel G, Tanswell P. Different receptors mediate the hepatic catabolism of tissue-type plasminogen activator and urokinase. *Biochem J* 1990; 267:647–52.

38. Fuchs HE, Berger HB, Pizzo SV. Catabolism of human tissue plasminogen activator in mice. *Blood* 1985;65:539–44.

39. Fong KL, Crysler CS, Mico BA, Boyle KE, Kopia GA, Kopaciewicz L, Lynn RE. Dose-dependent pharmacokinetics of recombinant tissue-type plasminogen activator in anesthetized dogs following intravenous infusion. *Drug Metab Dis* 1988; 16:201–6.

40. Korninger C, Stassen JM, Collen D. Turnover of human extrinsic (tissue-type) plasminogen activator in rabbits. *Thromb Haemostasis* 1981;46:658–61.

41. Mordenti J. Man versus beast: pharmacokinetic scaling in mammals. *J Pharmaceut Sci* 1986;75:1028–40.

42. Rijken DC, Otter M, Kuiper J, van Berkel TJ. Receptor-mediated endocytosis of tissue-type plasminogen activator (t-pa) by liver cells. *Thromb Res Suppl* 1990;10:63–71.

43. Smedsrod B, Einarsson M, Peroft H. Tissue plasminogen activator is endocytosed by mannose and galactose receptors of rat liver cells. *Thromb Haemostasis* 1988; 59:480–4.

44. Kuiper J, Otter M, Rijken DC, van Berkel TJ. Characterization of the interaction in vivo of tissue-type plasminogen activator with liver cells. *J Biol Chem* 1988; 263:18220–4.

45. Smedsrod B, Malmgren M, Ericsson J, Laurent TC. Morphological studies on endocytosis of chondroitin sulphate proteoglycan by rat liver endothelial cells. *Cell Tiss Res* 1988;253:39–45.

46. Hotchkiss A, Refino CJ, Leonard CK, O'Connor JV, Crowley C, McCabe J, Tate K, Nakamura G, Powers D, Levinson A. The influence of carbohydrate structure on the clearance of recombinant tissue-type plasminogen activator. *Thromb Haemostasis* 1988;60:255–61.

47. Bakhit C, Lewis D, Billings R, Malfroy B. Cellular catabolism of recombinant tissue-type plasminogen activator: identification and characterization of a novel high affinity uptake system on rat hepatocytes. *J Biol Chem* 1987;262:8716–20.

48. Krause J, Seydel W, Heinzel G, Tanswell P. Different receptors mediate the hepatic catabolism of tissue-type plasminogen activator and urokinase. *Biochem J* 1990; 267:647–52.

49. Datta-Mannan A, Witcher DR, Tnag Y, Watkins J, Wroblewski VJ. Monoclonal antibody clearance. Impact of modulating the interaction of IgG with the neonatal Fc receptor. *J Biol Chem* 2007;282(3):1709–17. http://www.jbc.org/cgi/doi/10.10741/jbc.M607161200

50. Richter WF, Gallati H, Schiller CD. Animal pharmacokinetics of the tumor necrosis factor receptor-immunoglobulin fusion protein lenercept and their extrapolation to humans. *Drug Meta Disp* 1999;27(1):21–5.

51. Kneer J, Dumont E, Birnbock H, Kusano T, Gallati H, Lesslauer W. A new TNF-neutralizing agent—lenercept—(TNFR55-IgG1, Ro 45–2081): pharmacokinetic/dynamic data over a 100-fold dose-range in healthy volunteers, and rheumatoid arthritis patients. *Rheumatol Eur* 1996;25 (Suppl 1) 52.

CHAPTER 13

Use of Animal Models of Disease in the Preclinical Safety Evaluation of Biopharmaceuticals

JOHAN TE KOPPELE, PhD, and RENGER WITKAMP, PhD

Contents

13.1 INTRODUCTION

The objective of the ICH S6 guidance for Preclinical Safety Evaluation of Biotechnology Derived Pharmaceuticals (biopharmaceuticals) [1] is a preclinical safety evaluation program that is based on relevant (animal) models. ICH S6 requires safety testing in a species in which the biopharmaceutical is pharmacologically active. In the absence of a relevant species, the use of transgenic animals expressing the human receptor or the use of homologous proteins should be considered. Animal models for human diseases may also be used. Although these models are mostly used to evaluate pharmacological

Preclinical Safety Evaluation of Biopharmaceuticals: A Science-Based Approach to Facilitating Clinical Trials, edited by Joy A. Cavagnaro

features of the product, they may be of value in evaluating the safety of biopharmaceuticals:

- To improve prediction of the toxicity or therapeutic index.
- To support the mechanistic interpretation of safety studies (as an alternative or a complement to toxicity studies in normal animals).
- To evaluate the undesirable disease progression.
- To predict a different kinetic behavior of the compound in healthy and diseased animals.

The FDA Critical Path Opportunities Report [2] recognizes that there is a need for "better animal disease or tissue injury models that could provide more accurate predictions of the toxicity of drugs, devices, and biological products that are used in ill or injured patients. Use of such models could also enhance our understanding of the potential toxic effects of compounds associated with many types of medical devices." It is important to note that the regulatory authorities will always require solid scientific justification for the use of these animal models for disease to support safety.

13.2   ANIMAL MODELS FOR DISEASE

Disease models include spontaneous models, induced models (e.g., treated with a compound, a microorganism or surgically), gene knockout(s), and transgenic animals (Table 13.1). Most such models are based on the effect of a certain stimulus that induces a pathological condition. Examples include the streptozotocin-mediated destruction of beta cells leading to type 1 diabetes [3], surgical dissection of the cruciate ligament resulting in osteoarthritis [4], or type II collagen-specific activation of the immune system, leading to arthritis [5]. A "stimulus leading to pathology" is essentially present in the spontaneous models. "Spontaneous pathologies" are often the result of the anatomical and/or metabolic makeup of a genetically distinct animal strain. For instance, aberrant hip architecture results in hip osteoarthritis in the German Shepherd dog [6]. Selective breeding resulted in the obese Zucker rat (fa/fa) [7,8]. This strain is considered a spontaneous model for obesity and type 2 diabetes because of its hyperglycemia, hyperinsulinemia, insulin-resistance, hypertriglyceridemia, and hypercholesterolemia. Alternatively, elimination of a gene may result in a loss of homeostasis, leading to disease. A particularly well-known general example is the loss of p53 tumor suppressor gene function in the majority of human cancers. In mice, the elimination of Apo lipoprotein E or low-density lipoprotein receptor (ApoE knockout and LDL receptor knockout) results in hyperlipidemic hypercholesterolemia and atherosclerosis [9,10,11].

Anti-sense oligonucleotides and, more recently, siRNA present exciting opportunities to eliminate specific genes or gene transcripts. There is widespread appreciation of siRNA not only for target validation and as a potential

TABLE 13.1 Categories of animal models for disease, illustrated with some examples

Category	Example	Reference
Spontaneous models	Spontaneous osteoarthritis: Dunkin Hartley	[36]
Mostly resulting from	guinea pigs, Shepherd dog	[6]
genetic, metabolic,	Diabetes/obesitas: zucker rat	[7,8]
developmental, or	Diabetes model in the cat	[37]
anatomical features		
of specific species		
and/or animal strains		
Induced models:	Porcine wound healing models	[38]
Surgically	Stenosis in the pig	[39]
	Osteoarthritis: Cruciate ligament transection in dogs	[4]
	Occlusion (e.g., to induce renal failure)	[33]
	Fractures (various species)	[40]
Induced models:	Chemically induced tumors: Mammary tumors, DMBA-rat model	[41]
Chemically	Urinary bladder tumors (N-butyl-N-(4-hydroxybutyl)nitrosamine-induced rat model)	[42]
	Diabetes: Streptozotocin, alloxan	[3]
	Chemically induced liver failure	[34]
	Parkinson's disease models (MPTP)	[43]
Induced models:	Arthritis: Collagen-induced arthritis	[5]
Immunological	Experimental autoimmune	[44]
	Encephalomyelitis (preclinical model for multiple sclerosis)	
	Inflammatory bowel disease/Crohn's disease	[45]
	Adoptive transfer of antibodies to the self-antigen, or immune cells to naive animals	[46,47]
Infection models	*Listeria monocytogenes* in mice	[29]
(bacterial, viral,	Pneumococcal infection model	[48]
fungal, protozoan,	HIV-infection models	[49]
parasitic, etc.)	Fungal infection models	[50]
Xenograft models	Tumor xenografts, various models	[51,52]
	Psoriasis xenografts on nude mice	[15]
Transgenic models:	Hyperlipidemia/hypercholesterolemia: ApoE knockout, LDL receptor knockout, ApoE-variant transgenes	[9,10]
Knockout, and		
knock-in	Diabetes/obesitas: Ob/ob mouse, db/db mouse	[7,53]

novel therapeutic approach but also as a tool for disease models, combining time- and tissue-controlled knockout with high transcript specificity.

There has been explosive growth in the number of disease models in recent decades, especially in the field of the knockouts and transgenic rodents. A description of the most frequently used models alone would take a separate volume, and even that would be outdated within no time. Information on the selection of models and background data can easily be found on the Internet. The US National Center for Research Resources (NCRR) provides overviews and links [12]. In addition the main providers of laboratory animals have very useful information on their Web sites. Readers looking for overviews on animal models per disease may find useful information in the *Drug Discovery Today: Disease Models* review journal (http://www.drugdiscoverytoday.com).

In our opinion there are a few important general considerations regarding the use of animal models for disease in this respect:

- A transgenic mouse is not automatically a model for disease. Most diseases are multifactorial. Aberrations and pathological imbalances are not limited to one mechanism, especially in the advanced stages of disease when more mechanisms are offset. In view of the complexity of biological systems it is increasingly recognized that the balanced modulation of multiple targets provides a better therapeutic effect, and a more favorable side-effect profile than the modulation of a single target.
- A disease model should be properly characterized by its phenotype, and enough background data should be available. This also applies for the more than 100,000 knockout mice that will become available over the next few years from large governmental programs (Canada, China, European Union, United States). In addition sufficient historical or reference data on the effects of chemical and biological compounds should be available.
- The model should ideally be available for comparison and be accessible to more than one party. For commercial models, options for noncommercial institutions to perform fundamental or mechanistic studies are recommended.

13.3 HUMANIZED MODELS FOR TRANSLATIONAL RESEARCH

Novel approaches for the design and development of in vivo models to predict drug safety in patients will become more and more relevant. In order to optimize prediction for the human situation, the models should be clearly defined, controllable, and as "humanized" as possible, for instance, using strategies based on novel technologies like siRNA-mediated gene knock-down and on systems enabling the tight and reliable control of human (trans) gene expression in a time- and tissue-specific manner. The so-called translational research to predict human safety (and efficacy) requires continual information exchange

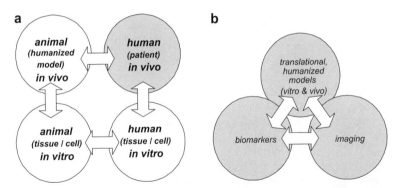

Figure 13.1 (*a*) Translational research strategies to predict human safety and efficacy based on in vitro studies (in animal and human cells) and animal studies. (*b*) Use of biomarkers and imaging techniques to increase the predictability of drug R&D.

between in vitro studies (animal and human cells) and animal studies (Figure 13.1*a*). New approaches for the design and development of safety assessment using human in vitro systems are becoming increasingly important for both biopharmaceutials and pharmaceuticals. Such tests are likely to comprise human stem-cell cultures, or co-cultures, combined with animal disease models. In addition to humanized translational test models, biomarkers and imaging are key to enhancing the predictability of drug research and development (Figure 13.1*b*). Ideally biomarkers are identical in animals and humans and measurable in vivo and in vitro.

In general, humanized models that aim for improved predictability for the human situation require the insertion of human features in animal-derived test models. Basically, this can be achieved at the gene, cell or even tissue level (Table 13.2). Insertion of human genes within in vitro test systems is relatively simple with the technology presently at hand. In vivo gene transfer is more complicated. Nowadays transgenic disease animals are considered essential to predict drug efficacy in humans. The ideal transgenic animals are those in which multiple genes can be overexpressed (or silenced) one by one, controllable per tissue/organ, and more important, controllable over time (on/off). This way local manipulation of human gene expression can be useful; overexpression can be achieved with locally administered or delivered vectors, and siRNA technology is full of promise as a suppressor of gene activity.

Human cells, tissues, or organs implanted or transplanted in animals present a relatively strong and valuable tool, provided that immune rejection of the human material can be avoided. Immune-deficient animals like mice may well be used to develop organ-like structures (teratomas) from transplanted stem cells [13] or with combinations of human cells or human tissue (e.g., synoviocytes and cartilage [14], and activated mononuclear cells and transplanted skin [15]).

TABLE 13.2 Types and examples of translational, humanized test models

		Example	Reference
	Transfer of human gene		
In vitro	Cell transfection		
In vivo local	Local delivery gene delivery by electroporation or a locally administered vector	Interleukin-10 knockout and overexpression on neointima formation in hypercholesterolemic (ApoE*3-Leiden) mice	[54]
In vivo systemic	Knock-in transgenic animal, preferably with time- and tissue-specific control of gene expression	hCETP combined with hApoE*3-Leiden	[10]
	Transfer of human cell/humanized cell		
In vitro	Cocultures of human and animal cells	Synovial fibroblast and articular cartilage	[14]
In vivo	Stem cell	Cancer growth in a human tissue microenvironment	[13]
	Immune competent cells	SCID mice transplanted with articular cartilage and synoviocytes	[14]
	Transfer of human tissue		
In vivo	Tissue engineering Tissue/organ tranplantation	Transplantation of tissue on immune-deficient mice: (e.g., [normal] skin from psoriasis patient in combination with administration of activated immune cells)	[15]

CASE EXAMPLE: TRANSGENIC HUMANIZED MOUSE MODELS FOR HYPERLIPIDEMIA

Cardiovascular disease models demonstrate aspects/features of humanized disease models. For hyperlipidemia-based atherosclerosis, there is a lack of a spontaneous in vivo mouse model because mice are resistant to (diet-induced) hyperlipidemia. Therefore a number of transgenic mice have been developed to better understand the pathogenesis in humans and obtain mouse models predictive of the human disease. Overexpression of ApoB, ApoE-variants, and knockout of ApoE, the LDL receptor or LPL (lipoprotein lipase), have enabled hyperlipidemic transgenic mice models to be developed. The spontaneous hypercholesterolemic ApoE knockout and the LDL receptor knockout are widely used as atherosclerosis models [9].

Given the multifactorial origin of atherosclerosis, combinations of knock-in and knockout transgenics have been produced. For instance, combining the ApoE*3Leiden transgenic, having a diet-controllable cholesterol profile, with the human CETP gene (cholesterol ester transfer protein) resulted in a transgenic model with human-like LDL as well as HDL profiles that are responsive to treatment with statins and fibrates (as in the human situation). [10] Figure 13.2

The humanized mouse model is used for safety assessment of drugs that affect lipid profiles as a side effect (and thereby possibly influence the risk of atherosclerosis and, subsequently, myocardial infarction). A typical example is the disturbed lipid profile and increased risk of myocardial infarction experienced by AIDS patients following the long-term use of HIV-1-protease inhibitors [16,17].

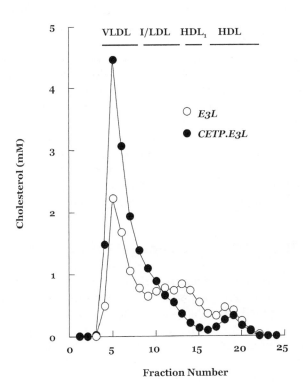

Figure 13.2 Effect of inserting a human CETP gene on cholesterol lipoproteins in E3L mice fed a Western-type diet containing 0.25% cholesterol. The E3L.hCETP mouse has shown to respond to statins, fibrates, and the new CETP inhibitor torcetrapib in a similar way as humans do, as manifested by decreased apoB-containing lipoproteins and increased HDL levels.

13.4   FROM PHARMACOLOGY TO TOXICOLOGY—WHAT IS PREDICTABLE?

"Exaggerated pharmacology" often poses an important biopharmaceutical safety issue. Most adverse effects of biopharmaceuticals are a direct consequence of their primary pharmacological action. Off-target effects, apart from hypersensitivity developing during repeated dosing, are rare. For many biopharmaceuticals the immune system is the intended target of the therapy, and the immunotoxicity observed is often exaggerated pharmacology. Biopharmaceuticals that are highly selective in their molecular target are likely to exert mechanism-based side effects if the target is expressed in/on other nontarget cell types. However, although biopharmaceuticals are generally very selective for their primary target, their effects can sometimes be highly pleiotropic. A recent well-known example is calamity with TGN1412, which produced a sudden and rapid release of pro-inflammatory cytokines in healthy volunteers, with severe consequences [18]. Therefore the safety assessment of a biopharmaceutical is critically dependent on an in-depth understanding of the pharmacology and physiology in order to anticipate the risks associated with the potentially intense effects on the target system and interaction with other biological systems. Another important difference between biopharmaceuticals and low molecular weight compounds is the dose–response relationship. Biopharmaceutical products may exhibit unusual dose–response curves that are nonlinear (saturation of target receptors at low dose), bell-shaped, and very steep with an apparent "on/off switch" [19,20]. Taken together, this supports the idea of combining pharmacology and safety studies in the case of biopharmaceuticals. If needed, exaggerated pharmacological effects can also be studied using the animal homologues of the human target. However, as also stated in the S6 guidance [1], the production process, range of impurities/contaminants, pharmacokinetics, and exact pharmacological mechanism(s) may differ between the homologous form and the product intended for clinical use.

13.5   WHY TEST SAFETY IN DISEASE MODELS?

It is well known that the response to a drug can differ between diseased and nondiseased individuals. For example, the expression of both pro- and anti-inflammatory mediators changes in many diseases and conditions such as rheumatic diseases, myocardial infarction, angina, aging, and obesity [21]. This may have an impact on toxicity and pharmacokinetics, and in particular, when the drug interacts with these mediators. In addition the pharmacokinetics of a drug can be affected by disease in general, a topic that is discussed later in this chapter.

Certain classes of drugs exhibit side effects that are characteristic of their group of compounds. In some cases, side effects are inherent to the pharmacological effect (exaggerated pharmacology, mechanism-based side effect). In other cases, side effects can differ among drugs belonging to a particular therapeutic class. For example, both infliximab (anti-TNFα monoclonal antibody) and etanercept (TNFα receptor p75Fc fusion protein) share an increased likelihood of opportunistic infections. However, there are indications that tuberculosis and some other granulomatous infections occur more frequently among patients treated with infliximab than among those treated with etanercept [22].

Based on specific disease knowledge, optimization of drug selection involves their common side effect (e.g., dyslipidemia, lipodystrophy of HIV protease inhibitors, [17]). In our laboratory we frequently use transgenic mice carrying the human apolipoprotein E3-Leiden variant gene ([11], see also the case example). These mice exhibit hyperlipoproteinemia and human-like lipoprotein profiles and develop atherosclerosis with all the characteristics of human pathology. In addition to investigating the effects of lipid-lowering drugs or diets, we are increasingly seeing requests to study indirect or side effects. Published examples are the side effect of dexamethasone as an inhibitor of venous graft thickening [23] and the impairment of plasma lipid profiles by Ritonavir [17]. In addition the model has proved its value for investigating the diabetogenic properties of certain drugs.

Despite the obvious demand for animal disease models in evaluating the safety of drugs [1,2], it is difficult to find examples for recently approved biopharmaceuticals or compounds under development. In the European Public Assessment Reports (EPARs) [24] very few registrations describe the use of animal disease models specifically for evaluating the safety of biopharmaceuticals. One illustrative example from the EPAR database is bevacizumab. It is a monoclonal antibody that binds to the human vascular endothelial growth factor (VEGF) to reduce the vascularization of tumors, thereby inhibiting tumor growth. Inasmuch as (VEGF-mediated) vascularization is essential to healing wounds, the concern was raised that the anti-VEGF activity of bevacizumab might delay the wound healing process in tumor patients undergoing biopsy procedures or surgery. A linear incision model (to mimic surgical incision) and a circular wound model (to mimic an ulcerative lesion) were used in rabbits to demonstrate that bevacizumab causes a reversible, dose-related delay in wound healing. Another group of growth factor therapeutics EGFR (epidermal growth factor receptor) inhibitors is used to treat colorectal and non–small-cell lung cancer. On limited occasions unique and dramatic dermatological side effects (skin rash) occurred because of the inhibition of EGFR-signaling pathways in the skin [25]. These two examples illustrate the mechanism-based side effects of the growth modulation factor or their receptors.

With the broadening of the therapeutic applications of biopharmaceuticals, new safety issues can be anticipated in the future. Since the late nineties, rituximab (anti-CD20 monoclonal antibody) has been used to treat non–Hodgkin's lymphoma. Recently studies on rituximab for the treatment of autoimmune diseases (renal disease and transplantation) have been initiated [26]. Yet another example are the studies performed with recombinant factor VIIa in animal models for trauma to show that rFVIIa was not associated with the systemic activation of coagulation or the microthrombosis of end organs [27].

13.6   DISEASE MODELS TO EVALUATE UNDESIRABLE DISEASE PROGRESSION

Immunosuppression is regarded as a potentially serious adverse effect of certain classes of biopharmaceuticals and may result in increased infection rates [22,28] or increased rates in primary or secondary malignancies. The ability to target and neutralize macrophage-derived inflammatory cytokines and pathways has proved to be one of the most important advances in the treatment of rheumatoid arthritis, Crohn's disease, and several other systemic inflammatory diseases. However, data that have emerged following the approval of infliximab, etanercept, and adalimumab show an increased likelihood of opportunistic infections caused by intracellular organisms including tuberculosis (*Mycobacterium tuberculosis*), *Listeria monocytogenes, Mycobacterium avium intracellulare*, and some fungal species [22]. There are indications that tuberculosis and some other granulomatous infections are likely to occur more frequently among patients treated with infliximab (monoclonal antibodies) than among those treated with etanercept (soluble TNF receptors) [22]. Animal models of tuberculosis have demonstrated the importance of TNFα in controlling and containing intracellular pathogens. An attractive mouse model to study the effects on host resistance to intracellular bacteria and potential differences between compounds is the *L. monocytogenes* model in mice [29]. In our laboratory this model has proved its value in studying the side effects of anti-TNF compounds as manifest by a difference in the *L. monocytogenes* clearance from the spleen. In addition to infections, an increase of malignancies is regarded as a potential side effect of biopharmaceuticals that interact with cytokine functioning. There is indeed some evidence of a dose-dependent increased risk of malignancies, in particular non–Hodgkin's lymphoma, in patients with rheumatoid arthritis treated with anti-TNF antibody therapy [30]. Associations with solid tumors seem to be less clear. Published reports on the effect of biopharmaceuticals on the relative tumor incidence in animal models could not be found. This is probably due to slow development of tumors and the development of antibodies in animals during treatment. In case of etanercept, mice and rats developed neutralizing antibodies within two to three weeks following initiation of twice-weekly administration. Therefore the CHMP (EMEA) concluded that there are probably no meaningful animal studies that can further evaluate the theoretical risk of increased malignancies resulting from chronic TNF inactivation. Instead, the company will conduct long-term surveillance for tumors in humans [24].

13.7   DISEASE MODELS TO EVALUATE ABNORMAL KINETIC BEHAVIOR OF THE COMPOUND

There are many examples of the abnormal kinetic behavior of drugs during disease. Obviously these effects are dependent on the nature of the compound and the pathophysiological condition. For example, generalized inflammation affects many physiological processes, including organ and peripheral blood flow, protein binding, and enzyme activity. Most data published so far are for low molecular compounds where the main focus has been on biotransformation and drug transporters, which is generally not relevant for biopharmaceuticals. During inflammation the expression of both pro- and anti-inflammatory mediators are changed. This can have pharmacokinetic consequences. Clearance of highly bound and efficiently eliminated drugs may be reduced in the presence of inflammation, resulting in increased circulating drug concentrations [21].

Sepsis, septic shock, and other critical conditions can have profound effects on the kinetics of compounds [31,32]. Drug absorption following intramuscular, subcutaneous, transdermal, and oral administration may decline due to a reduced perfusion of muscles, skin, and splanchnic organs. Compromised tissue perfusion may also affect drug distribution, resulting in a reduced distribution volume. On the other hand, the increase in capillary permeability and interstitial edema during sepsis and septic shock may enhance drug distribution. Changes in plasma protein binding, body water, tissue mass, and pH may also affect drug distribution. The kidneys are an important excretion pathway for many drugs. Renal failure, which often accompanies sepsis and septic shock, will result in the accumulation of both the parent drug and its metabolites. Studies with animal models for renal failure [33], hepatic failure [34], or sepsis may be indicated especially for those compounds that are intended for use in critically ill patients and/or those in intensive care settings.

Other diseases and conditions that can have an effect on the kinetics include cardiac failure, diabetes, and (severe) obesity [35]. Dermal disease and lesions can affect the absorption (unintended) of a compound through the skin. Therefore it may be useful to at least include safety endpoints when testing drugs for psoriasis and dermatitis in animal models.

13.8   IMMUNOGENICITY ISSUES

The immunogenicity issue is discussed in detail elsewhere in this book (see Chapter 20). However, in relation to the topics addressed above, the following issues are of specific interest here:

- It is important to know whether the pharmacokinetic behavior of the compound is affected by an immune response.
- The disease severity or progression should not be directly related to immunogenic properties of the compound in the test species. Immunogenicity may cause an effect similar to that observed with adjuvants. In preclinical animals models for rheumatoid arthritis, multiple sclerosis, and inflammatory bowel disease, activation of the immune system with adjuvant is applied to evoke an autoimmune response (e.g., against type II collagen in collagen-induced arthritis, or against myelin-peptides in experimental autoimmune encephalomyelitis as a model for multiple sclerosis).
- Vice versa, the disease may affect the immunogenicity of biopharmaceuticals. For instance, the activated immune system in diseases like rheumatoid arthritis, multiple sclerosis, and inflammatory bowel disease is likely to produce a faster and/or stronger response to biopharmaceuticals. Inasmuch as this applies to patients, the same issue may have relevance for safety testing; that is, application of a relevant inflammatory disease model may give greater insight and better predictability than healthy animals do.

13.9 CONCLUDING REMARKS

The application of animal disease models fits in well with the rational, science-based, case-by-case approach for preclinical safety evaluation of biopharmaceuticals [20]. Drug-related (class effects), disease-related, and therapeutic mechanism-based toxicity require the integration of safety and efficacy research, including kinetics and (if relevant) metabolism. The use of animal models of disease to assess in vivo activity together with safety is expected to provide a better understanding of the therapeutic index, and therefore improved clinical-dose selection. This is especially relevant for biopharmaceuticals inasmuch as their side effects often involve exaggerated pharmacology. Compared to new chemical entities, safety evaluation and pharmacology are less distinct from each other in the case of biopharmaceuticals. So far there are a limited number of examples of approved biopharmaceuticals that have been assessed for safety in animal models of disease. However, we expect a rapid increase in these figures when suitable models become available in greater numbers. It appears that many developers are including animal models of disease, if available, in current programs to answer specific questions.

Continued development and better application of humanized in vitro models (stem cells, cell lines, or ex vivo tissue, including transgenesis) and in vivo models (transgenesis and transplantation) that closely mimic the human situation should ultimately improve the predictive value of preclinical studies to human safety.

REFERENCES

1. ICH S6 Guidance. http://www.ich.org/
2. FDA Critical Path Opportunities Report. http://www.fda.gov/oc/initiatives/critical-path/reports/opp_report.pdf
3. Rees DA, Alcolado JC. Animal models of diabetes mellitus. *Diab Med* 2005;22: 359–70.
4. Brandt KD. Transection of the anterior cruciate ligament in the dog: a model of osteoarthritis. *Sem Arthritis Rheum* 1991;21:22–32.
5. Van den Berg WB. Lessons from animal models of arthritis. *Cur Rheum Rep* 2002;4:232–9.
6. Smith GK, Mayhew PD, Kapatkin AS, McKelvie PJ, Shofer FS, Gregor TP. Evaluation of risk factors for degenerative joint disease associated with hip dysplasia in German Shepherd Dogs, Golden Retrievers, Labrador Retrievers, and Rottweilers. *J Am Vet Med Assoc* 2001;219:1719–24.
7. Chen D, Wang MW. Development and application of rodent models for type 2 diabetes. *Diab Obes Metab* 2005;7:307–17.
8. Mathe D. Dyslipidemia and diabetes: animal models. *Diab Metab* 1995;2:106–11.
9. Huang Y. Transgenic and gene-targeted mice in the study of hyperlipidemia. In Xu Q, ed. *A Handbook of Mouse Models of Cardiovascular Disease*. New York: Wiley, 2006;33–41.
10. Westerterp M, van der Hoogt CC, de Haan W, Offerman EH, Dallinga-Thie GM, Jukema JW, Havekes LM, Rensen PC. Cholesteryl ester transfer protein decreases high-density lipoprotein and severely aggravates atherosclerosis in APOE*3-Leiden mice. *Arterioscl Thromb Vas Biol* 2006;26:2552–9.
11. van den Maagdenberg AM, Hofker MH, Krimpenfort PJ, De Bruijn I, Van Vlijmen B, Van der Boom H, Havekes LM, Frants RR. Transgenic mice carrying the apolipoprotein E3-Leiden gene exhibit hyperlipoproteinemia. *J Biol Chem* 1993; 268:10540–5.
12. National Center for Research Resources (NCRR). http://www.ncrr.nih.gov/comparative_med.asp
13. Tzukerman M, Skorecki KL. A novel experimental platform for investigating cancer growth and anti-cancer therapy in a human tissue microenvironment derived from human embryonic stem cells. *Meth Mol Biol* 2006;331:329–46.
14. Muller-Ladner U, Gay S. The SCID mouse—a novel experimental model for gene therapy in human rheumatoid arthritis. *Drugs Today (Barcelona)* 1999;35:379–88.
15. Caspary F, Elliott G, Nave BT, Verzaal P, Rohrbach M, Das PK, Nagelkerken L, Nieland JD. A new therapeutic approach to treat psoriasis by inhibition of fatty acid oxidation by Etomoxir. *Brit J Dermatol* 2005;153:937–44.
16. Carr A, Samaras K, Chisholm DJ, Cooper DA. Pathogenesis of HIV-1-protease inhibitor-associated peripheral lipodystrophy, hyperlipidaemia, and insulin resistance. *Lancet* 1998;351:1881–3.
17. den Boer MA, Berbee JF, Reiss P, van der Valk M, Voshol PJ, Kuipers F, Havekes LM, Rensen PC, Romijn JA. Ritonavir impairs lipoprotein lipase-mediated lipolysis and decreases uptake of fatty acids in adipose tissue. *Arterioscl Thromb Vas Biol* 2006;26:124–9.

18. Suntharalingam G, Perry MR, Ward S, Brett SJ, Castello-Cortes A, Brunner MD, Panoskaltsis N. Cytokine storm in a phase 1 trial of the anti-CD28 monoclonal antibody TGN1412. *N Engl J Med* 2006;355:1018–28.

19. Thomas PT. Nonclinical evaluation of therapeutic cytokines: immunotoxicologic issues. *Toxicology* 2002;174:27–35.

20. Cavagnaro JA. Preclinical safety evaluation of biotechnology-derived pharmaceuticals. *Nat Rev Drug Discov* 2002;1:469–75.

21. Kulmatycki KM, Jamali F. Drug disease interactions: role of inflammatory mediators in disease and variability in drug response. *J Pharm Pharmaceut Sci* 2005;16: 602–25.

22. Winthrop KL. Risk and prevention of tuberculosis and other serious opportunistic infections associated with the inhibition of tumor necrosis factor. *Nat Clin Pract Rheumatol* 2006;2:602–10.

23. Schepers A, Pires NM, Eefting D, de Vries MR, van Bockel JH, Quax PH. Short-term dexamethasone treatment inhibits vein graft thickening in hypercholesterolemic ApoE3Leiden transgenic mice. *J Vas Surg* 2006;43:809–15.

24. European Public Assessment Reports (EPARs) database. http://www.emea.europa. eu/htms/human/epar/eparintro.htm

25. Agero AL, Dusza SW, Benvenuto-Andrade C, Busam KJ, Myskowski P, Halpern AC. Dermatologic side effects associated with the epidermal growth factor receptor inhibitors. *J Am Acad Dermatol* 2006;55:57–70.

26. Salama AD, Pusey CD. Drug insight: rituximab in renal disease and transplantation. *Nat Clin Pract Nephrol* 2006;2:221–30.

27. Schreiber MA. Preclinical trauma studies of recombinant factor VIIa. *Crit Care* 2005;9:S25–8.

28. Giles JT, Bathon JM. Serious infections associated with anticytokine therapies in the rheumatic diseases. *J Intens Care Med* 2004;19:320–34.

29. Edelson BT, Unanue ER. Immunity to *Listeria* infection. *Curr Opin Immunol* 2000;12:425–31.

30. Bongartz T, Sutton AJ, Sweeting MJ, Buchan I, Matteson EL, Montori V. Anti-TNF antibody therapy in rheumatoid arthritis and the risk of serious infections and malignancies: systematic review and meta-analysis of rare harmful effects in randomized controlled trials. *JAMA* 2006;295:2275–85.

31. van Dalen R, Vree TB. Pharmacokinetics of antibiotics in critically ill patients. *Intens Care Med* 1990;16(Suppl 3):S235–8.

32. De Paepe P, Belpaire FM, Buylaert WA. Pharmacokinetic and pharmacodynamic considerations when treating patients with sepsis and septic shock. *Clin Pharmacokinet* 2002;41:1135–51.

33. Lieberthal W, Nigam SK. Acute renal failure. II. Experimental models of acute renal failure: imperfect but indispensable. *Am J Physiol Ren Physiol* 2000;278: F1–12.

34. Bélanger M, Butterworth RF. Acute liver failure: a critical appraisal of available animal models. *Metab Brain Dis* 2005;20:409–23.

35. Cheymol G. Effects of obesity on pharmacokinetics implications for drug therapy. *Clin Pharmacokinet* 2000;39:215–31.

36. Jimenez PA, Glasson SS, Trubetskoy OV, Haimes HB. Spontaneous osteoarthritis in Dunkin Hartley guinea pigs: histologic, radiologic, and biochemical changes. *Lab Animal Sci* 1997;47:598–601.

37. O'Brien TD. Pathogenesis of feline diabetes mellitus. *Mol Cell Endocrinol* 2002;197(1–2):213–9.

38. Sullivan TP, Eaglstein WH, Davis SC, Mertz P. The pig as a model for human wound healing. *Wound Repair Regener* 2001;9:66–76.

39. Kelly BS, Heffelfinger SC, Whiting JF, et al. Aggressive venous neointimal hyperplasia in a pig model of arteriovenous graft stenosis. *Kidney Int* 2002;62:2272–80.

40. Nunamaker DM. Experimental models of fracture repair. *Clin Ortho Rel Res* 1998;355S:S56–65.

41. Morse MA, Baird WM, Carlson GP. Distribution, covalent binding, and DNA adduct formation of 7,12-dimethylbenz(a)anthracene in SENCAR and BALB/c mice following topical and oral administration. *Cancer Res* 1987;47:4571–5.

42. Grubbs CJ, Moon RC, Squire RA, Farrow GM, Stinson SF, Goodman DG, Brown CC, Sporn MB. 13-cis-retinoic acid: inhibition of bladder carcinogenesis induced in rats by N-butyl-N-(4-hydroxybutyl)nitrosamine. *Science* 1977;198:743–4.

43. Yang SC, Markey SP, Bankiewicz KS, London WT, Lunn G. Recommended safe practices for using the neurotoxin MPTP in animal experiments, *Lab Animal Sci* 1988;38:563–7.

44. Nagelkerken L, Blauw B, Tielemans M. IL-4 abrogates the inhibitory effect of IL-10 on the development of experimental allergic encephalomyelitis in SJL mice. *Int Immunol* 1997;9:1243–51.

45. Hoffmann JC, Pawlowski NN, Kuhl AA, Hohne W, Zeitz M. Animal models of inflammatory bowel disease: an overview. *Pathobiology* 2002–2003;70:121–30.

46. Kim HY, Kim S, Chung DH. FcgammaRIII engagement provides activating signals to NKT cells in antibody-induced joint inflammation. *J Clin Invest* 2006;116:2484–92.

47. Rao P, Segal BM. Experimental autoimmune encephalomyelitis. *Meth Mol Med* 2004;102:363–75.

48. Orihuela CJ, Tuomanen EI. Models of pneumococcal disease. *Drug Discov Today Dis Mod* 2006;3:69–75.

49. Stoddart CA, Reye RA. Models of HIV-1 disease: a review of current status. *Drug Discov Today Dis Mod* 2006;3:113–9.

50. Steinbach WJ, Zaas AK. Newer animal models of Aspergillus and Candida infections. *Drug Discov Today Dis Mod* 2004;1:87–93.

51. Sausville EA, Burger AM. Contributions of human tumor xenografts to anticancer drug development. *Cancer Res* 2006;66:3351–4.

52. Golas JM, Lucas J, Etienne C, Golas J, Discafani C, Sridharan L, Boghaert E, Arndt K, Ye F, Boschelli DH, Li F, Titsch C, Huselton C, Chaudhary I, Boschelli F. FSKI-606, a Src/Abl inhibitor with in vivo activity in colon tumor xenograft models. *Cancer Res* 2005;65:5358–64.

53. Allen TJ, Cooper ME, Lan HY. Use of genetic mouse models in the study of diabetic nephropathy. *Curr Atheroscl Rep* 2004;6:197–202.

54. Eefting D, Schepers A, De Vries MR, Pires NM, Grimbergen JM, Lagerweij T, Nagelkerken LM, Monraats PS, Jukema JW, van Bockel JH, Quax PH. The effect of interleukin-10 knock-out and overexpression on neointima formation in hypercholesterolemic APOE*3-Leiden mice. *Atherosclerosis* 2007;193:335–42.

PART V

SAFETY/TOXICITY ENDPOINTS

Safety Pharmacology: Similarities and Differences between Small Molecules and Novel Biopharmaceuticals

EDWARD W. BERNTON, MD

Contents

Preclinical Safety Evaluation of Biopharmaceuticals: A Science-Based Approach to Facilitating Clinical Trials, edited by Joy A. Cavagnaro
Copyright © 2008 by John Wiley & Sons, Inc.

14.1 INTRODUCTION

Safety pharmacology studies were given regulatory definition in the 2001 ICH S7A guidance [1]. They were differentiated from primary and secondary pharmacodynamic studies used for exploration of structure–activity relationships and lead selection and validation, which generally are not directly supportive of safety of the proposed human uses and dose ranges. Safety pharmacology is defined as "those studies that investigate the potential undesirable pharmacodynamic effects of a substance ... in relation to exposure in the therapeutic range and above." The emphasis for small molecule drugs is on (1) identification of unsuspected "off-target" activities independent of the primary pharmacodynamic effect, (2) further investigation of adverse effects suspected from either clinical or preclinical studies, or (3) detailed investigation of adverse effects that are commonly associated with the specific therapeutic class of the drug candidate (i.e., potassium ion channel cardiac effects with neuroleptics). The safety evaluation of new biopharmaceuticals is often made more difficult by the higher percentage of novel drug targets, compared to small molecules, especially for monoclonal antibodies and soluble receptors. Target specificity is usually very high. For these products, safety pharmacology tends to be a more focused investigation of highly specific drug–target interactions, and an in-depth characterization of pharmacodynamic effects.

14.2 SAFETY PHARMACOLOGY REGULATORY REQUIREMENTS FOR SMALL MOLECULES AND BIOPHARMACEUTICALS

14.2.1 The "Core Battery" Approach for Small-Molecule Safety Pharmacology

The ICH S7A guidance recommends that the safety pharmacology studies be designed with specific consideration of the pharmacologic activities of the test article. It recognizes, however, that in early development, sufficient information may not be available to design such studies. In this case a more general approach to safety pharmacology is recommended, referred to as the "core battery."

The core safety pharmacology is designed to detect organ-based toxicities, with the emphasis on cardiovascular, central nervous, and respiratory systems, where even transient dysfunction secondary to drug exposure can be life-threatening. Other organ systems, such as the gastrointestinal, renal, or hematopoetic symptoms can be transiently impaired by adverse pharmacodynamic effects without causing irreversible harm.

A core battery is normally hierarchical in structure. Screening tests are suggested in section 2.7 of the guidance for CNS, cardiovascular, and respiratory systems. Examples are given of possible follow-up studies providing more detailed analysis of pharmacologic effects. For example, blood pressure, heart rate, and ECG, ideally by telemetry in an unrestrained animal, can provide initial cardiovascular safety assessment. If abnormalities are detected, then full analysis via cardiac catheterization might be performed to study cardiac output, ventricular contractility, vascular resistance, and interactions with endogenous mediators such as vagolytic or vagotonic agents, catecholamines, and so forth. In vitro testing such as the hERG screen for potential effects on the potassium channel cardiac repolarization can also be performed as safety pharmacology, if not performed as screens during the lead selection process. Typical CNS core batteries might be the Irwin behavioral battery in mice or rats, which can be expanded to include locomotor activity, rotatating rod tests of coordination, analgesia screens, PTZ seizure threshold, and/or more extensive characterization of dose–response curves if indicated.

The core safety pharmacology battery can also be performed with a small molecule's major metabolite, particularly if that metabolite is unique to human metabolism and the toxicology species did not have significant exposure to it.

All these studies should be performed in compliance with good laboratory practice (GLP) where feasible. The screening battery is frequently performed with full GLP. More complex or specialized studies should be well-designed, properly controlled, and carefully documented "when not in compliance." When safety pharmacology endpoints are incorporated into toxicology studies, not an uncommon situation, they should be conducted under GLP.

Certain information from commonly used lead selection screens may also suggest specific safety pharmacology screens for small molecules, such as the results of standardized receptor binding screens, cross-species plasma binding profiles, in vitro metabolism profiles, and in vitro studies on cell phenotype or function. It should be pointed out that standard single- and repeat-dose toxicology protocols and the usual in-life observations, clinical laboratory parameters, and histopathology are relatively insensitive means for detection of nonfatal abnormalities in the organ function of central nervous, respiratory, and cardiovascular systems, and in particular the immune system. Nonetheless, in general experience it is relatively uncommon for the routine safety pharmacology battery to disclose dose-limiting toxicities that can alter the design of human trials if these were not observed in primary and secondary pharmacology studies or in GLP toxicology studies. Additionally diseased patient populations may have increased sensitivity to pharmacodynamic effects of the test article (i.e., cancer patients or tumor-bearing test animals to circulatory effects of TNF-alpha and other cytokines, potentiation of hematotoxicity, nephrotoxicity, cardiotoxicity by other concurrent cancer therapies, safety in renal- or hepatic-impaired populations) not reflected in standard safety pharmacology.

14.2.2 Safety Pharmacology for Biopharmaceuticals

For biotechnology-derived pharmaceuticals, including proteins, polypeptides, virally vectored vaccines, or gene-therapy therapeutics, and oligonucleotides, safety pharmacology tends to be a more focused investigation of highly specific drug–target interactions. Interspecies variation in metabolism and metabolites, clearance, and protein-binding becomes less of an issue, but the frequent species specificity of both the target interaction (i.e., monoclonal antibodies, certain growth factors, and cytokines) and postreceptor signaling and effects, particularly for immunomodulators, makes selection of appropriate in vivo models more difficult.

Recognizing these issues, the S7A guidance states, "For biotechnology-derived products that achieve highly specific receptor targeting it is often sufficient to evaluate the safety pharmacology endpoints as part of toxicology and/or pharmacodynamic studies; therefore the safety pharmacology studies can be reduced or eliminated for these products." But because of the challenge that many biopharmaceuticals present, some quite species-specific in their binding interactions, for predictive toxicology and safety pharmacology, in 1997 the ICH published a consensus guidance for such preclinical safety evaluations. This S6 guidance, "Preclinical Safety Evaluation of Biotechnology-Derived Pharmaceuticals" [2], together with the ICH S8 guidance "Immunotoxicity Studies for Human Pharmaceuticals" [3] provides some further information relevant to safety pharmacology for biopharmaceuticals, many of which have immunomodulatory activities.

The safety evaluation of new biopharmaceuticals is made more difficult by the rising percentage of novel drug targets, compared to small molecules, especially for monoclonal antibodies. Often the function and even the distribution of these novel targets is incompletely characterized or understood. Thus the thorough delineation of pharmacologic effects and dose-limiting human toxicities can require an extremely thoughtful, individualized, and product-specific research program.

For biopharmaceuticals such as growth factors and cytokines with agonistic properties, transgenic knock-in mice which overexpress the murine homologue of the candidate molecule can provide useful information, particularly regarding chronic drug exposures and potential developmental effects of the candidate. Alternately, mice can be dosed with an active murine homologue of recombinant DNA origin, if the human protein lacks full activity in this test species. In the case of such surrogates for monoclonal antibody products with restricted species cross-reactivity, the model should be carefully validated by in vitro studies of mouse target binding affinities and pharmacodynamic activity, as described by Clarke et al. [4]. For soluble receptors and monoclonal antibody therapeutics designed to interfere with signaling via a specific receptor or ligand, siRNA can be used to silence the therapeutic target, both in vitro and in preclinical models, allowing investigation of the pharmacologic consequences in both healthy animals and models of disease [5].

Alternatively, a knockout transgenic mouse strain can be similarly utilized to understand the safety issues involved in target inhibition or neutralization. For example, the phenotype of CXCR5 and integrin beta 6 knockout mice helped characterize the pharmacodynamic and pathologic consequences of human monoclonal antibodies blocking both these receptors. CXCR5 null mice had defects in delayed-hypersensitivity responses but resistance to a common preclinical inflammatory bowel disease model. Integrin beta 6 null mice demonstrated chronic inflammation in the lung and skin but resistance to bleomycin-induced pulmonary fibrosis [6–8]. Various humanized transgenic mouse strains also can be used to investigate toxicity and pharmacodynamic responses of specific biopharmaceuticals interacting specifically with human immune-cell targets [9]. In preclinical disease models all of these strategies may be part of early target validation work, but such models also have great utility at a later point when utilized with a greater emphasis on safety pharmacology endpoints. As Green and Black state in their useful review of safety assessment for immunomodulatory biopharmaceuticals [10], "In this field of development, preclinical models often need to reflect recent technology innovations; therefore, these models are not always 'validated' in the conventional sense. Experience to date suggests that improved methods and approaches are needed as these agents are developed for use in lower or moderate risk patient populations."

In evaluating the suitability of animal test species for safety pharmacology, it is essential to confirm that the binding affinity of the product and its target is similar in the tissues of the test species and in human tissues. Similarly the distribution of the target of monoclonal antibody therapies should compare in tissue cross-reactivity studies in both human tissues and those from the test species. Primary cell cultures or cell lines derived from mammalian cells can be used to examine the effects of the biopharmaceutical on cell phenotype, signaling pathways, cytokine secretion, and proliferation, and these may provide useful information on the relevance or lack of sensitivity of a proposed in vivo safety species. The S6 guidance specifically states, "toxicity studies in nonrelevant species may be misleading and are discouraged." Examples of the validation of pharmacodynamic activity of the biopharmaceutic in toxicology and safety species are provided in publications by Hart et al. that review the preclinical studies for monoclonal antihuman IL-4 and IL-5 antibodies [11,12].

The species-specificity of activity for some biopharmaceuticals has immediate implications when one considers the dependence of the standard "core" and "extended" safety pharmacology batteries on rodent models, or in some cases dogs and minipigs, or when absolutely required, nonhuman primates [13]. For biopharmaceuticals with highly species-specific drug–target interactions, opportunities for traditional safety pharmacology screens can be highly constrained, and if primate studies are required, both expensive and time-consuming. Thus safety pharmacology studies for pharmaceuticals tend to be limited to those clearly required to further evaluate findings in standard toxicology studies or else clearly required by considerations such as mechanism of action or drug class.

The pharmacokinetic evaluation of biopharmaceuticals is generally simplified by the usual metabolism of products to small peptides and to amino acids, and thus classical biotransformation and metabolism studies are rarely necessary. Routine studies to assess mass balance are not useful. However, both single- and multiple-dose toxicokinetic data are essential in safety pharmacology asessments, and these can be complicated by two factors: (1) biphasic clearance with a saturable, initial, receptor-dependent clearance phase, which may cause nonlinearity in dose–exposure relationships and doseresponses [14] and (2) antibody production against an antigenic biopharmaceutical that can alter clearance or activity in more chronic repeat-dose safety studies in the preclinical model.

In general, both dose–exposure and exposure–response relationships tend to be less linear and predictable for many biopharmaceuticals than is seen with most small molecule drugs. This can involve saturable receptor-binding, upregulation of soluble receptors that alter clearance, stimulation of biologic cascades by agonists at immune cell receptors, and temporal disassociation of pharmacologic effects from plasma levels due to persistence and activity in nonplasma compartments or the delayed induction of secondary mediator release. All such factors make the prediction of both estimates of exposure and adverse effect profiles in humans generally less reliable than that based on allometric scaling from toxicokinetic studies of small molecules, and argue for conservative human starting doses and cautious dose escalation in the initial clinical studies of novel biopharmaceuticals.

The induction of antibody formation against biopharmaceuticals in animal test species is not highly predictive for the potential of antibody formation in humans. Humans may also develop antibodies to human or humanized proteins that may not necessarily abrogate a therapeutic response. However, in repeat-dose safety animal studies with a biopharmaceutical, it is imperative that the sponsor (developer) establish that any antibody response detected does not neutralize the biopharmceutical or significantly alter its clearance or the animal's exposure. Product sponsors should modify the interpretation of safety results to account for any such attenuation of exposure. In general, biopharmaceuticals given by an intravenous route can be expected to be less antigenic than those administered subcutaneously.

14.3 TESTING FOR QT LIABILITY AND TORSADOGENIC POTENTIAL OF NEW DRUGS

14.3.1 Background and History

Relationships between the whimsically named human ether-a-go-go related gene (hERG), drug-induced QT interval prolongation, and the torsades de pointes (TdP) arrhythmia are now a serious and constant theme in drug safety evaluation. hERG encodes the inward rectifying potassium channel (i(Kr)). Mutations in five cardiac potassium rectifier channel genes, including KCNQ1, HERG, SCN5A, KCNE1, and KCNE2, constitute the principal cause of inherited long-QT syndrome (LQTS). Typically each family carries its own private mutation, and the disease manifests with varying phenotype and incomplete penetrance, even within particular families. Individuals with a high-penatrance channel gene mutation have a prolonged QT interval on their electrocardiogram and have a propensity toward serious arrhythmias, including the often fatal TdP.

In the 1990s a pattern of sudden death and occurrence of TdP was noticed in patients taking a variety of commonly prescribed drugs, most notably terfenadine, astimazole, and cisipride. This was usually associated with a prolonged QT interval on the electrocardiogram. Further investigation found that these drugs could cause QT prolongation and subsequent arrhythmia, usually at elevated blood levels or in susceptible individuals. Virtually all drugs known to cause TdP block the rapidly activating component of the delayed rectifier potassium current (I(Kr)). Arrhythmias are more likely to occur if drug-induced QTc prolongation coexists with other risk factors, such as individual susceptibility, presence of congenital long-QT syndromes, heart failure, bradycardia, electrolyte imbalance, drug overdose of a QTc prolonging drug, female sex, restraint, old age, hepatic or renal impairment, or slow metabolizer status.

In particular, the interaction of ketoconazole, which inhibits CYP3A4 metabolism of terfenadine and cisipride, was found to be associated with higher risk of TdP. These discoveries led to withdrawal certain drugs from the market and black-box labeling of risk of QT prolongation and torsades for others. As a class effect, most class Ia and III antiarrhythmic drugs prolong QT, but unlike antihistamines or antireflux therapies, these are used to treat serious cardiac disease and titrated to effect with careful patient and ECG observation. Therefore these drugs have remained on the market. Other noncardiac drugs are now marketed with label warnings regarding QT liability. These include chloroquin, clarithromycin, domperidone, droperidol, erythromycin, haloperidol, methadone, pentamidine, and thioridazine. Patients with known long-QT syndrome are cautioned to avoid using them.

Nevertheless, the FDA considered a risk of fatal cardiac arrhythmias, in even a minuscule percentage of patients, to be a toxicity that needed to be exhaustively evaluated prior to marketing authorization of a new small molecule drug. In 2005 the agency published Guidance E14, "Clinical Evaluation of QT/QTc Interval Prolongation and Proarrythmic Potential for Nonantiarrhythmic Drugs." This guidance outlined the "definitive QT study" as a mandatory clinical evaluation for new drugs, as well as other practices for analysis of arrhythmagenic potential in phase 3 study data. The guidance established as a drug toxicity the drug effect on the QT interval as a surrogate for risk of TdP.

14.3.2 Preclinical Evaluation for QT Liability

In 2005 the FDA published Guidance S7B, "Nonclinical Evaluation of the Potential for Delayed Ventricular Repolarization by Human Pharmaceuticals," considered an extension of the S7A safety pharmacology guidance. The S7B guidance states, "the objectives of studies are to: (1) identify the potential of a test substance and its metabolites to delay ventricular repolarization, and (2) relate the extent of delayed ventricular repolarization to the concentrations of a test substance and its metabolites. The study results can be used to elucidate the mechanism of action and, when considered with other information, estimate risk for delayed ventricular repolarization and QT interval prolongation in humans."

The testing should include in vitro assays that evaluate drug effects on current through a native or expressed potassium rectifier channel protein, such as that encoded by hERG or measurement of ion currents in drug-exposed isolated animal or human myocytes or cultured cell lines. It should also include in vivo electrophysiologic studies of drug effects on the relationship between QT and RR intervals, using dog, monkey, swine, ferret, or rabbit. Use of mice or rats is not recommended, since the primary ion currents controlling repolarization are different than in humans. The guidance suggests that the in vivo assay can be integrated into the cardiovascular safety pharmacology study. The fact that high-sensitivity in vitro QT assays have relatively low specificity has led to the development of additional models for electrophysiologic studies, such as the arterially perfused rabbit ventricular wedge preparation [15,16].

In vitro studies need to be well-designed, with known QT-prolonging or TdP-associated drugs used as positive controls, and careful characterization of the test item dose–response. A drug's IC50 for hERG inhibition or for other measures of the effect on cardiac repolarization is usually compared to the effective therapeutic plasma concentration of the unbound drug (ETPC(unbound)). If the IC50/ETPC ratio is greater than 50 to 100, this generally predicts a lack QT liability of the drug when dosed in patients, and negative results in a definitive QT interval clinical study. However, lower values can be poorly predictive. For example, drugs withdrawn from the market due to TdP or drugs with a measurable incidence of TdP in humans have hERG IC50/ETPC ratios ranging from 0.1 to 31. For the majority of drugs with no reports of TdP in humans, the ratio is greater than 30 [17].

14.3.3 Clinical Evaluation of QT Liability—When Is It Applicable to Biopharmaceuticals?

The E14 guidance on clinical evaluation of the QT/QTc interval prolongation states: "an adequate premarketing investigation of the safety of a new pharmaceutical agent should include rigorous characterization of its effects on the QT/QTc interval." This evaluation should be performed at both the steady-state therapeutic exposure, and at three- to fourfold higher exposures, to model inadvertent overdose or impaired drug clearance. Sometimes preliminary clinical studies are required to establish the maximum tolerated steady-state exposure to be used in the definitive QT study. Studies must be double-blinded and placebo-controlled, and incorporate a positive control, such as moxifloxin, to establish the sensitivity of the trial to detect a 10 ms average effect on QTc. (QT interval corrected for heart rate). Study designs can involve a multiperiod crossover or parallel groups. When possible these studies are done in healthy volunteers. Careful attention must be given to replicate sets of ECGs to minimize inherent variability and QT hysteresis in QTc measurements, to provide an adequate ECG baseline to correct for circadian and meal effects, and to obtain adequate sampling of blood levels to document relationships of ECG changes with drug exposure. Usually a commercial "core ECG lab" is utilized to conduct the ECG analysis. All ECG tracings and the measurements made to determine the QT interval must be archived in a format suitable for submission to the FDA, using a digital file format.

Typically these studies cost from $1.5 to $3 million to conduct. Based on the perceived probability of a significant QT interval effect (based on preclinical studies, class effects, and ECG data from phase 1 studies) a decision must be made whether to conduct the definitive QT study prior to proceeding with a proof-of-concept study in patients, or whether to delay this study until the proof of concept (POC) has been demonstrated. Of note, for many biopharmaceutical products it would not be possible nor ethical to dose to steady state in healthy volunteers, to dose at two to four times anticipated therapeutic exposures, or to use a crossover design with reasonable washout periods. Thus a QT study performed with a biopharmaceutical may need to vary from the usual design and the E14 guidance, and may present great challenges for subject or patient recruitment.

Historically, therapy with biopharmaceuticals have not been felt to associated with risk of TdP. It was felt that the specificity of receptor interactions common to cytokines, growth factors, and monoclonal antibodies made high-affinity off-target interactions with ion channel proteins extremely unlikely. A theoretical exception to this might be certain neuropeptides, some of which are known to modulate certain neuronal ion channels. To this author's knowledge, no biologic therapy has been associated with TdP with the exception of vasopressin [18], where the arrhythmia was secondary to vasopressin-induced bradycardia. A search of the National Library of Medicine bibliographic database crossing either the term "torsades" or "arrhythmia" with the terms "interleukin," "monoclonal antibody," "TNF-alpha," "erythropoietin," "colony-stimulating factor," or "cytokine therapy" revealed only one report, which described the association of interleukin-11 therapy for thrombocytopenia in elderly patients with atrial fibrillation. However, in vitro electrophysiologic studies showed no direct cardiac membrane effects of therapeutic concentrations of IL-11 [19].

This is not to say that cardiotoxicity is not seen with biopharmaceuticals. Cardiomyopathy is now a well-recognized complication of trastuzumab and and has been reported with bevacizumab treatment, in particular in combination with other cytotoxic cancer therapies [20]. Myocarditis and pericarditis are a well-documented complications of vaccinia immunization [21], and could also complicate use of a pox-virus vector for other therapeutics. In 1995 Genetics Institute suspended phase 2 cancer trials of Interleukin-12 for serious toxicities including cardiac arrhythmia. However, such toxicities are best detected by incorporation of biomarkers for myocardial damage such as troponin-T into preclinical and early clinical studies, and continual ECG monitoring for arrhythmia in preclinical and early clinical studies, *not* by in vitro explorations of electrophysiology.

With the transfer of most biopharmaceutical INDs from CBER to CDER in 2003, there has been an increased tendency to apply the small-molecule paradigm for evaluation of QT liability to biopharmaceutical product candidates, and to request information on hERG assays or plans for definitive clinical QT studies. This does not seem reasonable based on the postmarketing safety data for biopharmaceuticals, nor on scientific grounds as discussed above. If these investigations become routinely required, they will only add significant time and costs to the process of biopharmaceutical product evaluation and have little ultimate impact on patient safety.

While the E14 guidance does not exempt biopharmaceuticals from the requirement for "rigorous characterization" of QT effects, in the past both scientific and practical considerations limited its application to these therapies. While there are no reports of TdP secondary to a biopharmaceutical, and currently a leading cardiac core lab provider knew of no definitive QT studies submitted for biologic products, it is clear that such a study will be required for at least one new biopharmaceutical, an erythropoietin. Regarding regulatory strategy, sponsors of new biopharmaceuticals must either inquire early (at a pre-IND meeting) if a definitive QT study will be required for marketing approval, and risk a positive answer in the absence of clear FDA policy, or wait until an end-of-phase-2 meeting, and plan such studies, if needed, in parallel with pivotal phase 3 trials. Given the extremely low probability of biopharmaceutical product development being limited by QT interval effects, this second strategy would appear more reasonable. While in the past the various CDER divisions frequently handled QTc questions with consults to the Cardiorenal Division, now the Interdiscplinary Review Team (IRT), provides this expertise for the primary review divisions, upon request.

14.4 ADDING PREDICTIVE SAFETY BIOMARKERS INTO STANDARD TOXICOLOGY PROTOCOLS FOR BIOPHARMACEUTICALS

The usual GLP 30- or 60-day repeat-dose toxicology study with a recovery group offers an opportunity to perform a more systematic investigation of the more subtle pharmacodynamic or toxicologic effects of biopharmaceuticals than those endpoints usually incorporated into such protocols. Some of these demand tissue samples, but many involve noninvasive biomarkers that can be carried forward into early phase human studies. These might include CNS assessments, inflammation and immune activation or suppression, cell proliferation or apoptosis in tissue samples, and end-organ toxicities.

14.4.1 CNS Assessments

An Irwin test at one or several study time points, for rodent studies, or a 24 hour period of actigraphy in a cage designed to measure spontaneous locomotor activity. In early clinical studies, clinical actigraphy with wrist-worn recording devices can detect not only hypo- or hyperactivity but changes in sleep latency, sleep fragmentation, and daytime sleep, often sensitive indicators of CNS side effects (www.ambulatory-monitoring.com/references.html).

14.4.2 Inflammation and Immune Activation or Suppression

While cytokine release may be localized both in tissue distribution and in time, secondary measurements can reflect cytokine release or resulting immune cell activation at time points with other scheduled safety labs. One of the most useful, with a long history of clinical use, is C-reactive protein (CRP), for which EIA kits are available for species including rodents, rabbits, and dogs. CRP is a serum acute-phase reactant, and levels can increase by over 2 logs driven mainly by release of IL-1, IL-6, and TNF-alpha. The peak increase usually lags cytokine release by 24 to 48 hours and can remain above baseline for several days to a week once the acute phase response is stimulated.

Neopterin is a metabolite of guanosine triphosphate that is produced and secreted by mainly by monocyte/macrophage/dendritic cells. Secretion is greatly upregulated when these cells are activated by cytokines, principally gamma-interferon, and serum blood levels are elevated with infections due to virus or intracellular pathogens, organ rejection, and other conditions associated with activation of mononuclear phagocytes. EIA methods to measure neopterin are readily available. The analyte is conserved across humans and all common toxicology species. Both CRP and neopterin can be more sensitive than clinical signs of immune activation (fever, weight loss, hypoactivity) in both NHP models and human studies. If CRP or neopterin prove to be dose-dependent biomarkers for an on-target pharmacodynamic effect, they can easily be incorporated as analytes into early-phase human trials. An example of the use of these markers in a FIH healthy volunteer single-dose safety and PK study is given in Table 14.1.

These biomarkers are most useful when they can be carried forward into phase 1 studies of novel products, where, particularly in healthy volunteer studies, a lack of therapeutic endpoints or surrogates (e.g., as viral load in HVB patients), makes pharmacodynamic information difficult to obtain. The first-in-human study results given in Table 14.1 demonstrate the utility of two biomarkers, CRP and neopterin, when carried forward into a first-in-human study of a novel toll-like receptor ligand in healthy volunteers. These biomarkers, while nonspecific, were a more sensitive indicator of biologic activity than other classical endpoints such as adverse events or routine safety laboratory monitoring. When biomarkers are incorporated into preclinical studies, as dose-ranging pharmacology studies, GLP toxicology studies, or "phase 0" preclinical studies, they can often provide robust information in the early phase of clinical development at little additional cost. CRP can be measured with commercially available kits in virtually any toxicology species.

Surface activation markers on circulating monocytes and T lymphocytes are also sensitive markers of immune activation secondary to either biopharmaceuticals or pathologic disease states. For lymphocytes, CD69, CD25, HLADR, and transferin receptor represent early-, late-, and proliferative-stage markers of activation. Lymphocyte CD69 can be upregulated as early as 4 to 8 hours after ex vivo stimulation of peripheral blood. Monocyte early activation also results in increased CD69 expression, as well as increased expression of CD14 receptors, CD11b, and HLADR, depending on the timing and stimulus. Human flow cytometry reagents can be used for blood samples from nonhuman primates, and reagents are also available for mouse and, to some extent, for other toxicology species. When immune cells are direct targets of immunostimulatory biopharmaceuticals, these activation markers have great utility (along with measurements of cytokine release) for in vitro studies to compare dose–response relationships between human cells and cells from toxicology species. When immune cells are targets of intentionally or potentially immunosuppressive therapeutics, these markers can also be used after stimulation and activation of cells to examine the dose–response relationships involved in inhibition of activation responses. An excellent example is the in vitro stimulation of monocytes with bacterial lipopolysacharide, using supernatant TNF-alpha accumulation as an endpoint. For development of anti-inflammatory PDE4 inhibitors, a lipid-A antagonist, and a p38 MAP kinase inhibitor, among others, this system was used not only for in vitro dose–response information but carried forward into phase 1 healthy volunteer studies as a pharmacodynamic marker (using ex vivo LPS stimulation of whole blood with TNF measurements). This allowed PK/PD correlations in the first-in-human trials [22–24].

TABLE 14.1 A first-in-human single-dose, dose-escalation study of biologic X, a putative TLR ligand and immune-response modifier in healthy volunteers

Subject Number/ Sex (Ranked by C_{max})	C_{max}, (ng/ml)	Adverse Events, 1–5 Days Post Dose	Elevated CRP Post Dose (ULN 3 mg/L)[a]	Elevated Neopterin (ULN 10 nM/L)[a]
103/M	750	Back pain, mild		
107/F	756			
106/M	1,253			
116/M	1,344		17.0/16.3	16/9.8
104/F	1,657			
103/M	1,659			
105/M	1,677			
110/M	1,783			
111/M	1,976			
108/F	2,008			
114/M	2,359			
125/F	2,667	Fever (38.0), mild nausea, Mild myalgia	9.2/8.4	28.2/21.4
120/M	2,704			
117/M	2,794			
124/M	2,951		3.8/2.8	
119/M	3,872		26.2/24.8	10.9/5.8
126/F	4,689	Mild somnolence, headache, anorexia		
127/M	5,318			
128/M	5,413		4.9/2.6	11.6/7.6
130/M	6,537		19.7/19.5	47.2/43.3
132/M	6,771			
133/F	8,992	Fever 37.8, chills, fatigue, chest discomfort, myalgia	12.0/11.6	17.4/11.9
135/F	9,107	Fever, myalgia	4.2/3.8	19.4/12.8
134/F	9,444			
115/M	15,108	Fever (38.8) × 12 h, myalgia, chills	34.0/33.5	28.9/21.9

Note: Dose cohorts of placebo (not shown) and 20, 50, 100, and 200 units of biopharmaceutical X, a putative TLR ligand and immunomodulator, dosed in healthy volunteers. Elevations of C-reactive protein and neopterin 48 hrs after dosing correlate with exposure and with dose emergent AEs. These nonspecific biomarkers appear more sensitive than symptoms or fever to detect biologic activity or reactogenicity.

[a]Value/change from baseline.

14.4.3 Cell Proliferation or Apoptosis in Tissue Samples

If segments of tissues harvested for routine histology from toxicology studies are snap frozen, a variety of informative endpoints can be examined in specific tissues. After pulsing of animals with the nucleotide analogue bromodeoxyuridine (BrdU), proliferative indexes can be calculated with fluorescent anti-BrdU antibodies, or by using antibodies to proliferating cell nuclear antigen (PCNA)-cyclin. Indexes of apoptotic cells can be calculated either by TUNNEL assay, UTP-nick translation, or fluorescent Annexin V binding to detect exposed phosphotidyl serine on cell membranes. Newer reagents such as fluorine-containing annexin analogues will allow in vivo imaging of apoptosis by micro PET techniques [25–27].

14.4.4 End-organ Toxicities

Serum creatinine and BUN, the most common indicators of renal function used in both clinical and preclinical safety laboratory panels, are relatively insensitive markers of injury, particularly for the renal tubules. Urinary measurements of alanine aminopeptidase and N-acetyl-beta-D-glucosaminidase and kidney injury molecule-1 (KIM-1) can provide much more sensitivity when nephrotoxicity is a potential safety concern [28,29]. These are also suitable for safety monitoring in early-phase human trials if preclinical studies validate such use to monitor product nephrotoxicity.

In a similar manner, troponin-T can greatly increase the sensitivity of safety labs to detect subclinical cardiac myotoxicity. Rat, dog, and pig troponin-T can all be determined using the automated Roche clinical diagnostic system for human Troponin-T [30]. This would have been of obvious relevance to the safety pharmacology of Herceptin®, where the association with cardiomyopathy was only established after widespread clinical use.

Likewise gene expression analysis utilizing DNA microarrays has established the new field of toxicogenomics, providing preclinical research with new predictive tools for organ toxicicity, including hepatotoxicity [31]. Of note, inflammation and immune activation has been shown to greatly potentiate the hepatotoxicity of certain small molecules which demonstrated sporadic hepatotoxicity in the postmarketing period, such as ranitidine. This may have implications for potential hepatotoxic interactions between small molecules and certain immunomodulatory biopharmaceuticals [32].

14.5 AN INTEGRATED APPROACH TO PRECLINICAL AND CLINICAL IMMUNOTOXICITY ASSESSMENTS

Immune system receptors and soluble signal proteins represent targets of a large group of biopharmaceuticals. *This means that immunotoxicity, defined as the unintended suppression or enhancement of immune function, is an impor-*

tant area of safety pharmacology for many biopharmaceuticals. It is complicated by the fact, which will be discussed below, that for a variety of reasons nonprimate species are not always suitable for safety pharmacology, and even nonhuman primates such as macaque monkeys and chimpanzees may have significant differences in their immune physiology and pharmacologic responses compared to humans.

14.5.1 Regulatory Guidances

The ICH S8 document, approved in 2005, provides general guidance on immunotoxicity studies for human pharmaceuticals, although the emphasis is on evaluation of small molecules for immunosuppressive effects. ICH S8 suggests that standard toxicity studies (STS) be reviewed for any evidence of immunotoxicity. Of special note would be findings from hematology, albumin/globulin ratios from clinical chemistry, weights of thymus and spleen, and histology of lymphoid organs (which may include Peyers patch, BALT, and bone marrow, when appropriate). The standard study design recommended for immunotoxicity assessments is a 28-day exposure in rodents, with a high dose that "should be above the NOAEL but below a level inducing changes secondary to stress (mediated by increased corticosteroid release)." Careful attention should be paid to the histopathology methods, as reviewed by the European Society of Toxicological Pathology in a 2005 publication [33].

The selection of immunotoxicity study endpoints should be based on any cause for concern raised by a "weight of evidence" review of various factors: for example, findings from STS, pharmacological properties of the drug, intended patient population, structural similarities to known immunomodulators, drug disposition, and/or clinical information. This S8 guideline allows for more flexible approaches; there is no given set of rules. Goals of more detailed immunotoxicology studies should be to characterize a relationship between exposure and altered immune endpoints and to sufficiently characterize the immunotoxicity profile to allow monitoring and management of such risks in human trials.

Additional possible preclinical immunotoxicity endpoints mentioned in the S8 guidance are as follows:

- The T cell dependent antibody response to immunization with SRBC or KLH.
- Immunophenotyping either by immunohistochemistry in lymphoid tissues or flow cytometry in blood samples to enumerate changes in specific leukocyte populations.
- NK cell activity assays.
- Host resistance studies, usually using murine challenge with pathogens such as influenza virus, CMV, *Listeria*, streptococcus, or tumor host resistance models with subcutaneous (sc). injection of tumor cell lines.

- In vitro or ex vivo macrophage/neutrophil functional assays including ADCC, phagocytosis, oxidative burst, and chemotaxis.
- Assays to measure cell-mediated immunity, with either in vivo sensitization and intradermal challenge (delayed-type hypersensitivity) or in vitro measurements of T cell responses to antigens or mitogens.

It should be noted that these recommended studies are all designed to detect suppression of normal immune responses, not inappropriate activation or dysregulation occurring in any compartment of the immune system. This represents one of the serious limitations of the S8 guidance. The suggested test systems also give little consideration to the difficulty of selecting a relevant test species for biopharmaceuticals that may be highly specific for a primate or human target.

The S8 guidance suggests that more comprehensive immunotoxicity studies (beyond the STS) should be completed "before the exposure of a large population of patients," which is usually phase 3. However, this suggestion is often not applicable to biopharmaceuticals. For many biopharmaceuticals the initial clinical development decision is whether a single-dose safety and pharmacokinetic study can be safely accomplished in healthy volunteers. Data are needed to guide dose selection and protocol design for these studies, or to determine whether the risk profile of the product requires first-in-human PK studies to be conducted in patients, who potentially can realize some current or future benefit. Such initial clinical pharmacology patient studies are frequently difficult to recruit, given that single-dose or short-term exposure to drug is not expected to result in near-term therapeutic benefit, only in safety and pharmacokinetic data that may enable future efficacy studies. Patients prefer participation in phase 2 or 3 trials offering more immediate potential benefit and provision of longer term medical care for their illness. Additionally initial PK and safety trials in patients may provide a less sensitive and accurate safety signal, complicated by variable comorbidities of concurrent illness and the frequent simultaneous treatment of disease with other therapeutics.

For these reasons, determining the nature, predictability, and reversibility of immune system effects become a critical factor in weighing the risk–benefit ration of an phase 1 trial in healthy volunteers, as well as the determining a safe starting dose, safe maximum dose, and methods for monitoring potential immunotoxicity in these subjects. Over the past decade single-dose PK and safety trials of biopharmaceuticals in healthy volunteers have often preceded initial patient studies, even for products with known immunomodulatory effects at the anticipated therapeutic chronic dose exposure.

While dozens of such healthy volunteer studies have been safely conducted, the catastrophic syndrome of T cell activation and depletion, cytokine release, and multi-organ failure seen in the 2006 Tegenero 1412 phase I study [34] reminded clinical investigators, sponsors, and regulatory agencies of the very real risks to healthy volunteers posed by inadequately and incompletely characterized biopharmaceuticals. Thus for many biopharmaceuticals, the preclinical investigations of potential immunotoxicity will occur prior to the first human trial, to inform the decision of whether the risk profile is suitable for a healthy volunteer trial. This is also becoming the case for many small-molecule noncytotoxic therapies for cancer. While traditional cytotoxic and potentially mutagenic cancer therapies were first studied clinically in cancer patients with progressive disease who were refractory to standard therapies, and doses then escalated to the maximum tolerated (and highly toxic) dose, it is now not uncommon for the PK, tolerability, and safety of a noncytotoxic cancer drug to first be investigated in healthy volunteers. This was the case for the oral kinase inhibitors gefitinib and erlotinib, where healthy volunteers were also used to characterize drug–drug interactions and it is becoming more common with biopharmaceuticals as well [35–37]. In such cases, just as with biopharmaceuticals, careful preclinical investigation of potential immunotoxicity is required.

14.5.2 New Techniques for Evaluating Immunosuppressive Activity

The assessment of immunosuppressive drug effects by ex vivo measurement of stimulated lymphocyte function in peripheral blood is becoming more informative. Ex vivo assays have been used to characterize the in vitro and in vivo interactions of immunosuppressive drugs such as cyclosporine, tacrolimus, mycophenolate mofetil, and FK778. These assays can be utilized to characterize pharmacodynamics in preclinical species, including the rat, carried forward into clinical pharmacology studies, and even utilized, in some cases, for therapeutic drug monitoring in patients. While often applied to small-molecule immunomodulators, some of these techniques are also applicable to biopharmaceuticals, preclinically and in phase 1 trials, especially for studying their interactions with approved small-molecule immunomodulators [38–40].

New techniques such as the Cylex photoluminescent detection of CD3 lymphocyte activation by mitogen or antigen, approved by the FDA for monitoring immunosuppression in transplant patients, are convenient, species nonspecific, and well suited for repeated measurements in preclinical and clinical studies of biopharmaceuticals [41]. This assay utilizes whole blood.

14.6 NOVEL PHARMACODYNAMIC MEASURES USING FLOW CYTOMETRY AND BLOOD MONONUCLEAR CELLS AS A SURROGATE FOR TISSUE RESPONSES

Over the past several years new techniques have vastly expanded the potential of flow cytometry to provide pharmacodynamic endpoints for a variety of pharmacotherapies, in a manner noninvasive enough to be carried forward from preclinical exposure–response studies into early-phase clinical pharmacology studies.

Intracellular signaling can now be visualized in peripheral blood lymphocytes with phosphospecific antibodies to MEK, ERK, p38 MAPK, STAT, JNK/SAPK, and other signal transducers. This allows pharmacodynamic monitoring of signal transduction agonists or inhibitors (especially when coupled with ex vivo T cell activation by phorbal esters or other agents, which can be performed in whole blood) [42–46].

Another interesting example is the ability of flow cytometric techniques to monitor histone acetylation levels of peripheral blood cells, and provide pharmacodynamic analysis of histone deacetylase inhibitors being utilized in oncology patient trials [47,48].

Currently flow-cytometric methods are also under development to examine effects of various inhibitors of PARP (poly(ADP-ribose)polymerase) that are in preclinical development or clinical trials and use native or stimulated PARP activity in peripheral blood mononuclear cells.

14.7 LOW PREDICTIVE VALUE OF CERTAIN TOXICITY STUDIES IN NONHUMAN PRIMATES

For biopharmaceuticals that are agonists at activation receptors on human immune cells (e.g., anti-CD3 or anti-CD4) or antagonists at inhibitory receptors, even safety studies in nonhuman primates may not accurately predict a product's pharmacodynamic effects and the exposure–response relationship in humans. For example, no clinical evidence of autoimmunity was seen in cynomolgus monkey studies of CTLA-4 blockade [49]. However, autoimmune phenomena, including colitis, dermatitis, vitiligo, panhypopituitarism, and thyroiditis, were among dose-limiting toxicities in trials of this product in melanoma patients [50]. In general, trials of various OKT3 or anti-CD3 antibodies in nonhuman primates have also underestimated the immune activation and cytokine-release syndromes seen in first-in-human trials.

The July 2006 report of the Joint ABPI/BIA Early Stage Clinical Trial Taskforce [51] provides useful guidance on assessing the adequacy of preclinical safety characterization and the safety of proposed human starting doses for novel biopharmaceuticals. The report states:

> Since toxicity usually arises from exaggerated pharmacological effects, sometimes combined with a narrow therapeutic range and/or a steep dose–response relationship from the NOAEL to toxicity, the pharmacologically active dose is often a more sensitive indicator of potential toxicity for biotechnology-derived pharmaceuticals (compared to the preclinical NOAEL adjusted by a safety

margin). The safety assessment should take due account of the dose–, concentration– and time–response relationships, receptor occupancy, relative potency in animals versus humans and, unless otherwise justified, the starting dose in the first-in-human study should be below the MABEL as predicted from all available preclinical data (i.e., in vitro data in humans and animals and in vivo data in animals).

The MABEL is the "minimum anticipated biologically effective level." In the case of the Tegenero monoclonal anti-CD28 "superagonist" antibody, in vitro incubation of the product with human T cells caused release of large amounts of TNF-alpha, gamma-interferon, and IL-2. Parallel in vitro studies with cynomolgus monkey T cells were not performed. These studies would likely have demonstrated a different pharmacodynamic profile in the safety species. In vivo studies in cynomolgus monkeys showed very limited release of cytokines after TGN1412 dosing [52]. This was used to justify a healthy volunteer FIH trial dose using 1/10 the NOAEL (5 mg/kg) as a maximum dose, and 1/500 of the claimed NOAEL as the starting dose (0.1 mg/kg) Despite this large safety margin versus the monkey NOAEL, life-threatening toxicities due to cytokine-release syndrome and profound T cell depletion were seen in the first human cohort that was dosed [53].

The ABPI/BIA taskforce recommendation of basing the first human dose on the MABEL, rather than solely on the NOAEL in a toxicology species, would have led to a lower and less hazardous human starting dose. These recommendations should guide design of future preclinical safety programs and future FIH clinical protocols, particularly for products with novel targets and mechanisms and pharmacodynamics and with restricted species specificity.

In a preclinical study of the immunosuppressive drug FK778, suppression of lymphocyte proliferation was studied with whole blood from four cynomolgus monkeys and four healthy human volunteers. This study showed the IC50 for FK778 to be lower in human than in monkey blood [54]. These and similar data were used to design the FIH trials, and this example provided guidance for extrapolations from in vivo preclinical safety studies.

With regards to glycosylated protein biopharmaceuticals, including monoclonal antibodies, it may be important to consider another distinction between protein therapeutics made in human and nonhuman mammalian cells, and between the human and nonhuman primate immune systems. One significant difference between humans and the Macaque monkeys typically used in safety studies, and between plasma-derived human immunoglobulins and recombinant antibodies produced in nonhuman mammalian cell lines, is the pattern of sialic acid usage. Most mammalian glycoproteins, including antibodies, display two major sialic acids, *N*-acetylneuraminic acid (Neu5Ac) and *N*-glycolylneuraminic acid (Neu5Gc). However, humans lack Neu5Gc on glycoproteins, because of a mutation in CMP-Neu5Ac hydroxylase, which occurred after evolutionary divergence from great apes [55]. Indeed this difference accounts for the resistance of monkeys and chimpanzees to human malarial infections [56].

SIGLEC family receptors, which recognize these sialic acids, serve to down-regulate macrophage activation induced via FcR interactions, as well as TCR-mediated lymphocyte activation, by signaling through intracellular tyrosine-based inhibitory motifs (ITIMs). Antibodies produced in CHO cells may have sialic acid residues that are not recognized efficiently by human SIGLECs, and thus may be poor ligands for these important inhibitory regulatory receptors [57]. The pattern of glycosylation and sialic acid usage, particularly in the Fc region, strongly affect the effector functions of antibodies [58]. For example, nonfucosylated MAbs produced in mutated CHO cells are far more potent inducers of ADDC in human cell systems than their homologues, which are highly fucosylated in normal CHO cells [59].

Additionally a recent article by Nguyyen et al. reports that human T cells give a much stronger proliferative response than chimpanzee T cells when activated via the TCR, although responses are similar after stimulation by the mitogen, PHA. This is correlated with the evolutionary loss in humans of the inhibitory Siglec-5 receptor on lymphocytes. Transfection of human T cells with chimpanzee Siglec-5 eliminated this increased responsiveness to TCR activation [60]. These data should help refute those that argue that more predictive preclinical safety studies of human biopharmaceuticals might, in the future, be performed using chimpanzees instead of monkeys. Indeed in terms of sialic acid and SIGLEC receptor usage, new world Aotus monkeys (unlike the chimpanzee) may more closely model human pharmacologic responses to immunomodulators [61].

However, nonhuman primates do overcome one significant limitation of nonprimate safety species, which is the lack of gamma-delta T cell populations. Part of the innate immune surveillance system, gamma-delta T cells are critical for clearance of intracellular bacterial pathogens, and they respond to low molecular weight nonpeptidic phospho-antigens in an MHC-unrestricted fashion. These cells express CD28, and other co-stimulatory receptors and can rapidly produce large amounts of TNF-alpha and gamma-interferon when activated. They are well represented in the T cell repertoire of nonhuman primates, and they appear to respond similarly to phosphoantigens [62]. Nevertheless, it is unknown whether differential expression of inhibitory SIGLEC receptors in monkeys compared to humans may alter gamma-delta T cell reactivity to potential biopharmaceuticals, which could target or stimulate these cells.

14.8 SUMMARY

The burden is on the clinical investigator, the biopharmaceutical sponsor, and the regulatory reviewer to be certain that the risk of exaggerated pharmacodynamic effects, off-target toxicities, and other harmful outcomes in first-in-human trials are reduced to the maximum extent possible, especially for healthy volunteer studies, which are now increasingly common for biopharmaceuticals. Novel therapeutics require a careful comparison of the pharmacodynamic effects in human cells and tissues and those of the safety model species, thoughtful and individualized design of safety pharmacology and immunotoxicity studies, and careful attention to selection of a safe starting dose and to pharmacodynamic monitoring in clinical protocols. Clinical investigators and institutional review boards should examine data carefully with this mandate in mind, and not rely exclusively on conclusions of the regulatory review process for first-in-human trials.

REFERENCES

1. ICH Guidance S7A.
2. ICH Guidance S6. Preclinical Safety Evaluation of Biotechnology-Derived Pharmaceuticals.
3. ICH Guidance S8. Immunotoxicity Studies for Human Pharmaceuticals.
4. Clarke J, Leach W, Pippig S, et al. Evaluation of a surrogate antibody for preclinical safety testing of an anti CD-11a monoclonal antibody. *Regul Toxicol Pharmacol* 2004;40(3):219–26.
5. Leung R, Whittaker P. RNA interference: from gene silencing to gene-specific therapeutics. *Pharmacol Ther*. 2005;107(2):222–39.
6. Dufour JH, Dziejman M, Liu MT, et al. IFN-γ-inducible protein 10 (IP-10;CXCL10)-deficient mice reveal a role for IP-10 in effector T cell generation and trafficking. *J Immunol* 2002;168:3195–3204.
7. Huang X, Wu J, Zhu W, Pytela R, Sheppard D. Expression of the human integrin beta6 subunit in alveolar type II cells and bronchiolar epithelial cells reverses lung inflammation in beta6 knockout mice. *Am J Respir Cell Mol Biol* 1998;19(4): 636–42.
8. Sheppard D. Integrin-mediated activation of transforming growth factor-beta(1) in pulmonary fibrosis. *Chest*. 2001;120(1 Suppl):49S–53S.
9. Herzyk D, Gore E, Polsky R, et al. Immunomodulatory effects of anti-CD4 antibody in host resistance against infections and tumors in human CD4 transgenic mice. *Infect Immun* 2001;69(2):1032–43.
10. Green J, Black, L. Overview of preclinical safety assessment for immunomodulatory biopharmaceuticals. *Hum Exp Toxicol* 200 19(4):208–12.
11. Hart TK, Blackburn MN, Brigham-Burke M, et al. Preclinical efficacy and safety of pascolizumab (SB 240683): a humanized anti-interleukin-4 antibody with therapeutic potential in asthma. *Clin Exp Immunol* 2002;130(1):93–100.
12. Hart TK, Cook RM, Zia-Amirhosseini P, et al. Preclinical efficacy and safety of mepolizumab (SB-240563), a humanized monoclonal antibody to IL-5, in cynomolgus monkeys. *J Allergy Clin Immunol* 2001;108(2):250–7.

13. *www.mdsps.com/over/MarketingMaterials/SafetyPharmacologyBrochure.pdf.*

14. Meijer R, Koopmans R, ten Berge I, Schellekens P. Pharmacokinetics of murine anti-human CD3 antibodies in man are determined by the disappearance of target antigen. *J Pharmcol Exp Ther* 2002;300(1):346–53.

15. Lawrence C, Pollard C, Hammond T, and Valentin J. Nonclinical proarrythmia models: predicting torsades de pointes. *J Pharmacol Toxicol Meth* 2005;52(1): 46–56.

16. Finlayson K, Witchel H, McCulloch J, and Sharkey J. Acquired QT interval prolongation and HERG: implications for drug discovery and development. *Eur J Pharmacol* 2004;500(1–3):129–42.

17. Redfern W, Carlsson L, Davis A, et al. Relationships between preclinical cardiac electrophysiology, clinical QT interval prlongation, and torsades de points for a broad range of drug: evidence for a provisional safety margin in drug development. *Cardiovasc Res* 2003;58(1):32–45.

18. Kupferschmidt H, Meier CH, Sulzer M, et al. Clinico-pharmacological case (2). Bradycardia and ventricular tachycardia of the torsades de pointes type as a side effect of vasopressin: 3 case reports. *Schweiz Rundsch Med Prax* 1996;85(11): 340–3.

19. Sartiani L, De Paoli P, Lonardo G, et al. Does recombinant human interleukin-11 exert direct electrophysiologic effects on. single human atrial myocytes? *J Cardiovasc Pharmacol* 2002;39(3):425–34.

20. Schneider JW, Chang AY, Garratt A. Trastuzumab cardiotoxicity: speculations regarding pathophysiology and targets. for further study. *Semin Oncol* 2002;29(3 Suppl 11):22–8.

21. Eckart RE, Love SS, Atwood JE, et al. Incidence and follow-up of inflammatory cardiac complications after smallpox vaccination. *J Am Coll Cardiol* 2004;44(1): 201–5.

22. Parasrampuria D, de Boer P, Desai-Krietger D, et al. Single-dose pharmacokinetics and pharmacodynamics of RWJ 67657, a specific p28 MAP kinase inhbitor: a first-in-human study, *J Clin Pharmacol* 2003;43(4):406–13.

23. Wong Y, Rossignol D, Rose, J, et al. Safety, pharmacokinetics, and pharmacodynamics of E5564, a lipid A antagonist, during an ascending single-dose clinical study. *J Clin Pharmacol* 2003;34(7):745–42.

24. Timmer W, Leclerc V, Birraux G, et al. The new PDE4 inhibitor roflumilast is efficacious in exercise-induced asthma and leads to suppression of LPS-stimulated TNF-alpha ex vivo. *J Clin Pharmacol* 2002;42(3):297–303.

25. Valenti MT, Azzarello G, Vinante O, et al. Differentiation, proliferation and apoptosis levels in human leiomyoma and leiomyosarcoma. *J Cancer Res Clin Oncol* 1998;124(2):93–105. *J Immunol Meth* 1995;184(1):39–51.

26. Vermes I, Haanen C, Steffens-Nakken H, et al. A novel assay for apoptosis: flow cytometric detection of phosphatidylserine expression on early apoptotic cells using fluorescein labelled Annexin V. *J Immunol Meth* 1995;184(1):39–51.

27. Damianovich M, Ziv I, Heyman SN, Rosen S, et al. ApoSense: a novel technology for functional molecular imaging of cell death inmodels of acute renal tubular necrosis. *Eur J Nucl Med Mol Imaging* 2006;33(3):281–91.

28. Verplanke AJ, Herber RF, de Wit R. Comparison of renal function parameters in the assessment Of cis-platin induced nephrotoxicity. *Nephron* 1994;66(3):267–72.

29. Ichimura T, Hung CC, Yang SA, et al. Kidney injury molecule-1: a tissue and urinary biomarker for nephrotoxicant-induced renal injury. *Am J Renal Physiol* 2004;286(3): F552–63.

30. Herman EH, Zhang J, Lipshultz SE, et al. Correlation between serum levels of cardiac troponin-T and the severity of the chronic cardiomyopathy induced by doxorubicin. *J Clin Oncol* 1999;17(7):2237–43.

31. Fielden MR, Pearson C, Brennan R, Kolaja KL. Preclinical drug safety analysis by chemogenomic profiling in the liver. *J Pharmacogenomics* 2005;5(3):161–71.

32. Waring JF, Liguori MJ, Luyendyk JP, Microarray analysis of lipopolysaccharide potentiation of trovafloxacin-induced liver injury in rats suggests a role for proinflammatory chemokines and neutrophils. *J Pharmacol Exp Ther* 2006;316(3): 1080–7.

33. Ruehl-Fehlert C, Bradley A, George C, et al. Harmonization of immunotoxicity guidelines in the ICH process—pathology considerations from the guideline committee of the European Society of Toxicological Pathology (ESTP). *Exp Toxicol Pathol* 2005;57(1):1–5.

34. Suntharalingam G, Perry MR, Ward S, et al. Cytokine storm in a phase 1 trial of the anti-CD28 monoclonal antibody TGN1412. *N Engl J Med* 2006;355(10): 1018–28.

35. Swaisland HC, Smith RP, Laight A, et al. Single-dose clinical pharmacokinetic studies of gefitinib. *Clin Pharmacokinet* 2005;44(11):1165–77.

36. Swaisland HC, Ranson M, Smith RP, et al. Pharmacokinetic drug interactions of gefitinib with rifampicin, itraconazole and metoprolol. *Clin Pharmacokinet* 2005;44(10):1067–81.

37. Frohna P, Lu J, Eppler S, et al. Evaluation of the absolute oral bioavailability and bioequivalence oferlotinib, an inhibitor of the epidermal growth factor receptor tyrosine kinase, in a randomized, crossover study in healthy subjects. *J Clin Pharmacol* 2006;46(3):282–90.

38. Barten MJ, Rahmel A, Garbade J, et al. C0h/C2h monitoring of the pharmacodynamics of cyclosporin plus mycophenolate mofetil in human heart transplant recipients. *Transplant Proc* 2005;37(2):1360–1.

39. Barten MJ, Streit F, Boeger M, et al. Synergistic effects of sirolimus with cyclosporine and tacrolimus: analysis of immunosuppression on lymphocyte proliferation and activation in rat whole blood. *Transplantation* 2004;77(8):1154–62.

40. Barten MJ, Dhein S, Chang H, et al. Assessment of immunosuppressive drug interactions: inhibition of lymphocyte function in peripheral human blood. *J Immunol Meth* 2003;283(1–2):99–114.

41. Zeevi A, Britz JA, Bentlejewski CA Monitoring immune function during tacrolimus tapering in small bowel transplant recipients. *Transpl Immunol* 2005;15(1): 17–24.

42. Perez O, Krutzik P, Nolan G. Flow cytometric analysis of kinase signaling cascades. *Meth Mol Biol* 2004;263:67–94.

43. Krutzik P, Hale M, Nolan G. Characterization of the murine immunological signaling network with phosphospecific flow cytometry. *J Immunol* 2005;175(4): 2366–73.

44. Krutzik PO, Clutter MR, Nolan GP. Coordinate analysis of murine immune cell surface markers and intracellularphosphoproteins by flow cytometry. *J Immunol* 2005;175(4):2357–65.

45. Grammer A, Fischer R, Lee O, et al. Flow cytometric assessment of the signaling status of human B lymphocytes from normal and autoimmune individuals. *Arthritis Res Ther* 2004;6(1):28–38.

46. Chow S, Hedley D, Grom P, Magari R, Jacobberger JW, Shankey TV. Whole blood fixation and permeabilization protocol with red blood cell lysis for flow cytometry of intracellular phosphorylated epitopes in leukocyte subpopulations. *Cytometry A* 2005;67(1):4–17.

47. Ronzoni S, Faretta M, Ballarini M, et al. New method to detect histone acetylation levels by flow cytometry. *Cytometry* 2005;66(1):52–61.

48. Chung EJ, Lee S, Sausville EA, et al. Histone deacetylase inhibitor pharmacodynamic analysis by multiparameter flowcytometry. *Ann Clin Lab Sci* 2005;35(4): 397–406.

49. Keler T, Halk E, Vitale L, et al. Activity and safety of CTLA-4 blockade combined with vaccines in cynomolgus macaques. *J Immunol* 2003;171(11):6251–9.

50. Ribas A, Camacho LH, Lopez-Berestein, et al. Antitumor activity in melanoma and anti-self responses in a phase I trial with the anti-cytotoxic T lymphocyte-associated antigen 4 monoclonal antibody. *J Clin Oncol* 2005;23(35):8968–77.

51. *http://www.abpi.org.uk/information/pdfs/BIAABPI_taskforce2.pdf*.

52. Tegenero. 1412 Investigators Brochure, 19 Dec 2005.

53. Suntharalingam G, Perry MR, Ward S, et al. Cytokine storm in a phase 1 trial of the anti-CD28 monoclonal antibody TGN1412. *N Engl J Med* 2006;355(10):1018–28.

54. Birsan T, Dambrin C, Klupp J, et al. Effects of FK778 on immune functions in vitro in whole blood from non-human primates and healthy human volunteers. *Transpl Immunol* 2003;11(2)164–7.

55. Gagneux P, Cheriyan M, Hurtado-Ziola N, et al. Human-specific regulation of alpha 2-6-linked sialic acids. *J Biol Chem* 2003;278(48):48245–50.

56. Martin MJ, Rayner JC, Gagneux P, Barnwell JW, Varki A. Evolution of human-chimpanzee differences in malaria susceptibility:relationship to human genetic loss of N-glycolylneuraminic acid. *Proc Natl Acad Sci USA* 2005;102(36):12819–24.

57. Scallon BJ, Tam SH, McCarthy SG, Cai AN, Raju TS. Higher levels of sialylated Fc glycans in immunoglobulin G molecules Can adversely impact functionality. *Mol Immunol* 2007;44(7):1524–34.

58. Hodoniczky J, Zheng YZ, James DC. Control of recombinant monoclonal antibody effector functions by Fc N-glycanremodeling in vitro. *Biotechnol Prog* 2005;21(6): 1644–52.

59. Niwa R, Hatanaka S, Shoji-Hosaka E, et al. Enhancement of the antibody-dependent cellular cytotoxicity of low-fucose IgG1 is independent of FcgammaRIIIa functional polymorphism. *Clin Cancer Res* 2004;10(18 Pt 1):6248–55.

60. Nguyen DH, Hurtado-Ziola N, Gagneux P, Varki A. Loss of Siglec expression on T lymphocytes during human evolution. *Proc Natl Acad Sci USA* 2006;103(20): 7765–70.

61. McConkey EH, Varki A. Genomics. Thoughts on the future of great ape research. *Proc Natl Acad Sci USA* 2005;102(36):12819–24.

62. Cairo C, Propp N, Hebbeler AM, et al. The Vgamma2/Vdelta2 T-cell repertoire in Macaca fascicularis: functional responses to phosphoantigen stimulation by the Vgamma2/Jgamma1.2 subset. *Immunology* 2005;115(2):197–205.

CHAPTER 15

Genetic Toxicology Testing of Biopharmaceuticals

DAVID JACOBSON-KRAM, PhD, DABT, and HANAN GHANTOUS, PhD, DABT

The potential for carcinogenic risk should be considered for all new pharmaceuticals especially those drugs that are intended for chronic use. In general, results from carcinogenicity testing are only available at the time of submission of a new drug application (NDA) or a biological license application (BLA). As a result hundreds or even thousands of individuals may be exposed during the drug development process without an understanding of potential for carcinogenicity. Phase 1 studies for new drugs are often performed in healthy volunteers for whom there is no obvious benefit. So risks for this population, in particular, should be exceedingly low.

Because carcinogenicity results are not available during the course of clinical trials, the FDA relies on the results of genotoxicity studies as a surrogate for potential cancer risk. The standard battery of assays recommended for small molecules as described in the ICH S2B guidance (A Standard Battery for Genotoxicity Testing of Pharmaceuticals) [1] was, however, not designed to include assessments of biopharmaceuticals. This is because in the absence of specific transport mechanisms, it was considered unlikely that large peptides and protein molecules would enter the cell and interact with cellular DNA or other chromosomal material to pose genotoxic risk. It is possible that large molecules enter a cell in a nonspecific manner, for example, through endocytosis. In fact externally applied restriction endonucleases have been shown to induce chromosomal aberrations in cultured cells [2,3].

In general, genotoxicity standard assays (e.g., bacterial reverse mutation assay [Ames test], in vitro chromosomal aberration assay, mouse lymphoma gene mutation assay, and rodent micronucleus assay) may not be suitable assays because the test cells do not contain the appropriate receptors to transport the product (i.e., not a relevant species) or because the biopharmaceutical

Preclinical Safety Evaluation of Biopharmaceuticals: A Science-Based Approach to Facilitating Clinical Trials, edited by Joy A. Cavagnaro

has an indirect mechanism that is not expressed in isolated in vitro systems. False positives have also been observed in the standard Ames test because of the presence of growth-promoting constituents in the test sample such as histidine or its precursors. In addition the genetic toxicity assays often rely on cytotoxicity to ensure assay validity, an effect difficult to reach with most biopharmaceuticals. Conducting these assays with large quantities of protein can sometimes confound the interpretation of the results.

General testing for genotoxic impurities may also not be appropriate, since the impurities and contaminants that may be contained in a biopharmaceutical product include residual host cell proteins and nucleic material, fermentation components, manufacturing process components such as column leachables and detergents, bacteria and viral particles, they do not include organic chemicals typically found in small-molecule manufacturing. However, genotoxicity testing of protein- or immunoconjugates (products containing organic chemical linkers) might be appropriate, particularly when a residual organic linker is found in the product because of the instability of the conjugate during storage or upon dilution in serum.

If genotoxicity appears to be a potential issue with a biologic product, it is uncertain whether the standard ICH battery would be adequate to assess this potential hazard. In a publication by Gocke et al. in 1999 [4], genotoxicity data for biologics were obtained from several sponsors. In summary, 4 of 78 biologic compounds assessed for genotoxicity (using a total of 177 assays) demonstrated genotoxic effects. These four were proteins: One was an antibody fragment conjugated to an organic chemical linker, and the positive effect was concluded to be produced by the linker. The second protein was positive in the mouse lymphoma test but not in the Ames test and the micronucleus test. However, no information was provided describing the compound, so no conclusion can be drawn. The third compound was a natural lipase, and the chromosomal aberrations observed with this product are most likely a result of the endonucleases released upon destruction of lysosomal membranes. This suggests that the protein was able to enter the cell in a nonspecific fashion. The fourth protein, glucagon, showed very weak and inconsistent positive signals with both endogenous and recombinant glucagon, and the effect is most likely attributed to its physiological activity.

In addition, and as discussed in the Draft guidance for biopharmaceuticals [5], a positive result in a genotoxicity assay of a biopharmaceutical may actually be the result of an exaggerated pharmacological response and not a direct DNA modification by the product, as is the case for lipase, glucagon, erythropoietin, and DNAse. DNAse was predictably positive in an in vitro clastogenicity assay only following electroporation. Recombinant and native erythropoietin increase the frequency of micronucleated polychromatic erythrocytes in bone marrow of mice but produce negative results in the bacterial reverse mutation tests and do not induce chromosomal aberrations in vitro in Chinese hamster ovary (CHO) cells or human peripheral blood lymphocytes. The induction of micronuclei was shown to be due to the accelerated proliferation and differentiation of erythrocytes and promotion of early release of polychromatic erythrocytes [6,7,8], an exaggerated effect of its mechanism of action. Therefore, in cases where it is deemed necessary to assess the ability of the biopharmaceutical to modify genetic material, careful attention should be given to the study design and to the interpretation of the results.

Twenty-seven out of 44 FDA-approved biopharmaceuticals have been tested in a battery of genotoxicity assays. Eighty-five different assays performed yielded negative results. The most commonly performed assays were the Ames test, the chromosomal aberration assay in human lymphocytes, the mouse lymphoma gene mutation assay, and the mammalian in vivo erythrocyte micronucleus test. Examples of the range of biopharmaceutical products tested include, dornase alfa (deoxyribonuclease I-DNAse), trastuzumab (mAb to human epidermal growth factor receptor 2), alteplase (tissue plasminogen activator), infliximab (mAb to the human tumor necrosis factor α).

In determining whether genotoxicity testing is appropriate and necessary, a variety of factors should be considered (see Figure 15.1 [5]):

- The properties of the biopharmaceutical.
- Whether the product is produced by fermentation or chemically synthesized.
- Presence of residual organic chemicals or small molecules used in modification of a protein or inclusion of transporter sequences that localize the biopharmaceutical to the nucleus during manufacturing.
- The stability of the product should be considered, whether the product is a protein- or immunoconjugate.
- The presence of a "free" organic linker in the product.
- The pharmacology and mechanism of action of the product.
- If the product alters DNA or RNA integrity, such as DNAses and ribozymes, the feasibility of the product and by-products interacting with nuclear material in intact cells under normal physiological conditions (i.e., in the absence of cell permeability enhancing agents and techniques) should be taken into consideration before performing standard genotoxicity tests.

The standard battery of genotoxicity tests or selected tests might be appropriate to determine the toxicity of conjugates or organic/chemical linkers in the molecule (e.g., Mylotarg). In these cases careful attention should be given to the study design of tests used to assess the potential for gene mutation, chromosome aberrations, and/or DNA damage.

Biopharmaceuticals may be nongenotoxic but have tumorigenic potential. For example, cytokines and growth factors may directly lead to cell proliferation as a function of drug receptor activation or may secondarily modulate growth as a result of production and activation of a complex cascade of cytokines and moieties (e.g., nitrous oxide). While the concerns for these types of

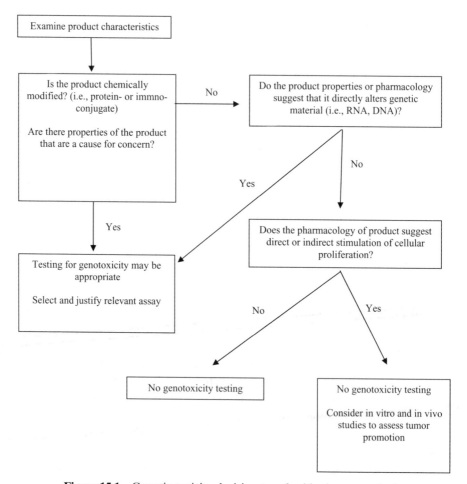

Figure 15.1   Genetic toxicity decision tree for biopharmaceuticals.

products in promoting tumor growth are valid, they cannot be addressed with genotoxicity assays. Appropriate in vitro and in vivo assays should, however, be considered (e.g., assessing the ability of the growth factor to stimulate tumor growth or alter the sensitivity of tumor cells to chemotherapy using in vitro and/or in vivo tumor xenograft models).

REFERENCES

1. ICH S2B. A Standard Battery for Genotoxicity Testing of Pharmaceuticals, 1997.
2. Obe G, Jonas R, Schmidt S. The restriction endonuclease Alu I induces chromosomal aberrations in human peripheral blood lymphocytes in vitro. *Mutat Res* 1986;163:271–5.

3. Vasudev V, Obe G. Evidence for a recptor-mediated endocytosis of Alu I in Chinese hamster ovary cells. *Mutat Res* 1988;197:109–16.

4. Gocke E, Albertini S, Brendel-Schwaab S, Muller L, Suter W, et al. Genotoxicity testing of biotechnology-derived products. Report of a GUM task force. *Mutat Res* 1999;436:137–56.

5. FDA Draft Guidance for Industry, Nonclinical Safety Evaluation of Biotechnology-Derived Pharmaceuticals (in preparation).

6. Yajima N, Kurata Y, Imai E, Sawai T, Takeshita Y. Genotoxicty of genetic recombinant erythropoietin in a novel test system. *Mutagenesis* 1993;8:231–6.

7. Yajima N, Kurata Y, Sawai T, Takeshita Y. Comparative studies in induction of micronuclei by three genetically recombinant and urinary human erythropoietins. *Mutagenesis* 2003;8:237–41.

8. Yajima N, Kurata Y, Sawai T, Takeshita Y. Induction of micronucleated erythrocytes by recombinant human erythropoietin. *Mutagenesis* 2003;8:221–9.

CHAPTER 16

General Toxicity Testing and Immunotoxicity Testing for Biopharmaceuticals

JEANINE L. BUSSIERE, PhD, DABT

Contents

16.1 INTRODUCTION

For general toxicity testing of biopharmaceuticals, the first step is identifying a "relevant" species (see Chapters 9 and 12). The choice of relevant species will determine the strategy for testing the general toxicity of the molecule. If the molecule is pharmacologically active in both rodent and nonrodent species, then the toxicology studies should be conducted in two species [1]. Often biopharmaceuticals are more restricted in their species cross-reactivity, and may only be pharmacologically active in nonhuman primates. In this case general toxicity testing in one species is sufficient, but the challenge is to conduct specialty studies in this relevant species such as reproductive toxicity,

Preclinical Safety Evaluation of Biopharmaceuticals: A Science-Based Approach to Facilitating Clinical Trials, edited by Joy A. Cavagnaro

immunotoxicity, or safety pharmacology. If the biopharmaceutical is only active in chimpanzees, then alternate strategies for assessing safety need to be considered. The strategies could include use of a surrogate molecule (i.e., the homologous protein in the animal species, or a monoclonal antibody that cross-reacts with the animal receptor/ligand) or use of a transgenic or knock-out mouse. These various options will be discussed in this chapter.

16.1.1   Molecule Is Pharmacologically Active in Rodents and Nonrodents

If the biopharmaceutical is pharmacologically active in rodents and nonro-dents, a more standard toxicology program can be used. In general, repeat-dose studies in both rodents and nonrodents are conducted to support first-in-human (FIH) trials, along with an assessment of safety pharmacology. The duration of repeat-dose studies is similar to those studies supporting the development of small-molecule pharmaceuticals and should follow the ICH M3 guidance [2]. In addition, if the biopharmaceutical is a monoclonal anti-body, then an in vitro tissue cross-reactivity study is conducted with a panel of human tissues as well as tissues from the species used in the toxicology studies (discussed in Chapter 10). Ideally the route and frequency of adminis-tration should mimic the clinical regimen as closely as possible. Cardiovascular safety pharmacology can be assessed in a stand-alone study in nonrodents, or these endpoints can be incorporated into the repeat-dose study. Respiratory and CNS activity can be assessed in separate studies in rats or incorporated into the repeat-dose study. Between the FIH study and the biological license application (BLA), additional toxicology studies will include subchronic and chronic studies (the duration of these studies are outlined in the ICH M3 and S6 guidances). Typically a duration of six months is acceptable for the chronic study [3]. In addition reproductive toxicology studies are conducted in rats (fertility, embryo-fetal development, peri/postnatal development) and rabbits (embryo-fetal development). For certain indications (i.e., oncology) reproduc-tive testing in one species is generally sufficient.

Immunogenicity is an important issue to consider for biopharmaceuticals as it can limit toxicity testing. An immune response to the biopharmaceutical is expected because the test agents are human proteins administered to animals, and the response can limit the duration of the toxicity studies. Antibodies to a test agent can neutralize its activity and thus reduce exposure. In addition antidrug antibodies can potentially cause toxicity such as deposition of immune complexes in the kidney. This issue is discussed further in Chapter 10.

Mainly because of species specificity and immunogenicity, carcinogenicity studies are generally not appropriate for biopharmaceuticals. However, in cases of immune suppressants or growth factors where there is cause for concern, assessment of carcinogenicity/tumorigenicity has been expected. If the biopharmaceutical is pharmacologically active in rodents, a carcinogenicity study can be conducted if needed, and if immunogenicity does not prevent exposure. In species-specific immune suppressants, the nonchronic toxicity study has been extended to 9 and 12 months to address this concern [3].

Immunotoxicity testing as outlined in the ICH S8 document [4] is not intended to cover biopharmaceuticals. However, many of the same assays can be used to assess immunologic effects of biopharmaceuticals [5,6]. These assays can help assess immunopharmacology as well as potential immunotoxicity as discussed later in this chapter.

16.1.2 Molecule Is Pharmacologically Active in Nonrodents Only

A typical toxicology program for a biopharmaceutical may be limited to repeat-dose studies in nonhuman primates (NHP) only (if that is the only species in which the drug is pharmacologically active), a safety pharmacology study, reproductive toxicology studies, and a tissue cross-reactivity study (for monoclonal antibodies only). Local tolerance of the test article can be evaluated in the repeat-dose toxicology study (histopathological evaluation of the injection site) or can be assessed in a stand-alone rabbit local tolerance test. Although the biopharmaceutical may not cross-react with the rabbit target, this test allows for the evaluation of the irritant potential of the clinical candidate.

The NHP has played an important role in the development of biopharmaceuticals by facilitating the general safety assessment and evaluation of these products in specialty disease areas. For example, aging primates are used to study geriatric diseases and osteoporosis, and for many ocular indications including macular degeneration, and retinopathy, or for testing retinal implants. Nonhuman primate models are also being developed to better understand the effects of drugs on the reproductive system and the immune system in order to better mimic effects that may be seen in humans. Several books have been published describing the various models in NHP and their use in drug development [7,8].

Nonhuman primate toxicity tests of biopharmaceuticals most often use macaques—primarily cynomolgus monkeys (*Macaca fasicularis*), although rhesus monkeys (*Macaca mulatta*) are also sometimes used. A large historical database exists for both rhesus and cynomolgus monkeys, and many contract research organizations (CROs) have experience with both strains. Some advantages of Macaques are that blood volume is not as limited as in rodents and many of the blood/serum-based markers of toxicity in NHP can then be used in clinical trials, allowing for direct comparison of the toxic effects of the drug in the preclinical studies with the effects seen in human patients.

Marmosets (*Callithrix jacchus*) may also be used and their small size (350–500 g) is both an advantage and a disadvantage. The advantages can include the small amount of test material needed and the relatively small amount of space required for suitable housing. The main disadvantage of small size is the low volume of blood that may be obtained. Also many biological therapeutics cross-react with cynomolgus or rhesus targets but not marmoset. Fewer CROs have experience with the marmoset and the historical database is more limited. However, certain CROs do have experience with toxicity testing in marmosets [9].

The age and size of the monkey are important considerations in the toxicity testing of biopharmaceuticals. Generally, animals should not be smaller than 2 kg as this limits the blood volume available for sampling. Younger animals are also less able to handle the stress of the various procedures on the study and may be more susceptible to GI effects (i.e., diarrhea), leading to confounding toxicities unrelated to the test article. In addition smaller animals are likely sexually immature and may respond to the drug differently than an adult animal. Evaluating effects on reproductive organs in the general toxicity studies is also problematic in these immature animals due to extensive variability or a lack of/exaggerated response. The appropriate age of the animals may further depend on the biological activity of the compound, and the age of the expected patient population. Most CROs have historical data ranges for clinical pathology parameters from animals of various age ranges as well as from various sources. Maintaining the same strain and source of animals throughout the drug development program, and not switching because of animal availability, is very important. Animals from different sources can vary significantly in hematology or immunophenotyping parameters, which can make interpretation across studies difficult.

Neonatal or juvenile monkey studies are difficult to conduct, but these studies may be necessary depending on the intended patient population. If a juvenile monkey study is to be conducted to support use of the therapeutic in pediatric patients, the appropriate age in the cynomolgus monkey, that closely matches the intended patient population, must be carefully considered. Unfortunately, the appropriate age may vary depending on the target organ of the therapeutic, and target organs of potential toxicity. For example, the age of a monkey that is appropriate to mimic neurologic developmental parameters in humans may be different than that to mimic immunologic or reproductive developmental parameters [10]. Neonatal studies can only be conducted by CROs that have breeding capabilities on site, as it is difficult to ship animals less than six months of age because of the stress of shipping, yet few CROs have a large enough population of young animals the same age to use for a toxicology study. For the development of new therapies for geriatric diseases (prostate disease, ocular pathology, osteoporosis, diabetes, Alzheimer's disease, etc.) it is important to understand how age-related disease and pathology develop. The cynomolgus monkey has been used for this type of testing and some CROs have special groups of older animals (generally 13 years of age and older). Ovarectomized cynomolgus monkeys are the most well-established model for osteoporosis [11], and ocular toxicity testing is also well-established in NHP [12–15].

The viral status of the monkeys is also important to test, especially prior to longer term studies (≥3 months duration). Many biological therapeutics are immune modulators, and latent viral infections can manifest in the chronic studies and confound the interpretation. Choosing B-virus negative animals is most important when an immunomodulatory compound is being tested.

Cardiovascular and CNS effects are often evaluated as part of the general toxicity program. ECGs can be measured in the repeated-dose toxicology studies although these are usually conducted in anesthetized animals. Stand-alone safety pharmacology studies (mainly cardiovascular/respiratory safety pharmacology studies) can be conducted in alert, telemetered animals. These are typically nonterminal single-dose studies, however, and additional data from anesthetized animals in repeated-dose studies can be valuable to look at potential multiple-dose effects. CNS safety pharmacology studies have not been validated in the NHP, but a small number of observations can be added to the cardiovascular/respiratory study. In addition, if the biopharmaceutical is a monoclonal antibody, an in vitro tissue cross-reactivity study is conducted with a panel of human and NHP tissues to address nonspecific binding of the monoclonal antibody.

Because the pharmacological action of biopharmaceuticals may occur at very low doses, a no observable effect level (NOEL) may not be seen in the repeated-dose toxicology studies. Testing the biological therapeutic at doses lower than the clinical range to try to achieve a NOEL does not add value to the clinical program. The no observable adverse effect level (NOAEL) is typically used in the safety studies. It can be difficult to determine what findings in the toxicology study are due to exaggerated pharmacology and when these findings become adverse and represent toxicity. Several considerations can be used to determine if these effects should be considered adverse, including a combined analysis of the biological and statistical effects, the presence of a dose–response relationship, whether the findings are seen in both sexes, whether the findings are outside the historical control range, and if related histopathological correlates exist. In addition, the clinical indication, the monitorability and reversibility of the effect, and the risk–benefit analysis for the patient population need to be considered. An adverse effect may be considered to be a change that may impair performance and generally have a detrimental effect on growth, development or life span, so it should be an effect that would be unacceptable if it occurred in a human clinical trial [16]. In addition, because the pharmacological activity of biopharmaceuticals may be very different in the disease state for which the test agent is being developed than in the healthy animals employed in the toxicology studies, adverse findings or exaggerated pharmacological effects may not be seen in the toxicology studies. If little to no toxicity is seen, it may not be possible to define a maximum tolerated dose (MTD). In such cases the use of a maximum feasible dose (MFD) or the use of reasonable multiples over the clinical doses has been sufficient to demonstrate safety. What constitutes "reasonable multiples" will depend on the clinical indication (life threatening vs. non–life threatening), the patient population (consideration of special populations i.e., children, elderly, women of child-bearing potential), chronic versus acute treatment, concomitant medications, alternative therapies, and so forth.

16.1.3 Molecule Is Pharmacologically Active in Humans and Chimpanzees Only

In certain cases the human protein has been so species-specific that it will only cross-react with human and chimpanzees (*Pan troglodytes*). Although safety studies can be conducted in chimpanzees, many limitations exist (no histopathology can be conducted, only small animal numbers can be used, limited CROs can conduct the studies and/or countries may have restrictions in use, limited historical control data exist, etc.) such that these studies are not generally conducted. In cases where the chimpanzee is the only relevant nonhuman species, alternative strategies could include testing a surrogate molecule (the rodent protein in rodents, a monoclonal antibody that cross reacts with the cynomolgus epitope, etc.) or using transgenic or knockout mice that overexpress or have a deletion of the targeted protein.

Surrogate Molecules One alternative to using nonhuman primates (or if the biopharmaceutical does not cross-react with nonhuman primates) is to use a surrogate (homologous, analogous) molecule. This would be the homologous protein (i.e., the murine protein for use in mice) or, for a monoclonal antibody therapeutic, an antibody that cross-reacts with the rodent or cynomolgus monkey target. This allows for the safety testing of the pharmacologic activity of the test agent, but it does not allow for testing of the clinical candidate itself. The surrogate molecule, however, should resemble the clinical candidate as much as possible with regards to the production process, range of impurities/contaminants, pharmacokinetics, binding affinity, and pharmacological mechanism. Making and characterizing a second molecule along with the clinical candidate results in the use of a great deal of additional resources. Additional assays must be developed to detect the product and antibodies that might form to the product. However, these efforts can allow for a greater understanding of the potential toxicities of the therapeutic candidate. Some toxicology programs have utilized this approach, for example, to assess reproductive and developmental toxicities with a murine surrogate of interferon-gamma [17] and with a monoclonal antibody surrogate [18,19].

Transgenic/Knockout Animals Knockout and transgenic mice are rapidly gaining acceptance as routine tools for mechanistic research, and they offer considerable promise for generating specific models of toxicological importance. Gene-targeted or "knockout" animals have been created using molecular and cellular genetic engineering techniques to specifically lack an endogenous gene [20]. Knockout mice have been used to assess drug specificity, to investigate mechanisms of toxicity, and to screen for mutagenic and carcinogenic activities of therapeutic candidates. Similarly the impact of novel therapeutic candidates can be estimated in knockout mice; generation of viable and fertile animals with null mutations for a potential target protein implies that pharmacological inhibition of the molecule in vivo will elicit no major adverse effects. Furthermore the apparent lack of an in vivo phenotype could be used in conjunction with substantial evidence of in vitro efficacy to support the selection of a likely NOAEL for use in preclinical pharmacology and toxicology studies. Knockout and transgenic mice, however, are often structurally normal even if functional abnormalities are apparent, while many engineered mice appear to lack both structural and functional defects. Subtle phenotypes (functional and/or structural changes resulting from the genetic engineering event) sometimes may be unmasked using pharmacological challenges or other physiological stressors [21,22].

Particular emphasis in future pharmacology and toxicology studies will likely be directed toward conditional knockout mice (to evaluate the impact of chemically mediated inhibition of a particular gene product at the relevant stage of life) and "humanized" knock-in animals (in which the endogenous mouse gene is replaced with the homologous human gene to examine its role in disease or drug metabolism). Humanized mice are of particular importance as these animals can be employed to evaluate the efficacy and toxicity of human proteins that are not pharmacologically active in normal rodents or that induce a neutralizing antibody response that limits long-term exposure. One particular criticism is that humanized mice manufacture one or a few human proteins of interest, but other proteins that interact with the human molecule are still of mouse origin. The physiological effect of human–mouse protein interactions may differ slightly—or substantially—from that of the normal human–human protein association. With the increasing number of species-specific biopharmaceuticals in development, it becomes even more important to demonstrate that the knockout mice are a viable alternative to testing in NHP and are relevant to the findings seen in humans.

16.2 IMMUNOTOXICITY TESTING

Immunotoxicity testing guidelines exist for small molecules where the toxicology is largely unpredictable and rodent species are typically used [4]. Despite the lack of a specific guidance on immunotoxicity evaluation until now, most biopharmaceuticals have assessed the immunotoxic potential of the biopharmaceutical as a part of general single- and/or repeat-dose toxicity studies [5,23].

The ICH guidance on immunotoxicity testing suggests a weight-of-evidence decision making approach. The general principles that apply to this guideline are as follows:

1. All new human pharmaceuticals should be evaluated for the potential to produce immunotoxicity.
2. Methods include standard toxicity studies and additional immunotoxicity studies conducted as appropriate. Whether additional immunotoxicity studies are appropriate should be determined by a weight of evidence review.

Data from standard toxicity tests could indicate an adverse effect on the immune system, including changes in hematology, alterations in immune organ weights or histology, changes in serum globulins, increased incidence of infections, or increased occurrence of tumors. If the weight of evidence suggests that additional testing is needed, then it is suggested that an immune function study be conducted, such as the T-dependent antibody response (TDAR) and immunophenotyping of leukocyte populations. For small molecule drugs, these studies are generally conducted in rodents in a 28-day study.

Although the ICH S8 guidance does not specifically apply to biopharmaceuticals, the same principals for understanding immunotoxicity can be applied. Additionally, for human biopharmaceuticals, the immune system is often the intended target of the therapy and the immunotoxicity observed may be exaggerated pharmacology. In this case NHP are generally used and the immune tests have been selected based on the known immunomodulatory properties of the drug. These assays have also been used as pharmacodynamic markers of drug activity or efficacy for the immune modulators. It is important to distinguish among immunopharmacology, where the immune system is the target organ of the therapeutic effect; immunotoxicity, where nontarget immune effects such as autoimmunity or immunosuppression may be observed; and immunogenicity, which represents an immune response to the drug.

Specialized immunotoxicity tests typically are not routinely conducted unless an effect on the immune system was seen in the general toxicity studies, or there is a known pharmacologic effect of the test agent on the immune system. Additional immunotoxicity testing are conducted if there is cause for concern. The current regulatory guidelines recommend that immunopathology be used as the initial screen to detect immunotoxicity, since standard hematology and histopathology are often sufficient to detect immune system alterations. Immunopathology can include total and differential white blood cell counts, and evaluation of the histopathology of lymphoid organs such as the thymus, spleen, lymph nodes, gut-associated lymphoid tissue (GALT), and the bone marrow. In addition more detailed measurements of any change in size and cellularity of immune cells, germinal center development, cortex–medulla ratio of the thymus, and immunohistochemistry of the lymphoid organs may be included. Again, these parameters are examined as part of general toxicity studies for biopharmaceuticals.

Several important factors should be considered when including immunotoxicity testing into GLP (good laboratory practice) toxicology studies, especially if they are conducted in nonhuman primates. These include (1) whether the assays have been validated, (2) whether to use the main study animals or a satellite group, and (3) the timing of these tests within the context of the GLP toxicology study. The advantages of using the "main" study animals instead of "satellite" animals for immunotoxicity testing are reduced animal use and correlation of any immunotoxicity findings with other toxicities seen in those same animals. The disadvantage of using main study animals is that the additional manipulations for immune testing (e.g., injection of an antigen for determining antibody response) may influence the toxicity or immunogenicity of the therapeutic agent. It is very important to include several baseline measurements because of the variability seen between animals, and even in the same animal over time. Because of the small number of NHP per group, it is important to reduce the variability in the assays as much as possible with regard to antigen source, technique, and so forth.

Flow cytometry is often included in a GLP toxicology study of immunomodulators to evaluate changes in lymphocyte subsets, including T cells (CD4$^+$, CD8$^+$), B cells (CD20$^+$), NK cells (CD16$^+$), and monocytes (CD14$^+$). These assays are typically conducted using peripheral blood, which allows for repeated sampling over time within the same animal. However, immunophenotyping can also be conducted on tissues to determine if there are effects on lymphocyte trafficking, although time points are limited to study termination unless serial biopsies can be performed (i.e., on lymph nodes). Serial biopsies may be difficult because they cannot be performed by all laboratories, and potential infections or other effects on the animals can affect data interpretation. Flow cytometry has also been used for more functional endpoints of immune competence, including lymphocyte activation, cytokine release, phagocytosis, apoptosis, oxidative burst, and natural killer (NK) cell activity. Any of these endpoints can be added if the mechanism of action of the drug suggests involvement of a particular function or type of immune cells.

In NHP the assay most commonly used to assess immune competence is the T cell dependent antibody response (TDAR). The ability to mount an antigen-specific antibody response requires a fully functioning immune system of T cells, B cells, antigen-presenting cells, cytokine production, and so forth. Animals are generally immunized with keyhole limpet hemocyanin (KLH) or tetanus toxoid (TT), and circulating antigen-specific antibody levels are measured by enzyme-linked immunosorbent assay (ELISA) or other methods. Immunization with KLH or TT should occur prior to drug treatment to assess the effects on the secondary antibody response (i.e., first immunization sc on day-7 and second immunization 14 days later), and the other antigen can be injected after two weeks of treatment to determine the effect on the primary immune response 7 to 10 days later. This immunization regimen allows for the assessment of both the primary and the secondary T cell dependent antibody response within the 28-day GLP toxicology study. For studies of longer duration, a booster immunization can be given at a later time point to assess the effect on the memory response, or to see if an altered response returns to normal during the recovery period.

Other immune parameters can be measured in the NHP such as cytokine measurements and delayed type hypersensitivity measurements, although these are less well characterized. Many human ELISA kits for cytokines can be used to measure cytokine levels in the NHP, but it is very important to determine if the reagents in these kits do truly cross-react with NHP cytokines. Whereas many of the human reagents do cross-react, exceptions exist, and the reagents need to be tested prior to use on a toxicology study.

Although immunomodulation can be assessed in the NHP, the assays are less well characterized than those used in the rodent. One issue is the lack of consistent protocols, and the timing of incorporating these assays into standard GLP toxicology studies varies. More historical control data are needed, and many assays have not been tested with an immunomodulatory control to confirm the level of sensitivity of the assay for detecting a mild/moderate immune modulator (both immunoenhancing and immunosuppressive activity). Currently there is an ILSI/HESI initiative to pool these types of data from numerous companies to improve our understanding of these assays in the NHP. Greater variability is inherent to NHP than in-bred rodents, and the animal number per group is generally much smaller than in rodent studies. It is therefore critical to find ways of reducing the variability in the assay to allow for more meaningful data interpretation. Strategies to improve study designs can include decreasing the inter-animal variability (using animals from the same source and of similar ages, decreasing stress during the study, increasing the number of baseline samples, etc.) and decreasing assay variability (standardizing the antigen source, assay technique, timing, etc.).

We are now at the stage at which assays of immunomodulation can be conducted in nonhuman primates, but unfortunately, we lack sufficient knowledge on the data generated across all the various developmental programs on biopharmaceuticals to date regarding which assays are the most useful in predicting immunomodulatory effects in humans. Assay methods thus need to be standardized so that we can truly compare the data to make that determination. Comparing data from the NHP with the immunotoxicity data in rodents would be useful to evaluate whether the NHP is more predictive of the human response. Additionally regulatory agencies should continue to treat the immunotoxicity testing of biological therapeutics on a case-by-case basis. However, immune testing in NHP for biopharmaceuticals goes beyond the estimation of immunotoxicity. Immune testing can be very valuable for understanding the pharmacology of an immune modulator and can help establish pharmacodynamic markers that can then be used in clinical trials. Combining all of the available data in NHP will allow for an improvement in the models and a better understanding of the value of these data. In addition differences have been seen in immune parameters (especially immunophenotyping) between cynomolgus monkeys from different geographical locations. It is therefore very important to keep the same source of animals for toxicology studies throughout the drug development program.

Recent adverse events reported with immunomodulatory monoclonal antibodies, such as Tysabri and TGN1412, highlight the need to improve the predictivity of immune effects in humans. During the clinical testing of a novel superagonist anti-CD28 monoclonal antibody, TGN1412, six healthy male volunteers suffered from a systemic inflammatory response characterized as a "cytokine storm" and became critically ill [24], a response that had not been predicted from the preclinical studies in NHP [25]. Despite the use of a battery of murine, NHP studies, and even ex vivo human cell assays [26], the immunological models used in TGN1412 preclinical testing were of insufficient predictive power to anticipate the serious adverse events in humans [27]. Cytokine release syndrome (CRS) has been seen with other monoclonal antibodies such as OKT3, a murine anti-CD3 monoclonal antibody [28]. A humanized anti-CD3 antibody, HuM291, with a modified Fc 28 domain was tested to see if the CRS could be eliminated [29]. Both antibodies were tested in chimpanzees, and there was no clinical evidence of CRS, although substantial cytokine secretion was detected. Clinical testing of HuM291 also showed that humans still experienced mild to moderate CRS. This suggests that even chimpanzees may not be the best model for assessing the clinical effects of cytokine release (or the side effects associated with anti-CD3 therapy in humans may not necessarily result directly from cytokine secretion) [30]. Evidence in vitro has also implicated CD16 and LFA-1 on NK cells in CRS [31].

Natalizumab (Tysabri), an anti-α4 integrin monoclonal antibody approved for the treatment of multiple sclerosis, was recently withdrawn from the market temporarily due to cases of progressive multifocal leukoencephalopathy, a demyelinating disease of the central nervous system associated with immunosuppression [32]. These cases highlight our incomplete understanding of the immune system and the translation of preclinical results to humans.

What could be done to better assess immunomodulatory effects in NHP that will be predictive of the outcome in humans? One important consideration comes back to the "relevance" of the animal species. Not only should the binding affinity and functionality at the target be considered, but the relative potency as well can be a critical factor. Understanding the dose-concentration–response relationships for receptor occupancy, receptor modulation and functionality, and target expression and distribution in comparison to normal human subjects and in disease state can help us to better assess risk to patients.

16.3 CONCLUSIONS

Toxicity testing of biopharmaceuticals is highly dependent on species specificity. Every program could be different in the type of studies that are needed to support safety assessment (i.e., case-by-case approach). If the biopharmaceutical cross-reacts with the rodent target, then general toxicity tests can be conducted in two species similar to what is done with pharmaceuticals. If the molecule is only pharmacologically active in nonrodents (usually nonhuman primates), than a more focused or targeted toxicology program (one species) is conducted. If the molecule is not active in nonhuman primates, then alternative strategies for conducting safety studies such as testing with surrogate (homologous animal protein) molecules, or using transgenic/knockout mice, need to be considered. These strategies have certain caveats that can be used to better understand the potential toxicities of the therapeutic candidate. Although immunotoxicity testing guidelines are not established for biopharmaceuticals, many of the same assays and methods have been used routinely to understand potential effects on the immune system (whether unintended or pharmacologic activity). Further work is needed to understand potential immune effects of biopharmaceuticals, especially in nonhuman primates, to improve our predictivity of safety in humans.

REFERENCES

1. International Conference on Harmonization of Technical Requirements for Registration of Pharmaceuticals for Human Use. S6. Preclinical Safety Evaluation of Biotechnology-Derived Pharmaceuticals, 1997.

2. International Conference on Harmonization of Technical Requirements for Registration of Pharmaceuticals for Human Use. M3. Maintenance of the ICH Guideline on Non-clinical Safety Studies for the Conduct of Human Clinical Trials for Pharmaceuticals, 2000.

3. Clarke J, Hurst C, Martin P, Vahle J, Ponce R, Mounho B, Heidel S, Andrews L, Reynolds T, Cavagnaro J. Duration of chronic toxicity studies for biotechnology-derived pharmaceuticals: Is six months still appropriate? *Regul Toxicol Pharmacol* 2008;50:2–22.

4. International Conference on Harmonization of Technical Requirements for Registration of Pharmaceuticals for Human Use. S8. Immunotoxicity studies for human pharmaceuticals, 2005.

5. Cavagnaro J. Immunotoxicity assessment of biotechnology products: a regulatory point of view. *Toxicology* 1995;105:1–6.

6. Cavagnaro JA, Mielach FA, Myers MJ. Perspectives on the immuntoxicological evaluations of therapeutic products: assessment of safety. *Meth Immunotoxicol* 1995;1:37–9.

7. Korte R, Weinbauer GF. Towards *New Horizons in Primate Toxicology*. Muenster: Waxmann, 2000;1–257.

8. Korte R, Vogel F, Weinbauer GF. *Primate Models in Pharmaceutical Drug Development*. Muenster: Waxmann, 2002;1–188.

9. Zuhlke U, Korte S, Niggermann B, Fuchs A, Muller W. The common marmoset (Callithrix jacchus) as a model in biotechnology. In Korte R, Vogel F, Weinbauer GF, eds. *Primate Models in Pharmaceutical Drug Development*. Muenster: Waxmann, 2002;119–25.

10. Mann DR, Fraser HM. The neonatal period: a critical interval in male primate development. *J Endocrinol* 1996;149:191–7.

11. Jerome C. Osteoporosis and aging: the nonhuman primate model. In Korte R, Vogel F, Weinbauer GF (eds), *Primate Models in Pharmaceutical Drug Development.* Waxmann Munster, 2002;85–90.

12. Dayhaw-Barker P. The eye as a unique target for toxic and phototoxic effects. In Korte R, Weinbauer GF, eds. *Towards New Horizons in Primate Toxicology.* Muenster: Waxmann, 2000;145–58.

13. Goralczyk R. Histological aspects of primate ocular toxicity with special emphasis on canthaxanthin-induced retinopathy in the cynomolgus monkey model. In Korte R, Weinbauer GF, eds. *Towards New Horizons in Primate Toxicology.* Muenster: Waxmann, 2000;159–74.

14. Niggerman B. Ocular toxicity investigations in primates and options for improvements. In Korte R, Weinbauer GF, eds. *Towards New Horizons in Primate Toxicology.* Muenster: Waxmann, 2000;189–201.

15. Zrenner E. Objective functional evaluation: electroretinography (ERG), electrooculography (EOG), visually evoked cortical potentials (VEP) and multifocal ERG. In Korte R, Weinbauer GF, eds. *Towards New Horizons in Primate Toxicology.* Muenster: Waxmann, 2000;175–88.

16. Dorato MA, Engelhardt JA. The no-observed-adverse-effect-level (NOAEL) in drug safety evaluation: Use, issues and definition(s). *Regul Toxicol Pharmacol,* 2005;42:265–74.

17. Bussiere JL, Hardy LM, Hoberman AM, Foss JA, Christian MS. Reproductive effects of chronic administration of murine interferon-gamma. *Reprod Toxicol,* 1996;10(5):379–91.

18. Clarke J, Leach W, Pippig S, Joshi A, Wu B, House R, Beyer J. Evaluation of a surrogate antibody for preclinical safety testing of an anti-CD11a monoclonal antibody. *Regul Toxicol Pharmacol* 2004;40:219–26.

19. Treacy G. Using an analogous monoclonal antibody to evaluate the reproductive and chronic toxicity potential for a humanized anti-TNF-alpha monoclonal antibody. *Hum Exp Toxicol* 2000;19(4):226–8.

20. Bolon B, Galbreath E, Sargent L, Weiss J. Genetic engineering and molecular technology. In Krinke G, ed. *The Laboratory Rat.* London: Academic Press, 2000; 603–34.

21. Doetschman T. Interpretation of phenotype in genetically engineered mice. *Lab Animal Sci* 1999;49:137–43.

22. Bolon B, Galbreath EJ. Use of genetically engineered mice in drug discovery and development: wielding Occam's razor to prune the product portfolio. *Int J Toxicol* 2002;21:55–64.

23. Brennan FR, Shaw L, Wing MG, Robinson C. Preclinical safety testing of biotechnology-derived pharmaceuticals. *Mol Biotechnol* 2004;27:59–74.

24. Ganesh Suntharalingam G, Perry MR, Ward S, Brett SJ, Castello-Cortes A, Brunner MD, Panoskaltsis N. Cytokine Storm in a Phase 1 Trial of the Anti-CD28 Monoclonal Antibody TGN1412. *N Engl J Med* 2006;355:1–11.

25. Hopkin M. Can super-antibody drugs be tamed? *Nature* 2006;440:855–6.

26. Wing MG, Waldmann H, Isaacs J, Compston DAS, Hale G. Ex-vivo whole blood cultures for predicting cytokine-release syndrome: dependence on target antigen and antibody isotype. *Ther Immunol* 1995;2:183–90.

27. Schneider CK, Kalinke U, Löwer J. TGN1412—a regulator's perspective. *Nat Biotechnol* 2006;24:493–6.

28. Abramowicz D, Schandene L, Goldman M, et al. Release of tumor necrosis factor, interleukin-2, and gamma-interferon in serum after injection of OKT3 monoclonal antibody in kidney transplant recipients. *Transplantation* 1989;47:606.

29. Hsu D, Shi JD, Homola M, Rowell TJ, Moran J, Levitt D, Druilet B, Chinn J, Bullock C, Klingbeil C. A humanized anti-CD3 antibody, HuM291, with low mitogenic activity, mediates complete and reversible T-cell depletion in chimpanzees. *Transplantation* 1999;68:545–54.

30. Norman DJ, Vincenti F, DeMattos AM, Barry JM, Levitt DJ, Wedel NI, Maia M, Light SE. Phase 1 trial of HuM291, a humanised anti-CD3 antibody, in patients receiving renal allografts from living donors, *Transplantation* 2000;70:1707–12.

31. Wing MG, Moreau T, Greenwood J, Smith RM, Hale G, Isaacs J, Waldmann H, Lachmann PJ, Compston A. Mechanism of first-dose cytokine-release syndrome by CAMPATH 1-H: involvement of CD16 (FcγRIII) and CD11a/CD18 (LFA-1) on NK cells. *J Clin Invest* 1996;98:2819–26.

32. Sheriden C. Third Tysabri adverse case hits drug class. *Nat Rev* 2005;4:357–8.

CHAPTER 17

Reproductive Toxicity Testing for Biopharmaceuticals

PAULINE L. MARTIN, PhD

Contents

17.1 INTRODUCTION AND BACKGROUND

The importance of evaluating the effects of pharmaceutical agents on the development of the embryo and fetus has been appreciated for at least 40 years following the thalidomide tragedy of 1957 to 1961. Since that time reproductive toxicity testing strategies have been developed for the evaluation of the reproductive and developmental toxicity of chemicals and medical products [1]. In 1966 the US Food and Drug Administration (FDA) published guidelines for Reproduction Studies for Safety Evaluation of Drugs for Human Use. The testing strategies were subsequently refined, and in 1994 the expert working group of the International Conference of Harmonization (ICH) of technical requirements for registration of pharmaceuticals for human use issued a final guideline for industry Detection of Toxicity to Reproduction

Preclinical Safety Evaluation of Biopharmaceuticals: A Science-Based Approach to Facilitating Clinical Trials, edited by Joy A. Cavagnaro
Copyright © 2008 by John Wiley & Sons, Inc.

for Medicinal Products—ICH S5A [2]. According to the ICH S5A guidance document, for most medicinal products a three-study design consisting of fertility and early embryonic development (preferred species rat), embryofetal development (preferred species rat and rabbit), and prenatal and postnatal development (preferred species rat) is considered to be adequate. The S5A guidance also states that other strategies or combinations of studies and study designs might be as valid or more valid as the three-study design depending on the circumstances. In addition S5A guidance states "if it can be shown by means of kinetics, pharmacological, and toxicological data that the species selected is a relevant model for the human, a single species can be sufficient. There is little value in using a second species if it does not show the same similarities to humans."

For issues unique to the nonclinical safety testing of therapeutic biological products the ICH S6 guidance, Preclinical Safety Evaluation of Biotechnology-Derived Pharmaceuticals, was developed and finalized in 1997 [3]. The S6 guidance describes reproductive toxicity testing briefly and states that the specific study design and dosing schedule may be modified based on issues related to species specificity, immunogenicity, biological activity, and/or a long elimination half-life. Importantly, one of the main principles of S6 is use of relevant species for toxicity assessments. S6 also states that there may be extensive public information available regarding potential reproductive and/or developmental effects of a particular class of compounds (e.g., interferons) where the only relevant species is the nonhuman primate. In such cases mechanistic studies indicating that similar effects are likely to be caused by a new but related molecule may obviate the need for formal reproductive/developmental toxicity studies. Both S5A and S6 guidances emphasize the need for flexibility in reproductive toxicity testing strategies.

For FDA product labeling, a pregnancy category is designated for each pharmaceutical based on the risk to the fetus. The categories are A, B, C, D, and X with A having proved safety in humans and X having proved adverse effects in humans (Table 17.1). Thalidomide and isotretinoin are category X drugs. Most pharmaceuticals fall into either category C or B. In the absence of well-controlled studies in humans, a pharmaceutical will be designated category C if animal studies have shown an adverse effect or if no animal studies have been conducted. Since the human risk is unknown for category C designated drugs, they should be used during pregnancy only when needed and if the potential benefit to the patient justifies the potential risk to the fetus. In general, for a category B designation, animal studies would need to reveal no evidence of harm to the fetus.

In the following sections the testing strategies that have been applied in support of the approved biopharmaceuticals are reviewed and discussed in terms of the relevance to the evaluations of human safety and the lessons that have been leaned for future reproductive developmental toxicity testing. All information provided in the following narrative, unless otherwise referenced, have been extracted from the FDA summary basis of approval information www.fda.gov, the European Medicines Agency (EMEA) centrally authorized

TABLE 17.1   FDA pregnancy category designations for product labeling

Category	Description
A	Adequate, well-controlled studies in pregnant women have not shown an increased risk of fetal abnormalities
B	Animal studies have revealed no evidence of harm to fetus; however, there are no adequate and well-controlled studies in pregnant women
	or
	Animal studies have shown an adverse effect, but adequate and well-controlled studies in pregnant women have failed to demonstrate a risk to fetus.
C	Animal studies have shown an adverse effect, and there are no adequate, well-controlled studies in pregnant women
	or
	No animal studies have been conducted, and there are no adequate, well-controlled studies in pregnant women
D	Studies, adequate, well-controlled, or observational, in pregnant women have demonstrated a risk to fetus. However, benefits of therapy may outweigh the potential risk
X	Studies, adequate, well-controlled, or observational, in animals or pregnant women have demonstrated positive evidence of fetal abnormalities; the use of the product is contraindicated in women who are or may become pregnant

product reviews (EPARs) www.emea.europa.eu, and the *Physicians Desk Reference* (PDR).

17.2   TESTING OF SMALL MOLECULAR WEIGHT DRUGS VERSUS LARGE MOLECULAR WEIGHT BIOPHARMACEUTICALS

In general, the reproductive and developmental testing strategies have not differed greatly for small molecular weight drugs and large molecular weight biopharmaceuticals. Small molecular weight drugs are generally not species specific and can therefore be tested using standard well-validated study designs in rodents and rabbits for which extensive databases are now available. Some biopharmaceuticals are also not species specific and can therefore be tested using the same testing strategies as those used for small molecules, with minor modifications to the study designs based on the route of administration and dosing regimen based on a longer half-life of the biopharmaceutical. The non–species-specific biopharmaceutics include recombinant forms of human insulin and human growth factor, erythropoietin and erythropoietin analogues, granulocyte colony stimulating factor, and various enzymes.

Although similar testing strategies can be applied to small molecular weight drugs and large molecular weight biopharmaceuticals, there are some notable differences between small molecules and large molecular weight biopharmaceuticals that need to be taken into consideration. Small molecular weight drugs can freely diffuse across membranes. The degree of diffusion across membranes depends on the physical properties of the molecule [4,5]. Therefore small molecular weight drugs can cross the placenta and produce direct exposure of the embryo/fetus to the drug. They can be secreted in the milk and be absorbed across the neonatal gut and can diffuse across the blood–testis barrier and have direct effects on spermatazoa. Therefore, because of their small size and their ability to diffuse across membranes, small molecules have the potential to affect many stages of reproduction and development.

Large molecular weight proteins and peptides, on the other hand, because of their large size, do not readily diffuse across membranes, and therefore any potential effects are more likely to be secondary effects of maternal or parental toxicity rather than direct effects on the fetus or the spermatozoa. For example, administrations of insulin, insulin analogues, or glucagon-like peptide 1 to pregnant animals, at doses that exceed the clinical dose, produce maternal hypoglycemia. Since the intended use of these hormones is to normalize blood glucose, the effects seen in the toxicology animals can be considered to be exaggerated pharmacological effects. Sustained maternal hypoglycemia leads to fetal malnutrition resulting in pre- and postimplantation losses and skeletal and visceral abnormalities [6,7]. The effects seen on the fetuses with the insulin analogues do not differ from that of regular human insulin when administered at suprapharmacological doses and do not differ from that of oral blood-glucose lowering drugs [8]. Similarly the erythropoeitic agents, at suprapharmacological doses, produce increases in maternal hematocrit and an increase in blood viscosity leading to impaired blood flow and oxygen delivery to various tissues in the developing fetus. As a consequence fetal growth retardation and decreased ossification are seen.

Therefore for large molecular weight biopharmaceuticals that have restricted biodistribution and have biological effects that are indistinguishable from that of the endogenous hormone, the effects on the fetus can be predicted by an understanding of the biology in the adult. The adverse effects on the fetus are not seen when maternal blood parameters are maintained within normal ranges. Because of the secondary effects seen on the fetus at suprapharmacological doses all the pharmacologically active molecules carry a pregnancy category of C except for insulin lispro, which failed to show maternal or fetal toxicity in rat and rabbit developmental studies and was designated as category B. It is, however, unlikely that insulin lispro is less toxic than the other insulin analogues since its pharmacological effects in animals are similar to that of normal human insulin. Therefore, for biopharmaceuticals that have poor penetration across biological membranes and have a well-defined biology in the adult animal, a single relevant species assessment of embryofetal development may be adequate. Some of the newer biotechnology derived therapeutics have been approved with reproductive/developmental toxicity assessments in a single species, rats (e.g., agalsidase beta and laronidase). No reproductive toxicity studies were performed for the platelet-derived growth factor (PDGF) whose intended route of administration is topical and showed limited systemic absorption.

The toxicity of small molecular weight drugs, however, cannot necessarily be predicted based solely on an understanding of the biology of the parent molecule in the maternal animals. Many small molecular weight drugs are susceptible to metabolic degradation, which may result in the formation of metabolites with different toxicity, biology, and distribution from that of the parent molecule. Since metabolic processes can differ across species, a two-species assessment of embryofetal development may be appropriate for most small-molecule drugs. For protein therapeutics, however, the expected consequence of metabolism is the degradation to small peptides and individual amino acids. Therefore for protein molecules that consist of only naturally occurring amino acids, the generation of toxic metabolites is unlikely and a single species assessment may be appropriate.

17.3 REPRODUCTIVE TESTING OF BIOPHARMACEUTICALS THAT SHOW LIMITED SPECIES CROSS-REACTIVITY

Some human specific proteins do not cross-react with rats and rabbits, and therefore alternate species need to be considered for the reproductive toxicity testing of these agents. The type I interferons are examples of this class of proteins. The type I interferons show a high degree of species specificity such that the macaque, and in some cases only the rhesus macaque, is a suitable biologically responsive species for toxicology testing. In addition the type I interferons are highly immunogenic in macaques. After about two weeks of dosing the dams develop neutralizing antibodies toward the human interferon that reduces maternal exposure and eliminates the pharmacological response. Therefore the design of the embryofetal development studies for these molecules has, in some cases, involved modification of study designs so that critical periods in development could be evaluated. The embryofetal development studies for these molecules showed an increased incidence of abortions. The abortions occurred early during gestation and were associated with decreased serum progesterone [9,10]. Since all the type I interferons have similar pharmacology, they all produced a similar early abortifacient effect. Treatment with the interferons was not associated with a tertatogenic effect in macaques or in patients with multiple sclerosis [11].

Because the type I interferons produced no adverse effects on embryofetal development and the early abortifacient effect could be predicted based on a measurement of female endocrine changes, the need to conduct additional macaque embryofetal development studies for type I interferons in nonhuman primates was considered unnecessary. Therefore, for the second-generation pegylated versions of the alpha interferons, only hormonal analysis was conducted in macaques. This is the only known example of where mechanistic studies have been accepted in place of developmental studies in accordance with ICH S6 guidance.

17.4 REPRODUCTIVE TOXICITY TESTING OF MONOCLONAL ANTIBODIES

The monoclonal antibodies represent a unique class of protein molecules with regard to developmental toxicity testing. Although antibodies are very large molecular weight proteins (~150 kDa), they are known to cross the placenta from mother to fetus [12]. The transfer of antibodies from mother to fetus occurs predominantly in the second and third trimesters in humans and in nonhuman primates and involves a specific transport mechanism. Because fetal exposure to therapeutic antibodies is likely if women are treated with therapeutic antibodies during pregnancy, the precaution sections of the product labels for each of the approved antibody products carries wording to this effect. The transport mechanism requires binding of the constant portion (Fc) of the antibody to a receptor (FcRn) on the placenta. Binding of antibodies to FcRn on endothelial cells is also involved in the antibody salvage pathway that results in serum persistence of antibodies [13,14]. Therefore all proteins that contain an intact Fc and can bind to FcRn will be transported across the placenta. This includes monoclonal antibodies and engineered proteins that contain the Fc antibody fragment in order to increase serum persistence of proteins, peptides, or drugs. Fab antibody fragments, such as abciximab, are not transported across the human placenta [15].

The approaches taken in the evaluation of the reproductive toxicity testing for monoclonal antibodies has varied greatly depending on the species cross-reactivity and immunogenicity of the antibody. The testing strategies employed and the results from these studies are summarized in Table 17.2.

For two of the approved monoclonal antibodies, infliximab and efalizumab, cross-reactivity was seen only to human and chimpanzee antigens. The chimpanzee is a protected species and therefore not appropriate for evaluating developmental toxicity. Since these monoclonal antibodies were being developed for non–life-threatening diseases, Crohn's disease, rheumatoid arthritis, and psoriasis, and included women of childbearing potential, an alternate strategy needed to be developed. In both cases surrogate monoclonal antibodies were developed that bound to the murine version of the antigen. With these surrogate antibodies all stages of reproduction, including embryofetal development, could be evaluated in the mouse [16,17]. However, the use of a surrogate (homologous) monoclonal antibody does not test the product intended for clinical use, and therefore these types of studies evaluate the potential risks associated with inhibition of a particular pathway rather than risks associated with administration of the clinical product. One alternative approach that has been employed is to develop a transgenic mouse that expresses the human antigen, thereby allowing the testing of the clinical product [18]. The disadvantages of this approach are that the biology in the transgenic mouse may not be the same as that in humans and the mice will likely develop an immune response to the human protein.

For most of the other monoclonal antibodies, species cross-reactivity has been limited to nonhuman primates. For these molecules the need to conduct reproductive and developmental studies has to be carefully considered on a case-by-case basis. S5A states that nonhuman primates are best used when the objective of the study is to characterize a relatively certain reproductive toxicant, rather than detect a hazard. The nonhuman primate reproductive toxicity studies are not powered to detect infrequent events.

For the antibodies intended to treat immune mediate diseases—adalimumab, natalizumab, and omilizumab—a macaque embryofetal development study was conducted. In these studies pregnant macaques were treated for a period including the period of organogenesis (gestation days 20–50, first trimester), and fetuses were examined at the end of the second trimester (gestation day-100). For the approved monoclonal antibodies only natalizumab and bevacizumab have shown cross-reactivity to species other than nonhuman primates. For natalizumab, a two-species embryofetal development assessment was conducted (macaque and guinea pig), whereas for bevacizumab, which was intended to treat cancer, only a single relevant species assessment was conducted (rabbit).

Fusion proteins that consist of recombinant forms of human proteins fused to the Fc portion of human IgG tend to be less species specific than monoclonal antibodies. Etanercept and abatacept showed cross-reactivity to rodents and rabbits, and therefore a full reproductive and developmental toxicity package could be obtained in rodents and rabbits for these agents. For alefacept species cross-reactivity was limited to the macaque.

For some monoclonal antibodies the epitope may only be present in the intended disease population. For example, the epitope may only be unregulated during disease, or the monoclonal antibody may target epitopes found only on viruses or bacteria. In such cases a single relevant species may be selected to assess off-target toxicity based on nonspecific binding to normal tissues. In these cases, however, unless there is nonspecific binding to reproductive organs, the nonhuman primate would not be a relevant species for assessing reproductive toxicity.

Reviews of the results from the reproductive toxicity testing for the approved monoclonal antibody biopharmaceuticals have shown very few incidences of harm to fetuses. The only notable effects that have been observed are hematologic changes in macaque fetuses exposed to natalizumab, skeletal abnormalities in rabbit fetuses exposed to bevacizumab, and immunological deficits in mice exposed to the efalizumab murine surrogate. In each of these examples the effects seen in the fetuses were predicable based on effects seen in the adult animals.

Natalizumab is a monoclonal antibody against the human $\alpha4$ integrins ($\alpha4\beta1$ and $\alpha4\beta7$). The $\alpha4$ integrins are expressed on leukocytes and hematopoeitic progenitor cells and mediate homing and adhesive functions. In disease states natalizumab prevents the migration of leucocytes into inflamed tissues and thereby suppresses inflammation [19]. In adult cynomolgus macaques the

TABLE 17.2 Summary of reproductive toxicity testing at time of approval for monoclonal antibodies and Fc-containing fusion proteins

Product (Approval Date)	Mechanism of Action	Indication	Reproductive/ Developmental Toxicity Test Species
Zenapax daclizumab (1997)	Anti-CD25 (IL-2R) (mAb-IgG1)	Acute organ rejection	Not done
Simulect basiliximab (1998)	Anti-CD25 (IL-2R) (mAb-IgG1)	Acute organ rejection	Cynomolgus, macaque (EFD)
Remicade infliximab (1998)	Anti-TNF (mAb-IgG1)	Crohn's disease, Rheumatoid arthritis	Mouse—murine homologue (F, EFD, PPD)
Humira adalimumab (2002)	Anti-TNF (mAb-IgG1)	Rheumatoid arthritis	Cynomolgus monkey (EFD)
Raptiva efalizumab (2003)	Anti-CD11a (T cells) (mAb-IgG1)	Psoriasis	Mouse—murine homologue (F, EFD, PPD)
Tysabri natalizumab (2004)	Anti-α4 integrin (mAb-IgG4)	Multiple sclerosis	Cynomolgus monkey (EFD), Guinea pig (F, EFD, PPD)
Xolair omalizumab (2003)	Anti-IgE (mAb-IgG1)	Asthma	Cynomolgus monkey (F, EFD)
Rituxan rituximab (1997)	Anti-CD20 (B cells) (mAb-IgG1)	Refractory non-Hodgkin's lymphoma	Not done
Herceptin trastuzumab (1998)	Anti-HER2 (mAb-IgG1)	Metastatic breast cancer	Cynomolgus monkey (F, EFD)

Effects in Adult Animals in Chronic Toxicity Studies	Doses Tested in EFD Study (NOAEL or highest dose tested)	Effects on Fertility, Pregnancy and Development	Clinical Dose	Pregnancy Category
Information not available	Not done	Unknown	1 mg/kg	C
Macaque None	5 mg/kg (GD20-50)	No harm to the fetus	20 mg (~0.3 mg/kg)	B
Mouse None	40 mg/kg (GD6-18)	↓ Male fertility? No harm to the fetus	3–5 mg/kg	B
Macaque ↓ thymus weight, ↓ spelnic follicular centers	100 mg/kg (GD20-97)	No harm to fetus	40 mg (~0.6 mg/kg)	B
Mouse ↓ humoral immune response, ↑ WBC, ↓ cellularity lymph nodes	30 mg/kg	No harm to the fetus, ↓ humoral immune response, ↓ cellularity lymph nodes	0.7 mg/kg	C
Macaque ↑ WBC, ↑ reticulocytes, ↑ spleen weight	30 mg/kg (GD20-70)	↓ Female fertility, mild anemia ↑ spleen weight, ↓ liver and thymus weight, no teratogenicity	300 mg (~4.3 mg/kg)	C
Macaque None	75 mg/kg (GD20-50)	No harm to the fetus	150–375 mg (~2–5 mg/kg)	B
↓ B cells	N/A	Unknown	375 mg/m^2 (~10 mg/kg)	C
None	50 mg/kg (GD20-50)	No harm to the fetus	2 mg/kg	B

TABLE 17.2 *Continued*

Product (Approval Date)	Mechanism of Action	Indication	Reproductive/ Developmental Toxicity Test Species
Campath alemtuzumab (2001)	Anti-CD52 (T and B cells) (mAb-IgG1)	Chronic lymphocytic leukemia	Not done
Erbitux cetuximab (2004)	Anti-EGF (mAb-IgG1)	Metastatic colorectal carcinoma	Not done
Avastin bevacizumab (2004)	Anti-VEGF (mAb-IgG1)	Metastatic colorectal cancer	Cynomolgus monkey (F) and rabbit (EFD)
Enbrel etanercept (1998)	TNFR:Fc IgG1 Anti-TNF	Rheumatoid arthritis, JRA, PsA	Rat (F, EFD, PPD) and rabbit (EFD)
Amevive alefacept (2003)	LFA3:Fc IgG1Anti-CD2 (T cells)	Psoriasis	Cynomolgus monkey (EFD, PPD)
Orencia abatacept (2006)	CTLA4:Fc IgG1(T-cells)	Rheumatoid arthritis	Mouse (EFD), rat (F, EFD, PPD), rabbit (EFD)
Reopro abciximab (1997)	Anti-GPIIb/IIIa Fab platelet inhibitor	Cardiac ischemic complications —PTCA	Not done

Source: All information included in this table and the accompanying text have been extracted from the US FDA summary basis of approval information www.fda.gov, the European Medicines Agency (EMEA) centrally authorized product reviews (EPARs) www.emea.europa.eu and the Physicians Desk Reference (PDR).

Note: F = fertility, EFD = embryofetal development, and PPD = pre and postnatal development.

only notable toxicological findings following natalizumab treatment were increased circulating leukocytes, increased reticulocytes, and increased spleen weights. These effects are most likely due to the primary pharmacological effect of natalizumab of decreased adhesion of leukocytes and hematopoetic progenitors. Treatment of pregnant macaques with natalizumab resulted in fetal effects consisting of mild anemia, reduced platelet counts, increased

Effects in Adult Animals in Chronic Toxicity Studies	Doses Tested in EFD Study (NOAEL or highest dose tested)	Effects on Fertility, Pregnancy and Development	Clinical Dose	Pregnancy Category
Information not available	N/A	Unknown	3-30 mg (~0.04– 0.4 mg/kg)	C
Macaque Skin/ epidermal toxicity	N/A	Unknown	400 mg/m^2 (~10 mg/kg)	C
Macaque ↓ Menstrual cycles, physeal dysplasia in adolescent males, ↓ body weight gain	≤10 mg/kg (GD6-18)	Impaired fertility ↓ fetal body weight skeletal alterations	5 mg/kg	C
None (15 mg/kg)	40 mg/kg (GD6-18)	No harm to fetus	50 mg (~0.7 mg/kg)	B
↓ T cells	5 mg/kg (GD20-birth)	No harm to the fetus	7.5 or 15 mg (0.1–0.2 mg/kg)	B
↓ Serum IgG, ↓ T and B cells activation ↓spelnic B cells	200 mg/kg (GD6-18)	No harm to the fetus, ↑ T-dependent Ab response, thyroid inflammation	10 mg/kg	C
	Not done	Not transported across human placenta in vitro	0.25 mg/kg	C

spleen weight, and reduced liver and thymus weight—associated with increased splenic extramedullary hematopoesis, thymic atrophy, and decreased hepatic hematopoiesis. These findings are generally consistent with the known pharmacological effects of natalizumab of decreased adhesion of hematopoetic progenitors and leukocytes and were completely reversible upon clearance of drug from the blood.

Bevacizumab is a monoclonal antibody against human vascular endothelial growth factor (VEGF). By inhibiting VEGF, bevacizumab inhibits tumor angiogenesis and thereby inhibits tumor growth. Toxicology studies conducted in young adult cynomolgus macaques showed bevacizumab treatment-related physeal dysplasia in immature animals with open growth plates and in mature females with reduced endometrial proliferation, an absence of corpora lutea, lower uterine weights, and decreased menstrual cycles [20]. In the six-month chronic toxicity study, decreased body weight gains were observed that were most likely due to decreased growth resulting from reduced angiogenesis in the bone growth plates. These effects are due to inhibition of VEGF that is required for normal physiological angiogenesis in the bone growth plates and in the ovaries. Bevacizumab showed cross-reactivity to cynomolgus macaque VEGF and to a lesser extent to rabbit VEGF. Because bevacizumab bound to rabbit VEGF, the rabbit was selected as an appropriate species for evaluating the developmental effects of bevacizumab. The lower sensitivity of the rabbit to bevacizumab was compensated for by increasing the dose levels and dose frequency relative to human dosing. Decreased fetal and maternal body weights were seen with an increase in the number of fetal resorptions and an increased incidence of specific gross and skeletal fetal alterations. These effects seen in the rabbit fetuses could be predicted based on the known biology of VEGF and the observations in the young adult animals.

Efalizumab is an antibody against the CD11a subunit of LFA-1 (lymphocyte function-associated antigen-1, a leukocyte cell surface protein); it inhibits the binding of LFA-1 to ICAM-1, 2, and 3 (intercellular adhesion molecules 1, 2, and 3). Efalizumab prevents the binding of LFA-1 on activated T lymphocytes to ICAM-1 on endothelial cells. Eflaizamab thereby inhibits immune-mediated processes involved in psoriasis. As mentioned previously, efalizumab does not bind to LFA-1 in any animal species suitable for conducting reproductive toxicity testing. Therefore the chronic toxicity studies and the reproductive toxicity studies were conducted with a murine surrogate of the human antibody referred to as muM17 [17]. In adult mice muM17 treatment-related effects consisted of increased circulating leukocytes, increased spleen weight, and decreased cellularity of the lymph nodes. These effects are most likely due to altered trafficking of white cells secondary to reduced adhesion. MuM17-treated adult animals showed a reduced primary antibody response to neoantigen challenge. In the developmental studies decreased antibody response was observed in the pups that was reversible by 25 weeks of age. Therefore the effects seen in the pups are consistent with the effects seen in the adults, and these effects are predictable based on the known biology of CD11a inhibition.

The other monoclonal antibodies shown in Table 17.2 produced either no toxicity or minimal biological effects in adult animals and no harmful effects to the fetus. One interesting observation is that even for those molecules that did show an effect in the fetuses, the effects that were observed were minor compared to effects that might be predicted based on observations in genetically deficient mice. Mice genetically altered to lack the α4 integrin are not viable. These knockout animals show cardiac and placental defects that are embryolethal [21]. Cardiac defects and embryo lethality is also seen in rats treated with certain small molecules inhibitors of α4 integrins [22]. However, the developmental studies conducted in macaques showed no cardiac toxicity, and fetuses and neonates were essentially normal except for the reversible hematologic changes. Mice genetically altered to lack VEGF are not viable because VEGF is essential to embryonic vasculogenesis [23]. However, in the rabbits treated with bevacizamab during pregnancy, most of the fetuses did survive and showed predominantly skeletal alterations. Mice genetically altered to lack tumor necrosis factor are viable but show disorganized lymphoid architecture and a reduced humoral immune response [24]. However, developmental studies conducted with two anti-TNFα antibodies and one TNFα receptor-IgG Fc fusion protein, infliximab surrogate (cV1q), adalimumab, and etanercept have failed to show any detrimental effect on the fetal or neonatal immune system.

One reason why monoclonal antibodies produce fewer developmental toxicological effects than would be predicted from the genetically deficient rodents and fewer effects than seen with certain small molecular weight drugs may be that embryonic exposure to monoclonal antibodies during the critical period of organogenesis is minimal in primates. In humans and nonhuman primates the transfer of antibodies increases throughout the second and third trimesters [25–27]. By the time of the cesarean sections in the nonhuman primate embryofetal development studies (gestation day-100, end of the second trimester), monoclonal antibody concentrations in the fetuses have reached only a fraction of the maternal levels (~25%). By the time of birth in macaques (gestation day-165), antibody levels in the neonates are similar to that of the mothers [28]. Therefore detection of monoclonal antibody in fetal blood at gestation day-100 does not imply that the embryo was exposed to the antibody during the period of organogenesis (GD 20–50). It is likely that only the dams were significantly exposed to the monoclonal antibody during the period of organogenesis. Therefore for monoclonal antibodies there is a very low likelihood of teratogenic effects occurring due to direct embryonic exposure during organogenesis. However, if the monoclonal antibody has a biological or toxicological effect on development, it is more likely to have an effect on growth and maturation during the fetal period where antibody exposure is high than on organogenesis where exposure is low.

Because the period of organogenesis for rodents and rabbit (50% and 38%, respectively) occupies a greater proportion of the total gestational period than in nonhuman primates (15%) or humans (13%), the likelihood of placental transfer occurring during organogenesis is higher in rodents and rabbits than in nonhuman primates or humans. Therefore, if rodents or a rabbits are selected as the toxicology species for developmental studies, they may overestimate the risk for humans. This has been demonstrated for a lymphotoxin β-receptor IgG1-Fc fusion protein that showed a lack of lymph node development in the F1 generation when administered to pregnant mice [29] but normal lymph node development when administered to pregnant macaques [30]. Therefore study design and choice of species are critically important for monoclonal antibodies.

Historically for the monoclonal antibodies intended to treat life-threatening diseases, such as oncology and organ rejection, reproductive toxicity studies have not routinely been conducted for all molecules prior to registration. The absence of this information resulted in the products being designated as pregnancy category C—namely the risk to the fetus is unknown. However, more recently approved oncology products have included embryofetal development toxicity studies either in cynomolgus macaques (trastuzumab) or in the rabbit (bevacizumab). With trastuzumab, which was developed to treat metastatic breast cancer and therefore included women of child-bearing potential, no adverse developmental effects were seen, allowing the product to carry a pregnancy category B. With bevacizumab the skeletal and visceral malformations that were seen resulted in the product remaining as a category C.

Cetuximab was approved in 2004 for the treatment of metastatic colorectal cancer. At the time of registration no developmental toxicology studies were conducted, consistent with that of many of the other oncology agents, and the product was designated as pregnancy category C. However, a macaque embryofetal development study was requested as a postmarketing commitment. Cetuximab is an antibody against epidermal growth factor receptor (EGFR). In adult macaques cetuximab produces skin toxicity due to the primary pharmacological action of EGF inhibition. Mice genetically altered to lack EGFR survive for up to eight days after birth and suffer from impaired epithelial development in several organs, including skin, lung, and gastrointestinal tract [31]. Therefore, based on the observations seen with the other monoclonal antibodies in macaques, it would be expected that the effects on the macaque fetus would be less than that seen in the genetically deficient animals and more consistent with that seen in the adult animals. Because epidermal toxicity can be expected in the fetuses, the product will likely retain its pregnancy category C designation.

One notable exception to this overall generalization for antibody therapeutics, that maternal biology predicts fetal biology (toxicity), is alefacept. Alefacept treatment produces profound depletions of T cells in adult animals due to its primary mechanism of action. However, in fetuses from macaques treated with alefacept during organogenesis and throughout pregnancy, no adverse effects on the immune system were seen even though fetal exposure was demonstrated. Therefore alefacept carries a pregnancy category of B.

17.5 REPRODUCTIVE TOXICITY TESTING OF NONTRADITIONAL BIOPHARMACEUTICALS

Most of the case studies described above are for recombinant forms of endogenous human proteins and human antibodies developed by traditional recombinant DNA technology. Newer technologies now have the ability to engineer molecules with specific desired properties that may deviate from naturally occurring sequences. For these agents the principles outlined in the S6 guidance document may not always apply. In addition conjugation of proteins with drugs in order to improve the targeting of the drug to certain sites in the body or to improve the serum half-life may result in molecules that have properties of both large molecular weight biopharmaceuticals and small molecular weight drugs. One example is that of toxin-conjugated antibodies where the antibody molecules functions to target a cytotoxic agent to a tumor cell. The scope of the toxicity testing for these agents may depend on the novelty of the toxin in addition to the species cross-reactivity of the antibody. Conjugation of biologically inert molecules such as polyethylene glycol, in order to increase serum half-life of the biotherapeutic or to reduce immunogenicty, has shown no adverse impact on the toxicity profile relative to the unconjugated versions. For the polyethyene glycol modified version of biopharmaceuticals a reduced reproductive and developmental toxicology package may be appropriate if the biological effects of the therapeutic can be shown not to be altered by the conjugation.

Oligonucleotides are a class of biopharmaceuticals that do not fall under the traditional biotechnology-derived pharmaceuticals as described in ICH S6 guidance. However, many of the principles of ICH S6 do apply to the oligonucelotides because consideration of species specificity does apply. While reproductive toxicology studies were performed with the clinical material for the approved oligonucleotide pegaptanib, many classes of oligonucleotides are specific for binding to human mRNA sequences and therefore are inactive in rodents. In these instances the generation of surrogate oligonucleotides toward the relevant rodent mRNA is the only meaningful way to establish the safety of these molecules [32].

17.6 DISCUSSION

Review of the reproductive/developmental toxicity studies that have been conducted in support of the approved biopharmaceuticals have shown that historically a flexible case-by-case approach has been applied. For biopharmaceuticals that cross-react only with nonhuman primates a limited reproductive toxicity testing strategy has been employed based on the patient population, the indication, and the proposed clinical use. The studies that have been performed have been sufficient to inform the patient populations of potential risk to the fetus.

Based on the very limited database of approved biopharmaceuticals, a few generalizations can be made. For pharmacologically active proteins that produce exaggerated pharmacology in the mothers, the toxicological effects seen in the fetuses are secondary effects of maternal toxicity rather than direct teratogenic effects. Large molecular weight protein cross the placenta very poorly, and therefore fetal exposure is minimal. For these agents the aim in the clinic is to maintain physiological parameters within normal limits and thereby avoid harm to the fetus. Because the fetal effects are secondary to exaggerated pharmacology in the mothers, the fetal effects can be predicted based on an understanding of the pharmacology in the adult animals. Therefore for molecules of a similar pharmacological class an argument could be made that mechanistic studies in adult animals could obviate the need to conduct formal developmental studies, as suggested by the S6 guidance document. In this way the number of animal studies need for the evaluation of developmental toxicity could be reduced. This approach is particularly important when the only relevant species is the nonhuman primate. However, the approach has been successfully applied only to the type I interferons.

The second generalization that can be made is that for monoclonal antibodies that produce biological effects in adult animals, similar biological effects are likely to occur in the F1 generation if the fetuses are exposed to the monoclonal antibody during the second and third trimesters and/or postnatally. Therefore, since a biological effect in the fetus is considered adverse, the product will most likely be labeled as category C. Monoclonal antibodies are unlikely to produce direct teratogenic effect in primates since exposure during the embryonic period is limited. Therefore, for these agents the need to conduct embryofetal development studies, especially when the only relevant species is the nonhuman primate, needs to be carefully considered.

It should be emphasized that the generalization made above are based on a very limited database of mostly traditional recombinant human proteins and monoclonal antibodies. However, these generalizations may not apply to second-generation molecules that contain components other than naturally occurring amino acids. Also the generalization that large molecular weight molecules, other than antibodies, do not cross the placenta may not be applicable to all molecules and may depend on the dose that is administered relative to clinical doses. If high enough doses are administered to pregnant animals, sufficient penetration may occur to produce a toxicological effect in the fetuses even if the fetal exposure relative to the maternal exposure is very low. Pegaptanib, an oligonucleotide-polyethylene glycol conjugate VEGF inhibitor with a molecular weight of 50kDa was shown at high doses to cross the placenta in mice in sufficient amounts to produce developmental defects in the fetus similar to those seen in rabbits with bevacizumab. However, possibly because the developmental effects occurred only at exposure levels that were vastly in excess of clinical exposures, the developmental effects are not described in the product label, which carries a pregnancy category of B. Smaller molecular weight oligonucleotides, when tested at lower doses, were shown not to cross the placenta in significant amounts in mice [32].

For biopharmaceuticals for oncology indications primate reproductive toxicity studies have not historically been conducted. The absence of a negative developmental toxicity study results in the product carrying a pregnancy category C designation that indicates the risk to the fetus as unknown, and therefore the use of the drug during pregnancy should be avoided unless the benefit to the patient outweights the risk to the fetus. For oncology indications the biopharmaceutical is frequently administered in combination with known teratogenic chemotherapeutic agents, for example, irinotecan, 5-fluorouracil or paclitaxel (pregnancy category D). Therefore a potential risk to the fetus exists for most drug–biopharmaceutical combinations. More recently, however, there has been a progression toward a requirement, or an expectation, that embrofetal development studies will be conducted for all biopharmaceuticals regardless of the indication or the species cross-reactivity. It is important to justify the use of animals in such cases for characterizing human risk.

For biopharmaceuticals that require developmental toxicity testing the design of the developmental studies should be adapted according to the type of molecule under investigation. The standard developmental protocols that have been developed for the evaluation of small molecular weight drugs may not be appropriate for all biopharmaceuticals. This is particularly important when the only relevant species is the nonhuman primate. If a primate developmental study is conducted, the design of the study should be based on good scientific judgment, as emphasized in the regulatory guidances, and not on a perceived regulatory requirement. The standard macaque embryofetal development study design has been adapted from the rodent and rabbit study designs in which pregnant animals are treated during the period of organogenesis and fetal examinations are conducted at a time when adequate anatomical evaluations can be conducted [33,34,10]. However, the macaque study design may need to be modified depending on the nature of the molecule being tested and the known biology of the molecule.

One important point about embryofetal development studies that needs to be emphasized is that traditionally an embryofetal development study examines only gross anatomical effects in the fetuses following exposure of the mothers to the drug during organogenesis. Histopathological examination of fetal tissues is not routinely conducted. Therefore for biopharmaceuticals that produce exposure during the fetal period, such as the antibodies, and therefore may have effects on the maturation of the immune system, for example, these effects would not be detected in a standard embryofetal development study unless additional immunological endpoints are incorporated. For rodent studies, functional and immunological endpoints are incorporated into the pre- and postnatal development studies. However, when the only relevant species is the nonhuman primate and only a single developmental study is planned, the study design should be modified to include additional clinically relevant endpoints and to cover the periods of greatest maternal and fetal exposure. These considerations, however, are no different than those for evaluating general toxicity where immune endpoints are routinely included in single- and/or repeat-dose toxicity studies to characterize toxicity (see Chapter 16).

The macaque embryofetal development study design has been shown to be appropriate for detecting the teratogenic effects of the small molecular weight drugs thalidomide and isotretinoin [35,36]. For large molecular weight biopharmaceuticals that do not cross the placenta the standard macaque embryofetal study design will only be able to detect maternal effects that may be just as readily detectable in nonpregnant females. Even for monoclonal antibodies that are known to cross the placenta, the design of the standard embryofetal development study may not be optimal for fully evaluating risk to the F1 generation. Although antibodies are transferred across the placental from mother to fetus, the transport is not consistent throughout pregnancy. In humans and nonhuman primates very little antibody exposure occurs during the first trimester. Antibodies are transported from mother to fetus during the latter part of pregnancy mostly during the third trimester [12]. It is unlikely that the embryo will be significantly exposed to an antibody during the dosing period if the dosing is restricted only to the first trimester. Therefore utilizing the "standard" study design for monoclonal antibodies examines maternal effects and at most the effect of minimal fetal exposure during a limited portion of the second trimester.

Although a three-segment approach to reproductive toxicity testing is routinely conducted for small molecular weight drugs and biopharmaceuticals that cross-react with rodents, the need to conduct a three-segment evaluation in primates for primate-specific biopharmaceuticals needs to be carefully considered. For nonhuman primates a single-study design that involves examination of neonates from dams dosed throughout pregnancy and lactation may be a more appropriate study design than conducting separate embryofetal development and postnatal development studies. A combined study could reduce the number of nonhumans primates and provide more meaningful information. It is not clear what additional information is gained from terminating macaque pregnancies midgestation. Important points for consideration for primate reproductive toxicity testing are the ethical consideration of using primates versus rodents and the duration of the nonhuman primate studies. An embryofetal development study in macaques can take approximately one year to complete, and a combined embryofetal development and postnatal development study can take up to two years to complete. Therefore, if these studies are considered to be essential for evaluating human risk, the timing of the studies relative to clinical testing may need to be adjusted to ensure timely access of therapeutics to patients with debilitating diseases.

Another question that needs to be considered is whether fertility studies conducted in nonhuman primates provide sufficient useful safety information for the patients to justify the use of the animals? The one aspect of the nonhuman primate fertility studies that cannot accurately be assessed is fertility. Nonhuman primates have a naturally low fertility rate [37] and high spontaneous abortion rate [38] such that the number of animals that would be required to demonstrate a meaningful effect on fertility would be too large to be practical or ethical. Therefore the "fertility" studies in nonhuman primates focus on evaluation of hormone levels and semen analysis. This limited information provides minimal safety information over and above the standard toxicology endpoints, and therefore the value of conducting these studies should be carefully considered.

In conclusion, as defined in the ICH S6 guidance, the reproductive/developmental toxicity testing for biopharmaceuticals needs to be justified on a case-by-case basis. No single testing strategy can be applicable to all types of molecules. The reproductive/toxicity testing strategy should be based on good science and a thorough understanding of the molecular class and the pharmacological and toxicological properties of the molecule.

REFERENCES

1. Collins TFX. History and evolution of reproductive and developmental toxicology guidelines. *Curr Pharmaceut Des* 2006;12:1449–65.

2. Guidance for Industry. Detection of Toxicity to Reproduction for Medicinal Products. ICH-S5A, 1994. www.fda.gov

3. Guidance for Industry. Preclinical Safety Evaluation of Biotechnology-Derived Pharmaceuticals. ICH-S6, 1997. www.fda.gov

4. Pacifici GM, Nottoli R. Placental transfer of drugs administered to the mother. *Clin Pharmacokinet Concepts* 1995;28:235–69.

5. Van der Aa EM, Peereboom-Stegeman JHJC, Noordhoek J, Gribnau FWJ, Russel FGM. Mechanisms of drug transfer across the placenta. *Pharm World Sci* 1997; 20:139–48.

6. Hofmann T, Horstmann G, Stammberger I. Evaluation of the reproductive toxicity and embryotoxcity of insulin glargine (LANTUS) in rats and rabbits. *Intl J Toxicol* 2002;21:181–9.

7. Tanigawa K, Kawaguchi M, Tanaka O, Kato Y. Sketelatal malformations in rat off spring: long-term effects of maternal-insulin induced hypoglycemia during organogenesis. *Diabetes* 1991;40:1115–21.

8. Baeder C. Embryotoxicological/teratological investigation, including effects on postnatal development, of the new oral antidiabetic glimepride after oral administration to rats and rabbits. *Clin Reprod* 1993;27:45–60.

9. Trown PW, Wills RJ, Kamm JJ. The preclinical development of Roferon®-A. *Cancer* 1986;57:1648–56.

10. Henck JW, Hilbish KG, Serabian MA, Cavagnaro JA, Hendrickx AG, Agnish ND, Kung AHC, Mordenti J. Reproductive toxicity testing of therapeutic biotechnology agents. *Teratology* 1996;53:185–95.

11. Sandberg-Wolheim M, Frank D, Goodwin TM, Giesser B, Lopez-Bresnahan M, Stam-Moraga M, Chang P, Francis GS. Pregnancy outcomes during treatment with interferon beta-1a in patients with multiple sclerosis. *Neurology* 2005;65:802–6.

12. Simister NE. Placental transport of immunoglobulin G. *Vaccine* 2003;21:3365–9.

13. Firan M, Bawdon R, Radu C, Ober RJ, Eaken D, Antohe F, Ghetie V, Ward ES. The MHC class I-related receptor, FcRn, plays an essential role in the maternofetal transfer of γ-globulin in humans. *Intl Immunol* 2001;13:993–1002.

14. Roopenian DC, Christianson GJ, Sproule TJ, Brown AC, Akilesh S, Jung N, Petkova S, Avanessian L, Choi EY, Shaffer DJ, Eden PA, Anderson CL. The MHC class I-like IgG receptor controls perinatal IgG transport, IgG homeostasis, and the fate of IgG-Fc-coupled drugs. *J Immunol* 2003;170:3528–33.

15. Miller RK, Mace K, Polliotti B, DeRita R, Hall W, Treacy G. Marginal transfer of ReoPro™ (Abciximab) compared with immunoglobulin G (F105), inulin and water in the perfused human placenta in vitro. *Placenta* 2003;24:727–38.

16. Treacy G. Using an analogous monoclonal antibody to evaluate the reproductive and chronic toxicity potential for a humanized anti-TNFα monoclonal antibody. *Hum Exp Toxicol* 2000;19:226–8.

17. Clark J, Leach W, Pippig S, Joshi A, Wu B, House R, Beyer J. Evaluation of a surrogate antibody for preclinical safety testing of an anti-CD11a monoclonal antibody. *Regul Toxicol Pharmacol* 2004;40:219–26.

18. Bugelski PJ, Herzyk DJ, Harmsen AG, Gore EV, Williams DM, Maleeff BE, Badger AM, Truneh A, O'Brien SR, Macia RA, Wier PJ, Morgan DG, Hart TK. Preclinical development of keliximab, a primatized anti-CD4 monoclonal antibody, in human CD4 transgenic mice: characterization of the model and safety studies. *Hum Exp Toxicol* 2000;19:230–43.

19. O'Connor P. Natalizumab and the role of alpha 4-integrin antagonism in the treatment of multiple sclerosis. *Expert Opin Biol Ther* 2007;7:123–36.

20. Ryan AM, Eppler DB, Hagler KE, Bruner RH, Thomford P, Hall J, Shopp RL, O'Neill CA. Preclinical safety evaluation of rhuMabVEGF, an antiangiogenic humanized monoclonal antibody. *Toxicol Pathol* 1999;27:78–86.

21. Yang JT, Rayburn H, Hynes RO. Cell adhesion events by α-4 integrins are essential in placental and cardiac development. *Development* 1995;121:549–60.

22. Crofts F, Pino M, DeLise B, Guittin P, Barbellion S, Brunel P, Potdevin S, Bergamann B, Hofmann T, Lerman S, Clark RL. Different embryo-fetal toxicity effects for three VLA-4 antagonists. *Birth Defects Res* 2004;71:55–68.

23. Ferrar N, Carver-Moore K, Chen H, Dowd M, Lu L, O'Shea KS, Powell-Braxton L, Hillan KJ, Moore MW. Heterozygous embryonic lethality induced by targeted inactivation of the VEGF gene. *Nature* 1996;380:439–42.

24. Pasparakis M, Alexopoulou L, Episkopou V, Kollias G. Immune and inflammatory responses in TNFα-deficient mice: A critical requirement for TNFα in the formation of primary B cell follicles, follicular dendritic cell networks and germinal centers, and in the maturation of the humoral immune response. *J Exp Med* 1996; 184:1397–411.

25. Malek A, Sager R, Kuhn P, Nicholaides KH, Schneider H. Evaluation of maternofetal transport of immunoglobulins during human pregnancy. *Am J Reprod Immunol* 1996;36:248–55.

26. Fujimoto K, Terao K, Cho F, Honjo S. The placental transfer of IgG in the cynomolgus monkey. *Jap J Med Sci Biol* 1983;36:171–6.

27. Coe CL, Kemnitz JW, Scneider ML. Vulnerability of placental antibody transfer and fetal complement synthesis to disturbance of the pregnant monkey. *J Med Primatol* 1993;22:294–300.

28. Coe CL, Lubach GR, Izard KM. Progressive improvement in the transfer of maternal antibody across the order primates. *Am J Primatol* 1994;32:51–5.

29. Rennert PD, Browning JL, Hochman PS. Selective disruption of lymphotoxin ligands reveals a novel set of mucosal lymph nodes and unique effects on lymph node cellular organization. *Intl Immunol* 1997;11:1627–39.

30. Martin PL. *Primate Models in Pharmaceutical Drug Development.* Muenster: Waxmann, 2002;105–18.

31. Miettinen PJ, Berger JE, Meneses J, Phung Y, Pedersen RA, Werb Z, Derynck R. Epithelial immaturity and multiorgan failure in mice lacking epidermal growth factor receptor. *Nature* 1995;376:337–41.

32. Henry SP, Denny KH, Templin MV, Yu RZ, Levin AA. Effects of human and murine antisense oligonucleotide inhibitors of ICAM-1 on reproductive performance, fetal development, and post-natal development in mice. *Birth Defects Res* 2004;71:359–67.

33. Weinbauer GF. *Primate Models in Pharmaceutical Drug Development*, Waxmann Verlag GmbH, 2002;49–66.

34. Buse E, Habermann G, Osterburg I, Korte R, Weinbauer GF. Reproductive/developmental toxicity and immunotoxicity assessment In the nonhuman primate model. *Toxicology* 2003;185:221–7.

35. Hendrickx AG, Makori N, Peterson P. Nonhuman primates: their role in assessing developmental effects of immunomodulatory agents. *Hum Exp Toxicol* 2000; 19:219–25.

36. Hendrickx AG. The sensitive period and malformation syndrome produced by thalidomide in crab-eating monkey (*Macaca fascicularis*). *J Med Primatol* 1973;2:267–76.

37. Meyer JK, Fitzsimmons D, Hastings TF, Chellman GJ. Methods for the prediction of breeding success in male cynomolgus monkeys (*Macaca fascicularis*) used for reproductive toxicology studies. *J Am Assoc Lab Animal Sci* 2006;45:31–6.

38. Hendrie TA, Peterson PE, Short JJ, Tarantal AF, Rothgarn E, Hendrie MI, Hendrickx AG. Frequency of prenatal loss in a macaque breeding colony. *Am J Primatol* 1996;40:41–53.

CHAPTER 18

Reproductive/Developmental Toxicity Assessment of Biopharmaceuticals in Nonhuman Primates

GERHARD F. WEINBAUER, PhD, WERNER FRINGS, PhD, ANTJE FUCHS, PhD, MICHAEL NIEHAUS, PhD, and INGRID OSTERBURG

Contents

18.1 INTRODUCTION

Assessment of developmental and reproductive toxicity (DART) is commonly done in rodents (mice and rats) and in rabbits (mainly developmental toxicity). These evaluations use standardized experimental designs described in detail in the respective ICH guidelines (Table 18.1). The entire spectrum of DART testing comprises three segments:

- Fertility and early embryonic development (segment 4.1.1)
- Prenatal and postnatal development (segment 4.1.2)
- Embryofetal development (segment 4.1.3)

Preclinical Safety Evaluation of Biopharmaceuticals: A Science-Based Approach to Facilitating Clinical Trials, edited by Joy A. Cavagnaro
Copyright © 2008 by John Wiley & Sons, Inc.

TABLE 18.1   Guidances for the conduct of developmental and reproductive toxicity studies and their effective dates

Guidance	Date
Detection of toxicity to reproduction for medicinal products (ICH S5A)	March 1994
Reproductive toxicology: male fertility studies (ICH S5B)	November 2000
Nonclinical studies for the safety evaluation of pharmaceutical excipients	May 2005
Safety testing of drug metabolites	June 2005
Considerations for developmental toxicity studies for preventive and therapeutic vaccines for infectious disease indications	February 2006
Nonclinical safety evaluation of pediatric drug products	February 2006
Nonclinical safety evaluation of drug and biological combinations	March 2006
Immunotoxicity studies for human pharmaceuticals (ICH S8)	May 2006

Beyond these three detailed developmental studies, a number of FDA guidelines can have a bearing on the need for the conduct of DART studies (Table 18.1).

Rodents and rabbits represent the standard DART species for small molecules and also for testing of biopharmaceuticals to which standardized designs can be applied. However, the development of biopharmaceuticals frequently necessitates the use of nonhuman primate models (NHP). A major reason for the requirement for NHP is species-specific cross-reactivity. Many therapeutic antibodies are highly specific and may not even recognize rodent, rabbit, or dog tissues. According to a recent survey "for the majority of MAbs (monoclonal antibodies) on the market cynomolgus monkeys have been used as the toxicology species and viewed by the regulators as the most relevant species" (National Centre for the Replacement, Refinement and Reduction of Animals in Research 2006, http://www.nc3rs.org.uk). Confined cross-reactivity might also render the marmoset as the relevant species. Another reason for using NHP is immunogenicity of the test item. Unlike for small molecules, large molecules bear the danger of eliciting an immune response and antibody formation. It can also happen that neutralizing antibodies to the test item are being produced, in which case the test item is rendered biologically ineffective or with diminished activity. For humanized antibodies (containing human sequences/fragments) and large "human" molecules, it is generally assumed that NHP are more appropriate for prediciting immunogenicity than rodent models. However, it must be borne in mind that there are cases where the NHP is not predictive at all and that the assumption above cannot be generalized [1–3].

Nonetheless, the need for DART studies using NHP is a frequent encounter with biopharmaceuticals, and rather than being an alternate approach, NHPs became an essential species for DART. Generally, NHPs offer several advantages over rodents and rabbits with regard to DART because of similarity to human, for example, with regard to endocrinology of testicular and ovarian function, endocrinology of early pregnancy, placental morphology and physiology, timing of implantation, and rates of embryonic development, and also because of similar responses to known human teratogens, for example, thalidomide and vitamin A [4]. The purpose of this contribution is to provide a state-of-the-art account on the feasibility and limitations of using NHPs for DART evaluation in the context of preclinical development of biopharmaceuticals.

18.2 WHICH NONHUMAN PRIMATE MODEL?

Reproductive and developmental physiologies have been described for a number of NHPs including Old World monkeys and New World monkeys. Notwithstanding this, among NHPs, the cynomolgus monkey model is now predominantly used for general and reproductive/developmental toxicity studies, followed by marmosets and rhesus monkeys. At our site the overall use of different NHPs in toxicology approximates 80% for cynomolgus monkey, 12% for marmoset, and 8% for rhesus monkey.

Cynomolgus monkeys *(Macaca fascicularis)* are sexually active and fertile throughout the entire year and are not considered to express distinct and significant reproductive seasonality. Under feral conditions, pregnant females were discovered throughout the entire year [5], and menstrual cyclicity was unrelated to seasonal environment [6,7]. Our own observations confirm the absence of ovarian seasonality in the cynomolgus monkey both under laboratory conditions and under natural light conditions [8]. For the cynomolgus monkey model well-established experimental designs for reproductive and developmental toxicity testing, and immunotoxicity assessment, are available [9,10]. The reproductive physiology and endocrinology have been extensively studied, and numerous publications demonstrate the relevance of the cynomolgus monkey as a preclinical model for human reproduction and development [11,12]. At present the cynomolgus monkey is the model of choice for DART assessment. Another advantage of the cynomolgus monkey resides in the fact that many assays for immune system evaluation are available for this species (see Chapter 16).

Rhesus monkeys *(Macaca mulatta)* are another species used for DART evaluation [4]. However, this species displays pronounced seasonality of reproductive activity for both sexes [13,14]. In this primate, reproductive functions are entirely shut off or severely diminished for approximately half of the year. In environments with distinct seasons sexual activity and gonadal activity are present roughly throughout October until March, but this may vary substantially for individual animals. It is crucial to consider that the annual rhythmicity of reproductive cycles can persist over years in captivity and under indoor artificial light pattern conditions [15]. Hence in indoor circumstances seasonality of reproduction may be uncoupled from the outdoor season, and eventually an animal may display periodic reproductive activation in unexpected months.

During the out-of-season periods, reproductive hormone secretion and gonadal activity are at a complete halt. Although the basic reproductive and developmental physiology appear similar to human in the rhesus monkey and many endpoint parameters are established, the distinct reproductive seasonality requires special timing and has practical implications for widespread use of this model for DART studies. With regard to immune system evaluation it can be assumed that most of the available tests for cynomolgus monkey will also be applicable to rhesus monkeys.

Marmosets *(Callithrix jacchus)* reside in the canopy of tropical forests and do not show reproductive seasonality of fertility or breeding. The basic reproductive and developmental features of the marmoset model are well described [16–19]. In general, reproductive physiology and endocrinology of the marmoset is substantially different from that of human and Old World monkeys [18] and the clinical relevance of the marmoset for reproductive toxicity assessment is unclear [20]. Among these differences are lack of menstrual bleeding, multiple ovulation (2–4 ova/cycle), twin/triplet pregnancies, common chorion/anastomoses leading to hematopoietic XX/XY chimerism, and the absence of key male fertility genes (e.g., DAZ = deleted-in-azoospermia gene) [17, 21–25]. Marmosets and tamarins seem to be the only anthropoid primate species that regularly exhibit multiple ovulation [26]. On the other hand, the sensitivity of marmosets to thalidomide derivates is well documented [27]. A totally unexpected difference between marmosets and Old World primates including human resides in the fact that marmosets lack luteinizing hormone (LH) [28]. Recent work suggests that this could even be a common feature of New World monkeys [25]. According to recent concepts the pituitary produces and releases chorionic gonadotropin (CG) instead of LH and CG stimulates gonadal steroid hormone production. Despite these differences a number of parameters are available for reproductive and developmental toxicity testing in this species (Tables 18.2, 18.3, 18.4 and 18.6). Aside from the different reproductive physiology, evaluation of immunotoxicity endpoints is somewhat limited in the marmoset model. Whereas standard techniques such as histology and hematology as well as immunophenotyping are available, further specific approaches to immune system evaluation are scarce. These tests comprise T cell dependent antibody responses (e.g., KLH) and limited determinations of immunoglobulins and cytokines. Analysis of NK cell activity is hampered by the limited blood volume available from marmosets.

18.3 FERTILITY AND EARLY EMBRYONIC DEVELOPMENT (SEGMENT 4.1.1)

Studies of fertility and embryonic development are designed to identify toxic effects resulting from treatment from before mating (both males and females) and continuing through mating and implantation. Unlike in rodents, the phase of conception until implantation is not evaluated in NHPs. These studies also

TABLE 18.2   Parameters for evaluation of female fertility in the nonhuman primate model

	Parameter
Oogenesis	Histology
Ovarian cyclicity	*Endocrinology* or vaginal smears
Endometrial changes	Biopsies, ultrasound
Ultrasound examination	Follicular growth, ovarian cysts
Endocrinology[a]	
Fertility	Mating

Note: Parameters refer to cynomolgus monkey. Italicized parameters are also available for the marmoset model. Since marmosets lack LH, the analysis of LH bioactivity reflects CG activity/levels.
[a]LH = luteinizing hormone, FSH = follicle-stimulating hormone, *CG = chorionic gonadotropin, prolactin, estrogens, progesterone, androgens*, inhibin A, inhibin B.

TABLE 18.3   Parameters for evaluation of male fertility in the nonhuman primate model

	Parameter
Spermatogenesis	Histology, DSP, spermatogenic stages, flow cytometry
Sperm maturation	Epididymis
Semen	
Testicular size	*Caliper or ultrasound*
Testis biopsy	
Endocrinology[a]	
Prostate status	Prostate volume, uroflow
Fertility	Mating

Note: Parameters refer to cynomolgus monkey. Italicized parameters are also available for the marmoset model. Since marmosets lack LH, the analysis of LH bioactivity reflects CG activity/levels.
[a]LH = luteinizing hormone, FSH = follicle-stimulating hormone, *CG = chorionic gonadotropin*, prolactin, *estrogens*, DHT = dihydrotestosterone, androstenedione, *progesterone, androgens*, inhibin A, inhibin B, SHBG = sex hormone binding globulin. DSP = daily sperm production.

assess potential changes in the estrous cycle of females and possible functional effects that may not be detected in acute toxicity testing by histological examinations of the male reproductive organs. Whereas the guidelines recommend physical mating for testing fertility—albeit feasible—this is not being done routinely in NHP mainly for two reasons: (1) Default litter size in macaques is one and checking for implantation sites is obsolete. Twin pregnancies/births are extremely rare in macaques with an overall twin live births incidence around 0.1% [7,29]. We encountered four twin pregnancies among more than 3600 pregnancies. (2) Spontaneous fertility rates in macaques are clearly below 100% (typically 40–70%) and pre-implantation loss in macaques is probably around 25% [30]. This scenario necessitates either large group sizes or

TABLE 18.4   Parameters for evaluation of postnatal development in the nonhuman primate model

	Parameter
TK/antibody analysis	Maternal milk/blood, infant blood
Mother–infant interaction	Video recording and analysis
Functional and behavioral test battery	>20 items
Growth and clinical signs	
Immune system	*Antibodies*
	Immunoglobulins
	Immunophenotyping
	NK cell activity[a]
	Lymphocyte proliferation
	TDAR and DTH[b]
	CD immunohistochemistry of lymphatic organs
	Cytokines
Hematology/clinical chemistry	
Organ weights	
Histopathology	
Optional	ECG, ocular investigations, skeletal growth (DEXA), blood gas analysis

Note: In case of continued maternal dosing, milk can be collected for further analysis. Parameters refer to cynomolgus monkey. Pre-/postnatal studies are considered feasible in the marmoset model (italicized parameters should be accessible in the marmoset model).
[a]NK = natural killer cell.
[b]TDAR = T cell dependent antibody response, DTH (=delayed-type hypersensitivity test) is problematic in NHP.

pronounced toxicity in order to be able to detect statistically significant effects on fertility via mating success. Compared to the sophisticated clinical parameters available (Tables 18.2 and 18.3), fertility test by mating is rather insensitive and is therefore not recommended except for specific indications that the test item might affect mating behavior. The request for physical mating in NHP fertility studies may be related to differential interpretation of ICH guidelines [31].

A large array of parameters is available for macaques for the evaluation of effects on male and female fertility (Tables 18.2 and 18.3). Most of these parameters correspond to clinical endpoints used by gynecologists and andrologists for diagnosis of infertility. For the marmoset the number of established fertility parameters is less comprehensive than for macaques (Tables 18.2 and 18.3). However, those parameters that are available for marmosets are considered sufficient to detect clear-cut effects on male and female fertility. Most important, no assays for the determination of inhibins are available for marmosets. This is unfortunate as inhibin B does represent a good marker for testicular toxicity [32] and inhibins are useful as markers of ovarian function [33].

18.4 PRENATAL AND POSTNATAL DEVELOPMENT (SEGMENT 4.1.2)

The set of prenatal and postnatal studies is designed to detect adverse effects on the conceptus and the offspring following exposure of the female from implantation through weaning. In the offspring, functional parameters such as behavior, maturation (puberty), and fertility are also tested. For the latter, the F1 generation is being mated to produce the F2 generation. Different from rodents and for feasibility considerations, the F1 infants are not observed throughout puberty and are not being mated for production of F2 in the NHP. Sexual maturity in cynomolgus monkeys occurs around 2.5 to 5 years of age. If F1 and F2 generation would be produced for cynomolgus monkeys according to the prevailing guidelines, such studies would require many monkeys and an estimated 5 to 8 years duration. Marmosets attain breeding maturity by 1.5 to 2 years of age. Yet, if marmosets would be used, a guideline-based study design would still require approximately 4 years.

Selection and enrollment of animals follow the same procedures used in an embryofetal development study. Dosing commences on gestational day (GD) 20 and lasts until termination of pregnancy. Duration of pregnancy in cynomolgus monkeys is around 160 days. For 167 control pregnancies the gestational duration ranged between 134 days and 184 days. It is possible to continue maternal dosing after delivery in order to evaluate transfer of test item to the newborn via breast milk. Transient antibody development of infants from mothers dosed with test item during lactation has been observed (confidential data not shown). A study design overview and a list of available parameters for infant evaluation are given in Figure 18.1 and Table 18.4.

A comprehensive test battery for behavioral and functional development is available for the cynomolgus monkey infant (Table 18.5). Many of these tests use the Brazleton-based human neonatal behavioral assessment scale, and the tests have been modified and adopted for use in NHP [34,35]. For mother–infant interaction, a video recording is evaluated quantitatively using a special computer program. Mother–infant pairs are videotaped in a home cage situation at 3 to 4 months of age. The tapes are scored for separations and reunions of the mother and infant, as well as which party initiates the separation/reunion and the reaction of the other party [36].

Whereas the experimental design is quite standardized regarding maternal aspects, the duration of postnatal infant assessments is rather variable between studies, for example, from 7 days to 720 days in our experience. Evidently there is a need for standardization of the timing and type of test batteries for infants and of the time period the infant should be raised. For behavioral tests, a postnatal observation period of 9 months appears essential since these tests can only by applied from the age of 6 months onward. For evaluation of immune system development, a period of 6 months appears mandatory since from that age onward blood volume is sufficient to conduct several tests, such as the T cell dependent antibody response (TDAR), NK cell

TABLE 18.5 Available test battery for assessment of behavioral and functional development in the cynomolgus monkey infant

Respiration rate
Muscle tonus[a]
Elicited state[a]
Dorsiflexion[a]
Grasp support[a]
Righting reflex[a]
Prone progression[a]
Clasp support[a]
Visual following[a]
Lip smack orient[a]
Sucking[a]
Rooting[a]
Snout reflex[a]
Glabellar tap[a]
Nystagmus[a]
Moro reflex[a]
Grip strength[b]
Pupillary reflex[c]
Learning ability
Mother-infant interaction (video-based)

Note: If a learning test is included in the test battery, the infants should be raised for at least 9 months as this test is used first at the age of 6 months.
[a]Performed on days 1 and 7 postpartum.
[b]Performed on day 28 postpartum.
[c]Performed on days 1 and 7 postpartum—if negative the test is repeated on day 14 postpartum or later.

activity test, lymphocyte proliferation test, and immunophenotyping. In the case of TDAR, a clear response was elicited at the age of 6 months and followed by an increased response to the second KLH injection at the age of 9 months (Figure 18.2). Finally, consensus is also needed as to whether or not to terminate the infant for full histopathological examination at termination of the study.

18.5 EMBRYOFETAL DEVELOPMENT (SEGMENT 4.1.3)

These studies are conducted in order to detect adverse effects on the pregnant female and the development of the embryo and fetus exposed in utero. Basically the period between implantation and closure of the hard palate is being investigated. In the NHP, however, only the period between postimplantation

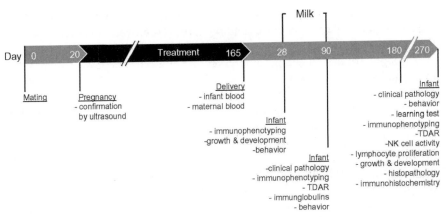

Figure 18.1 Study design for the pre- and postnatal development evaluation in the cynomolgus monkey. Maternal treatment is either discontinued at term or is continued into the lactation period in order to investigate transfer of test item to the infant. Transfer of biopharmaceuticals via milk has been observed in this species. The duration of the postnatal observation period is variable and not yet standardized. In our laboratory the longest postnatal observation period covered 720 days. A variety of parameters is available for testing infant development (see also Table 18.4 for details). For biopharmaceuticals, a minimum period of 6 months appears appropriate. If the behavioral test battery comprises learning tests that are recommended from the age of 6 months onward, infants should be observed for at least 9 months.

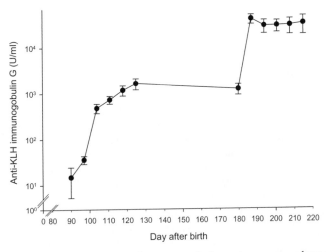

Figure 18.2 T-cell dependent antibody response in immature cynomolgus monkeys at various postnatal ages. Keyhole limpet hemocyanin (KLH) was administered intradermally at 100 μg in Freunds's incomplete adjuvant. Note that a clear antibody response is present at about 3 months of age followed by an increased response after second immunization at about 6 months of age. Data represent mean values ± SEM of 5 to 6 animals (males and females combined).

and closure of the hard palate is covered. Animals are then dosed throughout the entire phase of organogenesis and the fetus is removed by cesarean section for examination.

The standard design and parameters for an embryofetal development study in cynomolgus monkeys are detailed in Figure 18.3 and Table 18.6. It is well established that the cynomolgus monkey is a relevant model for detection of effects on embryofetal development [37,38]. Timed matings are achieved by vaginal smear-based monitoring of the ovarian cycle and pairing around the suspected time point of ovulation followed by ultrasound examination for pregnancy. Since ovarian cycles cannot be synchronized, every female animal—once pregnant—is on its own time line and it may take some time—depending on the colony size of regularly cycling female animals—until all animals are pregnant and enrolled into the study. Test items are normally administered during GD 20 to 50 followed by cesarean section on GD 100 ± 1. If biopharmaceuticals with defined targets in the immune system are being tested, it may be advisable to prolong the period of dosing. For example, fetal thymic CD3$^+$

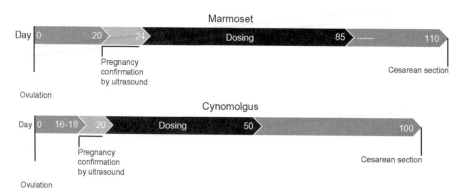

Figure 18.3 Comparison of study design for embryofetal development evaluation in the marmoset and in the cynomolgus monkey. Following mating, pregnancy confirmation is achieved by ultrasound in both species. Double-sided arrows indicate the length of the dosing period. Note that the dosing period starts later (day 25 vs. day 20) and last longer (until day 85/longer [dotted line] vs. day 50) in marmosets compared to the cynomolgus monkey. Palate fusion occurs during GD 75 to 80 in the marmoset monkey and during GD 45 to 50 in the cynomolgus monkey. Cesarean sections are performed routinely on GD 110 ± 1 in the marmoset model and on GD 100 ± 1 in the cynomolgus monkey. Duration of pregnancy is somewhat shorter in the marmoset (approx. 140 to 150 days) compared to the cynomolgus monkey (approx. 155 to 165 days). It is important to recognize that for the marmoset, the mated pair must be housed together throughout the entire study duration, whereas for the cynomolgus monkey, the male is removed upon mating and the female is housed singly. This fact has implications for the study conduct with biopharmaceuticals in that male marmoset blood should also be analyzed for the presence of test item upon termination of the study.

TABLE 18.6   Parameters for evaluation of embryofetal development in the nonhuman primate model

Maternal Parameters	Fetal Parameters
TK analysis	*Fetal examination*
Hematology/clinical chemistry	*Organ weights*
Immunophenotyping	*Histopathology*/CD immunocytochemistry of
Immunoglobulins	lymphatic organs
Antibodies	*Immunoglobulins*
	Morphometry
	Cardiac assessment
	Amniotic fluid
	Umbilical cord blood flow
	Umbilical cord blood for TK/blood gas analysis

Note: Parameters refer to cynomolgus monkey. Italicized parameters are also available for the marmoset model. Parameters for a placental transfer study in cynomolgus monkey and marmosets comprise TK/PK samples, such as maternal blood before (animal not sedated) or at (animal sedated) cesarean section, blood from umbilical cord, and collection of amniotic fluid.

cells appear on GD 60 [39] and immunoreactive B cells are only present from GD 85 onward [10]. Studies with interferons or cytokines used a dosing phase of GD 20 to 70 or GD 20 to 80 [4]. In our laboratory we extended the dosing period from GD 20 up to GD 90 in embryofetal development studies using specific biopharmaceuticals.

A study plan for assessing embryofetal development in the marmoset is available [40]. Earlier work demonstrated the sensitivity of marmosets to thalidomide derivates [27]. Since marmosets do not have menstrual bleedings, cycle monitoring and timed matings were the pattern of circulating progesterone concentrations [41]. Embryofetal development is slower compared to macaques or human [42] and—following pregnancy confirmation by ultrasound—the dosing period ranged from GD 25 up to GD 109. Cesarean sections were performed on gestational day 110 ± 1, and fetuses were removed for further examination. Figure 18.3 compares the basic design of an embryofetal development study in the cynomolgus monkey and the marmoset. The number of live fetuses at cesarean section ranged from one to four with 62% twins and 24% triplets. Moreover a compound with teratogenic activity induced malformations at a rate of 99% (confidential data not shown). A major concern with such marmoset studies is the lack of a sizable reference database. On the other hand, the presence of the same malformation in twin fetuses from a test item exposed mother animal would—in all likelihood—be considered as evidence for test item related embryofetal toxicity without the need to consult a reference database. Since, however, the available experience using the marmoset approach is very limited, judgments and assumptions may change with increasing usage and experience in that nonhuman primate species (Table 18.7).

TABLE 18.7 Presumed advantages and disadvantages of the marmoset model for embryofetal development evaluation

Advantages	Disadvantages
Body weight	Limited reference database
Litter size	Male presence required throughout study
Mating success	Animal supply
	Limited blood volume

Note: As the experience using this approach is currently very limited, our judgments, and assumptions may need to be modified with increasing usage of this NHP.

If there is concern whether the biopharmaceutical is able to cross the placental barrier, a placental transfer study can be undertaken both in cynomolgus monkey or marmoset. Animals receive a single high dose of test item on GD 100 (cynomolgus) or GD 110 (marmoset) followed by cesarean section at a time point determined by the half-life of the test item. Parameters to be studied comprise TK/PK samples such as maternal blood before (animal not sedated) or at (animal sedated) cesarean section, blood from umbilical cord, and collection of amniotic fluid for analysis of test item concentrations. The qualitative pattern of immunoglobulin G transfer across the placenta and relative to gestational duration appears comparable between human and cynomolgus monkey [10,43,44]. Immunoglobulin G levels increase during the last trimester with a prebirth peak followed by a postnatal decline [10].

18.6 REPRODUCTIVE FAILURE AND RELEVANCE FOR DEVELOPMENTAL TOXICITY STUDIES

Reproductive failure is significant among primates. A review of this aspect in nine macaque species concluded that overall reproductive failure comprises—on average—16.3% abortions, 9.9% stillbirths, 21.9% neonatal deaths, and 15.2% infant deaths [45]. More recently Hendrie et al. [7] reviewed the incidence of prenatal loss in macaque breeding colonies. Throughout a 8 to 9 years observation period, the annual prenatal loss rates varied between 13% to 23% in the rhesus monkey (seasonal breeder), 10% to 50% in the bonnet monkey (seasonal breeder), and 8.6% to 28% in the cynomolgus monkey (non-seasonal breeder). Small [45] described six studies in the cynomolgus monkeys in which abortion rates ranged from 11.7% to 30.2%.

The cumulative prenatal loss rate for cynomolgus monkey until GD 150 across a 9-year period (1984 to 1993) was 14.8 % (65 losses in 439 pregnancies) [7] (Table 18.8). In our experience, cumulative prenatal loss rate in control animals was 12.9% (40 losses in 311 timed pregnancies) until GD 150 in time-mated toxicity studies across a 10-years period (1994–2004). The vast majority of prenatal losses occurred prior to GD 100. Interestingly the frequency of

TABLE 18.8   Cumulative prenatal loss rates in timed-mated cynomolgus monkeys

Pregnancies	Losses	Percentage	Period	Data Source
439	65	14.8	1984–1993	Hendrie 1996 [7]
311	40	12.9	1994–2004	Covance[a]
330	29	8.8	1994–2004	SNBL[b]
217	30	13.8	—	CRL[c]
138	13	9.4	2004–2006	Covance[d]

[a]Combined data from control animals from studies with cesarean section on gestational days 100 or 150. Animals were dosed during variable periods of gestation (range: days 16 to 150) using various dose routes (oral, subcutaneous, intramuscular, intravenous).
[b]Shin Nippon Biomedical Laboratories November 1, 2004, brochure.
[c]Charles River Laboratories—data until pregnancy term (Reproductive Toxicology Historical Data CD, Society of Toxicology 2006, file 7HCD-Nevada from 27.02.2006).
[d]Data from untreated pregnant animals until gestational day 70.

pregnancy failure did not relate to variable housing or management conditions such as handling, shipping, relocation, parity, and indoor time-mated versus outdoor random-mated [7]. In a cohort of 138 pregnant animals in whom dosing started after GD 70, we encountered 13 (9.4%) losses until GD 70 (Table 18.8).

It is important to recognize, however, that cumulative prenatal loss rates do not reflect variability between studies and single experimental groups. Despite reasonably low cumulative prenatal loss rates, abortion rates within a study can vary considerably. For separate controlled mating studies, prenatal loss rates ranging from 0% to 20% have been reported for the cynomolgus monkey [46–49]. A retrospective analysis of 70 embryofetal development studies from our laboratory suggests that—in statistical terms—prenatal loss rates of 10% to 30% occurred in 50% of studies and prenatal loss rates of 0% or more than 45% occurred in 5% of studies, respectively. Clearly, for cynomolgus monkeys— like other primate species—prenatal loss is a physiological reality and should be taken into account when planning for group size in developmental toxicity studies. With regard to potential untoward effects of a test item on embryofetal development—aside from the prenatal loss rate—one should also consider the timing of prenatal loss and whether a dose-dependency is prevalent.

The incidence of prenatal loss in the marmoset was 17%, and losses were detected between GD 36 and GD 102 [40]. Prenatal loss consistently affected all embryos/fetuses per female. Heger and colleagues reported a 20% to 35% postimplantation loss in the marmoset [50].

As already described earlier, NHP also experience significant loss at term and shortly thereafter [45]. Hence in a pre-/postnatal toxicity study overall reproductive failure (prenatal loss, stillbirth, neonatal and infant death) can amount to 40% or even 50% losses in single experimental groups. For developmental toxicity studies naive animals are frequently requested. Female animals with proven fertility and breeding experience might improve this situation, in particular, with regard to their response to birth and thereafter. Interestingly, though, reproductive success appeared comparable between primiparous and multiparous cynomolgus monkeys [51] and rhesus monkeys/bonnet monkeys [7].

European guidelines are forthcoming that will recommend social housing of nonhuman primates whenever possible. Whether pair-housing or even group-housing will be feasible for pregnant nonhuman primates in toxicity studies remains questionable. Reports are available suggesting an increased prenatal loss and reproductive failure in pair-housed versus single-housed pregnant cynomolgus monkeys. Similarly production of viable offspring is more successful during individual housing compared to being exposed to groups of cage-mates.

18.7 PRENATAL AND POSTNATAL DEVELOPMENT OF THE IMMUNE SYSTEM

The pre- and postnatal development of the immune system in the cynomolgus monkey was studied using various approaches including detailed histological and immunohistochemical techniques [10,39]. Relative to pregnancy duration, the timing of crucial events—such as hematopoietic stem cell formation; cell migration to fetal thymus, liver, and bone marrow formation; preparedness for immune function and formation of memory cells—is strikingly similar between human and cynomolgus monkey but substantially different from mouse. It is evident that the prenatal and postnatal development and maturation of the immune system are largely comparable between human and cynomolgus monkey but are clearly different from rodents. The major difference relates to the fact, that in primates immune system maturation is generally more advanced relative to gestational and postnatal age compared to rodents.

Similar to humans [52,53], the CD4–CD8 ratio decreases during the postnatal phase in macaques. We observed a CD4–CD8 ratio reduction, on average, from 2.2 at one month of age to 1.3 at 12 months of age in the cynomolgus monkey and—in another study—a ratio decrease from 2.2 to 1.6 (Figure 18.4). Baroncelli et al. reported a ratio decrease from approx. 3.1 to 1.5 within 12 months in the same species [54]. A similar pattern was obtained for the rhesus monkey with a CD4–CD8 ratio decline from 3.5 in neonates to 0.7 in adult animals [55].

Data from KLH-vaccinated cynomolgus monkey infants show an evident TDAR in animals of 3 months of age and a pronounced secondary antibody response to a booster immunization approximately 3 months thereafter (Figure 18.2). Since TDAR requires functional antigen-presenting cells, T cells, and B cells (including the switch to antibody-producing plasma cells), it is supposed to be the most relevant functional assay for a general assessment of immunosuppression. Besides others, another functional assay to be considered for use in juvenile monkeys is a functional test of natural killer (NK) cell activity.

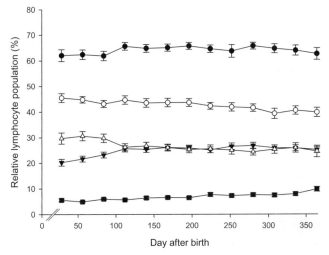

Figure 18.4 Postnatal distribution of lymphocyte subsets by immunophentyping analysis in immature cynomolgus monkeys. Typically CD4–CD8 ratio declines during postnatal development, (e.g., from 2.2 to 1.6 within 12 months in this data set). Others reported a ratio decrease of 3.1 to 1.5 within 12 months for the same species [54]. Data represent mean values ± SEM of 26 to 32 animals (males and females combined). ● CD3+, ○ CD4+, △ CD20+, ▼ CD8+, ■ CD16+.

However, it is known that the NK cell activity is low in neonatals of different species and that the ability to be activated by the functional stimulator inter-leukin IL-2 is reduced [56,57]. Therefore, and since a relatively high blood volume is required, this assay is recommended from the age of 6 months onward in the cynomolgus monkey.

18.8   CONCLUSION

DART evaluation of biopharmaceuticals frequently necessitates the use of NHP owing to species specificity. Cynomolgus monkey currently represents the most frequently used NHP. Fertility studies and embryofetal development studies are also feasible in the marmoset. A broad array of immune function tests is available for adult and infant cynomolgus monkeys. Primates experience significant prenatal losses and also losses around term, and this should be considered when planning group sizes. Whereas the study designs for male/female fertility and embryofetal development are established, a need for standardization prevails for the design duration of the postnatal phase in pre-/post-natal studies. The pre- and postnatal development of the immune system is similar between human and cynomolgus monkey but clearly different from rodents such as mouse. For biopharmaceuticals and immune system evaluation, a minimum postnatal observation period of 6 months is recommended.

If the behavioral test battery includes a learning test, a minimum of 9 months for postnatal evaluation is appropriate.

ACKNOWLEDGMENTS

We are greatly indebted to Shiela Srivastav and Jan Sternberg for their help during preparation of this chapter.

REFERENCES

1. Frings W, Cavagnaro JA. Predicting clinical immunogenicity: Intended or unintended. In Weinbauer G, Buse E, Muller W, Vogel F, eds. *New Developments and Challenges in Primate Toxicology*. Muenster: Waxmann, 2005;9–21.

2. Bugelski PJ, Treacy G. Predictive power of preclinical studies in animals for the immunogenicity of recombinant therapeutic proteins in humans. *Curr Opini Mol Ther* 2004;6(1):10–6.

3. Kropshofer H. Preclinical immunogenicity risk assessment of biotherapeutic proteins. In Weinbauer G, Vogel F, eds. *Novel Approaches towards Primate Toxicology*. Muenster: Waxmann, 2006;91–102.

4. Henck JW, Hilbish KG, Serabian MA, et al. Reproductive toxicity testing of therapeutic biotechnology agents. *Teratology* 1996;53(3):185–95.

5. Kavanagh M, Laursen E. Breeding seasonality among long-tailed macaques, Macaca fascicularis, in Peninsula Malaysia. *Int J Primatol* 1984;5:17–29.

6. Dang DC. Absence of seasonal variation in the length of the menstrual cycle and the fertility of the crab-eating macaque (*Macaca fascicularis*) raised under natural daylight ratio. *An Biolog Biochim Biophys* 1977;17:1–7.

7. Hendrie T, Peterson P, Short J, et al. Frequency of prenatal loss in a macaque breeding colony. *Am J Primatol*. 1996;40:41–53.

8. Niehoff M, Bergmann M, Müller W, Weinbauer GF. Effects of group housing on reproductive parameters. In Weinbauer G, Buse E, Muller W, Vogel F, eds. *New Developments and Challenges in Primate Toxicology*. Muenster: Waxmann, 2004;137–44.

9. Buse E, Habermann G, Osterburg I, Korte R, Weinbauer GF. Reproductive/developmental toxicity and immunotoxicity assessment in the nonhuman primate model. *Toxicology*. 2003;185(3):221–7.

10. Buse E. Development of the immune system in the cynomolgus monkey: the appropriate model in human target toxicology. *J Immunotoxicol* 2005;2:211–6.

11. ILAR. Nonhuman primate and other animal models of women's health. *Inst Lab Animal Res*. 2004;45:83–219.

12. Weinbauer G, Korte R. Reproduction in nonhuman primates—A Model Sytem for Human Reproductive Physiology and Toxicology. Muenster: Waxmann, 1999.

13. Herndon JG, Bein ML, Nordmeyer DL, Turner JJ. Seasonal testicular function in male rhesus monkeys. *Hormones Beh* 1996;30(3):266–71.

14. Ghosh D, Sengupta J. Patterns of ovulation and pre-implantation embry development, during the breeding season in rhesus monkeys kept under semi-natural conditions. *Acta Endocrinol* 1992;127:168–73.

15. Wickings EJ, Nieschlag E. Suppression of spermatogenesis over two years in rhesus monkeys actively immunized with follicle-stimulating hormone. *Fertility Sterility* 1980;34(3):269–74.

16. Luetjens CM, Weinbauer GF, Wistuba J. Primate spermatogenesis: new insights into comparative testicular organisation, spermatogenic efficiency and endocrine control. *Biol Rev Camb Phil Soc* 2005;80(3):475–88.

17. Hearn JP, Lunn SF. The endocrinology of the ovarian cycle and of pregnancy in the marmoset monkey, *Callithrix jaccus. J Endocrinol* 1975;65(3):1P.

18. Abbott DH, Barnett DK, Colman RJ, Yamamoto ME, Schultz-Darken NJ. Aspects of common marmoset basic biology and life history important for biomedical research. *Comp Med* 2003;53(4):339–50.

19. Li LH, Donald JM, Golub MS. Review on testicular development, structure, function, and regulation in common marmoset. *Birth Defects Res B Dev Reprod Toxicol.* 2005;74(5):450–69.

20. Zuhlke U, Weinbauer G. The common marmoset (*Callithrix jacchus*) as a model in toxicology. *Toxicol Pathol* 2003;31(Suppl):123–7.

21. Haig D. What is a marmoset? *Am J Primatol* 1999;49(4):285–96.

22. Gilchrist RB, Wicherek M, Heistermann M, Nayudu PL, Hodges JK. Changes in follicle-stimulating hormone and follicle populations during the ovarian cycle of the common marmoset. *Biol Reprod* 2001;64(1):127–35.

23. Gromoll J, Weinbauer GF, Skaletsky H, et al. The Old World monkey DAZDeleted in AZoospermia) gene yields insights into the evolution of the DAZ gene cluster on the human Y chromosome. *Hum Mol Genet* 1999;8(11):2017–24.

24. Jaquish CE, Tardif SD, Toal RL, Carson RL. Patterns of prenatal survival in the common marmoset (*Callithrix jacchus*). *J Med Primatol* 1996;25(1):57–63.

25. Muller T, Simoni M, Pekel E, et al. Chorionic gonadotrophin beta subunit mRNA but not luteinising hormone beta subunit mRNA is expressed in the pituitary of the common marmoset (*Callithrix jacchus*). *J Mol Endocrinol* 2004;32(1):115–28.

26. Tardif SD, Smucny DA, Abbott DH, Mansfield K, Schultz-Darken N, Yamamoto ME. Reproduction in captive common marmosets (*Callithrix jacchus*). *Comp Med* 2003;53(4):364–8.

27. Merker HJ, Heger W, Sames K, Sturje H, Neubert D. Embryotoxic effects of thalidomide-derivatives in the non-human primate *Callithrix jacchus*. I. Effects of 3-(1,3-dihydro-1-oxo-2H-isoindol-2-yl)-2,6-dioxopiperidine (EM12) on skeletal development. *Arch Toxicol* 1988;61(3):165–79.

28. Muller T, Gromoll J, Simoni M. Absence of exon 10 of the human luteinizing hormone (LH) receptor impairs LH, but not human chorionic gonadotropin action. *J Clin Endocrinol Metab* 2003;88(5):2242–9.

29. Resuello RG. Cynomolgus monkey twins. *Vet Rec.* 1987;121(7):155.

30. Binkerd PE, Tarantal AF, Hendrickx AG. Embryonic/fetal loss and spontaneous malformations In nonhuman primates. In Neubert D, Merker HJ, Hendrickx AG, eds. *Non-human Primates—Developmental Biology and Toxicology.* Wien-Berlin: Ueberreuter Wissenschaft, 1988;115–27.

31. Mineshima H, Endo Y, Ogasawara H, et al. Impact of globalization under the ICH guidelines on the conduct of reproductive toxicity studies—report on current status in Japan, Europe and the US by questionnaire survey. *J Toxicol Sci* 2004; 29(3):201–15.

32. Foppiani L, Schlatt S, Simoni M, Weinbauer GF, Hacker-Klom U, Nieschlag E. Inhibin B is a more sensitive marker of spermatogenetic damage than FSH in the irradiated non-human primate model. *J Endocrinol* 1999;162(3):393–400.

33. Fraser HM, Groome NP, McNeilly AS. Follicle-stimulating hormone-inhibin B interactions during the follicular phase of the primate menstrual cycle revealed by gonadotropin-releasing hormone antagonist and antiestrogen treatment. *J Clin Endocrinol Metab* 1999;84(4):1365–9.

34. Golub MS, Gershwin ME, Hurley LS, Hendrickx AG, Saito WY. Studies of marginal zinc deprivation in rhesus monkeys: infant behaviour. *Am J Clin Nutrit.* 1985; 42(6):1229–39.

35. Golub MS, Sassenrath EN, Chapman LF. Mother-infant interaction in rhesus monkeys treated clinically with delta-9-terahydrocannabiol. *Child Dev* 1981; 52:389–92.

36. Maestripieri D, Jovanovic T, Gouzoules H. Crying and infant abuse in rhesus monkeys. *Child Dev.* 2000;71(2):301–9.

37. Hendrickx AG, Binkerd P. Nonhuman primates and teratological research. *J Med Primatol* 1990;19:81–108.

38. Hendrickx AG, Tzimas G, Korte R, Hummler H. Retinoid teratogenicity in the macaque: verification of dosing regimen. *J Med Primatol* 1998;27(6):310–8.

39. Buse E, Habermann G, Vogel F. Thymus development in *Macaca fascicularis* (cynomolgus monkey): an approach for toxicology and embryology. *J Mol Histol* 2006;37(3–4):161–70.

40. Fuchs A, Weinbauer G. Feasibilty of embryofetal development studies in the marmoset (*Callithrix jacchus*). In Weinbauer G, Vogel F, eds. *Novel Approaches towards Primate Toxicology.* Muenster: Waxmann 2006;110–22.

41. Harlow CR, Gems S, Hodges KH, Hearn JP. The relationship between plasma progesterone and the timing of ovulation and early embryonic development in the marmoset monkey (Callithrix jacchus). *J Zool London* 1983;201:273–82.

42. Merker HJ, Sames K, Csato W, Heger W, Neubert D. The embryology of *Callithrix jacchus*. In Neubert D, Merker HJ, Hendrickx AG, eds. *Non-human Primates— Developmental Biology and Toxicology.* Wien-Berlin: Ueberreuter Wissenschaft, 1988;219–42.

43. Simister NE. Placental transport of immunoglobulin G. *Vaccine* 2003;21(24): 3365–9.

44. Fujimoto K, Terao K, Cho F, Honjo S. The Placental transfer of IgG in the cynomolgus monkey. *Jap J Med Sci Biol* 1983;36:171–76.

45. Small MF. Reproductive failure in macaques. *Am J Primatol* 1982;2(2):137–47.

46. Cukierski MA, Prahalada S, Zacchei AG, et al. Embryotoxicity studies of norfloxacin in cynomolgus monkeys: I. Teratology studies and norfloxacin plasma concentration in pregnant and nonpregnant monkeys. *Teratology* 1989; 39(1):39–52.

47. Tarantal AF, O'Brien WD, Hendrickx AG. Evaluation of the bioeffects of prenatal ultrasound exposure in the cynomolgus macaque (*Macaca fascicularis*): III. Developmental and hematologic studies. *Teratology* 1993;47(2):159–70.

48. Carlock L, Oneda S, Bussiere J. An assessment of the effects of human soluble IL-4 receptor on reproduction and neonatal development when administered intravenously to pregnant cynomolgus monkeys. *Toxicologist* 2003;72:327.

49. Hardy L, Ortega S, Rogers B, Sinicropi D, Clarke J, Oneda S. Recombinant human nerve growth factor is not teratogenic when administered subcutaneously to cynomolgus monkeys. *Toxicologist* 1998;42(1–S):259.

50. Heger W, Merker HJ, Neubert D. Frequency of prenatal loss in marmoset monkeys (*Callithrix jacchus*). In Neubert D, Merker HJ, Neubert D, eds. *Non-human Primates—Developmental Biology and Toxicology*. Wien-Berlin: Uebereuter Wissenschaft, 1988;120–40.

51. Boot R, Leussink AB, Vlug RF. Influence of housing conditions on pregnancy outcome in cynomolgus monkeys (*Macaca fascicularis*). *Lab Animals* 1985; 19(1):42–7.

52. Denny T, Yogev R, Gelman R, et al. Lymphocyte subsets in healthy children during the first 5 years of life. *J Am Med Assoc* 1992;267(11):1484–8.

53. Heldrup J, Kalm O, Prellner K. Blood T and B lymphocyte subpopulations in healthy infants and children. *Acta Paediat* 1992;81(2):125–32.

54. Baroncelli S, Panzini G, Geraci A, et al. Longitudinal characterization of CD4, CD8 T-cell subsets and of haematological parameters in healthy newborns of cynomolgus monkeys. *Vet Immunol Immunopathol* 1997;59(1–2):141–50.

55. DeMaria MA, Casto M, O'Connell M, Johnson RP, Rosenzweig M. Characterization of lymphocyte subsets in rhesus macaques during the first year of life. *Eur J Haematol* 2000;65(4):245–57.

56. Hodge S, GHodge G, Flower R, Han P. Cord blood leucocyte expression of functionally significant molecules involved in the regulation of cellular immunity. *Scand J Immunol* 2001;53(1):72–8.

57. Frings W, Weinbauer G. Flow-ytometry-based evaluation of lymphocyte subsets and natural killer cell activity in developing and adult cynomolgus monkeys. *Toxicologist* 2004;78(1–S):430.

CHAPTER 19

Preclinical Evaluation of Cancer Hazard and Risk of Biopharmaceuticals

JOY A. CAVAGNARO, PhD, DABT, RAC

Contents

Preclinical Safety Evaluation of Biopharmaceuticals: A Science-Based Approach to Facilitating Clinical Trials, edited by Joy A. Cavagnaro
Copyright © 2008 by John Wiley & Sons, Inc.

I am not so worried about a positive rodent bioassay because we usually explain it away; I am more worried about a negative one
                    —Professor Gerhard Zbinden (personal communication)

19.1   BACKGROUND

Carcinogenesis is the term used to denote the development of neoplasia that can be induced experimentally by exposure to exogenous agents or can occur spontaneously without intentional or active intervention [1]. Neoplasias result following a complex biological process consisting of multiple cellular mutations followed by the selective growth of mutated cells, and the eventual progression of cells to malignancy [1,2]. While most of the known carcinogenic agents act directly on the cell and damage somatic cell DNA as part of the multi-step process, changes in the rate of cell division and cell death are also be critical to the process of malignant transformation. The diverse modes of action (MOA) of carcinogenic agents in relation to their effects on specific stages in the natural history of cancer development allow for greater congruence of many theories on carcinogenesis [1].

Currently the basic experimental paradigm used to identify potential human carcinogens and estimate their potency is the rodent bioassay [3,4,5]. This assay is nearly universally applied to new molecular entities, and positive results have an important impact on the future of a drug, including its approvability. When needed, carcinogenicity testing is usually performed during a clinical development program once activity and safety have been demonstrated in the intended patient population. A positive tumor response in the rodent bioassay is a strong stimulus to toxicologists to attempt to fully understand the reasons for the response [6]. Mechanistic studies may be suggested to support the claim that effects are not relevant or not of great concern to humans under the conditions of clinical use. Even when rodent carcinogenicity findings do not prevent approval, the results can restrict marketing or otherwise reduce their perceived competitive utility based on the potential risks communicated in the label [7].

In the early 1960s the National Cancer Institute (NCI) developed procedures to formalize the process for the evaluation of the human risk of cancer from chemical exposures [8]. This approach was based on decades of research that demonstrated that chemicals that were known to cause cancer in humans could also induce cancer in laboratory animals. The bioassay was originally envisioned as a cancer screen useful for identifying agents that would be examined in human epidemiology studies, assuming that relatively few compounds would induce tumors in animals. Despite the fact that the approach by the NCI was only intended as an initial screening tool for carcinogenic activity the use of two rodent species exposed for two years as the primary means to identify potential human hazards was in widespread use by the early 1970s. In 1975 the approach was developed into a recommendation that formed the basis of regulatory guidance [9]. Rodent bioassays were subsequently expected for evaluating the safety of long-term chemical exposure and for the marketing of chronically administered drugs or those expected to have persistent effects. As such, the rodent bioassay became the "gold standard" for carcinogenicity assessment. The bioassay also evolved to occupy a primary role in the identification of agents considered "possible" or "probable" human carcinogens by the International Agency for Research on Cancer (IARC), and those "reasonably anticipated to be human carcinogens" by the National Toxicology Program (NTP) Report on Carcinogens [6].

Contemporary quantitative risk-assessment methodology for chemicals estimates cancer risks using slope factors derived from the rodent bioassay. These cancer-slope factors are based on, and intended to represent, the potency of the chemical under conditions of continuous lifetime exposure. However, in many situations for drugs used for chronic indications, exposure is not continuous over a lifetime but intermittent over short durations. When estimating risk from less-than-lifetime exposure, the assumption is usually made that cancer risk from exposure at a given rate decreases proportionally with decreasing exposure duration, and adjustments are made accordingly in the risk calculation. Although this approach represents a means to develop cancer risk estimates for limited exposure duration scenarios, its validity has never been well established [10]. One example that calls into question this paradigm is the recognized age differences in susceptibility to particular agents. If a carcinogen affects an animal or human primarily in a particular life stage, a short-term exposure during that stage may be very effective in producing cancer, while the same short-term exposure during a different life stage may be ineffective. When compared to continuous exposure over a lifetime, the apparent potency of the short-term exposure may be greater or less than that of continuous exposure, depending on when the short-term exposure occurs relative to the period of greatest susceptibility to the particular carcinogen [11].

Although sophisticated mathematical models are often relied upon for quantitative risk assessments, assessments have also been made on more qualitative evaluation of animal test data. In part this is because mathematical models are often based on assumptions on mutation rates and not all carcinogens are primary mutagens.

Over the past decade other concerns have been raised about the continued use of rodent data and its relevance for predicting human risk [11–16]. For example, more than half of the chemicals evaluated in the rodent bioassay have tested positive in one or more rodent species. One explanation has been that the large doses that are tested (i.e., maximum tolerated doses) may overwhelm the body's natural detoxification mechanisms. Cyclosporin A (CyA), a pharmaceutical used clinically as an immunosuppressant, is nongenotoxic (or equivalent in an in vitro mammalian cell assay) and negative in the rodent bioassay but in humans is associated with an increase in the development of B cell lymphomas and squamous cell carcinomas, particularly of the cervix [17]. CyA and other immunosuppressants such as anti-lymphocyte globulin (ALG) probably act by their therapeutic role of depressing immunity resulting in a loss of normal body defenses against spontaneous cancer-causing agents, oncogenic viral agents, and so forth. There is also increasing evidence that some chemicals produce cancer in rodents through species-specific mechanisms that are irrelevant to human physiology and thus may not necessarily predict human hazard. Examples include urinary bladder tumors in rats exposed to high doses of saccharin or melamine, male rat kidney tumors induced by compounds like d-limonene that produce a characteristic male rat hydrocarbon nephropathy, rat mammary tumors produced in response to β-adrenergic blocking agents, and mesovarial leiomyomas in rats exposure to β-agonists like salbutamol. Endocrine tumors in rats including thyroid tumors or gastric ECL-cell carcinoid tumors have also been shown to be rodent specific as well as peroxisome proliferators that cause rodent liver tumors [16,18]. These examples are where specific biochemical mechanisms have been elucidated.

An increased knowledge about carcinogenic differences in the mode of action and processes between rodents and humans coincides with an emerging view that cancer arises from fewer pathways then scientists once assumed. Consideration has therefore been given to refocusing cancer hazard identification to the specific aspects of the tumor response, including toxicity exhibited in an organ, the history of response of the tumor type in that organ to other substances, as well as any evidence of altered oncogene or tumor suppressor gene expression. Measures of cell proliferation, evidence of altered hormonal stimulation, structure activity relationships (SAR), comparative exposure and metabolism data, pharmacodynamic and mechanism of action information, are therefore being considered in addition to other alternative short-term bioassays. The relevance of the rodent tumors to human cancer hazard is also being considered through the application of a "mode of action" analysis [19]. The mode of action is sufficient evidence to draw a reasonable working conclusion regarding the influence of the test articles on key processes. The mode of action concept permits information on precursor events to be evaluated and incorporated in the risk-assessment process.

Gottman and colleagues compared 121 replicated rodent carcinogenicity assays from the NCI/NTP and the literature to estimate the reproducibility of the rodent carcinogenicity assays for SAR studies and risk assessment [20]. The results indicated a concordance of 57% between the overall rodent carcinogenicity classifications from the replicate bioassays. This value did not improve substantially when additional biologic information (species, sex, strain, target organs) was considered, suggesting that rodent carcinogenicity assays are much less reproducible than previously expected. Based on these findings the authors concluded that it is not only difficult to identify carcinogens in general, but also to identify reliably powerful multi-species and multi-organ carcinogens. Risk assessment of nongenotoxic carcinogens of importance for human safety from a statistical point of view is even more difficult due to the high spontaneous tumor background in a two-year study in rodents against which positive or negative effects can be missed.

Since drug-induced cancers are rare in human, the results of routine carcinogenicity testing may be misleading as an indication of risk to humans. Therefore the results need careful interpretation. Because of the increasing concerns regarding the relevance and reproducibility of the rodent bioassay, it has been suggested that the bioassay may not be needed in the future to predict carcinogenic risk of pharmaceuticals if sufficient information on the specific agent can be derived from other studies [18,21]. High-throughput screens based on genomic, proteomic, and metabolomic cancer biomarkers are increasingly being used to prioritize chemicals for long-term testing. Based on the major advances in computer technology, chemoinformatics, and predictive toxicology, the accumulated results of rodent carcinogenicity studies in public databases and regulatory files can be used to improve the scientific bases of regulatory and product development decisions. It has been proposed that over time with increased experience and confidence in carcinogenicity predictive software, it may be possible to reduce carcinogenicity testing for compounds that have molecular structures that are highly represented in well-defined carcinogenicity databases [7]. The additional information for risk assessment would include whether the test article is a direct-acting DNA mutagen, induces liver enzymes, causes hyperplasia or toxicity in particular organs, causes cell proliferation, is cytotoxic, immunosuppressive or causes hormonal perturbations [16].

In 2001 the International Programme on Chemical Safety (IPCS) Conceptual Framework for Evaluation (animal) Mode of Action for Chemical Carcinogens provided a framework for a generic approach to the principles commonly used for evaluating mode of action. It outlined a list of elements to be considered in analyzing whether available data support a particular mode of action. In 2006 this "Harmonization Project" completed work to extend the 2001 Framework to address the issue of human relevance. The IPCS Framework for Analyzing the Relevance of a Cancer Mode of Action for Humans was published in a special issue of *Critical Reviews in Toxicology*, Volume 36(10), November–December 2006. Ultimately it will be published as a WHO document. A technical working group focused on cancer hazard identification, operating under the umbrella of the Health and Environmental Sciences Institute (HESI) in Washington, DC, has recently been formed to explore the hypothesis that carcinogenic signals can be identified in short-term studies exclusive of the rodent bioassay. Another group, the Predictive Safety Testing Consortium (PSTC) carcinogenicity working group, is focused on identifying signatures of nongenotoxic carcinogenicity. The PSTC was formed in the United States in 2006 under the auspices of the Critical Path Institute (C-Path) to enable pharmaceutical companies to pool their monetary and data resources to develop biomarkers for preclinical safety testing. A similar initiative is ongoing under the European Commission's Sixth Framework

Programme (FP6). The FP6 is the framework for the EU activity in the field of science, research, and innovation. The main objective of the FP6 is to contribute to the creation of the European Research Area (ERA) by improving integration and coordination of research in Europe. One of seven priority thematic areas is Life Science, Genomics and Biotechnology for Health.

The ultimate question that must be answered during clinical development of a biopharmaceutical is, Does the proposed use of the biopharmaceutical carry a carcinogenic risk for humans in the intended patient population under the conditions of intended clinical use? The answer should consider whether the risk is real or theoretical based on knowledge of the particular product or product class. In selected instances human experience in long-term disease and genetic disorders may reveal the nature and magnitude of the clinical risk, such as the known propensity of patients with certain types of congenital immune disorders to develop lymphomas. The availability of appropriate preclinical models and study designs must also be considered not only to identify the hazard but also to support rationalization of the potential risk. A follow-up question could be asked as to whether animal data would alter the perception of risk. Determining optimal management of the potential risk through patient monitoring and follow-up and/or restrictions in use, as well as providing effective communication of the potential risk through informed consent and ultimately in the product label, are all critical components to the processes of human carcinogenic risk assessment and risk management.

19.2   HUMAN EXPERIENCE

Despite the high percentage of positive rodent carcinogens there are a relatively few pharmaceuticals demonstrated to be carcinogenic in humans [22]. The known human carcinogens have been genotoxic, immunosuppressive, hormonally active, or belong to a class of reactive dermatologicals (e.g., arsenicals) [17]. Unfortunately, it is very difficult to attribute cancer cases to a particular product unless the cancer occurs in a high percentage of individuals, the relationship of the cancer incidence has been studied rigorously (e.g., the associations of PUVA therapy and various skin neoplasms years later), or the product induces a rare form of cancer, as was the case for DES [23].

The time to occurrence of human malignancy varies widely. Most estimates suggest years of exposure are required. For many of the well-defined cancers arising in susceptible hosts, as well as for patients with known carcinogen exposures, the period before development of a malignant tumor is often measured in decades. The complex accumulation of factors influencing the development of neoplasms include viral infections, chronic antigenic stimulation, direct or synergistic carcinogenic effects of certain immunosuppressive agents, sunlight exposure, and other exogenous carcinogenic stimuli in addition to an individual's genetic susceptibility to certain cancers.

Some malignancies occur in association with a wide variety of immune suppression conditions such as inherited diseases of the immune system, acquired immunodeficiency disorders, disorders of immune dysregulation, and iatrogenic immunosuppression (e.g., patients receiving varying degrees of immunosuppressant therapies). These malignancies may occur within a few years. Regardless of how the immunodeficiency is produced, the malignancy is generally associated with an increased risk of certain cancers, namely B cell lymphomas, usually associated with Epstein-Barr virus (EBV), squamous cell carcinomas associated with human papilloma virus (HPV), particularly of the cervix, and Kaposi's sarcoma associated with herpes virus 8 (HHV-8) in patients with AIDS [24]. These tumors are predominantly associated with viral infections that cannot be kept under control because of the immunodeficiency. In such cases it is unlikely that the immunosuppressive therapies themselves are directly carcinogenic; rather, the carcinogenic stimulus is more likely due to induction of immunosuppression that leads to the specific viral-associated tumors [24].

The precise role of immunological surveillance in tumorigenesis is not well defined for the majority of malignancies. The occurrence of a unique spectrum of malignancies in immunosuppressed individuals suggests either that immune surveillance is only important in certain tumors or that the duration needed to see an increased incidence of many more common tumors (e.g., colorectal, breast, lung, or prostate carcinomas) is not reached. Suppression of T cell mediated immunity has, however, been unequivocally associated with an increased incidence of certain malignancies. In patients with profound defects in T cell immunity the time to tumor detection is often shorter than for cancers induced by other mechanisms.

The risk of developing lymphoproliferative disorders following immunosuppressive therapy is also associated with the duration and intensity of immunosuppression [25]. In early postmarketing surveillance following the approval of the first approved therapeutic monoclonal antibody, Orthoclone OKT®3 (muromonab CD3), a murine monoclonal antibody directed against the CD3 antigen on human T cells, the incidence of lymphomas was disproportionately higher in heart and lung transplant recipients when compared to renal transplant recipients, presumably due to the more intensive regimen (dose and duration) in the first two indications. Unfortunately, with transplant patients it is often difficult to evaluate the contribution of any specific agent because many are used in combination regimens for treatment of rejection. See below and Chapter 27 for a discussion of concerns with immunodulatory biopharmaceuticals.

19.3 DETERMINING THE NEED FOR PRECLINICAL CARCINOGENICITY ASSESSMENT

The need for carcinogenicity assessment of a biopharmaceutical is not different than that for a conventional pharmaceutical. The need is based on an intended duration of (i.e., ≥6 months of continual dosing or dosing frequently in an intermittent manner for a chronic or recurrent condition), cause for concern, indication and patient population including the nature of the disease and its effect on life span and overall patient health, route and exposure, and extent of systemic exposure when certain delivery systems may result in prolonged exposures. The need is also established if there is cause for concern based on the product class or if there is evidence of preneoplastic lesions in repeat-dose chronic studies. For pharmaceuticals an additional concern is long-term retention of parent compound or metabolite(s), which may result in local tissue reactions or other pathological responses (See Table 19.1) [26]. In most cases the rat and/or mouse have been deemed relevant species for assessment of conventional carcinogenic risk of conventional pharmaceuticals based on regulatory precedent.

In the early days of the production of human proteins by recombinant DNA technology using *E. coli* bacteria, there was considerable and reasonable concern about the presence of bacterial impurities that may be carried through the purification processes. Genotoxicity studies were widely used to ensure that these impurities were not mutagenic or clastogenic. However, with the development of improved methods of synthesis and purification, together with highly sophisticated and sensitive analytical techniques for detection of possible impurities, the need for genotoxicity studies has been greatly reduced. Despite this important progress, toxicologists in industry have continued to perform genotoxicity studies and/or the studies have been requested by regulatory agencies even though the data may not have apparent scientific relevance (see Chapter 15). Ironically, regardless of their lack of relevance, the absence of positive findings in the various genotoxicity assays have often been used as "scientific" justification for not needing to assess carcinogenic potential in vivo in animals

19.3.1   Peptide Hormones and Growth Factors

In the case of biopharmaceuticals the particular cause for concern for carcinogenic risk is raised by the action of peptide hormones and growth factors. These may directly promote cellular growth through direct activation of the drug receptor or through other factors involved in growth regulation [27]. Thus for growth factors, where one of the putative mechanisms of concern would be increased proliferation, an evaluation of this endpoint in the appropriate target tissue in in vivo studies in a relevant species is important in order to determine potential concern for tumorigenic risk. Although unidentified, target or nontarget tissues may also be a cause for concern.

19.3.2   Immunomodulatory Biopharmaceuticals

For biopharmaceuticals intentionally developed to target critical immune-signaling molecules, current in vitro and in vivo methods confirm

TABLE 19.1 Factors to consider for carcinogenicity testing of pharmaceuticals

Factors	Considerations When Rodent Bioassays Performed	Considerations When Rodent Bioassays Not Needed
Duration and exposure	• Expected clinical use continuous for 6 months • Expected to be used frequently in an intermittent manner in the treatment of chronic or recurrent conditions • For certain delivery systems which may result in prolonged exposures	• Used infrequently or for a short duration of exposure (e.g., anesthetics and radiolabeled imaging agents) if no cause for concern
Cause for concern	• Previous demonstration of carcinogenic (oncogenic) potential in the product class that is considered relevant to humans • Structure-activity relationship suggesting carcinogenic risk • Evidence of preneoplastic lesions in repeated-dose toxicity studies • Long-term tissue retention of parent compound or metabolite(s) resulting in local tissue reactions or other pathophysiological responses	
Genotoxicity	• Recommended ICH test battery • A single positive result in any assay for genotoxicity does not necessarily mean that the test compound poses a genotoxic hazard to humans (also concern for nongenotoxic carcinogens), although in vivo positive may be considered differently than in vitro positive	• Unequivocally genotoxic compounds, in the absence of other data, that are presumed to be transspecies carcinogens, implying a hazard to humans (chronic toxicity of up to 1 year may be needed if drug is intended to be used chronically to detect early tumorigenic effects)
Indication and patient population	• Expected to be completed before application for marketing approval (not needed prior to conduct of large-scale clinical trials unless cause for concern) • For pharmaceuticals that are intended for adjuvant therapy in tumor free patients or for prolonged use in noncancer indications (may be additional conditions for compounds especially designed for use in children)	• May be conducted postapproval if drug is intended for life-threatening or severely debilitating disease, especially where no satisfactory alternative therapy exists • Oncolytic agents intended for treatment of advanced disease (if treatment is successful, there may be later concerns regarding secondary cancers)

TABLE 19.1 Factors to consider for carcinogenicity testing of pharmaceuticals (*Continued*)

Factors	Considerations When Rodent Bioassays Performed	Considerations When Rodent Bioassays Not Needed
Route and exposure	• Route should be the same as the intended clinical route when feasible • Alternative route is acceptable if similar metabolism and systemic as well as target organ exposure (e.g., lung for inhalation agents) can be demonstrated (exposure may be derived from pharmacokinetic data)	
Extent of systemic exposure	• Pharmaceuticals applied topically (e.g., dermal and ocular routes of administration) if knowledge is already available from systemic exposure further local testing may not be necessary unless concentration or duration are very prolonged • Cause for concern for photocarcinogenic potential (dermal application generally in mice)	• Pharmaceuticals showing poor systemic exposure from topical route • Pharmaceuticals administered by ocular route unless cause for concern or unless there is significant systemic exposure • For different salts, acids, or bases of the same therapeutic moiety, where prior carcinogenicity studies are available (provided no significant changes in pharmacokinetics, pharmacodynamics, or toxicity) (When changes in exposure and consequent toxicity are noted, additional bridging studies may be used to determine whether additional carcinogenicity studies are needed) • For esters and complex derivatives, similar data would be valuable in assessing the need for an additional carcinogenicity study (determined on a case-by-case basis)

| Endogenous peptides and protein substances and their analogues | • Should be considered for endogenous peptides or proteins if indicated by treatment duration, clinical indication, or patient population (providing neutralizing antibodies are not elicited to such an extent in repeated-dose studies as to invalidate the results)
— for products where there are significant differences in biological effects to the natural counterpart(s)
— for products where modifications lead to significant changes in structure compared to the natural counterpart
— for products resulting in humans in a significant increase over the existing local or systemic concentration (i.e., pharmacological levels; concern is increased if principal action is to increase cell proliferation or to prolong cell survival; combination therapy with known carcinogenic stimulus) | • Endogenous substances given essentially as replacement therapy (i.e., physiological levels), particularly where there is previous clinical experience with similar products (e.g., animal insulins, pituitary-derived growth hormone, and calcitonin). |
| Need for additional testing | • Further research may be needed, investigating the mode of action (to confirm the presence or the lack of carcinogenic potential for humans)
• Mechanistic studies are useful to evaluate the relevance of tumor findings in animals for human safety | |

Source: Adapted ICH S1A, The Need for Long-term Rodent Carcinogenicity Studies of Pharmaceuticals (http://www.fda.gov/cder/guidance/index.htm).

immunosuppressant activity, rather than reveal a clinically useful designation of safe, "pharmacologically immunosuppressive," or toxic "adversely immuno-suppressive." Concerns following chronic treatment of immunosuppressive agents include the potential impairment leading to opportunistic infections and/or lymphoproliferative disorders. The pharmacological activity of thera-peutic immunosuppressive drugs is thought to make them highly likely to act as tumor promoters/co-carcinogens, even in the absence of genotoxic activity. For example, potent immunosuppressive agents may increase the risk of tumor promotion by impairing the endogenous tumor surveillance mechanism. As far as we know, cellular and humoral immunosuppression probably carry similar risks. Thus it is assumed that this class of drug would represent a cancer hazard in the absence of confirmatory standard bioassay [28] (see Chapter 27).

19.3.3 Cell Lines Used to Produce Biopharmceuticals

The international quality guidance document ICH Q5D requires tumorigenic-ity testing for products for which live cells cannot be excluded or products that have minimal downstream purification (e.g., conventional live virus vaccines) [29]. The guidance states that tumorigenicity testing of proteins is generally not needed provided that residual host cell DNA limits are established and met. These limits were based on careful consideration of the amount of DNA involved and evidence about the likelihood that it might transmit a viable oncogenic agent. The above-mentioned guidance does not require tumorige-nicity testing for cell lines that have been previously shown to be tumorigenic, but the sponsor may want to evaluate the previous results in light of current proposed indications. However, if the cell line is to be licensed as a nontumori-genic cell line, it has to be demonstrated by a negative result in tumorigenicity assays. Newer previously uncharacterized diploid cell lines should be evalu-ated for their tumorigenic potential by using cells from the master cell bank (MCB). The assessments should include comparison between the cell line under evaluation and a positive (tumorigenic) cell line used as a positive control. Animal models for assessing tumorigenicity include athymic mice (Nu/Nu), suckling mice or hamsters treated with antithymocyte serum, and/or irradiated and thymectomized mice reconstituted (T-B+) with bone marrow of healthy mice [29]. Additional considerations may also be applied to cells from nonmammalian sources used to produce therapeutic proteins.

19.3.4 Cellular-Based Therapies

Tumorigenicity studies are also needed for certain cell therapy products based on the specific product attributes and clinical indications. Somatic cell therapy includes cells from various sources such as adult cells derived from the indi-vidual being treated (autologous), cells donated from one human to another (allogeneic), and cells from an animal source and used for human treatment (xenogeneic). Stem cell therapy includes cells derived from a variety of adult human tissue, fetal tissue, and embryonic tissue. The two characteristics that distinguish stem cells for other types of cells are (1) stem cells can self-renew and (2) stem cells can differentiate into other types of cells. These specific stem cell proliferative properties raise concerns for the potential tumorigenicity of such products. Tumorigenicity studies are thus needed for human derived embryonic stems cells and may also be needed for fetal derived and adult tissue derived multipotent stem cells produced by extended culture. Embryonic stem cells have been shown to produce a benign tumor called a teratoma in immunosuppressed mice. Teratomas typically contain a mixture of many differentiated or partially differentiated cell types.

When performed, the clinically relevant route of administration should be used and appropriate animal species, including appropriate study design and duration, should be justified 6 months up to lifetime observation depending on the particular cell type. Positive controls are important for a number of reasons, including the potential technical errors related to tumor cell implantation, specimen processing, and analysis in order to ensure that findings from tumorigenicity study are interpretable. Importantly, unlike for other pharmaceuticals or biopharmaceuticals, the results of the tumorigenicity study must be available to support initiation of the initial clinical trial (see Chapter 33).

19.3.5 Gene Therapies

The concern regarding carcinogenicity of gene therapies is based on the theoretical potential for insertional mutagenesis of the vector and/or a direct effect of the expressed transgene. Concerns for potential insertional mutagenesis are also raised with DNA vaccines (see Chapter 31).

Reports of gene therapy associated leukemia related to insertional activation of proto-oncogenes by retroviral vectors have occurred and have raised serious concerns in the field of gene therapy [30]. Biodistribution studies are performed preclinically to determine whether there is vector integration and persistence of vector in tissues. Evaluation of tumorigenic potential takes into account vector-specific and patient-specific issues, including whether the vector is integrating or nonintegrating, as well as pediatric versus adult population and whether the disease being treated is serious or life threatening. As with most biopharmaceuticals the standard rodent bioassay is generally not appropriate as rodents may not be susceptible to the viral vector, daily administration of vector is not feasible, and/or host immune response to vector and/or transgene will likely limit toxicity and effects on tumor development. Alternative animal models will likely be more appropriate for specific integrating gene therapy vectors, such as genetically modified mice or neonatal mice including animal models of the intended disease state [31]. Importantly, a long-term follow-up is required of all clinical trial participants receiving gene therapy products in order to properly monitor for long-term adverse effects of gene therapy treatments and mitigate their potential impact on study participants [32]. (See also Chapters 31 and 32.)

19.4 ADDITIONAL CONSIDERATIONS FOR BIOPHARMACEUTICALS

Clinical indications for biopharmaceuticals have evolved from uses as replacement therapies and therapies for life-threatening diseases to uses as lifetime therapies for chronic diseases. Because of their short half-lives, conventional pharmaceuticals used to treat chronic disease are generally administered daily unless specifically designed for long-acting release. Most biopharmaceuticals, on the other hand, are slowly eliminated and thus dosed intermittently. However, in some cases, such a humanized monoclonal antibody, a single administration may lead to extended duration of exposure prolonging a biological response for days to months. In the extreme, hypothetically, a single administration of a gene therapy to correct a gene defect could result in lifetime reconstitution of the genetic defect and potential cure of the disease.

The international safety guidance ICH S6 offers a discussion about assessing carcinogenic potential, including the variety of approaches that should be considered. The utility of a single rodent species should be considered in those cases where a product is biologically active and nonimmunogenic in rodents and when other studies have not provided sufficient information to allow assessment of carcinogenic potential. In such cases careful consideration should be given to the selection of doses including the rationale for dose selection. The use of a combination of pharmacokinetic and pharmacodynamic endpoints with consideration of comparative receptor characteristics and intended human exposures represents the most scientifically based approach for defining appropriate doses [27].

The standard rodent bioassay is often inappropriate in large part due to species specificity and/or immunogenicity of human proteins in rodents. Most animals develop an immune response to foreign proteins. This cross-species immunogenicity of a human protein in a foreign host is an important component in the challenge of deciding how best to evaluate carcinogenicity in accepted preclinical animal models [33]. The development of neutralizing antibodies in various animal species has generally been the determining factor, limiting the duration of repeat-dose toxicity testing of recombinant derived human proteins due to potential alteration of PK/PD and influence on exposure. In some cases it has been advisable to continue dosing beyond documentation of the first presence of antibodies especially when the antibody response is not correlated with dose. In addition, when antibody responses are also observed in humans, treatment through the antibody response has been considered for repeat-dose animal toxicity assessment to mimic the human dosing regimen. The risk of anaphylaxis and immune complex disease in the test species should be recognized, since occurrence will also limit the feasibility of long-term testing. Antibody development will also be a problem for long-term repeat-dosing or lifetime exposure. For example, when renal function becomes impaired by age, immune complex deposition could be a more important issue. While nonhuman primates may be a relevant species for repeat-dose toxicity studies with biopharmaceuticals, dosing for a major part of their lifetime (~20 years or more) is impractical and no longer feasible.

The production and use of homologous proteins (also referred to as "analogous" or "surrogate" molecules) are useful for "proof of concept" decision-making and for providing an early understanding of mechanism of action during the development of human proteins. In a limited number of cases they have also been useful for safety assessment, for example, in the assessment of reproductive and chronic toxicity, and in particular, for the safety of humanized monoclonal antibodies [34,35]. In some cases, however, it may not be possible to derive and/or manufacture the homologous protein; for instance, the biology may be different among the various species despite a high sequence homology of the protein or receptor, the mechanism of action of the receptor may differ, or the homologous protein may also be immunogenic following repeat dosing. The challenge when considering chronic dosing with homologous proteins is to ensure their comparability with the human protein product with respect to purity, potency, and stability and also in manufacturing process. For example, the protein should be comparable with respect to production specifications, impurities and contaminants, formulation, stability, as well as ensuring appropriate level of GMP compliance [36]. A case can be made to assess carcinogenic potential with the homologous product if it can be determined that the product and pharmacological activity are comparable. In such cases as the clinical material is not being evaluated, a single rodent species should be acceptable for carcinogenicity assessment.

Products that may have the potential to stimulate growth or induce proliferation or clonal expansion of cell types, in particular, transformed cells, all processes that may eventually lead to neoplasia should be evaluated with respect to receptor expression in various malignant and normal human cells that are relevant to the patient population under study [27]. In such cases normal human cell lines and multiple human cancer cell lines expressing the relevant receptor, as well as primary cells derived from human tumor explants, should be used for in vitro assessment. When in vitro data demonstrate enhanced growth, further studies in relevant in vivo xenograft animal models with receptor expressing tumor cell lines may be needed. In addition incorporation of sensitive indexes of cellular proliferation in long-term repeat-dose toxicity studies may provide useful information.

19.5 PRECLINICAL APPROACHES FOR ASSESSING CARCINOGENIC POTENTIAL

The considerations above have been used to scientifically justify a relevant approach on a case-by-case basis for currently approved and marketed biopharmaceuticals. Table 19.2 outlines the various approaches currently used to assess the carcinogenic potential of pharmaceuticals and highlights the potential advantages and limitations of the specific models for

TABLE 19.2 Preclinical approaches for assessing carcinogenic potential

Model	Advantages	Limitations
	Validated/accepted models	
Two-year rodent bioassay	• Standardized • Large historical database	• Costly • Time-consuming • High animal numbers ($N = 50$ to 100/sex/group) • Variability exists between species and strains • May not detect weak carcinogens or promoters under standard protocol • Difficulty separating spontaneous geriatric findings from induced changes • Use of homologous protein is needed for species-specific proteins
Nonhuman primate bioassay	• Used to assess oral contraceptives	• Duration ≥20 years • Difficulties in interpretation due to low animal numbers • No longer feasible on ethical and welfare grounds
Tumorigenicity assessment in immunocompromised rodents	• Most commonly used for assessing tumorigenic potential of cell lines to produce biopharmaceuticals • Used to assess tumorigenic potential of categories of cellular products via intended route of administration • May allow use of clinical product	• Lack of available positive controls for recombinant proteins and monoclonal antibodies • Optimal study design, including adequate number of animals and study duration not established • Lack of knowledge on which genetic defect and which strain of rodent is most appropriate

Characterized/supportive models

Model	Advantages	Limitations
Initiation-promotion models in Rodent species • Mouse skin tumor assay • Rat liver focus assay	• Evaluates the two-stage concept of carcinogenesis (initiation and promotion) • Both systems are capable of evaluating tumor promotion	• Both systems are limited to one target tissue • Not validated for biopharmaceuticals • Use of homologous protein is needed for species-specific proteins
Syrian hamster embryo (SHE) cell transformation assay (In vitro) (SHE cells are used to evaluate the potential of a wide range of agents to induce morphological transformations. Following carcinogen exposure (1–7 days), SHE cells display a multistage pattern of neoplastic progression similar to that observed in vivo)	• Reduced cost and time • Used to study mechanisms of carcinogenesis • Evaluates potential to induce morphological transformation • Displays multistage pattern of progression similar to in vivo carcinogenesis • Useful for prioritizing genotoxic chemicals for further development • Good concordance with rodent bioassay	• Experimental difficulties • Unable to discriminate between genotoxic and nongenotoxic rodent carcinogens • Not useful in determining which nongentoxic rodent carcinogens are going to be human noncarcinogens • Limited if any data with biopharmaceuticals • Use of homologous protein is needed for species-specific proteins
Cell Transformation Assays (in vitro) (e.g., Balb/c 3T3, C3H10T1/2, Bhas 42 cells)	• Reduced cost and time • Screen for nongenotoxic carcinogens	• Experimental difficulties • Variation in sensitivity among laboratories • Refinement in protocol needed regarding test concentrations and re-examination when equivocal data are obtained • Limited if any data with biopharmaceuticals

TABLE 19.2   Preclinical approaches for assessing carcinogenic potential (*Continued*)

Alternative models (transgenic animals) "short term assays"/supportive models (activity often limited to one or a few tissues)

Model	Advantages	Limitations
−p53 +/− (expresses heterozygous inactivation of the p53 tumor suppressor gene, which is critical to cell cycle control and DNA repair)	• Reduced cost • Reduced time and number of animals • Semivalidated (biopharmaceuticals were not included in industry sponsored validation efforts)	• Defined inbred line and may be unlike random outbred species • Not suitable for evaluating nongenotoxic carcinogens • Better standardization of pathology evaluations is needed (e.g., distinguishing hyperplasia from adenoma) • Equivocal responses occur • Doubtful relevance for growth factors or immunomodulatory/immunosuppressive proteins • Limited data available with biopharmaceuticals • May require rodent homologue
Tg-AC (skin painting model; expresses a mutation of the v-ras proto-oncogene, which has been demonstrated to detect human carcinogens)	• Detects both genotoxic and nongenotoxic carcinogens • Semivalidated (biopharmaceuticals were not included in industry sponsored validation efforts)	• Defined inbred line and may be unlike random outbred species • No historical use of IV or SC route of administration (primarily topical and oral) • Limitations with respect to extrapolation of dose and organ specificity • Better standardization of pathology evaluations is needed (e.g., distinguishing hyperplasia from benign neoplasms) • Equivocal responses occur • Limited if any data available with biopharmaceuticals • May require rodent homologue

Model	Advantages	Disadvantages
Tg-Hras2 (carries human cH-ras proto-oncogenes driven by their own promoter region, which has been demonstrated to detect human carcinogens)	• Reduced cost • Reduced time and number of animals • Semivalidated • Detects spectrum of weakly to strongly genotoxic compounds • Appears to have greater sensitivity than nontransgenic mice to compounds that are human carcinogens but are Ames negative • Has be used to assess recombinant human growth factor (rhKFG) (biopharmaceuticals were not included in industry sponsored validation efforts)	• Defined inbred line and may be unlike random outbred species • Not suitable for evaluating nongenotoxic carcinogens • Better standardization of pathology evaluations is needed • Dependent on specific mechanism(s) • May not be susceptible to relevant tumor type • Equivocal responses occur • Limited historical database on background incidence • Limited if any data available with biopharmaceuticals • May require rodent homologue
XPA −/− (deletion across exons 3 and 4 of both XPA alleles, rendering cells totally defective in nucleotide excision DNA repair; animals comparable to human xeroderma pigmentosum)	• Reduced cost • Reduced time and number of animals • Semivalidated • Sensitive to genotoxic carcinogens that are reactive to the nucleotide excision repair pathway	• Defined inbred line and may be unlike random outbred species • Not suitable for evaluating nongenotoxic carcinogens • Better standardization of pathology evaluations is needed (e.g., distinguishing hyperplasia from adenoma) • Dependent on specific mechanism(s) • May not be susceptible to relevant tumor type • Equivocal responses occur • Limited historical database on background incidence • Limited if any data available with biopharmaceuticals • May require rodent homologue

TABLE 19.2 Preclinical approaches for assessing carcinogenic potential (*Continued*)

Model	Advantages	Limitations
Eμ-pim-1 (expresses the pim-1 proto-oncogene, which has been shown to increase the susceptibility to T and B cell lymphomas)	• Sensitive assay for carcinogens that target the lymphoid system	• Defined inbred line and may be unlike random outbred species • Clear results only for those carcinogens that are genotoxic • Limited validation • Better standardization of pathology evaluations is needed (e.g., distinguishing hyperplasia from adenoma) • Equivocal responses occur • No data available for biopharmaceuticals • May require rodent homologue

Alternative models (other)/ supportive models

Model	Advantages	Limitations
Neonatal rodent (utilizes the increased tumorigenic sensitivity of the new-born rodent. Model consists of a 28-day range-finding experiment and a 1 year-long tumorigenicity study. Test article is administered on days 8 and 15.	• Sensitive biological assay • Historical database (>40 years) • Detects moderately to strongly genotoxic carcinogens • Distinguishes between definite genotoxicity and weak to nongenotoxic potential • Multiple routes of administration have been used • May be able to use clinical product	• Uncertainty about its range of predictiveness of nongenotoxic carcinogens • Uncertainty about its range of predictiveness for genotoxic carcinogens • Limited historical database on background incidence • Inadequate data are available with biopharmaceuticals

Experimental/ developmental models

Model	Advantages	Limitations
Spontaneous/chemically induced tumors (increase in number, change in tumor types or earlier appearance of tumors)	• Potential opportunity to address potency • Decreased concern if no findings • May provide some information with respect to risk and level of concern	• Clinical product may be immunogenic • Limited historical database on background incidence • Variability in tumor induction rate • Limited data available with biopharmaceuticals • May require rodent homologue

Tumor host resistance in rodents (e.g., B16F10 melanoma)	• Used to assess immunotoxicity potential of test articles • May provide some information with respect to risk and level of concern • Has been used to assess impact of immunosuppressive biopharmaceuticals on host resistance to neoplasia	• Limited to disease promotion/progression • May require rodent homologue
Tumor xenograft in immunosuppressed mice	• Routinely performed for assessing efficacy of cancer drugs • May provide some information with respect to risk and level of concern • Has been used to evaluate the impact of growth factors on tumor growth and metastasis where the human tumor cells express the receptor for the growth factor	• Some difficulties in transferring standardized assays used to determine activity to new assays for safety assessment • Variability in models (nude, SCID, SCID-Beige, etc.) • Immunosuppression can either increase or decrease tumor growth
In vitro/ex vivo mitogenicity in human cell lines or animal cell lines (expressing receptor or transfected with human receptor)	• Test system sensitive for mitogenic and/or metabolic effects of test article • Provide data in nontumor as well as tumor tissues (containing aberrant receptors) • May predict in vivo effects under certain circumstances • Increased mitogenicity justifies request of in vivo data • "doable" • Can provide some information as to relative potency—cause for concern	• Limited data with respect to correlation of findings with in vivo effects • May be difficult to develop an in vivo model to validate findings

TABLE 19.2 Preclinical approaches for assessing carcinogenic potential (*Continued*)

Model	Advantages	Limitations
Transgenic knockout (chronic inhibition of target)	• Useful for assessing worst-case scenario	• May overestimate response—effects may differ from those of therapeutic agent • Difficult to extrapolate a positive response • Test article is not administered therefore no information with respect to dose and exposure
Transgenic knock-in (overexpression of protein)	• Useful for assessing worst-case scenario	• May overestimate response—effects may differ from those of therapeutic agent • Difficult to extrapolate a positive response • Test article is not administered therefore no information with respect to dose and exposure
Transgenic "humanized" mouse (human receptor)	• Allows testing of the clinical product	• May overestimate response • Difficult to extrapolate a positive response • May not have appropriate physiological regulation of gene expression • May not have appropriate physiological response to test article
Neonatal tolerance induction in rodents	• Option of dosing animals very early in life to produce animals tolerant to subsequent chronic administration of human proteins (potential to conduct rodent bioassay) • Use of clinical product	• No data on positive controls • Limited if any data on biopharmaceuticals
Chronic toxicity with proliferation endpoints	• Opportunity to determine carcinogenic potential earlier in development using sensitive biomarkers • May provide some information with respect to risk and level of concern	• Limited experience • Increased cell proliferation has been identified as a risk factor for carcinogenesis but is not a defining endpoint • May not be sufficient to use this data for human risk assessment in absence of tumor endpoint

biopharmaceuticals. Additional discussion on the various approaches used to assess the carcinogenic potential of pharmaceuticals is provided below.

19.5.1 Rodent Bioassay

As previously discussed, the rodent bioassay has recently been under scrutiny for its relevance for identifying the carcinogenic hazard of pharmaceutical products. The assays are the most costly (up to 800–1000 animals/test (500/species); approximately 2 million US dollars each for a rat and mouse study) and time-consuming (2 years of treatment; an additional 1–2 years for histopathological analysis and report writing) of the preclinical regulatory requirements [7]. It is especially important that the results provide value for predicting human risk. Recently a retrospective evaluation was made on 60 systemic two-year studies of pharmaceuticals reviewed in the Center for Drug Evaluation and Research (CDER) FDA between January 2002 and December 2004. Based on an evaluation of the CDER/FDA database, the authors concluded that additional information and data, beyond what are already being collected, are needed to better predict or obviate the need for two-year carcinogenicity studies. The authors further acknowledged that many of the mechanisms of carcinogenesis found with pharmaceuticals may not be amenable to early prediction at this time as many of the mechanisms identified to date for pharmaceuticals appear to be nongenotoxic in nature and thus may require the prolonged treatment to be expressed [37,38]. However, these mechanisms may not be associated with human tumor risk. Nevertheless, based on this initial review, the FDA does not currently support the idea that short-term studies accurately predict the potential neoplastic findings in long-term assays of pharmaceuticals [16].

19.5.2 Short-term Carcinogenicity Assays

As the International Conference on Harmonization (ICH) Expert Working Group on Safety has conducted discussions involving how best to assess potential human cancer risk of pharmaceuticals, important questions were raised regarding the added value of a second rodent species. Following review of various databases created and evaluated by the participants, it was suggested that under certain circumstances data from alternative short-term assays may prove of equal or greater value to the bioassay in a second rodent species, and those assays were presented as possible alternatives in the guidance document [39,40].

In 1996 a collaborative effort was subsequently initiated under the auspices of the Health and Environmental Sciences Institute (HESI) branch of the International Life Sciences Institute (ILSI) with the specific purpose of facilitating a focused systematic evaluation of several of the new alternative models proposed within the ICH guidance. Participation in this research collaboration was global in scope encompassing Europe, Japan, and the United States and included representatives from academe, industry, and governmental agencies. The effort was not undertaken to determine if the results of alternative assays correlated with the results obtained in the rodent bioassay, but rather, whether the data from these assay could add value to the process of human risk assessment. The research involved input from over 50 industrial, governmental (United States, Denmark, Netherlands, and Japan), and academic laboratories representing a financial commitment of approximately 33 million US dollars [41]. The focus of the ICH discussions was pharmaceuticals. Importantly, no biopharmaceuticals were included in the collaborative study. Therefore the validity of extrapolating the results to biopharmaceuticals is currently not known [42].

The research program was overseen by a Steering Committee of scientists drawn from academe and pharmaceutical companies. The models under consideration included the p53+/−, ras H2+/−, Tg.AC, Xpa−/−, Xpa−/−/p53+/− transgenic animal models, the neonatal mouse model, and the in vitro Syrian hamster embryo (SHE) assay. The protocols used were based on the existing knowledge of each model. Positive control chemicals were used to demonstrate that each testing laboratory could undertake and report a positive assay for the model under test. A number of articles have been published commenting on the utility of the alternative short-term bioassays for assessing the carcinogenic potential of pharmaceuticals [43–52].

The overall conclusion of the ILSI effort was that none of the models used was suitable as a definitive determinant of potential cancer risk, but they could serve as useful hazard identification models similar to the rodent bioassay. For those chemical compounds found positive in the rodent bioassay yet not considered carcinogenic in humans, there were fewer positive results in transgenic mouse models; that is, the models exhibit a better correlation with actual human data than the rodent bioassay. The lack of correlation between organ specificity and potential human carcinogenicity limits the information that can be gained with respect to mechanism of toxicity, especially for pharmaceuticals that are nongenotoxic. Additionally, because the positive responses were frequently only seen at the highest doses, the models are more limited for quantitative risk assessment and determination of a dose response. Since the neonatal mouse appeared only to detect chemicals that were moderate to strongly genotoxic carcinogens, the model was considered to be of limited usefulness. The data also suggested that the SHE assay was unable to discriminate between genotoxic and nongenotoxic chemicals or between rodent carcinogens versus noncarcinogens and thus would likely be less useful for predicting human carcinogenicity versus noncarcinogenicity.

The report concluded that a reasonable weight of evidence on the evaluation of potential risk to humans could be achieved if information from the short-term bioassay is used in conjunction with information from other sources such as the rat bioassay, the Ames assay, the chemistry of the test article, and the repeat-dose studies evaluating intermediate markers of malignancy from knowledge of the pharmacological activities of the test substance and from additional mechanistic research [41]. Consistent with the earlier recommendation [28], the usefulness of animal models in evaluating strongly immunosuppressive chemicals was questioned for providing any added value due to the expected result of viral tumors associated with the induction of immunosuppression. Further research was recommended to identify models with greater relevance to mechanisms of toxicity in humans as well as short-term in vivo models to evaluate nongenotoxic carcinogenesis and tumor promoters. These research efforts may provide models for identifying carcinogenic hazard that are more relevant for biopharmaceuticals.

19.5.3 Proliferation Indexes from Repeat-Dose Chronic Toxicity Studies

The ICH S6 guidance states that incorporation of sensitive indices of cellular proliferation in long-term repeated-dose toxicity studies may provide useful information [27]. Tumor cell proliferation is a key characteristic of stepwise neoplastic promotion and progression and is often detectable prior to the appearance of overt neoplastic changes. Detectable histological features related to tumor cell proliferation include Ki67expression and increased mitotic rate and growth phase of affected cells, sometimes with consequential changes in the morphology of affected tissues. The Ki67 protein is expressed in all phases of the cell cycle except G_0. It has therefore been suggested as a more sensitive biomarker for cellular proliferation than visualization of mitoses [53]. Immunochemical staining for Ki67 or proliferating cell nuclear antigen (PCNA) can be performed on formalin fixed tissues. However, these staining methodologies, which detect significant increases in proliferation, may not be able to assess small changes in proliferation as the rate of cell death could still have an effect on tumor formation, especially in tissues that have a low basal proliferative rate. While an increase in proliferation rate can result in an increase in mutation rate, the death of a cell sustaining a mutation will prevent progression to neoplasia. Thus a large increase in proliferation rate may sometime be of little or no consequence when the rate of cell death is equal or higher, especially when the cells affected undergo terminal differentiation. Conversely, no change in proliferation but a reduced rate of cell death can also have a significant effect on tumor formation. Thus, while information on proliferation potential can be of some value with respect to hazard identification, the correlation between proliferation and a tumor endpoint is not inevitable and needs to be evaluated in each case. It is difficult to prospectively evaluate all potential targets. This is difficult to do even when the target tissue is identified with a dedicated evaluation.

19.5.4 Tumor Host-Resistance Models

Host-resistance assays offer a way to determine the relative significance of a compound-related decrease in immune function, commonly one of such magnitude as to be associated with a change in the histological appearances of the lymphoid [54]. Implanted tumor cell host-resistance models have also been utilized in hazard identification and risk assessment in immunotoxicology [55]. Immunomodulators can be assessed for their potential to suppress host defense against experimental metastases and growth factors, and other agents can be assessed for their potential to directly accelerate the tumorigenic response via an immunological or other process. At the very least, such models may be able to demonstrate the relative potency of the compound in showing whether the compound is an immunomodulator or a strong immunosuppressant compound. The results obtained would then be of value in carcinogenic risk communication. Because animal host-resistance models can be comparable to and may reflect human disease, their greatest utility is in providing a perspective on how compound-related changes in immune function impact on host resistance to disease [54].

19.5.5   Transgenic Animals

In addition to spontaneous mutant strains of mice and rats, transgenic mice (knock-ins and knockouts) are frequently used as models to understand and confirm the biological activity of biopharmaceuticals. They have also been used to assess aspects of toxicity [56]. Humanized mice have been developed to express target cells with the human receptor to determine binding and its consequences of an agonist or antagonist. In such cases the clinical product binds to the intended receptor and can therefore be used to assess toxicity. Knock-ins have also been used to model a worst-case scenario of overexpression of a protein, for example, of an endogenous growth factor. Knockouts have been used to model a possible worst-case scenario of blocking a receptor, for example, a monoclonal antibody directed against a specific receptor. In these cases the clinical product is not evaluated, but the consequences of the extreme exaggerated pharmacological response of knocking in or knocking out a key signaling molecule that results in subsequent tumor formation may suggest a higher risk and subsequently require additional characterization. A negative response can also be used to better characterize and communicate potential risk.

In all cases where transgenic mice are used it is important to understand the limitations of the specific model in the context of the pathology demonstrated in order to optimize extrapolation of the results. Model attributes that may influence interpretation include epitope distribution, density, localization/compartmentalization, turnover, expression, function, regulation, comparability of signal transduction pathways/regulation, and natural life history. Divergent and even discrepant experimental results have been obtained in transgenic mouse models, depending on the transgene and the promoter used due to variation in promoter regulation and expression phenotype. The background genotype of the strain used may also be important, and variation in the sites of insertion of the transgene into the host genome may be difficult to control [42].

19.5.6 In vitro Cell Proliferation

Increased cell proliferation has been identified as a risk factor for carcinogenesis; therefore in vitro proliferation assays are generally useful. An understanding of receptor expression in normal and malignant cell lines is an important component to hazard identification. Mechanisms whereby cell growth might become disordered include (1) abnormalities of growth factor production, (2) abnormalities of growth factor receptors, (3) disturbance of postreceptor signal transmission and normal control of activation and reduced production of a growth inhibitory factor, and (4) sensitivity to such factors.

The risk of increased stimulation by a growth factor is generally decreased if the growth factor acts on committed cells with a limited life span and if the stimulated cells readily undergo terminal differentiation. The use of a variety of in vitro evaluations, including in vitro cell proliferation, proved to be important in characterizing the level of concern during the re-evaluation of the safety and dosing of erythropoiesis-stimulating agents (ESAs) in cancer patients with respect to increase mortality and/or tumor promotion (see Table 19.3) [58].

TABLE 19.3 Preclinical evidence of carcinogenic risk with erythropoiesis stimulating agents

Finding	Comment
Epo receptor (EpoR) is not an oncogene. The EpoR gene is not significantly amplified or over expressed in solid tumors and over expression of constitutively activated mutant forms of EpoR does not transform cells	If Epo-induced signaling could drive proliferation of cancer cells this would increase cause for concern
EpoR hyperactivating mutations result in polycythemia and are not a feature of malignancy. In addition in clinical conditions in which Epo is overexpressed (e.g., Chuvash polycythemia) or in which EpoR signaling is not controlled (EpoR truncations), polycythemia results but with no increase in tumors	The fact that EPO overexpression in humans is not associated with malignancy is reassuring
EpoR gene is transcribed in most tissues and cell lines at low to moderate levels. Levels of EpoR are rarely elevated in tumors and cell lines above that observed in the normal tissue of tumor origin	Molecules that deliver proliferative signals are frequently expressed at high levels by at least some tumors

TABLE 19.3 Preclinical evidence of carcinogenic risk with erythropoiesis stimulating agents (*Continued*)

Finding	Comment
EpoR protein synthesis does not necessarily correlate with cell surface expression or signaling of the EpoR Less than 1% of EpoR normally gets to the surface of the cell because of inefficient processing, protein degradation, requirements for limiting accessory molecules for trafficking to the surface, requirements for limiting accessory molecules for intracellular signaling, and short cell-surface half-life	In addition to low-level expression of EpoR on the cell surface, EPO does not bind to tissues other than those expressing EpoR
Studies of the direct role of Epo–EpoR in signaling, proliferation, migration, and survival of cancer cells have not yielded conclusive results	Effects of such treatments have been in models despite the fact that most have used levels of rHuEpo (>10 U/ml) that are unattainable in patients
All rodent tumor models (23 independent studies) have demonstrated that ESAs do not enhance tumor growth	ESAs have actually shown increase sensitivity of tumor cells to radiation and chemotherapy
ESAs do not mediated any consistent adverse effect on tumor angiogenesis in rodent tumor models	Increased tumor oxygenation actually reduces hypoxia-regulated VEGF levels and consequently tumor angiogenesis
Data do not support a meaningful effect of ESAs on mobilization of endothelial progenitor cells	Consistent with lack of an affect on tumor vascularization
Proliferative response to nonhematological cells is not altered in vitro or in vivo	Reassurance for lack of off-target effect
No tumorigenic or unexpected mitogenic response in any tissue type has been noted in 6-month chronic toxicity studies	In vivo support of in vitro data

Source: Adapted 2007 ODAC Meeting, Information Package Darbepoetin alfa (BLA#103951) and Epoetin alfa (BLA#103234)

19.6 CURRENT EXPERIENCE IN CARCINOGENICITY ASSESSMENTS OF BIOPHARMACEUTICALS

Examples of product class carcinogenicity hazard identifications and assessments and ultimate risk communications for biopharmaceuticals approved in the United States for chronic use or based on potential cause for concern are provided in Table 19.4a (products without carcinogenicity assessment) and Table 19.4b (products with carcinogenicity assessment). The data are derived from publicly available regulatory assessments and product labels. Specific examples are discussed below.

19.6.1 Immunomodulators

A variety of immumodulatory biopharmaceuticals have been approved spanning various degrees of immune modulation including intended marked immune suppression. A specific discussion on assessing carcinogenic risk of immunomodulatory biopharmaceuticals is presented in Chapter 27. It is of interest to review the individual product labels for their ultimate communication of carcinogenic risk. This important communication varies in a number of respects: for each product as well as products within a class, whether or not preclinical studies were performed, and the impact of these studies with specific findings on the label.

Abatacept   Abatacept is a T cell activation inhibitor. It is a fusion protein composed of the extracellular domain of T lymphocyte associated antigen 4 linked to the portion of IgG (human heavy chain fragment). T cell activation is implicated in the pathogenesis of rheumatoid arthritis. Abatacept is indicated for treating RA patients. The mouse carcinogenicity study for abatacept (CTLA4Ig) was conducted because of concerns related to prolonged immunosuppression. There were no "preneoplastic" lesions in the 6-month chronic toxicity studies. The treated mice in the carcinogenicity study developed mammary tumors and lymphomas (increased incidence after 6 months) at a higher incidence than controls, and a no effect dose level could be determined. The tumors were shown likely to be related to tumorigenic mouse retroviruses (MTV and MTLV). A chronic 12-month toxicity study in monkeys, however, did not replicate the effect, even though monkeys in the study had been previously exposed to an endogenous lymphocryptovirus. These viruses share a tropism for B lymphocytes and have a propensity to oncogenicity. A significant increase in the incidence of lymphoma, mammary tumors, or other tumors was not observed in the clinical studies. It could be argued then that the mouse was more sensitive or that the mouse confirmed the anticipated risk, namely prolonged immune suppression, which results in an increased incidence of immune suppression-related tumors under certain circumstances.

The human experience was not unlike that of the anti-TNFs with respect to an approximate 3- to 3.5-fold higher rate of lymphoma in the intended population (patients with RA) who are at higher risk for the development of lymphoma or lung cancer, particularly those with highly active disease. Similar is the statement that the role of the particular product and the development of human malignancies is not known or fully understood. There is also the added precaution to lessen the putative risk in patients to avoid use with other immunosuppressive agents.

Anakinra   Anakinra is likewise indicated for the treatment of patients with rheumatoid arthritis. Anakinra is the recombinant form of human IL-1 receptor antagonist (IL-1ra) and is identical to the naturally occurring, nonglycosylated form of the protein, with an additional N-terminal methionine residue. Binding of IL-1ra to the IL-1R1 receptor does not initiate IL-1 mediated cell signaling,

TABLE 19.4a Examples of communication of human carcinogenic risk without preclinical assessment of carcinogenic risk

Biopharmaceutical	Class	Mechanism of Action	Preclinical Studies	Human Experience/Product Label
		Immunomodulators		
Etanercept Enbrel®	• Recombinant DNA-derived dimeric fusion protein (anti-TNF) • Extracellular ligand binding portion of the human tumor necrosis f actor receptor linked to the Fc portion of IgG₁	• Binds tumor necrosis factor α (TNF-α) and blocks interaction with cell surface tumor necrosis receptors	• No rodent bioassay • Not genotoxic—in vitro and in vivo mutagenesis studies	• In the control and open-labeled portions of the clinical trials a threefold higher incidence of lymphomas was observed compared to the general population. While patients with RA or psoriasis, particularly those with active disease may be at high risk (up to sevenfold) for the development of lymphoma, the potential role of TNF-blocking therapy in the development of malignancies is not known *Warnings* • Malignancies • Use of Enbrel in patients receiving concurrent cyclophosphamide therapy is not recommended
Infliximab Remicade®	• Chimeric IgG₁κ monoclonal antibody (anti-TNF)	• Binds TNF-α	• No rodent bioassay • Not genotoxic (Ames, in vivo MN) • No findings in 6-month study with murine homologue (up to 8× human dose) • Significance to human risk unknown	• In the controlled portions of clinical trials of some TNF-blocking agents including Remicade, more malignancies (excluding lymphoma and nonmelanoma skin cancers) have been observed in patients receiving the TNF-blocker compared with control patients • The potential role of TNF-blocking therapy in the development of malignancies is not known. Rates in clinical trials of Remicade cannot be compared to rates in clinical trials of other TNF-blockers and may not predict rates observed in a broader patient population • Patients with Chron's disease, rheumatoid arthritis, or plaque psoriasis, particularly patients with highly active disease and/or chronic exposure to immunosuppressant therapies, may be at a higher risk (up to several fold) than the general population of lymphoma, even in the absence of TNF-blocking therapy • Caution should be exercised in considering Remicade treatment in patients with a history of malignancy or in continuing treatment in patients who develop malignancy while receiving Remicade

| Adalimumab Humira® | Fully human IgG$_1$ monoclonal antibody (anti-TNF) | • Neutralizes the biological activity of TNF-α by binding with high affinity to the soluble transmembrane form of TNFα and inhibits binding of TNFα with its receptors | • No rodent bioassay
• Not genotoxic (Ames or in vivo MN) | *Black box warning*
• Rare postmarketing cases of hepatosplenic T cell lymphoma reported. This rare type of T cell lymphoma has a very aggressive disease course and is usually fatal within 2 years of diagnosis
• All lymphomas occurred in patients on concomitant treatment with azothioprine or 6-mercaptopurine
• Causal relationship to hematosplenic T cell lymphoma remains unclear
• Malignancies including non-Hodgkin's lymphoma and Hodgkin's disease have been reported in patients following approval

Adverse reactions
• Neoplasia: adenoma, carcinomas such as breast, gastrointestinal, skin, urogenital and others; lymphoma and melanoma

Warnings and precautions
• In the controlled portions of clinical trials of some TNF-blocking agents, including Humira, more cases of malignancy have been observed among patients receiving TNF-blockers, compared to control patients
• Lymphoma rates were observed at approximately 3.5-fold higher than the expected general population
• Rates in clinical trials for Humira cannot be compared to rates of clinical trials with other TNF-blockers and may not predict the rates observed in a broader patient population
• Patients with rheumatoid arthritis, particularly those with higher active disease, are at a higher risk for the development of lymphoma |

Biopharmaceutical	Class	Mechanism of Action	Preclinical Studies	Human Experience/Product Label
Daclizumab Zenapax®	• Humanized IgG$_1$ monoclonal antibody (anti-CD25)	• Binds specifically to the alpha subunit of IL-2 receptor (TAC or CD 25) • Inhibits IL-2 mediated activation of lymphocyte, a critical pathway in the cellular immune response involved with allograft rejection	• No rodent bioassay • Not genotoxic (Ames or in vitro chromosomal aberrations assay (V79))	• Addition of Zenapax did not increase the number of posttransplant lymphomas up to 3 years posttransplant *Warnings* • While the incidence of lymphoproliferative disorders in the limited clinical trial experience was no higher in patients treated with Zenapax compared with placebo-treated patients, patients with immunosuppressive therapy are at higher risk for developing lymphoproliferative disorders and should be monitored accordingly
Basiliximab Simulect®	• Recombinant chimeric (murine/human) monoclonal antibody (IgG$_{1\kappa}$) (anti-CD25)	• Binds specifically to an blocking interleukin-2 receptor α-chain (CD25) on surface of activated T cells • Functions as an IL-2 receptor antagonist	• No rodent bioassay • Not genotoxic (Ames, V79 Chinese hamster cells)	• Overall incidence of malignancies among all patients in the controlled studies was not significantly different between Simulect and placebo-treated groups *Warnings* • While the incidence of lymphoproliferative disorders was not higher n the SIMULECT treated patients than in placebo-treated patients, patients on immunosuppressive therapies are at increased risk for developing these complications and should be monitored accordingly
Murumonab-CD3 Orthoclone OKT3®	• Murine monoclonal antibody to human CD3 T cells (anti-CD3)	• Early activation of T cells and premature release of cytokines (e.g., IL-6 and IL-10) followed by blocking of T cell function	• No rodent bioassay	*Warnings* • Serious and sometimes fatal neoplasias in patients • High risk of EBV related B cell neoplasms, skin cancer, melanoma, leukemia, breast cancer, adenocarcinoma • No apparent increase with drug combinations • Monitoring required

Peptide hormones

Somatropin Genotropin®	Recombinant somatropin (rDNA origin)	• Identical to human growth hormone of pituitary origin • Stimulates linear growth in patients who lack endogenous growth hormone also normalizes concentrations of IGF-1(insulin-like growth factor-1/somatamedin C)	• No rodent bioassay • Not genotoxic (Ames, gene mutations in mammalian cells grown in vitro (mouse L5178Y cells), in vivo chromosomal damage (BM cells in rats)

• Leukemia has been reported in a small number of pediatric patients treated with growth hormone, including growth hormone of pituitary origin and recombinant somatropin. The relationship, if any, between leukemia and growth hormone therapy is uncertain

Contraindications

• In general, somatropin is contraindicated in the presence of active malignancy. Any preexisting malignancy should be inactive and its treatment complete prior to instituting therapy with somatropin. Somatropin should be discontinued if there is evidence of recurrent activity. Since growth hormone deficiency may be an early sign of the presence of a pituitary tumor (or, rarely, other brain tumors), the presence of such tumors should be ruled out prior to initiation of treatment. Somatropin should not be used in patients with any evidence of progression or recurrence of an underlying intracranial tumor

Precautions

• Neoplasm has been reported in patients treated with somatropin after their first neoplasm. Intracranial tumors, in particular meingiomas, in patients treated with radiation to the head for their first neoplasm were the most common of these second neoplasms. In adults, it is unknown whether there is any relationship between somatropin replacement therapy and CNS tumor recurrence

• Patients should be monitored carefully for any malignant transformation of skin lesions

TABLE 19.4a Examples of communication of human carcinogenic risk without preclinical assessment of carcinogenic risk (*Continued*)

Biopharmaceutical	Class	Mechanism of Action	Preclinical Studies	Human Experience/Product Label
Somatropin Humatrope®	Recombinant somatropin (rDNA origin)	• Identical to human growth hormone of pituitary origin • Stimulates linear growth in patients who lack endogenous growth hormone also normalizes concentrations of IGF-1(insulin-like growth factor-1/somatamedin C)	• No rodent bioassay • No evidence of Humatrope-induced mutagenicity	• Leukemia has been reported in a small number of pediatric patients who have been treated with growth hormone, including growth hormone of pituitary origin as well as recombinant DNA origin (somatrem and somatropin). The relationship, if any, between leukemia and growth hormone therapy is unknown • There are also reports of association between acromegaly and colon cancer (not in label) *Contraindications* • In general, somatropin is contraindicated in the presence of active malignancy. Any preexisting malignancy should be inactive and its treatment complete prior to instituting therapy with somaptorpin. Somatropin should be discontinued if there is evidence of recurrent activity. Since growth hormone deficiency may be an early sign of the presence of a pituitary tumor (or, rarely, other brain tumors), the presence of such tumors should be ruled out prior to initiation of treatment. Somatropin should not be used in patients with any evidence of progression or recurrence of any underlying intracranial tumor

| Somatropin
Nutropin®

Recombinant
somatropin (rDNA
origin) | • Identical to human
growth hormone of
pituitary origin
• Stimulates linear
growth in patients
who lack endogenous
growth hormone
also normalizes
concentrations of
IGF-1(insulin-like
growth factor-1/
somatamedin C) | • No rodent assay
• No genotoxicity studies | *Precautions*
• Patients with preexisting tumors of growth hormone deficiency secondary to an intracranial lesion should be examined routinely for progression or recurrence of the underlying disease process. In pediatric patients, clinical literature has revealed no relationship between somatropin replacement therapy and central nervous system (CNS) tumor recurrence or new extracranial tumors. However, in childhood cancer survivors, an increased risk of a second neoplasm has been reported in patients treated with somatropin after their first neoplasm. Intracranial tumors, in particular meingiomas, in patients treated with radiation to the head for their first neoplasm, were most common of these second neoplasms. In adults, it is unknown whether there is any relationship between somatropin replacement therapy and CNS tumor recurrence
• Patients should be monitored carefully for any malignant transformation of skin lesions
• Leukemia has ben reported in a small number of GHD patients treated with GH. It is uncertain whether this increased risk is related to the pathology of GH deficiency itself, GH therapy, or other associated treatments such as radiation therapy for intracranial tumors. On the basis of current evidence, experts cannot conclude that GH therapy is responsible for these occurrences. The risk to GHD, CRI, or Turner syndrome patients, if any, remains to be established
• There are also reports of association between acromegaly and colon cancer (not in label) |

TABLE 19.4a Examples of communication of human carcinogenic risk without preclinical assessment of carcinogenic risk (*Continued*)

Biopharmaceutical	Class	Mechanism of Action	Preclinical Studies	Human Experience/Product Label
				Contraindications
				• In general, somatropin is contraindicated in the presence of active malignancy. Any preexisting malignancy should be inactive and its treatment complete prior to instituting therapy with somatropin. Somatropin should be discontinued if there is any evidence of recurrent activity. Since growth hormone deficiency may be an early sign of the presence of a pituitary tumor (or, rarely, other brain tumors), the presence of such tumors should be ruled out prior to initiation of treatment. Somatropin should not be used in patients with any evidence of progression or recurrence of an underlying intracranial tumor
				Precautions
				• Patients with preexisting tumors or growth hormone deficiency secondary to an intracranial lesion should be examined routinely for progression or recurrence of the underlying disease process. In pediatric patients, clinical literature has revealed no relationship between somatropin replacement therapy and central nervous system (CNS) tumor recurrence or new extracranial tumors. However, in childhood cancer survivors, an increased risk of a second neoplasm has been reported in patients treated with somatropin after their first neoplasm. Intracranial tumors, in particular meningiomas, in patients treated with radiation to the head for their first neoplasm, were the most common of these second neoplasms. In adults, it is unknown whether there is any relationship between somatropin replacement therapy and CNS tumor recurrence
				• Patients should be monitored carefully for any malignant transformation of skin lesions

Somatropin Omnitrope™ (first approved biosimilar)	Recombinant somatropin (rDNA origin)	• Identical to human growth hormone of pituitary origin • stimulates linear growth in patients who lack endogenous growth hormone also normalizes concentrations of IGF-1 (insulin-like growth factor-1/ somatamedin C)	• No rodent assay • No genotoxicity studies	• Leukemia has been reported in a small number of pediatric patients who have been treated with growth hormone, including growth hormone of pituitary origin and recombinant GH. The relationship, if any, between leukemia and growth hormone therapy is uncertain *Contraindications* • Omnitrope should not be used when there is any evidence of neoplastic activity. Intracranial lesions must be inactive and antitumor therapy complete prior to the institution of therapy. Omnitrope should be discontinued if there is evidence of tumor growth *Precautions* • Patients should be monitored carefully for any malignant transformation of skin lesions
Somatropin Valtropin® (approved as a biosimilar)	Recombinant somatropin (rDNA origin)	• Identical to human growth hormone of pituitary origin • Stimulates linear growth in patients who lack endogenous growth hormone also normalizes concentrations of IGF-1 (insulin-like growth factor-1/ somatamedin C)	• No rodent bioassay • Not genotoxic (Ames, in vitro Chinese hamster ovary and Chinese hamster lung cell chromosomal aberration assay, and the in vivo mouse micronucleus assay	• In published literature, leukemia has been reported in a small number of pediatric GHD patients treated with somatropin. It is uncertain whether this increased risk is related to the pathology of GHD, somatropin therapy, or other associated treatments such as radiation therapy for intracranial tumors. So far, epidemiological data have failed to confirm the hypothesis of a relationship between somatropin therapy and leukemia

TABLE 19.4a Examples of communication of human carcinogenic risk without preclinical assessment of carcinogenic risk (*Continued*)

Biopharmaceutical	Class	Mechanism of Action	Preclinical Studies	Human Experience/Product Label
				Contraindications
				• In general, somatropin is contraindicated in the presence of active malignancy. Any preexisting malignancy should be inactive and its treatment complete prior to instituting therapy with somatropin. Somatropin should be discontinued if there is evidence of recurrent activity. Since growth hormone deficiency may be an early sign of the presence of a pituitary tumor (or, rarely, other brain tumors), the presence of such tumors should be ruled out prior to initiation of treatment. Somatropin should not be used in patients with any evidence of progression or recurrence of an underlying intracranial tumor
				Precautions
				• Patients with preexisting tumors or growth hormone deficiency secondary to an intracranial lesion should be examined routinely for progression or recurrence of the underlying disease process. In pediatric patients, clinical literature has revealed no relationship between somatropin replacement therapy and central nervous system (CNS) tumor recurrence or new extracranial tumors. However, in childhood cancer survivors, an increased risk of a second neoplasm has been reported in patients treated with somatropin after their first neoplasm. Intracranial tumors, in particular meningiomas, in patients treated with radiation to the head for their first neoplasm, were the most common of these second neoplasms. In adults, it is unknown whether there is any relationship between somatropin replacement therapy and CNS tumor recurrence
				• Patients should be monitored carefully for any malignant transformation of skin lesions

Drug	Action	Testing	Warnings/Precautions
Insulin detemir Levemir®	• Recombinant human insulin analogue (rDNA origin) Long-acting basal insulin analogue	• Regulation of glucose metabolism	• No rodent bioassay • Not genotoxic (Ames, human lymphocyte peripheral blood lymphocyte chromosome aberration test, in vivo mouse micronucleus test) • Relative mitogenicity less than human insulin	• No malignancies reported in Adverse Reactions in clinical trials • No warnings or precautions regarding carcinogenic risk

Growth factors

Drug	Recombinant	Action	Testing	Warnings/Precautions
Filgrastim Neupogen®	• Recombinant derived human growth factor (rhG-CSF)	• Acts on cells of the hematopoietic cells by binding to specific cell surface receptors and stimulating proliferation, differentiation commitment, and some end-cell functional activation	• No rodent bioassay • Not mutagenic (Ames)	*Precautions* • Potential effect on malignant cells • The possibility that Neupogen can act as a growth factor for any tumor type cannot be excluded • Neupogen should not be administered in the period 24 hours before the administration of chemotherapy
Sargramstim Leukine®	• Recombinant derived human growth factor (rh GM-CSF)	• Stimulates proliferation and differentiation of hematopoietic progenitor cells	• No rodent bioassay • Leukine increases the cytotoxicity of monocytes toward certain neoplastic cell lines and activates polymorphonuclear neutrophils to inhibit the growth of tumor cells	*Precautions* • The possibility that Leukine can act as a growth factor for any tumor type, particularly myeloid malignancies, cannot be excluded • Because of the possibility of tumor growth potentiation, precaution should be exercised when using this drug in any malignancy with myeloid characteristics. Should disease progression be detected during Leukine treatment, therapy should be discontinued
Epoietin alpha Epogen®	• Recombinant derived humanized growth factor	• Stimulates red blood cell proliferation	• No rodent bioassay • Not genotoxic (Ames, in vitro chromosomal aberrations in mammalian cells, in vivo mouse MN, in vitro gene mutation of HGPRT locus)	*Warnings* • Increased mortality and/or tumor progression

437

Biopharmaceutical	Class	Mechanism of Action	Preclinical Studies	Human Experience/Product Label
Becaplermin Regranex® (topical)	• Recombinant-derived human growth factor (rh PDGFβ)	• Promotes the chemotactic recruitment and proliferation of cells involved in wound repair and enhancing the formation of granulation tissues	• No rodent bioassay • Not genotoxic (Ames, in vitro chromosomal aberrations, in vitro mammalian point mutations, DNA damage/repair, in vivo rodent MN and BM)	*Precautions* • Regranex administered every other day for 13 days displayed histological changes indicative of accelerated bone remodeling consisting of periosteal hyperplasia *Contraindications* • Known neoplasm(s) at the site(s) of application
			Cytokines	
Interferon alpha-2a Roferon®	• Recombinant-derived human cytokine (type 1 interferon)	• Direct antiproliferative activity against tumor cells, inhibition of virus replication, and modulation of the host immune response play important roles in antitumor antiviral activity	• No rodent bioassay • Not genotoxic (Ames, in vitro cytogenetic assay in human PBLs) • A chromosomal defect following the addition of human leukocyte interferon to lymphocyte cultures from a patient suffering form lymphoproliferative disease has been reported. Other studies have failed to detect chromosomal abnormalities following treatment of lymphocyte cultures form healthy donors	• No malignancies reported in Adverse Reactions in clinical trials • No warnings or precautions regarding carcinogenic risk

Pegylated interferon alfa-2a Pegasys®	• Covalent conjugate of recombinant alfa-2a interferon with monomethoxy polyethylene glycol (PEG) (type 1 interferon)	• Interferons bind to specific receptors on the cell surface, initiating intracellular signaling via complex cascades of protein–protein interactions leading to rapid activation of gene transcription • Interferon-stimulated genes modulate many biological effects including inhibition of viral replication in infected cells, inhibition of cellular proliferation and immunomodulation • Clinical relevance of these in vitro activities is not known	• No rodent bioassay • Not genotoxic (Ames, in vitro chromosomal aberrations)	• No malignancies reported in Adverse Reactions in clinical trials • No warnings or precautions regarding carcinogenic risk
Peginterferon PegIntron™	• Covalent conjugate of recombinant alfa-2b interferon with monomethoxyl polyethylene glycol (PEG) (type 1 interferon)	• See PEGASYS • Also upregulation of the TH1-helper cell subset in vitro • Clinical relevance of these findings are unknown		• No malignancies reported in Adverse Reactions in clinical trials • No warnings or precautions regarding carcinogenic risk

TABLE 19.4a Examples of communication of human carcinogenic risk without preclinical assessment of carcinogenic risk (*Continued*)

Biopharmaceutical	Class	Mechanism of Action	Preclinical Studies	Human Experience/Product Label
Interferon beta-1a Rebif®	• Recombinant derived interferon beta-1a (type 1 interferon)	• Binding of interferon beta to its receptor initiates a complex cascade of intracellular events that leads to the expression of numerous interferon-induced gene products and markers, including 2′, 5′-oligoadenylate synthetase, beta2-microglobulin, and neopterin, which may mediate some of the biological activities	• No rodent bioassay • Not genotoxic (Ames, in vitro cytogenetic assay in human lymphocytes)	• No malignancies reported in Adverse Reactions in clinical trials • No warnings or precautions regarding carcinogenic risk
Interferon beta-1a Avonex®	• Recombinant derived interferon beta-1a (type 1 interferon)	Modulates antiviral, antiproliferative and immunomodulatory activities	• No rodent bioassay • Not genotoxic (Ames, in vitro cytogenetic assay in human PBLs, does not directly bind DNA)	• No malignancies reported in Adverse Reactions in clinical trials • No warnings or precautions regarding carcinogenic risk

Interferon gamma-1b Actimmune®	• Recombinant derived interferon gamma-1b (type 2 interferon) • Interferon gamma binds to different cell surface receptors than alpha and beta • Specific effect of interferon gamma include enhancement of oxidative metabolism of macrophages, antibody-dependent cellular cytotoxicity, activation of natural killer cells, and expression of Fc and major histocompatibility antigens	• No rodent bioassay • Not genotoxic (Ames, in vivo mouse MN and mouse bone marrow)	• No malignancies reported in Adverse Reactions in clinical trials • No warnings or precautions regarding carcinogenic risk
Interferon alfacon-1 Infergen®	• Consensus interferon (type 1 interferon) • While all alpha interferon have similar biological effects, not all activities shared by each and in many cases the extent of activity various substantially for each interferon subtype	• No rodent bioassay • Not genotoxic (Ames, in vitro Chromosomal Aberrations in Human PBLs)	• No malignancies reported in Adverse Reactions in clinical trials • No warnings or precautions regarding carcinogenic risk

TABLE 19.4a Examples of communication of human carcinogenic risk without preclinical assessment of carcinogenic risk (*Continued*)

Biopharmaceutical	Class	Mechanism of Action	Preclinical Studies	Human Experience/Product Label
		Enzyme replacement therapies (ERTs)		
Imiglucerase Cerezyme®	• Recombinant human lysosomal glycoprotein enzyme β-glucocerebrosidase	• Catalyzes the hydrolysis of glycoplipid glucerebroside to glucose and ceremide	• No rodent bioassay • No genotoxicity studies	• No malignancies reported in Adverse Reactions in clinical trials • Studies have not be conducted in either animals or humans to assess the potential effects on carcinogenesis or mutagenesis • No warnings or precautions regarding carcinogenic risk
Agalsidase Fabryzyme®	• Recombinant human lysosomal α-galactosidase A enzyme	• Catalyzes hydrolysis of glubtriasyl ceramide and other α-galactyl-terminated neutral glycosphingolipids to ceremide dihexoside and galactose	• No rodent bioassay • No genotoxicity studies	• No malignancies reported in Adverse Reactions in clinical trials • There are no animal or human studies to assess carcinogenic or mutagenic potential • No warnings or precautions regarding carcinogenic risk
Laronidase Aldurazyme®	• Recombinant polymorphic variation of human α-L-iduronidase lysosomal hydrolase	• Catalyzes the hydrolysis of terminal α-L-iduronic acid residues of dermatan sulfate and heparin sulfate	• No rodent bioassay • No genotoxicity studies	• No malignancies reported in Adverse Reactions in clinical trials • Studies to assess mutagenic and carcinogenic potential have not been conducted • No warnings or precautions regarding carcinogenic risk

Drug	Description	Other	
Anakinra Kineret™	• Recombinant, nonglycosylated human interleukin-1 receptor antagonist (rhIL-1ra)	• Blocking activity of IL-1 by competitively inhibiting IL-1 binding to the interleukin-1 type I receptor (IL-1RI)	• No rodent bioassay • Not genotoxic in standard in vitro and in vivo battery • An assessment of carcinogenic risk was requested by European authorities; additional in vitro mitogenesis/cell proliferation data provided; literature search revealed no published data on increased tumorigenicity in transgenic or knockout animals	*Malignancies* • Lymphoma incidence rate was 3.6 fold higher than rate for general population • Thirty-seven malignancies other than lymphoma were observed. Of these, the most common were breast, respiratory system, and digestive system • While patients with RA, particularly those with active disease, may be at higher risk (up to several-fold) for the development of lymphoma, the role of IL-1 blockers in the development of malignancy is not known *Precautions* Immunosuppression • Impact of Kineret on the development of malignancies is not known
Omalizumab Xolair®	• Recombinant DNA-derived humanized IgG1k monoclonal antibody (anti-IgE)	• Inhibits binding of IgE to high affinity IgE receptor on surface of mast cells and basophils	• No rodent bioassay • Not mutagenic (Ames)	*Warnings* • Malignant neoplasms observed in 0.5% XOLAIR-treated compared to 0.2% in controls in clinical studies of asthma and other allergic disorders • Varity of types of tumors • Majority of patients were observed for <1 year • Impact of longer exposures or use in patients at higher risk for malignancy is not known
Pegaptanib Macugen® (ocular)	• Covalently conjugated oligonucelotide	• Selected vascular endothelial growth factor antagonist	• No rodent bioassay • Not genotoxic (Ames, in vitro chromosomal aberration, cell transformation) *E. coli* strain positive	• The safety and efficacy of Macugen beyond 2 years has not been demonstrated • No malignancies noted in AE profile

Source: Information based on product label or FDA Pharmacology/Toxicology Review for FDA Approved Drug Products (http://www.accessdata.fda.gov/scripts/cder/drugsatfda/); supportive information EPAR's for authorized medicinal products for human use (http://www.emea.europa.eu/htms/human/epar/a.htm).

443

TABLE 19.4b Examples of communication of human carcinogenic risk *with* preclinical assessment of carcinogenic risk

Biopharmaceutical	Class	Mechanism of Action	Preclinical Studies	Human Experience/Product Label
Immunomodulators				
Abatacept Orencia™	• Recombinant soluble fusion protein • Consists of the extracellular domain of human cytotoxic T lymphocyte associated antigen 4 (CTLA-4) linked to the modified Fc (hinge, CH2 and CH3) portion of human immunoglobulin G1 (IgG1) produced in a mammalian cell expression system (anti-CTLA-4)	• Selective co-stimulation modulator, inhibits T cell activation by binding to CD80 and CD86, thereby blocking the interaction of CD28 • Activation provides a co-stimulatory signal necessary for full activation of T cells	• In a mouse carcinogenicity study, weekly sc injections up to 84 weeks was associated with increased incidence of malignant lymphomas (0.8 to 3× MRHD) and mammary gland tumors in mid and high doses in females • Mice from this study were infected with MuLV and MMTV. These viruses are associated with an increased incidence of lymphomas and mammary gland tumors respectively, in immunsuppressed mice • In a one-year toxicity study in cynomolgus monkeys, at weekly doses up to 9× MRHD no morphologic changes were observed, despite the presence of a virus (lymphocryptovirus) known to cause these lesions in immunosuppressed monkeys within the time frame of this study • Relevance of this finding to the clinical use of Orencia is unknown	• In the placebo-controlled portion of the clinical trial the rate observed for lymphoma was approximately 3.5× higher than expected in the general population • Patients with RA, particularly those with highly active disease, are at higher risk for the development of lymphoma. Other malignancies were also observed • The role of Orencia in the development of malignancies in humans is unknown *Precautions* Immunosupression • Possibility exists for drugs inhibiting T cell activation, including Orencia to affect malignancies, since T cells mediate cellular immune responses. Impact of treatment with Orencia on the development and cause of malignancies is not fully understood

Drug	Description/Mechanism	Toxicity/Warnings
		• Not genotoxic (Ames, CHO/HGPRT forward point mutation assay, in vitro chromosomal aberrations in human PBLs)	• Orencia should not be administered with TNF agonists • Orencia is not recommended for use concomitantly with anakinra • No malignancies reported in Adverse Reactions in clinical trials • No warnings or precautions regarding carcinogenic risk
Natalizumab Tysabri®	Recombinant humanized IgG$_{4κ}$ antibody (anti-α4 integrin)	Selective adhesion molecule inhibitor produced in murine myeloma cells, binds to α4-submunit of human integrin which is highly expressed on the surface of all leukocytes, with exception of neutrophils and blocks the interaction with vascular cell adhesion molecule-1 (ICAM-1)	• No rodent bioassay • Tumor promotion potential was evaluated by first identifying human tumor cell lines that bind natalizumab in vitro • Tumor promotion potential was then evaluated by assessing tumor growth in athymic nude mice after tumor transplantation (sc) followed by treatment with natalizumab. Natalizumab did not show any tumor promoting potential on two α4 expression tumors (leukemia, melanoma) in a nude mouse xenograft model • Not genotoxic (Ames, in vitro chromosomal aberrations in human PBLs)
Alefacept Amevive®	• Recombinant dimeric fusion protein • Consists of intracellular CD2-binding portion of the human leukocyte function antigen-3 linked of the Fc portion of human IgG1 (anti-LFA-3/CD2)	• Interferes with lymphocyte activation by specifically binding to the lymphocyte antigen CD2, and inhibiting LFA-3/CD2 interaction	• No rodent bioassay • Not genotoxic (in vitro and in vivo studies)	*Warnings* • Animals (nonhuman primates) developed B cell hyperplasia and one animal developed lymphoma • Role of AMEVIVE in the development of lymphoid malignancy and hyperplasia

TABLE 19.4b Examples of communication of human carcinogenic risk *with* preclinical assessment of carcinogenic risk (*Continued*)

Biopharmaceutical	Class	Mechanism of Action	Preclinical Studies	Human Experience/Product Label
				observed in nonhuman primates and the relationship to humans is unknown
				• Immunodeficiency-associated lymphocyte disorders (plasmacytic hyperplasia, polymorphic proliferation and B cell lymphoma) occurs inpatients that have congenital acquired immunodeficiencies including those resulting form immunosuppressive therapies
				Precautions
				• Amevive may increase the risk of malignancies
				• Amevive should not be administered to patients with a history of systemic malignancy
				• Caution should be exercised when considering use in patients at high risk for malignancy
				• Advise discontinuation if patient develops a malignancy

Peptide hormones

Insulin glulisine Apidra®	• Recombinant human insulin analogue (rDNA origin). Rapid action insulin analogue	• Regulation of glucose metabolism	• No rodent bioassay • 12-month chronic rat study (up to 20× MRHD). There was a non–dose-dependent higher incidence of mammary gland tumors in female rats administered insulin glulisine compared to untreated controls. Incidence of mammary tumors for insulin glulisine and regular human insulin was similar. Relevance of these finding to humans is unknown • Not genotoxic (Ames, in vitro mammalian chromosome aberration test in V79 Chinese hamster cells, in vivo mammalian erythrocyte micronucleus test in rats) relative mitogenicity similar to human insulin	• No malignancies reported in Adverse Reactions in clinical trials • No warnings or precautions regarding carcinogenic risk
Insulin Exubera® (inhaled)	• Recombinant human insulin (rDNA origin)	• Regulation of glucose metabolism	• No rodent bioassay • Six-month chronic study (rats) (up to 8.3× MRHD based on body surface area) and 6-month chronic study (cynomolgus monkeys) (up to 1.4× MHRD based on body	• No malignancies reported in Adverse Reactions in clinical trials • No warnings or precautions regarding carcinogenic risk

TABLE 19.4b Examples of communication of human carcinogenic risk *with* preclinical assessment of carcinogenic risk (*Continued*)

Biopharmaceutical	Class	Mechanism of Action	Preclinical Studies	Human Experience/Product Label
			surface area)—both were maximum tolerated doses based on hypoglycemia. No effect evident on cell proliferation indexes in alveolar or bronchiolar area in the lung in either species	
Insulin glargine Lantus®	• Recombinant human insulin analogue (rDNA origin)	• Regulation of glucose metabolism	• Not mutagenic (Ames) • Standard 2-year bioassays performed in rats (up to 10× MRHD based on body surface area) and mice (up to 5× MHRD based on body surface area). Findings in female mice were not conclusive due to excessive mortality in all dose groups during the study. Histiocytomas found at injections sites in male rats (statistically significant) and male mice (not statistically significant) in acid vehicle containing groups. These tumors were not found in female animals, in saline control, or insulin comparator groups using a different vehicle • Relevance of these finding to humans is unknown	• No malignancies reported in Adverse Reactions in clinical trials • No warnings or precautions regarding carcinogenic risk

| Insulin aspart Novolog® | • Recombinant human insulin analogue (rDNA origin) Long-acting basal insulin analogue | • Regulation of glucose metabolism | • Not genotoxic (Ames and HGPRT tests, and in tests for detection of chromosomal aberrations (cytogenetics in vitro in V79 cells and in vivo in Chinese hamsters)
• Relative mitogenicity greater than human insulin
• No rodent bioassay
• 52-week chronic repeat dose study in rats (up to 32× MRHD based on body surface area). At highest dose Novolog increased the incidence of mammary tumors in females when compared to untreated controls. The incidence of mammary tumors was not significantly different than for regular human insulin. Relevance of these findings to humans is not known
• Not genotoxic (Ames, mouse lymphoma cell forward gene mutation test, human peripheral blood lymphocyte chromosome aberration test, in vivo micronculeus test in mice, ex vivo UDS test in rat liver hepatocytes
• Relative mitogenicity less than or equal to human insulin | • No malignancies reported in Adverse Reactions in clinical trials
• No warnings or precautions regarding carcinogenic risk |

TABLE 19.4b Examples of communication of human carcinogenic risk *with* preclinical assessment of carcinogenic risk (*Continued*)

Biopharmaceutical	Class	Mechanism of Action	Preclinical Studies	Human Experience/Product Label
Teriparatide Forteo™	• Recombinant human parathyroid hormone (1–34) Identical sequence to the 34N-terminal amino acids of the 84-amino acid human parathyroid hormone	• Primary regulator of calcium and phosphate metabolism in bone and kidney • Physiological actions of PTH include regulation of bone metabolism, renal tubular reabsorption of calcium and phosphate, and intestinal calcium absorption	• Two carcinogenicity bioassays were conducted in rats (3–60× MRHD). Treatment resulted in a marked dose-related increase in the incidence of osteosarcoma, a rare malignant bone tumor, in both male and female rats. Osteosarcomas were observed at all doses and the incidence reached 40–50% in the high-dose groups. Teriparatide also caused a dose-related increase in osteoblastoma and osteoma in both sexes. Bone tumors in rats occurred in association with a large increase in bone mass and focal osteoblast hyperplasia • Second 2-year study was carried out in order to determine the effect of treatment duration and animal age on the development of bone tumors. Female rats were treated for different periods between 2 and 26 months of age (at 3× to 20× MRHD based on body surface area). The	*Black box warning* • In male and female rats, teriparatide caused an increase in the incidence of osteosarcoma (a malignant bone tumor) that was dependent on dose and treatment duration. Effect was observed at systemic exposures to teriparatide ranging from 3 to 60 times the exposure in humans given a 20mcg dose. Because of the uncertain relevance of the rat osteosarcomas finding to humans, teriparatide should be prescribed only to patients for whom the potential benefits are considered to outweigh the potential risk. Teriparatide should not be prescribed for patients who are an increased baseline risk for osteosarcoma (including those with Paget's disease of bone or unexplained

study showed that the occurrence of osteosarcoma, osteoblastoma and osteoma was dependent on dose and duration of exposure. Bone tumors were observed when immature 2-month old rats were treated with 20× MRHD for 24 months or with 3× and 20× MRHD for 6 months. Bone tumors were also observed when mature 6-month-old rats were treated with 20× MRHD for 6 months or 20 months. Tumors were not detected when mature 6-month old rats were treated with 3× MRHD for 6 or 20 months. Results did not demonstrate a difference in susceptibility to bone tumor formation, associated with teriparatide treatment, between mature and immature rats. Relevance of these rat findings to humans is uncertain

elevations of alkaline phosphatase, open epiphyses, or prior radiation therapy involving the skeleton)

Warnings
• Patients with bone metastases or a history of skeletal malignancies should be excluded from treatment with Forteo

Precautions
• Safety and efficacy of Forteo have not been evaluated beyond 2 years of treatment. Consequently use of the drug for more than 2 years is not recommended

Information for patients
• Patients should be made aware that FORTEO caused osteosarcomas in rats and that the clinical relevance of these findings is unknown

Growth factors

Mecasermin
Increlex™

• Recombinant derived human insulin-like growth factor-1 (rhIGF-1)

• IGF-1 is the principal hormonal mediator of statural growth. In target tissues the type 1

• Two-year rat chronic bioassay in rodents was performed
• Increased incidence of adrenal medullary hyperplasia and pheochromocytoma observed

Contraindications
• Increlex is contraindicated in the presence of active or suspected neoplasia and therefore should be

TABLE 19.4b Examples of communication of human carcinogenic risk *with* preclinical assessment of carcinogenic risk (*Continued*)

Biopharmaceutical	Class	Mechanism of Action	Preclinical Studies	Human Experience/Product Label
		IGF-1 receptor, which is homologous to the insulin receptor is activated by IGF 1 leading to intracellular signaling which stimulates multiple processes leading to statural growth	in male rates at ≥1× MRHD (males) and ≥0.3× (females) the MRHD. Increased incidence of kertoacanthoma in the skin in rats ≥4× MRHD (males) and 7× MRHD (females). Increased incidence of mammary gland carcinoma in males and females at 7× MRHD. Based on excess mortality secondary to IGF-1 induced hypoglycemia in skin and mammary tumor findings only observed at greater than human MTD • *No interpretation provided as to relevance of findings above to humans* • Not clastogenic (in vitro chromosomal aberration assay and in vivo mouse MN)	discontinued if evidence of neoplasia develops • Increlex is not intended for use with chronic treatment of pharmacological doses of anti-inflammatory steroids
Peg-filgrastim Neulasta™	• Covalent conjugate of recombinant-derived human growth factor (rh G-CSF and monomethoxypolyethylene glycol)	• Acts on cells of the hematopoietic cells by binding to specific cell surface receptors and stimulating proliferation, differentiation commitment, and	• No rodent bioassay • No genotoxicity studies were performed • In a toxicity study of 6 months duration in rats given sc once weekly up to 1000 mc/kg (approx 23× MRHD) no precancerous or cancer lesions	*Precautions* • G-CSF receptor through which pegfilgrastim and filgrastim act has been found on tumor cell lines including some myeloid, T lymphoid, lung, head and neck and bladder tumor cell lines

	some end-cell functional activation	• Possibility that pegfilgrastim can act as a growth factor on any tumor type cannot be excluded
Darpopoetin alpha Aranesp™	• Recombinant human derived erythropoeisis stimulating protein closely related to erythropoietin	*Warnings* • Erythrocyte-stimulating agents increase mortality and/or tumor progression
	• Stimulates erythropoietin by same mechanism of action as endogenous erythropoietin	• No rodent bioassay • No tumorigenic or unexpected mitogenic response observed in any tissue type • No binding to human tissues other than those expressing the erythropoietin receptor • No alteration of proliferative response of non-hematological cells in vitro or in vivo • Not genotoxic (Ames, in vitro chromosomal aberration, in vivo mouse MN)
Palifermin Kepivance®	• Recombinant derived human growth factor (rhKFG)	• No rodent bioassay • Not clastogenic or mutagenic effects were observed but such studies are not informative for biological products • Tg,rasH2 model completed postapproval. The study is mentioned in the Summary of Product Characteristics (SPC) and the postapproval procedural steps summary
		Precautions • Kepivance has been shown to enhance the growth of human epithelial tumor cell lines in vitro ($15\times$ MRHD) and to increase the rate of tumor cell line growth in a human carcinoma xenograft model (25–$67\times$ MRHD)

TABLE 19.4b Examples of communication of human carcinogenic risk *with* preclinical assessment of carcinogenic risk (*Continued*)

Biopharmaceutical	Class	Mechanism of Action	Preclinical Studies	Human Experience/Product Label
				• In mice and rats, Kepivance enhanced proliferation of epithelial cells as measured by Ki67 immunohistochemical staining and BrDu uptake and demonstrated and increase in tissue thickness of the tongue, buccal mucosa and GI tract • Safety and efficacy of Kepivance has not been established in patients with non hematologic malignancies • Effects of Kepivance on stimulation of KGF-receptors-expressing non-hematopoietic tumors in patients are not known
Oprelvekin Neumega®	• Recombinant *E. coli* derived human growth factor (rhIL-11)	• Primary hematopoietic activity is stimulation of megakaryocytopoisis and thrombopoiesis	• No rodent bioassay • In vitro Neumega did not stimulate growth of tumor colony-forming cells harvested from patients with a variety of malignancies • Not-genotoxic (in vitro studies)	• Safety and efficacy of chronic administration has not been established • Treatment should be discontinued at least two days before staring the next planned cycle of chemotherapy

Cytokines

Interferon beta-1b Betaseron®	• Recombinant interferon beta-1b (Type I interferon)	• Binding of human interferon-1b to specific cell receptors induces the expression of a number of interferon-induced gene products (e.g., 2',5'-oligoandenylate synthetase, protein kinase, and indoleamine 2,3-dioxygenase that are believed to be mediators of the biological actions	• No rodent bioassay • Not genotoxic (Ames, Balb/3T3 mouse embryo transformation assay)	• No malignancies reported in Adverse Reactions in clinical trials • No warnings or precautions regarding carcinogenic risk

Other

Dornase alpha Pulmozyme®	• Recombinant enzyme (rhDNAse)	• Selectively cleaves DNA released by degenerating leucocytes that accumulate in response to infection in CF patients	• Two-year chronic bioassay was conducted in rats up to 28× human dose (no increase in benign or malignant neoplasms)	• No malignancies reported in Adverse Reactions in clinical trials • No warnings or precautions regarding carcinogenic risk

Source: Information based on product label or FDA Pharmacology/Toxicology review for FDA Approved Drug Products (http://www.accessdata.fda.gov/scripts/cder/drugsatfda/); supportive information EPAR's for authorized medicinal products for human use (http://www.emea.europa.eu/htms/human/epar/a.htm).

and therefore effectively competitively inhibits the biologic activity of interleukin-1. There was no discussion of the immunotoxic or carcinogenic potential of IL-1ra in the original published FDA pharm/tox review [58]. A comment was made that genotoxicity assays had been done, but they were not considered to be of particular value because they were designed to detect mutagenic effects of small-molecule drugs, chemicals, and environmental agents that cause direct damage to DNA molecules. As such they were regarded as inappropriate for protein biotherapeutics. An assessment of carcinogenic risk was requested by the European authorities [59]. In the scientific discussion of anakinra it was stated that the carcinogenic potential was evaluated with an emphasis on risk of direct tumor production, risk of tumor stimulation, and indirect effects on tumor growth. The risk of tumor production was considered unlikely due to lack of findings in the genotoxicity assays (see comment above regarding relevance) and lack of tumors found in the 6-month rat study. The risk of tumor stimulation was also considered to be low as binding of anakinra to IL-1 receptors did not cause signal induction and data were also presented indicating that anakinra did not appear to directly stimulate mitogenesis or cell proliferation. With respect to indirect effects on tumor growth, data were presented to support lack of immunosuppression in the rat and monkey toxicity studies. A literature search revealed no published data on increased tumorigenicity in transgenic or knockout mice with an analogous defect. In addition, information was provided based on seven years of experience by the director of the laboratory that produced IL-1ra overexpressing mice and IL-1ra mutant knockout, stating that that no increased carcinogenic risk in the mice was observed.

Again, the higher incidence rate of lymphomas in RA patients compared to the general population was communicated as a warning in the label as well as by the fact that RA patients, particularly those with active disease, may be at higher risk for the development of lymphoma, but the role of IL-blockers in the development of malignancy was not known.

Muromonab CD3 Orthoclone OKT® 3, the first US approved monoclonal antibody, is a murine monoclonal antibody directed against the CD3 antigen on human T cells. It was approved by the US FDA for the treatment of acute renal allograft rejection in June 1986. No formal preclinical carcinogenicity assessment was performed because the muromonab CD3 did not cross-react in rodents. Nevertheless, because of the expected risk of lymphoproliferative disorders following immunosuppressive treatment, the Center for Biologics Evaluation and Research, FDA required a commitment at the time of licensure for the manufacturer to perform specific postmarketing surveys on the incidence of lymphomas in humans in addition to routine postmarketing surveillance to determine the number of malignancies following Orthoclone OKT®3 treatment. Ultimately the risk of serious and sometimes fatal neoplasias in patients was communicated as a warning in the product label in context of the diseases being treated as well as concomitant treatments including other immunosuppressive agents.

19.6.2 Peptide Hormones

Growth Hormones In 1988 Watanabe et al. reported leukemia in patients receiving growth hormone (GH) therapy [60]. Over the next several years there were additional reports suggesting a GH-related increase in the incidence of leukemia. In 1997 Allen et al. reported that the incidence of leukemia in GH-treated patients without risk factors for leukemia was comparable to that in the general population of age-matched children using data form the National Cooperative Growth Study in the United States and Canada [61]. Nishi et al. followed with a report in 1999 based on data collected from more than 32,000 GH-deficient patients from 1975 through 1997. The authors concluded that the incidence of leukemia in GH-treated patients without risk factors is no greater than in the general population aged 0 to 15 years, and that a possible increased occurrence of leukemia with GH treatment appears to be limited to patients with risk factors (e.g., Fanconi's anemia, neoplasia, previous radiation, or chemotherapy). There was also no suggestion that longer periods of GH treatment were associated with more frequent development of leukemia [62].

Preclinical carcinogenicity assessment of growth hormones has not been performed for currently marketed growth hormones. In an effort to better understand the potential carcinogenic risk of growth hormone, rodent bioassays were recently performed using recombinant rat and mouse growth hormones (human homologues) in chronic rat and mouse bioassays [63]. It was difficult to compare exposure, but the levels at the high doses were higher than the basal or peak level in humans. The authors concluded that the lack of carcinogenic effects following chronic administration of GH in these two bioassays lends greater weight of evidence that high circulating levels of GH would not be associated with greater risk of tumors in subjects receiving GH replacement therapy. Unfortunately, the authors did not provide a justification for using two rodent species, especially since it was noted that there was a limited quantity of rmGH available for the mouse bioassay; therefore the high dose was lower than the dose needed to induce weight gain in mice in a 5-week study.

The current labels for growth hormones read "leukemia has been reported in a small number of pediatric patients who have been treated with growth hormone, including growth hormone of pituitary origin and recombinant somatropin. The relationship, if any, between leukemia and growth hormone is uncertain. Carcinogenicity studies have not been performed for the currently approved recombinant growth hormones."

The data using the homologous products did not show carcinogenic effects in rodents and thus can be used to support the position that there is a lack of convincing evidence for an increased risk of cancer in children receiving recombinant GH therapy. However, it is unclear whether the data are sufficient to modify the current labels for communicating carcinogenic risk. Furthermore, since the clinical data already seemed to support the lack of effect in GH-treated patients without risk factors, it could have been of interest to have included conditions in, for example, the rat bioassay that addressed the effect of previous chemotherapy or irradiation to better understand, in a well-controlled rodent animal model, the potential impact of known human risk factors on tumor formation.

Insulin Analogues Insulin, a polypeptide hormone produced by pancreatic islet β cells, was discovered in 1921. It was initially isolated from bovine/porcine glands up to the mid-1970s. Native human insulin has, in addition to its metabolic actions, a weak mitogenic effect. This effect has become important for the safety assessment of modified insulins, since structural modification of the insulin molecule could increase the mitogenic potency, possibly resulting in growth simulation of preexisting neoplasms.

Recombinant "normal" insulin has been produced since the 1980s. In the 1990s recombinant insulin analogues became available. The basic assumption that insulin was "safe" and not carcinogenic was not tested. However, results of carcinogenicity testing with the analogue AspB10 showed tumors in animals. In subsequent in vitro studies AspB10 insulin was found to possess a mitogenic activity that exceeded that of normal human insulin. It has now been shown that normal insulin can cause tumors in rats within one year of dosing at very high doses, implying a threshold for tumorigenicity.

In view of the life long exposure and large patient populations, insulins with increased mitogenic effect in relation to the unmodified human insulin in current use were thus considered to constitute a major public health concern. Therefore a thorough assessment of carcinogenic potential was recommended for all new modified insulins in 2001 [64].

In addition to the standard battery of genotoxicity studies, new insulin analogues are generally evaluated for in vitro and in vivo mitogenicity compared to normal insulin. The duration of the rodent study is based on an understanding of relative mitogenicity compared to normal insulin. Six-month repeat-dose studies have been sufficient if mitogenicity potential is low, and longer term studies are recommended if mitogenicity potential is high. In the later cases both normal insulin and ASP10 are generally included as study controls. Assessment of risk is based on cross-species pharmacology comparisons and the margin of safety compared to the intended clinical exposure.

To date, no malignancies have been reported as adverse reactions in clinical trials with insulin analogues. There are also no warnings or precautions regarding carcinogenic risk in the product labels for insulin analogues. The relevance of the findings in the rat bioassay to humans for insulin glargine, an insulin analogue with greater mitogenicity than insulin, was stated as unknown.

Insulin-like Growth Factor Human Insulin like growth factor (rhIGF-1) is identical to endogenous human IGF-1. The actions of IGF-1 as a "somatomedin" are obligate for growth hormone to be able to stimulate bone and body growth. In addition to mediating many of the activities of GH, IGF-1 also has "insulin-like" metabolic activities that support statural growth. The hormonal, cellular, and molecular mechanisms mediating the actions of rhIGF-1 on growth and metabolism are well characterized. IGF-1 concentrations are elevated in acromegaly, and there have been reports confirming that agromegaly predisposes to colonic neoplasia. While it seems probable that GH/IGF-1 may in some way be involved in the pathogenesis, it is unlikely to be an initiating carcinogen; other intraluminal local environmental influences may be important [65].

The package insert for rIGF-1 contains no interpretation or statements with respect to significance provided for the findings observed in a two-year chronic bioassay in rats with rhIGF-1 that showed an increase in tumors. Presumably this is because it was reasoned that the skin and mammary tumor findings were observed only at doses greater than the human maximum tolerated dose. Nevertheless, clinical dosing is contraindicated in the presence of active and suspected neoplasia, and discontinuation of dosing is recommended if neoplasia develops.

PTH and PTH Analogues   Parathyroid hormone and its analogues represent a new class of agents with anabolic effects on the skeleton. In two-year carcinogenicity studies of PTH (1-34) in two strains of rats and one strain of mice the animals developed osteosarcomas when given PTH and related peptides from weaning to 18 months of age. Many of the tumors were discovered by direct palpation and were often metastatic at the time of discovery, suggesting that they had been present for a long time. While there was a dose-related incidence in osteosarcomas, in some cases tumors occurred in animals at exposures equivalent to those commonly used in the clinical studies.

The relevance of the animal findings to the clinical administration is not currently known. The FDA subsequently developed a guidance to clarify the Agency's thinking regarding the impact of these preclinical findings on PTH drug development programs for the treatment and/or prevention of osteoporosis [66]. As a result of the concern about carcinogenicity, studies to evaluate carcinogenic potential should be performed for PTH and related peptides, although these studies could entail unique design features.

In an effort to improve the benefit-to-risk ratio of PTH in the context of the uncertain relevance of the findings in rodents, it was strongly recommended that participation in clinical studies be limited to adults with severe osteoporosis who have completed bone maturation. It was further advised that any case of osteosarcoma (or other bone tumor) be immediately reported and long-term follow-up be conducted for patients treated with PTH. Importantly, subjects in clinical trials of PTH and PTH analogues should be informed about the occurrence of osteosarcomas in rodents.

The current label for PTH(1-34) , the first approved PTH analogue, reports dose-related increase in osteosarcomas, osteoblastomas, and osteomas in two-rat carcinogenicity studies as well as results from a second two-year study in rats designed to determine the effect of treatment duration and animal

development of bone tumors. The study showed that the occurrence of osteosarcomas, osteoblastomas, and osteomas was dependent on dose and duration of exposure. However, tumors were not detected when mature 6-month old rats were treated with 3× the human dose for 6 or 20 months. Again, the label states that the relevance of the rat findings to humans is uncertain. The Medication Guide highlights the findings in a section entitled "What is the most important information I should know about Foreto™. The guide states that osteosarcomas in humans is a very serious but very rare cancer that occurs in about four out of every million older adults each year and that it is not known if humans treated with Forteo™ also have a higher chance of getting osteosarcoma.

Similar to concerns regarding the relative potency of insulin analogues, the relative carcinogenic potential of PTH and analogues will need to be compared to PTH (1-34). The actual details of the study design may need to be discussed with respective regulatory authorities. However, since osteosarcomas are due to exaggerated pharmacology, it is likely that the same regulatory and labeling standards will be applicable to all PTH and analogue products regardless of potency [67]. The question remains as to whether a two-year bioassay will be needed to communicate carcinogenic risk. Notably there is an apparent lack of osteosarcomas in humans with very long term PTH secreting tumors and in pseudohypothyroidism.

19.6.3 Growth Factors

Most growth factors are highly conserved molecules and demonstrate biological activity across species. With the exception of GM-CSF, which appears to be uniquely specific, most growth factors have been demonstrated to have activity in rodent species. There have been no rodent carcinogenicity studies reported to date and no findings of concern in short-term or chronic toxicity studies for approved growth factors: PDGF (topical), G-CSF, GM-CSF, KGF, or EPO. In addition no rodent bioassays have been reported for other growth factors that have been in clinical development, including NGF, BDNF, CNTF, EGF, TGF-α, and TGF-β. Growth factors have at least a theoretical risk for tumor promotion of cells with receptors that respond to the growth factor. These products are unlikely to be used for trivial indications; however, rodent carcinogenicity studies are unlikely to provide any useful information. The potential for tumorigenicity will likely best be determined in humans under the clinical conditions of use.

Becaplermin   Becaplermin is produced by recombinant DNA technology by insertion of the gene for the β chain of the platelet-derived growth factor (PDGF) into the yeast, *Saccharomyces cerevisiae*. Becaplermin has biological activity similar to that of endogenous platelet-derived growth factor, which includes promoting the chemotactic recruitment and proliferation of cells involved in wound repair and in enhancing the formation of granulation tissue.

Becaplermin is indicated for the topical treatment of lower extremity diabetic neuropathic ulcers that extend into the subcutaneous tissue or beyond and have an adequate blood supply.

In reviewing the data on becaplermin, the CPMP decided that there were no suitable tests that the applicant could employ to produce unequivocal evidence that becaplermin is or is not carcinogenic since no data were available in humans. The CPMP agreed that the risk of skin tumors or other malignancies was limited, although a theoretical concern remained since the active substance was a growth factor. The contraindications for use of the product considered known neoplasm at or near the site of application and urged caution in the use of the product in patients with known malignancies. Postmarketing follow-up to obtain additional long-term clinical safety data with particular emphasis on the incidence of tumor formation was also recommended [68].

The possibility that growth factors can act as growth stimulants for some tumor type will likely never be excluded and therefore should be communicated in product labels. However, it may be possible that the concern may be reduced through in vitro or in vivo short-term studies to better understand and characterize the potential risk.

Palifermin   Palifermin, a human keratinocyte growth factor (KGF), produced by recombinant DNA technology in *E. coli.*, targets epithelial cells by binding to specific cell-surface receptors, stimulating proliferation, differentiation, and upregulation of cytoprotective mechanisms. The first 23 N-terminal amino acids of KGF were deleted to improve protein stability. The key findings in toxicology studies performed in rats and monkeys were generally attributable to the pharmacological activity of palifermin, specifically, proliferation of epithelial tissue.

The effect of rHuKGF on the proliferation rate of 41 tumor lines was assessed as well as the effect on the growth of subcutaneous receptor positive human tumor xenografts in athymic mice. One tumor showed a statistically significant positive. The overall data to predict potential for tumor promotion in humans were deemed questionable.

The current product label, under precautions, states that the effects of Kepivance™ on stimulation of KGF receptor expressing, nonhematopoietic tumors are not known. Kepivance™ has been shown to enhance the growth of epithelial tumor cell lines in vitro and to increase the rate of tumor cell growth in a human carcinoma xenograft model. The label advises that patients should be informed of the evidence of tumor growth and stimulation in cell cultures and in animal models of nonhematopoietic human tumors. Of note, the mutagenicity sections states that although no clastogenic or mutagenic effects were observed, such studies are generally not informative for biological products.

Although not required for approval, a short-term bioassay, Tg-Hras2 model, was conducted postapproval and is mentioned in the Summary of Product Characteristics (SPC) and the postapproval procedural steps summary. There were no findings suggestive of tumor growth promotion in this study.

19.6.4   Cytokines

Interferons are uniquely species specific and are not active in rodents. In addition the class-specific product attributes, including the mechanisms of action of the respective subtypes, reduces cause for concern for carcinogenic risk. No malignancies have been reported under adverse reactions in clinical trials, and there are no warnings or precautions regarding carcinogenic risk in the product labels or adverse reports reported postmarketing.

19.6.5   Enzyme Replacement Therapies

A variety of enzyme replacement therapies have been approved including those listed in Table 19.4a. Despite the fact that these products are used chronically, no genotoxicity or carcinogenicity studies have been performed presumably based on specific product class attributes.

19.6.6   Other

Omalizumab   Omalizumab is a recombinant humanized monoclonal antibody that binds to human IgE that is indicated for use in adults and adolescents with moderate to severe persistent asthma who are inadequately controlled with inhaled corticosteroids and have a positive skin test or in vitro reactivity to a perennial aeroallergen. Omalizumab is not pharmacologically active in rodents. Studies in wild-type mice showed a different cell distribution of IgE affinity receptor (FcεR1) compared to humans and humanized (FcεR1) transgenic mice were not available during development. Tumor host resistance models (e.g., B16 melanoma) could have been used; however, this would have required development of a humanized FcεR1 transgenic model with appropriate FcεR1 cell distribution as well as an appropriate homologous anti-mouse IgE mAb. In addition to the considerations above the chemical structure of omalizumab did not represent a carcinogenic risk, and there was no clinical epidemiological data supporting the role of IgE in immunosurveillance. Therefore no additional studies were performed to assess carcinogenic risk. In the clinical trials of less then a year study duration, a slightly higher increase in malignant neoplasms compared to controls was reported. The label reads that the impact of longer exposures or use in patients at higher risk for malignancy is not known.

DNase   A rodent bioassay was conducted in rats based on the intended patient population (in large part children) as well as the relevancy and feasibility of the rodent to assess toxicity. No adverse findings were observed.

19.7   RATIONALE FOR NOT PERFORMING THE RODENT BIOASSAY

Some of the shortcomings of the rodent bioassay have been discussed above. There is an increasing body of evidence suggesting that the data necessary to identify potential human hazards may be obtained without the current reliance on the results of rodent bioassay(s) [17,18]. There are also various proposals suggesting what might constitute a relevant assessment of carcinogenic risk of pharmaceuticals. One proposed assessment includes an evaluation of a number of possible characteristics. The components of the assessment include in vitro and in vivo genotoxicity studies, a six-month rodent (or nonrodent study depending on the biologic activity of the molecule), additional pharmacologic assays to further assess pharmacodynamic or immunomodulatory effects and define dose–response relationships, pharmacokinetic studies to describe systemic exposure and dose–response behavior, and an alternative short-term carcinogenicity assay. A rodent bioassay would only be needed if all other data are inconclusive [18]. Another proposal includes conduct of a 13-week repeat dose study focusing on four endpoints: genotoxicity, immunosuppression, estrogenicity, and increased cell proliferation. These data would be combined with structure-activity models of chemical effects [17]. Short-term assessments of these effects are expected to provide predictive signals that would allow scientists to determine the likelihood of cancer in rodents, as well as the human relevance of the associated pathways. It is also important to consider human experience of spontaneous, often genetic diseases and diseases in humans or animals that may mimic potential effects of the biopharmaceutical with greater potency and specificity and that show what happens in the target species.

It is important to emphasize that while some scientists concur, in principle, that alternative assays may provide information for the integrative assessment of carcinogenic risk, they also admit that the assays may not provide a definitive answer. As previously discussed, the FDA is still considering the totality of the available data, including the results of rodent bioassay in most cases for identifying carcinogenic hazard of pharmaceuticals [16]. However, in the United States there is the opportunity to submit a waiver of carcinogenicity testing based on supported scientific rationale considering the specific product attributes, all available preclinical data and the intended patient population (see Table 19.5).

19.8 MANAGEMENT AND COMMUNICATING OF CARCINOGENIC RISK

Do animal data alter the perception of carcinogenic risk? Are the preclinical data adequate to support the clinical use of the product in patients? To what extent can we accept lack of experimental data before a product is used to treat humans? Should a study be done if the relevance of the test system is questionable? Can risks be communicated without "doing a study"? What and whose risk is it not "doing a study"?

The goal of preclinical safety testing, especially carcinogenicity studies, is to protect patients by helping to prevent toxic exposures or at least

**TABLE 19.5 Considerations supporting waiver of carcinogenicity studies for Fuzeon®
(enfuviritide, T-20)**

Sponsor Arguments	FDA Response	FDA Recommendation
Concerns related to product class		*Reasons to support conducting carcinogenicity testing of T-20*
• T-20 is a novel retroviral agent with respect to biological and chemical characteristics and therefore there is no concern based on carcinogenicity of other retroviral agents • Unique mechanism of action of T-20 involves a specific protein–protein interaction with the extracellular portion of the transmembrane glycoprotein gp41 of the HIV virus, thus blocking viral fusion with the T cell membrane • Polypeptides are not known to be carcinogenic	• Insofar as T-20 is a novel retroviral agent (there are no other products in its class), the argument is irrelevant whether other products in its class have not demonstrated carcinogenic activity • Question of whether there was evidence for T-20 tissue (protein-protein) interactions (that might suggest that T-20 stimulates cell division, or blocks cell apoptosis). (No data are available that looked at T-20-tissue interactions except that NIH had conducted a study of T-20 that produced unambiguous or difficult-to-interpret data) • There are polypeptides that are known to be carcinogenic. All those that were located are hormones or ones that demonstrated hormonal activity	• In some cases T-20 administration was shown to cause chronic irritation and inflammation at injection sites when administered by subcutaneous injection or infusion. In some cases, injection of T-20 caused hard masses at injection sites, suggesting that T-20 was not well-absorbed • Administration of T-20 is expected to exceed 6 months in some patients • T-20 is a new molecular substance
Structure-activity relationships		
• T-20 is expected to be metabolized into smaller peptides and amino acids. As such, there are no classical structural alerts suggesting a carcinogenic risk		

TABLE 19.5 *Continued*

Sponsor Arguments	FDA Response	FDA Recommendation

Concerns from repeated-dose toxicity studies

- In repeat-dose toxicity studies of T-20 (6 months in rats, 9 months in monkeys), hyperplasia and preneoplastic lesions have not been observed

- In a 28-day repeat-dose intravenous study of T-20 in monkeys, splenic hyperplasia was observed in most of the animals (all of the high-dose animals), and the severity of splenic hyperplasia was greater in T-20-injected animals than in control animals. One animal in the high-dose group had a spleen that was greater than 3% of its body weight. This hyperplasia likely resulted from an immune reaction to T-20. However, we do not believe it is correct to state that there is no evidence of treatment-related hyperplasia

Long-term retention of parent compound or metabolite

- Pharmacokinetic studies in rats after intravenous injection revealed a 2.4-hour half-life and low distribution (26.3 ml) suggesting that there is a little long-term retention of T-20 in rodents

- Studies where T-20 was administered by subcutaneous injection to rats or monkeys indicated poor absorption at the injection site in some instances, which in turn suggest long-term retention of T-20 is possible under some circumstances
- Studies of the rates of elimination of radioactivity in feces, urine, and air after a single intravenous injection of tritiated T-20 in the rat suggest catabolism of T-20 amino acids and reincorporation of radiolabel into body tissue proteins. Highest amount of radiolabel appeared in skeletal muscle 48 hours after T-20 administration. No systemic degeneration of muscle tissue was noted after chronic T-20 administration

**TABLE 19.5   Considerations supporting waiver of carcinogenicity studies for Fuzeon®
(enfuviritide, T-20) (*Continued*)**

Sponsor Arguments	FDA Response	FDA Recommendation
Genotoxicity		*Strongest arguments for NOT conducting carcinogenicity testing of T-20*
• There was no evidence of genotoxicity in the standard genotoxicity test battery bacteria reverse mutation (Ames) tests, forward gene mutations in mammalian (Chinese hamster ovary AS42) cells, or mouse bone marrow MN test	• Not all carcinogens are genotoxic	• T-20 did not induce tumor in 6-month repent-dose studies in rats and 9-month repeat-dose studies in monkeys • T-20 is a polypeptide comprised of naturally occurring L-amino acids. Some data indicate that T-20 is metabolized to amino acids and they, in turn, are incorporated into body tissues • T-20 was not mutagenic in the standard battery of mutagenicity studies • The only proteins that are carcinogenic in animals are proteins that demonstrate hormonal action. T-20 does not have hormonal action
Compounds producing chronic irritation/inflammation		
• Repeated twice-daily injection via sc administration of T-20 to rats or monkeys resulted in various degrees of inflammation and irritation at the injection sites. In the 6-month rat study, the incidence and severity of lesions was comparable to that observed in vehicle-treated animals. Evidence of an injection site reaction in primates was not common until week 17. Injection site reactions have been observed in humans, which vary in severity and rarely cause treatment discontinuation • Patients are instructed to rotate sites of injection to avoid chronic irritation/ inflammation at a single site	• Early studies of T-20 (e.g., rat 6-month repeat-dose study) were inconclusive as to whether injection site inflammation was solely a result of the procedure of the drug or some combination of the two. In retrospective review of data, it appears that inflammation is, at least in part, a reaction to the drug. It is irrelevant that microscopic evidence of an injection site reaction in primates was not common until week 17. In the same (9-month primate) study, increased eosinophils (compared with controls) were measured at 3 months (earliest postdosing hematological measurement), and inflammatory response were evident in the spleens (increased germinal centers and lymphocytic proliferation) and thymuses (cortical lymphocytic depletion) at 3 months. In the 28-day, repeat-dose primate study antibodies to T-20 were detected at day 7. Thus inflammation, while not clearly evident macroscopically until week 17 in the 9-month study, was microscopically evident earlier on	

TABLE 19.5 *Continued*

Sponsor Arguments	FDA Response	FDA Recommendation
	• Observations that injection site reactions in T-20 patients rarely cause treatment discontinuation, and that "patients are instructed to rotate sites of injection, thus avoiding chronic irritation/inflammation at a singe site" are irrelevant to the carcinogenic risk assessment but important to the potential carcinogenic risk assessment	
	Patient population	*Waiver granted*
• T-20 is intended for patients with advanced HIV infection, and will be tested in patients who have experienced all three classes of marketed antiviral drugs. These patients have limited treatment options • It is expected that patients may continue treatment of T-20 beyond 6 months, the treatment duration limit beyond which carcinogenicity studies for conventional pharmaceutical agents are generally needed. But, HIV patients have limited treatment options and the benefit–risk ratio for T-20 is considered extremely high, regardless of the outcome of animal carcinogenicity studies	• It is true that HIV infection is a life-threatening disease and that patients with advanced systemic HIV infection face limited treatment options. But, there are treatment options available to some patients. Since the advent of HAART regimens and the consequential decrease in mortality and increase in longevity of these individual, carcinogenic risk from anti-HIV drugs is a concern, especially for children. ICH guidance S1A states that where life expectancy in the indicated population is short (i.e., less than 2–3 years) long-term carcinogenicity studies may not be required. Many HIF-infected individuals are not living longer than 3 years, so this argument does not apply to all HIV-infected individuals who might receive T-20 • Treatment with T-20 beyond 6 months is a reason for conducting carcinogenicity testing. It is no longer true that carcinogenic risk is not a concern in the treatment of HIV-infected individual	• Most compelling reason to be concerned about carcinogenic potential of T-20 is that the subcutaneous administration of T-20 causes chronic inflammation. This adverse effect in humans can be monitored in humans • Rats have limited body surface area for subcutaneous injections sites and the procedure harms the rats • It is reasonable to grant the requested waiver unless there is a compelling reason to think that T-20 might be carcinogenic • Other evidence suggests that T-20 is not a carcinogen

**TABLE 19.5 Considerations supporting waiver of carcinogenicity studies for Fuzeon®
(enfuviritide, T-20) (*Continued*)**

Sponsor Arguments	FDA Response	FDA Recommendation
Relevance of carcinogenicity testing of polypeptides		
• Standard carcinogenicity bioassays may be in appropriate for compounds such as large molecular weight proteins and polypeptides	• Large molecular weight proteins are not mentioned in the ICH guidance documents referenced above	

Source: Adapted NDA No. 21–281 Pharmacology/Toxicology Review—William H. Taylor (http://www.accessdata.fda.gov/scripts/cder/drugsatfda/).

warn patients of the risks so that appropriate risk–benefit decisions can be made for the product and ultimately each patient. Despite the experimental uncertainties and limitations, appropriate communication of carcinogenic risk must be addressed. The initial guidance on the rodent bioassay for identifying carcinogenic hazard represented the best thinking of the time on how to accomplish the critical task of prospectively identifying chemicals that pose a carcinogenic risk to humans [18]. In the 40 years since this guidance was published, these recommendations continue to form the foundation of cancer risk assessment despite significant progress in our understanding of the biology of the carcinogenic response in animals and humans. However, the availability of large and extensive databases currently in development by various groups should support the development of a more rational, science-based approach to this process.

The specific product attributes of pharmaceuticals and biopharmaceuticals are blurring. Pharmaceuticals are increasing in molecular weight, including a variety of alternative scaffolds in efforts to extend half-lives and allow better efficacy and more convenient dosing regimens, while biopharmaceuticals are becoming smaller, focusing on more specific molecular interactions in efforts to improve efficacy and reduce immunogenicity and cost of goods. As is true for conventional pharmaceuticals, the cause for concern for tumorigenicity of biopharmaceuticals is heightened based on knowledge and plausibility of particular mode of action.

Special issues of concern following chronic treatment of immunomodulatory pharmaceuticals and biopharmaceuticals include the potential for immune impairment leading to opportunistic infections and/or lymphoproliferative disorders. Mitogenicity is a concern for exogenously administered biopharmaceuticals such as hormones and growth factors and may also be a concern for pharmaceuticals designed to stimulate their endogenous production. For DNA-based therapies, integration and the consequences of insertional muta-

TABLE 19.6   Factors to consider for carcinogenicity testing of biopharmaceuticals[a]

For Rodent Bioassay	Against Rodent Bioassay
Chronic use	Species-specific protein (rodent lacks receptor or epitope, receptor or epitope, is only upregulated in disease, product induces immune response in rodents)
Cause for concern based on product class (e.g., growth factor, immunomodulatory protein)	Relative risk is considered no greater than other products in the class (class label)
Studies have routinely been performed for pharmaceuticals intended for chronic use	Studies have not been previously performed with approved products in class
Feasibility is not an issue based on availability of the homologous test article determined to be comparable to the clinical product (e.g., recombinant protein or monoclonal antibody)	Homologous test article[b] may not be relevant (different pharmacological activity, different physiological regulation, product is otherwise not comparable, e.g., product quality issues)
Effecting the intended pathway may have expected consequences	Absence of findings in rodents would not necessarily preclude precaution or warning in label of potential human risk
Sponsor has an obligation in the label to provide an assessment of the potential carcinogenic effect of its product. (This obligation may be satisfied as a postmarketing commitment)	Alternative assays can be used to identify potential risk—together with thorough understanding of nature and biological properties of the product obtained from studies or literature references. Such information should be provided in the label
Regulatory expectation	Increased animal use with little predictive value for human risk (based on one or more of the above considerations); raising regulatory hurdles for similar products in the future

Note: [a]The testing is to provide meaningful information for human risk assessment and product labeling that informs physicians and patients about risks.
[b]The animal version of the human biopharmaceutical (e.g., rodent version of a recombinant protein or a monoclonal antibody).

genesis is a cause for concern, and for certain cell therapies based on specific product attributes there is an increased concern for the potential to cause tumors. Table 19.6 summarizes the factors for consideration of carcinogenicity assessment of biopharmaceuticals.

Bucher and Portier have suggested that "it is important for toxicologists to reevaluate our collective understanding of adverse biological responses in short-term in vivo and in vitro assays. That in spite of the recognized limitations, our understanding of carcinogenicity has advanced to the point that data from these assays could support decisions that are as protective of the public health as are current approaches relying on the results of the rodent bioassay "[6]. MacDonald concurs suggesting that with careful consideration from academic, regulatory, and industry scientists, and an appropriately rigorous process for decision making, a significant enhancement over the current process of carcinogenicity assessment can be envisioned. Further he notes that a prospective, comprehensive evaluation of the biologic effects of chemicals could better utilize our current understanding of the carcinogenic processes and could ultimately yield a more efficient and effective assessment of potential human risk [18].

Importantly, appropriate labeling is critical to communicating potential human risk and also when appropriate should be supported with a risk mitigation plan. As most assessments of carcinogenic risk are made on individual products, additional consideration may also be needed when patients are exposed to multiple products for treating the intended disease. The need for a prospectively defined pharmacovigilance plan is a final imperative for ensuring the availability of safe medicines [36].

ACKNOWLEDGMENTS

I would like to thank Drs. Richard Lewis, Michael McClain, James McDonald, and Professor Anthony Dayan for their critical reading of this chapter and thoughtful comments.

REFERENCES

1. Pitot HC, Dragan YP. Facts and theories concerning the mechanisms of carcinogenesis. *FASEB J* 1991;5:2280–6.
2. Yuspa SH. Overview of carcinogenesis: past, present and future. *Carcinogenesis* 2000;21:341–4.
3. Contrera JF, Jacobs AC, DeGeorge JJ. Carcinogenicity testing and the evaluation of regulatory requirements for pharmaceuticals. *Regul Toxicol Pharmacol* 1997; 25:30–45.
4. Jena GB, Kaul CL, Ramarao P. Regulatory requirements and ICH guidelines on carcinogenicity testing of pharmaceuticals: a review on current status. *Ind J Pharmacol* 2005;37:209–22.
5. Williams GM, Iatropoulos MJ. Principles of testing for carcinogenic activity. In Hayes AW, ed. *Principles and Methods of Toxicology*, 4th ed. Philadelphia: Taylor and Francis, 2001;1–42.
6. Bucher JR, Portier C. Human carcinogenic risk evaluation. Part V: The National Toxicology Program vision of assessing the human carcinogenic hazard of chemicals. *Toxicol Sci* 2004;82:363–6.
7. Contrera JF, MacLaughlin P, Hall LL, Kier LB. QSAR modeling of carcinogenic risk using discrimiant analysis and topological molecular descriptors. *Curr Drug Discov Technol* 2005;2:55–67.

8. Boorman GA, Maronpot RR, Eustis SL. Rodent carcinogenicity bioassay: past, present and future. *Toxicol Pathol* 1994;22(2):105–11.

9. Sontag JM, Page NP, Saffiotti U. Guidelines for Carcinogen Bioassay in Small Rodents. National Cancer Institute, NCI-CG-TR-1. DHEW Publ. No. (NIH) 76-801. Washington: US GPO.

10. Halmes NC, Roberts SM, Tolson JK, Portier CJ. Reevaluating cancer risk estimates for short-term exposure scenarios. *Toxicol Sci* 2000;58:32–42.

11. Crump KS, Howec RB. The multistage model with a time-dependent dose pattern: applications to carcinogenic risk assessment. *Risk Anal* 1984;4:163–76.

12. Weisburger JH, Williams GM. Carcinogen testing: current problems and new approaches. *Sci* 1981;214:401–7.

13. Huff J, Haseman J, Rall D. Scientific concepts, value and significance of chemical carcinogenesis studies. *Ann Rev Pharmacol Toxicol* 1991;31:621–52.

14. Benigni R, Zito R. The second National Toxicology Program comparative exercise on the prediction of rodent carcinogenicity: definitive results. *Muta Res* 2004; 566:49–63.

15. Gold LS, Slone TH, Ames BN. What animal cancer tests tell us about human cancer risk? Overview of analyses of the carcinogenic potency database. *Drug Metab Rev* 1998;30:359–404.

16. Jacobs A. Prediction of 2-year carcinogenicity study results for pharmaceutical products: How are we doing? *Toxicol Sci* 2005;88:18–23.

17. Cohen SM. Alternative models for carcinogenicity testing: weight of evidence evaluation across models. *Toxicol Pathol* 2001;29:183–90.

18. MacDonald JS. Human carcinogenic risk evaluation. Part IV: Assessment of human risk of cancer from chemical exposure using a global weight-of-evidence approach. *Toxicol Sci* 2004;82:3–8.

19. Meek ME, Bucher JR, Cohen SM, Dellarco V, Hill RN, Lehman-Mckeeman LD, Longfellow DG, Pastoor T, Seed J, Patton DE. A Framework for human relevance of information on carcinogenic modes of action. *Crit Rev Toxicol* 2004; 33(6):591–653.

20. Gottmann E, Kramer S, Pfahringer B, Helma C. Data quality in predictive toxicology: reproducibility of rodent carcinogenicity experiments. *Environ Health Persp* 2001;109:509–14.

21. Cohen SM. Human carcinogenic risk evaluation: an alternative approach to the two-year rodent bioassay. *Toxicol Sci* 2004;80:225–9.

22. IARC. Monographs on the Evaluation of Carcinogenic Risk to Humans. Vol. 50. Pharmaceutical Drugs. International Agency for Research on Cancer, Lyons, France, 1990.

23. Jacobs A, Jacobson-Kram D. Human carcinogenic risk evaluation. Part III. Assessing the cancer hazard and risk in human drug development. *Toxicol Sci* 2004; 81:260–2.

24. Cohen SM. Infection, cell proliferation and malignancy. In Parsonnet J, Henning S, eds. *Microbes and Malignancy: Infection as a Cause of Cancer*. New York: Oxford University Press, 1999:89–106.

25. Hutsch T, Kapp A, Spergel J. Immunomodulation and safety of topical calcineurin inhibitors for the treatment of atopic dermatitis. *Dermatology* 2005;211:174–87.

26. ICH S1A. International Conference on Harmonization ICH S1A (1995). Need for Carcinogenicity Studies of Pharmaceuticals, 1995. http://www.fda.gov/cder/guidance/index.htm

27. ICH S6. International Conference on Harmonization ICH S6. Preclinical Safety Evaluation of Biotechnology-derived Pharmaceuticals, 1997. http://www.fda.gov/cder/guidance/index.htm

28. Hastings KL. Assessment of immunosuppressant drug carcinogenicity: standard and alternative models. *Hum Exp Toxicol* 2000;19:261–5.

29. ICH Q5D Q5D. Quality of Biotechnological/Biological Products: Derivation and Characterization of Cell Substrates Used for Production of Biotechnological/Biological Products; Availability, 1998. http://www.fda.gov/cder/guidance/index.htm

30. Hacein-Bey-Abina S, Von Kalle C, Schmidt M, McCormack MP, Wulffraat N, Leboulch P, Lim A, Osborne CS, et al. LMO2-associated clonal T cell proliferation in two patients after gene therapy for SCID-X1. *Science* 2003;302(5644):415–9.

31. Shou Y, Ma Z, Lu T, Sorrentino BP. Unique risk factors for insertional mutagenesis in a mouse model of XSCID gene therapy. *Proc Nat Acad Sci USA* 2006;103(31): 11730–5.

32. Guidance for Industry. Gene Therapy Clinical Trials-Observing Subjects for Delayed Adverse Events, November 2006. http://www.fda.gov/cber/gdlns/gtclin.pdf

33. Claude JR. Difficulties in conceiving and applying guidelines for the safety evaluation of biotechnology-produced drugs: some examples. *Toxicol Lett* 1992; 64–64:349–55.

34. Clark J, Leach W, Pippig S, Joshi A, Wu B, House R, Beyer J. Evaluation of a surrogate antibody for preclinical safety tesing of an anti-CD11a monoclonal antibody. *Regul Pharmacol* 2004;40:219–26.

35. Treacy G. Using an analogous monoclonal antibody to evaluate the reproductive and chronic toxicity potential for a humanized anti-TNFalpha monoclonal antibody. *Hum Exp Toxicol* 2000;19:226–8.

36. Cavagnaro JA, Spindler P. Methods for predicting tumorigenicity of immunomodulatory pharmaceuticals. *Hum Exp Toxicol* 2000;19:213–5.

37. Melnick RL, Kohn MC, Portier CJ. Implications for risk assessment of suggested nongenotoxic mechanisms of chemical carcinogenesis. *Environ Health Persp* 1996;104(Suppl 1):123–34.

38. Lima BS, Van der Laan JW. Mechanisms of nongenotoxic carcinogenesis and assessment of the human hazard. *Regul Toxicol Pharmacol* 2000;32:135–43.

39. Van Oosterhout JP, Van der Laan JW, De Waal EJ, Olejniczak K, Hilgenfeld M, Schmidt V, et al. The utility of two rodent species in carcinogenic risk assessment of pharmaceuticals in Europe. *Regul Toxicol Pharmacol* 1997;25:6–17.

40. ICH S1B. International Conference on Harmonization ICH S1B. Testing for Carcinogenicity of Pharmaceuticals, 1997. http://www.fda.gov/cder/guidance/index.htm

41. Cohen SM, Robinson D, MacDonald J. Alternative models for carcinogenicity testing. *Toxicol Sci* 2001;64:14–19.

42. Rosenblum IY, Dayan AD. Carcinogenicity testing of IL-10: principles and practicalities. *Hum Exp Toxicol* 2002;21:347–58.

43. Contrera JF, DeGeorge JJ. In vivo transgenic biossays and assessment of the carcinogenic potential of pharmaceuticals. *Environ Health Persp* 1998;106:71–80.

44. Tenant RW, Spalding J, French JE. Evaluation of transgenic mouse bioassays for identifying carcinogens and noncarcinogens. *Mutat Res* 1999;265:119–27.

45. Gulzeian D, Jacobson-Kram D, McCullough CB, Olson H, Recio L, Robinson D, Storer R, Tennant R, Ward JM, Neumann DA. Use of transgenic animals for carcinogenicity testing: considerations and implications for risk assessment. *Toxicol Pathol* 2000;28:482–99.

46. Popp JA. Criteria for evaluation of studies in transgenic models. *Toxicol Pathol* 2001;29:20–3.

47. Ashby J. Expectations for transgenic rodent cancer bioassay models. *Toxicol Pathol* 2001;29:177–82.

48. MacDonald J, French JE, Gerson RJ, Goodman J, Inoue T, Jacobs A, Kasper P, Keller D, Lavin A, Long G, et al. The utility of genetically modified mouse assays for identifying human carcinogens: a basic understanding and path forward. *Toxicol Sci* 2004;77:188–94.

49. Flammang TJ, Von Tungeln LS, Kadlubar FF, Fu PP. Neonatal mouse assay for tumorigenicity: alternative to the chronic rodent bioassay. *Regul Toxicol Pharmcol* 1997;26:230–40.

50. Omen GS. Assessment of human cancer risk: challenges for alternative approaches. *Toxicol Pathol* 2001;29:5–12.

51. Goodman JI. A perspective on current and future uses of alternative models for carcinogenicity testing. *Toxicol Pathol* 2001;29:173–6.

52. Mauthe RJ, Gibson DP, Bunch RT, Custer L. The Syrian hamster embryo (SHE) cell transformation assay: review of the methods and results. *Toxicol Pathol* 2001; 29(Suppl):138–46.

53. Brown DC, Gatter KC. Ki67 protein: the immaculate deception? *Histopathology* 2002;40:2–11.

54. Wierda D. Can host resistance assays be used to evaluate the immunotoxicity of pharmaceuticals? *Hum Exp Toxicol* 2000;19:244–5.

55. Luster MI, et al. Risk assessment in immunotoxicology. II. Relationships between immune and host resistance tests. *Fund App Toxicol* 1993;21:71–82.

56. Bugelski PJ, Herzyk DJ, Rehm S, Harmsen AG, Gore EV, Williams DM, Maleeff BE, Badger AM, Truneh A, O'Brien SR, Macia RA, Wier PJ, Morgan DG, Hart TK. Preclinical development of Keliximab, a primatized anti-CD4 monoclonal antibody, in human transgenic CD4 mice: characterization of the model and safety studies. *Hum Exp Toxicol* 2000;19:230–43.

57. FDA Pharmacology/Toxicology review (anakinra) Kineret. http://www.fda.gov/cder/foi/nda/2001/103950-0_Kineret_Pharmr.PDF12

58. Sinclair AM, Todd MD, Forsythe MD, Knox SJ, Elliott S, Begley CG. Expression and function of erythropoietin receptors in tumors: implications for the use of erythropoiesis-stimulating agents in cancer patients. *Cancer* 2007;110:477–88.

59. EPAR Kineret. http://www.emea.europa.eu/humandocs/Humans/EPAR/kineret/kineret.htm12

60. Watanabe S, Tsunematsu Y, Komiyama A, Fujimoto J. Leukemia in patients treated with growth hormone (Letter). *Lancet* 1988;1:1159–60.

61. Allen DB. Safety of human growth hormone therapy: current topics. *J Pedia* 1996; 128:S8–13.

62. Nishi Y, Tanaka T, Takano K, Fujieda K, Igarashi Y, Hanew K, Hirano T, Yokoya S, Tachibana K, Saito T, Watanabe S. Recent Status in the Occurrence of Leukemia in Growth Hormone-Treated Patients in Japan. *J Clin Endocrinol Metab* 1999; 84:1961–5.

63. Farris GM, Miller GK, Wollenberg GK, Molon-Noblot S, Chan C, Prahalada S. Recombinant rat and mouse growth hormones: risk assessment of carcinogenic potential in 2-year bioassays in rats and mice. *Toxicol Sci* 2007;97:548–61.

64. Points to Consider on the Non-clinical Assessment of the Carcinogenic Potential of Insulin Analogues (CPMP/SWP/372/01), November 2001.

65. Jenkins PJ, Besser GM, Farclough PD. Colorectal neoplasia in acromegaly. *Gut* 1999;44:585–7.

66. Guidance for Industry. Development of Parathyroid Hormone for the Prevention and Treatment of Osteoporosis, May 2000.

67. Hodsman AB, Bauer DC, Dempster DW, Dian L, Hanley DA, Harris ST, Kendler DL, McClung MR, Miller PD, Olszynski WP, Orwoll E, Yuen CK. Parathyroid hormone and teriparatide for the treatment of osteoporosis: a review of the evidence and suggested guidelines for its use. *Endocrine Rev* 2005;26:688–703.

68. EPAR Regranex. http://www.emea.europa.eu/humandocs/PDFs/EPAR/Regranex/028799en6.pdf

■■■■ **CHAPTER 20**

Immunogenicity of Therapeutic Proteins and the Assessment of Risk

HUUB SCHELLEKENS, MD, PhD, and WIM JISKOOT, PhD

Contents

Preclinical Safety Evaluation of Biopharmaceuticals: A Science-Based Approach to Facilitating Clinical Trials, edited by Joy A. Cavagnaro
Copyright © 2008 by John Wiley & Sons, Inc.

20.1 INTRODUCTION

Nearly all therapeutic proteins induce an immune response, although the incidence differs [1,2]. Some proteins induce an immune response only very rarely, and others in the majority of patients. The antibodies may have a variety of consequences. Low level of binding antibodies have, in general, no effects, although they may sometimes decrease the half-life and biological activity. High levels of neutralizing antibodies may interfere with the efficacy of the therapeutic proteins. The antibodies may also neutralize endogenous proteins, which may have serious biological consequences. Antibodies may also modulate the side effects of the therapeutic proteins. With some products like interferon alpha-2 the reduction of side effects may be the first sign of an immunogenic response. With monoclonal antibodies the induction of antibodies may increase the symptoms of the side effects.

The immunogenic response in itself may also lead to complications such as skin reactions, anaphylaxis-like reaction, transfusion reactions, and serum sickness. These complications may also be the results of an immunogenic response to impurities and contaminants. Both the EMEA and the FDA expect the evaluation of possible biological and clinical consequences and the assay strategy of immunogenicity to be based on a risk based approach. The elements for a risk analysis and management are discussed in this chapter, and the factors influencing the probability of an antibody response and the consequences will be categorized.

20.2 DEFINITION OF RISK

The definition of risk is the probability times the consequences (Figure 20.1). So the probability of an immune response is not synonymous with its risk. A high risk can be associated with a relative high probability, but also with a low probability if the consequences are severe. For example, the probability of an immune response to epoetin is rather low, but one of the consequences, antibody-induced severe anemia, is severe [3]. This makes the risk of immunogenicity of epoetins relatively high.

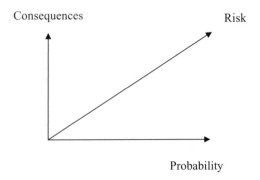

Figure 20.1 Risk as a combination of probability and consequences.

TABLE 20.1   Important considerations when assessing the possible consequences of immunogenicity

1. Absence of alternative treatments
2. Similarity with important endogenous factors
3. To be administered in high doses
4. Presence of allergenic structures

20.3 GRADING THE POSSIBLE CONSEQUENCES OF IMMUNOGENICITY

Table 20.1 lists important considerations when assessing the consequences of immunogenicity. A severe consequence of immunogenicity is the loss of efficacy of the product, if there is no alternative treatment and the product has a clinically important effect. Antibodies to factor VIII that inhibit its activity in hemophilia patients, for which there are no alternatives, are clearly severe, whereas inhibiting antibodies to Botox® used for cosmetic reasons will be considered low risk even without alternative treatment options. Loss of efficacy by the immune response may occur with any product independent whether the product is human (or derived from a human gene), nonhuman, or an artificial protein. Another severe consequence is the cross-neutralization of a biologically important endogenous factor by antibodies induced by the therapeutic protein. This can only occur if the protein drug is (partly) similar with the endogenous factor. An example is the megakaryocytic growth and differentiation factor (MGDF) that was under development for the treatment of thrombocytopenia. This truncated pegylated molecule induced antibodies in volunteers and cancer patients that cross-reacted with endogenous thrombopoetin, resulting in severe thrombocytopenia needing platelet transfusions [4].

Side effects such as anaphylaxis-like reactions and serum sickness are mainly caused by the formation of immune complexes seen with monoclonal antibodies administered in high doses. (See Chapter 21.)

20.4 PREDICTING THE PROBABILITY OF AN IMMUNE RESPONSE

There are two mechanisms by which therapeutic proteins induce antibodies: the classical activation of the immune system by foreign proteins and the breaking of B cell tolerance by human proteins. The two mechanisms differ in time of onset and response level as we have described extensively previously [2]. Also the immunological mechanisms behind the two types of immune activation differ fundamentally and therefore also the characteristics of the product that are involved in induction of antibodies.

20.4.1 Breaking B Cell Tolerance

By definition, we are immune tolerant to products that are copies of endogenous proteins such as interferons, colony stimulating factors, and epoetins. The products not necessarily need to be exact copies of the natural proteins to share this immune tolerance. When human therapeutic proteins induce antibodies, they are breaking B cell tolerance, which starts with the activation of autoreactive B cells. The probability of breaking B cell tolerance depends on several factors (Table 20.2). Presenting the self-epitopes in an array form is a very potent way to activate B cells [6,7]. This explains why aggregates of human proteins are the most important factor in induction of antibodies [8,9,10]. These aggregates may not be immediately present in the product but may appear during storage, making stability and formulation an important issue in predicting the immunogenicity. Some factors influence the formation of aggregates, such as the presence of oxidized therapeutic protein and the reduced solubility by the lack of glycosylation by expression of a glycoprotein in a prokaryotic host [11].

There are only a few studies in experimental model systems on the properties of the aggregates that break B cell tolerance, indicating that only multiple order aggregates (>trimers) are involved [8]. There are different methods to identify the presence of aggregates such as size exclusion chromatography and SDS-PAGE and Western blotting. However, these methods may miss immunogenic aggregates. Other methods such as analytical ultracentrifugation, field-flow fractionation, and light-scattering techniques have shown to be able to detect aggregates that go undetected by standard assays.

The only biological test to study the capacity of a protein product to break B cell tolerance are mice made transgenic for the specific protein [12,13]. These mice are immune tolerant, and there is a good correlation of an immune response in these mice and in patients. Although these models have helped to identify the factors important for breaking B cell tolerance and also have been useful in improving the formulation of products, there is not yet enough experience to use them as absolute predictors of immunogenicity of human proteins.

20.4.2 Classical Activation of the Immune System by Foreign Proteins

The classical activation of the immune system is driven by the presence of non–self-epitopes. If the therapeutic protein is of nonhuman origin like microbially derived streptokinase and asparaginase or bovine adenosine deamidase,

TABLE 20.2 **Most important factors increasing the probability of an immune response to human proteins**

1. Aggregates
2. Chronic treatment
3. Subcutaneous administration
4. Impurities
5. Breaking tolerance in immune tolerant mice

a strong immune response is highly likely, especially after subcutaneous administration (Table 20.3). If the product is a modified human protein, prediction becomes more difficult. The level of divergence of the human amino acid sequence is not very informative because the consequence of the sequence deviation is highly dependent on the type of amino acid change and the location of the change in the molecule. In some cases a single amino acid change has been reported to induce a complete new epitope [14]. In others, extensive amino acid exchanges have no effect on immunogenicity.

Also in the prediction of the introduction of new epitopes by protein modification immune-tolerant transgenic mice can be used. Mice transgenic for human insulin and tissue plasminogen activator have been used to identify new epitopes in products with amino acid modifications [14,15].

Antisera have also been used to monitor reduction in immunogenicity of a protein. A reduced binding with the modified protein by serum raised by the original product was considered to show reduced immunogenicity [16]. However, binding of antibodies is an antigenicity, which is a physical process. An antigenicity is different from an immunogenicity, the capacity to induce an immune response. Although in some cases these properties are related, in many cases proteins with a high antigenicity for neutralizing antibodies, proved to be non-immunogenic.

Also a number of in vitro stimulation and binding tests and computational models are promoted as predictors of immunogenicity [17]. However, all these tests have their limitations. T cell proliferation assays have the drawback that many products are capable of either inducing some level of T cell activation or inhibit cell proliferation, leading to false positive and negative effects. The computational algorithms that are claimed to predict T cell epitopes only give limited information on the interaction of the proteins with the immune system and underdetect epitopes. Although these assays and algorithms may help predict to some extent which parts of the proteins will be involved in immunogenicity, their limitations are also evident when they are used to reduce immunogenicity. There is hardly any convincing evidence of a clinically relevant reduction of antibody induction.

Glycoproteins produced in nonhuman cells such as plant cells and yeast cells may have a modified glycan structure. Although natural antibodies exist that react with nonhuman glycan structures [18], there is no example of an immune reaction that was mounted to modified glycan structure of a therapeutic protein.

TABLE 20.3 Most important factors increasing the probability of an immune response to foreign proteins

1. Level of non-self
2. Subcutaneous administration

20.4.3 Mixed Type Immune Reactions

In some cases therapeutic proteins induce antibodies both by breaking B cell tolerance and the vaccine-like activation of the immune system, depending on the level of immune tolerance of the patients. An example is the immune response induced by factor VIII in hemophilia patients [19]. The antibody response is related to the type of defect in the factor VIII gene in these patients. If the genetic defect leads to an inability to produce factor VIII, the patients lack immune tolerance, and they respond as to a foreign protein. In patients producing a nonfunctional but immunologically normal factor VIII, antibodies are produced by breaking B cell tolerance. It is likely, although not studied, that chimeric proteins consisting of both a human and nonhuman part such as chimeric and humanized monoclonal antibodies also will produce a mixed type of response.

20.5 OTHER FACTORS INFLUENCING THE ANTIBODY RESPONSE

20.5.1 Length of Treatment

Foreign proteins like streptokinase and asparaginase induce antibodies often after a single injection. Breaking B cell tolerance by human protein takes in general more than 6 months of chronic treatment. This illustrates the fundamental difference between a vaccine-like response to foreign proteins and breaking of immune tolerance against human proteins.

20.5.2 Route of Administration

The route of administration influences the likelihood of an antibody response independent of the mechanism of induction. The probability of an immune response is the highest with subcutaneous administration, less probable after intramuscular administration and intravenous administration is the least immunogenic route. There are no studies comparing parenteral and nonparenteral routes of administration. However, as both mucosal tissues and the skin are immune competent organs designed to keep invaders out of the body, intranasal, pulmonary, and transdermal administration of therapeutic proteins may increase the risk of an immune response as compared to parenteral routes.

20.5.3 Biological Activities of the Product

The biological activities of the product are influencing the immune response. An immune stimulating therapeutic protein is more likely to induce antibodies than an immune suppressive protein. Monoclonal antibodies targeted to cell bound epitopes are more likely to induce an immune response than monoclonal antibodies with a target in solution [20]. Also the Fc bound activities of monoclonal antibodies have an influence. A monoclonal antibody with a modified Fc part has been reported to be less immunogenic than the unmodified monoclonal antibody [21].

20.5.4   Presence of Impurities

Impurities may influence immunogenicity. The immunogenicity of products as human growth hormone, insulin, and interferon alpha-2 have declined over the years due to improved downstream processing and formulation, reducing the level of impurities. There are studies showing that the induction of antibodies by oxidized protein cross-reacted, with the unmodified product and host cell derived endotoxin acting as an adjuvant [22]. The probability of an immune response therefore increases with the level of impurities. Besides their possible role as adjuvant, impurities may also induce an immune response to themselves. Moreover they may be the cause of skin reactions, allergies and other side effects.

20.5.5   Product Modifications

Product modifications that are intended to enhance half-life potentially also increase the exposition of the protein to the immune system and may increase immunogenicity. In addition the modification may reduce biological activity necessitating more protein for the same biological effect.

Pegylation is claimed to reduce the immunogenicity of therapeutic proteins by shielding [23]. There is evidence that pegylation reduces the immunogenicity of nonhuman proteins like bovine adenosine deamidase and asparginase. Whether pegylation also reduces the capacity of human proteins to break B cell tolerance is less clear. There are reports of high immunogenicity of pegylated human proteins such as PEG-rhuMDGF, but the immunogenicity of unpegylated MDGF products is unknown.

20.5.6   Patient Characteristics

Gender, age, and ethnic background have all been reported to influence the incidence of antibody response to specific therapeutic proteins. However, the only patient characteristic that consistently has been identified for a number of different products is the disease that the patients suffer from. Cancer patients are less likely to produce antibodies to therapeutic protein than other patients. The most widely accepted explanation for this difference is the immune-compromised state of cancer patients, both by the disease as by anticancer treatment. Also the median survival of patients on treatment by therapeutic proteins may be too short to develop an antibody response. In any case, cancer reduces the probability of an antibody response to a protein considerably.

20.5.7   Impact of Concomitant Therapy

As the experience in cancer patients shows, immune suppressive therapy reduces the probability to develop an immune response to proteins. In addition immune suppressive drugs such as methotrexate are often used in conjunction with monoclonal antibodies and other protein drugs that further serves to reduce the immune reactions.

20.6 ASSAY STRATEGIES

A specifically designed assay strategy is an essential part of every risk analysis and management program for a new therapeutic protein. When validating the assays and also when evaluating the data on immunogenicity and their clinical impact, it is important that assays are not standardized and international reference and standard preparations are in general not available [25]. This makes it difficult to compare studies with similar products. That is, the same product studied in comparable patient populations may show a wide variety of antibody incidence. Also the different analyses differ in their criteria for considering a patient antibody positive. In some studies all patients with at least a single positive binding assay result were included in the antibody positive groups. Because it is unlikely that a transient level of binding antibodies has any biological effect, this type of analysis leads to an underestimation of the effects of antibodies.

The more logical approach is to categorize patients depending on the AUC of the neutralizing antibody levels. This type of analysis also allows study of the dose–response relation between antibody levels and clinical effects. In some cases the unpredictable disease progression, the lack of good efficacy markers and the extended effect after treatment has stopped, may complicate the evaluation of the clinical effects of immunogenicity.

Because of the lack of adequately designed studies and standardized assays for many products the consequences of their immunogenicity is unclear. So assuming a product to be non-immunogenic based on literature is impossible. In other words, every new protein should be assumed to be immunogenic unless proved otherwise with a well-designed and validated assay strategy.

Recently a number of papers have appeared written mainly by authors in the US biotechnology industry, and they are the basis of a growing consensus on the principles of immunogenicity testing [26,27,28]. One single assay is not considered sufficient to evaluate the immunogenicity of a new protein drug. Most antibody assay strategies are based on different stages approach: the first stage being a screening assay to identify the antibody positive sera and the second stage being the assay to evaluate whether the antibodies are neutralizing. This may be followed by assays to establish titer, affinity, and isotype of the antibodies.

20.6.1 Types of Assays

The screening assay is, in general, a binding assay, mostly an ELISA-type assay, or a radio-immune-precipitation method. Standard ELISA-type immunoassays are not always considered appropriate, however, for measuring binding antibodies because the circulating therapeutic protein may interfere with the assay. So a bridging assay, which in the ELISA plate is coated with the protein drug and anti-drug antibodies are detected with a labeled version of the drug, has been advocated as the best type of screening assay. A bridging assay detects all types of antibodies independent of type and species of origin. The bridging assay may miss low-affinity antibodies. Therefore, for the early immune response, the use of surface plasmon resonance technology as BIAcore is advocated rather than the ELISA type of assay methodology. However, the sensitivity of ELISAs and RIAs for high-affinity antibodies is generally higher than the BIAcore assays.

Screening assays are designed for optimal sensitivity to avoid false negatives. For new proteins defining an absolute sensitivity is impossible because of lack of positive sera. An alternative approach is to set the cut point for the assay at the 5% false positive level using a panel of normal human sera and/or untreated patient sera representative of the groups to be treated.

20.6.2 Assay Sensitivity

To get an idea of the sensitivity of the assay in quantitative terms, affinity purified animal sera are used. In general, these are obtained by immunization of rabbits by the therapeutic product. The rabbit serum diluted in normal human serum can also serve as a positive control or to provide a standard curve. Because the screening assays are tuned for high sensitivity and a predefined false positive rate, all initial positive sera need to be confirmed. A confirmation can be achieved by another binding assay based on another principle than the original assay. So, if an ELISA type of assay is used, the confirmation can be a radio-immune precipitation assay or a BIAcore assay. An initial positive can also be confirmed by doing a displacement step before doing the original assay. Product is added to the serum and should result in a predefined relative reduction in signal, such as 25% or 50%, or an absolute reduction based on a low positive control. Only the confirmed positives are labeled as positives and are then further analyzed. Confirmed positive sera should be tested for neutralizing antibodies that may interfere with the biological and clinical activity. Assays for neutralizing activity are based on the inhibition of the biological effect of the protein in vitro. Because every product has its own specific biological effect, assays for neutralizing activity need to be designed individually.

20.6.3 Measuring Neutralizing Antibodies

The assay for neutralizing antibodies is, in general, a modification of the potency assay of the therapeutic protein product. The potency assay is in most cases an in vitro cell based assay. A predefined amount of product is added to the serum and the reduction of activity is evaluated in the bioassay. Sometimes the assay is performed in two steps. An assay with the lowest dilution of serum and a minimal amount of protein is used to screen for neutralizing activity and, if any neutralization is identified, a full titration of the sera is performed.

An important issue in the neutralization assay is the amount of therapeutic protein product to add. This dose should be based on the dose–response curve of the protein in the assay. The reduction should be in the linear part of the curve and be significant enough to be reliably testable in the assay. The titer of the neutralization is often expressed in units. The highest dilution of the serum with a significant inhibition is defined to contain one neutralizing unit. Sometimes the activity is expressed in arbitrary units using an animal antiserum as reference. Further characterization of the antibodies may include evaluation of Ig isotype and affinity. Although alternative methods may be employed, the BIAcore assay has become the standard for these types of analyses.

20.6.4   Timing of Blood Sampling

Another important aspect when studying the immunogenicity of therapeutic proteins concerns the timing of the blood sampling. With products such as monoclonal antibodies that have a relative long half-life, the circulating product may interfere with the detection of induced antibodies. Sampling sera up to weeks after the last injection is then necessary to avoid the interference of circulating protein drug.

20.6.5   Evaluation of Impurities

In general, the evaluation of the immunogenicity of impurities is restricted to binding antibodies. Only in the case where the biological activity of the impurity is known and its inactivation is biologically relevant, a neutralization assay may be necessary.

The most important source of impurities is the host cells. And in nearly all biological products traces of host cells can be identified. Not all of them will raise antibodies. Based on the literature about the immunogenicity of a protein, it is general safe to assume that if the level of contaminant is below 0.5 μg per dose, the induction of antibodies is unlikely. For a proper binding antibody assay, the material resulting from a complete extraction and purification process of a mock production run of the host cells without the inserted gene (0 cells) should be used. This procedure should results in material containing the impurities as present in the product. The impurities that are co-purified with the therapeutic protein will also be present in the whole cell extract, but the presence of other substances can introduce interference in the binding assay. The 0-cell product can also be used in the confirmatory displacement assay and to immunize rabbits to obtain a positive control serum. The same material can also be used in an immunoblot or BIAcore assay, which can serve as confirmatory assays.

20.7 STUDYING THE CONSEQUENCES OF IMMUNOGENICITY

To evaluate the biological consequences of antibodies, patients with positive responses should be monitored for their impact on the pharmacokinetic and pharmacodynamic effect of the therapeutic protein. Also the effect on adverse events and possible neutralization of the endogenous protein, in cases where human proteins are administered at pharmacological doses, should be monitored. When the consequences of the immunogenicity are known, the risk can be established.

REFERENCES

1. Schellekens H. Immunogenicity of therapeutic proteins: clinical implications and future prospects. *Clin Ther* 2002;24(11):1720–40.
2. Schellekens H. Bioequivalence and the immunogenicity of biopharmaceuticals. *Nat Rev Drug Discov* 2002;1(6):457–62.
3. Casadevall N, Nataf J, Viron B, Kolta A, Kiladjian JJ, Martin-Dupont P, Michaud P, Papo T, Ugo V, Teyssandier I, Varet B, Mayeux P. Pure red cell aplasia and antierythropoietin antibodies in patients treated with recombinant erythropoietin. *New Engl J Med* 2002;346:469–75.
4. Vadhan-Raj S. Clinical experience with recombinant human thrombopoietin in chemotherapy-induced thrombocytopenia. *Semin Hematol* 2000;37(2 Suppl 4): 28–34.
5. Klastersky J. Adverse effects of the humanized antibodies used as cancer therapeutics. *Curr Opin Oncol* 2006;18(4):316–20.
6. Bachmann MF, Rohrer UH, Kundig TM, Burki K, Hengartner H, Zinkernagel RM. The influence of antigen organization on B cell responsiveness. *Science* 1993; 262:1448–51.
7. Chakerian B, Lenz P, Lowy DR, Schiller JT. Determinants of autoantibody induction by conjugated papillomavirus virus-like particles. *J Immunol* 2002;169: 6120–6.
8. Hermeling S, Schellekens H, Maas C, Gebbink MF, Crommelin DJ, Jiskoot W. Antibody response to aggregated human interferon alpha2b in wild-type and transgenic immune tolerant mice depends on type and level of aggregation. *J Pharm Sci* 2006;95(5):1084–96.
9. Moore WV, Leppert P. Role of aggregated human growth hormone (hGH) in development of antibodies to hGH. *J Clin Endocrinol Metab* 1980;51:691–7.
10. Braun KL, Labow MA, Alsenz J. Protein aggregates seem to play a key role among the parameters influencing the antigenicity of interferon alpha (IFN-alpha) in normal and transgenic mice. *Pharm Res* 1997;14:1472–8.
11. Runkel L, Meier W, Pepinsky RB, Karpusas M, Whitty A, Kimball K, Brickelmaier M, Muldowney C, Jones W, Goelz SE. Structural and functional differences between glycosylated and non-glycosylated forms of human interferon-beta (IFN-beta). *Pharm Res* 1998;15:641–9.

12. Hermeling S, Jiskoot W, Crommelin D, Bornaes C, Schellekens H. Development of a transgenic mouse model immune tolerant for human interferon Beta. *Pharm Res* 2005;22(6):847–51. Epub 2005 Jun 8.

13. Hermeling S, Crommelin DJ, Schellekens H, Jiskoot W. Structure-immunogenicity relationships of therapeutic proteins. *Pharm Res* 2004;21(6):897–903.

14. Ottesen NP, Jami J, Weilguny D, Duhrkop M, Bucchini D, Havelund S, Fogh JM. The potential immunogenicity of human insulin and insulin analogues evaluated in a transgenic mouse model. *Diabetologia* 1994;37:1178–85.

15. Stewart HPG, Hollingshead PG, Pitts SL, Chang R, Martin LE, Oakley H. Transgenic mice as a model to test the immunogenicity of proteins altered by site-specific mutagenesis. *Mol Biol Med* 1989;6:275–81.

16. Elliott S, Chang D, Delorme E, Dunn C, Egrie J, Giffin J, Lorenzini T, Talbot C, Hesterberg L. Isolation and characterization of conformation sensitive antierythropoietin monoclonal antibodies: effect of disulfide bonds and carbohydrate on recombinant human erythropoietin structure. *Blood* 1996;87:2714–22.

17. Flower DR, Doytchinova IA. Immunoinformatics and the prediction of immunogenicity. *Appl Bioinformatics* 2002;1(4):167–76.

18. Buzas EI, Gyorgy B, Pasztoi M, Jelinek I, Falus A, Gabius HJ. Carbohydrate recognition systems in autoimmunity. *Autoimmunity* 2006;39(8):691–704.

19. Lee CA, Lillicrap D, Astermark J. Inhibitor development in hemophiliacs: the roles of genetic versus environmental factors. *Semin Thromb Hemost* 2006;32(Suppl 2):10–4.

20. Pendley C, Schantz A, Wagner C. Immunogenicity of therapeutic monoclonal antibodies. *Curr Op in Mol Ther* 2003;5:172–9.

21. Presta LG. Engineering of therapeutic antibodies to minimize immunogenicity and optimize function. *Adv Drug Deliv Rev* 2006;58(5–6):640–56. Epub 2006 May 23.

22. Milner RDG, Flodh H. In *Immunological Aspects of Human Growth Hormone: Proceedings of a Workshop*, London, 12 November 1985. Medical Education Services, Oxford (1986).

23. Veronese FM, Pasut G. PEGylation, successful approach to drug delivery. *Drug Discov Today* 2005;10(21):1451–8.

24. Rutgeerts P, Van Assche G, Vermeire S. Optimizing anti-TNF treatment in inflammatory bowel disease. *Gastroenterology* 2004;126(6):1593–610.

25. Schellekens H, Ryff JC, van der Meide PH. Assays for antibodies to human interferon-alpha: the need for standardization. *J Interferon Cytokine Res* 1997; 17(Suppl 1):S5–8.

26. Neyer L, Hiller J, Gish K, Keller S, Caras I. Confirming human antibody responses to a therapeutic monoclonal antibody usinga statistical approach. *J Immunol Meth* 2006;315(1–2):80–7. Epub 2006 Aug 7.

27. Geng D, Shankar G, Schantz A, Rajadhyaksha M, Davis H, Wagner C. Validation of immunoassays used to assess immunogenicity to therapeutic monoclonal antibodies. *J Pharm Biomed Anal* 2005;39(3–4):364–75.

28. Mire-Sluis AR, Barrett YC, Devanarayan V, et al. Recommendations for the design and optimization of immunoassays used in the detection of host antibodies against biotechnology products. *J Immunol Meth* 2004;289:1–16.

■■■■ CHAPTER 21

Assessment of Autoimmunity and Hypersensitivity

JACQUES DESCOTES, MD, PharmD, PhD, and THIERRY VIAL, MD

Contents

21.1 INTRODUCTION

The immune system is an extremely complex network of closely interacting regulatory and effector cells and molecules, whose primary function is the discrimination of self from non-self in order to maintain homeostasis in living organisms. The renewal, differentiation, and activation of immunocompetent cells ensure an adequate level of immune responsiveness under the control of many mechanisms with either redundant or conflicting outcome. It is important to bear in mind, however, that not all immune responses are beneficial to the host. Some may result in autoimmunity when directed against self-constituents of the body, or in hypersensitivity when directed against "innocent" foreign antigens (allergens) [11]. Biopharmaceuticals, either via

Preclinical Safety Evaluation of Biopharmaceuticals: A Science-Based Approach to Facilitating Clinical Trials, edited by Joy A. Cavagnaro
Copyright © 2008 by John Wiley & Sons, Inc.

their (immuno)-pharmacological mechanism of action, or their chemical structure (foreign proteins), most often have the potential for inducing autoimmunity and/or hypersensitivity reactions in treated human subjects. Therefore autoimmunity and hypersensitivity are critical issues to be considered during the preclinical as well as the clinical safety evaluation of most, if not all biopharmaceuticals.

21.2 OVERVIEW OF THE CLINICAL EXPERIENCE

There is a growing body of clinical evidence demonstrating that autoimmunity and hypersensitivity are relatively common and potentially severe adverse effects of biopharmaceuticals [26,37,41].

21.2.1 Autoimmunity

Autoimmunity is still largely a mystery. It consists of specific immune responses involving antibodies and T cells directed against self-antigens. Importantly, physiological autoimmune responses are relatively common as most healthy individuals normally produce autoantibodies. Autoimmune diseases occur when autoreactive T cells and/or autoantibodies cause tissue damage resulting in overt pathological conditions [8]. They are relatively common diseases as 5% to 8% of the US population have been estimated to be affected. Autoimmune diseases can target any organ system, and occur at nearly any age. Approximately 80 diseases have been described. They are usually classified into organ-specific and systemic diseases, depending on the affected organ(s), even though this classification does not necessarily reflect a common pathophysiology. A number of predisposing factors are strongly thought to be involved, especially genetic predisposition and environmental exposures, including drug therapy.

Autoimmune diseases have been reported to be more frequent in human subjects treated with several recombinant cytokines [38]. For instance, increased titers or the new occurrence of autoantibodies have been observed in hepatitis C patients treated with the recombinant interferons-alpha (IFNα). Quite a few clinical case reports describe the development of organ-specific as well as systemic autoimmune diseases including systemic lupus erythematosus, insulin-dependent type I diabetes mellitus, autoimmune thrombocytopenia, autoimmune hemolytic anemia, myasthenia gravis, and autoimmune thyroiditis in patients under IFNα therapy. Although the mechanism involved is not fully elucidated, the available data support the pathogenic potential of IFNα in autoimmunity [31]. In contrast, autoimmune effects associated with IFNβ therapy are thought to be of lesser concern based on the current clinical evidence [38]. Thyroid autoimmunity in contrast to other autoimmune diseases is frequent in patients treated with recombinant interleukin-2 (rIL-2). Thus, among 281 previously euthyroid cancer patients treated with rIL-2, up to 41%

developed thyroid dysfunction [16]. However, rIL-2 therapy rather rarely exacerbates other latent autoimmune diseases, including diabetes mellitus, myasthenia gravis, and rheumatoid arthritis [38]. Autoimmunity has also been reported to be an adverse event of antitumor necrosis factor-alpha (TNFα) therapy involving either the monoclonal antibody infliximab or the fusion protein etanercept [2]. Although autoimmune diseases, such as rheumatoid arthritis or Crohn's disease are their primary therapeutic targets, autoimmune complications, such as systemic lupus erythematosus have been described [9], and this emphasizes the complex interplay of the cytokine and immune cell networks in the development of autoimmunity [21].

21.2.2   Hypersensitivity

Because the word allergy has so often been used misleadingly, hypersensitivity is the recommended term to refer to those adverse drug events mediated by inadvertent immune responses that develop in a small number of human subjects [14]. Typically hypersensitivity reactions involve either specific antibodies or T lymphocytes directed against a given drug antigen. They can affect nearly every organ or tissue of the body, but one organ or tissue is often a predominant target. They are the consequence of the exquisite capacity of the immune system to recognize structural elements (epitopes) of non-self molecules, and mount specific responses involving the immunological memory [11].

Since the vast majority of biopharmaceuticals are large foreign molecules, they have the potential to act as direct immunogens; that is to say, they can directly both sensitize the treated host and then trigger an adverse clinical reaction upon a subsequent rechallenge. Virtually all therapeutic proteins, including human therapeutic proteins, humanized or human monoclonal antibodies, are immunogenic to some extent [15]. The most common finding in relation to the immunogenicity of biopharmaceuticals is the development of specific antibodies whose clinical consequences range from no apparent adverse effects to potentially life-threatening complications. Indeed specific antibodies can be neutralizing and result in altered pharmacokinetics or reduced clinical response, or they can evoke hypersensitivity reactions such as immune complex-associated diseases and acute hypersensitivity reactions [12]. The incidence and characteristics of these antibodies are dependent on several criteria, which include the product, the dose and duration of treatment, the frequency of dosing, the route of administration, the immune status, and/or genetic profile of the patient, the disease type, and the functional activities of the protein. For instance, the rate of anti-IFNα antibody formation ranges from zero to more than 50% of patients across clinical studies. Although no obvious clinical consequence are associated with anti-IFNα antibodies in most patients, changes in pharmacokinetics due to neutralizing antibodies are sometimes noted, but reduced clinical response has rarely been documented. Anti-IFNα antibodies have so far not been associated with immune complex-associated diseases nor hypersensitivity reactions, and no IgE-mediated reactions to

IFNα have ever been reported to the best of our knowledge [38]. Similarly anti-IFNβ antibodies have commonly been detected in the sera of treated patients. Neutralizing antibodies seem to be more frequent with IFNβ than IFNα. The former may be associated with a higher relapse rate or shortened time to first relapse in patients with multiple sclerosis [33], and worsening of the disease has been suggested to be correlated with persistent high titers of neutralizing antibodies [19]. Nevertheless, extremely rare hypersensitivity reactions to IFNβ have so far been reported. The clinical experience gained with recombinant IL-2 confirms that only a relatively small fraction of specific antibodies are neutralizing and that ensuing hypersensitivity reactions are exceptional [38].

Predicting the consequences of specific antibodies to therapeutic proteins is in fact extremely difficult, as exemplified by the recombinant hemophilia factors VIII and IX. While specific antibodies to factor VIII have been detected in the sera of up to 30% to 50% of treated patients, resulting in transient inhibition and hemorrhage risk, neutralizing antibodies to factor IX have been detected in only 1% to 3%; these antibodies were associated with severe ana-phylactic reactions in approximately 50% of the affected patients [18]. Specific antibodies against therapeutic monoclonal antibodies are also commonly reported. For instance, antibodies to the anti-TNFα agent infliximab, a chime-ric monoclonal IgG_1 antibody, have been detected in the sera of 10% to 60% of patients and are not uncommonly associated with reduced efficacy. Impor-tantly, anti-infliximab antibodies have been associated with an increased inci-dence of infusion reactions [4]. Although the majority of infusion reactions are not IgE-mediated, true anaphylactic reactions have been described [6].

To date, the most severe immune-mediated adverse event associated with specific antibodies to a therapeutic protein is erythropoietin-associated pure red cell aplasia [17]. Hundreds of cases have been described with a majority involving patients with chronic kidney disease receiving subcutaneous injec-tions of erythropoietin-α. There is a major concern that therapeutic proteins used as replacement therapy in case of deficiencies affecting a natural protein of the body can trigger a specific immune response, the most likely manifesta-tion of which is the production of neutralizing antibodies as described above. By inhibiting the biologic effects of both the recombinant and natural protein, neutralizing antibodies can result in severe complications as exemplified by pure red cell aplasia in patients where neutralizing antibodies eradicated any residual release of erythropoietin, the hormone required for erythrocyte pro-duction. Because erythropoietin-specific antibodies are involved, but the immune response was initially mounted against the potentially "slightly dif-ferent," recombinant erythropoietin, used as a therapeutic agent compared to endogenous erythropoietin, pure red cell aplasia can be defined as a hyper-sensitivity reaction as well as an autoimmune reaction.

Finally, it should be emphasized that drug-induced hypersensitivity reactions can be either immune mediated (e.g., anaphylaxis) or non–immune mediated [43]. Infusion reactions associated with a number of therapeutic monoclonal antibodies are a typical example of non–immune-mediated hypersensitivity reactions. Indeed the majority of reported infusion reactions are not associated with the detection of specific IgE. A nonspecific activation of the complement cascade is an attractive hypothesis as demonstrated with rituximab, a chimeric anti-CD20 monoclonal antibody [34].

21.3 REGULATORY GUIDANCE

Not much progress has been made in the area of predictive methods for autoimmunity and hypersensitivity induced by biopharmaceuticals since Gerhardt Zbinden's review published in 1990 [44]. Not surprisingly, regulatory guidance is very scarce at the present time. There are no comprehensive guidelines on the approaches recommended or required for predicting hypersensitivity during product development, and absolutely none on the prediction of autoimmunity. This presumably reflects the current lack of adequately standardized and validated animal models and assays that can be used during preclinical safety evaluation to predict either risk potential [3,10].

Although the ICH S6 guideline on the preclinical safety evaluation of biotechnology-derived pharmaceuticals clearly identified immunogenicity as a critical safety issue for biopharmaceuticals, and states that "the expression of surface antigens on target cells may be altered, which has implications for autoimmune potential," the document states "testing strategies may require screening studies followed by mechanistic studies to clarifly this issues." No specific recommendation was provided regarding practical modalities that could be helpful to predict either autoimmunity or hypersensitivity reactions associated with biopharmaceuticals basedon the lack of adequately standardized and validated animal models and assays, as mentioned above. This may also be the reason that ICH S8 Guideline on Immuntoxicology Studies for Human Pharmaceuticals (2006) specifically excludes guidance on drug-induced hypersensitivity and autoimmunity.

21.4 PRECLINICAL EVALUATION OF THE POTENTIAL OF BIOPHARMACEUTICALS FOR AUTOIMMUNITY

Our currently poor understanding of the mechanisms leading to autoimmunity and autoimmune diseases following drug therapy is a major hurdle. To date, no animal model or assay can reliably predict the potential, of biopharmaceuticals or pharmaceuticals, for inducing autoimmunity reactions in human subjects.

The search for autoantibodies in the sera of treated animals during standard toxicity testing cannot be recommended as it has proved to be usually negative or inconclusive [36]. Autoantibodies have sometimes been detected in the sera of animals treated with various compounds (either pharmaceuticals or chemicals) suspected to induce autoimmunity in animals and/or human subjects. However, the design of such studies was overtly inconsistent, and results were obtained in animal strains that are not conventionally used in "regulatory toxicity" studies, such as Brown Norway (BN) rats or C57BL/6, BALB/c, and AKR mice.

The popliteal lymph node assay (PLNA) has long been proposed as a tool to investigate and predict drug and chemically induced autoimmunity [29]. In the direct PLNA, mice or rats are injected with the test article subcutaneously into one footpad and with the vehicle into the contralateral footpad. Popliteal lymph nodes are typically removed on day +7, then weighted and a weight index is calculated. The assay is considered to be positive when the weight index is ≥ 2. The increase in weight of the treated popliteal lymph node has been assumed to reflect a pseudo-graft versus host reaction mimicking a systemic autoimmune response. Although over 100 compounds have been tested, there is no firm evidence at the present time that the direct PLNA is a reliable predictor of drug-induced autoimmunity. Importantly, no biopharmaceutical has seemingly ever been tested in this assay. The early direct PLNA procedure was subsequently refined, but the databases using any of these refinements are always quite small. The latest procedure—the modified PLNA—has been proposed as a predictive tool for drug-induced immunostimulation or sensitization [23]. Although many similarities can be found in the pathophysiological mechanisms of sensitization and autoimmunity, it is unclear to what extent, if any the modified PLNA can be useful to predict drug-induced autoimmunity.

In the clinic, autoimmunity associated with biopharmaceuticals is usually reflected by more frequent autoimmune diseases as mentioned previously. Although the mechanism(s) involved is not elucidated, an immunopharmacological effect that would reveal an underlying predisposition toward autoimmunity or a latent autoimmune disease is an attractive hypothesis. A number of rodent strains including (NZB/NZW) F_1, non-obese diabetic (NOD), and MRL-*lpr/lpr* mice, BN and bio-breeding (BB) rats have long been shown to develop more frequent autoimmune diseases spontaneously [30]. There is some evidence that immunomodulatory biopharmaceuticals may accelerate or exacerbate the natural course of the spontaneous disease. Thus IFNα [20] and the interferon inducer tilorone [39] were shown to accelerate lupus-associated mortality in (NZB/NZW) F_1 mice, whereas IFNβ was found to accelerate autoimmune type I diabetes in NOD mice [1]. However, major discrepancies were also noted between responses in these animal models and the clinical data. Although autoimmune type I diabetes has been reported to be an adverse effect of IFNα in human subjects [38], IFNα was found to inhibit the development of diabetes in autoimmune-prone NOD mice [32]. Similarly rIL-2, which is associated with more frequent autoimmune diseases in treated patients [38], did not exacerbate the lupus disease in (NZB/NZW) F_1 mice [28]. Our limited understanding of the pathophysiology of the spontaneous animal disease as well as uncertainties regarding the immunopharmacological mechanism of the tested compound that may be dissimilar in animals compared to humans account for these discrepancies. In any case, this does not lend much support to the routine use of these models for predicting the potential of biopharmaceuticals to increase the incidence of autoimmune diseases in human subjects.

21.5 PRECLINICAL EVALUATION OF THE POTENTIAL OF BIOPHARMACEUTICALS FOR HYPERSENSITIVITY REACTIONS

Preclinical immunogenicity testing is most often limited to monitoring antibody formation in rodents and nonhuman primates, even though immune responses to therapeutic proteins in conventional animal models poorly predict immunogenicity in humans [5,42]. Indeed immunogenicity is detected in animal studies even if the protein is minimally immunogenic in humans. For instance, specific antibodies have been detected in less than 5% of patients treated with the anti-TNFα fusion protein etanercept, whereas antibodies are present in 80% to 100% of animals in preclinical toxicity studies [7]. Similarities between animal and human antibody responses, however, have also been reported. For instance, the immunogenicity of three recombinant and pituitary human growth hormones was notably similar in rhesus monkeys and in humans [45]. However, such similarities are far too much inconsistent to be considered as a reliable predictor of risk for hypersensitivity reactions in humans.

A variety of assays have been designed and validated to measure specific antibodies in the sera of treated animals. In addition efforts have been paid to minimizing the immunogenicity of therapeutic proteins. As these issues are addressed comprehensively in another chapter of this volume, the focus here will be on predicting problems that may ensue from the presence of such antibodies, namely hypersensitivity reactions. Presumably because allergic reactions have long been considered to be nonreproducible in animal models, limited efforts have been paid to designing predictive animal models until recently. Unexpectedly, the consequence is that no adequately standardized and validated model is available at the present time.

Anaphylactic models in guinea pigs have long been used [35]. In systemic anaphylaxis models guinea pigs are sensitized by one or several subcutaneous or intradermal injections of the test article sometimes mixed with an adjuvant, such as aluminum hydroxide, and then after a rest period of variable duration (usually 1–3 weeks), the animals are challenged intravenously with a non–acutely toxic dose. Clinical signs, primarily difficulties in breathing, develop within minutes after the intravenous injection and death may ensue rapidly. In cutaneous passive anaphylaxis, the pooled serum of sensitized guinea pigs is injected intradermally to naive animals and the test article mixed with a dye, such as Evan's blue, is injected intravenously. When specific antibodies are present in the pooled serum, the local antigen–antibody reaction is evidenced by a blue spot arising within a few hours. The diameter of the blue spot can be used as a quantitation of antibody titers. Both systemic and cutaneous passive anaphylaxis models have been designed in other species as well, such as mice. Despite their extensive use for the past 40 years, these models have several major limitations. They are unsuitable for predicting hypersensitivity reactions to small molecules, namely the vast majority of pharmaceuticals, because they have to bind covalently to a carrier protein to become immunogenic (haptenization), and no procedure is available to reproduce this spontaneous phenomenon experimentally. Although large molecules, such as proteins, can act as direct immunogens and induce anaphylaxis in sensitized animals, proteins of human origin that are not immunogenic in humans consistently induce severe anaphylaxis in guinea pigs, and thus anaphylaxis guinea pig models are not at all relevant to predict the potential of human or humanized biopharmaceuticals for inducing hypersensitivity reactions in humans. The same conclusion applies whatever the animal species.

Because predicting the risk of biopharmaceuticals for inducing hypersensitivity reactions is so crucial, efforts are currently being paid to designing animal models and assays that could prove more predictive. Genetically engineered mice are promising models [22]. They include either knockout (KO) or transgenic mice. In KO mice the deletion of a gene expressing a cytokine or a chemokine considered to be pivotal in hypersensitivity responses may provide a more predictive model. KO mouse models are increasingly used in contact hypersensitivity research [40]. Transgenic mice overexpress a gene of interest, including human genes. Transgenic mice expressing the human insulin gene in pancreatic β cells were found unable to produce human insulin-specific antibodies and helpful to evaluate the potential immunogenicity of several insulin analogues [25]. Similarly a mouse model transgenic for the human IFNβ gene could be used to evaluate the immunogenicity of novel IFNβ analogues [13]. Although genetically engineered mouse models are widely thought to be promising, a number of hurdles have to be overcome before they can be recommended for routine use in the prediction of the potential of biopharmaceuticals to induce hypersensitivity reactions. Overall, these models are poorly standardized. No historical database is available, so interpreting results obtained with any new compound can be tricky. Finally, these models have been suggested to be helpful to evaluate immunogenicity, but it is not known whether these or other models can predict the risk of hypersensitivity reactions. It is indeed important to bear in mind that the clinical experience clearly showed that immunogenicity evidenced by specific antibodies in the sera of treated patients does not necessarily result in clinically patent hypersensitivity reactions.

21.6 CONCLUSION

Overall, autoimmunity and hypersensitivity reactions associated with drug therapy are of major concern in drug development and beyond [24,27]. Such adverse events have been described in association with biopharmaceuticals. This overview of current animal models and assays demonstrates that predicting this risk during preclinical safety evaluation is hardly possible for the time being. Current research efforts in the field of hypersensitivity may result in more predictive models within a reasonable time frame. In contrast, significant progress in the field of autoimmunity is likely to take much more time.

Today, whatever the findings during animal studies of novel biopharmaceuticals, it is impossible to provide any reassurance regarding the safety of such compounds in human subjects as far as autoimmunity and hypersensitivity reactions are concerned. Therefore biopharmaceuticals should be considered high-risk compounds. Adequate follow-up of treated patients and risk management are absolutely essential. Assessing the potential of biopharmaceuticals for inducing autoimmunity and hypersensitivity reactions should not be restricted to clinical trials. Indeed, because pure red cell aplasia associated with recombinant erythropoietins was identified only after several years of clinical use, long-term postmarketing surveillance (pharmacovigilance) is crucial.

REFERENCES

1. Alba A, Puertas MC, Carrillo J, Planas R, Ampudia R, Pastor X, Bosch F, Pujol-Borrell R, Verdaguer J, Vives-Pi M. IFN beta accelerates autoimmune type 1 diabetes in nonobese diabetic mice and breaks the tolerance to beta cells in nondiabetes-prone mice. *J Immunol* 2004;173:6667–75.

2. Atzeni F, Turiel M, Capsoni F, Doria A, Meroni P, Sarzi-Puttini P. Autoimmunity and anti-TNF-alpha agents. *Ann NY Acad Sci* 2005;1051:559–69.

3. Bala S, Weaver J, Hastings KL. Clinical relevance of preclinical testing for allergic side effects. *Toxicology* 2005;209:195–200.

4. Baert F, Noman M, Vermeire S, Van Assche G, D'Haens G, Carbonez A, Rutgeerts P. Influence of immunogenicity on the long-term efficacy of infliximab in Crohn's disease. *N Engl J Med* 2003;348:601–8.

5. Bugelski PJ, Treacy G. Predictive power of preclinical studies in animals for the immunogenicity of recombinant therapeutic proteins in humans. *Curr Opin Mol Ther* 2004;6:10–16.

6. Cheifetz A, Mayer L. Monoclonal antibodies, immunogenicity, and associated infusion reactions. *Mount Sinai J Med* 2005;72:250–6.

7. Chirino AJ, Ary ML, Marshall SA. Minimizing the immunogenicity of protein therapeutics. *Drug Discov Today* 2004;9:82–90.

8. Davidson A, Diamond B. Autoimmune diseases. *N Engl J Med* 2001;345:340–50.

9. De Bandt M, Sibilia J, Le Loet X, Prouzeau S, Fautrel B, Marcelli C, Boucquillard E, Siame JL, Mariette X, Club Rhumatismes et Inflammation. Systemic lupus erythematosus induced by anti-tumour necrosis factor alpha therapy: a French national survey. *Arthritis Res Ther* 2005;7:R545–51.

10. Descotes J. Autoimmunity and toxicity testing. *Toxicol Letts* 2000;112–3:461–5.

11. Descotes J, Vial T. Immune response in human pathology: hypersensitivity and auto-immunity. In Nijkamp FP, Parnham M, eds. *Textbook of Immunopharmacology*, 2nd ed. Basel: Birkhäuser Verlag, 2005;117–29.

12. Frost H. Antibody-mediated side effects of recombinant proteins. *Toxicology* 2005;209:155–60.

13. Hermeling S, Jiskoot W, Crommelin D, Bornaes C, Schellekens H. Development of a transgenic mouse model immune tolerant for human interferon beta. *Pharmaceut Res* 2005;22:847–51.

14. Johansson SG, Bieber T, Dahl R, Friedmann PS, Lanier BQ, Lockey RF, Motala C, Ortega Martell JA, Platts-Mills TA, Ring J, Thien F, Van Cauwenberge P, Williams HC. Revised nomenclature for allergy for global use: report of the Nomenclature Review Committee of the World Allergy Organization, October 2003. *J Allergy Clin Immunol* 2004;113:832–6.

15. Koren E, Zuckerman LA, Mire-Sluis AR. Immune responses to therapeutic proteins in humans—clinical significance, assessment and prediction. *Curr Pharmaceut Biotechnol* 2002;3:349–60.

16. Krouse RS, Royal RE, Heywood G, Weintraub BD, White DE, Steinberg SM, Rosenberg SA, Schwartzentruber DJ. Thyroid dysfunction in 281 patients with metastatic melanoma of renal carcinoma treated with interleukin-2 alone. *J Immunother* 1995;18:272–8.

17. Lim LC. Acquired red cell aplasia in association with the use of recombinant erythropoietin in chronic renal failure. *Hematology* 2005;10:255–9.

18. Lusher JM. Inhibitor antibodies to factor VIII and factor IX: management. *Sem Thromb Hemost* 2000;26:179–88.

19. Malucchi S, Sala A, Gilli F, Bottero R, Di Sapio A, Capobianco M, Bertolotto A. Neutralizing antibodies reduce the efficacy of beta IFN during treatment of multiple sclerosis. *Neurology* 2004;62:2031–7.

20. Mathian A, Weinberg A, Gallegos M, Banchereau J, Koutouzov S. IFN-alpha induces early lethal lupus in preautoimmune (New Zealand Black x New Zealand White) F1 but not in BALB/c mice. *J Immunol* 2005;174:2499–506.

21. Miossec P. Cytokines and autoimmune diseases: from the control of autoimmune diseases with anti-cytokine treatment to the induction of autoimmunity with cytokine treatment. In House RV, Descotes J, eds. *Cytokines in Human Health: Immunotoxicology, Pathology and Human Health*. Totowa NJ: Humana Press, 2007; 233–58.

22. Moser R, Quesniaux V, Ryffel B. Use of transgenic animals to investigate drug hypersensitivity. *Toxicology* 2001;158:75–83.

23. Nierkens S, Pieters R. Murine models of drug hypersensitivity. *Curr Opin Allergy Clin Immunol* 2005;5:331–5.

24. Olsen NJ. Drug-induced autoimmunity. *Best Pract Res Clin Rheumatol* 2004;18:677–88.

25. Ottesen JL, Nilsson P, Jami J, Weilguny D, Duhrkop M, Bucchini D, Havelund S, Fogh JM. The potential immunogenicity of human insulin and insulin analogues evaluated in a transgenic mouse model. *Diabetologia* 1994;37:1178–85.

26. Pichler WJ. Adverse side-effects to biological agents. *Allergy* 2006;61:912–20.

27. Ratajczak HV. Drug-induced hypersensitivity: role in drug development. *Toxicol Rev* 2004;23:265–80.

28. Ravel G, Christ M, Ruat C, Burnett R, Descotes J. Effect of murine recombinant IL-2 on the course of lupus-like disease in (NZBxNZW) F1 female mice. *Immunopharmacol Immunotoxicol* 2002;24:409–21.

29. Ravel G, Descotes J. Popliteal lymph node assay: facts and perspectives. *J Appl Toxicol* 2005;25:451–8.

30. Ravel G, Descotes J. Animal models of autoimmune diseases and their use in safety evaluation studies. *Persp Exp Clin Immunotoxicol* 2007;1:30–9.

31. Selmi C, Lleo A, Zuin M, Podda M, Rossaro L, Gershwin ME. Interferon alpha and its contribution to autoimmunity. *Curr Opin Invest Drugs* 2006;7:451–6.

32. Sobel DO, Ahvazi B. Alpha-interferon inhibits the development of diabetes in NOD mice. *Diabetes* 1998;47:1867–72.

33. Sorensen PS, Ross C, Clemmesen KM, Bendtzen K, Frederiksen JL, Jensen K, Kristensen O, Petersen T, Rasmussen S, Ravnborg M, Stenager E, Koch-Henriksen N. Clinical importance of neutralising antibodies against interferon beta in patients with relapsing-remitting multiple sclerosis. *Lancet* 2003;362:1184–91.

34. Van der Kolk LE, Grillo-Lopez AJ, Baars JW, Hack CE, Van Oers MH. Complement activation plays a key role in the side-effects of rituximab treatment. *Brit J Haematol* 2001;115:807–11.

35. Verdier F, Chazal I, Descotes J. Anaphylaxis models in the guinea-pig. *Toxicology* 1994;93:55–61.

36. Verdier F, Patriarca C, Descotes J. Autoantibodies in conventional toxicity testing. *Toxicology* 1997;119:51–8.

37. Vial T, Choquet-Kastylevsky G, Descotes J. Adverse effects of immunotherapeutics involving the immune system. *Toxicology* 2002;174:3–11.

38. Vial T, Descotes J. Clinical adverse effects of cytokines on the immune system. In House RV, Descotes J. eds. *Cytokines in Human Health: Immunotoxicology, Pathology and Human Health*. Totowa NJ: Humana Press, 2007;319–48.

39. Walker SE. Accelerated mortality in young NZB/NZW mice treated with the interferon inducer tilorone hydrochloride. *Clin Immunol Immunopathol* 1977;8: 204–12.

40. Wang B, Esche C, Mamelak A, Freed I, Watanabe H, Sauder DN. Cytokine knock-outs in contact hypersensitivity research. *Cytokine Growth Factor Rev* 2003;14: 381–9.

41. Weber RW. Adverse reactions to biological modifiers. *Curr Opin Allergy Clin Immunol* 2004;4:277–83.

42. Wierda D, Smith HW, Zwickl CM. Immunogenicity of biopharmaceuticals in laboratory animals. *Toxicology* 2001;158:71–4.

43. Yates AB, DeShazo RD. Allergic and nonallergic drug reactions. *South Med J* 2003;96:1080–7.

44. Zbinden G. Safety evaluation of biotechnology products. *Drug Safety* 1990;5 (Suppl 1):58–64.

45. Zwickl CM, Cocke KS, Tamura RN, Holzhausen LM, Brophy GT, Bick PH, Wierda D. Comparison of the immunogenicity of recombinant and pituitary human growth hormone in rhesus monkeys. *Fund Appl Toxicol* 1991;16:275–87.

PART VI

SPECIFIC CONSIDERATIONS BASED ON PRODUCT CLASS

CHAPTER 22

Current Practices in the Preclinical Safety Assessment of Peptides

SHAWN M. HEIDEL, DVM, PhD, and TODD J. PAGE, PhD

Contents

22.1 INTRODUCTION

Peptides constitute the earliest class of biopharmaceutical medicines and, perhaps, the most studied to date. Insulin has been an effective diabetes therapy for more than 75 years in the United States. Insulin has gone through an evolution that began with its isolation from animal pancreata and continues with numerous analogues being manufactured with state-of-the-art bacterial, mammalian, and yeast recombinant technology [1]. There has been an explosion of peptides in drug development, and there are currently dozens of marketed therapeutic peptides [2]. This chapter reviews the preclinical development experience across this class of important biopharmaceuticals, highlighting what has gone before and some considerations for the future.

A specific definition of what constitutes a peptide is difficult to find. Most people involved in developing biopharmaceuticals would define a peptide as

Preclinical Safety Evaluation of Biopharmaceuticals: A Science-Based Approach to Facilitating Clinical Trials, edited by Joy A. Cavagnaro

a small biopharmaceutical or a traditional biopharmaceutical, but would then elaborate on development issues for peptides manufactured by recombinant rather than synthetic chemical processes. For the purposes of this chapter, and the peptides surveyed in Table 22.1, peptides are defined as those biopharmaceuticals with 5 to 100 amino acids. A distinction will also be made with regard to recombinant versus chemical manufacturing and will be discussed with respect to available guidance, or lack thereof, and experience.

The road map for developing peptides is by association to existing biopharmaceutical and/or new chemical entity guidance documents rather than a guidance that is specific for peptides. The International Conference on Harmonization (ICH) has published a guidance specific for preclinical development of biopharmaceuticals (ICH S6), which is appropriate for most peptides. However, other safety guidance, including regional guidance, may need to be considered dependent on the manufacturing process, the inclusion of unnatural amino acids, or the intended patient population. For instance, there is regional guidance for insulin and parathyroid hormone in Europe and the United States, respectively [3,4]. Regulatory approaches to biopharmaceuticals in Japan are covered in separate chapter (Chapter 5). A review of approved peptide products revealed preclinical studies or parameters that are a blend of typical biopharmaceutical and new chemical entity (NCE) programs (Table 22.1). Therefore there is a blend of studies recommended for peptides based on guidances developed for biopharmaceuticals that includes ICH S6 and those for NCEs (e.g., ICH S1-S5, S7-S8, and M3) (see www.ich.org and www.fda.gov).

22.2 SPECIES SELECTION

Species selection for most peptides has taken into account the pharmacological activity of the peptide in the test species, which is the primary concern for species selection of biopharmaceuticals. Species selection for NCEs is based mostly on in vitro metabolite comparisons between the preclinical species and humans with an assumption of comparable cross-species biologic activity. In contrast to NCEs, biopharmaceuticals are degraded to naturally occurring amino acids rather than metabolized by p450 enzymes to xenobiotic metabolites. Therefore in vitro metabolism studies are not done early in development for peptides. Rather, in vitro or in vivo pharmacology studies are conducted to demonstrate species relevance prior to preclinical toxicology studies. For example, measuring a reduction in glucose following insulin administration would be a demonstration of pharmacological activity. In many cases pharmacology is not as simple as measuring a decrease in glucose levels. When the mechanism of action is more complex, in vitro cell based assays can be used to demonstrate pharmacology. Using a larger, protein biologic to provide an example, interference with a cytokine-induced cell proliferation assay can be used to demonstrate cross-species pharmacology. In this model an antibody

TABLE 22.1 Overview of studies used to support peptide development

Peptide	Class	Safety Pharmacology[a]/Chronic Toxicity	Carcinogenicity Testing	Genetic Toxicity	Method of Manufacture	Approval Date
Bivalrudin (Angiomax, Angiox) [10,11]	Cardiac	Safety pharmacology studies appear to have been done separately 1 month (rat) 1 month (cyno)[c]	No	Standard battery[b]	Synthetic	FDA-2000 EMEA-2004
Cetrorelix (Cetrotide) [26,27]	Hormone	Safety pharmacology studies appear to have been done separately 6 month (rat) 6 month (dog)	No	Standard battery	Synthetic	FDA-2000 EMEA-1999
Eptifibatide (Integrelin) [12,13]	Cardiac	Separate safety pharmacology studies One month (rat) One month (cyno)	No	Standard battery	Synthetic	FDA-1998 EMEA-1999
Enfuvirtide (Fuzeon) [15,16]	Antiviral	Safety pharmacology included in toxicology studies 6 month (rat) 9 month (cyno)	No	Standard battery	Synthetic	FDA-2003 EMEA-2003
Nesiritide (Natrecor) [28]	Cardiac	Cardiac safety pharmacology separate 2 week (rat) 2 week (monkey)	No	Ames only	Recombinant	FDA-2001

TABLE 22.1 *Continued*

Peptide	Class	Safety Pharmacology[a]/Chronic Toxicity	Carcinogenicity Testing	Genetic Toxicity	Method of Manufacture	Approval Date
Ziconotide (Prialt) [29,30]	Pain	Non-GLP safety pharmacology studies, GLP toxicology studies used to support non-GLP studies 14 day (monkey) 28 day (rat) 42 day (dog)	No	Standard battery	Synthetic	FDA-2004 EMEA-2005
Exenatide (Byetta) [31,32]	Hormone	Separate CNS study (mice), separate CV study (monkey) 182 day (mouse) 91 day (rat) 273 day (monkey)	104 week (rat), benign thyroid C cell adenoma 104 week mouse	Standard battery	Synthetic	FDA-2005 EMEA-2006
Leuprolide (Lupron-Depot) [33]	Hormone	ND	2 year (rats, mice), benign pituitary hyperplasia and adenoma (rat, 24 months, 100× clinical dose)	ND	Synthetic	FDA 1997
Calcitonin-Salmon (Fortical, Forcaltonin) [34,35]	Hormone	ND	1 year (SD and Fisher rats) nonfunctioning pituitary adenomas (130–160× clinical dose)	Standard battery	Recombinant	FDA-2005 EMEA-1999
Octreotide (Sandostatin) [36]	Hormone	ND	99 weeks (mice) 116 weeks (rats)	Were performed, specifics not given	Synthetic	FDA-1988

Drug	Type	Safety pharmacology	Carcinogenicity	Genotoxicity		Approval
rhPTH(1-34) (Forteo, Forsteo) [37,38]	Hormone	Separate safety pharmacology studies in rat and dog, studies in cyno were included in chronic tox 6 month (rat) 12 month (monkey)	2 year (rat) Observed malignant metastatic osteosarcoma.	Standard battery	Recombinant	FDA-2002 EMEA-2003
Insulin lispro (Humalog) [39]	Insulin analogue	Safety pharmacology studies appear to have been done separately. 12 month (rat) 12 month (dog)	No in vitro studies to assess DNA synthesis stimulation using HepG2 cells	Standard battery	Recombinant	FDA-1996 EMEA-1996
Insulin glulisine (Apidra) [7,8]	Insulin analogue	Separate CV and respiratory studies 12 month (rat) 6 month (dog)	No, but the 12-month chronic study was designed to investigate the carcinogenic potential of the compound	Standard battery	Recombinant	FDA-2004 EMEA-2004
Insulin glargine (Lantus) [40,41]	Insulin analogue	Separate safety pharmacolgy. CNS, CV, pulmonary, renal 6 month (rat) 6 month (dog)	2 year (mouse) 2 year rat	Standard battery	Recombinant	FDA-2000 EMEA-2000
Insulin detemir (Levemir) [6,20]	Insulin analogue	6 month (rat) 12 month (dog)	No in vitro mitogenic potential (CHO-K1, MCF-7, human osteosarcoma, L6-hIR) No Although mammary tumors were observed in the 12 month (rat) study	Standard battery	Recombinant	FDA-2005 EMEA-2004
Insulin aspart (NovoLog, NovoRapid) [42,43]	Insulin analogue	12 month (rat) 12 month (dog)		Standard battery	Recombinant	FDA-2000 EMEA-1999

Source: All data for this table was taken from Label, FDA Summary Basis for Approval, and EPAR (European Public Assessment Report) documents.

[a] Safety Pharmacology ICHS7.

[b] Genetic Toxicity Standard Battery ICHS2A.

[c] Cynomolgus monkey (cyno).

to the human cytokine is assessed for its ability to bind to the intended test species cytokine homologue by measuring inhibition of cytokine-induced cell proliferation. This demonstration of pharmacology is usually sufficient to justify the use of the test species for preclinical safety evaluation of the anti-human cytokine antibody.

Toxicology testing for peptides is typically completed in two species. In the peptide development programs that were reviewed, rats were the most common rodent and nonrodents were about equally split between monkeys and dogs. All of the 12 peptides where data were available were tested in at least two species. In some cases three species were evaluated (e.g., exenatide, ziconatide) (Table 22.1). This is consistent with ICH S6, which indicates two species should be used, if appropriate. However, many biopharmaceuticals are evaluated only in nonhuman primates because of the lack of pharmacology or the development of a significant immune response in rodents. If a peptide is pharmacologically active in only a single species, then it is appropriate to use only that species for toxicology testing. Conducting studies in a species that lacks pharmacology would not provide useful information, and may in fact complicate the extrapolation of the animal data to humans. For example, an absence of findings in a species that is not pharmacologically responsive may be misinterpreted as a lack of potential safety issues, even though high-dose pharmacology was not evaluated. Like other biopharmaceuticals, pharmacology in the test species should be the key determinant of species selection for peptides primarily because peptides are not metabolized like NCEs.

22.3 GENETIC TOXICOLOGY

Genetic toxicology studies were completed for almost all peptides in the survey, which is a requirement for NCEs (per ICH S2) but not necessary and/ or appropriate for most biopharmaceuticals (per ICH S6) (see Chapter 3). The main reason that these studies are not needed for biopharmaceuticals is the inability of biopharmaceuticals to cause direct DNA damage. Most biopharmaceuticals do not cross cell or nuclear membranes to access DNA. Moreover direct DNA damage is caused by chemically reactive molecules that bind or associate with DNA, which is not expected for peptides. While scientific rationale and current guidance documents clearly indicate that genetic toxicology tests are not required for biologics, they have been completed for most approved peptides. The likely reason for this paradox is that most tests were completed prior to the implementation of ICH S6 in 1997. However, these tests have been completed for some more recently approved peptides. The rationale for this is not clear.

A pivotal publication of 78 biopharmaceuticals provides data supporting the lack of positive genotoxicity with peptides. The publication concluded, "genotoxicity testing is generally inappropriate and unnecessary" [5]. Additional support for this position comes from the regulatory agencies; in a 2004 review the EMEA stated, "Although not applicable to biotechnology-derived pharmaceuticals, insulin detemir was tested for gene mutations in bacteria and for chromosome aberrations in vitro and in vivo. As expected, there was no evidence of genotoxic potential in any of these tests" [6]. If impurities from the manufacturing process have not been previously evaluated in genetic toxicology studies, they may need additional testing. In those cases it is appropriate to test only the impurity rather than the peptide. This does not imply that genetic toxicology studies are necessary for all synthetically produced peptides, only that it needs to be evaluated with consideration given to impurities from the manufacturing process rather than the peptide. The lack of genetic toxicity risk of the peptide is the same regardless of whether the peptide is produced by recombinant or synthetic methods. Based on good scientific rationale and data, genetic toxicology studies should not be routinely conducted for peptides.

Genetic toxicology testing of peptides containing "nonnatural" amino acids has been controversial. One conceivable genetic risk would be incorporation of these unique amino acids into proteins. Even if this were possible, the likelihood of incorporation into a protein critical for DNA replication or repair seems remote. In addition incorporation of a nonnatural amino acid into host protein(s) in and of itself would not be sufficient for concern. Malfunction of the protein to increase inherited mutations would also be required. Another conceivable risk of the nonnatural amino acid is the potential metabolism of the unique amino acid to a genotoxic metabolite. Although these rationale may provide a scientific justification for not performing genetic toxicity testing, in many cases studies may still be needed to support regulatory concerns like those in Japan (see Chapter 5). Given the potential scientific and regulatory concerns, it may be prudent to complete genetic toxicology testing of nonnatural amino acids.

Some biopharmaceuticals may cause cellular proliferation that could increase the likelihood of inheriting a spontaneous mutation. However, genetic toxicology studies are not designed to evaluate these concerns. The potential for inducing a mitogenic response can be addressed in other toxicology studies.

22.4 SAFETY PHARMACOLOGY

Separate safety pharmacology studies were completed for many peptides in the survey. Separate safety pharmacology studies are usually performed for NCEs but not biopharmaceuticals. Since rodents are typically used for stand-alone central nervous system and respiratory studies, the usefulness of these studies for NCEs is based on the assumption that rodents are pharmacologically responsive or have some of the same metabolites as would be expected in humans. The lack of concern for metabolism and the significant reduction or absence of pharmacology in rodents with most biopharmaceuticals eliminates the relevance of these studies. In contrast to the larger biopharmaceuticals, many of which are species specific, peptides are frequently pharmacologically active in rodents, and therefore useful data can be generated in separate safety pharmacology studies. However, as with large biopharmaceuticals, an absence of pharmacological activity of the peptide in rodents should similarly preclude conduct of these studies. When rodent studies are not appropriate, evaluations are usually done within a repeated dose toxicology study in nonrodents. For example, quantitative electrocardiograms (ECGs), detailed neurologic and behavioral evaluations, and qualitative measurements of respiratory rate and depth assess effects on the cardiovascular, central nervous system, and respiratory systems, respectively. Pharmacological activity should determine the appropriate species for safety pharmacology studies, which is consistent with ICH S6 as well as other ICH guidance.

Findings in safety pharmacology evaluations of peptides are generally consistent with anticipated pharmacology. Because the pharmacology of most peptides would not be predicted to affect safety pharmacology, no findings were observed in most studies. Other findings, such as decreased blood pressure, heart rate, breathing rate, and increased QTc for insulins were due to hypoglycemia and considered exaggerated pharmacology based on predicted pharmacology [7,8].

22.5   CHRONIC TOXICITY TESTING

The duration of chronic toxicity testing for peptides is driven primarily by their intended indication and duration of treatment. Of the peptides studied, the duration of the pivotal repeat dose toxicology studies, ranges from a low of two weeks, for neseritide, to a high of one year for many of the insulin analogues. For the 9 chronic use peptides included in our analysis, chronic toxicology studies of 6, 9, or 12 month durations were completed for 3, 2, or 4 of them, respectively. This is more consistent with guidance for NCEs, which typically have 9- or 12-month durations due to ICH S4 guidance. Most other chronic use biopharmaceuticals have completed chronic studies of 6-month duration, which is consistent with ICH S6 guidance [9].

Eptifibatide and bivalrudin, two peptides tested for 28 days in the chronic toxicity studies, provide interesting case studies [10–13]. Bivalrudin is a linear 20 amino acid peptide that is derived from hirudin, an anticoagulant found in the saliva of leeches, and is intended for use during invasive intravascular procedures. Eptifibatide is a cyclic heptapeptide that is an RGD (arginine, glycine, aspartic acid) mimetic that acts as an inhibitor of platelet aggregation and is indicated for the treatment of acute coronary syndrome. As a class of drugs, RGD mimetics are based on a sequence (RGD) found in fibronection that mediates its interactions with the integrins [14]. These observations illustrate that it is not the structure (linear vs. cyclic) or the origin (nonhuman vs. human) that determines the length of the chronic toxicology studies for peptides but the intended indication and duration of treatment.

One of the most striking observations that can be made of the peptides as a class is their remarkable safety profile. Of all of the peptides currently on the market that were investigated for this analysis (Table 22.1), there was only one observation in the chronic toxicology studies that was not linked to exaggerated pharmacology. Admittedly, our analysis is biased by the fact that only approved compounds were included; however, this data set is still very instructive. The observation in question was from enfuvirtide, a 36 amino acid linear peptide derived from the HIV-1 glycoprotein gp41 [15,16].

Enfuvirtide interferes with viral attachment and entry into target cells by disrupting the interaction of viral gp120 with target cell receptors (CD4, CXCR4, CCR5). In the repeat-dose toxicology studies thymic lymphocyte depletion was observed in a 9-month cynomolgus study. However, this finding was not considered to be adverse as it was attributed to exaggerated pharmacology. Additionally, microgranuloma and inflammatory loci were observed in the lungs of rats after 28 days of treatment. Presumably, these findings were related to the affinity of the peptide for the formyl peptide receptor (FPR), which has been demonstrated to mediate an inflammatory response at the site of bacterial infection via the recruitment of phagocytic cells. The pharmacological basis for these observations is being investigated by the manufacturer postapproval.

As our analysis demonstrates, in almost all cases the toxic effects of peptides can be predicted from their inherent pharmacological properties. It would follow then that one of the most important steps in the successful development of a peptide is selection of the appropriate pharmacologically responsive species for testing. Moreover, since the pharmacological effects of biologics are usually predictable and observed in studies of 6-month duration or less, the utility of longer studies is not readily apparent.

22.6 CARCINOGENICITY TESTING

The pharmacology of the peptide, duration of treatment, and patient population should be taken into consideration in designing and/or evaluating the need for carcinogenicity testing. As previously discussed, peptides are not expected to be genotoxic and therefore are not considered complete carcinogens [17]. The main concern for peptides is the potential for mitogenesis or tumor promotion.

ICH S6 indicates that carcinogenicity studies are not generally needed for endogenous substances given essentially as replacement therapy, particularly where there is previous clinical experience with similar products. The issue of carcinogenicity testing for peptides is complicated by the fact that most approved peptide drugs are hormone or hormone analogues. Supraphysiological doses of a hormone or biopharmaceutical with hormonal properties would be anticipated to cause hyperplasia, and therefore there would be a cause for concern for neoplasia.

Human parathyroid hormone (1-34) is an example of a peptide that is administered at supraphysiological doses compared to naturally secreted human parathyroid hormone (PTH). Substantial increases in bone mass, consistent with the pharmacology of PTH 1-34, were observed in a two-year carcinogenicity study in rats. In addition bone tumors were observed at all doses [18]. The data from this initial study suggested that the tumors resulted from the long duration of treatment coupled with the exaggerated pharmacological response in rats to daily treatment with PTH 1-34. Therefore a second study was conducted to more fully characterize the dose–response and duration of treatment on the formation of bone tumors. This study identified a no-effect level and quantified the effect on bone mass using computed tomography and histomorphometry [19]. These studies provided data indicating important differences between the pharmacological response in rats compared to human clinical data, which suggests the increased incidence of bone neoplasia in rats is likely not predictive of an increased risk of bone cancer in adult osteoporotic humans treated with PTH 1-34 for a limited duration. Moreover these studies demonstrate the importance of understanding the species differences for interpreting human risk.

In cases where exaggerated pharmacology might be predicted to give rise to positive findings in carcinogenesis studies, it can be very helpful, when available, to include the natural human analogue that the peptide drug is derived from for comparison purposes. This will assist in determining the relative risk of the novel peptide analogue compared to the normal analogue. This approach has been important for the development of many insulin analogues because of the propensity for mammary gland hyperplasia. For example, there was an observation of increased proliferation in the mammary gland of rats treated with suprapharmacological doses of insulin detemir [6,20]. When the study was repeated using suprapharmacological doses of human insulin as a comparator, it was found that the increases in mammary gland proliferation were similar between human insulin and insulin detemir. Therefore the risk assessment for tumors with this insulin analogue was the same as that for normal insulin, demonstrating the usefulness of including the normal human orthologue as a comparator.

In vitro studies are frequently useful for evaluating the mitogenic properties of peptides. The European guidance for insulin analogues promotes in vitro testing to determine the mitogenicity of new analogues compared to normal human insulin and AspB10, an analogue with increased mitogenicity and tumorigenic properties [21,22]. The absence of an increase in mitogenicity would decrease the cause for concern and likely eliminate the need for a two-year carcinogenicity study with the novel analogue. In cases where a peptide is not pharmacologically active in rodents, in vitro mitogenic assays may be critical for the assessment for tumor promotion. Another useful test for determining the ability to promote tumors is to evaluate multiple tumor types for the receptor target. If tumors do not contain the receptor, then there would be no risk of tumor promotion. If tumors contain the receptor, it would be important to evaluate the ability of the peptide to promote mitogenesis in comparison with the normal human orthologue, as was done with insulin analogues. Comparable mitogenicity would indicate limited risk with novel analogues given at physiological levels as replacement therapy.

The Carcinogenicity Assessment Committee (Enfuvirtide, Summary Basis for Approval, Pharmacology, 2003, http://www.fda.gov/cder/foi/nda/2003/021481_fuzeon_review.htm) notes in the FDA approval documents for enfuviritide highlight considerations for carcinogenicity testing. The strongest arguments not to test were (1) the lack of structural alerts in a peptide, (2) the absence of hyperplasia in the chronic toxicity studies, and (3) the polypeptides with known carcinogenic properties that are hormones or demonstrate hormonal activity [16]. The arguments to test were (1) chronic inflammation was observed at the injection site, (2) the indication was chronic use, and (3) the product is a new therapeutic. The most compelling reason for testing was thought to be chronic inflammation, but this is easily monitored and would be managed in the clinic. Other points to consider are whether the peptide binds a cell-surface receptor to elicit signal transduction. The lack of signal transduction or immunosuppression would decrease the cause for concern for carcinogenicity. One theoretical example would be a peptide that binds a plasma-derived cytokine with little consequence for immunity. The final FDA decision was to waive the need for carcinogenicity testing with enfuviritide.

Even therapies that are potent immunosuppressive agents present challenges for carcinogenicity assessment. This is mainly due to their pharmacology, which makes it highly likely that they will act as tumor promoters. Therefore it could be assumed that these therapies would present a carcinogenic risk without a two-year study. In addition completing a full two-year study in rodents at clinically relevant doses has proved difficult because of rodent sensitivity to the pharmacological effects, which results in low survival. The pharmacological properties coupled with difficulties in completing lifetime studies in rodents has led to the suggestion that alternative models to two-year carcinogenicity studies might be more appropriate for risk assessment of immunosuppressive drugs [23].

A threshold for the carcinogenicity of hormones is widely accepted by regulatory agencies [24,25]. Therefore using historical practices for peptide hormones is not appropriate for establishing broad guidelines on the need for carcionogenicity testing for all peptides. While it is difficult to understand a scientific rationale for carcinogenesis testing for classes of peptides that do not have mitogenic properties (e.g., antiviral, cardiac peptides), in other cases it would seem to be warranted because the downstream pharmacology may be mitogenic (GnRH analogues) as demonstrated by multiple tumors in 2-year rodent carcinogenicity studies with analogues, such as Leu prolide [33]. For these reasons the need for carcinogenicity testing needs to carefully evaluated, primarily taking into account the expected pharmacology of the molecule.

Carcinogenicity testing of chronic use peptides has been evaluated in a number of ways, ranging from in vitro assays coupled with an evaluation of hyperplasia in repeat-dose studies (insulin detemir) to full two-year studies (i.e., PTH 1-34). The type of carcinogenicity assessment is dependent on the accumulated database for the therapeutic class, including data from positive and negative controls that can be used to gauge risk.

22.7   RECOMBINANT VERSUS SYNTHETIC PEPTIDES

The differences between the manufacture of recombinant and synthetic peptides typically should not result in a different battery of toxicology studies. Pharmacology should be the primary determinant of the appropriate studies and thus the preclinical development programs would be expected to be similar regardless of the method of manufacture. A notable exception would be the level of process-related impurities that might be introduced during synthetic production. In those cases the impurities may need to be qualified in genetic toxicology tests and/or other tests. In the absence of novel impurities, the development considerations should be the same for either manufacturing method and should primarily focus on potential toxicities associated with exaggerated pharmacology.

22.8   CONCLUSIONS

Peptides are a unique class of biopharmaceuticals and have been developed with a battery of toxicology studies that is a blend of those traditionally used for NCEs and biopharmaceuticals. Historically peptides were developed much like NCEs, probably owing to the experience of the sponsor and the various regulatory agencies, which was predominantly NCE focused. The pharmacology of the peptide should be the primary consideration for toxicology testing. This is mainly due to the lack of potentially reactive metabolites or competition for metabolic clearance that are important drivers of NCE testing. Exaggerated pharmacology is the main concern for peptides and thus should be the main determinant in selecting the appropriate battery of toxicology studies.

The development of peptides will likely continue to appear somewhat different from larger biopharmaceuticals. This is mostly driven by the rodent being a pharmacologically responsive species for many peptides. Therefore many peptides will continue to have repeat-dose toxicology studies, separate safety pharmacology studies, and carcinogenicity assessments in rodents. The rationale for not performing similar studies with larger biopharmaceuticals is often based on the absence of pharmacology in rodents and/or the induction of an immune response that eliminates exposure needed for a meaningful evaluation. Pharmacology in rodents has led to the majority of the differences in toxicology studies for peptides compared to other biopharmaceuticals.

Many marketed peptides are chronic use hormones that have undergone carcinogenicity testing. The potential for superpharmacologic hyperplasia is a common concern for hormones and emphasizes the need for assessment of carcinogenic potential. This has led to full two-year carcinogenicity assessments for some peptide hormones. Recent advances in the understanding of specific pharmacological classes, such as insulin analogues, have provided in vitro tools to assess the risk of mitogenicity without completing a two-year study. As knowledge and technical capabilities progress, new methods for carcinogenicity assessments will arise and should be considered. Many other biopharmaceuticals do not have specific pharmacology requiring an extensive two-year carcinogenicity bioassay. Examples are those peptides that do not bind cell-surface receptors or are used only for acute treatment. The most appropriate assessment for carcinogenic potential of peptides should be justified and may not include a two-year study in rodents.

As classes of peptides have evolved, it has become clear that sponsors and regulatory agencies consider pharmacological activity as the primary concern and therefore follow the principles outlined in the ICH S6 guidance. This approach is science-driven based on the lack of potentially reactive metabolites and the emphasis on exaggerated pharmacology as the primary concerns for improving the predictive value of safety evaluation programs. For new peptide classes in development, as with any new medicine, the key is to develop the appropriate hypotheses that dictate the appropriate scientific considerations and studies.

REFERENCES

1. Chance RE, Frank BH. Research, development, production, and safety of biosynthetic human insulin. *Diabet Care* 1993;16(Suppl 3):133–42.

2. Marx V. Watching Peptide Drugs Grow Up. *Chem Eng News* 2005;83(11):17–24.

3. EMEA. Points to consider document on the non-clinical assessment of the carcinogenic potential of insulin analogues, 2001. http://www.emea.europa.eu/pdfs/human/swp/037201en.pdf

4. FDA. Development of Parathyroid Hormone for the Prevention and Treatment of Osteoporosis, 2000. http://www.fda.gov/cder/guidance/3789dft.htm

5. Gocke E, Albertini S, Brendler-Schwaab S, Muller L, Suter W, Wurgler FE. Genotoxicity testing of biotechnology-derived products: report of a GUM task force. Gesellschaft fur Umweltmutationsforschung. *Mutat Res* 1999;436(2):137–56.

6. Insulin Detemir. Summary Basis for Approval, EPAR, 2006. http://www.emea.europa.eu/humandocs/PDFs/EPAR/levemir/093604en6.pdf

7. Insulin Glulisine. Summary Basis for Approval, Pharmacology Review, 2004. http://www.fda.gov/cder/foi/nda/2004/21-629_Apidra.htm

8. Insulin Glulisine. Summary Basis for Approval, EPAR, 2006. http://www.emea.europa.eu/humandocs/PDFs/EPAR/apidra/121804en6.pdf

9. Clarke J, Hurst C, Martin P, Vahle J, Ponce R, Mounho B, Heidel S, Andrews L, Reynolds T, Cavagnaro J. Duration of chronic toxicity studies for biotechnology-derived pharmaceuticals: Is six months still appropriate? *Regul Toxicol Pharmacol* 2008;50:2–22.

10. Bivalrudin. Summary Basis for Approval, Pharmacology Review, 2000. http://www.fda.gov/cder/foi/nda/2000/20873_Angiomax.htm

11. Bivalrudin. Summary Basis for Approval EPAR, 2004. http://www.emea.europa.eu/humandocs/PDFs/EPAR/angiox/103304en6.pdf

12. Eptifibatide. Summary Basis for Approval, Pharmacology Review, 1998. http://www.fda.gov/cder/foi/nda/98/20718_Integrilin.htm

13. Eptifibatide. Summary Basis of Approval, EPAR, 2004. http://www.emea.europa.eu/humandocs/PDFs/EPAR/Integrilin/110099en6.pdf

14. Humphries MJ, Olden K, Yamada KM. A synthetic peptide from fibronectin inhibits experimental metastasis of murine melanoma cells. *Science* 1986; 233(4762):467–70.

15. Enfuvirtide. Summary Basis for Approval, Pharmacology Review, 2003. http://www.fda.gov/cder/foi/nda/2003/021481_fuzeon_review.htm

16. Enfuvirtide. Summary Basis for Approval, EPAR, 2004. http://www.emea.europa.eu/humandocs/PDFs/EPAR/fuzeon/169503en6.pdf

17. Pitot HC, Dragan YP, *Casarett and Doull's Toxicology*, 6 ed. Klaassen C, ed. 2001; 266–78.

18. Vahle JL, Sato M, Long GG, Young JK, Francis PC, Engelhardt JA, Westmore MS, Linda Y, Nold JB. Skeletal changes in rats given daily subcutaneous injections of recombinant human parathyroid hormone (1–34) for 2 years and relevance to human safety. *Toxicol Pathol* 2002;30(3):312–21.

19. Vahle JL, Long GG, Sandusky G, Westmore MS, Ma YL, Sato M. Bone neoplasms in F344 rats given teriparatide [rhPTH(1–34)] are dependent on duration of treatment and dose. *Toxicol Pathol* 2004;32(4):426–38.

20. Insulin Detemir. Summary Basis for Approval, Pharmacology Review, 2005. http://www.fda.gov/cder/foi/nda/2005/021-536_LevemirTOC.htm

21. Dideriksen LH, Jorgensin LN, Drejer K. Carcinogenic effect on female rats after 12 months administration of the insulin analogue B10 Asp. *Diabetes* 1992;41:143A.

22. Milazzo G, Sciacca L, Papa V, Goldfine ID, Vigneri R. ASPB10 insulin induction of increased mitogenic responses and phenotypic changes in human breast epithelial cells: evidence for enhanced interactions with the insulin-like growth factor-I receptor. *Mol Carcinog* 1997;18(1):19–25.

23. Hastings KL. Assessment of immunosuppressant drug carcinogenicity: standard and alternative animal models. *Hum Exp Toxicol* 2000;19(4):261–5.

24. Jacobs A, Jacobson-Kram D. Human carcinogenic risk evaluation. Part III: Assessing cancer hazard and risk in human drug development. *Toxicol Sci* 2004; 81(2):260–2.

25. Silva Lima B, Van der Laan JW. Mechanisms of nongenotoxic carcinogenesis and assessment of the human hazard. *Regul Toxicol Pharmacol* 2000;32(2);135–43.

26. Cetrorelix. Summary Basis for Approval, Pharmacology Review, 2000. http://www.fda.gov/cder/foi/nda/2000/21-197_Cetrotide.htm

27. Cetrorelix. Summary Basis for Approval, EPAR, 2003. http://www.emea.europa.eu/humandocs/PDFs/EPAR/Cetrotide/297998en6.pdf

28. Nesiritide. Summary Basis for Approval, Pharmacology Review, 2001. http://www.fda.gov/cder/foi/nda/2001/20-920_Natrecor.htm

29. Ziconatide. Summary Basis for Approval, Pharmacology Review, 2004. http://www. fda.gov/cder/foi/nda/2004/21-060_Prialt.htm

30. Ziconatide. Summary Basis for Approval, EPAR, 2006. http://www.emea.europa. eu/humandocs/PDFs/EPAR/Prialt/14122704en6.pdf

31. Exenatide. Summary Basis for Approval, Pharmacology, 2005. http://www.fda.gov/ cder/foi/nda/2005/021773_ByettaTOC.htm

32. Exenatide. Summary Basis for Approval, EPAR, 2006. http://www.emea.europa. eu/humandocs/PDFs/EPAR/byetta/H-698-en6.pdf

33. Leuprolide. Label, 1993. http://www.fda.gov/cder/foi/label/2004/20263slr024_ lupron_lbl.pdf

34. Calcitonin. Summary Basis of Approval, EPAR, 1999. http://www.emea.europa.eu/ humandocs/PDFs/EPAR/Forcaltonin/238798en6.pdf

35. Calcitonin. Label, 2005. http://www.fda.gov/cder/foi/label/2005/021406lbl.pdf

36. Octreotide. Label, 2005. http://www.fda.gov/cder/foi/label/2005/019667s050lbl.pdf

37. Forsteo. Summary Basis For Approval, EPAR, 2004. http://www.emea.europa.eu/ humandocs/PDFs/EPAR/forsteo/659802en6.pdf

38. Forteo. Summary Basis For Approval, Pharmacology Review, 2002. http://www.fda. gov/cder/foi/nda/2002/21-318_FORTEO_Pharmr_P1.pdf

39. Insulin Lispro. Summary Basis for Approval, EPAR, 2004. http://www.emea.europa. eu/humandocs/PDFs/EPAR/Humalog/060195en6.pdf

40. Insulin Glargine. Summary Basis for Approval, Pharmacology Review, 2000. http:// www.fda.gov/cder/foi/nda/2000/21081_Lantus.htm

41. Insulin Glargine. Summary Basis for Approval, EPAR, 2003. http://www.emea. europa.eu/humandocs/PDFs/EPAR/Lantus/061500en6.pdf

42. Insulin Aspart. Summary Basis for Approval, Pharmacology Review, 2000. http:// www.fda.gov/cder/foi/nda/2000/20-986_NovoLog.htm

43. Insulin Aspart. Summary Basis for Approval, EPAR, 2004. http://www.emea. europa.eu/humandocs/PDFs/EPAR/Novorapid/272799en6.pdf

CHAPTER 23

Enzyme Replacement Therapies

LAURA ANDREWS, PhD, DABT, and
MICHAEL O'CALLAGHAN, DVM, PhD, MRCVS

Contents

23.1   INTRODUCTION

Enzyme replacement therapy (ERT) is a therapeutic approach in which the specific enzyme that is absent or inactive in affected individuals is replaced with a functional enzyme molecule. Pancreatic enzyme preparations of porcine or bovine origin have been available in the United States for treatment of exocrine pancreatic insufficiency (EPI) in children and adults with cystic fibrosis and chronic pancreatitis since before the enactment of the Federal Food, Drug and Cosmetic Act of 1938 (ref FDA guidance on EIP April 2004). A

Preclinical Safety Evaluation of Biopharmaceuticals: A Science-Based Approach to Facilitating Clinical Trials, edited by Joy A. Cavagnaro
Copyright © 2008 by John Wiley & Sons, Inc.

modified version of adenosine deaminase (ADA), polyethylene modified ADA (PEG-ADA), was approved in 1990 as an enzyme replacement therapy for immunodeficiency due to ADA deficiency. This chapter addresses the issues facing development of enzyme replacement treatments for the specific group of mutational conditions termed lysosmal storage diseases (LSDs). First, some of the pathophysiological features of LSDs will be described, with a discussion of the obstacles to delivering therapeutic proteins to diseased lysosomes. The patchy past history of attempts to treat these long considered "untreatable" conditions will be covered, before moving to the most recent decade of significant advances in enzyme replacement therapy (ERT) that has opened up a new era of hope for LSD sufferers. Some of the key advances that have led to successful commercial production of enzymes for ERT will be addressed. Particular attention will be given to production scale up and the challenges of providing in vitro and in vivo verification of product consistency through the period from preclinical studies to mature commercial production. The changing regulatory framework that has governed the development of ERTs with reference to obtaining worldwide licensure, a necessity for participating companies if these therapies are to be commercially viable, will be covered. We will address some of the unique issues posed by LSDs, in particular, the emerging recognition that substrate load in animal models and patients significantly complicates the translation of preclinical safety (and other) findings into a human risk–benefit equation. In addition we will attempt to illustrate some of the most pertinent challenges and developments that have led to the recent expansion of therapeutic options for many LSD patients who once faced a uniformly dire prognosis on diagnosis of their disease. Finally, we will address the current status of ERTs as they pertain to the LSDs as a group, noting alternative and emerging ancillary therapies such as chaperones and gene therapy. We will also discuss two major remaining obstacles: notably the problem of how to gain access to the central nervous system for the more than 50% of LSDs with neurologic manifestations, and how the biopharmaceutical industry and regulatory agencies are to address the ever-diminishing pool of patients with rarer LSDs now that effective treatments are available for the relatively more populous conditions, Gaucher, Fabry, MPS I and II, and Pompe.

23.2   HISTORICAL BACKGROUND

LSDs are deceptively classified as a single group of diseases, based simply on the common finding of accumulated macromolecular material in the lysosomes of various tissues. While there are some similarities among certain LSDs such as the mucopolysaccharidoses (MPSs1-7) most of the named LSDs are highly dissimilar by pathophysiology, organ involvement, and therapeutic challenge. Until the advent of recombinant gene technology these diseases were essentially untreatable; however, hints of potentially successful approaches were provided by pioneering work in bone marrow transplantation, and more recently, delivery of tissue-extracted enzymes such as Ceredase® [1].

23.2.1 Pathophysiology of LSDs

LSDs comprise a collection of approximately 50 rare conditions characterized by abnormal and varying accumulation of metabolic substrates in the lysosomes of many cell types and tissues. Substrate accumulation is the result of impairment (total absence, partial absence, and structural distortion) of specific lysosomal hydrolases essential for degradation of macromolecular cellular components. Individual LSDs are the result of fortuitous pairings of random parental mutations in the genes for a particular lysosomal enzyme. Clinical manifestations of the individual LSDs vary widely as a result of the cell types most affected by abnormal accumulation of substrate. Typically many cell types throughout the body accumulate the misdigested lysosomal material, but the degree of accumulation is not always the determining factor in whether a particular organ or system is seriously impaired. For example, substantial accumulation of substrate in neurons is common to many LSDs, but this accumulation may not be manifest clinically in some (Pompe disease, MPS IV and VI), whereas others present with severe and rapidly progressive neurologic impairment (MPS I, II, III, and VII) [2]. Similarly in other organs the degree of dysfunction is not correlated with degree of accumulation in particular cells, but rather the impairment that the substrate imparts on the particular cell type. For example, in the kidneys of Fabry patients accumulation of globotriaocyl-ceramide in podocytes is uniformly intense, but with only moderate consequences for glomerular filtration. The severe renal (and CNS) pathology in Fabry disease rather arises from relatively modest substrate accumulation in the endothelium, resulting in significant pro-inflammatory upregulation, with numerous downstream pathologic consequences [3].

Most LSDs have a short rapid course, beginning in early childhood, progressing to premature death within a few months or years. A few, such as Fabry disease, have more prolonged courses characterized by predominantly subclinical progression of the underlying pathology (other signs of the disease may, however, be present), only progressing to significant clinical decline in the third or fourth decade with death usually occurring in middle age. Several LSDs (e.g., MPS-I, Pompe) are also well recognized for having distinct and different subsets of clinical phenotypes, varying by clinical onset and progression. These range from severe, rapid-onset infantile forms with early death to more slowly progressive or late-onset adult forms of the disease. This variability of phenotype in such small patient populations complicates the task of defining clinical trial cohorts. More than half of the LSDs have severe neurologic phenotypes, some with devastatingly rapid progression. The difficulty of effectively delivering therapies across the blood–brain barrier remains a significant obstacle for these conditions.

Etiologies for most of the LSDs have been well documented, some for almost a century. The unique variations of phenotype, age at onset, clinical progression, and severity of the individual LSDs, depend on the degree of enzymatic deprivation, determined principally by whether the mutational mix results in complete absence of the lysosomal enzyme (null) or variable partial reduction or dysfunction of the protein (misfolding, missing sections of the enzyme, etc.). As a result therapeutic approaches to the LSDs, while possessing some common themes, must allow for individually tailored strategies.

23.2.2   Therapies for LSDs

The first successful efforts to treat LSDs came in the form of allogeneic bone marrow transplants aimed at providing at least residual levels of circulating enzyme from the grafted cells of normal, closely matched donors (often a sibling or family member)[2]. While bone marrow transplants remain an option for some LSDs still lacking viable therapies, they rarely achieve the necessary blood levels of enzyme and exposure for full- or long-term reversal of the disease phenotype.

The first major breakthrough in providing significant and sustained therapy for any of the LSDs came in the form of Ceredase® (alglucerase), an ERT for Gaucher disease developed by Genzyme and approved for commercialization in 1991. Ceredase® was the native human enzyme extracted from large numbers of human placentas and purified on an unprecedented manufacturing scale. While this product proved to be highly effective in treating the predominant macrophage-based pathology of Gaucher disease, the long-term logistics and commercial challenge of maintaining this type of product was daunting. However, Ceredase® established the therapeutic credibility of ERT, such that alternative manufacture of lysosmal enzymes by bioreactor technology became an immediate and potentially viable alternative [1]. As a result Ceredase® was quickly surplanted by a follow-on bioreactor product Cerezyme® in 1997, although a few patients are still maintained on Ceredase® treatment as a result of immunological intolerance to the recombinant enzyme.

In the mid-1980s rapid expansion of recombinant protein production techniques ushered in an explosion of protein and antibody-based therapies for many unmet diseases [4] However, commercial development of ERTs for rare diseases was not possible without one other simultaneous development—passing of the US Orphan Drug Act in 1983, later emulated by similar legislation in Japan (1993) and Europe (1999). By providing exclusive marketing rights for a period of several years to the company first able to obtain approval for a viable therapy (defined as diseases with less than 200,000 affected individuals in the US Orphan Drug Act), there was an incentive to engage in the long and risky business of developing therapies for rare diseases. Absence of direct competition also permitted pricing practices and revenue generation that could not have arisen in the open market. As a result there are now eight approved ERTs (Ceredase®, Cerezyme®, Fabrazyme®, Replagal®, Aldurazyme®, Naglazyme®, Myozyme®, and Elaprase®), with several others in various stages of development. This has been an important advance, the basis for which, bioreactor-produced enzymes, will be reviewed below.

23.2.3 LSDs and Models

What is evident immediately on attempting to develop a therapy for any particular LSD is the scant (and for many LSDs, virtually absent) information on disease pathophysiology. Beyond recognition of the enzyme deficiency responsible for the disease and the biochemistry of the accumulating substrate, much of the literature is in the form of case reports on individuals or small patient sets, often with minimal characterization of disease pathology. The paradox is that a more complete body of literature only develops after an effective treatment becomes available (e.g., Gaucher and Fabry diseases). Considerable initial research is therefore needed by any company seeking a successful therapeutic for a specific LSD.

Experience gained from developing the different ERTs (and in some cases their predecessors) has highlighted the individual complexities of providing drug exposure to the relevant tissues for a particular LSD. To characterize enzyme kinetics, drug exposure, inter- and intracellular transport, and substrate elimination, numerous molecular biology tools and in vivo strategies have been developed, specific to LSD biology. An obstacle has largely been the mismatch between animal models (mostly knockout or transgenic mice, or naturally occurring mutations in various species) and the human counterpart of the LSD in question. For Gaucher disease, at the time of developing Ceredase®, and later Cerezyme®, no suitable animal model was available since the murine knockout was embryonically lethal. For Fabry disease, there was a viable knockout mouse, however, alternative metabolic pathways in key cell types (endothelium, podocytes, cardiomyocytes) meant that only proof-of-principle pharmacodynamic data could be obtained from affected tissues (liver, vascular smooth muscle), thus severely limiting the value of the model. For Pompe disease, the opposite was true: there were two very suitable models, a naturally occurring mutation in quail (with significant functional impairment) and a knockout mouse with many of the pathologic features of the disease, thus allowing for significant preclinical investigation and development of a relatively complete preclinical dossier. Other development programs such as Aldurazyme® for MPS I relied on data from a naturally occurring dog model of the disease with the inherent difficulty of small data sets and inability of developing an all encompassing preclinical program. The generation of a nonlethal mouse model for Niemann Pick disease has allowed for detailed and relevant investigation into the safety of ERT in a model that has substrate accumulation.

23.2.4 Delivering ERTs

In healthy individuals lysosomal enzymes are transported from the endoplasmic reticulum to the lysosome via mannose-6-phosphate (M6P) mediated vesicles or other receptor-mediated transporters [5]. The phosphate-labeled enzyme in the case of M6P-mediated transport is released to the lysosome by clipping the phosphate and recyling the M6P vesicle to the endoplasmic reticulum. Some vesicles are also cycled to the cell membrane as part of a mechanism for mopping up enzyme that may have escaped into the interstitial space [6]. ERT is dependent on this latter mechanism of plasma membrane receptor cycling for capture of therapeutically delivered enzyme. The efficiency of enzyme uptake in the target tissue of specific LSDs depends on a complex interplay of receptor mediated mechanisms. This interplay begins with the delivery of the enzyme to the intravascular space by infusion. The unique relative combinations of exposed N-glycosylated sugars (mannose, mannose-6-phosphate, sialic acid, galactose) on the glycosylation sites of the enzyme is crucial to tissue targeting of the enzyme. It is the combination of relative organ blood flow, absolute receptor density, and relative receptor mix that ultimately determines exposure, uptake, and potency for any particular cell type/tissue. Organs such as the liver with multiple, densely populated receptor systems and high blood flow take up the bulk of delivered enzyme, an advantage in a disease such as Gaucher in which the liver is a key player. The opposite can be said for Pompe disease in which the skeletal muscle is poorly endowed with the relevant M6P receptor, thereby suffering from relatively poor exposure.

Since base glycosylation pattern and secondary decoration of the glycosylation sites can be manipulated by bioreactor conditioning or posttranslational chemistry respectively, manufacturers can significantly influence the therapeutic behavior of their products. Such flexibility, however, also produces the potential for unpredictable product variability and the need for very tight controls on bioreactor conditions and verification of product specifications. Delivered enzymes are therefore a controlled mix of enzyme species decorated with varying combinations of mannose, mannose-6-phosphate, sialic acid, and galactose moieties (among others). For example, based on the seven glycosylation sites of Myozyme®, and the combination and permutations of the oligosaccharide species potentially able to occupy these sites, several hundred thousand different versions of the enzyme are possible products of the individual cells in a bioreactor.

23.2.5 Defeating the Pathophysiology of LSDs

The final link in the therapeutic chain is delivery of the enzyme to the lysosome, enzyme activation, and processing of the substrate. Unlike small-molecule therapeutics, the delivery and eventual fate of the enzyme is a one-way street—once delivered to the lysosme, little if any recycling (or re-diffusion) occurs. This is a particular pharmacokinetic model that perplexes some regulators as well as some developers more used to small-molecule therapeutics. What occurs in the lysosome in many ERTs remains only partially understood. In the case of Myozyme®, for example, there is considerable processing (clipping and re-arrangement of the enzyme) into two successive, and active, multi-subunit complexes of the enzyme over several days [7]. Further the manner in which the substrate is processed, or in some cases fails to be processed (e.g., GL-3 in cardiomyocytes of Fabry patients, glycogen in the skeletal muscle of the most severely affected Pompe infants), is only partially understood. Considerable ongoing effort is focused on improving the yield of substrate removal, particularly when these failures negatively impact the best outcomes of ERT [8].

23.3 CURRENT TECHNOLOGIES

Since the early 1980s production of most therapeutic human proteins was performed in bioreactors containing well-characterized bacteria or yeasts [4]. More recently immortalized mammalian cell lines such as CHO (Chinese hamster ovary) and some human cell lines have increasingly been employed, particularly for more complex proteins [4]. Mammalian cell lines, while more demanding to produce and maintain, are necessary when correct glycosylation and appropriate folding behavior are required of the protein. Such is the case for most lysosomal enzymes, although new methods of engineering yeasts to produce humanized glycosylation patterns by selective knockouts and knock-ins of specific genes has recently provided a potentially more economic bioreactor alternative [9]. Cells in the bioreactor have been genetically modified to produce and secrete the desired human protein. Harvesting of the secreted protein is conducted either at the end of each culture run by processing the entire contents of the bioreactor before starting again (batch mode) or in the case of bioreactors equipped with cell microcarriers, in perfusion mode, by siphoning off culture medium in a continuous process. While a detailed description of bioreactor management is not the subject of this chapter, several features of the manufacturing process have a direct impact on preclinical testing. One is that significant control can be exerted over the composition of the protein, and more particularly the glycosylation pattern, by manipulating growth and culture conditions at several points in the manufacturing process. The second is that each scale-up to bigger reactors to meet patient demand changes the culture conditions and proportionality, resulting in a potentially different mix of enzyme species extracted from the bioreactor. These changes in composition, while relatively minor in most cases, can significantly alter the pharmacokinetics and potency of the product and are closely monitored by regulatory agencies. To place these challenges in context, we include a brief description of the bioreactor steps that most commonly impact product characteristics.

In general, the first step in producing bioreactor enzymes involves selecting the most appropriate cDNA from which to generate the protein. The gene for the human protein (enzyme in the case of ERT) is then inserted into a suitable vector (usually a plasmid), and transfected into the cell line intended for use in the bioreactor. Numerous transfected cell lines are tested for replication efficiency (clonal selection), based on activity/expression levels in high-throughput, plate format screens. During clonal selection, manipulation of the culture system with methotrexate or other gene expression modifiers may be employed to force expression in favor of a particular glycosylation pattern. A small number of candidates may be chosen from this process for benchtop flask culturing, from which the first more complete analysis of protein product can be performed by assays such as SDS-PAGE. At this stage the final candidate clone is selected to move forward into early production runs.

During the next stage a series of parallel activities accompanies progressive expansion of culturing into benchtop bioreactors (8 L), thence up to roughly 30 L systems. These include progressive purification steps and the development of more sophisticated assays to characterize the protein, including antibody-based assays (ELISAs, Westerns). The purpose at this stage is to produce sufficient purified enzyme to begin in vivo testing and to more accurately characterize the enzyme, particularly the glycosylation pattern and other characteristics that could determine in vivo behavior. Further modification of the enzyme product can be introduced in this midstage. One method is to introduce back into the cell culture media chemicals such as kifunensin that induce remodeling of the oligosaccharide side chains by promoting sialidases to clip certain sugars. The other way to modify the decorating oligosaccharides is to treat the purified product posttranslationally with enzymes specific for their activity on sialic acid, galactose, mannose, or glucosamine residues. This way the oligosaccharide complexes can be clipped to expose a different and more beneficial selection of signaling sugars. Each of these steps requires an array of assays to characterize each step and the resulting product. One further potential modification is open to the manufacturer. This involves taking the final glycoslyated product through a series of biochemical steps to restructure and adorn the oligosaccharides with the desired species (e.g., bisphosphorylation of a particular group of mannose terminations).

Bioreactor scale-up remains a considerable challenge for producers of ERTs. One reason is that pivotal trials for LSDs are conducted on small numbers of patients, using quantities of enzyme that can be produced in smaller bioreactors, before the need to scale up quantities of product (and bioreactor size) to meet commercial demand. This is a conundrum that places considerable pressure on sponsors. The pitfall is that different scales may change the product profile and pharmacokinetics characteristics sufficiently that regulators require duplication of preclinical safety studies and even clinical trials after the pivotal phase 3 trials have been completed. This places an undue burden on sponsors seeking registration for these rare conditions.

23.4 REGULATORY GUIDANCE

Little regulatory guidance was in place during development of the early recombinant human enzymes. Ceredase® and Cerezyme® were developed in the absence of the ICH S6 document, and therefore safety packages for these enzymes were a combination of traditional safety studies as well as specific studies to address the unique properties of a recombinant human protein. Studies for the recombinant human enzymes were designed to establish a safety margin above the clinical dosing regimen and to identify any possible effects of the administered protein. Since these enzymes are naturally occurring human proteins, the likelihood of side effects was low. However, understanding the pharmacokinetics, biodistribution, and exposure was key to establishing the safety profile of the enzymes.

With acceptance and implementation of the ICH S6 guidance document, more consistent development of the recombinant human proteins was possible. Similar studies were performed to assess the short- and long-term safety of administered proteins. Challenges induced by immunogenicity and the ability to dose normal animals for sufficient duration became the biggest issue. The utility of long-term dosing in rodents became questionable due to the anticipated generation of antibodies to the recombinant human protein. A major consideration was the relevance of the animal model, and which study would enable prediction of safety outcomes in patients. As more and more recombinant enzymes reached the development phase, the best studies and relevant endpoints were increasingly challenged. It was necessary to conduct studies for appropriate lengths of time, but also to deliver the protein in a manner similar to the clinical program. For ERTs this meant hour-long infusions in an animal considered likely to display the appropriate safety signals without exhibiting the hypersensitivity associated with administration of a human protein. Despite the lack of utility and predictability of many of these safety studies, they were still considered necessary for the safety assessment of products such as Fabrazyme® and Aldurazyme®.

Several recombinant human proteins have been approved over the last 10 years for use as long-term ERT in patients. Because of the specificity of the individual enzymes for particular lysososmal storage products, demonstration of a clear pharmacodynamic effect can only be performed in genetically modified animal models lacking the enzyme of interest (or, in rare naturally occurring disease models). Many genetically induced animal models are embryonic lethal or have alternative compensatory mechanisms such that the pathology of the disease is not consistent with the human disorder. In addition, as a result of significant antibody responses in some knockout mouse models, administration of recombinant human proteins may preclude meaningful interpretation. Long-term studies of the human protein are often not achievable in these animal models. Unfortunately, toxicology studies in normal animals are limited by the presence of native enzyme and the absence of pathologic substrate accumulation, both features that we now recognize can significantly impact safety of the product. While development programs for some of the enzyme replacement therapies were conducted prior to the ICH S6 document, many were nonetheless consistent with the guidance. The challenges and relevance of some of the development programs are described below.

It is important to remember that as a class of proteins, ERTs are expected to be relatively safe because of their specific targeting via mannose or mannose

6 phosphate receptors, their endogenous protein nature, and their relatively little activity at a physiologic pH. Since these are compelling arguments, safety evaluations for some early programs were very brief and limited to only a single species. Further, until recently, all of the safety studies conducted to support clinical used normal animals. In light of recent developments (see below) the relevance of this approach, and the relevant species, need to be reconsidered for development work.

23.4.1 Cerezyme®

Imiglucerase (Cerezyme®) was approved in 1997 for use as long-term enzyme replacement therapy in patients with confirmed diagnoses of non-neuropathic (type 1) or chronic neuropathic (type 3) Gaucher disease. Gaucher disease, also called gluocosylceramide lipidosis or β-glucocerebrosidase (GCR) deficiency, is the most common of the sphingolipidosis or lipid storage diseases, and is inherited in an autosomal recessive manner. Imiglucerase catalyses the breakdown of glucocerebrosidase, thereby preventing the buildup glucocerebroside. Imiglucerase is the recombinant form of alglucerase. Alglucerase (Ceredase®), derived from human placental tissue, was the first mannose-terminated-B-glucocerebrosidase.

The clinical features of Gaucher disease include anemia and thromoboctyopenia due to splenic sequestration, and bone marrow displacement by accumulating Gaucher cells. Hepatomegaly, spenomegaly, and osteonecrosis are common symptoms in type 1 and 3 Gaucher disease. The neuropathic forms also manifest neurological abnormalities such as seizures, dementia, spasticity, ataxia, and loss of intellectual function. Imiglucerase is given by infusion over 2 to 3 hours every two weeks, starting at a specified dose that can be lowered as therapy (and clinical response to treatment) progresses.

The efficacy of imiglucerase was not studied in an in vivo preclinical model because there is was no satisfactory animal model of Gaucher disease. Receptor binding was characterized in vitro using rat alveolar macrophages. Data from preclinical studies showed similar pharmacodynamic actions of imiglucerase and alglucerase. Three-month repeated intravenous dose toxicity studies were performed in rats and monkeys to support clinical trials and approval. Anti-imiglucerase antibodies were detected in all dose groups in rats. However, the onset of the antibody response and the number of animals responding was dose dependent. Interestingly, the anti-imiglucerase antibody response was more prominent in monkeys than in rats. The most common clinical side effect is hypersensitivity. Because humans can develop antibodies that may affect efficacy, it is recommended that patients be monitored for any allergic reaction during their first year of treatment.

There are some interesting and important features of the development strategy adopted for this product which differ from more conventional approaches. It seems reasonable to assume that a nature-identical human protein produced by rDNA technology will be inherently safe if administered to humans. Therefore it seems reasonable to conclude that risk assessment of proteins that are not nature-identical should focus on differences from the natural product, since such differences might affect important processes such as primary biological action, tissue distribution, storage, metabolism, clearance, and immune response.

Imiglucerase differs from the native glycoprotein in two important respects. First, there is a single amino acid substitution in the primary sequence, which arose in the cloning process. Second, the glycosyl moiety of the protein is deliberately modified to increase the affinity of rGCR for the mannose receptors of macrophages. The philosophy used in the risk assessment program was, first, to compare the rDNA product with the natural protein and, second, to investigate directly the preclinical safety of imiglucerase. It is important to recognize that the pivotal 13-week toxicity study in the primate was performed with material from a 2000 L batch, which is effectively the clinical marketed finished product. This lot was a prevalidation lot manufactured by the same process, as the 2000 L validated process, and although full characterization was not conducted, it did meet all release specifications and therefore should be indicative of the clinical/market material at the 2000 L scale. The data from this animal study were therefore central to interpretation of potential human risk. Because no satisfactory animal model of Gaucher disease existed, it was not possible to predict the efficacy of Cerezyme® from animal studies.

The development program was designed to elucidate the fundamental biological properties and action of imiglucerase. However, in comparison to the preclinical toxicology plan, which is generally presented for low molecular weight pharmaceuticals, there were several obvious differences.

Broadly, there was no study of clastogenicity, only one species was used in the evaluation of acute toxicity, and no studies of potential effects on reproductive function or oncogenic potential were performed. In contrast, detailed studies of the biologically important receptor binding and macrophage uptake were presented together with detailed assessments of the kinetic processes defining receptor binding and plasma clearance.

Macrophage mannose receptor binding is a particularly important issue in the assessment of rGCR as an enzyme replacement therapy because macrophages are the predominant cell type that accumulates lipid in Gaucher patients. In addition demonstrating that the recombinant protein behaved virtually identically to the naturally occurring protein would provide reassurance in the risk assessment process.

A series of pharmacokinetic and ADME studies was performed with imiglucerase in order to assess clearance and targeting of imiglucerase in vivo. Because there was no suitable animal model for Gaucher disease, these studies were performed in normal animals.

Three toxicology studies were conducted: an acute study in rats and two 13-week studies in rats and monkeys. Most findings in these studies could be attributed to infusion of large amounts of exogenous protein that directly or indirectly (through an immune response) effected changes. As would be expected, repeated administration of Cerezyme® to rats and monkeys elicited a dose-dependent antibody response in more than 50% of the animals exposed to the test article. Since this antibody response against imiglucerase was demonstrated in the rat and monkey, it was considered that additional longer term toxicology studies were not justified as potential target organ exposure to the test article could not be quantified. In view of minimal, subchronic toxicity findings this was considered an acceptable safety package for marketing approval. An Ames test was also performed.

23.4.2 Fabrazyme®

In 2003 agalsidase beta (Fabrazyme®) was approved for use in patients. Agalsidase beta is a recombinant human α-Galactosidase A enzyme with the same amino acid sequence as the native enzyme. In Fabry disease an X-linked inherited deficiency in α-Galactosidase (αGAL) leads to progressive lysosomal accumulation of globotriasylceramide (GL-3) in most tissues of the body. As a recombinant equivalent of naturally occurring α-Galactosidase, recombinant human α-Galactosidase (r-hαGAL) was also expected to reduce GL-3 accumulation in tissue, and thereby ultimately to alleviate the clinical consequences of GL-3 accumulation. Pharmacodynamic studies were designed to evaluate the potential for r-hαGAL to clear GL-3 substrate from tissues of an αGAL SV129 knockout mouse model. The use of the mouse model is justified as it provides the only biochemical model for Fabry Disease.

A safety pharmacology study in dogs assessed cardiovascular and respiratory toxicity. Neurological toxicity was not assessed as part of the safety pharmacology study since r-hαGal is a large protein and unlikely to cross the blood–brain barrier. In accordance with the International Conference on Harmonization (ICH) S7 guideline, Safety Pharmacology Studies for Human Pharmaceutics, secondary pharmacology studies are not warranted as available information from toxicology studies and clinical studies, including 24 months of safety information from patients in the phase 3 trial who have continued on treatment but have not identified a cause for concern such that secondary pharmacology studies would be required.

Biodistribution studies were performed in Balb/C mice, the αGAL SV129 knockout mouse model and Sprague–Dawley rats to assess the uptake and stability of r-hαGAL in target organs. Additionally pharmacokinetic analyses were performed across three species (rat, dog, and monkey) with either single-dose or repeat-dose administration of r-hαGAL. Accumulation studies were conducted in rats and monkeys.

In the toxicity studies the maximum administered dose was identified as the NOAEL. A traditional lethal dose study was not performed. Instead, the relationship between dose levels and toxicity were evaluated. These studies demonstrated that r-hαGAL had extremely low toxicity. It was unlikely that a clear toxic dose could have been identified for r-hαGAL given that r-hαGAL cannot be sufficiently concentrated to deliver a lethal dose and test animals will not tolerate the volume required to deliver a less concentrated lethal dose. This approach is consistent with the International Conference on Harmonization (ICH) S6 guideline, Preclinical Safety Evaluation of Biotechnology Derived Pharmaceuticals, which states that for some classes of products with little to no toxicity, it may not be possible to define a specific maximum dose, so consideration should be given to the volume that can safely and humanely be administered to the test animal.

Both single-dose and repeat-dose toxicity studies were conducted in two species, rat and dog, and rat and monkey, respectively. In developing plans for the toxicity studies, the Sprague–Dawley rat was selected as a relevant species to test. A 27-week repeat-dose toxicity study in SD rats was conducted to evaluate the long-term safety profile of r-hαGAL. Given the lifelong use of r-hαGAL in Fabry patients, it was recognized that data from a second species at high doses would be useful. A second long-term safety study was therefore conducted in cynomolgus monkeys. The ICH guideline provides that in principle, the dosing duration for the toxicity study may be six months even in the case of a test substance for which the expected period of clinical use exceeds six months. In addition long-term administration of a compound that is known to be immunogenic in an animal model is unlikely to give relevant safety information. Due to the immunogenic nature of the recombinant protein in the nonhuman primate, dosing for a period of nine months was unlikely to provide any additional information over dosing to six months. Conduct of a long-term infusion study was the most technically achievable in the nonhuman primate.

Additionally antigenic studies were performed in two species (rat and monkey) and an embryofetal development study was conducted in rats. Sperm morphology evaluation, conducted as part of the 25-week repeat-dose toxicology study in monkeys was inconclusive due to the immature age of the monkeys. A segment 1 study in rats was also conducted. Perinatal development studies have not been conducted, and the recommendation that r-hαGAL should not be used during pregnancy, unless clearly necessary, is adequately reflected in the proposed labeling. Given that r-hαGAL is a nature-identical human protein, and based on the therapeutic indication and patient population, studies to assess effects of r-hαGAL on mutagenic and carcinogenic potential were not considered necessary as part of the development program.

There were no significant treatment-related findings in any of these studies. The only finding consistent with administration of test article was a hypersensitivity response seen in the rat study. As predicted, antibodies to agalsidase beta were detected in both chronic studies, but the antibodies did not have an impact on safety assessments or pharmacokinetics of the therapeutic.

In the clinical setting, infusion reactions occurred in many patients treated with agalsidase beta, and some of these reactions were severe. Infusion reactions occurred in some patients after receiving antipyretics, antihistamines, and oral steroids.

23.4.3 Aldurazyme®

Laronidase (α-l-iduronidase) is intended for the treatment of mucopolysac-charidosis I (MPSI). The MPS disorders are caused by deficiencies of specific lysosomal enzymes required for the catabolism of glycosaminoglycans (GAGs). Accumulation of GAG substrates occurs in a variety of tissues and is depen-dent on the location of the affected substrates and their rate of turnover. Deficiency of α-l-iduronidase results in accumulation of dermatan and heparan sulfate in many tissues, particularly connective tissue, leading to chronic pro-gressive loss of joint function, disordered skeletal growth, organomegaly, and neurologic impairment in more affected cases.

Canine MPS I was discovered in a Plott hound that presented with corneal clouding [10]. Studies by Shull and Neufeld showed that the dogs were defi-cient in α-l-iduronidase [11]. Being null, MPS I dogs are genetically similar to the most severe form of MPS I in humans, but clinically they more closely resemble moderately affected patients. These animals provide a valuable bio-chemical/clinical model for MPS I disease. Since they have no confounding residual enzyme activity, they accumulate GAGs in relevant tissues, and their clinical phenotype closely resembles the human disease.

MPS I dogs were used to evaluate the biodistribution of rh-iduronidase, pharmacodynamic reduction of tissue GAGs and in vivo efficacy. Pharmaco-kinetics and the effects of various doses and regimens of rh-iduronidase were also evaluated in this model. Heterozygote dogs from the MPS I colony, referred to as normal carriers, were used to derive normal tissue levels of α-l-iduronidase activity and GAG storage.

The pharmacokinetics of rh-iduronidase were characterized in two studies, along with five pharmacodynamic studies in which pharmacokinetics, biodis-tribution, or both, were determined. The pharmacodynamic studies were con-ducted in the MPS I dog evaluating reduction of tissue and urine GAG levels. These studies ranged from short-term (5–12 days) to long-term studies lasting up to 74 weeks. Multiple-dose levels were tested to determine the effect of dose on levels of α-l-iduronidase activity and GAG in tissues and urine. The effects of dosing regimen, including once and three times weekly, as well as continuous infusion, were also tested. In the long-term studies, assessments were made of the effects of treatment on the clinical symptoms of the disease. Two additional toxicokinetic studies were conducted as part of an acute single-dose intravenous (IV) infusion toxicity study in normal dogs and as part of a 26-week IV infusion toxicity study in cynomolgus monkeys.

There were no significant treatment-related findings in any of these studies. The only test article related finding was a hypersensitivity response seen in a few of the animals treated. Antibodies to laronidase were detected in the chronic studies, but the antibodies did not have an impact on the safety assessment or pharmacokinetics of the therapeutic. In addition there were no findings at six months that had not been noted at the three-month time points.

In the clinical studies the most common adverse events observed with laronidase treatment were upper respiratory tract infection, rash, and injection site reaction. The most common adverse reactions requiring intervention were infusion-related reactions (IRRs), particularly flushing. Those requiring intervention were offset by slowing the infusion rate, temporarily stopping the infusion, and/or administering additional antipyretics and/or antihistamines.

23.4.4 Myozyme®

In 2006 recombinant alglucosidase alfa (Myozyme®) received approval in the United States and Europe for the treatment of Pompe disease in all patients. While the development program of alglucosidase alfa was in consideration of the ICH S6 document, and with further consideration to conduct studies in the most relevant species with the greatest predictability, additional pressure was placed on this program for the establishment of safety in animal studies.

The GAA knockout mice used for the nonclinical program were generated by Raben et al. [12,13]. The model was produced by inserting a neomycin-resistance (neo) gene, into exon 6 of the murine GAA gene, resulting in disruption of the coding region. Mice homozygous for this disruption ($6^{neo}/6^{neo}$) lack enzyme activity, accumulate lysosomal glycogen, and "recapitulate(s) critical features of both the infantile and the adult forms of the disease at a pace suitable for the evaluation of enzyme or gene replacement" [12]. By 3 weeks of age, homozygous $6^{neo}/6^{neo}$ mice begin to accumulate glycogen in cardiac and skeletal muscle lysosomes due to the lack of GAA enzyme activity. However, they grow normally, reach adulthood, and remain fertile. By 8 to 9 months of age, obvious muscle wasting and a weak and waddling gait develops, and, by 18 to 19 months of age, they have severe progressive muscle-wasting resembling advanced late-onset Pompe disease. At this age, they have pronounced glycogen accumulation in multiple organs (including skeletal muscle, diaphragm, heart, and brain), as well as cardiomyopathy, hypotonia, severe motor disability, and profound muscle weakness and wasting [12].

Glycogen accumulation and extent of muscle pathology in GAA knockout mice is not as striking as that noted in infantile-onset Pompe patients. Based on life span $6^{neo}/6^{neo}$ GAA mice more closely resemble late-onset Pompe disease in humans. Despite these differences GAA knockout mice provided a valuable tool for preclinical studies. Since they lack GAA enzyme activity, they can be used to evaluate the pharmacokinetics and biodistribution of GAA activity following administration of clinically relevant doses of rhGAA. Moreover, since the heart and skeletal muscle of GAA knockout mice contain accumulated glycogen, they can also be used to evaluate the pharmacodynamic effects of rhGAA dose and dosing regimens on glycogen depletion. Since most pharmacodynamic studies were conducted on asymptomatic mice less than 6 months of age, we were unable to determine if rhGAA could reverse or stabilize the clinical phenotype.

While useful for evaluating substrate reduction and tissue distribution, the knockout mouse also presented specific challenges to the preclinical development program. After repeated administration of rhGAA, a predictable hypersensitivity response to the recombinant human protein was observed. Frequently this reaction resulted in morbidity and mortality associated with test article administration. This hypersensitivity reaction responded to diphenhydramine prior to, and as necessary, during dosing; however, such intervention complicated interpretation of toxicity studies.

In vivo, single- and repeat-dose pharmacodynamic studies were conducted in GAA knockout mice to evaluate the efficacy of rhGAA. Most of these studies were designed to assess depletion of glycogen from target tissues, while others assessed the time course of glycogen depletion and re-accumulation following administration of rhGAA. Tissue glycogen content was measured by biochemical assay and histomorphometric analysis. In addition a safety pharmacology study was performed in beagle dogs.

A series of pharmacokinetic studies were performed to assess absorption of rhGAA across single- and repeat-dose administration, species (mouse, rat, dog, and monkey), dose, formulation, and process scale. Process scale-up to larger reactors to accommodate the high dose and rapid expansion of patient numbers has placed an especially demanding pharmacokinetic burden on this program, even postapproval. Biodistribution studies were performed in GAA knockout mice to assess the uptake and tissue residence time of rhGAA in target organs.

Toxicity studies were designed to establish a maximum tolerated dose and safety profile in mice, rats, dogs, and cynomolgus monkeys. Two single-dose acute toxicity studies in rats and dogs, two repeat-dose subchronic toxicity studies in rats, one repeat-dose subchronic toxicity study in mice, and two repeat-dose chronic toxicity studies in cynomolgus monkeys were performed to evaluate the safety of rhGAA administered intravenously (IV). Furthermore three reproductive toxicity studies were conducted in mice to assess the effect of rhGAA on fertility, early embryonic development and embryofetal development.

23.4.5   Acid Sphingomyelinase

Niemann–Pick disease is caused by partial or complete absence of the lysosomal enzyme acid sphingomyelinase, resulting in lysosmal accumulation of sphingomyelin in numerous tissues, but particularly in cells of the macrophage lineage and in neurons. Clinically patients suffer from progressive hepatosplenomegaly and associated pathology, and many eventually succumbing to pulmonary complications and pneumonia in late childhood to middle age (Niemann–Pick type B). Recent characterization of Niemann–Pick type B populations suggests significant pathophysiology related to high cholesterol profiles, resulting in many early deaths from vascular disease. In the most severe classification of the disease (Niemann–Pick type A) rapidly progressive neurologic disease claims individuals in early childhood.

An appropriate knockout mouse model for Niemann–Pick disease is available. This ASMKO mouse was produced by inserting a neomycin-resistant gene (neo) into exon 2 of the *ASM* gene resulting in disruption of the coding region [14]. Mice homozygous for this disruption lack acid sphingomyelinase activity and develop a clinical condition resembling Niemann–Pick A disease. Born normal, these mice develop trembling and ataxia by 8 weeks of age, progressing through lethargy to severe ataxia by 4 months and death between 6 and 8 months of age. Progressive accumulation of sphingomyelin occurs in macrophage lineage cells, the lungs, and the CNS in a manner closely resembling the human disease. This model has allowed for significant preclinical development efforts and disease-related characterization.

As discussed previously, relevant animal models and predictability of safety have become significant issues. Recent experience with developing ERT for Niemann–Pick disease has highlighted the potential risk of relying on standard toxicity models and not identifying the most relevant test species.

To establish the safety profile for recombinant human acid sphingomyelinase (rhASM), several animal models were evaluated including normal rats and dogs. Findings from three single- and repeat-dose toxicity studies resulted in a no-observable-effect level (NOEL) of the highest doses tested. However, in parallel efforts to maximize efficacy of rhASM in different organ systems, unexpected deaths occurred in ASMKO mice at several dose levels, all well below the previously determined NOEL. Signs of toxicity included lethargy, hypothermia, and death, symptomatic of clinical shock. Subsequent characterization of this response established that the toxicity is directly related to substrate load, but the load can be managed pharmacodynamically by initially dosing at low levels to deplete the most labile substrate. Doses can then be increased to the therapeutic levels necessary to maintain control of substrate in all tissues. Appropriate adjustments to the clinical dosing regimen have been incorporated in our phase 1 protocol to manage this risk. The fact that toxicity occurred only in knockout animals indicates that for LSDs (and perhaps other diseases with substrate accumulation) future toxicological studies may need to be conducted in animal models of the disease to ensure that the most sensitive species has been included.

23.5 CONCLUSION

Recombinant enzymes manufactured from mammalian cell-based bioreactors have established a solid treatment paradigm for several lysosomal storage diseases, a class of rare diseases until recently considered untreatable. While small clinical populations, variable animal models, and the need to upscale manufacturing during and after approval have provided formidable regulatory challenges, the fact that eight separate enzyme therapies have emerged in little over a decade is remarkable. Credit must go to the companies that have committed to this risky field, and also to the foresight of legislatures that established critical orphan drug laws and to the regulatory bodies in many countries open to creative approaches by sponsors. The examples presented of successful preclinical programs demonstrate the importance of flexibility based on unique aspects of the individual diseases and the availability of relevant animal models to address specific safety concerns, consistent with the ICHS6 science-based approach.

New challenges resulting from this decade of cumulated experience are, however, placing increasing pressure on maintaining this momentum. Among the most pressing are (1) the troubling antibody responses to recombinant human enzymes in patients—nearly impossible to investigate effectively in animal models; (2) the recent discovery that the substrate load (in some LSDs) may impart unique toxicity risks that cannot be explored in normal animals; and (3) increasing evidence that despite predictable dose–responses in relevant models, some patients (and some tissues) are not pharmacodynamically (and clinically) responsive even at elevated doses. These, among others, continue to impose increasingly complex preclinical and CMC regulatory obligations at a time when increasingly rare LSDs invariably dictate more restrained investment. When combined with the absence of a clear pathway to accessing the CNS, the prospect for the next decade of ERT development is less certain. Based on recent small-molecule approaches to substrate inhibition and chaperone-assisted refolding for certain mutations, the next wave of development for LSDs, including those with neurologic involvement, may come through small-molecule therapies (possibly in combination with proteins). Gene therapy with long-lived vectors, and in combination with tissue-specific delivery, remains a viable but complex option. On the positive side are the increasingly creative animal models and laboratory technologies available to support these more complex paradigms—there is no doubt that they will be needed!

REFERENCES

1. Pastores GM, Sibille AR, Grabowski GA. Enzyme therapy in Gaucher disease type 1: dosage efficacy and adverse effects in 33 patients treated for 6 to 24 months. *Blood* 1993;82(2):408–16.
2. Watts W, Gibbs D, eds. *Lysosomal Storage Diseases: Biochemcial and Clinical Aspects*. London: Taylor and Francis, 1986.
3. Thurberg BL, Rennke H, Colvin RB, Dikman S, Gordon RE, Collins AB, Desnick RJ, O'Callaghan M. Globotriaosylceramide accumulation in the Fabry kidney is cleared from multiple cell types after enzyme replacement therapy. *Kidney Int* 2002;62(6):1933–46.
4. Alcamo E. *DNA Technology: The Awesome Skill*. San Diego: Academic Press, 1996.
5. Kornfeld S. Structure and function of the mannose 6-phosphate/insulinlike growth factor II receptors. *Annu Rev Biochem* 1992;61:307–30.

6. Griffiths G, Hoflack B, Simons K, Mellman I, Kornfeld S. The mannose 6 phosphate receptor and the biogenesis of lysosomes. *Cell* 1988;52(3):329–41.

7. Moreland RJ, Jin X, Zhang XK, Decker RW, Albee KL, Lee KL, Cauthron RD, Brewer K, Edmunds T, Canfield WM. Lysosomal acid alpha-glucosidase consists of four different peptides processed from a single chain precursor. *J Biol Chem* 2005;280(8):6780–91.

8. Fukuda T, Ewan L, Bauer M, Mattaliano RJ, Zaal K, Ralston E, Plotz PH, Raben N. Dysfunction of endocytic and autophagic pathways in a lysosomal storage disease. *Ann Neurol* 2006;59(4):700–8.

9. Hamilton SR, Davidson RC, Sethuraman N, Nett JH, Jiang Y, Rios S, Bobrowicz P, Stadheim TA, Li H, Choi BK, Hopkins D, Wischnewski H, Roser J, Mitchell T, Strawbridge RR, Hoopes J, Wildt S, Gerngross TU. Humanization of yeast to produce complex terminally sialylated glycoproteins. *Science* 2006;313(5792): 1441–3.

10. Shull RM, Munger RJ, Spellacy E, Hall CW, Constantopoulos G, Neufeld EF. Canine alpha-L-iduronidase deficiency. A model of mucopolysaccharidosis I. *Am J Pathol* 1982;109(2):244–8.

11. Spellacy E, Shull RM, Constantopoulos G, Neufeld EF. A canine model of human alpha-l-iduronidase deficiency. *Proc Natl Acad Sci USA* 1983;80(19):6091–5.

12. Raben N, Nagaraju K, Lee E, Kessler P, Byrne B, Lee L, LaMarca M, King C, Ward J, Sauer B, Plotz P. Targeted disruption of the acid alpha-glucosidase gene in mice causes an illness with critical features of both infantile and adult human glycogen storage disease type II. *J Biol Chem* 1998;273(30):19086–92.

13. Raben N, Nagaraju K, Lee E, Plotz P. Modulation of disease severity in mice with targeted disruption of the acid alpha-glucosidase gene. *Neuromuscul Disord* 2000; 10(4–5):283–91.

14. Horinouchi K, Erlich S, Perl DP, Ferlinz K, Bisgaier CL, Sandhoff K, Desnick RJ, Stewart CL, Schuchman EH. Acid sphingomyelinase deficient mice: a model of types A and B Niemann-Pick disease. *Nat Genet* 1995;10(3):288–93.

CHAPTER 24

Toxicology of Oligonucleotide Therapeutics and Understanding the Relevance of the Toxicities

ARTHUR A. LEVIN, PhD, DABT, and SCOTT P. HENRY, PhD, DABT

Contents

24.1 INTRODUCTION

This chapter will describe the existing practices for assessing the toxicity of oligonucleotide therapeutics and the rationale for these practices. The only

Preclinical Safety Evaluation of Biopharmaceuticals: A Science-Based Approach to Facilitating Clinical Trials, edited by Joy A. Cavagnaro
Copyright © 2008 by John Wiley & Sons, Inc.

537

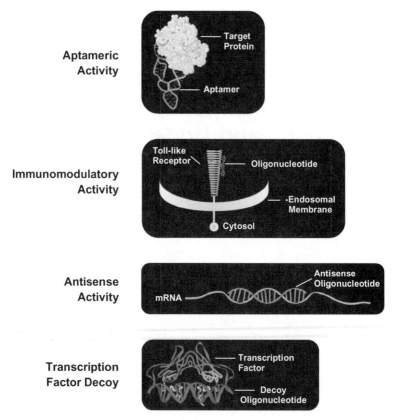

Figure 24.1 Cartoon depicting the mechanism of action of oligonucleotide molecules for aptameric interactions with proteins, interactions with specific receptors of the innate immunity, target mRNAs through hybridization, and transcriptional activators as transcription decoys. Note siRNA works through a hybridization dependent mechanism as depicted for antisense. See color insert.

way to discuss the practices is to put them into the context of the existing body of knowledge on the toxicity of these novel therapeutic entities. In this regard the authors are indebted to those institutions that have shared their scientific findings in the open literature allowing the science behind the application of therapeutic oligonucleotides to be shared and advanced.

There are at least four categories of oligonucleotide therapeutics: single-stranded oligonucleotides that work through RNAse H or steric effects, double-stranded RNAs that work through the dicer pathway, immunostimulatory oligonucleotides that work by stimulating innate immunity, and aptamers that work by binding to proteins and modifying their function (Figure 24.1). (A fifth group, transcription factor decoys, is not going to be covered in this review.) These are a diverse group of agents, with widely differing chemistries.

Because of such diversity the testing strategies that work for some compounds may not be applicable to all, or in some cases there are insufficient published data to know whether a strategy works.

24.2 CHEMISTRY

24.2.1 Aptamers

Aptamers are nonnaturally occurring nucleic acid derived molecules that bind to protein and peptide targets with high affinity and specificity. A typical therapeutic aptamer comprises 15 to 40 nucleotides, folds into a unique secondary and/or tertiary structure that allows specific target recognition, and contains a substantial number of nucleotides with modifications (e.g., 2′-methoxy) that prevent degradation by serum nucleases. Aptamers are often derivatized site specifically with high molecular weight polyethylene glycol (PEG) to increase their effective size, decrease renal filtration, and increase circulating half-life in vivo. Most commonly aptamers are used to target extracellular protein interactions. That way the mechanisms of action of aptamers are more comparable to monoclonal antibodies or traditional drugs than to antisense ODNs or siRNAs that act by hybridization to mRNAs intracellularly.

24.2.2 Immunostimulatory Oligonucleotides

Immunostimulatory CpG oligodeoxynucleotides are approximately 20 to 30 nucleotides in length, with phosphorothioate or occasionally phosphodiester linkages. Phosphorothioate linkages replace the more labile phosphodiester linkages that increase the resistance of the oligonucleotide to nucleases. The distinguishing features of these oligonucleotides are their palindromic hexamer motifs that stimulate receptors in the innate immune system through interaction with TLR9 receptor. The compounds that Coley Pharmaceuticals, Dynavax, and others are currently developing share a great deal of similarity with the early first generation phosphorothioate oligodeoxynucleotides used as antisense agents: that is to say, they are roughly 6000 to 7000 Da molecular weight with around 20 to 30 negative charges. Because each phosphorothioate linkage is a chiral center, there are 2^{N-1} stereoisomers possible (where N = number of nucleotides). The phosphorothioate linkages tend to increase protein binding compared to the phosphodiester linkages of endogenous nucleic acids. The increase in protein binding has important effects on distribution and toxicity of these drugs (reviewed in [1]).

Newer classes of immunostimulatory oligonucleotides that are composed of RNA and bind different receptors are now being identified. Single- and double-stranded RNA have the potential to be proinflammatory, but the receptor and sequence-dependence are distinct from CpG oligonucleotides. These RNA oligonucleotides tend to bind to TLR3, 7, and 8 as well as the more recently characterized soluble cytoplasmic receptors such as RIG-1 (see below). Like antisense DNA, the proinflammatory effects of RNA are a property to potentially be exploited for immunomdulatory effects or minimized in the case of siRNA.

24.2.3   Single-Stranded Oligonucleotides Used for Antisense Activity

For simplicity we will concentrate on two classes of single-stranded antisense oligonucleotides (ASOs) . The first are those with phosphorothioate backbones. These compounds can have both deoxy ribose and ribose sugars. Oligonucleotides that employ RNase H to cleave the target mRNA require at least a portion of the molecule to be DNA-like because the RNase H recognizes a RNA/DNA duplex. These compounds are approximately 20 nucleotides in length with 19 negative charges and 2^{19} stereoisomers. These compounds differ from endogenous DNA (or RNA) by the substitution of a sulfur for a nonbridging oxygen in each phosophodiester linkage. In addition some oligonucleotides are modified at the 2′ position of the ribose with methoxyethyl (second-generation ASOs) or methoxy groups. This modification increases affinity for the mRNA target and slightly alters protein binding. Most important, it markedly reduces the susceptibility of the oligonucleotide to exonuclease cleavage, and methoxyethyl modifications tend to slightly diminish the binding of the phosphorothioate oligonucleotide to proteins. Even this small change in protein binding has significant consequences to the pharmacokinetic and toxicologic properties (reviewed in [1]).

The second class of single-stranded ASO are the morpholinos. These compounds have the typical heterocyclic bases attached to a substituted morpholino ring system. These are linked together with dimethylamino phosphinyldeoxy functions. These compounds bind and act through steric action on the mRNA. The morpholinos differ from immunostimulatory oligonucleotides and from RNase H-utilizing oligonucleotides because they are uncharged. The absence of a charge diminishes protein binding significantly, which has important implications for toxicities and for distribution. Binding to plasma proteins has the beneficial effect of protecting the oligonucleotide from glomerular filtration, and enhancing binding to cells and cell uptake. Without charges, the morpholinos are more susceptible to rapid excretion in urine. On the other hand, the minimal protein binding of morpholinos reduces their potential to have toxicities associated with protein binding, for example, changes in activated partial thromboplastin time (aPTT) [2].

24.2.4   Double-Stranded RNAs–siRNA

These oligonucleotides differ from the other classes of nucleotides described above in that they are duplexes rather than single stranded. Because this class of nucleotides is relatively new and because there are two strands that can be modified chemically, it is more difficult to generalize about the chemistry of this class. Because unmodified RNA is so labile, some chemical modifications or protection from nucleases are needed to reduce degradation in plasma and tissues in order to be effective in vivo. Some siRNAs utilize phosphorothioate linkages, and others do not. Sugar modification such as 2' O-methyl and 2' flouro have also been used to improve durability and affinity for targets, often in complex repeating patterns in either the sense or antisense strand of the duplex (reviewed in [3]). What is critical to this chapter is that the duplexed oligonucleotide has different physical properties than a single-stranded nucleic acid and a molecular weight that is twofold greater. The increase in molecular weight and the duplex nature significantly affect the cell uptake of these compounds. Unlike single-stranded antisense oligonucleotides, these double-stranded oligonucleotides do not readily penetrate cells. This has led some researchers to conjugate them with small lipophilic molecules like cholesterol: a modification that may have significant consequences for the toxicity profile. Liposomal formulations are the other approach that has been taken to improve cell uptake with siRNA therapeutics. The use of complex formulations sets siRNA apart from the other classes of oligonucleotide therapeutics.

24.3 PHARMACOKINETICS

24.3.1 Assessing the Pharmacokinetics of Oligonucleotide Drugs

On the surface the assessment of the pharmacokinetics of oligonucleotide therapeutics is not entirely different than the assessment of the pharmacokinetics of traditional drugs. The simplest assessment of oligonucleotide pharmacokinetics can be obtained by using radiolabeled compounds with nonexchangeable tritium on one or more of the heterocycles [4,5]. Mass balance experiments with compounds so labeled provided the first data on terminal elimination half-lives and organ distribution. In addition, depending on site of the radiolabel, it is possible to follow the labeled heterocycle through catabolism to the end product CO_2. Phosphorothioate oligonucleotides can be labeled on the sulfur atom, but these can be labile and the resultant products are low molecular weight entities found in urine, possibly in the form of sulfate, thiophosphate, or low molecular weight thiated oligonucleotide fragments.

With the advent of sensitive bioanalytical assays like capillary gel electrophoresis, hybridization-dependent ELISA [6] and LC/MS [7–9], it is now possible to perform toxicokinetic analyses as part of toxicity studies either in satellite groups or in study animals without the use of radiolabel [10]. These techniques provide a basis of assessing the exposure of target organs in toxicology studies and allow for the determination of critical concentrations for the production of morphologic or functional changes. These relationships can be used to design dose and schedule for clinical trials [11].

One strategy being used for a full assessment of the pharmaco/toxicokinetics of oligonucleotide therapeutics is to perform a mass balance study with radiolabeled material followed by quantitation with combustion of tissues and scintillation counting or with whole body autoradiography. This type of study provides an understanding of distribution and routes of clearance. It is possible to also collect information on the metabolic fate of the oligonucleotide, but more often metabolite identification and toxicokinetics can be performed on samples from animals dosed with nonradiolabeled material using HPLC, CGE, or LC/MS [10].

If a novel oligonucleotide chemistry or route of administration is being tested for the first time in a species, it is advantageous to understand the tissue kinetics to design dose regimens for toxicity studies. However, in most cases it is possible to estimate what the kinetics of a novel oligonucleotide sequence are based on data from other sequences with related chemistry. In those cases the pharmacokinetics studies can be performed in conjunction with subchronic studies. A strategy employed by our group uses a satellite group in large animal studies to assess tissue levels after a single dose, after a loading regimen, and then at specified intervals after the completion of the loading regimen. This design allows us to understand first-dose kinetics, as well as multiple-dose kinetics and finally drug clearance from plasma and tissues. Properly spaced sampling allows for the estimation of tissue half-lives in large animals with relatively small numbers of animals. In the animals in the toxicology study groups, we also analyze plasma and tissues samples for drug and metabolite levels at the end of the treatment and recovery periods. It is these results that allow us to relate tissue/plasma concentrations of drug and metabolites with histopathologic or functional changes.

24.3.2 A Brief Summary of the Pharmacokinetics of Oligonucleotide Drugs

Aptameric Oligonucleotides The pharmacokinetics of aptameric oligonucleotides is highly dependent on the chemical modifications. In most cases these compounds are modified to have long residence time in plasma by the addition of pendants to the backbone structure consisting of polyethylene glycol. With these pendants plasma residence time can be substantially prolonged, often to a time scale of hours or days. The pharmacokinetics of a particular drug can be tailored by the modifications to yield an optimal clearance rate. For this class of drugs protein binding is essential for both prolonging half-life as well the actual activity of the drug. Longer half-lives in plasma are beneficial for aptamers that have intracellular sites of activity as they seem to increase tissue uptake [12,13]. Like PS ODNs aptamers accumulate in renal proximal tubular cells, and in resident macrophages in various organs, and are visible when stained with hematoxylin.

Phosphorothioate Oligonucleotides Single-stranded phosphorothioate ODNs (PS ODN), either immunostimulatory or ASO, administered parenterally appear rapidly in plasma where they are bound to hydrophilic sites on plasma proteins, and are thus protected from glomerular filtration. These binding sites are not the hydrophilic sites where lipophilic drugs bind, and there is little competition for plasma protein binding by ODNs [14]. Plasma kinetics are polyphasic with a short distribution phase that is on the order of hours, and then a terminal elimination phase that has half-lives on the order of days or weeks (reviewed in [11,15,16]). The initial distribution phase may also be influenced by plasma metabolism. Depending on the chemistry of the PS ODN, there can be metabolism by nucleases in plasma, or if the PS ODN is protected from exonuclease metabolism with 2′ modifications, then there is little or no metabolism in plasma.

The initial distribution phase is primarily related to binding to and distribution into tissues, with liver, kidney, lymph nodes, and spleen being the sites of highest binding and uptake. For PS ODN little renal clearance occurs because of the binding of the PS ODN to plasma proteins. However, at very high doses plasma protein binding can be saturated and spillage into urine is more likely (reviewed in [17]). Uptake into tissues is also saturable, and therefore the distribution kinetics are dose dependent, with clearance rates slowing and AUC increasing with increasing doses [16,18–20]. Once bound to cells, PS ODNs transit into cells by moving down concentration gradients from extracellular compartments to intracellular compartments, probably by shuttling from one protein binding site to another, across cell membranes. PS ODNs in cells bind to available targets, but the majority of the PS ODN in cells is probably bound to intracellular proteins (reviewed in [1]).

Within cells, tissues, and plasma, ubiquitous nucleases metabolize (or catabolize) PS ODN drugs, and not the cytochrome P450 enzymes that typically metabolize low molecular weight drugs. PS ODNs therefore do not compete with traditional drugs for metabolic processes, reducing the potential for drug–drug interactions. Whole body elimination is the result of metabolism in tissues, and a re-equilibration of metabolites and parent drug out of tissues and into circulation, where they are ultimately excreted in the urine. These processes are very similar in laboratory animals and humans. In fact the processes are similar enough that for a given chemistry (e.g., PS ODNs or second-generation PS ODNs) doses scale from species to species on the basis of body weight, not surface area, allowing for good extrapolations from laboratory animals to humans [21,22]. In these extrapolations, mice are outliers compared to rats, rabbits, dogs, monkeys, and humans. This later point is key for assessing the relevance of findings in animal studies to humans, and for the design of early clinical trials. For a given sequence and route of administration it is possible to predict plasma levels in human subjects directly from data in monkeys with a high level of confidence in PS ODNs, and to some extent it is possible to generalize from sequence to sequence, albeit with less precision than within a single sequence.

After subcutaneous or intravenous administration, PS ODNs tend to accumulate in kidney, liver, spleen, bone marrow, and lymph nodes (reviewed in [1]). While the kidney generally accumulates the greatest concentration of oligonucleotide, the liver with its greater mass accumulates a greater total burden. Approximately 20% to 30% of the total dose accumulates in liver. At the cellular level oligonucleotide can be found in all cell types in the liver, with the phagocytically active Kupffer cells accumulating it in phagolysomes. When these cells are stained with hematoxylin, the oligonucleotides appear as basophilic granules. Similarly the phagocytically active proximal tubular cells also tend to accumulate oligonucleotide in basophilic granules [23,24]. As dose is increased, liver and kidney concentrations tend to saturate and that leads to greater distribution to the spleen, bone marrow, and other lower avidity organs [18].

Single-Stranded Morpholino Oligomers   The phosphorodiamindate morpholino oligomers (PMOs), because of their low level of protein binding, have very different kinetics than all of the other classes of oligonucleotide therapeutics. Limited protein binding makes these compounds more rapidly excreted in urine than other oligonucleotides, and initial clearance is therefore less dependent on tissue uptake than it is on glomerular filtration. Clearances for PMOs from plasma in rats is between 1 and 33 ml/min with a volume of distribution of 0.4 to 56 L/kg [2]. The plasma elimination half-life is variable, with sequence and tissue half-lives in liver and kidney reported to be as long as 7 to 14 days. Metabolism does not appear to be a key factor in terminal elimination of PMOs, with greater than 95% of the dose recovered intact. Because of the lack of charge, sequence plays a much greater role in determining the pharmacokinetics of the oligomers than it does for the charged PS ODNs or siRNAs. In those molecules the polyanionic nature tends to dominate over the chemical characteristics associated with differences in sequence. For PMOs then there is less predictability from drug to drug, which is a key disadvantage relative to PS ODN.

In the clinic a single slow bolus injection of 90 mg of AVI 4126 had a multiphasic distribution plasma kinetics with half-lives of approximately 1 and 11 hours, but no data were reported on elimination half-life. The volume of distribution was roughly 250 ml/kg, somewhat different than those seen in rats. Metabolites were not detected in plasma [25].

Double-Stranded RNA-Based Therapeutics   The pharmacokinetics of unmodified double-stranded RNAs is largely a product of rapid degradation, urinary filtration, and tissue uptake. The role of enzymatic degradation can be minimized through modifications to the backbone, often 2′ F or 2′ O-methyl groups [3]. Unmodified double-stranded RNA and double-stranded RNA with one of the two strands a full diester and the other strand a full phosphorothioate (PO/PS duplex), distribute rapidly to the liver and kidney after injection, peaking at 5 minutes, with radiolabel appearing in bladder urine over the same time frame. Oligonucleotides labeled with ^{125}I on the 3′-termini administered by intravenous injection and radiolabel can be found in the kidney and liver as soon as 1 hour and as late as 72 hours (the first and last observations). The highest concentrations is observed in kidney. The more stable PO/PS duplex accumulated slightly more in spleen, lung, and heart, and slightly less to liver and kidney [26].

24.4   TOXICITY OF OLIGONUCLEOTIDE THERAPEUTICS

24.4.1   Overview

All the oligonucleotide therapeutic agents discussed in the review are synthesized chemically and none are produced in biological reactions. As a result these compounds have been regulated not as biologics, but as "drugs." Oligonucleotide-based therapeutics are biotechnology-dervied products and could be covered by ICH S6. Some aspects of oligonucleotide therapeutic agents are much more akin to biologics. For example, the chemical characterization of these compounds often shows that they have complex profiles more similar to a biologic agent than a traditional drug [27]. Additionally their metabolism is more akin to catabolism in that they are reduced to nucleotides by nucleases much the same as biologics are catabolized to amino acids. However, because oligonucleotides were synthetically derived, they have been tested in nonclinical assays like small molecules, with complete toxicity characterizations in genotoxicity, safety pharmacology, genotoxicity, subchronic, and, when appropriate for the indication, chronic toxicity and carcinogenicity assays.

When trying to understand the toxicity of oligonucleotide therapeutics, it is useful to classify the sources of toxicity. An oligonucleotide therapeutic can produce toxicity either through a hybridization-dependent or hybridization-independent mechanism.

Hybridization-Dependent Toxicities   Toxicity can be induced through hybridization in two ways. First, through exaggerated pharmacology: hybridization reduces the expression of the target mRNA and produces toxicity related to the intended gene product. This type of toxicity is possible, but is usually discovered in preclinical pharmacology studies. The easiest way to avoid this type of toxicity is to carefully select pharmacology (gene) targets that are not critical for cell survival. As is obvious but bears stating, the only way to induce exaggerated pharmacology in a toxicology study is to have an active oligonucleotide. Because mRNA sequences are often species specific, that means that it may be necessary to test different sequences in the toxicology models in addition to, or in place of, the sequences that will be used in human clinical trials. While it is possible to select oligonucleotide sequences that have activity across species, it often happens that specific surrogate (homologous) oligonucleotides are needed for one or more of the animal species used in toxicity studies. A broader discussion of surrogate drugs appears below.

The second mechanism of hybridization-dependent toxicity is related to the reduction in expression of an unintended target by an antisense mechanism.

These so-called off-target effects are uncommon, on the basis of the low probability of having a perfect match to a 20-mer sequence two places in the genome. The probability of having an off-target effect can be further reduced by performing the appropriate blast searches for matches in other known genes in the expressome and selecting sequences for drugs that are unique.

There may be marked differences on the potential for the different classes of oligonucleotide drugs to have hybridization-dependent off-target effects. Aptamers are generally decorated with PEG groups, so they may have reduced affinity for complementary sequences and, more important, a reduced propensity for entering cells. On the other hand, because aptamers are designed to interact with specific proteins, it is possible for off-target effects with aptamers to be related to off-target protein binding.

The potential for off-target effects with siRNAs is just becoming recognized. The molecular basis for siRNA activity makes off-target phenomena more likely to occur with siRNA than with oligonucleotides that work through RNase H. There are three primary reasons for the greater potential for hybridization-dependent off-target effects [28]. First, in an siRNA two different sequences are being administered, the "sense" and "antisense" strands. Second, there is greater tolerance of mismatches with this mechanism. Only a portion of the 3′ region of the antisense strand of the siRNA needs to be a perfect match. The so-called seed region matches allow for many more potential binding sites than would be allowed if full complementarity (of the 20-mer) was required for the cleavage of a target mRNA [28]. Third, it has been reported that siRNA can induce changes in the methylation state of genomic DNA and thereby alter gene expression (either silence or activate off-target genes through an interaction with the RNA-induced initiation of transcriptional gene silencing—the RITS complex) [29]. Thus, because siRNA can produce more than just specific reductions in target protein expression, this mechanism brings with it the greater potential for hybridization-dependent off-target effects than RNaseH mediated antisense activity. However, this issue has been identified early in the understanding of siRNA mechanisms, and therefore it can be addressed as these drugs advance in toxicity studies and clinical trials.

Hybridization-Independent Toxicities   Many, if not most, of the toxicities that have been observed with PS ODN and other oligonucleotide classes are related to the hybridization-independent effects. These class effects are related to the chemistry, and many are known to be related to the interaction of oligonucleotides with proteins (reviewed in [17,30,31] [1]). Toxicities such as the prolongation of aPTT, the activation of complement, and immunostimulation are all examples of oligonucleotide protein interactions that are independent of hybridization. Thus reducing protein binding also reduces the likelihood of some of these toxicities, but that comes at a cost. Reduced protein binding reduces uptake into cells and increases the fraction of the drug that gets filtered by the kidney (and it may increase renal concentrations). So protein binding is a factor that needs to be understood, not just avoided.

Some hybridization-independent toxicities are sequence-dependent. The most obvious example of this is CpG oligonucleotides that have specific sequence motifs that make them more immunostimulatory through interactions with Toll-like receptors or protein components of innate immunity (reviewed in [32]). While immunostimulatory effects are the basis of the pharmacologic activity for a whole class of oligonucleotides, for single-stranded antisense compounds and compounds that work via antisense or through the siRNA pathways, stimulating innate immunity is considered an undesirable effect [33,34]. The CpG motifs have been well characterized as motifs that control hybridization-independent effects of oligonucleotides. Whether there are other motifs that have there own unique "toxic" or pharmacologic effects remains to be determined.

In our experience with PS ODNs, there may be quantitative variation in potency for some toxicities, but there are a great number of qualitative similarities in toxicity profiles. A number of the toxicities may be considered common to the chemical class. The responses from one PS ODN sequence to the next are similar within a single species. We and others have found that there are striking differences in the responses of rodents and nonhuman primates.

Surrogate Oligonucleotide Drugs   Because of species-dependent sequence differences, siRNA and ASOs may not hybridize with the mRNA for the target gene in the animal species used in toxicity studies. With oligonucleotide therapeutics (excluding aptamers) it is possible to design and synthesize species-specific compounds that are perfectly complementary to the mRNA for the target gene in a specific species. Not only is it possible, but from what we know about the synthetic process and what is understood about synthesis-related impurities, we can predict that species-specific oligonucleotides will have similar chemistry manufacturing and controls as the sequence used in clinical trials. These animal-specific drugs (surrogates) can be tested alongside the human sequence in toxicity studies to establish if there are biologic effects (exaggerated pharmacology) associated with downregulating the target gene. This concept has been part of the toxicity profiling of antisense drugs for the last decade [35,36]. One of the reasons that this approach is viable is that the class-related toxicity profiles and the pharmacokinetics are so similar from sequence to sequence. Thus, if there is a unique toxicity profile in the surrogate drug, it most likely arises from the effects on the expression of the target. For PS ODNs, this differentiation is useful because there are a number of class-related toxicities like the propensity for immunostimulation and mononuclear cell infiltrates in rodents that are not clinically relevant. Using surrogates allows one to distinguish between these "nonrelevant" toxicities and toxicities related to reductions in target expression. In the toxicity assessment of low molecular weight drugs or some biopharmaceuticals, investigators simply increase the dose if the pharmacologic effects of a drug are weaker in animals than in humans. For siRNA and ASOs, simply overdosing will not produce an antisense effect through hybridization. So unlike low molecular weight drugs, overdosing is not a practical solution for overcoming low activity. There are, of course, exceptions, and these need to be considered. For example, if there are one or two mismatches near the termini of an antisense or siRNA construct, it is possible that there would be an antisense effect. The degree of activity depends on the placement of the mismatches and is sometimes target specific. In these cases we would propose that there is no need for using a surrogate drug sequence to characterize exaggerated pharmacology, but including a nonactive control group might be considered for comparison purposes to distinguish class-related effects from exaggerated pharmacology.

In practice, there are times when surrogates need not be used simply because the target does not exist in the toxicity study species (or has a completely different function) or the target is related to an infectious agent not normally present in the toxicity study species. Aptamers may represent a unique challenge in this regard. It may not always be possible to develop species-independent aptamer, and because aptamer design is more empirical than antisense and siRNA, the choice of a surrogate is not clear, nor is there any assurance that an aptamer surrogate would have the same molecular mechanism. Thus the surrogate approach is not as rational for aptamers.

The scope of the toxicity studies when surrogate molecules have been used includes pharmacology studies, subchronic and chronic studies, reproductive toxicity studies, immunotoxicity studies, and even carcinogenicity studies. Short-term assays like safety pharmacology studies are too short for there to be an antisense effect, so we have not used the surrogate approach in these assays. However, when safety pharmacology endpoints are included in subchronic or chronic studies, surrogates are assessed.

When designing a toxicity study with a surrogate drug, for practical purposes, it is necessary to decide whether to run a full dose-response curve for the surrogate or for the human sequence. We have elected to use a single dose of the surrogate, one that is known to produce significant (if not maximal) pharmacologic activity. This dose is often not equivalent to the high dose in the study because the high dose is generally associated with marked nonspecific effects. One could argue for a full dose–response analysis for the surrogate, but for practical purposes and humane reasons a well-selected single-dose group should be sufficient unless there is marked toxicity associated with the reduction in the target protein.

24.4.2 Genotoxicity

Assessing the Genotoxicity   Most of the published data on the genotoxicity of oligonucleotide therapeutic agents is for the PS ODNs. PS ODNs have been routinely examined in the standard battery of genetic toxicology assays that include the Ames bacterial mutagenicity assay, the CHO cell chromosomal aberrations assay, the L5178Y/TK (+/−) mouse lymphoma mammalian gene mutation assay, and the mouse micronucleus assay. Because these compounds are highly soluble and have low cytotoxicity, most in vitro assays have been run at or near the limit concentration of 5000 μg/ml. While there is little published data on the other classes, because they have been accepted for clinical trials, we assume that the findings with the other classes of oligonucleotide therapeutics are not markedly genotoxic.

Genotoxic Potential of Oligonucleotide Therapeutics   Published data from genotoxicity assays for a number of different PS ODNs indicate that there is little or no genotoxic potential. Additionally ISIS has tested more than 10 unique sequences, all routinely negative (Table 24.1).

Representative example of these assays have been thoroughly reviewed and published for PS ODN [37]. Included in these assays are both the demonstration of cytotoxicity and the demonstration of cellular uptake of the test compounds, such that there is clear evidence for exposure of cells to oligonucleotide and any metabolites that might be formed.

There was concern that metabolism of these compounds at the high concentrations used in genotoxicity assays would produce changes in the nucleotide pools. This was unfounded as the compounds have been routinely negative for the 2′-methoxyethyl modified PS ODNs even with the presence of modified nucleosides. However, in the testing of several 2′-MOE ASOs, no genetic toxicity has been observed. It turns out that the 2′-O-methoxyethyl modified nucleotides are highly resistant to exonuclease cleavage, so little 2′-MOE modified nucleotide is released.

Because of the uniform negativity of in vitro genotoxicity assays, EMEA has published guidance on the genetic toxicity potential for antisense oligonucleotides [38]. The document has two primary concerns: (1) the potential for base mispairing due to liberation of metabolites, resulting in point mutations in newly synthesized DNA, and (2) site-specific mutations resulting from triplex formation with DNA [39]. The traditional gene mutation and clastogenicity assays are considered of suitable specificity and sensitivity to address the first potential issue. However, based on the negative response in these assays, in light of the documentation of exposure and metabolism, the EMEA concluded that PS ODN were not likely to pose a genotoxic hazard by this mechanism. As a result the report suggested that in vitro testing of novel antisense inhibitors in these assays was not necessary. The FDA has not accepted similar arguments, so in practice, for drug registration in the United States, it is still necessary to do the in vitro tests.

In vivo genotoxicity studies or clastogenicity studies are not mentioned in the EMEA guidance, and PS ODNs have been routinely tested in the mouse micronucleus assay. Again, even when exposure to the bone marrow is well documented, the assays are routinely negative. Other assays like unscheduled

TABLE 24.1 Summary of genetic toxicity assays

	Bacterial Mutagenesis			In vitro Assays			In vivo Assay
Isis Compound Number	Salmonella	E. coli	Cytogenetics (Chromosomal Aberation)	Mouse Lymphoma Mammalian Mutagenesis	CHO/HGPRT Mammalian Mutagenesis	Rat Hepatocyte UDS	Mouse Micronucleus
First generation							
2,105	Neg	—	Neg	—	Neg	Neg	Neg
2,302	Neg	Neg	Neg	Neg	—	—	Neg
2,922	Neg	Neg	Neg	Neg	—	—	Neg
3,521	Neg	Neg	Neg	—	—	—	Neg
5,132	Neg	Neg	Neg	—	—	—	Neg
Second generation							
107,248	Neg	Neg	—	Neg	—	—	—
112,989	Neg	Neg	—	Neg	—	—	—
104,838	Neg	Neg	—	Neg	—	—	Neg
113,715	Neg	Neg	—	Neg	—	—	—
301,012	Neg	Neg	—	Neg	—	—	Neg
325,568	Neg	Neg	—	Neg	—	—	—

DNA synthesis assays have been run occasionally for PS ODNs and have been negative.

The PS ODNs are metabolized to nucleotides that are identical to endogenous nucleotides. It is possible, and perhaps even likely, that as oligonucleotide therapeutics move further away from building oligonucleotide therapeutics from the endogenous nucleotides to building the oligomers from synthetically modified nucleotides and heterocycles (bases), and that mutagenic components will be accidentally or intentionally included. The result could be a drug or metabolic product that is mutagenic. For that reason when new chemistries are included in oligonucleotide therapeutics, it is important that they be tested in the genotoxicity assays that are appropriate.

24.4.3 Safety Pharmacology

Assessing the Safety Pharmacology of Oligonucleotide Therapeutic Agents   The battery of safety pharmacology studies for oligonucleotide compounds can be ascertained from the ICH guidance on the topic.

> The purpose of the safety pharmacology core battery is to investigate the effects of the test substance on vital functions. In this regard, the cardiovascular, respiratory and central nervous systems are usually considered the vital organ systems that should be studied in the core battery. In some instances, based on scientific rationale, the core battery may need to be supplemented (see also section 2.8) or may not need to be implemented (see also section 2.9).

> The exclusion of certain test(s) or exploration(s) of certain organs, systems or functions however should be scientifically justified.

The safety pharmacology of oligonucleotide therapeutics should include application of the generally recognized guidance where there is scientific rationale. Clearly, understanding the effects of oligonucleotides on vital organ functions is an important part of all toxicologic assessments. What is less clear is whether there is a requirement for tests for which there is little scientific rationale. For example, oligonucleotide therapeutics administered by subcutaneous, intravenous, or oral routes do not cross the blood–brain barrier, and there is little or no accumulation in the brain. As such, these compounds might be expected to have no CNS effects. Under conditions where there is little or no exposure, is there a sufficient rationale to justify the study? Other batteries of safety pharmacology studies are more easily justified scientifically.

There are other complex issues with regard to the assessment of safety pharmacology studies. With the oligonucleotide therapeutics that modulate the translation of mRNA to proteins, like antisense/siRNA, there is a lag between administration of the drug and the pharmacologic activity that is mediated by reduction in protein levels. This lag is related to the mechanism of action and how long it takes for a reduction in protein synthesis to be reflected in reduced protein levels. Because of this lag it is probably better to perform as much of the safety pharmacology battery as part of repeated-dose toxicity studies as possible, and not as acute studies.

Cardiovascular Safety Effects on vascular tone have received the most attention, as a result of toxicities that were identified very early in the development of the first systemically administered PS ODNs. We showed that there was correlation between complement activation and the reported alterations in blood pressure and heart rate in monkeys treated with high doses of PS ODN [40–42]. The observation appears to be unique or at least more prominent in monkeys, and that has actually driven the need to characterize the toxicity of oligonucleotide therapeutics in monkeys as the nonrodent species. (Note that complement activation has not proved to be a significant issue in the clinic, although in clinical studies we strive to avoid plasma levels that might be associated anaphylactoid responses in monkeys.)

Because the monkey is the most sensitive species for the effects on complement, we have opted to perform cardiovascular safety studies as part of subchronic study protocols using implanted telemetry units in selected monkeys (two/sex in at least two different treatment groups, including the high dose) to measure ECG, mean arterial pressure, heart rate, and body temperature. These parameters are then recorded at frequent intervals for a 24-hour period prior to treatment to establish circadian fluctuations and normal response to various stimuli encountered during the day. This technique enables us to assess both acute alterations related to complement activation after single doses and chronic safety after repeated administration.

The in vitro hERG assay has become the standard for testing for effects on QT prolongation. Various PS ODNs have been tested against the human ether-a-go-go channels, and under the conditions of the assays there is no apparent affect up to 1050 µg/ml reviewed in [43]). These concentrations are many-fold higher than the concentrations attained in hearts in animals in toxicity studies. Thus, based on the very large margins of safety, there is little concern for QT prolongation in patients. This is not surprising, considering the chemical nature of the oligonucleotides as polyanionic molecules being approximately 7000 Da. Most of the compounds that have typically been associated with alteration of ion channel function have been small compounds capable of interacting with the ion channel. We would therefore recommend that the hERG assay be eliminated from the battery of safety pharmacology studies.

Renal Safety Pharmacology Oligonucleotides accumulate in the kidney, particularly in the proximal convoluted tubular epithelial cells. At high doses in monkeys the kidney is a target organ for toxicity. Thus assessment of renal function for oligonucleotide therapeutics is essential. The concerns for renal toxicity are largely attributed to the concentration of oligonucleotide in tissue over time, and therefore it is probably inappropriate to examine renal function in the context of the typical single-dose experiments used in safety pharmacology assays. It is more relevant to examine renal function as part of the repeat-dose toxicology studies. For renal safety, monkeys, with their pharmacokinetics similarities to humans, are considered by the authors to be the most relevant species. Evaluation of renal function relies primarily on routine serum chemistry, urinalysis, and histopathology. In addition quantitative urine total protein and creatinine ratios can be employed. Protein–creatinine ratios are a well-accepted biomarker in human clinical trials. Other measures of tubular function have occasionally been examined such as renal blood flow, glomerular filtration, urine, glucose, urine amino acids, measurement of specific low molecular weight proteins in urine, and enzyme markers of epithelial cell damage in urine. These assays are designed to assess tubular transport or the viability of the proximal tubular epithelium. Markers like α-glutathione-S-transferase, N-acetylglucose aminidase, and retinol-binding protein levels have all been applied to nonclinical and clinical assessment of renal function of oligonucleotide therapeutics. Because of difficulties in obtaining clean urine samples for these analyses, cystocentisis samples are preferable, but cage pan collections have been used. In general, no changes in these markers have been observed even when kidneys are stressed by glucose load or under conditions requiring the concentration of urine. The most reliable measure of renal changes has been total urine protein or protein–creatinine ratios.

Pulmonary and Gastrointestinal Safety Pharmacology Pulmonary and gastrointestinal function studies have been performed for PS ODNs and are uniformly negative in the typical rodent assays. In one experiment a collection of PS ODN sequences were administered to rats, and CNS, pulmonary, and cardiovascular function were evaluated. Included in this group of compounds were both active and inactive compounds for the rat. The results show that the compounds are uniformly negative in this series of short-term safety pharmacology studies, suggesting that as a class these compounds do not affect these parameters (Isis Pharmaceuticals, unpublished data).

For pulmonary safety pharmacology studies, some laboratories are collecting the pulmonary safety data as part of subchronic or chronic toxicity studies by collecting data on respiratory rates and blood gases. Using subchronic treatment may be both more relevant and may reduce the numbers of additional studies and animals to perform the assessment. Although the preponderance of the data suggest that with the current PS ODNs, including 2'-MOE modified compounds, there are no acute pharmacologic effects for the class. Obviously collecting additional data will provide a rationale for only doing scientifically relevant assays.

CNS Safety Pharmacology CNS safety pharmacology studies do not appear to be necessary based on our understanding of the biodistribution of PS ODNs. These drugs, because of their polyanionic nature, do not cross the blood–brain barrier; therefore, after administration by intravenous or subcutaneous injections, there is little or no accumulation in the brain. Some have argued that there are low accumulations in brain from analyses of whole brain homogenates and therefore it is not unreasonable to perform CNS safely pharmacology. However, quantitative whole body autoradiographs suggest that the neuronal tissue is not accumulating oligonucleotide.

For ASOs injected or infused directly into the CNS, the situation is quite different Neurons are known to take up PS ODNs, and antisense activity in CNS can be shown after local injections or intraventricular infusions. For PS ODNs that are administered locally to the CNS, safety pharmacology studies should be performed. For systemically administered PS ODNs, the scientific rationale is weak.

24.4.4   Acute Toxicity

Oligonucleotide therapeutics have a relatively low order of acute toxicity, with the notable exception of the polyanionic PS ODNs, which have been known to activate complement through the alternative pathway in monkeys. Because these compounds do not cross the blood–brain barrier nor accumulate in cardiac muscle, and because the uptake of these compounds is dependent on saturable processes, very high doses of oligonucleotides tend not to produce central effects or acute organ failure, thus lowering the potential for acute lethality.

Assessing Acute Toxicity   Assessment of acute toxicity can be performed in rodents as a stand-alone study, as part of acute toxicity screens, or as part of the dosing ranging process for the mouse micronucleus assay. Acute studies in nonrodent species have not generally been performed for PS ODNs because of the well-understood activation of a complement cascade that can result in an anaphylactoid-like response. This response will be similar for each sequence. For phosphorothioate oligodeoxynucleoitdes without 2′ modifications, there is a remarkably reproducible threshold plasma concentration for the drug that is associated with activation of the complement. The same threshold was observed for multiple sequences. PS ODNs that are partially modified with 2′-methoxyethyl groups share properties, though the threshold is greater than for unmodified PS ODNs (reviewed in [31]). Because of this reproducible toxicity and the well-understood nature of the complement activation, acute toxicity studies for PS ODNs in primates are difficult to justify.

If one uses a novel chemistry, a pyramiding dose escalation type of study in primates may provide useful information for dose selection. However, the class similarities in the toxicity profile, short of using a novel chemistry, suggest that such study would be of limited value for most PS ODN therapeutics.

Acute Toxicities   The estimated lethal doses in mice of various PS ODNs with and without 2′-MOE modifications are all approaching 1 g/kg, indicating a low level of acute toxicity in mice (Table 24.2). In monkeys, a high-dose administration of PS ODNs results in the inhibition of factor H of the alternative complement cascade. Factor H is a endogenous inhibitor of the

TABLE 24.2 Estimated dose required to produce 50% mortality in mice injected intravenously

	Sequence	LD50 (mg/kg)
First generation	ISIS 2105	890
	ISIS 2922	720
	ISIS 2302	>1000
	ISIS 3521	500
	ISIS 5132	>1000
Second generation	ISIS 104838	2000
	ISIS 301012	>2000

complement cascade, and removing this "brake" from the system may promote complement activation and the anaphylactoid-like response that has been so well characterized [40–42]. When plasma concentrations of unmodified PS ODNs exceed 50 to 75 μg/ml, there is activation of the cascade in monkeys. The end result is the release of anaphylatoxins C3a and C5a. In vitro assays with human plasma indicate that humans may be less susceptible to the activation of the complement cascade, and it appears that in human plasma the cascade may be more susceptible to inhibitory effects of PS ODN (reviewed in [31]). The complement activation is directly responsible for the cardiovascular collapse observed acutely in nonhuman primates. This relationship was definitively demonstrated using a specific complement inhibitor CAB2 [42]. Because of this clear mechanistic relationship, acute toxicity studies in monkeys with PS ODNs simply reproduce what is already known about complement activation and add little to our understanding of the toxicity of a particular sequence.

Another effect associated directly with plasma concentrations is related to a transient concentration-related inhibition of the tenase complex by PS ODNs [44–46]. The inhibition results in a prolongation of aPTT, but has little or no effect on PT. Only one arm of the clotting cascade is affected, and the effects are transient. We have demonstrated in both clinical trials and in nonclinical trials that there is less than a 1 second increase in aPTT per μg/ml. Typical concentrations of PS ODNs after intravenous infusion of 3 mg/kg in monkeys or humans are in the range of 10 to 20 μg/ml, suggesting that at C_{max} there might be a transient increase in aPTT of 10 to 20 seconds [47,48]. This inhibitory effect is directly proportional to plasma concentrations so that, as plasma is cleared of PS ODN, the inhibition reverses. With a distribution half-life of less than 1 hour, this effect is transient and is almost completely reversed within 3 hours. When oligonucleotides are administered by the subcutaneous route, C_{max} is blunted and typical peak plasma concentrations after a dose of 3 mg/kg are in the range of 3 to 5 μg/ml.

Thus for subcutaneously administered PS ODNs the prolongation is not clinically significant. Even in monkeys treated with high doses of PS ODN there has been no indication of hemorrhage, though at very high doses (~50 mg/kg) bruising has been observed [49]. In our clinical experience dosing more the 3000 patients, no significant adverse effects have ever been reported related to prolongation of aPTT.

Some oligonucleotide therapeutics (aptamers) have been designed specifically to inhibit clotting, and for those compounds the anticoagulant effects are more pronounced, as intended. The doses used in toxicity studies are designed to characterize the superpharmacology of these agents.

Because PMOs are not charged and do not contain the phosphorothioate linkages, they do not have the same potential for these acute effects. However, they will have their own unique toxicities. To date, PMOs have not been published in any detailed form.

The double-stranded siRNA chemistries that are being employed include some of the modifications (e.g., phosphorothioate) that result in protein binding and are therefore charged and capable of binding to plasma proteins. Acute toxicity data for these compounds have not been reported at this time. Because they consist of two 20-mer strands, they still have the potential to produce similar kinds of toxicities as other PS ODNs.

By encapsulating oligonucleotides in liposomes, it is possible to reduce the acute effects of siRNA compounds. This was demonstrated for a PS ODN in a "stealth" liposome formulation [50]. These types of delivery systems are being increasingly employed with siRNA. Oligonucleotide formulations can reduce the propensity to produce the typical PS ODN effects, but it will be necessary to characterize their acute effects.

24.4.5 Subchronic and Chronic Toxicity

The protocols for performing subchronic and chronic studies with oligonucleotide therapeutics are not dissimilar to those used for low molecular weight drugs, with a few exceptions. Much of what is done today to characterize the toxicity of this class of drugs is relatively unchanged from the Points-to-Consider documents on oligonucleotide therapies, by Black and others [35,36]. Additional understanding and experience gained in the past decade make it appropriate to reconsider some of these points.

Assessing Subchronic and Chronic Toxicity Subchronic and chronic toxicity studies for oligonucleotides have been performed primarily in rodents (often mice) and monkeys. Most other small-molecule drugs are characterized in rats and dogs. The choice of species is based on a number of factors. For small molecules, species are often selected on the basis of similarities in metabolism, pharmacokinetics, or frankly, tradition. For oligonucleotides, the catabolic pathways for degradation of the oligonucleotides are very similar from species to species. Because metabolism was not an issue, the ability of the test species to mimic responses in humans became the driving force for the selection of nonhuman primates. Selection of a relevant species to mimic the human response is also the driving force for species selection for biopharmaceuticals. Mice were generally used as the rodent species for early studies on the toxicity of oligonucleotides because many of the pharmacology models are in mice, and therefore surrogate molecules were readily available. In hindsight, this was a fortuitous decision (vide infra). Monkeys were selected originally because they were thought to be more representative of humans than dogs. Again in hindsight, that was a good decision because the pharmacokinetics of oligonucleotide drugs appear to be very similar in monkeys and humans. In fact, at similar doses on a milligram per kilogram basis, plasma levels of a given sequence administered by the same route of administration are nearly identical in monkeys and humans. Clearance, volume of distribution, initial distribution half-lives and terminal elimination half-lives are all similar between monkeys and humans. Compared to rodents, the toxicity profiles in monkeys may be more predictive of those in humans.

The selection of mice over rats was fortuitous because rats treated with PS ODNs develop a low-grade low molecular weight proteinuria. It is dose-dependent (usually observed at doses ≥10 mg/kg) and independent of sequence. Most important, proteinuria is *not* seen in mice, monkeys, or man. Proteinuria may be related to decreases in tubular reabsorption of low molecular weight proteins. This effect may be attributed to a simple competitive interaction for a particular receptor or receptors on tubular epithelium between the oligonucleotide and low molecular weight proteins. Competition for a receptor may explain why these changes are readily reversible and are not associated with other changes in kidney function. Why rats are more sensitive is not known, but may be related to the greater susceptibility of rats to development of renal abnormalities (i.e., proteinuria). Male rats are notoriously sensitive to kidney insult as evidence by the aging rat nephropathy that develops in this gender and species, and rats show unusual sensitivity to agents, like the nephropathy associated with puromycin treatment. Rats also normally excrete far more protein in their urine than monkeys or humans. Understanding of the relative species specificity of this effect and the potential mechanistic basis would not have been possible before a relatively large database of safety information was available in mice, monkeys, and humans to interpret the species specificity.

Whether dogs can be used to characterize the toxicity of oligonucleotide therapeutics is an open question. In preliminary studies, pharmacokinetics of PS ODNS in the dog appear similar to monkey and human. The dog may be a suitable model for toxicity studies, but our experience is limited and the limited genomic information available for dogs makes designing surrogate molecules more challenging. It is possible to show reductions in target protein expression in dogs with oligonucleotide sequences that are homologus to multiple species. One interesting observation is that dogs did not appear to have the same complement activation response with PS ODNs, seen in primates (Isis, unpublished observations). Thus single-dose studies in monkeys need to be performed to characterize the potential of a new sequence to activate the complement cascade. With the acute toxicity associated with complement activation characterized in the most sensitive species (monkey), separate subchronic studies could be performed in dogs. Dog studies have been used to successfully support INDs for locally and orally administered oligonucleotide therapeutics. This strategy would provide a complete characterization of toxicity.

Subchronic and Chronic Effects

Basophilic Granules   One of the hallmarks of exposure to oligonucleotide therapeutic agents is the appearance of basophilic granules in cells and tissues that accumulate oligonucleotides. These basophilic granules are often found in phagocytically active cells, like macrophages, Kupffer cells, and epithelial cells and the proximal convoluted tubule of the kidney (Figure 24.2). Hematoxylin stains synthetic oligonucleotides like it stains endogenous oligonucleotides, and the accumulation of oligonucleotides in phagolysomes results in this distinct punctuate appearance. We have confirmed that the basophilic material consists of oligonucleotide using immunohistochemistry and fluorescently labeled oligonucleotides [23,24]. Electron microscopic examination of the tissues with granules reveals that these granules are membrane bound as would be expected if they are the product of phagocytosis or endocytosis. These granules are common to all of the oligonucleotide therapeutic classes that are taken up into cells.

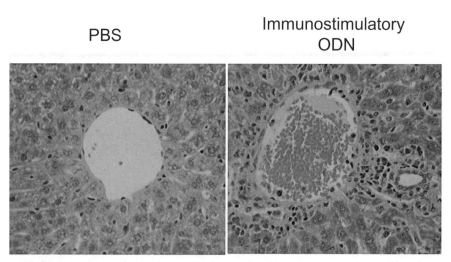

PBS   Immunostimulatory ODN

Figure 24.2   Photomicrograph of the renal cortex of a monkey treated with 40 mg/kg/wk for 5 weeks with a typical second generation 20-mer oligonucleotide modified with methoxyethyl groups on the 5 residues at each terminus. Stained with hematoxylin and eosin. The arrows point toward basophilic granules in the cells of the proximal convoluted tubules that are abundant throughout the renal cortex at this dose. See color insert.

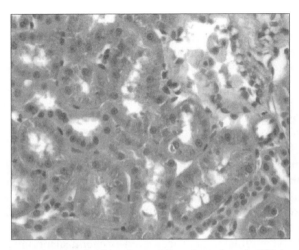

Figure 24.3   Photomicrograph of sections of liver from female CD-1 mice treated by subcutaneous injection with either saline (PBS) or an immunostimulatory oligodeoxy-nucleoitde at 4 mg/kg ever other day for 1 week. Lymphohystiocytic infiltrates are apparent adjacent to the central vein in the section from the ODN-treated mouse. See color insert.

Lymphohistiocytic Infiltrates   The other hallmark of exposure that is common in rodents treated with PS ODNs are lymphohistiocytic infiltrates in numerous organs (Figure 24.3). These mononuclear cell infiltrates have been described in liver, kidney, salivary glands, pancreas, uterus, urinary bladder, as well as other tissues. These infiltrates will resolve after treatment is ceased, but the clearance of them is prolonged (reviewed in [43]). They have been described as perivascular in some tissues with mononuclear cells appearing to migrate from the vasculature. They are not a prominent feature in other species.

Histocytosis is often also present in lymph nodes and spleen. This effect is related to the pro-inflammatory effects of PS ODNs. These effects are primarily observed in rodents and are associated with cytokine and chemokine release. The uncharged PMOs have also reported increases in lymph node macrophages [2].

The CpG oligonucleotides selected to be highly immunostimulatory are many-fold more potent at producing these effects than are some of the sequences selected for their antisense activity. It was in fact shown early on that by excluding CpG motifs and by replacing cytosines with 5-methyl cytosines, the proinflammatory potential of the sequence can be minimized. The CpG oligonucleotides work through Toll-like 9 receptors of innate immunity, but non-CpG oligonucleotides may work through other as yet unidentified receptors [51].

Mononuclear cell infiltrates have been occasionally observed in the high-dose groups in monkey studies; primarily at the site of subcutaneous injection, the severity and the incidence is much lower than in rodents. In rodents, depending on the sequence and chemistry, infiltrates have been observed after doses as low as 1 mg/kg and perhaps lower for oligonucleotides designed to be immunostimulatory. The rodents are much more sensitive to these effects than primates and that sensitivity is unrelated to pharmacokinetic differences. In primate studies, tissue concentrations of PS ODNs often exceed those observed in rodents. Rodents appear to overpredict for other species, including humans, presumably.

The siRNAs also produce pro-inflammatory responses and release of cyokines like interferons through Toll-like receptor 3, 7, and or 8 [33,34,52]. More siRNA and single-stranded RNAs with 5′ phosphates interact with the retinoic acid inducible protein (RIG-1) in the cytosol and stimulate innate immunity as part of antiviral mechanisms [53,54]. For this activity there is no currently identified sequence motif; rather, it is the presence of exogenous RNA that is apparently being recognized as foreign (viral). How this stimulation of innate immunity will be modulated or exacerbated by chemical modifications remains to be seen. For now, siRNAs like the single-stranded oligonucleotide therapeutics have the potential for proinflammatory effects.

Cardiovascular   In rodents, lymphohistiocytic infiltrates have been observed in the heart and in the perivascular space in various organs. Tissue macrophages in the heart can contain basophilic granules. In monkeys, no changes in ECG, heart rate, or blood pressure have been observed with numerous oligonucleotides. Under conditions when complement is activated, changes in blood pressure and cardiovascular collapse due to hypotension have been observed [55], but we have shown this to be related to complement activation rather than a direct effect on the cardiovascular system. (Of course, other mechanisms for hypotension could occur with other chemistries. For example, if an oligonucleotide formulation or its metabolic products chelates calcium, reductions in ionizable calcium could also produce a hypotensive crisis.) For most PS ODNs the most likely cause of hypotension is complement activation as demonstrated with complement inhibitors.

Hematologic   Dosing mice with high doses of PS ODNs can result in slight reductions in red cell parameters, probably the result of increased destruction of cells because of the slight splenomegaly seen at higher doses. The reduction in red cell parameters does not appear to be related to synthesis as the morphology of marrow is generally unremarkable in mice. With highly immunostimulatory oligonucleotides, when treatment causes significant splenomegaly, we have often observed reductions in platelets that follow the time course of the splenomegaly, beginning with the first increases in spleen weights and reversing only when the splenic enlargement reverses. Production of platelets in these mice appears normal as there is no diminution of megakaryocyte number or size. The reduction in platelets is nevertheless often accompanied by extramedullary hematopoiesis featuring megakaryocytes, suggesting that production is still active.

In monkeys treated with some sequences of PS ODNs at doses more than 20 mg/kg/wk, reductions in platelets have been observed. Reductions in platelets are not common to all sequences; rather, the reduction seems to be related to specific sequences and not others. This effect is unlikely to be related to pharmacology because it has been observed for compounds with diverse targets. These sequence-dependent reductions in platelets have generally been observed in high-dose monkeys, and some reductions in platelets have occasionally been observed in human subjects treated with the same sequences. In both monkeys and in humans the reduction in platelets appears to be reversible over the course of weeks or months depending on the half-life of the sequence. This reduction in platelets is distinct from transient sequestration of platelets that has been observed during constant intravenous infusions of PS ODNs: an effect probably related to the polyanionic nature and one that reverses within minutes or hours as the plasma is cleared of oligonucleotide.

Immunologic As discussed above, the most obvious immunologic effects in mice are the lymphohistiocytic infiltrates commonly observed in the parenchyma of numerous organs. These collections of histiocytes can sometimes be observed perivascularly and have been at times found in clusters, giving the appearance of microgranulomas. As would be expected, the increase in mononuclear cells in tissues is sometimes associated with increases in circulating monocytes, and plasma cytokine and chemokines concentrations.

The uptake of oligonucleotide drugs by the tissue macrophages causes their enlargement and gives them the appearance of being activated, though we have not determined if specific markers of activation are displayed on these engorged cells. Studies characterizing the immunotoxicity of oligonucleotides do not provide any evidence of macrophage dysfunction in mice. The engorgement of tissue macrophages occurs in monkeys as well as mice, but again, no indications of altered macrophage function have been recorded. Specific studies to address the consequences of loading macrophages with oligonucleotide need to be performed with each of the classes of oligonucleotide drugs.

Administration of oligos to rodents can induce the production of immunoglobulins in a nonspecific way [56,57]. These increases in immunoglobulins are not directed specifically toward the oligonucleotide, but rather, they represent a polyclonal expansion of B cells probably secondary to direct mitogenic effects on B cells associated with PS ODNs. In general, there is little or no evidence that oligonucleotides currently being used in clinical trials are antigenic. It is possible to reduce the proinflammatory effects of oligonucleotides by avoiding the stimulatory motifs and by chemical modifications. Modifications like the inclusion of 5-methyl cytosine and the addition of 2′ alkoxy groups can reduce the mitogenic potential of PS ODNs [58].

Hepatic Liver is the organ that contains the second highest oligonucleotide concentration in all species studied [11,70]. Liver is the organ that accumulates the greatest quantity of oligonucleotide. Concentrations in renal cortex may be higher, but the greater size of the liver makes it the organ that accumulates the greatest quantity of oligonucleotide for PS ODNs. PS ODNs are present in all the cell types within liver [23,24,59], but aptamers and siRNA may have more limited distribution. The presence of oligonucleotide in hepatocytes makes those cells good targets for antisense activity. Antisense activity has also been demonstrated in Kupffer cells [60,61]. Much of the toxicity for PS ODNs has already been reviewed [31]. In mice treated with PS ODNs, the mononuclear infiltrates and the associated single-cell necrosis result in slight increases in serum transaminases. These are reversible after the removal from treatment, and there is ample literature suggesting that the more potent the proinflammatory effects of a sequence the greater likelihood that there will be increases in transaminases [31,58,62,63]. The rat is somewhat less sensitive to the hepatic effects of PS ODNs than mouse. In monkey, increases in transaminases are not generally observed, and there are few hepatic effects at clinically relevant doses and even at doses 10-fold greater than those in clinical trials. This includes dose regimens for several different 2'-MOE ASO that ranged up to 140 mg/kg/wk for 5 weeks, or 80 mg/kg/wk for 13 weeks (Isis Pharmaceuticals, Inc., unpublished observations).

Consistent with the monkey data, PS ODN and 2'-MOE ASO have been largely absent of hepatotoxicity in clinical trials [47,48,64,65]. The only notable exception was the report of mild and transient increases in ALT of patients treated with anti-HIV PS ODN, GEM 91 [66]. This was also likely attributable to the proinflammatory effects that were present for this early generation of ASO comprised of 27 nucleotide residues along with CpG motifs.

Renal Kidney is the organ that contains the highest oligonucleotide concentration after oligonucleotide administration, and it is a target organ for toxicity in monkeys and rats. Oligonucleotide in kidney accumulates as a result of re-uptake of solutes by the kidney: a normal function of the kidney. Oligonucleotide is filtered at the glomerulus and is readily reabsorbed by the proximal tubular epithelium [67]. The oligonucleotide is then taken up into these cells by endocytosis, like other solutes [68]. The majority of oligonucleotide in proximal tubular epithelium resides in membrane-bound endosomes and lysosomes, generally oriented toward the luminal (apical) surface.

At high concentrations of oligonucleotide there are histologic changes in the proximal tubular cells [49,69]. The preferential uptake of oligonucleotide by proximal tubular epithelium and processing into endosomes and lysosomes is similar in mice, rats, and monkeys, though mice take up less oligonucleotide into kidney than other species.

In the absence of changes in cell morphology, these basophilic granules are considered not toxicologically significant. Often associated with basophilic granules are cytoplasmic vacuoles in the tubular epithelial cells [70]. The size and incidence of these vacuolar changes can be variable depending on the fixative, processing, and other unknown variables. The vacuoles are typically single-to-multiple large clear cytoplasmic vacuoles, often with small amounts of basophilic material in them. In rare instances when the concentrations of oligonucleotide are high enough, there can be swelling and rupture of cells, but again this is not solely determined by concentration but rather by a combination of factors like fixation conditions and preservation. Vacuolation, and the mild degenerative changes, are reversible after treatment is withdrawn. The vacuoles are not associated changes in renal tubular function [70].

The vacuoles result from the localized high concentrations of hydroscopic material in phagolysosomes. Oligonucleotides are highly water soluble molecules that could easily be extracted if they are not completely cross-linked by fixative in tissues. Because of these properties it is also possible that high concentrations of oligonucleotide contained in membrane-bound subcellular compartments would be osmotically active upon fixation, particularly in slower fixation processes such as immersion in formalin. The vacuoles in the proximal tubular cells of monkeys treated with oligonucleotides differ from classical tubular vacuolar degeneration. Vacuolar degeneration is characterized by generalized organelle swelling, but this is *not* manifested in the tubules in oligonucleotide-treated monkeys.

Other changes in renal morphology associated with oligonucleotide treatment include dose- and concentration-dependent degenerative changes in the proximal tubular epithelium and regenerative changes. Degeneration is characterized as minimal reductions in the height of the brush border and height of the proximal tubular cells. Tubular cell regeneration is characterized by more active-looking nuclei. As concentrations increase, focal tubular epithelial cell degeneration, and finally, frank epithelial cell degeneration, can occur. The concentrations that produce these effects are highly dependent on the chemistry of the oligonucleotide that is accumulating in the tubule. For unmodified PS ODNs, concentrations above 2000 to 3000 µg/g of tissue can produce frank tubular cell degeneration [71]. For oligonucleotides that are modified with 2'-MOE, the concentrations required to produce these changes in morphology are nearly twice as high.

It is only at these very high renal concentrations that some functional changes begin to occur. The dose required to produce these changes are at or exceed 40 mg/kg/wk. At this dose the only functional changes noted occasionally in monkeys are slightly increased urinary protein levels [70,71]. The effect of renal accumulations of oligonucleotide accumulations in granules and vacuoles on renal function was studied in monkeys treated with a 2'-MOE ASO administered at 40 mg/kg/wk (administered on days 1, 3, 5, 7, 14, 21, and 28). This regimen produced a typical pattern of vacuoles and minimal proximal tubular degeneration after a month of treatment [70]. A battery of renal functional assessment was performed including BUN, creatinine, creatinine clearance, amino acid secretion, GFR, and inulin clearance. In addition renal functional stress tests were performed to look at the how well treated monkeys could concentrate urine, and respond to a glucose load. The only change associated with these histologic changes at the higher doses was a low incidence of mild increases in urinary protein secretion. Protein-creatinine ratios increased from approximately 0.2 at baseline to just above the upper limit of normal, 1.2, and the increase was tubular in origin [70] (unpublished, Isis Pharmaceuticals, Inc.).

There were no other functional changes observed. No changes in mean serum creatinine or BUN and no changes in electrolytes were measured. Effective renal plasma flow rate and glomerular filtration rate were unchanged in treated monkeys, and there were no changes in excretion of substrates for tubular reabsorption, including glucose, amino acids, or β2-microglobulin [70]. Typical markers of tubular damage like *N*-acetyl glucosaminidase (NAG) were unaffected. Even with this detailed assessment of renal and tubular epithelial cell function, no tubular functional changes were induced by treatment with 40 mg/kg/wk of a second-generation oligonucleotide. There were no indications of changes in glomerular function, nor were there changes in an ultrastructural assessment of morphology.

With the information that is available from these types of studies, it is possible to define concentration–response relationships for each of the morphologic changes observed in the kidneys of monkeys. A qualitative plot of these relationships demonstrates that concentrations predicted for therapeutic doses of oligonucleotide produce renal cortex concentrations well below those associated with any significant renal morphologic findings (Figure 24.4). The existing data suggest that renal effects are more a function of concentration than

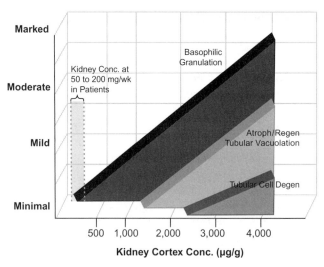

Figure 24.4 Schematic representation of the relationship between renal cortex concentration and morphologic changes present in the kidneys of monkeys dosed with second-generation antisense oligonucleotides.

they are of duration of exposure, and renal morphologic changes do not appear to progress in monkeys treated from one to three months. We are collecting data on longer term exposures.

The atrophic and regenerative changes, as well as the vacuolar changes, are all reversible after treatment is removed. The rate of reversal is related to the half-life of the drug, so that unmodified phosphorothioate oligonucleotides with their shorter half-lives reverse faster than the compounds modified to have prolonged half-lives. A thorough understanding of the dose–response and concentration–response relationships, markers like urinary protein-to-creatinine ratios to monitor for renal functional changes, and the reversibility of the changes are all important factors that need to be characterized in the toxicity program for any systemically administered oligonucleotide therapeutic.

24.4.6   Reproductive and Endocrine

Reproductive toxicity studies with PS ODNs have been performed with both human-specific sequences as well as species-specific sequences. Like chronic studies, this combination of human drug and surrogate provides insight into whether any effects observed are class related or target related.

Fertility, fetal development, and development and reproductive function of off-spring receiving PS ODNs have been assessed in mice, rats, and rabbits. To our knowledge, no reproductive toxicity studies have been performed in primates treated with oligonucleotides. Traditional embryonic and fetal exposure protocols have been used for these studies. In these studies we have included assessments of placental and embryonic exposure to the drugs. Even at doses that produce maternal toxicity, there have been no definitive indications of direct effects on in utero development. This is most likely the result of the absence of significant exposure to the conceptus. Placental concentrations of oligonucleotide are very low, and little or no oligonucleotide can be found in fetal tissues even when the oligonucleotide is administered by constant infusion over the course of development [72]. Fetal kidney concentrations are less than 1% of those of the maternal kidney and most fetal tissues contain oligonucleotide concentrations below the limits of detection or quantitation for capillary gel electrophoresis. The low levels of placental uptake and transfer reduce the exposure and the potential effects of oligonucleotide therapeutics in the developing embryo and fetus.

Fertility assessments performed on male rodents treated with PS ODNs have also been uniformly negative. This finding is consistent with the pharmacokinetics of this class. The highly charged and water-soluble oligonucleotide therapeutics are effectively excluded from the seminiferous tubules by the blood–testes barrier. The interstitial cells of the testes can accumulate oligonucleotide, but detailed autoradiography and immunohistochemistry suggest that there is none in the seminiferous tubules or in the developing sperm.

The female reproductive organs like the uterus and ovaries are not in privileged sites in that they will accumulate oligonucleotides after treatment, and they are sites where mononuclear cell infiltrates can be seen in rodents treated with high doses of PS ODNs. High-dose treatment of mice with at least one sequence has produced reductions in reproductive performance, most likely secondary to local inflammation in the ovaries or the uterus. This effect on ovaries was associated with a dose-dependent decrease in the fertility index in mice at doses at or over 20 mg/kg/wk. These same proinflammatory effects have also been shown to induce premature labor and abortion in rodents treated with maternal toxic doses of PS ODNs. This phenomenon has been observed in both mice and rabbits treated with PS ODNs at maternal toxic doses. For this reason it is unlikely that this phenomenon is clinically relevant.

There are several examples where investigators have used antisense inhibitors to study the effects on reproductive function. The most notable was the use of a 2'-*O*-methyl modified oligonucleotide targeted to VEGF. In this study antisense treatment produced a 50% inhibition of VEGF mRNA and was associated with developmental abnormalities similar to that observed in the VEGF-deficient mice [73]. These effects were attributed to the inhibition of VEGF because of both the similarity of the phenotype and the lack of effect on VEGF expression or fetal development of a 5-base mismatched control. While these effects are clearly related to the targeted pharmacology, it does raise important points about the accessibility of fetus to antisense inhibitors during development. It is possible that the exposure of the vascular endothelium to the VEGF inhibitor in placenta is sensitive to antisense inhibition at least at certain points in development, or it is possible these effects were related to inhibition of maternal VEGF systemically during an important phase of development. In any case, the assessment of fetal effects as well as extra-fetal effects of novel therapeutic agents is critical, and careful assessment of oligonucleotide therapeutic agents should be performed with active agents when possible, despite the absence of significant transfer to the developing conceptus.

24.4.7 Immunotoxicity

The most obvious effect on the immune system with oligonucleotide administration is the tendency to stimulate a pro-inflammatory reaction in some species (reviewed in [31,74]). Whether this is a true immunotoxicity is one of the questions that needs to be addressed for oligonucleotide therapeutics.

Assessing the Immunotoxicity Currently the assessment of the immunotoxicity of oligonucleotide therapeutics is performed using the typical tiered set of rodent assays. We have assessed both the human oligonucleotide and the surrogate "rodent-specific" sequences. Unfortunately, these batteries of tests are much more relevant to the assessment of immunosuppressive drugs and are not particularly well adapted to immunostimulatory compounds like oligonucleotides. While there have been discussions of how to monitor and assess immune-stimulating drugs, there are still no well-accepted guidelines.

Immunotoxicity of Oligonucleotide Therapeutics   The pro-inflammatory activity of the ASOs produces a constellation of effects, which includes splenomegaly, lymphoid hyperplasia, and multi-organ lymphohistiocytic cell infiltrate driven by the production of pro-inflammatory cytokines [57,63,75]. Incorporation of immunostimulatory sequences like unmethylated CG dinucleotides mimic bacterial DNA [76]. Unmethylated CG dinucleotides interact with receptors of the innate immune system such as TLR9 to produce a shift toward T-helper type 1 immunity [77,78]. Oligonucleotides with these motifs modulate the immune system. We have recently reported on a direct evaluation for effects on immune function.

In these studies ISIS 2302 (a PS ODN inhibitor of human ICAM-1 with no CG motifs) was administered to normal mice, and the effects of the drug on both the humoral and cellular immune functions were assessed by a battery of commonly used tests. As expected, treatment with high doses produced an increase in splenic weight that was accounted by increased splenocyte numbers, including increases in B cell numbers, which appeared to cause a shift in the population leading to decreased relative numbers of T cells but no decrease in absolute T cell numbers. There were no meaningful changes in antibody response in a sheep red blood cell assay, and the response to mitogens was not diminished. Consistent with an increase in total B cells, previously published information on this class of compound has documented an increase in total IgG and/or IgM [79,80]. No antibodies specific to dsDNA or ISIS 2302 were detected in sera. Oligonucleotides have been shown to elicit their proinflammatory effects directly on cells of the innate immune system producing a polyclonal increase in B cells, and therefore specific antibody responses are absent [32,74]. This is a key finding for the technology. Polyclonal expansion including IgG and IgM secretion is expected in rodents (and perhaps other species), and this occurs in the absence of antibodies directed toward the oligonucleotide and with no greater specificity to DNA than would be expected on the basis of chance.

Cellular responses, as measured by a mixed-lymphocyte reaction, cytotoxic T lymphocyte response, and NK cell activity, were all undiminished, and if anything, there was a slight increase in CTL and NK responses. As would be expected by the histologic profile and the known increases in cytokine and chemokine production associated with the administration of PS ODNs in rodents, in this series of experiments there was no diminution in immune response. Administering a mouse-specific ICAM-1 inhibitor produced reductions in mixed lymphocyte reactions. This inhibition was expected as this is one of the desired pharmacologic effects of reducing ICAM-1 expression.

Relevance of Immunotoxicity Findings to Humans   Monkeys, unlike rodents, do not display the same constellation of effects associated with the proinflammatory effects of PS ODNs. Human responses are thought to be more like the monkey. The human response differs from the monkey response in a few ways. First, at high doses of PS ODNs (>5 mg/kg) some subjects experience fever chills and rigors, that are readily reversible and treatable with nonsteroidal anti-inflammatory drugs. This particular toxicity has been dose limiting in some studies. These same doses have been associated with elevations in cytokine levels [65]. This febrile response has not been recorded in monkeys, though some increases in cytokines have been observed in monkeys. The second difference is that in humans, there is a characteristic local response to subcutaneous injections. This response is a relatively mild local erythematous area typically with blanching in the central region. After a subcutaneous injection of over 100 mg in one milliliter, these reactions are approximately 2 to 3 cm in diameter, are reddened but not painful, not pruritic, and not raised. They generally resolve in three to seven days. Slight erythema has been described in monkeys receiving subcutaneous injections; these reactions differ from those seen in human subjects in that they do not feature the central blanching and annular appearance.

24.4.8 Carcinogenicity

Oligonucleotides are not genotoxic in traditional in vitro and in vivo assays, and as such, they are not thought to be classical carcinogens. No reports of carcinogenesis with oligonucleotides are in the literature. Lifetime exposure of rodents to PS ODNs, with their propensity to cause mitogenesis and proliferation of stroma and mononuclear cells, is expected to have some potential for inducing hyperplastic or even neoplastic changes. Neoplasias have been observed in one study with a PS ODN administered by subcutaneous injections on alternate days for two years to mice (Isis, unpublished observations). The systemic pro-inflammatory effects combined with the local irritation produced by injections resulted in neoplastic transformation of some of the infiltrating cells. The histiocytic sarcomas that were observed were dose related. A less immunostimulatory PS ODN was administered in parallel, and it did not produce that same neoplastic change. If the treatment was intermittent, allowing for the injection sites to heal between dosing cycles, there also was no neoplastic change. These later results clearly support the PS ODN treatment having promoter-like effects, *not* initiator effects. If the neoplastic changes are associated with repeated administration to highly inflamed sites and local and systemic mononuclear infiltrates, then it is likely that this positive bioassay for a PS ODN does not have clear clinical relevance.

24.5 SUMMARY

The toxicology of oligonucleotides was at one time thought to be a real limitation to the technologies. To date, careful assessment of toxicity in the types of studies described here have demonstrated that it is likely that there may be attractive therapeutic indexes, particularly with the second-generation antisense oligonucleotides. The other classes of oligonucleotide therapeutics are also moving forward, and all of them will have distinctive hurdles to overcome. With strong scientific commitment to the assessment of toxicity and understanding mechanisms of toxicity, it is likely that these classes with continue to advance through preclinical studies and clinical trials as well.

ACKNOWLEDGMENTS

The authors would like to acknowledge the editorial comments and discussions with Dr. Christopher Horvath of Archemix. In addition they would like to acknowledge Lori Cooper for her help in the preparation of this manuscript and Robert Saunders for his expertise with EndNote.

REFERENCES

1. Levin AA, Yu RZ, Geary RS. Basic PrInciples of the PharmacokInetics Of antisense Oligonucleotide drugs. In Crooke ST, ed. *Antisense Drug Technology*. New York: Dekker, 2007.

2. Iversen PL. Morpholinos. In Crooke ST, ed. *Antisense Drug Technology*. New York: Dekker, 2007.

3. Manoharan M. Harnessing RNA interference pathways for therapeutics utilizing chemistry: chemically modified siRNAs, drug delivery systems and antagomirs. In Crooke ST, ed. *Antisense Drug Technology*. New York: Dekker, in press.

4. Cossum PA, Sasmor H, Dellinger D, Truong L, Cummins L, Owens SR, Markham PM, Shea JP, Crooke ST. Disposition of the 14C-labeled phosphorothioate oligonucleotide ISIS 2105 after intravenous administration to rats. *J Pharmacol Exp Therapeut* 1993;267(3):1181–90.

5. Cossum PA, Troung L, Owens SR, Markham PM, Shea JP, Crooke ST. Pharmacokinetics of a ^{14}C-labeled phosphorothioate oligonucleotide, ISIS 2105, after intradermal administration to rats. *J Pharmacol Exp Therapeut* 1994;269(1):89–94.

6. Yu RZ, Baer B, Chappel A, Geary RS, Chueng E, Levin AA. Development of an ultrasensitive noncompetitive hybridization-ligation enzyme-linked immunosorbent assay for the determination of phosphorothioate oligodeoxynucleotide in plasma. *Anal Biochem* 2002;304(1):19–25.

7. Gaus HJ, Owens SR, Winniman M, Cooper S, Cummins LL. On-line HPLC electrospray mass spectrometry of phosphorothioate oligonucleotide metabolites. *Anal Chem* 1997;69(3):313–9.

8. Griffey RH, Greig MJ, Gaus HJ, Liu K, Monteith D, Winniman M, Cummins LL. Characterization of oligonucleotide metabolism in vivo via liquid chromatography/electrospray tandem mass spectrometry with a quadrople ion trap mass spectrometer. *J Mass Spec* 1997;32:305–13.

9. Murphy AT, Brown-Augsburger P, Yu RZ, Geary RS, Thibodeaux S, Ackermann BL. Development of an ion-pair reverse-phase liquid chromatographic/tandem mass spectrometry method for the determination of an 18-mer phosphorothioate oligonucleotide in mouse liver tissue. *Eur J Mass Spec* 2005;11(2):209–15.

10. Yu RZ, Geary RS, Levin AA. Application of novel quantitative bioanalytical methods for pharmacokinetic and pharmacokinetic/pharmacodynamic assesments of antisense oligonucleoutides. *Curr Opin Drug Discov Dev* 2004;7(2):195–203.

11. Yu RZ, Geary RS, Levin AA. Pharmacokinetics and pharmacodynamics of antisense oligonucleotides. In Meyers RA, ed. *Encyclopedia of Molecular Cell Biology and Molecular Medicine*, Weinheim, Germany: Wiley-VCH, 2007.

12. Boomer RM, Lewis SD, Healy JM, Kurz M, Wilson C, McCauley TG. Conjugation to polyethylene glycol polymer promotes aptamer biodistribution to healthy and inflamed tissues. *Oligonucleotides* 2005;15(3):183–95.

13. Healy JM, Lewis SD, Kurz M, Boomer RM, Thompson KM, Wilson C, McCauley TG. Pharmacokinetics and biodistribution of novel aptamer compositions. *Pharmaceut Res* 2004;21(12):2234–46.

14. Watanabe TA, Geary RS, Levin AA. Plasma protein binding of an antisense oligonucleotide targeting human icam-1 (ISIS 2302). *Oligonucleotides* 2006;16(2):169–80.

15. Geary RS, Yu RZ, Siwkowski A. Pharmacokinetic/pharmacodynamic properties of phosphorothioate 2'-O-(2-methoxyethyl) modified antisense oligonucleotides in animals and man. In Crooke ST, ed. *Antisense Drug Technology*. New York: Dekker, 2007.

16. Geary RS, Yu RZ, Leeds JM, Ushiro-Watanabe T, Henry SP, Levin AA, Templin MV. Pharmacokinetic properties in animals. In Crooke ST, ed. *Antisense Drug Technology: Principles, Strategies, and Applications*. New York: Dekker, 2001; 119–54.

17. Levin AA, Geary RS, Leeds JM, Monteith DK, Yu RZ, Templin MV, Henry SP. The pharmacokinetics and toxicity of phosphorothioate oligonucleotides. In Thomas JA, ed. *Biotechnology and Safety Assessment*. Philadelphia: Taylor and Francis, 1998;151–75.

18. Phillips JA, Craig SJ, Bayley D, Christian RA, Geary RS, Nicklin PL. Pharmacokinetics, metabolism and elimination of a 20-mer phosphorothioate oligodeoxynucleotide (CGP 69846a) after intravenous and subcutaneous administration. *Biochem Pharmacol* 1997;54(6):657–68.

19. Geary RS, Ushiro-Watanabe T, Truong L, Freier SM, Lesnik EA, Sioufi NB, Sasmor H, Manoharan M, Levin AA. Pharmacokinetic properties of 2'-O-(2-methoxyethyl)-modified oligonucleotide analogs in rats. *J Pharmacol Exp Therapeut* 2001;296(3):890–7.

20. Geary RS, Yu RZ, Levin AA. Pharmacokinetics of phosphorothioate antisense oligodeoxynucleotides. *Curr Opin Invest Drugs* 2001;2(4):562–73.

21. Geary RS, Holmlund J, Kwoh TJ, Yu RZ, Dorr FA. Dosing of antisense oligodeoxynucleotides (ODNS) by ideal body weight, rather than actual body weight, may be preferred. Paper presented at Proceedings of the 11th NCI-EORTC-AACR Symposium, 2000.

22. CDER. Guidance for industry—estimating the maximum safe starting dose in initial clinical trials for therapeutics in adult healthy volunteers. In Center for Drug Evaluation and Research (U.S. Department of Health and Human Services), 2005; 1–27.

23. Butler M, Stecker K, Bennett CF. Cellular distribution of phosphorothioate oligodeoxynucleotides in normal rodent tissues. *Lab Invest* 1997;77(4):379–88.

24. Butler M, Stecker K, Bennett CF. Histological localization of phosphorothioate oligodeoxynucleotides in normal rodent tissue. *Nucleosides Nucleotides* 1997; 16(7–9):1761–4.

25. Devi GR, Beer TM, Corless CL, Arora V, Weller DL, Iversen PL. In vivo bioavailability and pharmacokinetics of a c-myc antisense phosphorodiamidate morpholino oligomer, AVI-4126, in solid tumors. *Clin Cancer Res* 2005;11(10):3930–8.

26. Braasch DA, Paroo Z, Constantinescu A, Ren G, Oz OK, Mason RP, Corey DR. Biodistribution of phosphodiester and phosphorothioate siRNA. *Bioorg Med Chem Letts* 2004;14(5):1139–43.

27. Capaldi DC, Scozzari AN. Manufacturing and analytical processes. In Crooke ST, ed. *Antisense Drug Technology*. New York: Dekker, 2007.

28. Jackson AL, Burchard J, Schelter J, Chau BN, Cleary M, Lim L, Linsley PS. Widespread siRNA "off-target" transcript silencing mediated by seed region sequence complementarity. *RNA* 2006;12:1179–87.

29. Verdel A, Jia S, Gerber S, Sugiyama T, Gygi S, Grewal SI, Moazed D. RNAI-mediated targeting of heterochromatin by the RITS complex. *Science* 2004; 303(5658):672–6.

30. Levin AA, Monteith DK, Leeds JM, Nicklin PL, Geary RS, Butler M, Templin MV, Henry SP. Toxicity of oligodeoxynucleotide therapeutic agents. In Crooke ST, ed. *Antisense Research and Application*. Heidelberg: Springer, 1998;169–215.

31. Levin AA, Henry SP, Monteith D, Templin M. Toxicity of antisense oligonucleotides. In Crooke ST, ed. *Antisense Drug Technology*. New York: Dekker, 2001; 201–67.

32. Krieg AM. CpG motifs in bacterial DNA and their immune effects. *Ann Rev Immunol* 2002;20:709–60.

33. Schlee M, Hornung V, Hartmann G. SiRNA and isRNA: two edges of one sword. *Mol Ther* 2006;14(4):463–70.

34. Kariko K, Bhuyan P, Capodici J, Weissman D. Small interfering RNAs mediate sequence-independent gene suppression and induce immune activation by signaling through Toll-like receptor 3. *J Immunol* 2004;172(11):6545–9.

35. Black LE, DeGeorge JJ, Cavagnaro JA, Jordan A, Ahn C-H. Regulatory considerations for evaluating the pharmacology and toxicology of antisense drugs. *Antisense Res Dev* 1993;3:399–404.

36. Black LE, Farrelly JG, Cavagnaro JA, Ahn C-H, DeGeorge JJ, Taylor AS, DeFelice AF, Jordan A. Regulatory considerations of oligonucleotide drugs: updated recommendations for pharmacology and toxicology studies. *Antisense Res Dev* 1994;4:299–301.

37. Henry SP, Monteith DK, Matson JE, Mathison BH, Loveday KS, Winegar RA, Lee PS, Riccio ES, Bakke JP, Levin AA. Assessment of the genotoxic potential of ISIS 2302: a phosphorothioate oligodeoxynucleotide. *Mutagenesis* 2002;17(3):201–9.

38. EMEA. CHNP SWP Reflection Paper on the Assesment of the Genotoxic Potential of Antisense Oligodeoxynucleotides. EMEA/CHNP/SWP/199726/2004 (2005).

39. Wang G, Seidman MM, Glazer PM. Mutagenesis in mammalian cells induced by triple helix formation and transcription-coupled repair. *Science* 1996;271(5250): 802–5.

40. Henry SP, Giclas PC, Leeds J, Pangburn M, Auletta C, Levin AA, Kornbrust DJ. Activation of the alternative pathway of complement by a phosphorothioate oligonucleotide: potential mechanism of action. *J Pharmacol Exp Therapeut* 1997; 281(2):810–6.

41. Henry SP, Jagels M, Hugli T, Giclas P. Species and pathway-specific activation of complement by a phosphorothioate oligonucleotide. Paper presented at Immunopharmacology.

42. Henry SP, Beattie G, Yeh G, Chappel A, Giclas PC, Mortari A, Jagels MA, Kornbrust DJ, Levin AA. Complement activation is responsible for acute toxicities in rhesus monkeys treated with a phosphorothioate oligodeoxynucleotide. *Intl J Immunopharmacol* 2002;2(12):1657–66.

43. Henry SP, Kim T-W, Kramer-Stickland K, Zanardi TA, Fey RA. Toxicologic properties of 2′-methoxyethyl chimeric antisense inhibitors in animals and man. In Crooke ST, ed. *Antisense Drug Technology*. New York: Dekker, in press.

44. Henry SP, Novotny W, Leeds J, Auletta C, Kornbrust DJ. Inhibition of coagulation by a phosphorothioate oligonucleotide. *Antisense Nucl Acid Drug Dev* 1997;7: 503–10.

45. Sheehan JP, Lan H-C. Phosphorothioate oligonucleotides inhibit the intrinsic tenase complex. *Blood* 1998;92(5):1617–25.

46. Sheehan JP, Thao PM. Phosphorothioate oligonucleotides inhibit the intrinsic tenase complex by an allosteric mechanism. *Biochemistry* 2001;40(16):4980–9.

47. Leeds JM, Mant TG, Amin D, Kisner DL, Zuckerman JE, Geary RS, Levin AA, Shanahan WR, Jr., Glover JM. Phase I safety and pharmacokinetic profile of an intercellular adhesion molecule-1 antisense oligodeoxynucleotide (ISIS 2302). *J Pharmacol Exp Therapeut* 1997;282(3):1173–80.

48. Sewell LK, Geary RS, Baker BF, Glover JM, Mant TGK, Yu RZ, Tami JA, Dorr AF. Phase i trial of isis 104838, a 2′-methoxyethyl modified antisense oligonucleotide targeting tumor necrosis factor-alpha. *J Pharmacol Exp Therapeut* 2002; 303(3):1334–43.

49. Henry SP, Bolte H, Auletta C, Kornbrust DJ. Evaluation of the toxicity of isis 2302, a phosphorothioate oligonucleotide, in a 4-week study in cynomolgus monkeys. *Toxicology* 1997;120:145–55.

50. Yu RZ, Geary RS, Leeds JM, Ushiro-Watanabe T, Fitchett JR, Matson JE, Mehta R, Hardee GR, Templin MV, Huang K, et al. Pharmacokinetics and tissue disposition in monkeys of an antisense oligonucleotide inhibitor of ha-ras encapsulated in stealth liposomes. *Pharmaceut Res* 1999;16(8):1309–15.

51. Senn JJ, Burel S, Henry SP. Non-CpG containing antisense 2′ MOE oligonucleotides activate a proinflammatory response independent of TLR-9 or myd88. *J Pharmacol Exp Therapeut* 2005;314:972–9.

52. Reynolds A, Anderson EM, Vermeulen A, Fedorov Y, Robinson K, Leake D, Karpilow J, Marshall WS, Khvorova A. Induction of the interferon response by siRNA is cell type- and duplex length-dependent. *RNA* 2006:12(6):988–93.

53. Hornung V, Ellegast J, Kim S, Brzozka K, Jung A, Kato H, Poeck H, Akira S, Conzelmann KK, Schlee M, et al. 5′-triphosphate RNA is the ligand for RIG-1. *Science* 2006;314:935–6.

54. Pichlmair A, Schulz O, Tan CP, Naslund TI, Liljestrom P, Weber F, Reis e Sousa C. RIG-1-mediated antiviral responses to single-stranded RNA bearing 5'-phosphates. *Science* 2006;314(5801):997–1001.

55. Henry SP, Geary RS, Yu R, Levin AA. Drug properties of second-generation antisense oligonucleotides: How do they measure up to their predecessors? *Curr Opin Invest Drugs* 2001;2(10):1444–9.

56. Liang H, Nishioka Y, Reich CF, Pisetsky DS, Lipsky PE. Activation of human B cells by phosphorothioate oligodeoxynucleotides. *J Clin Invest* 1996;98(5): 1119–29.

57. Klinman DM, AE-Kyung Y, Beaucage SL, Conover J, Krieg AM. CpG motifs present in bacterial DNA rapidly induce lymphocytes to secrete interleukin 6, interleukin 12, and interferon γ. *Proc Nat Acad Sci USA* 1996;93:2879–83.

58. Henry SP, Stecker K, Brooks D, Monteith D, Conklin B, Bennett CF. Chemically modified oligonucleotides exhibit decreased immune stimulation in mice. *J Pharmacol Exp Therapeut* 2000;292(2):468–79.

59. Graham MJ, Crooke ST, Monteith DK, Cooper SR, Lemonidis KM, Stecker KK, Martin MJ, Crooke RM. In vivo distribution and metabolism of a phosphorothioate oligonucleotide within rat liver after intravenous administration. *J Pharmacol Exp Therapeut* 1998;286(1):447–58.

60. Ponnappa BC, Israel Y. Targeting kupffer cells with antisense oligonucleotides. *Frontiers Biosci* 2002;7:e223–33.

61. Ponnappa BC, Israel Y, Aini M, Zhou F, Russ R, Cao QN, Hu Y, Rubin R. Inhibition of tumor necrosis factor alpha secretion and prevention of liver injury in ethanol-fed rats by antisense oligonucleotides. *Biochem Pharmacol* 2005;69(4): 569–77.

62. Henry SP, Zuckerman JE, Rojko J, Hall WC, Harman RJ, Kitchen D, Crooke ST. Toxicological properties of several novel oligonucleotide analogs in mice. *Anticancer Drug Des* 1997;12:1–14.

63. Zhao Q, Temsamani J, Zhou R-Z, Agrawal S. Pattern and kinetics of cytokine production following administration of phosphorothioate oligonucleotides in mice. *Antisense Nucl Acid Drug Dev* 1997;7:495–502.

64. Kastelein JJP, Wedel MK, Baker BF, Su J, Bradley JD, Yu RZ, Chuang E, Graham MJ, Crooke RM. Potent reduction of apolipoprotein B and low-density lipoprotein cholesterol by short-term administration of an antisense inhibitor of apolipoprotein B. *Circulation* 2006;114:1729–35.

65. Kwoh JT. An overview of the clinical safety experience of first and second generation antisense oligonucleotides. In Crooke ST, ed. *Antisense Drug Technology*. New York: Dekker, 2007.

66. Schechter PJ, Martin RR. Safety and tolerance of phosphorothioates in humans. In Crooke ST, ed. *Antisense Research and Applications*. Berlin, Heidelberg: Springer-Verlag, 1998;231–41.

67. Oberbauer R, Schreiner GF, Meyer TW. Renal uptake of an 18-mer phosphorothioate oligonucleotide. *Kidney Int* 1995;48:1226–32.

68. Rappaport J, Hanss B, Kopp JB, Copeland TD, Bruggeman LA, Coffman TM, Klotman PE. Transport of phosphorothioate oligonucleotides in kidney: implications for molecular therapy. *Kidney Int* 1995;47:1462–9.

69. Monteith DK, Levin AA. Synthetic oligonucleotides: The development of antisense therapeutics. *Toxicol Pathol* 1999;27(1):8–13.

70. Henry SP, Johnson M, Zanardi TA, Fey R, Auyeung D, Lappin PB, LevIn AA. Renal uptake and tolerability of a 2′-*O*-methoxyethyl modified antisense oligonucleotide (ISIS 113715) in monkey. *Toxicol Sci* (in press).

71. Monteith DK, Horner MJ, Gillett NA, Butler M, Geary RS, Burckin T, Ushiro-Watanabe T, Levin AA. Evaluation of the renal effects of an antisense phosphorothioate oligodeoxynucleotide in monkeys. *Toxicol Pathol* 1999;27(3):307–17.

72. Soucy NV, Riley JP, Templin MV, Geary R, de Peyster A, Levin AA. Maternal and fetal distribution of a phosphorothioate oligonucleotide in rats after intravenous infusion. *Birth Defects Res B Dev Reprod Toxicol* 2006;77(1):22–8.

73. Driver SE, Robinson GS, Flanagan J, Shen W, Smith LEH, Thomas DW, Roberts PC. Oligonucleotide-based inhibition of embryonic gene expression. *Nat Biotechnol* 1999;17:1184–7.

74. Krieg AM. The role of CpG motifs in innate immunity. *Curr Opin Immunol* 2000; 12(1):35–43.

75. Sparwasser T, Hultner L, Koch ES, Luz A, Lipford GB, Wagner H. Immunostimulatory CpG-oligodeoxynucleotides cause extramedullary murine hemopoiesis. *J Immunol* 1999;162:2368–74.

76. Klinman DM. Immunotherapeutic uses of CpG oligodeoxynucleotides. *Nat Rev Immunol* 2004;4(4):249–8.

77. Takeshita F, Leifer CA, Gursel I, Ishii KJ, Takeshita S, Gursel M, Klinman DM. Cutting edge: role of Toll-like receptor 9 in CpG DNA-induced activation of human cells. *J Immunol* 2001;167:3555–8.

78. Krieg AM. Antitumor applications of stimulating Toll-like receptor 9 with CpG oligodeoxynucleotides. *Curr Oncol Rep* 2004;6(2):88–95.

79. Branda RF, Moore AL, Hong R, Mccormack JJ, Zon G, Cunningham-Rundles C. B-cell proliferation and differentiation in common variable immunodeficiency patients produced by an antisense oligomer to the rev gene of hiv-1. *Clin Immunol Immunopathol* 1996;79(2):115–21.

80. Branda RF, Moore AL, Lafayette AR, Mathews L, Hong R, Zon G, Brown T, McCormack JJ. Amplification of antibody production by phosphorothioate oligodeoxynucleotides. *J Lab Clin Med* 1996;128(3):329–38.

CHAPTER 25

Preclinical Safety Evaluation of Biological Oncology Drugs

THERESA REYNOLDS, BA, DABT

Contents

25.1 BACKGROUND

The development of biopharmaceuticals in oncology began in 1986 with the introduction of IFN-α-2a (Roferon A) and IFN-α-2b (Intron A) for the treatment of hairy cell leukemia, a subtype of chronic lymphoid leukemia that accounts for approximately 2% of all leukemia cases in the United States [1]. These initial marketing approvals were followed by labels for AIDS-related Kaposi's sarcoma (1988), and hepatitis C (1995). The introduction of protein-derived therapeutics to small but significant areas of unmet medical need followed by expansion to new indications has evolved in parallel with our understanding of underlying biological mechanisms of disease. Since the introduction of the interferons to the practice of oncology, the pace of marketing approvals for protein therapeutics has continued to accelerate, and new products for cancer treatment have kept pace (Figure 25.1). In the 20 years since

Preclinical Safety Evaluation of Biopharmaceuticals: A Science-Based Approach to Facilitating Clinical Trials, edited by Joy A. Cavagnaro
Copyright © 2008 by John Wiley & Sons, Inc.

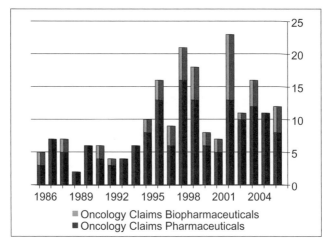

Figure 25.1 US FDA approvals in oncology from 1986 to 2006 (2006 data reported through July 24, 2006).

the introduction of IFN-α, a number of new and novel therapies have emerged from the biotechnology sector that have made a significant impact on disease outcomes and patient care. The proven benefit and future promise of oncology treatments derived from biotechnology is reflected in the proliferation of new biopharmaceuticals that are under study in clinical and preclinical settings.

25.2 THERAPEUTIC TARGETS AND MOLECULAR CLASSES

As of 2006 the US FDA has granted marketing approval to 22 biotechnology-derived pharmaceuticals with varying applications to oncology practice (Table 25.1). Some common mechanistic themes are as follows:

- Expansion of specific cell populations to replace those lost to cytotoxic chemotherapy (erythropoietin, G-CSF, GM-CSF, IL-11), or to enhance immunocompetence (IL-2, IFN-α).
- Targeted destruction of malignant cells via specific receptor binding by antibodies (anti-HER2, anti-EGF, anti-CD20, anti-CD52).
- Use of specific receptors to target delivery of a toxin to malignant cells (immunoconjugates, fusion proteins, antibody drug conjugates).
- Alteration of the local microenvironment to starve cells of essential nutrients (anti-VEGF, L-asparaginase enzymes).

Biotechnology has made significant contributions to supportive care in oncology, developing recombinant growth factors to replenish cell populations vulnerable to the dose-limiting neutropenia, anemia, and thrombocytopenia

TABLE 25.1   Biopharmaceuticals approved by US FDA for use in oncology from 1986 to 2006

Generic Name	Trade Name	Description	Type	Approval Date
Aldesleukin	Proleukin	rh IL-2	Growth factor	5/5/1992
Alemtuzumab	Campath	hu Anti-CD52	MAb	5/7/2001
Asparaginase	Elspar	rh L-asparaginase	Enzyme	8/1/2002
Bevacizumab	Avastin	hu Anti-VEGF	MAb	2/26/2004
Darbepoetin alpha	Aranesp	rh Novel erythropoetic stimulating protein	Growth factor	9/17/2001
Denileukin diftitox	Ontak	r Diphtheria toxin + IL-2	Fusion protein	2/5/1999
Epoetin alpha	Epogen	rh Erythropoetin	Growth factor	7/26/1999
Cetuximab	Erbitux	Chimeric (hu/mu) anti-epithelial growth factor receptor	MAb	2/12/2004
Filgrastim	Neupogen	Recombinant human G-CSF	Growth factor	2/20/1991
Gemtuzumab Ozogamicin	Mylotarg	Humanized anti-CD33 + calicheamicin	ADC	5/17/2000
IFN-α-2a	Roferon A	IFNα-2a	Cytokine	6/4/1986
IFN-α-2b	Intron A	IFNα-2b	Cytokine	6/4/1986
Ibritumomab tiuxetan	Zevalin	mu Anti-CD20 + Y-90 & In-111	Immunoconjugate	2/19/2002
Palifermin	Kepavance	rh Keratinocyte growth factor	Growth factor	12/15/2004
Oprelvekin	Neumega	rh IL-11	Growth factor	11/25/1997
Pegaspargase	Oncaspar	Pegylated r L-asparaginase	Enzyme	2/1/1994
Pegfilgrastim	Neulasta	Pegylated rh G-CSF	Growth factor	1/31/2002
Rasburicase	Elitek	r Urate oxidase	Enzyme	7/12/2002
Rituximab	Rituxan	Chimeric (hu/mu) anti-CD20	Chimeric Mab	11/26/1997
Sargramostim	Leukine, Prokine	rh GM-CSF	Growth factor	11/7/1996
Tositumomab	Bexxar	Chimeric (hu/mu) anti-CD20 + I-131	Immunoconjugate	6/27/2003
Trastuzumab	Herceptin	hu Anti-HER2	MAb	9/25/1998

Source: See US FDA [3]. 2006 data reported through July 24, 2006.

Note: ADC: antibody drug conjugatehu; hu: humanized; IFNα: interferon alpha; MAb: monoclonal antibody; Mu: murine; r: recombinant; Rh: recombinant human.

associated with cytotoxic chemotherapy, and an enzyme (rasburicase) to deplete plasma uric acid secondary to therapeutic-induced tumor lysis.

Although biotechnology-derived imaging agents and vaccines are part of the oncology armamentarium, they will not be discussed in detail in this chapter as they have less in common with the molecular entities listed above. The imaging agents are single use and are not designed for therapeutic benefit, while vaccines have their own specialized regulatory path (see Chapter 31).

25.3   CONSIDERATIONS FOR PRECLINICAL SAFETY ASSESSMENT OF ONCOLOGY PRODUCTS

Although the molecular structures and therapeutic indications vary, there is a consistent approach to characterization of the preclinical safety profile that requires consideration of a number of factors:

- *Clinical application*: Duration of treatment, current standard of care, and patient population.
- *Drug attributes*: Mechanism of action, species cross-reactivity, availability of pharmacodynamic markers for evidence of activity, long drug half-life, potential for drug accumulation, and immunogenic potential.
- *Material production*: Evolution of production methods and appropriate bridging studies.

These assessments are discussed broadly in other chapters. This section will address their application as it pertains to preclinical safety for oncology indications.

25.3.1   Clinical Application

Phase 1 studies with biopharmaceuticals for oncology indications have typically been conducted in cancer patients rather than in healthy volunteers, due in large part to product specific concerns including the potential for an anti-drug antibody response to treatment that could preclude future therapy, or expression of a tumor-specific antigen that is not present in nontumor-bearing individuals thus potentially impacting pharmacologic activity and/or pharmacokinetic parameters. With the early enrollment of patients in the course of clinical development comes the hope of an earlier indication of therapeutic benefit, resulting in multiple-dose phase 1 trials designed to assess disease activity in terms of progression, stable disease, or patient benefit. Phase 1 clinical trials of three-months' exposure (with an option to extend treatment in patients who benefit) are increasingly common and assist in recruiting patients to experimental therapies that may alter the course of their disease. However, because patients cannot be subjected to an experimental therapy when an established standard of care (SOC) with proven efficacy exists, patients enrolled into phase 1 programs are usually those whose disease has not been responsive to standard therapy. While phase 1 studies are generally single-agent studies of the experimental therapeutic, pivotal clinical trials to support product approval must demonstrate benefit over the existing standard of care. As a result pivotal clinical studies typically compare patients treated according to SOC with those given SOC plus experimental drug.

The earliest impact of the intended clinical application on the preclinical safety program is on the duration of the IND-enabling multiple-dose toxicity study. As is true with other therapeutic indications, the duration of the supporting preclinical study must be equal to the duration of the planned clinical study. Because oncology trials allow for extended (and often indefinite) treatment of patients who benefit, the key component to the determination of the duration of the preclinical safety study is *the point at which the clinical protocol specifies that determination of patient benefit will be made in order to extend treatment.* The preclinical study must support the "protocol-specified" duration of treatment in the clinical protocol. In the case of a 3-month treatment period for phase 1, a preclinical safety study with a three-month treatment period would be advisable. Extension of treatment for patients with responsive disease can occur following negotiation with regulatory authorities, and this is a familiar attribute of clinical trials in oncology. At a March 2006 Oncology Drugs Advisory Committee Meeting, the FDA acknowledged the value of expediting development of novel oncology products, and noted that most sponsors start out with 1-month toxicology studies in support of phase 1 trials while seeking regulatory authorization for patient treatment in excess of the treatment duration supported by the toxicology program. In the absence of 3-month animal safety data, the FDA requested sponsors to limit patient treatment, and requested 3-month toxicology studies prior to allowing patient treatment for extended durations. Continuation of clinical dosing beyond the nonclinical testing period has been approved based on the acceptability of toxicities (e.g., reversibility, degree of potential harm) and the ability to monitor anticipated toxicity endpoints. Furthermore potential patient risk–benefit must be weighed against the toxicologic profile characterized in animal studies when sponsors seek regulatory authorization for indefinite extension of patient treatment. [4,5].

While phase 1 trials often include patients of different treatment backgrounds and, depending on the mechanism of action of the experimental therapeutic, may include many different tumor types (e.g., an "all-comers" scenario), pivotal clinical trials are more tightly controlled in order to maximize the opportunity to detect an efficacy signal. As mentioned previously, the earliest pivotal clinical trials compare SOC alone and SOC in combination with experimental therapy to determine whether the experimental therapeutic provides additional patient benefit. Once this incremental benefit is demonstrated, additional clinical trials may be conducted to determine whether the experimental therapy is beneficial in earlier stage disease (e.g., the adjuvant

TABLE 25.2 Single-dose pharmacokinetic/safety interaction study for Herceptin®

Group	Test Materials[a]	Dose (mg/kg)
1	Trastuzumab	1.5
2	Paclitaxel	4.0
3	Doxorubicin	1.5
4	Doxorubicin + cyclophosphamide	1.5 + 15
5	Trastuzumab + paclitaxel	1.5 + 4.0
6	Trastuzumab + doxorubicin	1.5 + 1.5
7	Trastuzumab + doxorubicin + cyclophosphamide	1.5 + 1.5 + 15

Source: See [6].

[a]Multiple test materials (Groups 4-7) were administered in the order shown. Group size: Three female monkeys/group.

setting). Assessment of the preclinical safety of combination therapy requires that likely mechanisms of interaction, (e.g., biological or pharmacokinetic data) be taken into consideration.

Whereas small molecules employ p450 activation/inhibition profiles to elucidate metabolic interactions/antagonisms, there is no comparable tool to model the potential interactions of multiple biologics or between biologics and cytotoxics. To assess potential interactions between a protein therapeutic and cytotoxic chemotherapy SOC, one approach is to conduct a single-dose PK interaction study to assess the impact of the protein therapeutic on the PK of the SOC cytotoxics in a pharmacologically relevant species (Table 25.2; [7,8]). The objective of these studies is to determine whether the protein therapeutic has an effect on the PK, particularly the peak concentration (C_{max}) and/or time of peak concentration (T_{max}) that might result in potentiation of the toxicity of the cytotoxic, or reduced efficacy associated with decreased exposure.

Cause for concern related to additive or synergistic mechanisms of activity or toxicity should be addressed in a scientifically appropriate manner in consultation with regulatory authorities as necessary. Because of the broad distribution of potential combinations and mechanisms of activity/toxicity, and the complexity of species-specificity, there is not a one size fits all approach that can be applied. Current FDA regulatory guidance in this area is limited to combination products, with the intent to co-package and/or co-market as a defined treatment [9].

25.3.2 Drug Attributes

The impact of the drug attributes of biopharmaceuticals on preclinical safety assessment programs for oncology products is not unique to this therapeutic area. As is true for all biopharmaceuticals, species cross-reactivity must be determined prior to selection of an appropriate animal model for safety evaluation. The nature of cross-reactivity can be based on a combination of pharmacologic activity, receptor homology, and target tissue binding, as appropriate. The value of highly human-specific and tumor-specific cell targeting in cancer treatment is unequivocal, but the impact of highly specific targeted human therapies on the selection of appropriate animal models is significant. Often the more targeted the therapy, the more limited is the choice of animal model; in many cases species cross-reactivity is limited to nonhuman primates (NHPs). For biopharmaceuticals that target a receptor (or biological process) that is expressed (or active) at very low levels in normal human tissue, and detected at even lower levels in normal NHP tissue, there is likely to be little opportunity to assess toxicities associated with exaggerated pharmacologic activity. The availability of pharmacodynamic markers for evidence of activity in preclinical safety studies is a useful tool in differentiating pharmacologic activity from suprapharmacologic toxicity and providing a meaningful therapeutic index. For example, potential clinical toxicities such as cytokine release associated with tumor lysis syndrome will not be evident in preclinical safety studies. In the case of highly selective biopharmaceuticals an apparent lack of toxicity in preclinical models may not be predictive of subsequent clinical experience.

Although biopharmaceuticals must be administered parenterally, their relatively large size, from roughly 15 kd for proteins such as recombinant human IL-2 (Proleukin®) to roughly 150 kd for monoclonal antibodies such as Herceptin®, confers a long half-life. The pharmacokinetic properties of biopharmaceuticals must be taken into account when determining dose and frequency of administration to reduce the potential for drug accumulation and potential toxicities secondary to suprapharmacologic exposure in vast excess of clinical relevance, and/or activation of endogenous scavenging mechanisms associated with massive protein overload. Either scenario can complicate interpretation of preclinical safety signals and extrapolation of appropriate clinical doses.

The immunogenic potential of biopharmceuticals is assessed in preclinical safety studies through careful monitoring of anti-therapeutic antibodies during the course of the treatment and recovery periods. An appropriate recovery period must be included for drug washout so that anti-drug antibodies can be measured in the absence of drug interference. Although it is generally agreed that there is little relevance to clinical safety of an observed anti-drug antibody response in preclinical safety studies, the generation of anti-drug antibodies can antagonize drug effect or result in untoward immune-mediated events that can confound the interpretation of the data.

25.3.3 Material Production

During the course of a drug development program, improvements in production methods, including cell line yield, process improvements, and formulation modification evolve to fit the scale and scope of the clinical trials, and ultimately the marketplace. For each change, appropriate bridging studies are conducted. Depending on the nature of the change, and the data generated during comparability testing, further comparative studies in animals or even humans may be warranted. This topic is discussed in Part III (see Chapter 8).

25.4   APPLICATION OF STANDARD TOXICOLOGY MODELS

Many of the standard toxicology models apply to oncology programs, and there are some additional points worthy of consideration. Systemic toxicity studies have been discussed previously in the context of the duration of preclinical studies supporting clinical development, and these studies are essential for characterizing the safety profile of a biopharmaceutical. Given that most clinical development plans include multiple dosing in phase 1, the utility of single-dose animal studies for anything other than dose ranging or overt tolerability is questionable and should be supported scientifically. If the scientific hypothesis for clinical efficacy requires consistent exposure to drug over time, then single-dose animal studies as part of an IND-enabling program provide little information regarding potential human risks associated with clinical administration. As discussed previously, the treatment period for multiple-dose systemic toxicity studies must equal the protocol-specified treatment period of clinical trials. An exception to this exists for chronic toxicity studies conducted to support chronic treatment in patients; these studies are generally conducted in support of licensing authorizations but may be conducted earlier in the clinical development life cycle as needed to support clinical trials of six months' duration or greater. In general, chronic toxicity studies of six months are sufficient to support chronic treatment in oncology, which is consistent with ICH S6. In a "white paper" authored by a working group of BioSafe (a subcommittee of the Regulatory Affairs Committee of the Biotechnology Industry Organization, BIO) an analysis of publicly available data to determine the extent to which data from chronic studies was predictive of human response and whether the six-month duration was appropriate. The authors concluded that the six-month duration was generally appropriate to support chronic clinical dosing, although there may be specific circumstances that might warrant longer term studies [10].

With regard to safety pharmacology endpoints it is standard practice to include cardiovascular and respiratory endpoints as part of the multiple-dose systemic toxicity studies. For biopharmaceuticals lacking cross-reactivity in rodents, it is possible to conduct limited neurobehavioral assessments of peripheral and central nervous system function in nonhuman primates, but with the caveat that unlike humans or even dogs, these wild animals are most likely to mask any physical deficit that would place them at a selective disadvantage in their natural habitat. In addition to incorporating safety pharmacology endpoints into systemic toxicity studies, these studies can be further maximized by assessing local tolerance at the sites of drug administration, thereby eliminating the need for a separate study of local tolerance in rabbits.

The standard battery of genetic toxicity studies is considered irrelevant for biopharmaceuticals per ICH S6. However, exceptions are made in cases where cause for concern exists, such as the presence of an organic linker molecule in a not yet approved conjugated protein product, or where new and appropriate testing systems are developed to elucidate genotoxic risk. For biopharmaceuticals that received marketing approval prior to the finalization of ICH S6 in 1997, it is not unusual to note the presence of a full battery of genetic toxicity studies as a component of the approval package. Likewise the rodent bioassay for carcinogenic potential is generally considered to be inappropriate for biopharmaceuticals due to species-specificity and immunogenic potential of human/humanized protein products in rodents.

Reproductive toxicity studies may be conducted, depending on the mechanism of action of the biopharmaceutical. In cases where NHPs represent the suitable animal model for safety testing, a full battery of male and female fertility, embryonic and developmental toxicity, and well as late-stage gestational, parturition, placental and lactational drug transfer and infant developmental studies have been applied in the preclinical safety evaluation of protein therapeutics. These studies are lengthy and complex, and unlike systemic toxicity studies where all animals begin and end treatment at the same time, female animals are enrolled on study as their pregnancy and/or hormonal status permits, creating a rolling study start and estimated times of study completion. A novel study design for assessing the potential embryonic and developmental toxicity in rabbits that were expected to mount an anti-drug antibody response to treatment has been used to successfully identify toxicities associated with drug treatment (Table 25.3). Rabbits had been demonstrated to be a cross-reactive species to the experimental therapeutic (tenecteplase), and it was anticipated that dose administration throughout the period of organogenesis would result in the formation of anti-drug antibodies that would impact

TABLE 25.3   Embryofetal toxicity study using divided dosing

Group	Dosing Days
Control	DG 6–18
Low	DG 6–10
Mid	DG 6–10
High	DG 6–10
Low	DG 11–14
Mid	DG 11–14
High	DG 11–14
Low	DG 15–18
Mid	DG 15–18
High	DG 15–18

Source: See [11].

Note: DG: day of gestation; 18 rabbits/group.

exposure. In that model the period of organogenesis (gestation days 6–18) is divided into discrete dosing intervals, and separate groups of animals receive drug for one of the three 4- to 5-day intervals. This study satisfied ICH tripartite guideline stages C and D of the reproductive process in a nonrodent species.

Constructing a scientific rationale for the preclinical safety testing strategy in support of a clinical development plan for oncology products is a key component of drug development. The scientific rationale should take into consideration a number of factors, including the clinical patient population and duration of exposure, species-specificity, available and appropriate in vitro and in vivo models, maximizing the value of each systemic toxicity study for responsible animal use, immunogenicity and impact on exposure, and an awareness of drug production changes that can impact the ability to rely on the foundation of previously conducted preclinical safety studies. This is consistent with the thinking that should be applied to the creation of a preclinical safety plan regardless of the therapeutic indication for which a biopharmaceutical is being studied.

25.5   SUMMARY AND CONCLUSION

Despite meaningful clinical advances over the past two decades, a great deal of unmet medical need remains in oncology. Our increasing understanding of the biological mechanisms of cancer has enabled the development of highly specific, targeted therapies that are rewriting the cancer descriptors from "tissue of origin," as in breast lung, colon, and prostate cancer, to the underlying mechanisms of pathology, as in HER2 overexpression. Hybrid molecular entities such as antibody–drug conjugates, fusion proteins, and one-armed antibodies, once considered novel and unusual are becoming more prevalent as the physical attributes of each biopharmaceutical are engineered to meet a particular therapeutic need—a classic case of the basic engineering principle of "form follows function (see Chapters 28 and 29). As our understanding of common pathologic processes has evolved, biopharmaceuticals that were initially developed as oncology treatments have provided benefit in other areas of unmet medical need. For example, since the introduction of the IFN-α in 1986 for the treatment of a small, but significant subset of chronic lymphoid leukemias, a critical role for IFN-α therapy in hepatitis was established. Rituxan®, a chimeric monoclonal antibody to the CD-20 receptor of B cells, was initially approved for the treatment of non-Hodgkin's lymphoma, and is now approved for the treatment of patients with rheumatoid arthritis.

Additional safety studies may be required to support the movement into new indications, and the complex "designer" biopharmaceuticals will continue to require creative approaches to safety assessment. In either case, the requirement for, and design and execution of, those studies should be driven by sound scientific rationale. Ultimately, the objective of preclinical safety evaluation is well articulated in ICH S6:

- Identification of an initial safe starting dose and dose escalation scheme for clinical trials.
- Identification of potential target organs of toxicity and reversibility of effect.
- Identification of safety parameters for clinical monitoring.

These objectives are best fulfilled through thoughtful planning and significant cross-functional generation of clinical development assumptions by toxicologists, clinicians, researchers, pharmacokineticists, bioanalytical assay scientists, and the scientists and engineers responsible for making and formulating the biopharmaceutical drug product. The design and implementation of scientifically appropriate in vitro and in vivo studies that are integrated into the support of a well-articulated clinical plan will best allow us to expeditiously move promising new therapies forward to patients in need while judiciously applying the human, animal and financial resources required.

REFERENCES

1. Saven A, Ellison DJ, Piro, LD. *Clinical Oncology*. New York: Churchill Livingstone Inc. 1995;2023–34.
2. www.accessdata.fda.gov/scripts/cder/onctools/yearlistclaim.cfm
3. www.accessdata.fda.gov/scripts/cder/onctools/yearlistclaim.cfm
4. Pilaro A. Nonclinical perspective on initiating phase 1 studies for biological oncology products—Case studies. Oncology Drugs Advisory Committee, March 13, 2006.
5. Green M. Pre-clinical requirements for phase 1 studies—biological oncology products. Oncology Drugs Advisory Committee, March 13, 2006.
6. Reynolds T, Baughman S, Schofield C, Palazzolo M, Dalgard D, Thomas DA. A 3-week interaction study of rhuMAb HER2 with doxorubicin, cyclophosphamide and paclitaxel in rhesus monkeys. *Toxicologist* 1996;30(1):36.
7. Modi NB, Lin YS, Reynolds T, Shaheen A, Christian BC. Pharmacokinetics of Xubix, an orally active IIbIIIa antagonist, in the presence of heparin, aspirin and rt-PA in beagles. *J Cardiovas Pharmacol* 1998;32:397–405.
8. Gaudreault J, Shiu V, Bricarello A, Christian BJ, Zuch CL, Mounho B. Concomitant administration of bevacizumab, irinotecan, 5-fluorouracil, and leucovorin: nonclinical safety and pharmacokinetics. *Intl J Toxicol* 2005;24:357–63.
9. 21 CFR part 3.2(e), Docket No. 2004N-0194, Federal Register, Vol 70, No. 164, 8/25/05.
10. Clarke J, Hurst C, Martin P, Vahle J, Ponce R, Mounho B, Heidel S, Andrews, L, Reynolds T, Cavagnaro J. Duration of chronic toxicity studies for biotechnology-derived pharmaceuticals. *Regul Toxicol Pharmcol* 2008;50:2–22.
11. Gross MC, Leach W, Prince W, Hoberman A, Barnett J, O'Neill C. Embryotoxic and teratogenic evaluation of TNK-tPA in rabbits: a study around antigenicity issues. *Toxicologist* 2000;54(1):397.

CHAPTER 26

Preclinical Safety Evaluation of Monoclonal Antibodies

GEORGE TREACY, MS, and PAULINE MARTIN, PhD

Contents

26.1 INTRODUCTION

Monoclonal antibodies (mAbs) are populations of identical, monospecific antibodies with defined specificity and affinity for a target antigen. The high degree of specificity for their target is the property that makes monoclonal antibodies so valuable clinically. As such, they can be used not only therapeutically to treat and prevent disease but also to diagnose a wide variety of diseases, and to detect drugs, abnormal proteins, viruses, and bacteria. Monoclonal antibodies are produced by the daughter cells of a single antibody-producing lymphocyte, often using an immortal hybridoma cell line grown in vitro. Monoclonal antibodies can also be constructed synthetically and produced as engineered recombinant proteins. In both cases cells can be grown continually in culture to produce large amounts of protein.

Preclinical Safety Evaluation of Biopharmaceuticals: A Science-Based Approach to Facilitating Clinical Trials, edited by Joy A. Cavagnaro
Copyright © 2008 by John Wiley & Sons, Inc.

Since the approval of the first therapeutic monoclonal antibody in 1986, considerable advances have been made in antibody technology [1,2]. With the improvement in antibody technology an increase in the clinical success of this group of molecules has been seen [3].

Monoclonal antibodies exhibit the same general structural and functional characteristics as naturally acquired antibodies, and they can be of any antibody class (IgG, IgM, IgD, IgE, or IgA) or isotype within a class. The most commonly developed monoclonal antibodies are of the IgG class, and they are tetrameric proteins consisting of two identical heavy chains and two identical light chains (Figures 26.1 and 26.2). Each IgG molecule contains two antigen combining sites formed by the N-terminal regions of the heavy and light chains, which determine the antigen recognition and binding properties of the monoclonal antibody. The specificity of a given monoclonal antibody is determined by the precise amino acid sequences of the heavy and light protein chains in the antigen-combining region (complementary-determining region,

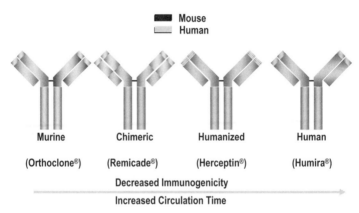

Figure 26.1   Structure of a monoclonal antibody and its interaction with antigen. See color insert.

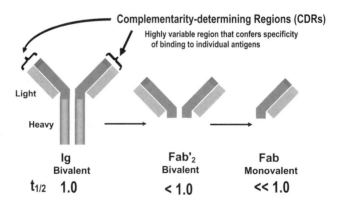

Figure 26.2   Examples of various classes of monoclonal antibodies. See color insert.

CDR); the sequences of this region are therefore somewhat variable among monoclonal antibodies of different specificities. The antigen-combining region is also known as the variable region because of this sequence variation. The remainder of the molecule is relatively constant in sequence among different monoclonal antibodies, and it functions to allow interactions with other immune system components. This region of the monoclonal antibody determines the class and isotype of the antibody, and is known as the constant region or Fc region.

Monoclonal antibodies can be grouped according to their potential use: (1) binding to a cell surface target, with recruitment of immune response and target cell lysis; (2) binding to a cell surface receptor causing apoptosis; (3) cross-linking to a cell-killing reagent (e.g. immunotoxin); (4) binding to a target to block an interaction (antagonist); (5) binding to a receptor to stimulate a downstream process (agonist); and (6) catalysis (catalytic antibodies).

Many monoclonal antibodies have now been approved for the diagnosis or treatment of various diseases. The target antigens include soluble factors such as tumor necrosis factor (TNFα), vascular endothelial growth factor (VEGF) and IgE, cell surface antigens on lymphocytes (CD3, CD20, CD25, CD52, CD11a, CD49d), antigens upregulated on tumor cells (HER2, EGFR), and viral specific antigens RSV (see Chapter 25). Antibodies have also been used to deliver toxins or radioactivity to tumor cells and imaging agents to tumors (see Chapter 29). In addition to a high degree of specificity and affinity for the target antigen, monoclonal antibodies exhibit in vivo pharmacokinetic properties similar to those of naturally acquired antibodies.

26.2 FC BINDING OF MONOCLONAL ANTIBODIES

Besides the binding of the variable region (Fab) of the monoclonal antibody to the target antigen, some monoclonal antibodies also require binding of the constant region to receptors on effectors cells. These receptors, referred to as Fcγ receptors (FcγR), are expressed on immune cells and consist of three distinct classes FcγRI (CD64), FcγRII (CD32), and FcγRIII (CD16). Binding to FcγR can lead to antigen-dependent cellular cytotoxicity (ADCC), phagocytosis, or other cellular effects. ADCC can be beneficial when the target antigen is present on a tumor cell. However, when the target antigen is present on lymphocytes, ADCC may be detrimental. For example anti-CD3 and anti-CD4 antibodies can lead to T cell depletion. Also binding of monoclonal antibodies to immune cell antigens may lead to cytokine release syndrome that may result in side effects of fever, nausea, and bronchospasm. IgG1 antibodies have greater potential effector function than IgG2 and IgG4 antibodies. However, IgG1 antibodies can be modified to have reduced or enhanced effector function, depending on the desired therapeutic effects [4,5].

Effector function can also be eliminated by removing the Fc portion of the molecule to produce a Fab molecule (e.g., abciximab). However, Fab molecules have very rapid elimination from the circulation relative to full-length molecules, and for certain clinical indications this may not be desirable. The reason for the shorter half-life of Fab molecules relative to full-length antibodies is that binding of the Fc portion of the antibody to another type of Fc receptor found on endothelial cells (FcRn) leads to antibody internalization and recycling, resulting in enhanced serum persistence. Therefore molecules that show poor binding to FcRn are rapidly eliminated from the serum.

26.3   FULLY MURINE MONOCLONAL ANTIBODIES

The first therapeutic monoclonal antibodies developed were fully murine sequence antibodies. These antibodies were developed by immunizing mice with a human antigen. Antigen-specific B cells were isolated from the immunized mice and were fused to an immortal cell line to generate monoclonal hybridomas secreting fully murine mAbs. (Figure 26.3). The first approved monoclonal antibody was muromomab-CD3, which is a murine monoclonal antibody against human CD3 on T lymphocytes. This antibody was developed for the treatment of acute transplant rejection. The main disadvantage of using murine monoclonal antibodies to treat human diseases is that because the antibodies contain murine sequences, they can be highly immunogenic in humans. Humans treated with muromomab-CD3 develop human anti-murine antibodies (HAMA) that result in reduced exposure to the antibody and a

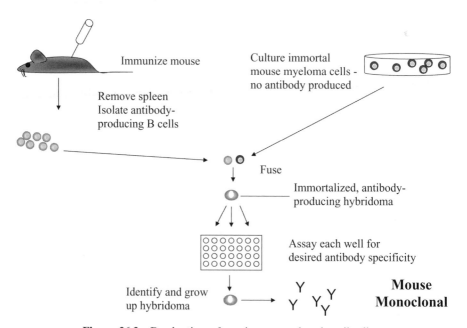

Figure 26.3   Production of murine monoclonal antibodies.

loss of efficacy even in the presence of concomitant immune suppression. Muromomab and other antibodies that bind to T cell receptors and activate the T cell can also cause cytokine release, which produces a systemic inflammatory response characterized by hypotension, pyrexia, and rigors [6]. The cytokine release can cause life-threatening pulmonary edema. Deaths due to cytokine release syndrome have been reported with OKT3. Cytokine release can be anticipated then for monoclonal antibodies that activate T cells and can usually be treated appropriately.

In addition to the immunogenic potential of murine monoclonal antibodies, another disadvantage of murine antibodies is their rapid elimination from the circulation relative to human antibodies. Muromomab has an elimation half-life of about 18 hours, whereas human antibodies have half-lives of weeks. Human antibodies have long serum persistence because they are recycled by endothelial cells. The Fc portion of murine monoclonal antibodies binds very poorly to human FcRn, and therefore murine antibodies are not recycled resulting in their poor serum persistence [7]. The converse, however, is not true. Human Fc binds well to murine FcRn, and therefore human antibodies have long serum persistence in mice. The lack of FcRn binding in combination with a HAMA response results in rapid clearance from the serum.

Because of these limitations murine antibodies have had very limited clinical use. The other murine antibodies include two radiolabeled versions of anti-CD20 antibodies that have been developed for the treatment of non-Hodgkins lymphoma and an anti-PSMA antibody-imaging agent for visualizing prostate tumors (Table 26.1). These antibodies are intended for short-term use and are administered at low doses. For these antibodies the short serum half-life and the potential to develop HAMA are not considered a limitation for therapy. Interestingly, since ibritumomab tiuxetan and tositumomab-I[131] are B cell depleting therapies, their mechanism of action reduces the immune response [8].

TABLE 26.1   Summary of approved fully murine monoclonal antibodies

Generic Name	Trade Name	Sponsor Company	Mechanism	Antibody Isotype	Indication	Approval Date
Muromonab-CD3	Orthoclone® OKT3	Ortho Biotech	Anti-CD3	IgG2a	Transplant rejection	1986
Abciximab	ReoPro®	Centocor	Anti-GPIIb/IIa	Fab	Cardiovascular	1997
Capromab pendetide	ProstaScint®	Cytogen Corp	Anti-PSMA	IgG1 kappa	Oncology imaging	1996
Ibritumomab tiuxetan	Zevalin®	Biogen Idec	Anti-CD20-Yttrium 90	IgG1 kappa	Oncology	2002
Tositumomab-I[131]	Bexxar®	Corixa	Anti-CD20 Iodine 131	IgG2a Lambda	Oncology	2003

TABLE 26.2 Summary of approved chimeric monoclonal antibodies

Generic Name	Trade Name	Sponsor Company	Type	Antibody Isotype	Indication	Approval Date
Rituximab	Rituxan®	Genentech	Anti-CD20	IgG1 kappa	Oncology	1997
Basiliximab	Simulect®	Novartis	Anti-CD25	IgG1 kappa	Transplant rejection	1998
Infliximab	Remicade®	Centocor	Anti-TNFα	IgG1 kappa	Immune-mediated diseases	1998
Cetuximab	Erbitux®	Imclone	Anti-EGFR	IgG1 kappa	Oncology	2004

26.4 CHIMERIC MONOCLONAL ANTIBODIES

Because of the limitations seen with the fully murine monoclonal antibodies the next generation of antibodies were chimeric antibodies (Table 26.2, Figure 26.2). Chimeric antibodies are constructed from variable regions derived from a murine source and constant regions derived from a human source. The chimeric antibodies show less of an immunogenic response than the fully murine antibodies, but human anti-chimeric antibody (HACA) rates can still be high with these antibodies. The chimeric antibodies nevertheless have relative long serum half-lives (9.5 days for infliximab) relative to the fully murine antibodies because the Fc portion is human and can therefore bind to human FcRn in a manner similar to that of native antibodies.

26.5 HUMANIZED MONOCLONAL ANTIBODIES

Humanized antibodies are constructed with only antigen binding regions (CDRs) derived from a mouse, and the remainder of the variable region derived from a human source. The humanized monoclonal antibodies represent the largest group of the currently approved monoclonal antibodies (Table 26.3, Figure 26.2). These antibodies have been highly successful in the clinic, and few serious immune-mediated adverse reactions have been observed. Two of the approved humanized monoclonal antibodies are IgG4 antibodies, gentuzumab ozogamicin and natalizumab. The remainder of the humanized antibodies are IgG1 antibodies. IgG4 antibodies have the potential advantage over IgG1 antibodies in certain situations because they lack effector function.

26.6 FULLY HUMAN MONOCLONAL ANTIBODIES

As of 2006 only two fully human monoclonal antibodies had been approved (Table 26.4). Adalimumab is a fully human antibody against human TNFα that

TABLE 26.3   Summary of approved humanized monoclonal antibodies

Generic Name	Trade Name	Sponsor Company	Mechanism	Antibody Isotype	Indication	Approval Date
Daclizumab	Zenapax®	Hoffman-La Roche	Anti-CD25	IgG1	Transplant rejection	1997
Palivizumab	Synagis®	MedImmune	Anti-RSV	IgG1 kappa	Anti-viral	1998
Trastuzumab	Herceptin®	Genentech	Anti-HER2	IgG1 kappa	Oncology	1998
Gemtuzumab ozogamicin	Mylotarg®	Wyeth-Ayerst	Anti-CD33 immunotoxin	IgG4 kappa	Oncology	2000
Alemtuzumab	Campath®	Millennium/LEX	Anti-CD52	IgG1 kappa	Oncology	2001
Omalizumab	Xolair®	Genentech	Anti-IgE	IgG1 kappa	Asthma	2003
Efalizumab	Raptiva®	Genentech	Anti-CD11a	IgG1 kappa	Psoriasis	2003
Bevacizumab	Avastin®	Genentech	Anti-VEGF	IgG1	Oncology	2004
Natalizumab	Tysabri®	Biogen idec	Anti-α4-integrin	IgG4	Multiple sclerosis	2004

TABLE 26.4   Summary of approved fully human monoclonal antibodies

Generic Name	Trade Name	Sponsor Company	Mechanism	Antibody Isotype	Indication	Approval Date
Adalimumab	Humira®	Abbott	Anti-TNFα	IgG1 kappa	Immune-mediated diseases	2002
Panitumumab	Vectibix™	Amgen	Anti-EGFR	IgG2 kappa	Oncology	2006

was developed from phage display technology. However, even though adalimumab is a fully human antibody, it has shown a significant human antihuman antibody (HAHA) response in patients [8]. Therefore fully human antibodies may not necessarily be an advantage from an immunogenicity perspective.

26.7 PRECLINICAL DEVELOPMENT PROGRAMS WITH MONOCLONAL ANTIBODIES

The design of preclinical safety evaluation of monoclonal antibodies is based on the class of monoclonal, the target epitope, and the clinical indication. Safety evaluation programs are then developed based on the availability of relevant species and specific attributes of the product on a "case-by-case" basis. Prior to issuance of regulatory guidance documents by the FDA and ICH [9,10] safety evaluations have included the use of nonrelevant assays (e.g., gentoxcity assays) and nonrelevant species. The nonclinical development programs have also included the use of murine homologues (surrogate monoclonal antibodies) when warranted. See Table 26.5 for examples of development programs for some nononcology indications.

The property of monoclonal antibodies that makes them highly desirable as therapeutics, namely the high degree of specificity for their target, also makes then a challenge from a preclinical development perspective. The earliest monoclonal antibodies were so specific for binding to their human target protein that they did not bind to the analogous target protein in any animal species except for chimpanzees. The chimpanzee is not an appropriate species for toxicology testing because the amount of nonclinical safety information that can be acquired from the chimpanzee is severally limited. Infliximab and efalizumab are examples of monoclonal antibodies developed to treat chronic non–life-threatening indications that bound only to their target in humans and chimpanzees. The preclinical safety program using the human monoclonal antibody was therefore restricted to limited nonterminal safety studies in chimpanzees and to in vitro tissue cross reactivity to a panel of human tissues.

In vitro tissue cross-reactivity studies are a key component of the safety assessment of monoclonal antibodies. These studies are required by regulatory authorities, and they need to be conducted on a panel of human tissues [9,10,11]. The purpose of these studies is to identify potential binding of the monoclonal antibody to nontarget tissues. A comparison of the in vitro cross-reactivity to human tissues and to tissues from one or more animal species may be performed to help determine species relevance for subsequent toxicology evaluation. In some cases tissue cross-reactivity alone has been used as a criterion for species selection for toxicology. Demonstration of a similar binding profile in human and animal tissues alone is, however, not usually considered to be an adequate means for selecting a toxicology species. The monoclonal antibody should be shown not only to bind to the analogous protein in the animal but also to produce a similar biological response in the human and in the animal. However, for some monoclonal antibodies that target tumor-associated antigens or virus (e.g., RSV) there will be no biological assay to show bioactivity between human and animal.

Because of the limited safety information provided by the chimpanzee studies and the in vitro human tissue cross-reactivity study, the need to develop an alternate strategy to evaluate safety for the human/chimpanzee specific monoclonal antibodies was appreciated. The ICH S6 guidance document for the preclinical safety testing of biotechnology-derived pharmaceuticals includes a provision for using a surrogate monoclonal antibody in such cases [9]. In both the infliximab and efalizumab examples anti-murine monoclonal antibodies were developed that could be tested in the mouse [12,13]. With these surrogate molecules chronic toxicity studies as well as reproductive toxicity studies were conducted. However, even though the monoclonal antibody being tested in these studies was not the same monoclonal antibody that was being evaluated in clinical trials, this alternate approach is considered to be acceptable. The preclinical safety program for infliximab was initiated

TABLE 26.5 Example preclinical safety evaluation programs with monoclonal antibodies

Product Name	Species Specificity	Initial Clinical Indication	Types of Studies to Support Approval
Infliximab (anti-TNFα) Remicade®	Chimpanzee specific	Crohn's disease	Tissue cross-reactivity: human Genetic toxicity: Ames,[a] in vitro chromosomal abberations human lymphocyte (CAHL),[a] mouse micronucleus (MM)[a] Toxicity: single dose—chimpanzee, rat;[b] repeat dose—chimpanzee, rat,[b] mouse[c] Fertility: mouse[c] Embryofetal development: mouse[c] Pre- and postnatal development: mouse[c]
Efalizumab (anti-CD11a) Raptiva®	Chimpanzee specific	Psoriais	Tissue cross-reactivity: human, chimpanzee, mouse[c] Toxicity: single dose—chimpanzee; mouse;[c] repeat dose—chimpanzee, mouse[c] Immunotoxicity: chimpanzee, mouse[c] Fertility: mouse[c] Embryofetal development: mouse[c] Pre- and postnatal development: mouse[c]
Adalimumab (anti-TNFα) Humira®	Reacts with cynomolgus macaque, no cross-reactivity with rodents	Rheumatoid arthritis	Tissue cross-reactivity: human, chimpanzee, cynomolgus, marmoset, rhesus, baboon, rat Genetic toxicity: Ames,[a] MN[a] Toxicity: single dose—mouse[b] and rat;[b] repeat dose—mouse[b] and cynomolgus[b] Embryofetal development: cynomolgus[b]

TABLE 26.5 *Continued*

Product Name	Species Specificity	Initial Clinical Indication	Types of Studies to Support Approval
Omalizumab (anti-IgE) Xolair®	Reacts with cynomolgus macaque, no cross-reactivity to rodents	Asthma	Tissue cross-reactivity: human, cynomolgus; Genetic toxicity: Ames[a]; Toxicity: single dose—mouse,[b] cynomolgus; repeat dose—cynomolgus; Fertility: cynomolgus; Embryofetal development: cynomolgus
Palivizumab (anti-RSV) Synagis®	Reacts with antigen on RSV No cross-reactivity to human or animal antigens	Prophylaxis of serious lower respiratory tract disease caused by RSV	Tissue cross-reactivity: human, cynomolgus; Toxicity: single dose—cynomolgus[b] and rabbit;[b] repeat dose—rat[b]; Virus challenge model: cotton rat

Note: All information included in this table and the accompanying text have been extracted from the US FDA summary basis of approval information (www.fda.gov) the European Medicines Agency (EMEA) centrally authorized product reviews (EPARs; www.emea.europa.eu) and the *Physicians Desk Reference* (PDR).

[a]Nonrelevant test system.

[b]Nonrelevant species.

[c]Use of murine homologue (surrogate antibody).

before the issuance of the ICH S6 guidance document, and consequently some studies, now considered to be unnecessary, were conducted with infliximab. For example, gentoxicity studies are now considered not to be appropriate for biopharmaceuticals and studies in biologically nonrelevant species are not considered to be appropriate. The only example where studies in a nonrelevant species may be appropriate is where similar nontarget binding of the monoclonal antibody is demonstrated to human tissues and to tissues in a biologically nonrelevant species.

Omalizumab and adalimumab are examples of monoclonal antibodies, developed for chronic non–life-threatening indication, that showed cross-reactivity to cynomolgus macaques as well as to humans. This broader species cross-reactivity allowed for a more thorough preclinical safety evaluation of the human monoclonal antibody developed for human use in the cynomolgus macaque. In the case of omalizumab, fertility studies and developmental toxicitiy studies were conducted in macaques in addition to the chronic toxicity studies. For adalimumab, no reproductive and developmental toxicity studies were conducted. The value of conducting fertility and developmental studies in macaques with monoclonal antibodies is described in Chapter 17.

The last example shown in Table 26.5 is palivizumab, a monoclonal antibody against an antigen expressed on a virus (RSV). Since this antigen does not exists in any animal species, including humans, all toxicology species are considered equally nonrelevant. The only relevant species is one that is infected with the virus. This example provides an interesting case where animal disease models could be considered more relevant than normal animals. Nevertheless, for palivizumab single-dose acute toxicity studies were performed in rats, rabbits, and macaques.

26.8 FUTURE OF ANTIBODY DEVELOPMENT

Recombinant DNA technologies can be used to manipulate monoclonal antibody sequences to produce monoclonal antibodies with improved properties, such as higher affinity, increased functional activity, and reduced immunogenicity for in vivo applications. Human sequence antibodies from transgenic mice, phage display, ribosome display, yeast display libraries, monoclonal antibody fragments, single-chain Fv, single-domain fragments, diabodies, minibodies (scFv fused to CH3 domain of mAbs), bispecific and multivalent mAb toxin-conjugates, and immunocytokines [2]. It is now possible to engineer monoclonal antibodies to have desired properties such as optimal serum half-life, reduced immunogenicity, and reduced or enhanced ADCC and CDC activities. It is also possible to engineer some monoclonal antibodies that will cross-react with multiple species, including rodents. The development of these monoclonal antibodies could allow more extensive toxicology evaluation than could be conducted with the species restricted monoclonal antibodies, assuming they are not immunogenic in the animals.

26.9 SUMMARY

Monoclonal antibodies have proved to be value therapeutic and diagnostic agents. In general, the clinical safety of monoclonal antibodies has been good. The high degree of specificity of monoclonal antibodies for their targets has contributed to the high success rate in the clinic. However, their high degree of specificity has also restricted the nonclinical safety testing that can be conducted with these molecules. The nonclinical development programs for monoclonal antibodies have been developed on a case-by-case basis depending on the clinical indication, the intended clinical use, and an understanding of the biology of the targeted antigen. In the future the advancement in monoclonal antibody technology may lead to monoclonal antibodies that do not behave like natural antibodies and may be less species restricted. In these cases the nonclinical safety testing may differ from that of the currently approved monoclonal antibodies.

REFERENCES

1. Weiner LM. Fully human therapeutic monoclonal antibodies. *J Immunother* 2006; 29:1–9.
2. Prezta LG. Engineering of therapeutic antibodies to minimize immunogenicity and optimize function. *Adv Drug Deliv Rev* 2006;58:640–56.
3. Reichert JM, Rosensweig CJ, Faden LB, Dewitz MC. Monoclonal antibody successes in the clinic. *Nat Med* 2005;23:1073–8.
4. Armour MR, Clark AG, Hadley LM, Williamson LM: Recombinant human IgG molecules lacking Fc gamma receptor I binding and monocyte triggering activities, *Eur J Immunol* 1999;29:2613–24.
5. Sheilds RL, Namenuk AK, Hong K, Meng J, Rae J, Briggs J, Xie D, Lai J, Stadlen A, Li B, Presta LG. High resolution mapping of the binding site on human IgG1 for FcγRI, FcγRII, FcγRIII and FcRn and design of IgG1 variants with improved binding to the Fcγ. *J Biol Chem* 2001;276:6591–604.
6. Sgro C. Side effects of a monoclonal antibody, muromomab CD3/orthoclone OKT3. *Toxicology* 1995;105:23–9.
7. Ober RJ, Radu CG, Ghetie V, Ward ES. Differences in promiscuity for antibody-FcRn interactions across species: implications for therapeutic antibodies. *Intl Immunol* 2001;13:1551–9.
8. Hwang WYK, Foote J. Immunogenicity of engineered antibodies. *Methods* 2005; 36:3–10.
9. United States-Food and Drug Administration (CBER). Points to Consider in the Manufacture and Testing of Monoclonal Antibody Products for Human Use, 1997. http://www.fda.gov/cber/gdlns/ptc_mab.pdf
10. ICH Harmonized Tripartite Guideline. S6 Preclinical Safety Evaluation of Biotechnology-Derived Pharmaceuticals, 1997. http://www.ich.org/pdfICH/s6.pdf

11. European Medicines Evaluation Agency (EMEA) Guideline. Production and Quality Control of Monoclonal Antibodies, Directive 75/318/EEC, 1995. http://www.q-one.com/guidance/emea.htm

12. Treacy G. Using an Analogous Monoclonal Antibody to Evaluate the Reproductive and Chronic Toxicity Potential for a Humanized Anti-TNFα Monoclonal Antibody. *Hum Exp Toxicol* 2000;19:226–9.

13. Clark J, Leach W, Pippig S, Joshi A, Wu B, House R, Beyer J. Evaluation of a surrogate antibody for preclinical safety testing of an anti-CD11a monoclonal antibody. *Regul Toxicol Pharmacol* 2004;40:219–26.

CHAPTER 27

Immunomodulatory Biopharmaceuticals and Risk of Neoplasia

PETER J. BUGELSKI, PhD, FRCPath, CLIFFORD SACHS, PhD, DABT, JOEL CORNACOFF, DVM, PhD, DABT, PAULINE MARTIN, PhD, and GEORGE TREACY, MS

Contents

27.1 INTRODUCTION

A number of immunomodulatory biopharmaceuticals (IMBPs), such as peptides, recombinant proteins, soluble receptors, and monoclonal antibodies, have been approved or are currently in development to treat chronic inflammatory diseases. These agents may be administered daily or, if long-acting,

Preclinical Safety Evaluation of Biopharmaceuticals: A Science-Based Approach to Facilitating Clinical Trials, edited by Joy A. Cavagnaro
Copyright © 2008 by John Wiley & Sons, Inc.

intermittently. For IMBP, two immunologic characteristics are important: (1) immunogenicity due to the response to a foreign protein and (2) the intended pharmacologic effects. These two properties may interact and facilitate achieving adequate exposure in toxicity studies. That is, the higher doses employed in toxicity studies may result in suppressed immunogenicity and thus possibly revealing clinically relevant, immunosuppressant activity or dose correlates [1]. Special issues or concerns following chronic treatment with IMBPs include the potential for immune impairment leading to opportunistic infections and/or lymphoproliferative disorders [2]. As is true for conventional pharmaceuticals, in addition to duration of therapy, the cause for concern for tumorigenicity (malignancy) may be heightened based on knowledge and plausibility of the mechanism of drug action, especially if an IMBP is administered with overtly immunosuppressive drugs. However, despite years of experience with testing environmental contaminants, food additives, and pharmaceuticals, predicting and quantitating an increased risk of neoplasia in patients receiving therapeutic doses of IMBPs remains a daunting task. Moreover, because the risk of neoplasia is a multifactorial issue, no "one size fits all" approach is likely to have much value.

The discussion in this chapter will focus on well-characterized, high-purity protein biopharmaceuticals derived from conventional recombinant expression systems that modulate immune function. Specifically, the points we raise are relevant to monoclonal antibodies, fusion proteins, and soluble receptors directed toward cytokines, cells, and receptors that regulate immune function. Also the discussion will include biopharmaceuticals that downmodulate immune function (e.g., a monoclonal antibody that neutralize a cytokine) or the "naked" antibody intended to selectively eliminate a specific immune cell population (e.g., an anti-CD4 antibody), that is, "naked" as the term is used to discriminate among nonconjugated antibodies and immunotoxins or radioimmunotherapeutics. Excluded from consideration will be biopharmaceuticals that cause sustained, polyclonal expansion of lymphoid cells, express growth factor-like effects on non-immune cells, or bear chemical modifications that can introduce genotoxic moieties. Nevertheless, our discussion will be germane to monoclonal antibodies that are intended to direct an immune response toward a non-immune cellular target, such as a tumor antigen. As with most issues concerning the safety of biopharmaceuticals, for any specific agent a science-driven, case-by-case approach that is consistent with the principles set forth in ICH S6 and is developed in the context of our growing experience with biopharmaceuticals in general and our knowledge base on that specific biopharmaceutical will be required for a proper risk assessment.

Implicit to our recommendation for IMBPs is that viral expression system derived DNA or excipient derived contaminant carcinogens are no longer an issue. Although, for example, host cell DNA can be a risk factor for neoplasia [3], the current stringent biochemical characterization, purification, and virus inactivation steps taken with all well-characterized biopharmaceuticals adequately mitigate any potential risk from these sources.

27.2 CLINICAL EXPERIENCE WITH IMMUNOSUPPRESSIVE AGENTS AND IMBP

It is well understood that cancer is no single disease. Each cell or tissue of origin likely has its own cause of neoplasia and, in turn, expresses a different disease. What is relevant for one tumor type, such as breast cancer, may have little relevance for another, such as lymphoma. Similarly not all agents that increase the risk of neoplasia are likely to act through the same mechanism or cause the same tumors. To set the stage for discussing predicting risk of neoplasia for patients receiving IMBPs, we should understand what neoplasms are relevant for those patients. Because clinical data on IMBPs are limited, to do this, we will turn to the more extensive data on small-molecule pharmaceuticals (xenobiotics).

For a number of overt, "broad spectrum" immunosuppressive xenobiotics (e.g., azathioprine) there is sufficient clinical experience to indicate the types of neoplasms for which there is an increased risk. These tumor types are listed in Table 27.1. Also listed are the tumors that occur in the unfortunate "experiment of nature," namely patients infected with human immunodeficiency virus type 1 (HIV-1) and the tumors that may occur at higher incidence with more selective yet strong immunosuppressants (e.g., cyclosporin, sirolimus, and tacrolimus). Compared to the broad spectrum immunosuppressive agents listed above, most IMBPs express a highly selective regulatory influence on the immune system; modulating the activity of host defense systems rather than mediating frank immunosuppression.

As shown by Table 27.1, the list of tumor types relevant to immunosuppression is surprisingly short. Although there are isolated case reports of a number of other tumor types, such as lung cancer [4,5], in patients receiving broad spectrum immunosuppressive therapies or in HIV-infected patients, the tumor types listed in Table 27.1 account for the vast majority of neoplasms associated with immunosuppression and IMBPs. Notably the major tumor types afflicting humans—colon, breast, and prostate—are not included because, as will become clear from our discussion, the increased risk of neoplasia posed by immunosuppression and especially IMBPs cannot be generalizabled to all neoplasms. The strategy we adopt for hazard identification and risk assessment for IMBPs therefore does not address the increased incidence of all possible tumor types. For all tumor types listed either as viral or radiation based in their etiology (Table 27.2), the strategy we adopt for hazard identification and risk assessment for IMBPs will not address the potential mechanisms of carcinogenesis.

27.3 IMMUNOMODULATORY BIOPHARMACEUTICALS ARE UNLIKELY TO BE COMPLETE CARCINOGENS

As noted above, the increased risk of neoplasia due to immunosuppression or IMBPs is limited to tumor types where a defined viral or radiation-based

TABLE 27.1   Human neoplasms associated with immunosuppression

Tumor Type	Immunosuppressant with Increased Incidence	Reference	Putative Carcinogen(s)	Reference
Non-Hodgkin's lymphoma	Cyclosporin Azathioprine and 6-mercaptopurine Sirolimus Human immunodeficiency virus (HIV) infection	Mougel et al. [40], Kwon and Farrell [42] Ibanez et al. [45], Schulz et al. [46]	Epstein-Barr virus (EBV) Human T cell leukemia virus-I (HTLV-I) Human Herpes Virus 8 (HHV-8)	Ahmed and Heslop [41], Jarrett [43] Malnati et al. [44]
Hodgkin's lymphoma	Sirolimus	Martin–Gomez et al. [47]	Epstein-Barr virus (EBV)	Ahmed and Heslop [41]
Kaposi's sarcoma	Cyclosporin HIV infection	Catatani et al. [48], Schulz et al. [46]	HHV-8	Chang et al. [49]
Non-melanoma skin cancers	Azathioprine Cyclosporin Prednisone and azathioprine Tacrolimus Infliximab (anti-TNFα) Efalizumab (anti-CD11a) HIV infection	Moloney et al. [50], Tiu et al. [52], Fortina et al. [53] Euvrard et al. [55], Esser et al. [56] Leonardi et al. [57], Schulz et al. [46]	Human papilloma viruses (HPV) Ultraviolet (UV) radiation	Purdie et al. [51] Madan et al. [54]
Hepatocarcinoma	Azathioprine	Vivarelli et al. [58]	Hepatitis virus B and C	Robinson [59], Koike et al. [60]

TABLE 27.2   Carcinogenic mechanisms for the neoplasms relevant to IMBPs

Carcinogen	Putative Mechanism of Carcinogenesis	Reference
Epstein–Barr virus (EBV)	Expression of EBV nuclear antigens 1–6	Li and Minarovits [61]
Human T cell leukemia virus-I (HTLV-I)	p40 Tax-mediated transcription of viral promoter, deregulation of cell cycle and genomic instability	Mahieux and Gessain [62]
Human herpes virus 8 (HHV-8)	Activation of oncogenes and expression of a virally encoded VEGF receptor	Flaitz and Hicks [63]
Human papilloma viruses	Genomic instability due to E6/E7 oncogenes	Snijders et al. [64]
Hepatitis virus B and C	Activation of oncogenes and suppression of growth control	Feitelson [65]
Ultraviolet radiation	DNA damage	Bachelor and Bowden [17]

process is at play. Because these processes are sufficient to cause neoplasia and so tumors can occur without immunosuppression, it is evident that immunosuppression, per se, is neither necessary nor sufficient to be carcinogenic. Were this not so, immunosuppression would be expected to be associated with a wider variety of tumor cell types and a wider variety of sites of origin. Moreover, if immunosuppression or imune modulation were carcinogenic, one would expect a higher incidence of tumors. For example, some of the constituents of tobacco smoke are well-recognized carcinogens. In a recent study of 8622 smokers of more than 30 cigarettes a day, the incidence of lung cancer in was 3.4% [6]. In contrast, the incidence of squamous cell cancer of the head and neck in a series of 1515 liver transplant patients receiving potent immunosuppressive treatment was only 0.86% [7]. Similarly the incidence of nonmelanoma skin cancer in a series of 15,789 rheumatoid arthritics receiving prednisone or TNF inhibitors was only 0.02% [8].

Finally, several of the diseases likely to be treated with IMBPs are associated with an increased incidence of the tumor types whose incidence is increased by immunosuppression even in the absence of immunosuppression. For example, studies of arthritis [9] and polymyalgia rheumatica/giant cell arteritis [10] found an increased incidence of lymphoma over population controls but failed to find evidence of an increased risk with immunosuppressive therapy. Taken together, these findings suggest that IMBPs are unlikely to be complete carcinogens, so we need to look to other steps in carcinogenesis where they may act.

27.4 IMMUNOMODULATORY BIOPHARMACEUTICALS ARE UNLIKELY TO BE CONVENTIONAL TUMOR PROMOTERS

Carcinogenesis can be considered in three steps: initiation, promotion, and progression [11]. In this model, initiation is believed to be the result of heritable changes (mutations) in the genome of a cell. Initiators (or their metabolites) must gain access to the genome and through chemical or radiochemical interactions with DNA result in mutations. This is exemplified by the classic "complete" carcinogens, such as 3-methylcholanthrene, and it is also probably the case with azathioprine as this potent immunosuppressant has been shown to be genotoxic [12]. Because IMBPs are non-DNA reactive proteins of generally greater than 30,000 kDa molecular weight, there is no evidence that they can gain access to the genome to interact with DNA. Moreover the metabolites of IMBPs are oligopeptides and ordinary amino acids, and they are thus very unlikely to be initiators. In sum, it is unlikely that IMBP act at tumor initiators.

In the process of neoplastic transformation, it is considered unlikely that a single mutation can result in the multiplicity of phenotypic changes associated with malignancy [13,14]. For full malignant transformation to occur, a cell must survive in its native milieu, accumulate a number of mutations, and expand its numbers as a nascent neoplastic clone. At this stage the nascent clone can be considered neoplastic, but it is not yet malignant. For a malignancy to occur, the nascent clone must continue to accumulate transformed phenotypes so as to include the ability to invade, disseminate, and escape destruction outside its native milieu (i.e., in the interstitial space, the lymphatic system, or the blood stream). Collectively these steps can be considered as tumor promoting.

In the classic model of initiation and promotion, conventional tumor promoters (CTP) inhibit the intracellular mechanisms that can eliminate the nascent clone, facilitate accumulation of the mutations necessary for full malignant transformation, or disrupt intercellular signaling [15]. A classic example of a CTP is 12-O-tetradecanoylphorbol-13-acetate (TPA, also referred to as phorbol myristate acetate, PMA). The mechanisms proposed for CTP that are relevant for the tumor types associated with immunosuppression, such as nonmelanoma skin tumors and lymphomas, are listed in Table 27.3. The table is limited to mechanisms of promotion and does not include tumor initiation mechanisms, namely those that directly or indirectly damage DNA (e.g., free radicals mediated by metabolism of ethanol) [16] or are mechanisms of neovasularization (e.g., angiogenesis in response to UV-A and B) [17]. The table also excludes mechanisms of CTP that have only been studied in the context of irrelevant tumors, such as TCDD in hepatocarcinogenesis [18].

As shown in Table 27.3, the mechanisms for CTP believed to be relevant in skin tumors and lymphomas act on the initiated cell, and notably, there are five mediated within the cytoplasm. These mechanisms are unlikely to be relevant to IMBPs because, as proteins, IMBPs (or their oligopeptide metabolites) cannot gain access to DNA in the nucleus. The remaining putative mechanisms of CTP—disruption of gap junctions, activation of protein kinase

TABLE 27.3   Mechanisms of conventional tumor promotion in neoplasms relevant to IMBPs

Putative Mechanism of Promotion	Tumor Type	Site of Action	Reference
Inhibition of protein phosphatases	Skin tumors	Cytoplasm	Slaga et al. [15]
Hypermethylation of tumor suppressor genes	Skin and lymphoma	Cytoplasm	Van Doorn et al. [66], Pini et al. [67]
Loss of pRb tumor suppressor activity	Skin and lymphoma	Cytoplasm	Flaitz and Hicks [63]
Loss of p53 tumor suppressor activity	Lymphoma	Cytoplasm	Fesus et al. [68]
Hypomethylation of genomic DNA	Skin and lymphoma	Cytoplasm	Bachman et al. [69], Pini et al. [67]
Loss of gap junction mediated intercellular communication	Skin tumors	Cytoplasm or cell surface	Trosko and Tai [11]
Activation of protein kinase C	Skin tumors	Cytoplasm or cell surface	Slaga et al. [15]
Hyperplasia secondary to inflammation	Skin tumors	Cytoplasm or cell surface	Marks et al. [70], Bachelor and Bowden [17]

C, and inflammation—can be mediated from the cell surface. However, as highly selective downregulators of the immune function, IMBPs are unlikely to mediate tumor promotion via these mechanisms.

27.5   IMMUNOMODULATORY BIOPHARMACEUTICALS AS ATYPICAL TUMOR PROMOTERS

In an alternate form of tumor promotion, referred to as atypical tumor promoters (ATPs), elimination of the nascent clones may be blocked by inhibiting apoptosis [19], by failure to eliminate nascent transformed cells, or by failure to control an active infection (or activation of a latent viral infection [20]) of a carcinogenic virus. Host defense mechanisms are primarily responsible for regulating extrinsic apoptosis, cytotoxicity, and control of viral infections. If an IMBP were to mediate tumor promotion, it would be acting through such a mechanism.

There are a number of host defense effector mechanisms, both humoral and cellular, that, when inhibited, have the potential to mediate atypical tumor promotion. These are listed in Table 27.4. As shown in the table, essentially all the effector cells of the immune system, with the exception of granulocytes, have the potential to eliminate nascent transformed cells or influence the

TABLE 27.4 Host defense effectors where inhibition by biopharmaceutical may mediate atypical tumor promotion

Defense Mechanism	Putative Mechanism of Atypical Tumor Promotion	Reference
Natural killer cells	Failure to control virus infection. Failure to eliminate nascent transformed cells and clones in situ. Failure to eliminate cells in lymphatics and in blood stream	Barao and Ascensao [71]
Macrophages	Failure to control virus infection. Failure to eliminate nascent transformed cells and clones in situ. Failure to eliminate nascent colonization.	Salek-Ardakani et al. [72], Andreesen et al. [73]
B lymphocytes	Failure to control virus infection. Failure to present tumor or viral-antigens to T cells.	Capello et al. [74] Guinana et al. [75]
Dendritic cells	Failure to control virus infection. Failure to present tumor or viral antigens to T cells.	Lund et al. [76], Qu et al. [77]
T lymphocytes	Failure to control virus infection. Failure to eliminate virally infected cells. Failure to eliminate nascent transformed cells and clones in situ. Failure to eliminate cells in lymphatics. Failure to eliminate nascent colonization.	Maini et al. [78], Yu and Fu [79]
Lymphokines	Failure to control virus infection. Failure to mediate extrinsic apoptosis. Failure to mediate cytotoxicity.	See Table 27.5

course of viral infections. Thus IMBPs directed toward the effector cells have the potential to act as ATPs. The role of granulocytes in eliminating tumor cells is more controversial. Although there is some work that suggests that granulocytes can kill tumor cells [21], there is also work that suggests that granulocytes (via production of free radicals) can act as tumor initiators or promoters [22].

Cytokines and interleukins are proteins produced by a variety of immune and non-immune cells that bind receptors on their target cells and elicit a variety of responses. As of 2008, 35 interleukins have been described [23]. The principle source of interleukins are immune cells (macrophages and lymphocytes), but they are also produced by a number of immune cells, e.g., Interleukin-6 (IL-6) in a variety of cell types [24], and they are sometimes referred to by the more general term cytokines. Cytokines, because of their ability to affect the activity of a large number of cells and cell types, can amplify an

TABLE 27.5 Lymphokines/cytokines with antitumor activity whose inhibition may mediate atypical tumor promotion

Cytokine	Reference
Tumor necrosis factor-α	Hori et al. [80]
Defensins	Kagan et al. [81]
Interferons	Brandacher et al. [82]
	Rees [83]
	Chada et al. [84]
CXC and C-C chemokinesIP-10, MCP-3, MIG and SDF-1α)	Chada et al. [84]
IL-1α and β	Veltri and Smith [85]
IL-2	Kuhn and Dou [26]
IL-3	Hansen [86]
IL-4	Maini et al. [87]
IL-6	Maini et al. [87]
	Kurebayashi [88]
IL-7	Appasamy [89]
IL-12	Chada et al. [84]
IL18	Pages et al. [90]
IL-21	Roda et al. [91]
IL-23	Oniki et al. [92]
IL-24	Chada et al. [84]
IL-27	Oniki et al. [92]
IL-28 α and β	Zitzmann et al. [25]
IL-29	Zitzmann et al. [25]
IL-32	Goda et al. [93]

immune response, and thus they may play a central role in host defense against neoplasia. Antitumor activity has been ascribed to a majority of cytokines (Table 27.5). Antitumor activity can be either direct (e.g., IL-29 inducing apoptosis of tumor cells [25]) or indirect (e.g., by activating cytotoxic immune cells or by IL-2 activating cytotoxic T cells [26]). Thus IMBPs directed toward cytokines by anticytokine monoclonal antibodies or soluble receptors have the potential to act as ATPs.

27.6 IMMUNOMODULATORY BIOPHARMACEUTICALS AS POTENTIAL TUMOR PROGRESSORS

To be clinically significant, the nascent transformed clone(s) must not only survive but grow locally (so as to damage or destroy the adjacent normal tissue) or disseminate and grow at distant sites as metastases. These steps can be considered tumor progression [11]. At the cellular level the mechanisms by which host defense can inhibit the ability of a malignant clone to grow locally or colonize a distant site have already been described in Table 27.4. An additional step in tumor progression is the ability to call up a new blood supply

TABLE 27.6   Host defense effector mechanisms whose inhibition may inhibit tumor promotion and/or progression

Antibodies against Host Defense Effector	Potential Effect of Inhibition on Tumor Progressor Activity	Reference
Anti-TNFα	Down regulation of tumor-promoting genes	Devoogdt et al. [94]
Anti-IL-4	Shift Th1/Th2 balance favoring tumor immunity	Becker [95]
Anti-IL-6	Shift Th1/Th2 balance favoring tumor immunity	Becker [95]
Anti-IL-8	Inhibition of angiogenesis	Melnikova and Bar-Eli [96]
Anti-IL-10	Shift Th1/Th2 balance favoring tumor immunity	Frumento et al. [97]
Anti-IL-26	Inhibition of activation of STAT 1 and 3 in tumor cells	Hor et al. [98]
Anti-IL-31	Inhibition of Jak1, Jak2, STAT1, −3, −5 Pi3 signaling pathways in tumor cells	Diveu et al. [99]
Anti-regulatory T cells (e.g., anti-CD25)	Shift Th1/Th2 balance favoring tumor immunity	Frumento et al. [97]
Anti-cytotoxic T cell antigen-4 (CTLA-4) antibodies	Rejection of established tumors and enhanced tumor immunity in mice	Leach et al. [100]
Anti-B cell antibodies	Decrease in tumor-promoting IgGs	Barbera-Guillem et al. [101]

(angiogenesis). Without angiogenesis, although a neoplastic clone may survive and even expand as a diffuse cellular infiltrate, metastasis as discrete space occupying or tissue destructive lesions cannot occur [27]. In this context host defense mechanisms can be a double-edged sword, and in contrast to their conventional role in inhibiting tumor growth, some can act as tumor progressors. In this case inhibition of host defense may have a paradoxical beneficial effect. These are listed in Table 27.6.

27.7   CRITICAL REVIEW OF MODEL SYSTEMS FOR IDENTIFICATION AND CHARACTERIZATION OF ATYPICAL PROMOTERS AND TUMOR PROGRESSORS

As mentioned above, the mechanisms by which IMBPs are likely to act as atypical tumor promoters are all centered on their desired, albeit exaggerated, pharmacology. Put another way, if IMBPs are acting as tumor promoters, it is likely due to a "toxic" effect on the immune system, meaning immunotoxicity. There are numerous approaches to the study of immunotoxicity, but it is beyond the scope of this chapter to discuss the pros and cons of the various purely mechanistic approaches to the study of IMBP as putative tumor promoters. The reader is therefore directed to Chapter 16, which reviews immunotoxicity for treatment of in vitro model systems that can be used to identify and characterize the specific pharmacology of IMBPs that can lead to tumor promotion. Here the discussion will focus on systems that directly address tumor promotion.

27.7.1 In vitro Mechanism-Based Systems

As shown in Table 27.7, a variety of in vitro systems have been used to study both CTP and ATP (in some cases the target of an IMBP has been studied and not the IMBP). One of the principal advantages for all these systems is that they can utilize human cells. (It should be noted that not all the systems cited in Table 27.7 use human cells, but likely depend on the "equivalent" non-human systems.) It is widely accepted (and codified in ICH6) that to have scientific relevance and meaning, the test article (in this case the IMBP) must be pharmacologically active in the test system. As reviewed by Green and Black [1], most IMBPs directed toward human targets are inactive in rodent systems. For this reason IMBPs are tested in vivo almost exclusively in nonhuman primates. Thus the IMBPs in development can be tested in the systems like those listed in Table 27.7, and there is no need for a homologous (also sometimes referred to "analogous" or "surrogate") IMBPs. (The issues with surrogate systems will be discussed below.)

The principal disadvantage of the systems listed in Table 27.7 is due to their very sophistication: they test for effects on a specific gene or phenotype, and generally do not test multiple mechanisms simultaneously. This concern could be partially mitigated by conducting a battery of such tests. However, because of the multiplicity of mechanisms involved in tumor promotion and progression, it is unlikely that an adequate battery of tests would be practical to design and validate to fully define the potential hazard posed by a specific IMBP. Another disadvantage inherent to the types of tests listed in Table 27.7 is the difficulty in translating the hazard identified by in vitro findings into a risk assessment for patients receiving therapeutic doses of an IMBP. No conceivable in vitro system could ever replicate the complexity of the intact immune network or the influences of pharmacokinetics. Thus, while in vitro approaches can identify and partially characterize the hazard posed by IMBPs, they have limited value in the final risk assessment for patients.

27.7.2 In vivo Systems

A number of in vivo systems have been used to evaluate CTP and ATP. These are listed in Tables 27.8, 27.9, and 27.10. The lists, although largely

TABLE 27.7 In vitro model systems for identification and characterization of atypical tumor promoters and tumor progression

In vitro Systems	Example for Conventional Tumor Promoters	Reference	Example for Atypical Tumor Promoters or Their Targets	Reference
Expression of specific tumor promoter genes	Enhanced expression of secretory leukocyte protease inhibitor by TPA	Schlingemann et al. [102]	Enhanced expression of secretory leukocyte protease inhibitor by TNFα	Devoogdt et al. [94]
Expression of viral tumor promoter genes	Enhanced expression of Epstein–Barr early antigen	Ohmori et al. [103]	Upregulation of HPV oncoproteins by a variety of cytokines	Lembo et al. [104]
Adhesion	Inhibition of integrin-mediated adhesion	Chang and Chambers [105]	Antitumor antibodies inhibit adhesion	Blumenthal et al. [106]
Invasion	Enhanced invasion of model extracellular matrix	Fridman et al. [107]	Antitumor antibodies inhibit invasiveness	Blumenthal et al. [106]
Cell–ell communication	Inhibition of gap junction communication	Noguchi et al. [108]	Inhibition of gap junction communication by IL-1	Hu and Xie [109]
Intracellular signaling	Increased protein kinase C activity or decreased protein phosphatase activity	Slaga et al. [15]	Anti-CD3 activates mitogen-activated kinase Erk2	Von Willebrand et al. [110]
Apoptosis	Inhibition of apoptosis	Fesus et al. [68]	Anti-IL-2 antibodies inhibit Fas mediated apoptosis	Algeciras–Schimnich [111]

complete in terms of model systems, are only exemplary and are not intended to be an exhaustive review of the entire literature on CTP or ATP in such systems.

Listed in Table 27.8 are what can be termed mechanistic approaches. Genetic defect and knockout mice where the gene or gene product has been shown to be involved in carcinogenesis (e.g., p53 heterozygous knockout mice) have been used rather extensively with complete carcinogens and some CTP, and these systems show some promise for replacing the standard two-year bioassay in mice [28]. Use of mice has, however, received much less attention for tumor promoters, and we have found no examples for use of mice genetically deficient in a gene shown to be involved in carcinogenesis with IMBP. In part, this observation likely reflects the lack of cross-reactivity of most IMBPs with murine targets due to species specificity.

In another form, the gene defect or knockout is directed toward immune cells or cytokines that are the targets for IMBPs. What are now classic examples are CD4 deficient "nude" mice, and severe combined immunodeficient SCID mice [29]. These systems have been shown to reveal the roles that various cells and cytokines may play in neoplasia and are thus proving to be an invaluable research tool. For hazard identification for IMBP, such systems can provide an important "proof of concept" that the target of the IMBP may play a role in emergence of spontaneous neoplasms. However, because there is no treatment per se, there can be no "dose response," and because the deficit is present throughout development and life, its role in risk assessment is currently limited. In the future, as technology advances and conditional knockouts where the gene product is downregulated in a controlled fashion become available, this situation will likely change. Although phenotype issues in KO mice may suggest potential toxicology issues, they often don't predict in vivo toxicity. In addition to the gene of interest, the phenotype of KO mice is influenced by traits that are unique to the background strain and by unpredictable interactions arising from strain-specific traits and elimination of the gene of interest that can lead to unexpected results. Even when high doses of an anti-cytokine monoclonal antibody (mAb) are administered, drug properties of disposition, pharmacodynamics, and pharmacokinetics are essential determinants of toxicity that cannot be evaluated in KO mice.

The remaining models listed in Table 27.8 are not measures of tumorigenesis but rather measures of host defense against neoplasia and/or tumor progression. The principal advantage of these systems is that they are in vivo models and, if they utilize murine cells, can be run in intact mice. The principal disadvantages are similar to those described for the in vitro systems listed in Table 27.7. Additionally, and of great importance, these systems are rodent based and no nonhuman primate form of the assay has been defined. Because most IMBPs are human or primate specific, most murine models cannot be run in a meaningful fashion with the actual IMBP, and a murine homologue (analogue) IMBP must be used. As will be discuss below, the reliance on surrogate IMBPs limits the usefulness of such systems.

TABLE 27.8   Critical review of mechanism based in vivo model systems for identification and characterization of atypical tumor promoters and tumor progression

Model System	Example for Conventional Tumor Promoters	Reference	Example for Atypical Tumor Promoters	Reference	Advantages	Disadvantages
Genetic defects and Knockout systems	Estradiol increased the incidence of ethylnitrosourea induced uterine tumors in p53 knockout mice.	Gray et al. [112]	Interferon-γ deficient mice are more susceptible to methylcholanthrene-induced tumorigenesis.	Blankenstein and Qin [113]	May be already available and well studied. Can be created for most cytokines or effector cells. May provide strong proof of concept.	May alter expression of "bystander" genes. Compensatory effects may mask deficit. "All or nothing" effect may overestimate hazard.
Experimental metastasis	Exposure to B16F1 cells to PMA in vitro and subsequent IV injection increases lung metastases.	La Porta and Comolli [114]	Metastases increased with B16 melanoma in human CD4 transgenic mice treated with anti-asialoGM1, anti-thy-1, or anti-CD4.	Herzyk et al. [31]	Test system is readily available. Database is limited.	Usually requires murine surrogate.
Immunization/ rejection	Treatment of tumor-bearing mice with PMA and subsequent transplantation results in tumor growth in immunized mice.	Kadhim et al. [115]	Anti-IL-12 (but not anti-TNFα) antibodies inhibits secondary cytotoxic lymphocyte response to β-gal transfected ES cells.	Mahnke and Schirrmacher [116]	Test system is readily available. Database is limited.	Usually requires murine surrogate.

Occasionally, however, the actual IMBP will be active in a murine system. Abatacept, a soluble fusion protein that consists of the extracellular domain of human cytotoxic T lymphocyte-associated antigen 4 (CTLA-4) linked to the modified Fc (hinge, CH2, and CH3 domains) portion of human immuno-globulin G1 (IgG1), is a unique example of a IMBP that was evaluated in a standard two-year carcinogenicity studies [30]. Unlike most IMBPs, abatacept is pharmacologically active in mice. In a mouse carcinogenicity study, following weekly subcutaneous injections of 20, 65, or 200 mg/kg of abatacept for up to 84 and 88 weeks in males and females, abatacept was associated with increases in the incidence of malignant lymphomas (at all doses) and mammary gland tumors in females at doses ≥65 mg/kg. Importantly, the mice from this study were infected with murine leukemia and mouse mammary tumor viruses, which increase incidence of lymphomas and mammary gland tumors, respectively, in immunosuppressed mice. Although in the cumulative abatacept clinical trials the rate observed for lymphoma is approximately 3.5-fold higher than expected in an age- and gender-matched general population, the RA population is known to have overall a higher incidence of lymphoma than the general population. Thus the relevance of the carcinogenicity findings to the clinical observation of increased lymphoma in patients receiving abatacept is unknown.

An other notable example is the work described by Herzyk et al. [31] where the effects of a Primatized® antihuman CD4 monoclonal antibody on experimental metastases with B16 melanoma cells was studied, and an increase in the number of lung colonies was found. Enabling this work, a murine CD4 knockout mouse reconstituted with human CD4 had been described in the literature and was available for license by the sponsor [32]. Moreover, in these mice, murine CD4 was faithfully replaced on T cells by human CD4, and the human protein mediated its physiologic function as an accessory binding protein in cellular and humoral immunity.

The work by Herzyk et al. [31], however, appears to be unique. To date, there have been no other reports of a human knock-in system being used in risk assessment of neoplasia, and similarly the literature on the use of tumor immunization/rejection models to evaluate the effects on IMBP on neoplasia is very scant. Because of the paucity of data, and because the anti-CD4 antibody studied by Herzyk et al. was never marketed and thus never used widely in patients, it is currently impossible to judge the predictive power of these systems for an increased risk of neoplasia in patients receiving IMBPs.

If a homologue IMBP must be used, a number of issues need to be addressed prior to embarking on studies to support registration. Some of these are listed in Table 27.9. And, while most of these issues will not be insurmountable, addressing them will not be trivial and will take significant time and effort. Moreover in some cases it may not be practical to conduct studies with homologue IMBP that comply with good laboratory practices. Given these issues, and the limited relevance of data from homologous systems to patients

TABLE 27.9   Potential issues with the applicability of homologous IMBPs

Attribute	Potential Issue
Role of target in immune function	Therapeutic target may not subserve the same function in rodents and humans.
Immunogenicity	Rodent homologue may be immunogenic in rodents.
Efficacy	Epitope bound by the rodent homologue mAb may not express the same functional activity as the human IMBP.
Fc functionality	Rodent homologue may not express the same Fc functionality as the human IMBP.
Stability	Rodent homologue may not have sufficient stability to allow testing.
Formulation	May be impossible to formulate the rodent homologue at a high enough concentration to allow testing.
Purity	May be impractical to produce the homologue with sufficient purity to allow testing.
Influence of expression system	Glycosylation pattern of the homologue may not reflect that of the human IMBP influencing exposure.

receiving therapeutic doses of an IMBP, the value of homologous systems is questionable.

Listed in Table 27.10 are the standard approaches to evaluating the carcinogenic potential of chemicals. As shown in the table, there are examples of the use of these systems for CTP and cyclosporin and, in the case of the two-year bioassay, an IMBP (abatacept, a cytotoxic lymphocyte antigen-4 (CTLA-4)-Ig fusion protein). Also as shown in the table, each model system has advantages and disadvantages. The primary drawback shared by these systems is that they rely on what can be referred to as "adventitious" or "environmental" initiation; that is, unlike the neoplasms clinically relevant to IMBPs where a viral or radiation initiator is likely, there is no defined tumor initiator. Issues with sometimes ill-defined background rates of tumorigenesis, irrelevant tumor sites, and strain and gender differences also pose very serious problems in experimental design and interpretation. In addition, as described by Hastings [33], rodents typically have been especially responsive to the pharmacological/toxicological effects of immunosuppressants, making it difficult to conduct lifetime bioassays at doses reasonably equivalent to those that would be used clinically. Taken together, these issues make false negative findings likely (i.e., by failure to show that an IMBP is an ATP). When coupled with the specific disadvantages listed in Table 27.10, the scientific rationale for the transgenic systems, neonatal mouse and two-year bioassay is quite poor.

Listed in Table 27.11 are a number of co-carcinogenesis models that have been used with CTP and in some cases APT. As with the models listed in

TABLE 27.10 Critical review of in vivo model systems relying on serendipitous initiation for identification and characterization of atypical tumor promoters and tumor progression

Model System	Example for Conventional Tumor Promoters	Reference	Example for Atypical Tumor Promoters	Reference	Advantages	Disadvantages
Transgenic systems	RasH2 mice show increased tumors with a variety of nongenotoxic carcinogens	Yamamoto et al. [117]	RasH2 mice show increased tumors with cyclosporin	Yamamoto et al. [117]	Some test systems available but expensive Custom systems very expensive and can take years to obtain in adequate numbers Limited but appreciable data on chemical carcinogens and promoters	Usually requires murine surrogate May not be susceptible to relevant tumor type (e.g., lymphoma) Dependent on specific mechanism(s) Limited background tumor database makes ensuring statistical power problematic Fail to detect immunosuppressive drugs

TABLE 27.10 *Continued*

Model System	Example for Conventional Tumor Promoters	Reference	Example for Atypical Tumor Promoters	Reference	Advantages	Disadvantages
Neonatal mouse	TPA increases skin tumors in two-stage model	Furstenberger [118]	Cyclosporin failed to increase tumors	McClain et al. [119]	Test system readily available Not dependent on specific mechanism Dose-dependent effects	Usually requires murine surrogate Neither designed nor powered to detect promoters Limited background tumor database makes ensuring statistical power problematic Immunogenicity of test article (even murine monoclonals) may confound assay
Two-year bioassay	Tumor promoter chlorophene increased tumors in mice but not rats	Yamarik [120]	Increased lymphoid neoplasms with cyclosporin Abatacept (CTLA-4-Fc fusion protein) increased lymphomas in mice	Ryffel [121] Anon. [30]	Test system is readily available Large background database Not dependent on specific mechanism Dose-dependent effects	Usually requires murine surrogate Neither designed nor powered to detect promoters Immunogenicity of test article (even murine monoclonals) may confound assay

TABLE 27.11   Critical review of in vivo initiation-promotion model systems for identification and characterization of atypical tumor promoters and tumor progression

Model System	Example for Conventional Tumor Promoters	Reference	Example for Atypical Tumor Promoters	Reference	Advantages	Disadvantages
Chemical carcinogenesis	Promotion of chemically induced skin tumors by phorbolesters	Marks et al. [70]	Azathioprine shortened tumor latency period when administered prior to exposure to 3-methylcholanthrene	De Jong et al. [122]	Test system readily available Large database on chemical carcinogens and promoters	Usually requires murine surrogate May express irrelevant tumor types
Radiation carcinogenesis	Promotion of ionizing radiation initiation by phorbolester in mouse skin	Bowden et al. [123]	Cyclosporin increases incidence of lymphomas in irradiated mice	Yabu et al. [124]	Test system readily available Limited database	Usually requires murine surrogate May express irrelevant tumor types

TABLE 27.11 *Continued*

Model System	Example for Conventional Tumor Promoters	Reference	Example for Atypical Tumor Promoters	Reference	Advantages	Disadvantages
Photocarcinogenesis	Increase in skin tumors induced by low-dose UV by phorbolesters	Yamawaki et al. [125]	No examples found		Test system readily available / Relies on relevant tumor initiator	Usually requires murine surrogate / May not express all relevant tumor types (e.g., lymphoma) / Limited database
Viral carcinogenesis	Cyclosporin increases incidence of lymphomas in murine herpes virus 68 infected mice	Sunil–Chandra et al. [39]	Abatacept (CTLA-4-Fc fusion protein) increased lymphomas in mice infected with murine leukemia virus	Anon. [30]	Test system readily available / Can be designed to rely on a relevant tumor initiator	Usually requires murine surrogate / May not express all relevant tumor types (e.g., skin tumors) / Murine virus may not be relevant to human (e.g., murine mammary tumor virus, MMTV) / Limited database

Table 27.8 and 27.9, in most cases the human directed IMBP will not be active in a rodent test system and the use of a surrogate IMBP is required. As described above, this limits their relevance for most IMBPs. Moreover, although these systems may be likely to demonstrate the ATP activity of the homologous IMBP and thus demonstrating that a hazard exists, one is still faced with the difficulty in extrapolating to humans exposed to the human virus (or relevant dose of UV) and receiving therapeutic doses of the actual IMBP. Again, as with all rodent models, while hazard identification may be more or less straightforward, risk assessment is likely to be problematic. An interesting example of testing the actual IMBP in primates is the finding that alphacept (an LFA-3-Fc fusion protein) leads to reactivitation of Epstein–Barr virus infection in primates, which ultimately leads to lymphomas. However, like the models listed in Table 27.10, this was a serendipitous finding rather than the result of a deliberate experiment.

27.8 CLASSIFICATION OF THE HAZARD POSED BY IMBP AND RISK ASSESSMENT

In the preceding sections the case that IMBPs are associated with a limited range of neoplasms, that these neoplasms are by and large associated with a recognized tumor inititiator (i.e., viruses or ultraviolet radiation), that IMBPs are likely acting as atypical tumor promoters, rather than complete carcinogens, and that atypical tumor promotion is likely to be an inherent immunotoxicologic consequence of the intended pharmacologic activity of the IMBP has been laid out. What remains is how to evaluate the risk posed by IMBPs to patients and how that risk can be quantitated and communicated.

IMBPs intended for use in preventing allograft rejection in transplant patients or as disease modifiers in rheumatoid arthritis or psoriasis are likely to be administered chronically. Thus it is normally expected that sponsors would have conducted preclinical studies to determine the carcinogenic potential of candidate compounds. For small molecule pharmaceuticals, this would mean that rodent carcinogenicity bioassays would be performed under most circumstances. However, immunosuppressant drugs, in general, and IMBPs, in particular, present unique challenges with respect to the issue of carcinogenicity bioassays.

As described above, the pharmacological activity of IMBPs (even in the absence of genotoxic activity) may allow them to act as atypical tumor promoters. Thus, even in the absence of confirmatory standard rodent bioassay data, it can be assumed that this class of drug would pose an increased risk of neoplasia to patients receiving chronic dosing. As suggested by Hastings [33] and Cohen [34], rather than embarking on what would be a very expensive (in terms of both monetary and animal resources) and—given the nonvalidated nature of chronic testing of ATP and the probability of false negative or

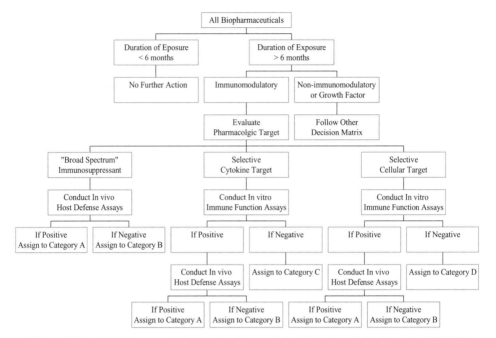

Figure 27.1 Decision matrix for evaluation and classification of the hazard of IMBP acting as atypical tumor promoters.

spurious findings—a possibly fruitless standard approach, alternative models might be more appropriate for risk assessment with this class of drug.

One such alternative approach is to stipulate that IMBPs pose a hazard, then to characterize the hazard experimentally by classifying the nature of the hazard, and finally, to make a risk assessment based on that classification. A scheme for characterizing and classifying the hazard posed by IMBPs is shown in decision tree form in Figure 27.1. It should be noted that the purpose of classifying the risk posed by IMBPs is not to diminish recognition of the hazard. As reviewed by Melnick et al. [35] and Perera [36], some "nongenotoxic carcinogens" are in fact genotoxic, some nongenotoxic pharmacologic activities can result in oxidative damage to DNA, and for receptor mediated effects, a threshold tumor response is not "inevitable." Thus, a classification approach may not be meaningful for all agents. Rather, the purpose is to ensure that the hazard is recognized and that the relative risk can be communicated to the physicians prescribing and the patients receiving IMBPs.

As seen in Figure 27.1, the first step in characterizing the hazard posed by an IMBPs is to determine the duration of its intended use. For short-term exposures, namely less than six months, in keeping with long-established guidelines, no further action is required. The next step is to determine if, based on its known pharmacologic activity, the agent in question fits the definition of an IMBP. If not, another decision matrix is required. This circumstance will not be discussed further in this chapter.

Having established that the agent is an IMBP that will be used for longer than six months, the next step is to evaluate the agent for suspicious structures or pharmacologic activity. This should include one or more in silico or "on paper" evaluations for known genotoxic or carcinogenic moieties [37], hormone-like effects [38], growth factor-like effects. If the agent has any of these characteristics, another decision matrix is then required. Again, this circumstance will not be discussed further in this chapter. However, for the vast majority of IMBPs, there will be no pharmacologic evidence of growth factor-like activity and no structural evidence of a genotoxic hazard. Thus there will be no scientific rationale for conducting genotoxicity testing on an IMBP.

The next step is to sort the IMBPs on the basis of their intended pharmacologic effects. If an IMBP is broadly active against multiple cell types or inhibits the activity of multiple cytokines, it can be considered a "broad spectrum" IMBP. Although this is the case with some pharmaceuticals such as cyclosporin, it will likely be a rare finding with an IMBP. Should this circumstance arise, it is likely that the agent will be active in in vitro immune function assays. And, rather than conduct in vitro assays whose outcome is almost forgone, the agent should be tested in in vivo host defense assays. These could include a viral challenge model (e.g., murine gamma herpes virus 68 as described by Sunil-Chandra et al. [39] or an experimental metastases model as described by Herzyk et al. [31]). Data generated from knockout systems may also be useful at this juncture. It must be noted, however, that the conduct of such models is not a trivial undertaking, and in most cases reliance will have to be placed on surrogates with their inherent limitations (see above). That being said, in vivo host defense models can play a pivotal role in the final classification of the hazard and the risk assessment for an IMBP and the outcome of the host defense assays can be used in classifying the IMBP as class A or B.

For IMBPs with more narrowly defined mechanisms of pharmacologic action, be they directed toward immune effector cells or cytokines, in vitro immune function assays may be a useful intermediate step. In many cases in vitro assays can be conducted with human cells, avoiding the need for a surrogate IMBP. Also, during the discovery phase for most IMBP some type of in vitro immune function assays will likely have been conducted. Moreover, for most drug targets a literature on the role of the target cell or cytokine in the immune function will likely exist. If in vitro data relevant to host defense already exists, and the IMBP or its target is known to modulate functions important in host defense, there is little rational for repeating in vitro assays, and one can go directly to in vivo host defense assays. It is expected that this would be the usual case, and depending on the outcome of the host defense assays, the IMBP would be assigned to class A or B.

Under more unusual circumstances an IMBP, when tested in a limited number of in vitro assays, would fail to show evidence that it can adversely affect host defense against neoplasia. These circumstances may pose a dilemma.

How much in vitro testing would be required to assign an IMBP to class C or D? There is likely no simple answer to this question. It may be answered on a case-by-case basis, as determined by the nature of the target for the IMBP and its intended clinical use. Alternatively, it may be more practical to go directly to in vivo host defense assays and assign the IMBP to class A or B.

Having classified the IMBP based on its effects on immune function, the next and final step would be to make a risk assessment and to communicate the risk to physicians and to the patients receiving therapeutic doses of the IMBP. This can be accomplished through the existing mechanisms of the Investigator's Brochure, Informed Consent documents, and ultimately, the product label.

27.9 CONCLUSIONS

In conclusion, IMBPs by virtue of their intended pharmacologic activity may act as atypical tumor promoters and thus pose a hazard for developing certain tumor types, especially lymphomas and skin cancer. Although conducting preclinical studies to identify this hazard is more or less straightforward, determining the relative risk to patients is and is likely to remain problematic. Traditional approaches that are used with pharmaceuticals are unlikely to be of much value. One alternative option may be to classify and label IMBPs based on their mechanism of action, for example, IMBPs that have an expected potential for increasing infection or lymphoproliferative disorders. This statement of the potential consequences would not be supported by lifetime animal data. One could also consider defining relative immunomodulation/immune suppression based on results of immunotoxicity assays. A product class label could later be defined based on a better understanding of the mechanism of action of the particular product and/or human data. In any event, the need for a prospective pharmacovigilance program to monitor carcinogenic risk is imperative for the clinical development program of IMBPs, including subsequent postmarketing commitments for products, especially if no animal studies can be performed.

REFERENCES

1. Green JD, Black L. Overview. Status of preclinical safety assessment for immunomodulatory biopharmaceuticals. *Hum Exp Toxicol* 2000;19:208–12.
2. Cavagnaro JA, Spindler P. Methods for predicting tumorigenicity of immunomodulatory biopharmaceuticals. *Hum Exp Toxicol* 2000;19:213–5.
3. Dorant PM, Classen IJ, van Kreyl CF, Van Steenis G, Wester PW. Risk assessment on the carcinogenic potential of hybridoma cell DNA: implications for residual contaminating cellular DNA in biological products. *Biologicals* 1997;25:381–90.

4. Pham SM, Kormos RL, Landreneau RJ, Kawai A, Gonzalez-Cancel I, Hardesty RL, Hattler BG, Griffith BP. Solid tumors after heart transplantation: lethality of lung cancer. *Ann Thoracic Surg* 1995;60:1623–6.

5. Engels EA, Brock MV, Chen J, Hooker CM, Gillison M, Moore RD. Elevated incidence of lung cancer among HIV-infected individuals. *J Clin Oncol* 2006;24: 1383–8.

6. Haiman CA, Stram DO, Wilkens LR, Pike MC, Kolonel LN, Henderson BE, Le Marchand L. Ethnic and racial differences in the smoking-related risk of lung cancer. *N Engl J Med* 2006;354:333–42.

7. Scheifele C, Reichart PA, Hippleer-Benscheidt M, Neuhaus P, Neuhaus R. Incidence of oral, pharyngeal and laryngeal squamous cell carcinomas among 1515 patients after liver transplantation. *Oral Oncol* 2005;41:670–6.

8. Chakravarty EF, Michaud K, Wolfe F. Skin cancer, rheumatoid arthritis and tumor necrosis factor inhibitors. *J Rheumatol* 2005;32:2130–215.

9. Franklin J, Lunt M, Bunn D, Symmons D, Silman A. Incidence of lymphoma in a large primary care derived cohort of cases of inflammatory arthritis. *Ann Rheumat Dis* 2006;65:617–22.

10. Askling J, Klareskog L, Hjalgrim H, Baecklund E, Bjorkholm M, Ekbom A. Do steroids increase lymphoma risk? A case-control study of lymphoma risk in polymyalgia rheumatica/giant cell arteritis. *Ann Rheumat Dis* 2005;64:1765–8.

11. Trosko JE, Tai MH. Adult stem cell theory of the multi-stage, multi-mechanism theory of carcinogenesis: role of inflammation on the promotion of initiated stem cells. *Contribut Microbiol* 2006;13:45–65.

12. Smith CC, Archer GE, Forster EJ, Lambert TR, Rees RW, Lynch AM. Analysis of gene mutations and clastogenicity following short-term treatment with azathioprine in MutaMouse. *Environ Mol Mutagen* 1999;34:131–9.

13. Boukamp P. Non-melanoma skin cancer: What drives tumor development and progression? *Carcinogenesis* 2005;26:1657–67.

14. Pettit SJ, Seymour K, O'Flaherty E, Kirby JA. Immune selection in neoplasia: towards a microevolutionary model of cancer development. *Brit J Cancer* 2000;82:1900–6.

15. Slaga TJ, DiGiovanni J, Weinberg LD, Budnova IV. Skin carcinogenesis; characteristics, mechanisms and prevention. *Prog Clin Biol Res* 1995;391:1–20.

16. Mufti SI. Alcohol acts to promote incidence of tumors. *Cancer Detect Prev* 1992;16:157–62.

17. Bachelor MA, Bowden GT. UVA-mediated activation of signaling pathways involved in skin tumor promotion and progression. *Sem Cancer Biol* 2004;14: 131–8.

18. Schrenk D, Schmits H-J, Bohnenberger S, Wagner B, Worner W. Tumor promoters as inhibitors of apoptosis in rat hepatocytes. *Toxicol Letts* 2004;149:43–50.

19. Peter ME, Legembre P, Barnhart BC. Does CD95 have tumor promoting activities? *Biochim Biophys Acta* 2005;1755:26–36.

20. van den Bosch CA. Is endemic Burkitt's lymphoma an alliance between three infections and a tumor promoter? *Lancet Oncol* 2004;5:738–6.

21. Di Carlo E, Forni G, Lollini P, Colombo MP, Modesti A, Musiani P. The intriguing role of polymorphonuclear neutrophils in antitumor reactions. *Blood* 2001;97: 339–45.

22. de Visser KE, Eichten A, Coussens LM. Paradoxical roles of the immune system during cancer development. *Nat Rev Cancer* 2006;6:24–37.

23. Collison LW, Workman CJ, Kuo TT, Boyd K, Wang Y, Vignali KM, Cross R, Sehy D, Blumberg RS, Vignali DA. The inhibitory cytokine IL-35 contributes to regulatory T-cell function. *Nature* 2007;450(7169):566–9.

24. Seghal PB. Interleukin-6: molecular pathophysiology. *J Investig Dermatol* 1990; 94(Suppl):2S–6S.

25. Zitzmann K, Brand S, Baehs S, Goke B, Meinecke J, Spottl G, Meyer H, Auernhammer CJ. Novel interferon-lambdas induce antiproliferative effects in neuroendocrine tumor cells. *Biochem Biophys Res Commun* 2006;344:1334–41.

26. Kuhn DJ, Dou QP. The role of interleukin-2 receptor alpha in cancer. *Frontiers Biosci* 2005;10:1462–74.

27. Herbst RS. Therapeutic options to target angiogenesis in human malignancies. *Expert Opin Emerg Drugs* 2006;11:635–50.

28. Mitsumori K. Evaluation on carcinogenicity of chemicals using transgenic mice. *Toxicology* 2002;181–2, 241–4.

29. Kelland LR. Of mice and men: values and liabilities of the athymic nude mouse model in anticancer drug development. *Eur J Cancer* 2004;40:827–36.

30. Anonamous. Orencia® (abatacept) package insert. Bristol-Myers Squibb Company, Princeton, NJ, 2007.

31. Herzyk DJ, Gore ER, Polsky R, Nadwodny KL, Maier CC, Liu S, Hart TK, Harmsen AG, Bugelski PJ. Immunomodulatory effects of anti-CD4 antibody in host resistance against infections and tumors in human CD4 transgenic mice. *Infect Immunity* 2001;69:1032–43.

32. Bugelski PJ, Herzyk DJ, Rehm S, Harmsen AG, Gore EV, Williams DM, Maleeff BE, Badger AM, Truneh A, O'Brien SR, Macia RA, Wier PJ, Morgan DG, Hart TK. Preclinical development of keliximab, a Primatized® anti-CD4 monoclonal antibody, in human CD4 transgenic mice: characterization of the model and safety studies. *Hum Exp Toxicol* 2000;19:230–43.

33. Hastings KL. Assessment of immunosuppressant drug carcinogenicity: standard and alternative models. *Hum Exp Toxicol* 2000;19:261–5.

34. Cohen S. Human carcinogenic risk evaluation: an alternative approach to the two-year bioassay. *Toxicol Sci* 2004;80:225–9.

35. Melnick RL, Kohn MC, Portier CJ. Implications for risk assessment of suggested nongenotoxic mechanisms of chemical carcinogenesis. *Environ Health Persp* 1996; 104(Suppl 1):123–34.

36. Perera FP. Perspectives on the risk assessment for nongenotoxic carcinogens and tumor promoters. *Environ Health Persp* 1991;94:231–5.

37. Matthews EJ, Kruhlak NL, Cimino MC, Benzm RD, Contrera JF. An analysis of genetic toxicity, reproductive and developmental toxicity, and carcinogenicity data: II. Identification of genotoxicants, reprotoxicants, and carcinogens using in silico methods. *Regul Toxicol Pharmacol* 2006;44:97–110.

38. Devillers J, Marchand-Geneste N, Carpy A, Porcher JM. SAR and QSAR modeling of endocrine disruptors. *SAR & QSAR Environ Res* 2006;17:393–412.

39. Sunil-Chandra NP, Arno J, Fazakerley J, Nash AA. Lymphoproliferative disease in mice infected with gammaherpesvirus 68. *Am J Pathol* 1994;145:818–26.

40. Mougel F, Dalle S, Balme B, Houot R, Thomas L. Aggressive CD30 large cell lymphoma after cyclosporine given for putative atopic dermatitis. *Dermatology* 2006;213:239–41.

41. Ahmed N, Heslop HE. Viral lymphomagenesis. *Curr Opin Hematol* 2006;13: 254–95.

42. Kwon JH, Farrell RJ. The risk of lymphoma in the treatment of inflammatory bowel disease with immunosuppressive agents. *Crit Rev Oncol Hematol* 2005;56:169–78.

43. Jarrett RF. Viruses and lymphoma/leukemia. *J Pathol* 2006;208:176–86.

44. Malnati MS, Dagna L, Ponzoni M, Lusso P. Human herpesvirus 8 (HHV-8/KSHV) and hematologic malignancies. *Rev Clin Exp Hematol* 2003;7:375–405.

45. Ibanez JP, Monteverde ML, Goldber J, Diaz MA, Turconi A. Sirolimus in pediatric renal transplantation. *Transplant Proc* 2005;37:682–4.

46. Schulz TF, Boshoff CH, Weiss RA. HIV infection and neoplasia. *Lancet* 1996; 348:587–91.

47. Martin-Gomez MA, Pena M, Cabello M, Burgos D, Gutierrez C, Sola E, Acedo C, Bailen A, Gonzalez-Molina M. Posttransplant lymphoproliferative disease: a series of 23 cases. *Transplant Proc* 2006;38:2448–50.

48. Cattani P, Capuano M, Graffeo R, Ricci R, Cerimele F, Cerimele D, Nanni G, Fadda G. Kaposi's sarcoma associated with previous human herpesvirus 8 infection in kidney transplant recipients. *J Clin Microbiol* 2001;39:506–8.

49. Chang Y, Cesarman E, Pessin MS, Lee F, Culpepper J, Knowles DM, Moore PS. Identification of herpesvirus like sequences in AIDS-associated Kaposi's sarcoma. *Science* 1994;266:1865–9.

50. Moloney FJ, Comber H, O'Lorcain P, O'Kelly P, Conlon PJ, Murphy GM. A population based study of skin cancer incidence and prevalence in renal transplant recipients. *Brit J Dermatol* 2006;154:498–504.

51. Purdie KJ, Surentheran T, Sterling JC, Bell L, McGregor JM, Proby CM, Harwood CA, Breuer J. Human papillomavirus gene expression in cutaneous squamous cell carcinomas from immunocompromised and immunocompetant individuals. *J Investig Dermatol* 2005;125:98–107.

52. Tiu J, Li H, Rassekh C, van der Sloot P, Kovach R, Zhang P. Molecular basis of posttransplant squamous cell carcinoma: the potential role of cyclosporine A in carcinogenesis. *Laryngoscope* 2006;116:762–9.

53. Fortina AB, Piaserico S, Caforio AL, Abeni D, Alaibac M, Angelini A, Iliceto S, Peserico A. Immunosuppressive level and other risk factors for basal cell carcinoma and squamous cell carcinoma in hear transplant recipients. *Arch Dermatol* 2004;140:1079–85.

54. Madan V, Hoban P, Strange RC, Fryer AA, Lear JT. Genetics and risk factors for basal cell carcinoma. *Brit J Dermatol* 2006;154(Suppl 1):5–7.

55. Euvrard S, Ulrich C, Lefrancois N. Immunosuppressants and skin cancer in transplant patients: focus on rapamycin. *Dermatol Surg* 2004;30:628–33.

56. Esser AC, Abrill A, Fayne S, Doyle JA. Acute development of multiple keratoacanthomas and squamous cell carcinomas after treatment with infliximab. *J Am Acad Dermatol* 2004;50(5 Suppl):S75–7.

57. Leonardi CL, Toth D, Cather JC, Langley RG, Werther W, Compton P, Kwon P, Wetherill G, Curtin F, Menter A. A review of malignancies observed during efalizumab (Raptiva) clinical trials for plaque psoriasis. *Dermatology* 2006;213:204–14.

58. Vivarelli M, Cucchetti A, Piscaglia F, La Barba G, Bolondi L, Cavallari A, Pinna AD. Analysis of risk factors for tumor recurrence after liver transplantation for hepatocellular carcinoma: key role of immunosuppression. *Liver Transplant* 2005;11:497–503.

59. Robinson WS. The role of hepatitis B virus in the development of primary hepatocellular carcinoma: Part I. *J Gastroenterol Hepatol* 1992;7:622–38.

60. Koike K, Moriya K, Kimura S. Role of hepatitis C virus in the development of hepatocellular carcinoma: transgenic approach to viral hepatocarcinogenesis. *J Gastroenterol Hepatol* 2002;17:394–400.

61. Li H, Minarovits J. Host-cell dependent expression of latent Epstein-Barr virus genomes: regulation by DNA methylation. *Adv Cancer Res* 2003;89:133–56.

62. Mahieux R, Gessain A. HTLV-1 associated adult T-cell leukemia/lymphoma. *Rev Clin Exp Hematol* 2003;7:336–61.

63. Flaitz CM, Hicks MJ. Molecular piracy: the link to viral carcinogenesis. *Oral Oncol* 1998;34:448–53.

64. Snjiders PJ, Steenbergen RD, Heideman DA, Meijer CJ. HPV-mediated cervical carcinogenesis: concepts and clinical implications. *J Pathol* 2006;208:152–64.

65. Feitelson MA. Parallel epigenetic and genetic changes in the pathogenesis of hepatitis virus-associated hepatocellular carcinoma. *Cancer Letts* 2006;239:10–20.

66. van Doorn R, Gruis NA, Willemze R, van der Velden PA, Tensen CP. Aberrant DNA methylation in cutaneous malignancies. *Sem Oncol* 2005;32:479–87.

67. Pini JT, Frachina M, Taylor JM, Kay PH. Evidence that general genomic hypomethylation and focal hypermethylation are two independent molecular events of non-Hodgkin's lymphoma. *Oncol Res* 2004;14:399–405.

68. Fesus L, Szondy Z, Uray I. Probing the molecular program of apoptosis by cancer chemopreventive agents. *J Cell Biochem* 1995;22(Suppl):151–61.

69. Bachman AN, Curtin GM, Doolittle DJ, Goodman JI. Altered methylation in gene-specific and GC-rich regions of DNA is progressive and nonrandom during promotion of skin tumorigenesis. *Toxicol Sci* 2006;1:406–18.

70. Marks F, Fürstenberger G, Heinzelmann T, Müller-Decker K. Mechanisms in tumor promotions: guidance for risk assessment and cancer chemoprevention. *Toxicol Letts* 1995;82/83:907–17.

71. Barao I, Ascensao JL. Human natural killer cells. *Arch Immunol Ther Exp* 1998; 46:213–29.

72. Salek-Ardakani S, Arrand JR, Mackett M. Epstein-Barr virus encoded interleukin-10 inhibits HLA-class I, ICAM-1, and B7 expression on human monocytes: implications for immune evasion by EBV. *Virology* 2002;304:342–51.

73. Andreesen R, Hennemann B, Krause SW. Adoptive immunotherapy of cancer using monocyte-derived macrophages: rationale, current status, and perspectives. *J Leukocyte Biol* 1998;64:419–26.

74. Capello D, Rossi D, Gaidano G. Post-transplant lymphoproliferative disorders: molecular basis of disease histogenesis and pathogenesis. *Hematol Oncol* 2005; 23:61–7.

75. Guinan EC, Gribben JG, Boussiotis VA, Freeman GJ, Nadler LM. Pivotal role of the B7:CD28 pathway in transplantation tolerance and tumor immunity. *Blood* 1994;84:3261–82.

76. Lund JM, Linehan MM, Iijima N, Iwasaki A. Cutting edge: plasmacytoid dendritic cells provide innate immune protection against mucosal viral infection in situ. *J Immunol* 2006;177:7510–4.

77. Qu M, Muller HK, Woods GM. Chemical carcinogens and antigens contribute to cutaneous tumor promotion by depleting epidermal Langerhans cells. *Carcinogenesis* 1997;18:1277–9.

78. Maini MK, Boni C, Ogg GS, King AS, Reignat S, Lee CK, Larrubia JR, Webster GJ, McMichael AJ, Ferrari C, Williams R, Vergani D, Bertoletti A. Direct ex vivo analysis of hepatitis B virus-specific CD8(+) T cells associated with control of infection. *Gastroenterology* 1999;117:1386–99.

79. Yu P, Fu YX. Tumor-infiltrating T lymphocytes: friends or foes? *Lab Investig* 2006;86:231–45.

80. Hori K, Ehrke MJ, Mace K, Maccubbin D, Doyle MJ, Otsuka Y, Mihich E. Effect of recombinant human tumor necrosis factor on the induction of murine macrophage tumoricidal activity. *Cancer Res* 1987;47:2793–8.

81. Kagan BL, Ganz T, Lehrer RI. Defensins: a family of antimicrobial and cytotoxic peptides. *Toxicology* 1994;87:131–49.

82. Brandacher G, Winkler C, Schroecksnadel K, Margreiter R, Fuchs D. Antitumoral activity of interferon-gamma involved in impaired immune function in cancer patients. *Curr Drug Metab* 2006;7:599–612.

83. Rees RC. MHC restricted and non-restricted killer lymphocytes. *Blood Rev* 1990; 4:204–10.

84. Chada S, Ramesh R, Mhashilkar AM. Cytokine- and chemokine-based gene therapy for cancer. *Curr Opin Mol Ther* 2003;5:463–74.

85. Veltri S, Smith JW Jr. Interleukin 1 trials in cancer patients: a review of the toxicity, antitumor and hematopoietic effects. *Stem Cells* 1996;14:164–76.

86. Hansen F. Hemopoietic growth and inhibitory factors in treatment of malignancies. A review. *Acta Oncol* 1995;34:453–68.

87. Maini A, Morse PD, Wang CY, Jones RF, Haas GP. New developments in the use of cytokines for cancer therapy. *Anticancer Res* 1997;17:3803–8.

88. Kurebayashi J. Regulation of interleukin-6 secretion from breast cancer cells and its clinical implications. *Breast Cancer* 2000;7:124–9.

89. Appasamy PM. Biological and clinical implications of interleukin-7 and lymphopoiesis. *Cytokines Cell Mol Ther* 1999;5:25–39.

90. Pages F, Berger A, Lebel-Binay S, Zinzindohoue F, Danel C, Piqueras B, Carriere O, Thiounn N, Cugnenc PH, Fridman WH. Proinflammatory and antitumor properties of interleukin-18 in the gastrointestinal tract. *Immunol Letts* 2000;75: 9–14.

91. Roda JM, Parihar R, Lehman A, Mani A, Tridandapani S, Carson WE 3rd. Interleukin-21 enhances NK cell activation in response to antibody-coated targets. *J Immunol* 2006;177:120–9.

92. Oniki S, Nagai H, Horikawa T, Furukawa J, Belladonna ML, Yoshimoto T, Hara I, Nishigori C. Interleukin-23 and interleukin-27 exert quite different antitumor and vaccine effects on poorly immunogenic melanoma. *Cancer Res* 2006;66: 6395–404.

93. Goda C, Kanaji T, Kanaji S, Tanaka G, Arima K, Ohno S, Izuhara K. Involvement of IL-32 in activation-induced cell death in T cells. *Intl Immunol* 2006;18:233–40.

94. Devoogdt N, Revets H, Kindt A, Liu YQ, De Baetselier P, Ghassabeh GH. The tumor-promoting effects of TNF-α involves the induction of secretory leukocyte protease inhibitor. *J Immunol* 2006;177:8046–52.

95. Becker Y. Molecular immunological approaches to biotherapy of human cancers—a review, hypothesis and implications. *Anticancer Res* 2006;26:1113–34.

96. Melnikova VO, Bar-Eli M. Bioimmunotherapy for melanoma using fully human antibodies targeting MCAM/MUC18 and IL-8. *Pigmented Cell Res* 2006;19: 395–405.

97. Frumento G, Piazza T, Di Carlo E, Ferrini S. Targeting tumor-related immunosuppression for cancer immunotherapy. *Endocrine, Metab Immune Disord Drug Targ* 2006;6:233–7.

98. Hor S, Pirzer H, Dumoutier L, Bauer F, Wittmann S, Sticht H, Renauld JC, de Waal Malefyt R, Fickenscher H. The T-cell lymphokine interleukin-26 targets epithelial cells through the interleukin-20 receptor 1 and interleukin-10 receptor 2 chains. *J Biol Chem* 2004;279:33343–51.

99. Diveu C, Lak-Hal AH, Froger J, Ravon E, Grimaud L, Barbier F, Hermann J, Gascan H, Chevalier S. Predominant expression of the long isoform of GP130-like (GPL) receptor is required for interleukin-31 signaling. *Eur Cytokine Net* 2004; 15:291–302.

100. Leach DR, Krummel MF, Allison JP. Enhancement of antitumor immunity by CTLA-4 blockade. *Science* 1996;271:1734–6.

101. Barbera-Guillem E, May KF Jr, Nyhus JK, Nelson MB. Promotion of tumor invasion by cooperation of granulocytes and macrophages activated by anti-tumor antibodies. *Neoplasia* 1999;1:453–60.

102. Schlingemann J, Hess J, Wrobel G, Breitenbach U, Gebhardt C, Steinlein P, Kramer H, Furstenberger G, Hahn M, Angel P, Lichter P. Profile of gene expression induced by the tumour promoter TPA in murine epithelial cells. *Intl J Cancer* 2003;104:699–708.

103. Ohmori K, Miyazaki K, Umeda M. Detection of tumor promoters by early antigen expression of EB virus in Raji cell using fluorescence miniplate-reader. *Cancer Letts* 1998;132:51–59.

104. Lembo D, Donalisio M, De Andrea M, Cornaglia M, Scutera S, Musso T, Landolfo S. A cell-based high-throughput assay for screening inhibitors of human papillomavirus-16 long control region activity. *FASEB J* 2006;20:148–50.

105. Chang PL, Chambers AF. Transforming JB6 cell exhibit enhanced integrin-mediated adhesion to osteopontin. *J Cell Biochem* 2000;78:8–23.

106. Blumenthal RD, Hansen HJ, Goldenberg DM. Inhibition of adhesion, invasion, and metastasis by antibodies targeting CEACAM6 (NCA-90) and CEACAM5 (Carcinoembryonic Antigen). *Cancer Res* 2005;65:8809–17.

107. Fridman R, Lacal JC, Reich R, Bonfil DR, Ahn CH. Differential effects of phorbol ester on the in vitro invasiveness of malignant and non-malignant human fibroblast cells. *J Cell Physiol* 1990;142:55–60.

108. Noguchi M, Nomata K, Watanabe J, Kanetake H, Saito Y. Changes in gap junction intercellular communication in renal tubular epithelial cell in vitro treated with renal carcinogens. *Cancer Letts* 1998;122:77–84.

109. Hu VW, Xie HQ. Interleukin-1 alpha suppresses gap junction-mediated intercellular communication in human endothelial cells. *Exp Cell Res* 1994;213: 218–23.

110. Von Willebrand M, Jascur T, Bonnefoy-Berard N, Yano H, Altman A, Matsuda Y, Mustelin T. Inhibition of phosphatidylinositol 3-kinase blocks T cell antigen receptor/CD3-induced activation of the mitogen-activated kinase Erk2. *Eur J Biochem* 1996;235:828–35.

111. Algeciras-Schimnich A, Griffith TS, Lynch DH, Paya CV. Cell cycle-dependent regulation of FLIP levels and susceptibility to Fas-mediated apoptosis. *J Immunol* 1999;162:5205–11.

112. Gray LE, Ostby J, Farrell J, Rehnberg G, Linder R, Cooper R, Goldman J, Slott V, Laskey J. A dose–response analysis of methoxychlor-induced alterations of reproductive development and function in the rat. *Fund Appl Toxicol* 1989; 12:92–108.

113. Blankenstein T, Qin Z. Chemical carcinogens as foreign bodies and some pitfalls regarding cancer immune surveillance. *Adv Cancer Res* 2003;90:179–207.

114. La Porta CA, Comolli R. Angiogenic capacity and lung-colonizing potential in vivo is increased in weakly metastatic B16F1 cells and decreased in highly metastatic BL6 cells by phorbol esters. *Clin Exp Metast* 1998;16:399–405.

115. Kadhim S, Burns BF, Birnboim HC. In vivo induction of tumor variants by phorbol 12-myristate 13-acetate. *Cancer Letts* 1987;38:209–14.

116. Mahnke YD, Schirrmacher V. Characteristics of a potent tumor vaccine-induced secondary anti-tumor T cell response. *Intl J Oncol* 2004;24:1427–34.

117. Yamamoto S, Urano K, Nomura T. Validation of transgenic mice harboring the human prototype c-Ha-ras gene as a bioassay model for rapid carcinogenicity testing. *Toxicology Letts* 1998;102–3:473–8.

118. Furstenberger G, Schweizer J, Marks F. Development of phorbol ester responsiveness in neonatal mouse epidermis: correlation between hyperplastic response and sensitivity to first-stage tumor promotion. *Carcinogenesis* 1985;6:289–94.

119. McClain RM, Keller D, Casciano D, Fu P, MacDonald J, Popp J, Sagartz J. Neonatal mouse model: review of methods and results. *Toxicol Pathol* 2001;29(Suppl): 128–37.

120. Yamarik TA. Safety assessment of dichlorophene and chlorophene. *Intl J Toxicol* 2004;23(Suppl 1):1–27.

121. Ryffel B. The carcinogenicity of ciclosporin. *Toxicology* 1992;73:1–22.

122. De Jong M, Coppee MC, De Halleux F, Deckers C, Maisin H. Immunosuppression and carcinogenesis: effects of azathioprine on induction of sarcomas by 3-methylcholanthrene. *Neoplasma* 1977;24:139–46.

123. Bowden GT, Jaffe D, Andrews K. Biological and molecular aspects of radiation carcinogenesis in mouse skin. *Rad Res* 1990;121:235–41.

124. Yabu K, Warty VS, Gorelik E, Shinozuka H. Cyclosporine promotes the induction of thymic lymphomas in C57BL/6 mice irradiated by a single dose of gamma-radiation. *Carcinogenesis* 1991;12:43–6.

125. Yamawaki M, Katiyar SK, Anderson CY, Tubesing KA, Mukhtar H, Elmets CA. Genetic variation in low-dose UV-induced suppression of contact hypersensitivity and in the skin photocarcinogenesis response. *J Investig Dermatol* 1997;109: 716–21.

■■■■■■ CHAPTER 28

Strategy Considerations for Developing the Preclinical Safety Testing Programs for Protein Scaffold Therapeutics

STANLEY A. ROBERTS, PhD, DABT, GARY WOODNUTT, PhD, and
CURT W. BRADSHAW, PhD

Contents

28.1 INTRODUCTION

A number and variety of conjugated peptides/proteins are currently being developed as potential therapeutic agents. The objective of this chapter is to discuss some of the key issues that contribute to the design of the preclinical safety assessment program for an emerging group of biopharmaceuticals that we have designated as protein scaffold therapeutics. These new compounds are diverse and include several different protein scaffolds such as monoclonal antibodies, transferrin, and albumin. Small pharmacologically active molecules

Preclinical Safety Evaluation of Biopharmaceuticals: A Science-Based Approach to Facilitating Clinical Trials, edited by Joy A. Cavagnaro
Copyright © 2008 by John Wiley & Sons, Inc.

633

(i.e., pharmacophores) are attached to the scaffolds so that these therapeutics can have many potential modes of intended pharmacologic action. The first-generation antibody-based scaffolds were immunotoxin conjugates directed toward cell surface receptors that acted as delivery systems for cytotoxic radionuclides (e.g., Bexxar® and Zevalin®) or chemical toxins (Mylotarg®). The antibody-directed specificity (e.g., CD33 for Mylotarg®, CD20 for Bexxar® and Zevalin®) allowed the cytotoxic activity to be preferentially directed toward the target cells. In the case of Mylotarg® the conjugated molecule is internalized via a receptor, after which the cytotoxin is released intracellularly to kill the targeted cell. Several of these conjugated therapeutics have proved to be clinically successful, with only relatively minor side effect profiles related to either the proteinaceous nature of the drug (e.g., antigenicity or hypersensitivity) or to the pharmacology of the conjugate (e.g., anemia, myelosuppression, tumor lysis syndrome). Collectively these data also suggest that administration of a protein conjugate per se does not increase the potential for systemic toxicity and in fact can provide significant improvement over the pharmacophore alone.

The targeted delivery of cytotoxins to neoplastic cells represented a significant step forward in improving the safety and efficacy of cancer therapy. Recently a new class of protein scaffold therapeutics has been developed where the role of the macromolecular scaffold (antibody, F_c, albumin, transferrin, etc.) is to improve the pharmacokinetics by providing protection for the active moiety (small molecule or peptide) from metabolic or urinary clearance. For these compounds the pharmacophore that is attached to the protein scaffold provides the desired pharmacologic target activity. The pharmacophore can either be produced as a fusion protein or it can be chemically linked to a specific site on the scaffold. An interesting feature of this latter technology is the specific stoichiometry for the macromolecule and pharmacophore combination, which allows for a precise characterization of the final drug product.

For this chapter we will specifically focus on protein scaffold therapeutic agents where the primary objective is to improve the pharmacokinetics of the pharmacophore. Other chapters in this book will specifically discuss immunotoxin conjugates [1]. The various protein scaffold therapeutics that are currently being advanced through late-stage discovery and/or clinical development are detailed in Table 28.1. As previously discussed, the biological activity of these agents is derived from the pharmacophore through which the pharmacological activity (e.g., inhibition or activation) is achieved. For example, GLP-1 (glucagon-like-peptide 1) analogues have been attached to albumin or transferrin and angiopoietin-2 binding peptides have been appended to F_c domains of antibodies. Interestingly the pharmacological potency of the conjugated peptides is often lower after the protein scaffold therapeutic has been created. Presumably this reduction in activity may be the result of steric hindrance of the pharmacophore in binding to the target or from alterations in the conformation of the peptide.

TABLE 28.1 Protein scaffold therapeutics under development

Scaffold	Company	Products	Pharmacophore	Clinical Status	Noteworthy Details
Albumin	Human genome sciences	Albuferon	Interferon-alpha	Phase 3	Yeast
		Albugon	Glucagon-like peptide-1	Phase 1	
		Albuleukin	Interleukin-2	Phase 1 (no longer active)	
		Albutropin	Human growth hormone	Phase 1 (no longer active)	
	Conjuchem	CJC-1134	Exendin-4	Phase 2	Albumin from yeast with chemical conjugation
		CJC-1295	Growth hormone	Phase1 (clinical hold)	
		CJC-1131	Glucagon-like peptide-1	Phase 2 (no longer active)	
		CJC-1008	Dynorphin	Phase 2 (no longer active)	
Fc	Amgen	Enbrel	Tumor necrosis factor receptor	Launched	Peptibodies (bacterial expression)
		AMG-531	Thrombopoietin mimetic	Phase 3	
		AMG-386	Angiopoietin antagonist	Phase 1/2	
		AMG-623	BAFF antagonist	Phase 1	
		AMG-403	Nerve growth factor	Phase 1	
	Genentech	BR3-Fc	BR3 receptor	Phase 1	
	EMD Lexigen	Fc-epo	Erythropoietin	Preclinical	
Antibody	CovX	CVX-045	Thrombospondin-1 mimetic	Phase 1	Mammalian expression
		CVX-060	Angiopoietin-2 antagonist	Phase 1	
		CVX-096	GLP-1 receptor agonist	Preclinical	
Transferrin	BioRexis	Transferrin-GLP-1	Glucagon-like peptide-1	Phase 1	Yeast expression
		Transferrin-interferon beta	Interferon beta	Preclinical	

The protein scaffolds are generally considered to be pharmacologically inert. The primary function for these scaffolds is to provide biological stability to prevent the pharmacophores from being rapidly cleared from the body. Scaffolds based on the F_c domain also remove the potential for ligand binding to the variable domain which may reduce the need for conducting certain studies (i.e., tissue cross-reactivity) during the preclinical safety assessment of these new agents. Other antibody scaffolds have F_{ab} domains that are specifically created to interact with synthetic linkers and not receptors or other ligands. However, the potential still does exist for some F_c specific function for these types of molecules. Nevertheless, not all of these agents are antibody based; albumin and transferrin are examples of other scaffolds that are currently under evaluation.

The normal physiological roles for albumin include maintaining the osmolarity of the blood and aiding in the transport of fatty acids and hormones. While it can be presumed that these functions would not be appreciably altered by the fusion process that creates the biopharmaceutical agent, the potential implications on safety are not known. However, the protein load provided by dosing an albumin conjugate would be minor in comparison to the overall albumin pool in the body, which could reduce the potential safety implications. On the other hand, the possible interaction of a transferrin fusion protein with its specific receptor could theoretically alter the internalization process and the subsequent endosomal acidification release of transported iron. The impact of this type of conjugate on the distribution and availability of iron throughout the body has not been reported. Thus the potential does exist for some protein scaffold therapeutics to have safety implications that would require specialized testing (i.e., monitoring of normal physiological activities) to accurately assess the preclinical safety of the new therapeutic agent.

Consistent with the case-by-case paradigm, the potential direct or secondary effect(s) of any scaffold should be carefully considered and monitored if judged necessary. An additional issue with these natural scaffolds is that each of these fusion proteins could be considered "foreign" by the immunological surveillance network. While the complex structure of these macromolecules may disguise the active pharmacophore moiety to some extent, it is still possible for immunogenicity and hypersensitivity reactions to result from this alteration of the scaffold. The extent to which this occurs will, in all likelihood, be dependent on the individual molecule and will not necessarily be entirely predictable for a particular scaffold. The inability to predict animal or human immunogenicity of these agents has been already been demonstrated by the diversity of antigenicity responses to various human protein therapeutics [2,3].

28.2 SAFETY ASSESSMENT PROGRAM STRATEGY DEVELOPMENT

The strategies to develop the preclinical safety assessment programs for biotechnology-derived therapeutics have often been characterized as case by case. Historically this customization has resulted from the need for flexible strategy designs from a variety of different challenges that have included rapid metabolism, inappropriate tissue distribution, poor chemical stability, and absence of the target or lack of efficacy in the animal species that were planned for use in the pharmacology or toxicology studies. In contrast, the preclinical toxicology and drug metabolism studies necessary for the regulatory approval of new drug candidates for small molecules (NCEs) have been standardized for decades [4], in part, the result of the perceived chemical and biological similarity of these molecules. Since 1991 these developmental strategies and study designs have been the subject of International Conference on Harmonization (ICH) activities [5]. Guidances have been issued for a number of toxicological, pharmacokinetic, and drug metabolism studies that are conducted for small molecule NCEs. In contrast, only the ICH S6 guidance for biotechnologically related molecules has been published [6].

As previously discussed, the common goal for protein scaffold therapeutics is to extend the duration of pharmacologic action of the pharmacophore by increasing the circulating half-life. The development strategies required for regulatory submission and approval of these fusion molecules could represent a combination of the studies conducted for traditional small molecule NCEs and biopharmaceuticals. These programs may be expected, however, to be relatively similar to biopharmaceuticals for the pharmacological, ADME/PK (absorption, distribution, metabolism, excretion/pharmacokinetics), and toxicological characteristics of the various components of the molecule.

28.3 CHOICE OF ANIMALS

A number of considerations can alter the design of the preclinical safety program for new pharmaceuticals whether they are traditional small-molecule NCEs or biotechnology derived. One of the earliest choices that can be made is the selection of animal species for the toxicology program. This decision can often be made a number of months prior to the filing of the IND. For the development of small-molecule NCEs the general criteria for selecting the rodent and nonrodent toxicology species include the presence of the pharmacological target, demonstration of efficacy, and a similarity to humans (in vitro) for ADME and PK characteristics. In an effort to develop more successful small-molecule drug candidates, many pharmaceutical companies now expend considerable effort in identifying new drug candidates for which the ADME and PK characteristics have been optimized prior to selection of a lead candidate for development. The predictability of this research over the last few years has become increasingly successful thanks to tremendous advances in analytical methodologies, pharmacokinetic modeling capabilities, and the increased availability of animal and human tissues [7]. As a result a considerable knowledge base of ADME and PK characteristics will have often been established for small-molecule NCEs in several animal species by the time that the IND is filed.

Based on the primary objective of improving the pharmacokinetic profile, a new protein scaffold therapeutic candidate will also have generally been selected for development following optimization of ADME and PK characteristics. Other critical candidate selection issues may also include the potential immunogenicity of the therapeutic molecule, the possible induction of autoimmunity, and the comparability between animals and humans for tissue cross-reactivity. The immunogenicity potential of a new therapeutic agent can be viewed as a potential mechanism for increased clearance, which could result in the dramatically reduced exposure to the drug during a multiple-dose toxicity study (e.g., subchronic studies of one to six months in length). This type of response could effectively disqualify an animal species from longer term toxicology testing because of the reduced drug exposure. It is also possible for the expression of antidrug antibodies to have other profound toxicologic effects that can theoretically include deposition of immune complexes in the kidney.

Considerable efforts are often expended on the quantification and characterization of the ability of the toxicology test species to build an antibody response to biopharmaceuticals. While this may help explain some effects seen in animal toxicology studies, these antigenicity results are often extended to an attempt to predict the response in humans. However, the immunogenicity of human proteins in animals is not a perfect predictor for the production of human antihuman antibodies in clinical studies [2,8]. While altered physiological states in humans, including disease-induced immunosuppression, may play a role in this lack of correlation, it does remain that antigenicity in humans is a poorly understood process. Therefore the observation of rodent antihuman antibodies or primate antihuman antibodies may have more relevance to the interpretation of the results from the animal toxicology studies than the potential to predict immunogenicity in humans.

The choice of animals for the toxicology testing of protein scaffold therapeutics therefore may depend on a potentially complex case-by-case decision-making process. All relevant information related to the expected (or known) efficacy against the target, ADME/PK characteristics, immunogenicity, and toxicity of these molecules must be utilized in the design of the toxicology program. This informational database should include all that is known about the chemistry and biological actions of the macromolecular scaffold and the pharmacophore. For successful regulatory development, it is expected that all new candidate drugs use both a rodent and nonrodent species in the preclinical safety programs [4,9]. For small NCE drug candidates, the most commonly used rodent species is the rat, with the beagle dog being the most frequently used nonrodent [9,10]. These two species are usually chosen based on a combination of factors that include ease of use, widespread availability, economics, historical database of toxicological and pathological parameters, historical predictability of animal to human toxicities [10], and as previously indicated, their pharmacological appropriateness and ADME/PK comparability to humans.

Since several of the scaffolds for protein scaffold therapeutics are based on endogenous proteins, the potential for antigenicity is anticipated to be low in humans [8]. However, since these scaffolds are based on human molecules, they are expected to be immunogenic in animals particularly in rodents. While rats are commonly used in most safety assessment programs, they often develop antibodies to human-derived proteins [8]. Therefore their use in a preclinical safety assessment program, as previously discussed, could be seriously compromised by the reduction in systemic drug exposure. Nevertheless, rats are always given serious consideration as a species for use in preclinical safety assessment because of their well-described historical database, relatively modest size (and reduced need for bulk drug) and their ease of use and care.

At the beginning of a new drug development program, it will probably be necessary to conduct some multiple-dose studies in rats to evaluate the immunogenic potential of the new molecule. If the result is positive, then the option to use another rodent species could include mice as the choice for subchronic or chronic toxicity studies. Although mice are infrequently used as the second species in preclinical safety assessment programs, they are often utilized in the efficacy studies for biotechnology-derived molecules. While animal husbandry issues may be somewhat challenging for some strains of mice, their small size can make them a potentially valuable species for safety assessment. As with rats the potential would seem to be high for mice to develop antibodies to a human-based protein. It would therefore be valuable to conduct the appropriate studies prior to including mice in a safety assessment program. On the other hand, if neither rats nor mice are considered appropriate, it may then be justified that only nonrodents be used in the toxicology program.

When considering the potential challenges with using rodents for protein scaffold therapeutics, it is clear that the preferred species will probably be nonhuman primates. The primary species currently used is the cynomolgous monkey, although rhesus monkeys have been used in a number of toxicology programs. Either species would seem appropriate provided that they respond pharmacologically to the drug. Protein scaffold therapeutics should also have the potential for reduced immunogenicity in primates, since the protein scaffolds and pharmacophores are directly derived from, or are similar to, those found in humans. The dramatically improved access to healthy captivity-raised cynomolgus and rhesus monkeys over the past two decades have supported the dramatic upturn in their use for biological molecule testing. However, due to continuing concerns about the contagious diseases carried by nonhuman primate species and the high bulk drug product requirements, the search has continued for primate toxicology species that carry fewer dangerous contagions, are easier to handle, and have lower body weights. Marmosets have been of interest in this regard but a commercially viable breeding program has not yet been established that could meet the needs for the worldwide development of even a few new biological products. Their relative lack of availability has not allowed a comprehensive data base to be developed that could be used to evaluate their more widespread use in toxicology development programs. It should also be noted that dogs are seldom used in the toxicity testing for biopharmaceuticals for a variety reasons that include their perceived propensity to develop antihuman antibodies and high susceptibility to anaphylaxis. In addition there is a scarcity of immunologic reagents available for dogs, and their large body weight would require significantly higher quantities of the active pharmaceutical ingredient.

The species selection process for targeted biopharmaceuticals such as monoclonal antibodies and protein scaffold therapeutics may use tissue cross-reactivity studies as a critical component in the decision-making process. These studies can be conducted using a variety of tissues from humans and the toxicology program animal species [11]. The objective of these studies is to determine the potential presence of target-based binding and to gain at least a semiquantitative estimation of the degree of binding in these tissues. Additionally the results observed in the animals are compared to those found in human tissues. Based on the knowledge and experience of the researchers, these results may be extended to hypothesize upon the potential mechanism(s) of pharmacological and/or toxicological action of the agent. Whether this binding results from a direct and specific interaction with an intended receptor/epitope or against unintended targets may need to be determined by subsequent experiments. It is important to remember that these studies can often produce results for which the human relevancy is not well understood, so substantial challenges can exist for projecting the safety of the new molecule in humans when the importance of these studies is too heavily weighted [11].

Tissue cross-reactivity experiments should be initiated with caution, as they may add only minimal scientific value to the safety assessment process but may create considerable challenges. Clearly, the choice of the primary animal species for protein scaffold therapeutics should be one that expresses the appropriate receptor/epitope. This could be established by a variety of efficacy-based experiments both in vivo and/or in vitro. The tissue cross-reactivity studies of a new therapeutic agent would then be conducted in the preferred toxicology species, with the results being compared to the binding seen in normal human tissues. One of the primary challenges with these studies can be that the pharmacologic target may, or may not, be found in the animal models of human disease or in the normal animals that would be used for toxicology studies. For a species to be considered appropriate in a toxicology program, the presence of target-directed binding in animals would be expected. In an appropriately qualified species, off-target binding could be interpreted as being suggestive of the potential for toxicity. However, apparent off-target binding should not be used as an unequivocal indicator of toxicity. Instead, it may be beneficial to further explore the potential nature of this binding in various animal models so that this observation can be placed in its proper perspective.

It is also possible that some targets may only be expressed in humans, and then any binding observed in animals would be off-target related. In these circumstances animal toxicology studies could, and should, still be conducted. However, this type of program would not be ideal as it would only be able to provide a generalized toxicity assessment before the human clinical studies are conducted. Depending on the nature of any effects seen in animals (and their reversibility), it should still be possible to conduct human phase 1 trials provided that these studies are carefully and thoughtfully designed. Some important factors that could improve the clinical study design for this scenario might include a low starting dose, dosing only one patient at a time, and having ready access to emergency medical equipment and staff [12].

If an appropriate species cannot be identified based on the lack of the target or poor efficacy, it has also been proposed that toxicology studies could be conducted using homologous molecules. This type of experiment has proved quite useful for anti-sense molecules [13]. However appealing this approach might be, it should not be universally applied to all types of biopharmaceuticals. Because of the high potential for this type of study to produce misleading or poorly understood results, it would seem that this strategy should only be used if the pharmacology of the homologous molecule is very well understood. While endogenous pharmacophores may be highly conserved across various species, the biological control mechanisms could be substantially different from one animal species to another. This could include scenarios where the pharmacology of the agent is similar but the balance of signaling and control pathways would be substantially different. Alternatively, it is possible that an individual pharmacophore could have completely different biochemical or physiological roles in different animal species. It would seem that unless the overall biological control of the pharmacophore system is well understood, or can be determined without exhausting time and resources, these studies could prove to be of very little practical value.

In summary, the choice of animal species to use for the toxicological testing of protein scaffold therapeutics will continue to be a complex decision-making process. In general, rats and monkeys will probably continue to be the initial species to be considered for the safety assessment program for a protein scaffold therapeutic provided that they possess the appropriate pharmacological target. However, because of potential immunogenicity issues in rodents, the primary species for testing will continue to be the nonhuman primate. The choice of a second species for toxicology testing, or an alternative strategy such as homologous pharmacophores, must be given careful consideration as an incorrect choice could provide the potential to significantly hinder or delay the safety assessment process.

28.4 DURATION AND TYPES OF STUDIES

One of the practical challenges in developing a new therapeutic (pharmaceutical or biopharmaceutical) is to conduct the appropriate length and type of toxicology study that will support an ongoing clinical program. Numerous cost pressures exist for all new pharmaceutical agents so that only those candidate drugs with the highest potential for success should proceed into and through development. Some of these economic factors also produce challenges to time lines for the conduct and reporting of toxicology studies. The first animal toxicology studies for the development of new pharmaceuticals are usually acute and/or short-term dose-range finding studies. After these initial studies are completed, the IND-enabling studies are initiated to support the regulatory submissions. The four week (i.e., one-month) study is usually the first conducted, and it is used to support the phase 1 or 2 human clinical studies for which the duration of continuous dosing must be equal to or less then four weeks. If standard development programs are conducted, the four-week animal toxicology study is then followed by studies that are three and six months in length.

As a new drug advances through the development process it is necessary for the animal toxicology studies to be equivalent, or longer, in duration than the human clinical studies. This strategy is generally referred to as the one-for-one dosing duration concept, and it can be a challenge for an aggressive human clinical research program that can easily outpace the ongoing animal toxicology studies. This is particularly true for the extension of dosing for human patients in phases 1 and 2. Because of the lengthy time required to order animals and conduct these toxicology studies, the proper planning and communication with clinical research teams and project management can ensure that these human clinical trials are not delayed. If a new agent is promising, and appropriate resources (e.g., bulk pharmaceutical product) can be identified, it may be desirable to accelerate the conduct of the three- or six-month toxicology studies by conducting them in parallel with the one-month study. From an operational viewpoint, the two studies can be conducted using a single protocol with the one-month study being an "interim" necropsy. Each of these studies incorporates the appropriate number of animals as if these studies were conducted separately. Therefore while these studies may provide some minimal cost savings from an administrative view, this strategy does require some "front loading" of resources, which includes the often limited supplies of the bulk active pharmaceutical ingredient. This strategy also incurs more initial risk, so it can be challenging for smaller companies or for any whose resources are limited or carefully controlled. In a recent Oncologic Drugs Advisory Committee meeting, a senior Food and Drug Administration official indicated that three-month toxicology studies would be sufficient to support a clinical program of new drugs prior to approval provided there are no overriding safety concerns [14]. This strategy could provide some advantages for promising new drugs, including protein scaffold therapeutics, that are being developed for critical diseases for which there are no currently available cures.

Another important consideration is whether developmental and reproductive toxicity studies and carcinogenicity studies should be conducted for protein scaffold therapeutics. As discussed in ICH S6, the decision to conduct these studies should be based on the nature of the product, its biological/ pharmacological actions, the clinical indication, and the intended patient population [6]. In addition the challenges elicited by the potential immunogenicity of the new drug in animals would be an important consideration. Because antidrug antibodies have the potential to decrease the circulating drug levels during the multiple day-dosing paradigms required for development or reproductive safety assessment studies, this can seriously complicate the interpretation of these studies; in fact it would question their value in the overall risk assessment process. Additionally the studies should not be required unless there are specific biological, pharmacological, or toxicological alerts that are suggestive of toxicity to the fetus, neonate, or mother.

Other factors that could impact the potential conduct of these studies may include the potential for class labeling. Recently the antidiabetic agent Byetta® was designated as a class C pregnancy hazard [15]. While the mechanisms for these effects on fetal development have not been reported, it is possible that there will ramifications for future therapeutic agents in this class. As with all types of safety assessment studies, the scientific rationale for the developmental and reproductive toxicity program should be carefully considered for protein scaffold therapeutics. Appropriate studies can then be conducted so that direct discussions with regulatory agency scientists can be held to achieve consensus.

The conduct of most in vitro genetic toxicology studies for biopharmaceutical molecules would generally not be necessary as indicated in ICH S6 [6]. Simply based on their size and physicochemical properties, it would not be expected that protein scaffold therapeutics would interact with genetic or chromosomal materials. Unless there are specific structural alerts, cellular or organ-specific toxicities, or other factors that increase concern, genetic toxicology tests should not, per se, be required for protein scaffold therapeutics. These same criteria would also apply for the animal carcinogenicity testing of protein scaffold therapeutics.

28.5 DOSAGE SELECTION

The dosage selection process can be challenging for any type of toxicology program, whether it be for small-molecule NCEs or biopharmaceutical derived molecules. The primary goals of such studies include identification of target organs, the no effect dosage level (NOEL), no adverse effect level (NOAEL), and the maximally tolerated dosage (MTD). For orally administered small-molecule NCEs it is often necessary to demonstrate that absorption and distribution are sufficiently adequate to allow the characterization of the toxicological potential of the molecule. In cases where the absorption is poor, it is often necessary to administer very high dosages to achieve reasonable safety multiples for systemic exposure (i.e., blood AUC levels). Most biopharmaceuticals will not be administered orally, so simple questions of absorption are not relevant. However, more challenging questions related to the disposition of a biopharmaceutical may come into play especially when novel parenteral dosage forms or routes are used. That is, the molecule could encounter bioavailability challenges from the site of injection due to differential dissolution or solubility characteristics that could be exacerbated by high drug concentrations in the formulation.

Ultimately the fundamental question for all classes of molecules may eventually become "how much is enough"? That is, for any relatively nontoxic molecule it may not be possible to achieve toxicologically significant evidence of effects, including toxicity, even after very high and even heroic dosages. However, simple physicochemical characteristics such as test article solubility can limit the amount of active agent that can be administered via parenteral administration. It is also possible that a poorly soluble test article may require the need to exceed the maximum volume of vehicle that can be safely administered during the conduct of an animal toxicology study. While this limitation can be at least partially overcome by multiple daily administrations, or even continuous daily infusion, it is still possible to reach a point at which no higher dosages of the drug or vehicle can be given. For low toxicity small-molecule drugs, a suggested limit of 25-fold over the clinical human exposure has traditionally been used. The magnitude of this safety factor would certainly seem reasonable as it would ensure that the potential of significant toxicities would be explored in animals. If any effects were to be observed, they could then be used to help establish the maximally suggested starting dosage in humans.

Because of the pharmacological specificity that is designed into protein scaffold therapeutics, it can be anticipated that any toxicities would be minimal and/or would probably be related to exaggerated pharmacology. It is possible that any observed biological effects may be directly related to the desired effects of the compound, or they may result from secondary effects. Pharmacodynamic effects may even play a greater role in establishing the toxicology dosages for protein scaffold therapeutics than what has been used for small-molecule NCEs. A potential complication may be that the normal animals used for toxicology experiments may only minimally express the necessary targets integral for the pharmacological mechanism of action. In these cases it may be necessary to require that arbitrary safety factors be reached to establish the upper limits of guided therapeutic toxicology studies. Whether this should be established via a body surface area normalized dosage or via anticipated systemic exposure (i.e., AUCs), it would seem reasonable to continue to use a 25-fold safety factor as the maximum limit. It is ironic to note that the "safer" (i.e., less overtly toxic) agents may need to be tested at substantially higher concentrations or dosages than compounds that are "less safe."

In conclusion, the ability to define the dosages of a protein scaffold therapeutic to be used in toxicology studies may prove to be difficult. Because the potential exists for these compounds to produce minimal toxicity, the dose selection process may rely more heavily on exaggerated pharmacodynamic effects than traditional small molecules have historically used.

28.6 METABOLISM AND PHARMACOKINETICS

To file an IND for a small-molecule NCE drug candidate, it is expected that the ADME (absorption, distribution, metabolism, and excretion) and PK characteristics would be generally understood prior to the human phase 1 study. At this early stage of drug development, these studies would be conducted in the animal species that were used for the pharmacology and toxicology studies. Typically the pharmacokinetics of small molecules would be determined in the relevant rodent and nonrodent species by the administration of nonradiolabeled drugs via both the intravenous and oral (if intended) routes of administration. These studies would allow the comprehensive determination of many PK characteristics including half-life ($T_{1/2}$), volume of distribution (V_d), time to maximum blood levels (T_{max}), bioavailability (F), exposure (AUC), and potentially the route of excretion. Additional data could also have been gathered on the metabolic pathways of these new compounds using ^{14}C- or ^{3}H-radiolabels, animal and human tissues, and new techniques in qualitative and quantitative mass spectrometry.

For biopharmaceuticals, the pharmacokinetic and drug metabolism expectations for filing an IND are much less extensive than for small molecules. The pharmacokinetic studies should utilize the same route of administration and include the animal species used in the pharmacology and toxicology studies. The basic pharmacokinetic characteristics from the intravenous route should include; alpha and beta $T_{1/2}$, C_{max}, AUC, and V_d. If other parenteral routes of administration are used (i.e., subcutaneous, intramuscular), it would also be important to determine the T_{max} and bioavailability. For biopharmaceuticals it is possible that various formulations would need to be investigated to define the effect on PK parameters. This could also necessitate the conduct of pharmacokinetic bridging studies in the selected toxicology species to ensure equivalent exposure that would result from sustained or delayed release formulations.

If all of the components of a protein scaffold therapeutic are naturally occurring or endogenous (e.g., proteins), then no classic drug metabolism, disposition, biotransformation or excretion studies would generally be required. That is, the metabolism, distribution, and excretion of these materials would be well understood and would not require further experimentation. Similarly, if some of these fundamental components (e.g., amino acids) are not naturally occurring but the metabolic disposition has been well-described, then no additional ADME studies should be necessary. However, this decision would depend on the chemical, physiological, and potential toxicological nature of the component. Because of their macromolecular nature, protein scaffold therapeutics would generate myriad metabolites, and the technical complexities involved in their analysis would require substantial resources with minimal scientific gain. Therefore, if the parent molecules are stable in the presence of serum or the appropriate tissue matrix, then the need to characterize the potentially innumerable metabolites would generally not warrant the potentially considerable expenditure of scientific or labor resources required. The impact of nonnaturally occurring components on the safety assessment of protein scaffold therapeutics would require a careful assessment of the scientific needs. For instance, if the candidate molecule contained non-natural amino acid components but the parent was stable in the presence of blood or tissues, then the need for traditional ADME studies would seem to be unnecessary. However, structural alerts and/or significant instability of the molecule with the subsequent potential release of these components would necessitate the need for a more detailed examination of ADME characteristics, particularly as the development of the compound proceeded. An important consideration in determining the necessity for additional studies being conducted would be the actual dose of these nonnatural components. Since these macromolecules will be quite large, it is probable that any single non-natural amino acid or other component would be dosed at a vanishingly low amount that would be without biological consequence.

28.7 BIOMARKERS AND INDICATORS OF TOXICITY

The ability to successfully detect and quantify toxicity in animal studies is a critical goal for the safety assessment of pharmaceuticals and biopharmaceuticals. Generalized or target organ specific toxicities in animals have typically been evaluated by a variety of different parameters, including clinical observations, body weight, food consumption, hematology, clinical chemistry, urinalysis, tissue histopathology, specific organ system functionality, and target-specific biochemical/organ markers. Based on safety concerns and resource utilization issues, it is advantageous to identify an undesirable drug as early as possible in a discovery or development program. The ability to predict or detect toxicities has dramatically changed over the past decade as advancements in analytical chemistry, molecular pathology, genomics, and proteomics have become widely available. However, the continuing need in drug discovery and development remains to minimize the false negative or false positive drugs so that resources can be successfully directed to the best candidate compounds. Therefore expanding the use of new technologies should be encouraged to better screen for animal toxicities and to identify undesirable candidate therapeutics early in the discovery phase before regulatory-based studies are initiated. As the screening and predictive capabilities of these technologies are improved for animals, it would obviously be valuable to develop the ability to extrapolate these data to better prediction of human toxicities.

Protein scaffold therapeutics represent a wide variety of chemical families and pharmacological classes. As such, it is difficult to propose a "one size fits all" guiding strategy for assessing their safety. The monitoring of traditional parameters or markers of toxicity and pathology should continue to be used as the primary screening tools for assessing the safety of protein scaffold therapeutics. However, because of their nature, protein scaffold therapeutics may produce few classic manifestations of toxicity except for exaggerated pharmacology. This will necessitate the need to establish the dosages for the toxicology studies based on pharmacological effects that would then require monitoring of the appropriate pharmacodynamic marker(s). These data would be used to support or validate the dose-limiting effects in the actual toxicology study. Depending on their nature and composition, protein scaffold therapeutics should also be examined for specific scaffold based toxicity. For example, monoclonal antibody scaffolds might require an assessment of effector function in vitro and/or an appraisal of all of the appropriate target tissues during a complete histopathological assessment in an animal toxicology study. Other scaffolds such as albumin or transferrin molecules would focus on an examination for disturbances of fluid or electrolyte balance or alterations in iron storage or metabolism, respectively.

It may be inappropriate or misleading to conduct some standard toxicology assays for protein scaffold therapeutics. For instance, the hERG assay is a common screening assay that is used to determine the potential for small-molecule NCEs to prolong the QT interval. However, this assay is sensitive to changes in protein and buffer concentrations [16]. Since many protein scaffold therapeutics are high molecular weight protein fusion or conjugate molecules, it would be difficult to adequately control for the addition of these large quantities of protein in this assay. It would probably be of greater value to monitor instead the cardiovascular system by conducting ECGs and doing blood pressure measurements during the nonrodent (e.g., primate) good laboratory practice toxicity study. It is also possible to monitor a number of additional physiological systems in nonhuman primates during a toxicology study, including the central nervous system (clinical signs), autonomic control (body temperature), and lung function (respiration rate) as would provide a generalized assessment of the safety pharmacology of this molecule.

The choice of assays or biomarkers that are used for assessing the safety of protein scaffold therapeutics should only be made after careful and thoughtful review. Specialized testing should be conducted for the scaffold or pharmacophore only after careful consideration has been given to the chemical structures and/or potential physiologic or pharmacologic actions.

28.8 CONCLUSIONS

In summary, protein scaffold therapeutics represent a new class of drugs that has been designed to improve the pharmacokinetic profile of smaller and more rapidly metabolized pharmacophores. As a result of the unique chemical and pharmacological nature of these therapeutic agents the case-by-case customized design of toxicology and ADME/PK studies will continue to be an evolving area of experimental design. The development strategies of each new drug will require a careful individual evaluation so that the appropriate experiments can be conducted. As the knowledge base increases for individual therapeutic agents and/or various compound classes, the preclinical program may require frequent adjustments to improve the risk assessment process for the human patient. One example is that some compound or pharmacological classes may require similar preclinical study strategies for regulatory approval, which would include monitoring common markers and conducting similar studies and assays. At the other extreme, most compounds for the foreseeable future will probably require a case-by-case assessment that will best be designed by a fully integrated collaboration with regulatory scientists. It would therefore be encouraged for each sponsor company to have frequent and detailed communications with scientists at the regulatory agencies to ensure the successful development of new therapeutic agents.

REFERENCES

1. Brown J, Entwistle J, Glover N, MacDonald GC. Preclinical safety evaluation of immunotoxins. In Cavagnaro JA, ed. *Preclinical Safety Evaluation of Biopharmaceuticals*, New York: Wiley, 2006;649–67.
2. Armin T, Carter G. Immunogenicity issues with therapeutic proteins. *Curr Drug Discov* 2004;4:20–9.
3. Shellekens H. Immunogenicity of therapeutic proteins. *Nephrol Dial Transplant* 2003;18:1257–9.
4. Goldenthal EI. Current views on safety evaluation of drugs. *FDA papers* 1968; 13–18.
5. Office Website for ICH. http://www.ich.org
6. ICH S6 Preclinical Safety Evaluation of Biotechnology-Derived Pharmaceuticals. http://fda.gov/cder/guidance/index.htm
7. Granneman RG, Marsh KM, Roberts SA. 2005, Unpublished results.
8. Bugelski PJ, Treacy G. Predictive power of preclinical studies in animals for the immunogenicity of recombinant therapeutic proteins in humans. *Curr Opin Mol Ther* 2004;6:10–16.
9. Dorato M, Vodicnik M. *The Toxicological Assessment of Pharmaceutical and Biotechnology Products*. New York: Taylor and Francis, 2001;243–83.
10. Olson H, Betton G, Robinson D, Thomas K, Monro A, Kolaja G, Lilly P, Sanders J, Sipes G, Bracken W, Dorato M, Von Deun K, Smith P, Berger B, Heller A. Concordance of the toxicity of pharmaceuticals in humans. *Regul Toxicol Pharmacol* 2000;32:56–67.
11. Hall W, Price-Schiavi SA, Wicks J, Rojko JL. Design and analysis of tissue cross reactivity studies. In Cavagnaro JA, ed. *Preclinical Safety Evaluation of Biopharmaceuticals*. New York: Wiley, 2006.
12. Expert Scientific Group on Phase One Clinical Trials Final Report 30 November 2006. www.tsoshop.co.uk
13. Levine A. The toxicology of oligonucleotides therapeutics and understanding the relevance of the toxicities. In Cavagnaro JA, ed. *Preclinical Safety Evaluation of Biopharmaceuticals*. New York: Wiley, 2006;357–74.
14. ODAC March 13, 2006 meeting minutes. http://www.fda.gov/ohrms/dockets/AC/06/minutes/2006-4203M1.pdf
15. Byetta® Product Label. http://www.fda.gov/cder/foi/label/2005/021773lbl.pdf
16. Gintant G. *Personal Communication*, Abbott, Abbott Park IL, 2006.

CHAPTER 29

Preclinical Safety Evaluation of Immunotoxins

JENNIFER G. BROWN, PhD, JOYCELYN ENTWISTLE, PhD, NICK GLOVER, PhD, and GLEN C. MACDONALD, PhD

Contents

29.1 INTRODUCTION

Chemotherapy represents the most common approach in the treatment of cancer. However, the overall clinical success of chemotherapeutics is often limited by drug resistance and nonselective targeting resulting in dose-limiting toxicities. The preference for highly potent anticancer molecules that specifically target tumor cells while demonstrating minimal toxicity toward normal

Preclinical Safety Evaluation of Biopharmaceuticals: A Science-Based Approach to Facilitating Clinical Trials, edited by Joy A. Cavagnaro
Copyright © 2008 by John Wiley & Sons, Inc.

tissue guides the rational design of the next generation of anticancer therapeutics.

Cancer immunotherapy became possible with the identification of tumor-associated antigens as well as the discovery of monoclonal antibodies (MAbs) that have the intrinsic properties of high affinity and specificity for their target antigen [38]. Antibodies exert their biological effector functions (e.g., antibody-dependant cellular toxicity (ADCC) or complement-dependant cellular toxicity (CDC)) once the antibody has bound to its target antigen. Despite the unique specificity of MAbs, in many cases the clinical benefit has been marginal prompting the search for more potent tumor-selective drugs that possess a different mechanism of action. The coupling of a cytotoxin to a MAb (or Mab fragment) has resulted in the generation of immunotoxins that derive their unique specificity from the antibody and impart a potent cell death signal to the targeted cells. Immunotoxins are emerging as important therapeutic agents for the treatment of a number of carcinomas and haematologic cancers [28]. In addition they are also being investigated for other diseases such as HIV [39,53], graft versus host disease [62], and autoimmune diseases [63].

This chapter will outline the development of immunotoxins and describe the preclinical development required for advancing VB4-845, an anti-EpCAM targeting scFv linked to a truncated form of *Pseudomonas* exotoxin A(252-608), into the clinic.

29.2 IMMUNOTOXIN DEVELOPMENT

The potency of an immunotoxin is dependent on the biochemical properties of both the antibody and toxin moieties. Of paramount importance are the characteristics of the target antigen and the antibody affinity for that antigen, rate of internalization into the cell, as well as the efficiency of the intracellular processing and the type of toxin.

29.2.1 Target Antigens

The development of a successful immunotoxin is clearly dependent on the choice of the antigen [7]. Prerequisites would be an antigen having a medium to high density of expression and a relatively homogeneous distribution on the tumor cell surface. As most toxins exert their mechanism of action in the cytosol by catalytically disrupting protein synthesis, an internalizing antigen is a necessity. Antigens that are shed from the cell surface, such as the carcino-embryonic antigen (CEA) and the non-Hodgkin's lymphoma (NHL) idiotype, do not represent optimal targets as free antigen would be competing with antigens displayed on cancer cells for the immunotoxin [64]. If shedding antigens are to be targeted, higher doses of drug would be required to remove the competing antigen from the circulation [36,45].

A number of solid tumor targets that are preferentially expressed on cancer cells have been identified such as the epithelial cell adhesion molecule

(EpCAM), HER2/neu (c-erbB-2), EGFR, cytokine receptors, mesothelin, as well as the carbohydrate-associated antigens such as LewisY that are highly expressed in many epithelial tumors [52]. Similarly many differentiation antigens have been identified for hemapoietic malignancies, including CD19, CD22, CD25, CD30, CD33, and CD56 [28].

29.2.2 Toxins

Certain plants, fungi, and bacteria produce pathogenic peptide toxins that are able to kill mammalian cells. Examples of these include ricin, gelonin, saporin, bryodin, pokeweed antiviral protein, and bouganin derived from plants, the fungal-derived toxins such as restrictocin and mitogillin, and the bacterially derived toxins diptheria toxin (DT) and *Pseudomonas* exotoxin A (ETA/PE). Although many of these toxins, as well as several other more exotic varieties, have been used for the construction of immunotoxins, the ones most commonly used have been ricin [32,33] from castor bean (*Ricinus communis*), diptheria toxin [23,61] from *Corynebacteriun diphtheria*, and *Pseudomonas* exotoxin A [46,47] from *Pseudomonas aeruginosa*. Toxins such as DT and ETA are extremely potent in killing tumor cells, and they exert their effect in the cytosol by interrupting protein synthesis, resulting in cell death [27].

29.3 RATIONAL DESIGN OF IMMUNOTOXINS

In general, first-generation immunotoxins consisted of chemically conjugating toxins to full-length antibodies. However, many of these toxins, such as ricin, naturally contain a cell-binding domain that targets normal tissue and proved unsuccessful in both animal models and in the clinic due to their nonspecific binding to normal tissue. In one case the attachment of ETA to the intact anti-TAC antibody that binds to CD25 on T cells and T cell malignancies resulted in severe liver toxicity in a phase 1 trial [16,46].

The design of immunotoxins has become more sophisticated, and efforts have been made to engineer safer, more efficacious molecules through a better understanding of the biochemistry of the toxins and antibodies as well as the physiological limitations surrounding effective delivery. For example, immunotoxins have been constructed with the cell-binding domain removed [25,55], thereby reducing toxicity and ensuring targeting through the antibody moiety. In addition genetically engineered fusion constructs containing antibody fragments with increased stability have been generated to enhance tumor penetration and to maximize serum half-life.

29.3.1 Immunogenicity and Toxicity

Despite the recent advances in immunotoxin design, there remain two major obstacles still to be resolved, namely immunogenicity and toxicity. Although the humanized or fully human antibody moiety of an immunotoxin has limited recognition by the immune system, toxins are highly immunogenic and rapidly elicit an immune response upon administration to patients. Further many people have been immunized against diptheria and already possess neutralizing antibodies against the toxin. Up to 20% of the general population possesses anti-*Pseudomonas* antibodies as a consequence of *Pseudomonas* infections, and this number can be as high as 80% in long-term hospitals patients (VBI, unpublished data). Similarly patients who have been exposed to castor oil may have developed anti-ricin antibodies. Although considerable success has been achieved in the treatment of patients with leukemias and lymphomas [48] due in part to the immunosuppressive nature of these diseases, this is not the case for immunocompetent patients with solid tumors who may rapidly develop antibodies precluding repeat systemic administration of the immunotoxin [20,26,44].

Another serious side effect of immunotoxin treatment and a consideration in designing a preclinical program for immunotoxins is vascular leak syndrome (VLS). VLS is a nonspecific, non–antigen-related toxicity characterized by fluid leakage from the capillaries into the tissue resulting in low blood pressure and reduced blood flow to internal organs. Major symptoms are low blood pressure, edema, and low levels of albumin. VLS symptoms have been observed in many immunotoxin trials, and although these symptoms are generally manageable, reports of vascular collapse have been reported with certain ricin-based immuntoxins [14]. In order to abrogate vascular damage, several ricin A chain constructs, with mutations in the VLS-associated motif, have been engineered and are currently being evaluated [3,59].

29.3.2 VB4-845

VB4-845 is a recombinant fusion protein consisting of a tumor-targeting humanized single-chain antibody fragment, 4D5MOCB, specific for epithelial cell adhesion molecule (EpCAM) linked to a truncated form of *Pseudomonas* exotoxin A (ETA) that lacks the cell-binding domain, ETA(252-608). EpCAM is a cell surface marker that is highly expressed on carcinoma cells of epithelial origin, but has limited expression on normal cells [37,51,65]. Once inside the cell, ETA is a potent inhibitor of protein synthesis that induces cell death [15]. VB4-845 is a single 70 kDa protein, produced in E104 *E. coli* cells and is being developed for intratumoral injection for patients suffering from squamous cell carcinoma of the head and neck (SSCHN).

As with other immunotoxins, immunogenicity and toxicity are two of the major challenges that limit the use of VB4-845 in the clinic. Direct administration of VB4-845 into the tumor offers a number of advantages over systemic delivery. The intratumoral route provides a higher concentration of drug to the tumor than could be achieved by intravenous injection. Moreover, since the interstitial protein concentration is minimal relative to the circulation, in particular for protein in excess of 60 kDa, the concentration of antibodies preexisting or generated over the course treatment would be low relative to the administered dose, thereby minimizing the neutralizing effects of an anti-immunotoxin response. As well, since immunotoxin uptake by the tumor should be maximized due to intratumoral injection, this route of delivery is predicted to limit the interaction of the immunotoxin with nontarget tissue and thus minimize the likelihood of dose-limiting toxicity.

29.3.3   Mechanism of Action

It has been wellestablished that ETA irreversibly inhibits protein synthesis in mammalian cells by adenosine di-phosphate (ADP)-ribosylation of elongation factor 2 [29,49]. To demonstrate that the activity of VB4-845 is consistent with that of ETA by the inhibition of protein synthesis, the uptake of [3H]leucine was measured in EpCAM positive and EpCAM negative tumor cell lines, following the addition of VB4-845 to the cell cultures. VB4-845 inhibited protein synthesis in EpCAM positive SW2 cells with an IC_{50} of 0.01 pM but not in the EpCAM negative control cell line RL over the range of concentrations tested (0.0001–100 pM) [12]. The activity of VB4-845 was shown to be due to the inhibition of protein synthesis and is consistent with the mechanism of action of ETA (Figure 29.1). Results also indicate that EpCAM is required on the cell surface for treatment with VB4-845 to result in pharmacological activity (VBI, unpublished data).

To examine the requirements to take an immunotoxin into the clinic, the preclinical developmental strategy of VB4-845 is described to examine the challenges encountered to progress this antibody from bench to clinic by following the ICH S6 guidelines.

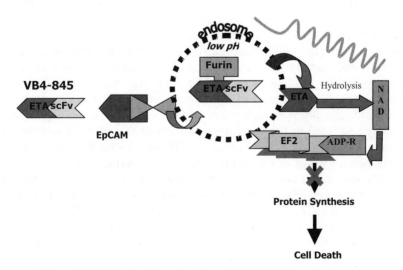

Figure 29.1   Mechanism of action of VB4-845. See color insert.

29.4 IMMUNOTOXIN EVALUATION USING THE ICH S6 GUIDELINES

Each immunotoxin is evaluated in a series of stages. These include assessment of specificity, cytotoxicity, and serum stability; selection of a relevant animal species and route of drug administration; and finally safety evaluation.

29.4.1 Specificity, Cytotoxicity, and Serum Stability

Initially immunotoxins are tested in vitro for specificity, cytotoxicity, and serum stability. The specificity of VB4-845 for EpCAM expressing tumor cells was demonstrated by flow cytometry and cell growth analyses of various epithelial-derived tumor and normal cell lines originating from different tissue types. VB4-845 showed strong cell surface reactivity to EpCAM positive tumor cell lines such as Cal 27, a squamous cell carcinoma of the tongue, but not to the colon-derived, EpCAM negative cell line, Colo-320. The specificity of VB4-845 was further highlighted by assessing cytotoxicity against a panel of cell lines exhibiting varying degrees of EpCAM expression. As predicted by the binding data, all EpCAM positive tumor cell lines were sensitive to killing by VB4-845, with IC_{50} values ranging from 0.001 to 1.84 pM. Normal cell lines, on the other hand, either were not affected by VB4-845 ($IC_{50} > 500$ pM) or were anywhere between 50- to 1000-fold less sensitive to VB4-845 than their counterpart tumor cell lines. For example, VB4-845 displayed potent activity against the bladder tumor cell line, TCCSUP ($IC_{50} < 0.005$ pM) but displayed no activity against the normal bladder cell line, HMVEC-bd ($IC_{50} > 500$ pM). This differentiation was also demonstrated in EpCAM positive and negative efficacy models [12].

Because immunotoxins are specifically targeted therapies, toxicities due to binding to receptors/antigens present on normal tissues occur at a much lower frequency than toxicities experienced with other anticancer drugs such as chemotherapy. According to FDA specifications [13], all antibodies are required to be tested for immunoreactivity against a human tissue panel of 33 normal frozen human tissues using immunohistochemistry (IHC). The in vitro immunoreactivity binding pattern of VB4-845 was membrane-associated in epithelial tissues, as is consistent with the detection of EpCAM expression by other antibodies [4]. Although normal epithelial cells express EpCAM, it is generally restricted to the basolateral portion of the cell [42], and therefore minimal in vivo binding is expected by VB4-845. To further ensure minimal patient toxicity, VB4-845 will be directly administered into SCCHN tumors. It should be noted that although tumor-reactive antibodies preferentially target cancer cells, they often cross-react with certain normal tissues that have limited expression of the target antigen, giving rise to significant toxicities. This does not preclude the use of such molecules as therapeutics. However, it underscores the requirement for testing the immunotoxin in a suitable animal model to determine its degree of interaction with critical normal tissues in the body.

Serum stability is another important attribute of immunotoxins as each immunotoxin must be sufficiently stable to progress from the blood into the tissues and be capable of penetrating into a tumor in a sufficient concentration to result in tumor cell death [8,12]. Examination at 37 °C showed that VB4-845 was a stable immunotoxin [12].

Although extensive in vitro testing is performed on each immunotoxin to assess its cytotoxicity and specificity, it is animal model studies that ultimately determine the serum half-life, serum stability, as well as the efficacy of an immunotoxin. A compilation of the in vitro and in vivo data enables a decision to be made on the potential of each immunotoxin to be an effective and safe therapeutic and to determine whether human clinical trials are warranted.

29.4.2 Selection of Animal Model and Route of Administration

As part of evaluating a new biopharmaceutical, the drug should be administered in a relevant animal species in which it is pharmacologically active. For an immunotoxin the drug should bind to the intended receptor or epitope expressed in the animal model. However, this result may not always be possible. In the case of VB4-845, cross-reactivity using IHC was examined in several animal species commonly used for toxicology studies: mouse, rat, dog, cynomolgus and rhesus monkeys, as well as the chimpanzee. No cross-reactivity was observed in any tissues of animals normally used for toxicology studies. Some cross-reactivity was observed in chimpanzee tissue, but because the pattern was not the same as that observed in human tissues, it was not considered to be a relevant species.

The use of nonrelevant animal species is discouraged as the results of such studies may be misleading (per ICH S6). Therefore the next option, when available, is to substitute a relevant transgenic animal model for a pharmacologically relevant species. Transgenic animal models for human EpCAM have been developed, but they either have a different tissue expression pattern from that seen in humans [41,43] or the model has not been validated [40], making them unsuitable for the evaluation of the safety of anti-EpCAM immunotherapeutics.

While safety evaluation programs require studies to be conducted in two species to characterize drug toxicity, should no viable option exist for a relevant species to conduct toxicology studies, the FDA suggests that toxicity be assessed in a single species [13]. Although no animal model system was available to examine possible binding of VB4-845 to EpCAM receptors, numerous studies have examined ETA-conjugated immunotoxins. It is well documented that the intravenous administration of ETA immunotoxins to rats results in symptoms that resemble VLS as seen in human immunotoxin trials [20,57]. Thus the choice of the Sprague–Dawley rat for toxicological testing was made for the well-known effects of immunotoxins in this animal model.

The route and treatment regimen in toxicology studies are expected to be as close as possible to that in the clinic. Single-dose studies aid in selecting the route of administration for a toxicology study if the intended human route of administration can not be mimicked in the animal. For VB4-845, the chosen route of administration in the clinic was intratumoral. While intratumoral administration was successfully demonstrated in a preclinical efficacy mouse model [12], this mode is not a viable option in toxicology studies. Therefore intradermal drug administration was used as a surrogate route of administration. Intravenous dosing, although not intended in the clinic, was used in the toxicology study with the rat as a comparison to examine the possible "worst case" effect of systemic exposure.

29.4.3 Safety Assessment

Single-Dose Toxicology Studies   Drug dosage in an animal model should be conducted so that a dose–response relationship may be examined. This may range from a no observed effect level (NOEL) and no observed adverse effect level (NOAEL) all the way to a maximum tolerated dose (MTD) of the drug. The dose response in a single-dose study will assist to determine the dose levels to be selected for a repeated-dose toxicology study. These levels will also aid in determining the first-dose level of the drug in humans as well as the therapeutic index and the margin of safety when dosing humans. When considering dosage in test animals, the volume must also be considered. Ethical maximum volumes have been determined for different species, which may mean that if there is a limitation to the drug concentration, a maximum feasible dose will be determined instead of an MTD.

Clinical signs noted in the dose-ranging study conducted in Sprague–Dawley rats administered VB4-845 locally (intradermal, ID) and systemically (intravenous, IV) were related to injection site lesions that exhibited a dose-dependent effect. There were no other findings in animals locally dosed. Animals that were systemically dosed had an increase in red blood cell parameters, total red blood cell counts, hemoglobin, and hematocrit and a decrease in albumin, total protein, and albumin–globulin ratio. While all these findings were dose dependent, these variations were within the normal physiological range.

Single-dose studies also help to determine whether dosing modifications are required based on the bioavailability or pharmacokinetics of the drug in the test species. Route of administration may also be modified if the drug has limited bioavailability by the chosen clinical route, or else treatment regimen may be changed to compensate for high clearance or low drug exposure.

Repeated-Dose Toxicology Studies   The repeated-dose toxicity study is expected to be a toxicology study under GLP conditions [17], which examines clinical signs, hematology, clinical biochemistry, urinalysis, and bone marrow to evaluate the effect of the drug during and after administration. Additional animal groups are required so that drug effect can be examined immediately after dosing in one group of animals and then later in another group of animals to determine whether any observed effects are reversible or in some cases whether the drug effects are delayed. Safety pharmacology, toxicokinetics, and immunogenicity may also be examined in this study for immunotoxins.

Based on the injection site reactions in the single-dose studies, it was anticipated that there would be difficulties dosing the Sprague–Dawley rat via the ID route. Therefore a subcutaneous (SC) route of administration was used as another representative route of local administration. Injection site reactions (slight erythema, edema, superficial necrosis, ulcerations, and scab formation) attributable to VB4-845 that were dose-related and noted at or above 5.0 μg/kg in most cases had resolved by the end of the observation period. Dose-dependent but transient changes were noted in hematology, coagulation parameters, and serum chemistry and were most likely due to acute tissue injury and inflammation at the injection sites. Liver enzyme levels were elevated in rats at upper-dose levels but returned to the normal physiological range by the end of the observation period. Systemic administration of VB4-845 (77.8 μg/kg) in rats resulted in microvascular injury and pulmonary edema, with subsequent hypoxia; these findings were consistent with VLS previously observed in rats exposed to ETA-based immunotoxins [22,56].

Examination of the various parameters may identify markers that vary with dose and may be used to examine drug effects in human studies. For example, although few effects were attributable to the local administration of VB4-845 in Sprague–Dawley rats, liver enzyme levels were elevated in rats at upper-dose levels. This provides a marker to follow drug response in clinical patients. As there was no evidence of toxicity following local administration at any of the dose levels tested, no NOAEL was attained at the highest dose tested (77.8 μg/kg), and it can be assumed that higher doses may be possible. In contrast, the animals treated systemically with VB4-845 experienced lethal toxicity at the same dose (77.8 μg/kg), thus illustrating a lower NOAEL for this route of delivery.

While animal studies are used for safety assessment prior to administration to humans, preclinical testing may not always predict human effect. For example, continuous-infusion therapy with 260F9 monoclonal antibody-recombinant ricin A chain resulted in severe neurotoxic effects in humans that were not demonstrated in monkey toxicology studies [21]. In such cases where suitable animal models are not available for safety testing it is important to consider the application of an appropriate safety factor to provide a margin of safety for protection of humans receiving the initial clinical dose [11,18].

Immunogenicity   Immunogenicity is a significant complicating factor surrounding the administration of immunotoxins to humans [19]. Immunogenicity can arise from either the antibody or toxin portions if they are foreign proteins. The shift from murine to humanized or human antibodies has reduced the immune response due to the antibody portion [10,35]. However, immune responses are still expected because the toxins employed are either of bacterial or plant origin and are thus inherently highly immunogenic.

The immune responses to VB4-845 by both the intended local route and systemic route of administration were investigated. Not surprisingly, a dose-dependent anti-drug antibody response was observed to both the antibody and toxin portions of the construct and a similar level antibody titer was induced regardless of sex. The VB4-845 titer following local administration was significantly higher than that observed after systemic administration at the same dose level, a phenomenon that has been demonstrated to be due to the use of different routes of delivery [50].

Although relatively high serum antibody titers were produced against VB4-845, this is not expected to have a negative impact on drug administration. Local administration of drug is expected to ensure a high local drug concentration in the tumor before coming into contact with anti-VB4-845 antibodies in the circulation. This point was illustrated with scFv(FRP5)-ETA, where a patient had a complete clinical response to intratumoral treatment (second administration) even though an immune-response was generated that completely neutralized the immunotoxin [2].

Drug Exposure Evaluation Immunotoxin exposure is largely dependent on the antibody portion used for targeting [10]. While whole IgGs may have half-lives up to 36 hours [5], scFv single-chain fragments can have a half-life as short as an hour or less. Although larger antibody portions are more stable and may prolong drug exposure, a larger sized molecule has more difficulty in tumor penetration [1]. A smaller sized antibody portion may not have as long a half-life, but it may permit better access to tumor cells and is able to leave the circulatory system more quickly, thereby reducing the exposure time of the endothelia to the toxin, and perhaps decrease VLS toxicity. F_{ab} antibody fragments or pegylation of the molecule increases the protein size, making it more stable but still small enough for cell entry.

As no relevant species exists, biodistribution studies were conducted in xenograft mice bearing EpCAM positive and negative tumors. This study confirmed that VB4-845 was retained in EpCAM positive tumors [12]. Although there was some detection in EpCAM negative tumors, this was most likely due to increased tumor vascularization. The biodistribution study also indicated that other organs may be targeted. However, toxicology studies did not result in any toxicity findings, indicating that the accumulation of radioactivity did not reflect binding or internalization of the immunotoxin within these tissues [12].

Toxicokinetic (TK) analysis of VB4-845 indicated that there was no gender difference. Nevertheless, different profiles were generated based on the mode of administration. Local administration resulted in a maximum VB4-845 plasma concentration of 50 ng/ml 4 h after administration (Figure 29.2). The subcutaneous dose appeared to be incompletely absorbed into the circulation, resulting in low bioavailability (13%) upon sampling (Table 29.1). Systemic administration resulted in a maximum VB4-845 plasma concentration of 1000 ng/ml after 10 minutes. The disappearance profile following the systemic

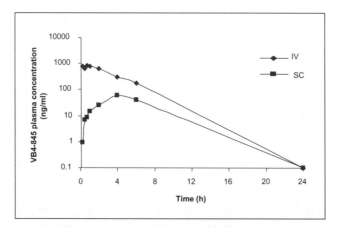

Figure 29.2   Mean plasma concentration-time curves following either systemic (intravenous) or local (subcutaneous) administration of VB4-845 on day 1. VB4-845 was not detected at 24 hours in either mode of drug administration.

TABLE 29.1   Toxicokinetic profile of VB4-845 administered SC or IV in Sprague–Dawley rats

Route	C_{max} (ng/ml)	AUC_{0-inf} (ng·h/ml)	k (h^{-1})	Ka (h^{-1})	$t_{1/2}$ (h)	CL (ml/kg/h)	V_d (ml/kg)	%F
SC	50 at 4 h	421	NC	0.31	NC	NC	NC	13
IV	1000 at 10 min	3242	0.3	NC	2.3	24	80	NC

Abbreviations: AUC_{0-inf} = area under the curve, CL = clearance, C_{max} = maximum plasma concentration, %F = bioavailability, k or Ka = elimination constant, NC = not calculated, $t_{1/2}$ = half-life, V_d = volume of distribution. The pooled data set from male and female rats was used for calculations.

dose was consistent with a one-compartment distributional model and first-order elimination with a half-life of 2.3 hours.

Comparison of plasma concentrations between days 1 and 7 showed no difference with local injections. However, concentrations following systemic injections were much lower on day 7 as compared to day 1. A dramatic enlargement of the distribution space, or possibly an unspecified bioadaptation is suggested, or more likely, the observed immune response depleted the blood plasma concentration. As mentioned earlier, an immune response raised against immunotoxins can affect the TK profile of a drug. The antibodies raised against the response bind to the antibody portion of the immunotoxin, causing it to be cleared at a quicker rate. This can decrease the half-life of the drug and, in most cases, is the stopping point for re-administration of the drug. Low bioavailability after local administration will not be an issue as VB4-845 is directly targeted to the tumor but rather indicates that there will be low systemic exposure to the immunotoxin.

Toxic effects of metabolites from drug degradation do not need to be monitored for immunotoxins (per IHC S6). As a recombinant protein, immunotoxins entering the human body are quickly degraded to small peptides and amino acids in the blood by proteases that specifically target foreign proteins and are cleared by the kidney.

Safety Pharmacology Safety pharmacology is important to assess the drug's effect on physiological functions through in vitro and in vivo assessment of central nervous, cardiovascular, and respiratory systems. These studies are required for biotechnology-derived biopharmaceuticals and assist to establish the type of monitoring parameters that may be required in clinical studies. However, because immunotoxins are specifically targeted drugs, these studies do not need to be conducted as individual studies but may be combined with toxicology studies that evaluate safety pharmacology endpoints.

Clinical signs observed in VB4-845 toxicology studies allowed for an in vivo assessment of the central nervous system and functional ability of the dosed rats. Animals dosed locally exhibited normal behavior, whereas those dosed systemically exhibited neurological symptoms (wobbly gait) and respiratory difficulties (dyspnea). Full safety pharmacology studies have not been conducted with VB4-845 because they are not required prior to the first administration in humans for anticancer drugs examined in end-stage cancer patients (per ICH S7A). VB4-845 has progressed to pivotal clinical trials, and therefore safety pharmacology studies examining cardiovascular and respiratory response are planned.

Immunotoxicity Studies Immunotoxicology studies are required for pharmaceuticals that may affect the immune system through suppression, enhancement, or sensitivity (per ICH S8). In general, immunotoxins do not have an effect on the immune system, and standard testing batteries are not recommended for biotechnology-derived pharmaceuticals. However, examination of hematology results together with detailed histopathological assessment of immune organs from single- or repeated-dose toxicology studies are routinely performed with biopharmaceuticals, and these evaluations provide initial information on whether the immune system has been affected.

Reproductive Performance and Developmental Toxicology Studies The assessment of reproductive performance and developmental toxicity is dependent on the clinical indication and patient population. The majority of immunotoxins in development are currently used for the treatment of cancer, a patient population that tends to be an older, nonreproductive population. As well, potential reproductive concerns for the patients in ongoing clinical trials are usually addressed in the clinical trial protocols.

Although VB4-845 will never be administered systemically and does not bind to human placenta, studies are planned as a step for marketing registration. Because a relevant species has not been identified, and the rat is unsuitable for use because it cannot be dosed systemically, embryofetal development will be examined in time-mated female rabbits to determine placenta binding and potential for transplacental passage. A formal study will not be conducted unless fetal effects are observed.

Genotoxicity Studies While the majority of the principles of the ICH S6 apply to immunotoxins, because they are a biotechnology-derived biopharmaceutical, certain tests such as genotoxicity and carcinogenicity studies do not directly apply.

Examination of genotoxicity of pharmaceuticals is required to assess the interaction of the drug with DNA. These studies are generally not applicable to immunotoxins. Unlike chemotherapeutics that cause cell death through DNA interaction, immunotoxins mediate cell death by preventing protein synthesis. However, immunotoxins use a linker to connect the toxin to the antibody that may need to be examined if it is an organic linker and has the ability to bind DNA (per ICH S6). The majority of immunotoxins use either a nonreducible thioether linker for intact toxins or a disulfide bond for A chains and ribosome-inactivating proteins and do not interact with DNA.

Carcinogenicity Studies Immunotoxins, in general, do not have the ability to transform cells or promote the growth of transformed cells. Therefore carcinogenicity bioassays are considered inappropriate. This is in contrast to toxins fused to growth factors that may promote tumor growth under certain circumstances if, for example, a less than toxic dose were administered. Should the immunotoxin interact with growth factors or cytokines, in vitro studies may be required to examine whether growth is promoted in transformed cells.

29.5 PROGRESS OF IMMUNOTOXIN THERAPEUTICS

Cancers of hematologic origin are more accessible to immunotoxin therapy and thus more amenable to treatment than solid tumors. One of the most promising immunotoxins, currently in development is BL22 used for the treatment of hairy cell leukaemia. BL22 is comprised of an anti-CD22 dsFv linked to truncated PE, and it has been evaluated in a phase 1 clinical trial of patients with B cell malignancies [31] and ongoing in phase 2 clinical trials [30]. Of the 32 patients treated in the phase 1 study, 16 hairy cell leukaemia patients responded with 11 patients having a complete remission and 2 having a partial remission. Neutralizing antibodies were only observed in 4 of the 16 patients. Although VLS was observed in some patients, the dose-limiting toxicity was the cytokine release syndrome. A variety of immuntoxins have undergone clinical testing, and the testing has been comprehensively reviewed by Kreitman [28] and Schaede and Reiter [54].

Currently two immunoconjugates have been approved by the FDA for clinical use in the treatment of cancer. Mylotarg® (Gemtuzumab ozogamicin,

Wyeth-Ayerst Laboratories) is a CD33 antibody conjugated to a calicheamicin, a cytotoxic antibiotic and Ontak® (denileukin diftitox, Ligand Pharmaceuticals, Inc.) is an IL-2 cytokine conjugated to the toxin DT. Both drugs target hematological cancers. While Mylotarg® is not conjugated to a toxin, it provides a good example of the progress of an antibody immunoconjugate from preclinical development to regulatory approval for market.

The targeted antigen, CD33, of Mylotarg® is not expressed in any other species besides humans and large primates; therefore a cross-reactive species was not available for Mylotarg® [9]. Instead, repeated-dose toxicology studies were conducted in Sprague–Dawley rats and cynomolgus monkeys that indicated hepato, renal, and hematopoietic toxicities due to drug administration. Mylotarg® was more immunogenic in rats than monkeys and had a slow clearance rate in both species, three and seven days, respectively. Safety pharmacology conducted in dogs resulted in minor changes in blood pressure and cardiac output that were noted at 16-fold above human starting dose with changes in ECG and heart rate noted at 52-fold above human dose. Reproductive toxicology was not conducted; however, histopathological changes were noted in rat testes and atrophy in the mammary gland. Developmental toxicology studies conducted in rats showed dose-related development effects with decreases in fetal weights, increases in embryo/fetal mortality, and fetal digital malformations, with reabsorptions at the highest dose. The cytotoxic antibiotic used in Mylotarg®, calicheamicin, kills cells by interacting with DNA and causing breakage. Therefore genotoxicity studies were conducted using an in vivo mouse micronucleus assay and confirmed that it was clastogenic. Mylotarg® was determined to have an acceptable toxicity profile in clinical trials and few patients developed antibodies to the drug. Infusion reactions were observed that sometimes occur with monoclonal antibody infusions. Preclinical studies predicted the liver toxicity observed in patients, which for the most part was transient and reversible [9]. The preclinical studies together with the response rate in clinical trials were satisfactory for approval of Mylotarg® for CD33 positive acute myeloid leukemia patients in first relapse who are 60 years of age or older. Since then, additional studies indicate further use of Mylotarg® with combination therapy [58] as well as other population groups [6].

29.6 SUMMARY

Immunotoxins continue to be actively investigated as viable alternatives to conventional therapies for a variety of diseases. An array of different recombinant, antibody formats are now available for use in immunotoxins. While these design changes have improved the overall in vitro and preclinical in vivo efficacy of immunotoxins, increased potency does not address either of the two major concerns for drugs of this type: immunogenicity and toxicity. As such, immunotoxins in their current form may have limited application other than to those disease conditions either where the patients are immunocompromised, as in the case for leukemia, or where the drug can be delivered directly, as was demonstrated for VB4-845 in the treatment of SCCHN and transitional cell carcinoma of the bladder. In order to expand the utility of immunotoxins to achieve a comparable safety profile, design considerations will be required to minimize immunogenicity and toxicity. To this end, pegylation [34,60] or T and/or B cell epitope depletion [24] from the toxin portion of the immunotoxin may be an alternative means to minimize an immune response while the discovery of newer toxins with better safety profiles may minimize nonspecific toxicities. In addition increasing the safety profile of immunotoxins through the discovery of new and more selective tumor targets will only serve to broaden their clinical use in the treatment against cancer.

REFERENCES

1. Adams GP, Schier R. Generating improved single-chain Fv molecules for tumor targeting. *J Immunol Meth* 1999;231:249–60.

2. Azemar M, Djahansouzi S. Regression of cutaneous tumor lesions in patients intratumorally injected with a recombinant single-chain antibody-toxin targeted to ErbB2/HER2. *Breast Cancer Res Treat* 2003;82:155–64.

3. Baluna R, Coleman E. The effect of a monoclonal antibody coupled to ricin a chain-derived peptides on endothelial cells in vitro: insights into toxin-mediated vascular damage. *Exp Cell Res* 2000;258:417–24.

4. Balzar M, Winter MJ, de Boer CJ, Litvinov SV. The biology of the 17-1A antigen (Ep-CAM). *J Mol Med* 1999;77:699–712.

5. Behr T, Becker W, Hannappel E, Goldenberg DM, Wolf F. Targeting of liver metastases of colorectal cancer with IgG, F(ab')2, and Fab' anti-carcinoembryonic antigen antibodies labeled with 99mTc: the role of metabolism and kinetics. *Cancer Res* 1995;55:5777s–85s.

6. Brethon B, Auvrignon A, Galambrun C, Yakouben K, Leblanc T, Bertrand Y, Leverger G, Baruchel A. Efficacy and tolerability of gemtuzumab ozogamicin (anti-CD33 monoclonal antibody, CMA-676, Mylotarg) in children with relapsed/refractory myeloid leukemia. *BMC Cancer* 2006;6:172.

7. Brinkmann U. Recombinant immunotoxins: protein engineering for cancer therapy. *Mol Med Today* 1996;439–46.

8. Brinkmann U. Recombinant antibody fragments and immunotoxin fusions for cancer therapy. *In vivo* 2000;14:21–8.

9. Bross PF, Beitz J, Chen G. Approval summary: gemtuzumab ozogamicin in relapsed acute myeloid leukemia. *Clin Cancer Res* 2001;7:1490–6.

10. Colcher D, Goel A, Pavlinkova G, Beresford GW, Booth B, Batra SK. Effects of genetic engineering on the pharmacokinetics of antibodies. *Quart J of Nucl Med* 1999;43:132–9.

11. DeGeorge JJ, Ahn CH, Andrews PA, Brower ME, Giorgio DW, Goheer MA, Lee-Ham DY, McGuinn WD, Schmidt W, Sun CJ, Tripathi SC. Regulatory considerations for preclinical development of anticancer drugs. *Cancer Chemother Pharmacol* 1998;41:173–85.

12. Di Paolo C, Willuda J, Kubetzko S, Lauffer I, Tschudi D, Waibel R, Pluckthun A, Stahel RA, Zangemeister-Wittke U. A recombinant immunotoxin derived from a humanized epithelial cell adhesion molecule-specific single-chain antibody fragment has potent and selective antitumor activity. *Clin Cancer Res* 2003;9:2837–48.

13. FDA. Points to consider in the manufacture and testing of monoclonal antibody products for human use. *J-Immunother* 1997;20:214–43.

14. Fidias P, Grossbard ML, Lynch T. A phase II study of the immunotoxin N901-blocked ricin in small-cell lung cancer. *Clin Lung Cancer* 2002;3:219–22.

15. FitzGerald D, Pastan I. Pseudomonas exotoxin: recombinant conjugates as therapeutic agents. *Biochem Soc Transact* 1992;20:731–4.

16. FitzGerald DJ, Waldmann TA, Willingham MC, Pastan I. Pseudomonas exotoxin-anti-TAC. cell-specific immunotoxin active against cells expressing the human T cell growth factor receptor. *J Clin Invest* 1984;74:966–71.

17. Food and Drug Administration. Good Laboratory Practice for Nonclinical Laboratory Studes. 21 Code Federal Regulation 1996;58.

18. Food and Drug Administration. Estimating the Safe Starting Dose in Clinical Trial for Therapeutics in Adult Healthy Volunteers, 2002.

19. Frankel AE. Reducing the immune response to immunotoxin. *Clin Cancer Res* 2004;10:13–15.

20. Frankel AE, Kreitman RJ, Sausville EA. Targeted toxins. *Clin Cancer Res* 2000; 6:334.

21. Gould BJ, Borowitz MJ, Groves ES, Carter PW, Anthony D, Weiner LM, Frankel AE. Phase I study of an anti-breast cancer immunotoxin by continuous infusion: report of a targeted toxic effect not predicted by animal studies. *J Natl Cancer Inst* 1989;81:775–81.

22. Haggerty HG, Warner WA. BR96 sFv-PE40 Immunotoxin: Nonclinical safety assessment. *Toxicol Pathol* 1999;27:87–94.

23. Herschman HR, Simpson DL, Cawley DB. Toxic ligand conjugates as tools in the study of receptor-ligand interactions. *J Cell Biochem* 1982;20:163–76.

24. Jones TD, Phillips WJ, Smith BJ, Bamford CA, Nayee PD, Baglin TP, Gaston JS, Baker MP. Identification and removal of a promiscuous CD4+ T cell epitope from the C1 domain of factor VIII. *J Thromb Haemost* 2005;3:991–1000.

25. Kondo K, FitzGerald DJ, Chaudhary V. Activity of immunotoxins constructed with modified pseudomonas exotoxin a lacking the cell recognition domain. *J Biol Chem* 1988;263:9470–5.

26. Kreitman RJ. Immunotoxins in cancer therapy. *Curr Opin Immunol* 1999; 11:570–8.

27. Kreitman RJ. Recombinant toxins for the treatment of cancer. *Curr Opin Mol Ther* 2003;5:44–51.

28. Kreitman RJ. Immunotoxins for targeted cancer therapy. *AAPS J* 2006; 8:E532–51.

29. Kreitman RJ, Pastan I. Accumulation of a recombinant immunotoxin in a tumor in vivo: fewer than 1000 molecules per cell are sufficient for complete responses. *Cancer Res* 1998;58:968–75.

30. Kreitman RJ, Pastan I. BL22 and lymphoid malignancies. *Best Pract Res Clin Haematol* 2006;19:685–99.

31. Kreitman RJ, Wilson WH, Bergeron K, Raggio M, Stetler-Stevenson M, FitzGerald DJ, Pastan I. Efficacy of the anti-CD22 recombinant immunotoxin BL22 in chemotherapy-resistant hairy-cell leukemia. *N Engl J Med* 2001;345:241–7.

32. Krolick KA, Uhr JW, Slavin S, Vitetta ES. In vivo therapy of a murine B cell tumor (BCL1) using antibody-ricin A chain immunotoxins. *J Exp Med* 1982;155:1797–809.

33. Krolick KA, Villemez C, Isakson P, Uhr JW, Vitetta ES. Selective killing of normal or neoplastic B cells by antibodies coupled to the A chain of ricin. *Proc Natl Acad Sci USA* 1980;77:5419–23.

34. Kubetzko S, Balic E, Waibel R, Zangemeister-Wittke U, Pluckthun A. PEGylation and multimerization of the anti-p185HER-2 single chain Fv fragment 4D5: effects on tumor targeting. *J Biol Chem* 2006;281:35186–201.

35. Kuus-Reichel K, Grauer L. Will immunogenicity limit the use, efficacy and future development of therapeutic monoclonal antibodies. *Clin Diagnost Lab Immunol* 1994;365–72.

36. Levy R, Miller RA. Therapy of lymphoma directed at idiotypes. *J Natl Cancer Inst Monogr* 1990;61–8.

37. Litvinov SV, Velders MP, Bakker HA, Fleuren GJ, Warnaar SO. Ep-CAM: a human epithelial antigen is a homophilic cell-cell adhesion molecule. *J Cell Biol* 1994;125:437–46.

38. Maynard J, Georgiou G. Antibody Engineering. *Annu Rev Biomed Eng* 2000;2:339–76.

39. McHugh L, Hu S, Lee BK, Santora K, Kennedy PE, Berger EA, Pastan I, Hamer DH. Increased affinity and stability of an anti-HIV-1 envelope immunotoxin by structure-based mutagenesis. *J Biol Chem* 2002;277:34383–90.

40. McLaughlin PM, Harmsen MC, Dokter WH, Kroesen BJ, van der MH, Brinker MG, Hollema H, Ruiters MH, Buys CH, de Leij LF. The epithelial glycoprotein 2 (EGP-2) promoter-driven epithelial-specific expression of EGP-2 in transgenic mice: a new model to study carcinoma-directed immunotherapy. *Cancer Res* 2001;61:4105–11.

41. McLaughlin PM, Kroesen BJ, Dokter WH, van der MH, de Groot M, Brinker MG, Kok K, Ruiters MH, Buys CH, De Leij LF. An EGP-2/Ep-CAM-expressing transgenic rat model to evaluate antibody-mediated immunotherapy. *Cancer Immunol Immunother* 1999;48:303–11.

42. Momburg F, Moldenhauer G. Immunohistochemical study of the expression of a Mr 34,000 human epithelium-specific surface glycoprotein in normal and malignant tissues. *Cancer Res* 1987;47:2883–91.

43. Mosolits S, Campbell F. Targeting human Ep-Cam in transgenic mice by anti-idiotype and antigen based vaccines. *Int J Cancer* 2004;112:669–77.

44. Pai LH, Wittes R, Setser A, Willingham MC, Pastan I. Treatment of advanced solid tumors with immunotoxin LMB-1: An antibody linked to Pseudomonas exotoxin. *Nat Med* 1996;2:350–3.

45. Parker BA, Vassos AB, Halpern SE, Miller RA, Hupf H, Amox DG, Simoni JL, Starr RJ, Green MR, Royston I. Radioimmunotherapy of human B-cell lymphoma with 90Y-conjugated antiidiotype monoclonal antibody. *Cancer Res* 1990;50:1022s–8s.

46. Pastan I. Immunotoxins containing pseudomonas exotoxin A: a short history. *Cancer Immunol Immunother* 2003;52:338–41.

47. Pastan I, FitzGerald D. Pseudomonas exotoxin: chimeric toxins. *J Biol Chem* 1989; 264:15157–60.

48. Pastan I, Hassan R, FitzGerald DJ, Kreitman RJ. Immunotoxin Treatment of Cancer. *Annu Rev Med* 2007;58:221–37.

49. Perentesis JP, Miller SP, Bodley JW. Protein toxin inhibitors of protein synthesis. *Biofactors* 1992;3:173–84.

50. Porter S. Human immune response to recombinant human proteins. *J Pharm Sci* 2001;90:1–11.

51. Proca DM, Niemann TH, Porcell AI, DeYoung BR. MOC31 immunoreactivity in primary and metastatic carcinoma of the liver: report of findings and review of other utilized markers. *Appl Immunohistochem Mol Morphol* 2000;8:120–5.

52. Reiter Y. Recombinant immunotoxins in targeted cancer cell therapy. *Adv Cancer Res* 2001;81:93–124.

53. Saavedra-Lozano J, Cao Y, Callison J, Sarode R, Sodora D, Edgar J, Hatfield J, Picker L, Peterson D, Ramilo O, Vitetta ES. An anti-CD45RO immunotoxin kills HIV-latently infected cells from individuals on HAART with little effect on CD8 memory. *Proc Natl Acad Sci USA* 2004;101:2494–9.

54. Schaedel O, Reiter Y. Antibodies and their fragments as anti-cancer agents. *Curr Pharm Des* 2006;12:363–78.

55. Siegall CB, Chaudhary V. Functional analysis of donaims II, Ib and III of pseudomonas exotoxin. *J Biol Chem* 1989;264:14256–61.

56. Siegall CB, Liggett D. Characterization of vascular leak syndrome induced by the toxin component of pseudomonas exotoxin-based immunotoxin and its protential inhibition with nonsteroidal anti-inflammatory drugs. *Clin Cancer Res* 1997;3: 339–45.

57. Siegall CB, Liggitt D. Prevention of immunotoxin-mediated vascular leak syndrome in rats with retention of antitiumor activity. *Proc Natl Acad Sci USA* 1994; 91:9514–18.

58. Sievers EL, Larson RA, Stadtmauer EA, Estey E, Lowenberg B, Dombret H, Karanes C, Theobald M, Bennett JM, Sherman ML, Berger MS, Eten CB, Loken MR, van Dongen JJ, Bernstein ID, Appelbaum FR. Efficacy and safety of gemtuzumab ozogamicin in patients with CD33-positive acute myeloid leukemia in first relapse. *J Clin Oncol* 2001;19:3244–54.

59. Smallshaw JE, Ghetie V, Rizo J, Fulton JRJ, Trahan L, Ghetie MA, Vitetta E. Genetic engineering of an immunotoxin to eliminate pulmonary vascular leak in mice. *Nat Biotechnol* 2003;21:387–91.

60. Tsutsumi Y, Onda M, Nagata S, Lee B, Kreitman RJ, Pastan I. Site-specific chemical modification with polyethylene glycol of recombinant immunotoxin anti-Tac(Fv)-PE38 (LMB-2) improves antitumor activity and reduces animal toxicity and immunogenicity. *Proc Natl Acad Sci USA* 2000;97:8548–53.

61. Uchida T, Pappenheimer AM, Jr, Harper AA. Diphtheria toxin and related proteins. II. Kinetic studies on intoxication of HeLa cells by diphtheria toxin and related proteins. *J Biol Chem* 1973;248:3845–50.

62. van Oosterhout YV, Van EL, Schattenberg AV, Tax WJ, Ruiter DJ, Spits H, Nagen-gast FM, Masereeuw R, Evers S, de WT, Preijers FW. A combination of anti-CD3 and anti-CD7 ricin A-immunotoxins for the in vivo treatment of acute graft versus host disease. *Blood* 2000;95:3693–701.

63. van Vuuren AJ, Van Roon JA, Walraven V, Stuij I, Harmsen MC, McLaughlin PM, Van de Winkel JG, Thepen T. CD64-directed immunotoxin inhibits arthritis in a novel CD64 transgenic rat model. *J Immunol* 2006;176:5833–8.

64. White CA, Weaver RL, Grillo-Lopez AJ. Antibody-targeted immunotherapy for treatment of malignancy. *Annu Rev Med* 2001;52:125–45.

65. Willuda J, Honegger A, Waibel R. High thermal stability is essential for tumor tar-geting of antibody fragments: engineering of a humanized anti-epithelial glycopro-tein-2 (epithelial cell adhesion molecule) single-chain Fv fragment. *Cancer Res* 1999;59:5758–67.

Preclinical Safety Evaluation of Blood Products

RICHARD M. LEWIS, PhD

Contents

30.1 INTRODUCTION

The historical development of blood products, in particular, plasma derivatives, reflects the development of "traditional" biological products. The early products were derived from donated blood. Their development through the 1960s and '70s consisted primarily of refining purification techniques. Because they are necessarily sourced from human materials, the issue of disease transmission has always been a concern. Along with improvements in purification came better donor selection, better donor testing, and manufacturing methods designed to separate and inactivate infectious agents. Later the implementation of manufacturing steps introduced specifically to reduce possible viral contaminants became important. The biotechnology revolution using cell culture methods allowed the consistent production of large amounts of

Preclinical Safety Evaluation of Biopharmaceuticals: A Science-Based Approach to Facilitating Clinical Trials, edited by Joy A. Cavagnaro
Copyright © 2008 by John Wiley & Sons, Inc.

products without the concern of human-derived infectious agents. The field has further progressed with advancing science to the consideration of gene therapy applications for many of the disorders that were previously treated using replacement therapy. Although current products under development primarily address diseases associated with single gene mutations or a single protein's lack of activity, the possibility of curing individuals using a biological therapy seems possible.

The Office of Blood Research and Review (OBRR) in CBER has a long history of review and approval of biological products. Many of the earliest blood products were not evaluated using what is now considered to be conventional preclinical and toxicological evaluations. This is in part because the Bureau of Biologics and its predecessor, Division of Biologics Control (transferred from NIH to FDA in 1972) [1] regulated products under a different mandate and in part because the blood products are often meant to replace or supplement levels of existing biologic factors. Albumin, fibrinogen, and gamma globulin were first purified from plasma using ethanol fractionation described by Cohn in 1940 [2]. It has been the assumption that the supplementing of normal plasma derivatives, with material isolated from plasma, does not cause classical toxicity. That is not to say that these products were not evaluated for harmful effects but that evaluation was most often linked to determination of effects of inherent activity or activity associated with changes in molecular structure. Changes such as cleavage of proteins in the product could result in generation of enzymatic activity. For example, such activity might subsequently result in lack of stability, increase in pro-thrombotic potential, or other effects caused by active fragments. An important case of such an incident was the association of hypotension with the administration of purified protein derivative, a product composed primarily of albumin [3]. Currently such molecular changes are evaluated and, as in all biological products, the issue of immunogenicity is also addressed and will be discussed.

The use of animals for the preclinical evaluation of blood derivatives primarily encompassed evaluation for activity [4], and later for viral contamination, but little from the perspective of actual toxicological endpoints. Many of the hemophiliacs who were treated with early versions of antihemophilic factor (AHF) and Factor IX became infected with hepatitis [5]. This provided the major reason for developing viral inactivation methods for AHF concentrates. The hepatitis agents were referred to as non-A, non-B hepatitis (NANB). The preclinical demonstration that the active virus had been inactivated required the use of chimpanzees, which were injected with the AHF concentrate. During the early 1980s plasma fractionators used chimpanzee studies to demonstrate the effectiveness for the reduction of HBV and NANB hepatitis infectivity [6]. Ultimately, previously untreated patients were evaluated in clinical trials that demonstrated the utility of a number of viral reduction methods for what was by then known as hepatitis C [7].

More recently some of the focus of preclinical evaluation of blood products has shifted to toxicological evaluations. This has come with the development of recombinant materials or biochemically modified molecules to address specific disease states. In the case of the hemoglobin-derived oxygen carriers, with extensive toxic characteristics, many aspects of preclinical assessment have been employed as will be discussed below.

Conventional preclinical studies are those using principles similar to those for toxicological assays of traditional drug products and used to determine such parameters as absorption, distribution, metabolism and excretion (ADME), no adverse effect level (NOAEL), maximum tolerated dose (MTD) levels, and determination of relevant animal species. These studies are generally conducted in concentrations based on multiples of the proposed human dose. Evaluation endpoints usually include mortality, clinical signs, body weight, food consumption, clinical chemistry, hematology, gross pathology, and histopathology.

The FDA refers to a few official documents for guidance in accomplishing a valid preclinical development program. These include International Conference on Harmonization (ICH) accepted guidances as well as US FDA guidance documents:

- Guidance for Industry: S6 Preclinical Safety Evaluation of Biotechnology-Derived Pharmaceuticals (1997)
- Guidance for Industry: M3 Nonclinical Safety Studies for the Conduct of Human Clinical Trials for Pharmaceuticals (1997)
- Guidance for Industry and Reviewers: Estimating the Safe Starting Dose in Clinical Trials for Therapeutics in Adult Healthy Volunteers

Additional biological product specific advice is provided in other documents:

- Points to Consider in the Manufacture and Testing of Monoclonal Antibody Products for Human Use (1997)
- Guidance for Industry: Guidance for Human Somatic Cell Therapy and Gene Therapy (1998)
- Guidance for Industry and Reviewers: Estimating the Safe Starting Dose in Clinical Trials for Therapeutics in Adult Healthy Volunteers

The ICH S6 document should be used in conjunction with the ICH M3 guidance, which provides the appropriate timing and duration of general toxicology studies as they relate to the proposed clinical trials. The principles and use of these various guidance documents are discussed in depth elsewhere in this volume. The intent in this chapter is to describe some of the preclinical programs that are publicly known and to offer suggestions for the development of plans for various groups of products regulated in the Office of Blood and Blood Products, the CBER, and the FDA.

30.2   HEMOGLOBIN-BASED OXYGEN CARRIERS

Although often referred to as blood substitutes, the major intent of hemoglobin-derived products has been for use as oxygen carriers. The hemoglobin-based oxygen carriers (HBOCs) represent a unique, and what has proved to be a difficult, class of blood product. The majority of products in this class have used the oxygen-binding characteristic of hemoglobin while attempting to avoid the toxicities associated with the molecule when not presented in the red cell. Early clinical studies using stroma-free human hemoglobin showed renal dysfunction, hypertension and severe abdominal pain [8]. This class of products demonstrated extreme toxicity in initial studies and changes to formulation and molecular structure have been made in attempts to address the toxicity [9]. One of the primary challenges to the developers of novel hemoglobin products is this demonstration of lack of toxicity.

Because there are a variety of methods that attempt to address the toxicities of hemoglobin [10], each novel material requires investigations into all of the various toxicities. Since it is known that hemoglobin causes renal, neural, and cardiac toxicity, a novel modification that is intended to remove or reduce these toxicities must be tested to address the effects on each of these target organs.

Although the HBOCs have attempted to find utility in different clinical settings where the risk–benefit profiles are different than for use as "blood substitutes," many aspects of the toxicities must still be addressed. For all of these reasons the most extensive requirements for preclinical safety information for therapeutics regulated as blood products have been for the hemoglobin-derived products. Because the hemoglobin-based oxygen carriers are viewed as a class, the FDA has taken the approach that each hemoglobin therapeutic candidate should address the issues of the others. The FDA draft guidance lists numerous toxicities that should be addressed [11]. These include vasoactivity, gastrointestinal toxicity, neurotoxicity, and cardiac toxicity as well as activity in vascular tone, oxidative stress, synergy with endotoxin, and enzymatic indications of pancreatic and liver toxicity. The guidance is very prescriptive regarding physicochemical characterization, estimation of in vitro activity, as well as some of the animal models that should be used to address particular toxicities. As in most preclinical safety tests, doses sufficient to observe toxicity are suggested, and at least one study in large animals should be used. The FDA draft guidance also encourages the use of animal models of disease to address many of the possible toxicities for a "complete safety profile." For example, a fully instrumented animal model study resembling the proposed clinical use should be used to measure cardiac, renal, and pulmonary function. Also recommended is an extensive list of laboratory data to be collected during these studies, such as effects on microvasculature, enzymes, histological and physical tests to evaluate renal function, and a collection of clinical chemistry parameters. One example of a preclinical program included studies on cardiovascular effects (3 species), genotoxicity (3 in vitro models), gastrointestinal effects

(3 species), hemorrhagic shock (3 species), hemostasis (1 specie), toxicology (5 studies in 3 species), oxygen delivery (1 specie), PK (1 specie), renal effects (1 specie), and reproductive toxicology (1 specie).

30.3 THERAPIES FOR DISEASES OF GENETICALLY DEFICIENT PROTEINS

As mentioned above, one of the primary uses of plasma-derived products is to replace missing proteins, in particular, genetic deficiencies such as hemophilia or immune deficiency. These products are administered intravenously. The development program for most of these products has not included extensive preclinical animal evaluation. Often animal models have been used to demonstrate product effectiveness prior to clinical trials. However, other more recent development programs have included toxicology assessments. For example, in the case of one particular non-enzyme plasma-derivative product deficient in some individuals, the toxicology program that was recommended included single- and multiple-dose toxicity studies. These were to be evaluated in rodents. The single-dose study incorporated a determination of the maximum tolerated dose as well as clinical observations and complete histopathology.

Another program recently recommended for a product with novel modifications included single-dose studies in a rodent and a nonrodent as well as another study in a higher mammal as a means to enter phase 1 trials. However, multiple-dose animal studies would be necessary and could probably be done in parallel to the single-dose human trials.

Although coagulation factor deficiency such as factor VIII and Factor IX is found only in males, any product that might be administered to females should include reproductive toxicology studies and follow the ICH S5A outline for segment 2 evaluation. Because deficient products are normally proteins, fertility and perinatal reproductive toxicology studies can be seen scientifically as extremely unlikely to provide any information. Teratology studies might reveal effects on organogenesis that occur as a result of complement or coagulation system changes or immunologic mediators, so such studies are recommended.

Homologous recombinant proteins have had to undergo a more extensive evaluation preclinically. For example, a recombinant factor VIII product was evaluated in acute and subacute studies in mice, rats, rabbits, dogs, and nonhuman primates over a range of concentrations and dose frequency [12].

30.4 IMMUNE GLOBULINS

Although there is no specific FDA document that provides guidance for preclinical studies for immune globulins, there is a draft guidance for safety, efficacy, and pharmacokinetic clinical trials to support licensure of intravenous immune globulin [13]. The guidance recommends that in clinical trails safety data be collected to include capture of adverse effects (AEs) regardless of determination of association with the product (temporal association is primary consideration). The characteristics of the particular infusion associated with an AE, as well as statistical consideration for evaluation of all AEs, should be included in any marketing application.

The efficacy of the product should be determined using the subject's bacterial infection rates and the pharmacokinetics of product, including the relationship of PK and infection. The ability of many of these products to block infection has been demonstrated.

In the future the FDA may develop guidance for preclinical toxicology studies but one has not been published at this time. The guidance recommending design of clinical studies can be used to model animal studies to support the various clinical trials.

A recent presentation by an FDA reviewer noted that for a number of immune globulin products surveyed, no preclinical animal studies were presented in the INDs [14]. The immune globulins surveyed included immune globulin (intravenous), as well as hyperimmune globulins both intravenous and intramuscular forms. This situation is likely due to the long history of these products and the similarities in their manufacturing.

Regarding the use of hyperimmune globulins such as used for treatment of bacterial, viral, or toxin diseases, the safety data from other immune globulins from the same manufacturer provide most of the information and assurance of safety. If one manufacturer has an approved immune globulin, the material isolated for a hyperimmune most likely will be manufactured in the same way except that a larger portion of the source plasma will have the specific immune globulin. As such, there is a high degree of confidence in the safety of the material from the previous nonspecific immune globulin.

In contrast, a literature report of a new IGIV discusses limited animal studies in preparation for human trials [15]. The development of this product, produced by Baxter, has used a series of preclinical animal testing methods to address concerns for the use of a plasma derivative. Although it would not be considered a "classical" toxicology program, acute toxicity was evaluated along with the application of a number of models in order to gain insight into the in vivo characteristics of the product. An in vivo assay was used to show protection from *Klebsiella pneumoniae* and *Streptococcus pneumoniae*. Bronchospastic activity in anesthetized guinea pigs was chosen to evaluate the potential for anaphylactoid reactions after rapid arterial injection, and the potential for changes in blood pressure was evaluated in the hypotensive rat model. Dog studies were used to evaluate possible cardiovascular, respiratory, and coagulation reactions. Thrombogenicity was measured in rabbits. Pharmacokinetic characteristics were studied in rats. Acute toxicity studies in mice and rats were used to determine the NOAEL.

30.5 COAGULATION FACTORS FOR REPLACEMENT THERAPY

As mentioned above, preclinical pharmacology and toxicology for plasma derivatives has not included preclinical assessments commonly employed for small-molecule drug products. Most preclinical development involves comparative pharmacokinetics and the use of animal models has been an important component of this evaluation. The coagulation factors have shown the potential for efficacy in animal models such as the von Willebrand swine and hemophilic dog [16,17].

These animal models of disease should be considered early on as potentially providing some of the data necessary for initiation of human studies. Besides utility as proof of concept, they can add to understanding dose response as well as help evaluate some safety endpoints. New products resulting from improved manufacturing can be compared with previously produced material using pharmacokinetic parameters.

In one "second-generation" recombinant factor VIII product, ReFacto®, hemophilic dogs were used to demonstrate utility for bleeding time correction, association with von Willebrand's factor, and evaluating pharmacokinetics [18]. A plasma-derived factor VIII was used for comparison. In another study that used a dog model, a recombinant von Willebrand factor was evaluated [19]. Pharmacokinetic data were collected as well as pharmacodynamic measurements of platelet aggregation support (ristocetin cofactor activity) and cuticle wound blood flow. An important component of these studies was the suitability of the model. These models were chosen because of the biochemical deficiency of the particular factors and the parallel clinical syndromes. Such in vivo data can help in determining activity and dosing when such a product is first used in human trials. The Refacto® molecule was also studied in rats and monkeys to determine its no observed adverse effect level, that was more than 10 times normal circulating levels. The major toxicity observed was the development of antibodies to the molecule that blocked activity and resulted in an acquired hemophilia syndrome. Similar findings were demonstrated when plasma-derived material was injected into monkeys [20].

30.6 IMMUNOGENICITY

Current regulatory concerns with protein therapies include the possibility of induction of autologous antibodies that interact with the therapeutic agent or, worse, with the subject's own residual analogous factor [21–23]. With the use of some bovine thrombin products, there has in fact been an association with coagulopathies and autologous antibodies [24–26]. Therefore the immunogenic potential needs to be addressed in the development program of every new product as well as manufacturing changes or with changes in excipient. The concern of immunogenicity has been expressed by US and European authorities and the Australian authorities have accepted the EMEA position [27–29]. Even prior to the development of recombinant affector proteins, an important consideration for the safety of the subjects using the plasma-derived coagulation factor therapies was the development of "inhibitors" to coagulation enzymes [30–32]. The development of these inhibitors, so named because of their ability to block activity and not initially known to be antibodies, was a serious event. The induction of this immune response was tragic for hemophiliacs because it drastically changed the ability to treat bleeding episodes or to provide prophylactic therapy [33].

Because of the unknown component of biotechnologically derived factors, evaluation of the development of such inhibitors was an important concern in their development [34,35]. In some cases, the hematopoietic compounds induced autologous antibodies, not only toward the biological drug but also toward the patient's own biological factor, leaving them with severe anemia [17–19].

Major regulatory agencies have developed guidance to specifically address immunogenicety in preclinical studies, if possible. Certainly sponsors should collect and present data on immunogenicity from clinical trials [36]. The FDA has particularly addressed the issue of antibodies to clotting factors at a public meeting [12]. The discussion at that meeting suggested possible future use of mouse models for inhibitor testing, including transgenic mice and hemophilia mice. In other venues the FDA has encouraged the development of in vitro immunological response testing [37]. Other methods for establishing an estimate of immunogenicity have included the use of immunochemical (ELISA) assays to compare response and to evaluate cross-reactivity for products that have changed formulation or manufacturing. The FDA has accepted the use of such immunochemical evaluations in some cases as part of product characterization. However, to date, the best method of detecting changes in immunogenicity of novel products or improved manufacturing is a clinical study with previously treated patients. Certainly some estimation of antigenicity should be done preclinically. Immunogenicity has also been a concern for gene therapy studies as mentioned below (also see Chapters 16 and 20 in this volume addressing immunogenicity).

30.7   RECOMBINANT BIOTECHNOLOGY-DERIVED COAGULATION FACTORS

The first therapeutic recombinant DNA-derived coagulation protein licensed by the FDA was factor VIII for treatment of hemophilia A in 1992 [38]. This step forward was a landmark in hemophilia therapy. This biotechnology process reduced the theoretical risk of human-derived viruses and seemed to provide for an unlimited market supply although other human and animal proteins were often used in the manufacturing and formulation of many recombinant products. Plasma-derived factors are still manufactured for a number of reasons, including cost and availability, but the use of recombinant factors is recommended by the Medical and Scientific Advisory Council of the Hemophilia Foundation [39]. The current virus reduction methods for plasma-derived concentrates are considered extremely safe and have virtually eliminated product-derived infections of HIV and hepatitis [40]. Additional manufacturing methods are also effective in reducing the chances of a parvovirus infection. Nevertheless, the use of recombinant coagulation factors has revolutionized not only manufacturing but patient therapy [41–43].

As discussed above, animal models have played an important part in characterizing recombinant molecules. Nevertheless, more classical toxicological evaluations are being applied in the preclinical setting. Research continues on the recombinant factor VIII and Factor IX using molecular techniques to improve the molecules as therapeutics. Modifications that increase activity, increase half-life, and increase expression are being investigated. In fact modifications that would make these genes better candidates for gene therapy are also being evaluated [44–46].

30.8   GENE THERAPY FOR THE TREATMENT OF COAGULATION DISORDERS

The concept of a cure for hemophilia has been a goal of scientists and practitioners for many years and studies are currently underway to address this goal [47]. As in the history of these products, the use of animal models as a proof of concept has been central to preclinical testing [48,49]. The specific aspects of the toxicology evaluation of gene therapy, in general, is addressed in Chapter 32, but some discussion of these animal models as they relate to hemophilia is pertinent here. As in all current studies, the issue of immunogenicity is an important consideration whose evaluation should be included in gene therapy product studies. In animal models, some have demonstrated the induction of an immune reaction to the expressed protein even after delivery of the gene by adenovirus [50]. Increased expression, decreased toxicity from viral elements, and decreased immunogenicity of the expressed proteins had been a formidable goal and has shown some progress as evaluated in animal models [51–54].

30.9   CONCLUSION

The preclinical assessment of blood products has been based on studies designed to answer specific questions on product-specific attributes with a consideration of the intended patient population. In many cases relevant animal models of the disease have been used to assess safety in addition to providing proof-of-concept information to support clinical development.

REFERENCES

1. Bren L. The Road to the Biotech Revolution: Highlights of 100 Years of Biologics Regulation, 2006. FDA Consumer. http://www.fda.gov/fdac/106_toc.html

2. Cohn EJ, Strong LE, Hughes WI, et al. Preparation and properties of serum and plasma proteins. IV. A system for the separation into fractions of the protein and lipoprotein components of biological tissue and fluids. *J Am Chem Soc* 1946; 68:459–75.

3. Alving BM, Hojima Y, Pisano JJ, Mason BL, Buckingham RE, Mozen MM, et al. Hypotension associated with prekallikrein activator (Hageman factor fragments) in plasma protein fraction. *N Engl J Med* 1978;299:66–70.

4. Graham JB, Buckwalter JA, Hartley LJ, Brinkhous KM. Canine hemophilia. Observations of the course, the clotting anomaly, and the effects of blood transfusions. *J Exp Med* 1949;90:97–111.

5. Mannucci PM. AIDS, hepatitis and hemophilia in the 1980s: memoirs from an insider. *J Thromb Haemost* 2003;1:2065–9.

6. Leveton L, Sox HC, Stoto MA. HIV and the blood supply: an analysis of crisis decision-making. Executive summary. *Transfusion* 1996;36:919–27.

7. Brettler DB, Alter HJ, Dienstag JL, Forsberg AD, Levine PH. Prevalence of hepatitis C virus antibody in a cohort of hemophilia patients. *Blood* 1990;76: 254–6.

8. Savitsky J, Doczi J, Black J, Arnold J. A clinical safety trial of stroma-free hemoglobin. *Clin Pharmacol Ther* 1978;23:73–80.

9. Stowell CP. What ever happened to blood substitutes? *Transfusion* 2004; 44:1403–4.

10. Buehler PW, Alayash AI, Toxicities of hemoglobin solutions: in search of in vitro and in vivo model systems. *Transfusion* 2004;44:1516–30.

11. Guidance for Industry. Criteria for Safety and Efficacy Evaluation of Oxygen Therapeutics as Red Blood Cell Substitutes. Draft Guidance. http://www.fda.gov/cber/gdlns/oxytherbld.htm

12. FDA, CBER, Workshop on Factor VIII Inhibitors, 2003. http://www.fda.gov/cber/minutes/fctrviii112103t.htm

13. Guidance for Industry. Safety, Efficacy, and Pharmacokinetic Studies to Support Marketing of Immune Globulin Intravenous (Human) as Replacement Therapy for Primary Humoral Immunodeficiency. Draft Guidance. http://www.fda.gov/cber/gdlns/igivimmuno.pdf

14. Preclinical Data to Support Human Studies of Immune Globulin Products. Annual FDA Science Forum, April 2006. http://www.accessdata.fda.gov/scripts/oc/science-forum/sf2006/Search/preview.cfm?abstract_id=952&backto=author

15. Teschner W, Butterweck HA, Auer W, Muchitsch EM, Weber A, Schwarz H-P. Biochemical and Pre-clinical Characterization of a New10% Liquid Triple Virally Reduced Human Intravenous Immune Globulin (IGIV, 10% TVR). http://www.bo-conf.com/ppb05/PPB05_reports.pdf

16. Giles AR. Use of an animal model to evaluate hemophila therapies, 184. *Prog Clin Biol Res* 1984;150:265–76.

17. Giles AR, Tinlin S, Hoogendoorn H, Fournel MA, Ng P, Pancham N. In vivo characterization of recombinant factor VIII in a canine model of hemophilia a (factor VIII deficiency). *Blood* 1988;72:335–9.

18. Brinkhous K, Sandberg H, Widlund L, Read M, Nichols T, Sigman J, et al. Preclinical pharmacology of albumin-free b-domain deleted recombinant factor VIII. *Sem Thromb Hemostasis* 2002;28:269–72.

19. Schwarz HP, Dorner F, Mitterer A, Mundt W, Schlokat U, Pichler L. Turecek PL. Preclinical evaluation of recombinant von Willebrand factor in a canine model of von Willebrand disease. *Wien Klin Wochenschr* 1999;111:181–91.

20. Summary Basis for Approval, 2000. Antihemophilic Factor (recombinant) Refacto®. http://www.fda.gov/cber/sba/ahfgen030600S.pdf

21. Bunn HF. Drug-induced autoimmune red-cell aplasia. *N Engl J Med* 2002;346: 522–3.

22. Casadevall N, Nataf J, Viron B, Kolta A, Kiladjian JJ, Martin-Dupont P, Michaud P, Papo T, Ugo V, Teyssandier I, Varet B, Mayeux P. Pure red-cell aplasia and antierythropoietin antibodies in patients treated with recombinant erythropoietin. *N Engl J Med* 2002;346:469–75.

23. Gershon SK, Luksenburg H, Cote TR, Braun MM. Pure red-cell aplasia and recombinant erythropoietin. *N Engl J Med* 2002;346:1584–6.

24. Zehnder JL, Leung LL. Development of antibodies to thrombin and factor V with recurrent bleeding in a patient exposed to topical bovine thrombin. *Blood* 1990;76:2011–6.

25. Rapaport SI, Zivelin A, Minow RA, et al. Clinical significance of antibodies to bovine and human thrombin and factor V after surgical use of bovine thrombin. *Am J Clin Pathol* 1992;97:84–91.

26. Lawson JH, Lynn KA, Vanmatre RM, et al. Antihuman Factor V Antibodies after use of relatively pure bovine thrombin. *Ann Thorac Surg* 2005;79:1037–8.

27. Guideline on Comparability of Medicinal Products containing Biotechnology-Derived Proteins as Active Substance: Non-clinical and Clinical Issues. http://www. tga.gov.au/docs/pdf/euguide/emea/309702en.pdf

28. Committee for Medicinal Products for Human Use (CHMP), 2003. Guideline on Comparability of Medicinal Products Containing Biotechnology-Derived Proteins as active Substance: Quality Issues. http://www.emea.eu.int/pdfs/human/bwp/ 320700en.pdf

29. Committee for Medicinal Products for Human Use (CHMP), 2006. Concept Paper on Guideline on Immunogenicity assessment of Therapeutic Proteins. http://www. emea.eu.int/pdfs/human/biosimilar/24651105en.pdf

30. Schwarzinger I, Pabinger I, Korninger C, et al. Incidence of inhibitors in patients with severe and moderate hemophilia A treated with factor VIII concentrates. *Am J Hematol* 1987;24(3):241–5.

31. Ehrenforth S, Kreuz W, Scharrer I, et al. Incidence of development of factor VIII and factor IX inhibitors in hemophiliacs. *Lancet* 1992;339(8793):594–8.

32. Peerlinck K, Arnout J, Gilles JG, Saint-Remy JM, Vermylen J. A higher than expected incidence of factor VIII inhibitors in multitransfused haemophilia A patients treated with an intermediate purity pasteurized factor VIII concentrate. *Thromb Haemost* 1993;69:115–18.

33. Key N. Inhibitors in congenital coagulation disorders. *Br J Haem* 2004;127: 79–391.

34. Lusher JM, Arkin S, Abildgaard CF, et al. Recombinant factor VIII for the treatment of previously untreated patients with hemophilia A: safety, efficacy, and development of inhibitors. *N Engl J Med* 1993;328(7):453–9.

35. Scharrer I, Bray GL, Neutzling O. Incidence of inhibitors in haemophilia A patients—a review of recent studies of recombinant and plasma-derived factor VIII concentrates. *Haemophilia* 1999;5(3):145–54.

36. Committee for Medicinal products for Human Use (CHMP), 2006. Concept paper on Guideline on Immunogenicity assessment of Therapeutic Proteins. Doc. Ref. EMEA/CHMP/BMWP/246511/2005. http://www.emea.eu.int/pdfs/human/biosimilar/24651105en.pdf

37. Comparability Studies for Human Plasma-Derived Therapeutics, 2002. http://www.fda.gov/cber/minutes/plasma053002.htm

38. Lusher J, Abildgaard C, Arkin S, Mannucci PM, Zimmermann R, Schwartz L, Hurst D. Human recombinant DNA-derived antihemophilic factor in the treatment of previously untreated patients with hemophilia A: final report on a hallmark clinical investigation. *J Thromb Haemost* 2004;2:574–83.

39. Medical and Scientific Advisory Council of the Hemophilia Foundation, Recommendation #177. http://www.hemophilia.org/NHFWeb/MainPgs/MainNHF.aspx?menuid=57&contentid=693

40. Tabor E. The epidemiology of virus transmission by plasma derivatives: clinical studies verifying the lack of transmission of hepatitis B and C viruses and HIV type 1. *Transfusion* 1999;39:1160–8.

41. Kurachi K. Recombinant antihemophilic factors. *Biotechnology* 1991;19:177–95.

42. Limentani SA, Roth DA, Furie BC, Furie B. Recombinant blood clotting proteins for hemophilia therapy. *Semin Throm Hemost* 1993;19:62–72.

43. Lusher JM. Recombinant clotting factor concentrates. *Baillieres Clin Haematol* 1996;9:291–303.

44. Saenko E, Ananyeva N, Shima N, et al. The future of recombinant coagulation factors. *J Thromb Haem* 2003;1:922–30.

45. Pipe S. Coagulation factors with improved properties for hemophilia gene therapy. *Semin Thromb Hemost* 2004;30:227–37.

46. Pipe S. The promise and challenges of bioengineered recombinant clotting factors. *J Thromb Haemost* 2005;3:1692–701.

47. High K. Clinical gene transfer studies for hemophilia B. *Semin Thromb Hemost* 2004;30:257–67.

48. VandenDriessche T, Collen D, Chuah M. Gene therapy for the hemophilias. *J Thromb Haem* 2003;1:1550–8.

49. Scallan C, Lillicrap D, Jiang H, et al. Sustained phenotypic correction of canine hemophilia A using an adeno-associated viral vector. *Blood* 2003;102:2031–7.

50. Chuah M, Schiedner G, Thorrez L, et al. Therapeutic factor VIII levels and negligible toxicity in mouse and dog models of hemophilia A following gene therapy with high-capacity adenoviral vectors. *Blood* 2003;101:1734–43.

51. Thorrez L, VandenDriessche L, Collen D, Chuah M. Preclinical gene therapy studies for hemophilia using adenoviral vectors. *Semin Thromb Hemost* 2004; 30:173–83.

52. Rawle F, Lillicrap D. Preclinical animal models for hemophilia gene therapy: predictive value and limitations. *Semin Thromb Hemost* 2004;30:205–13.

53. Chuah M, Collen D, Vandendriessche T. Preclinical and clinical gene therapy for haemophilia. *Haemophilia* 2004;10(s4):119–25.

54. Nathwani A, Davidoff A, Tuddenham E. Prospects for gene therapy of haemophilia. *Haemophilia* 2004;10:309–18.

CHAPTER 31

Preclinical Safety Evaluation of Viral Vaccines

A. MARGUERITE DEMPSTER, PhD, DABT, and RICHARD HAWORTH, FRCPath, DPhil

Contents

31.1   INTRODUCTION

For nearly a century vaccines have proved to be one of the most important and effective medical treatments. Because of successful vaccination the

Preclinical Safety Evaluation of Biopharmaceuticals: A Science-Based Approach to Facilitating Clinical Trials, edited by Joy A. Cavagnaro
Copyright © 2008 by John Wiley & Sons, Inc.

smallpox virus has been virtually eradicated. In addition to smallpox, vaccines continue to prevent millions of deaths worldwide and protect children from a variety of serious diseases such as diphtheria, pertussis, measles, tetanus, rubella, and mumps [1]. As effective as currently marketed vaccines are, diseases caused by other viruses such as human immunodeficiency virus type 1 (HIV-1), human papillomavirus (HPV), and hepatitis C virus (HCV) are not presently controlled by vaccination, and they clearly represent a significant unmet medical need. For example, according to the United Nations program on AIDS, approximately 40 million people worldwide were living with HIV by the end of 2006, approximately 4 million were newly infected and 3 million had lost their lives to AIDS [2]. It is believed that at least 20 million people have died of AIDS since the first cases of AIDS were identified in 1981 [2,3].

The purpose of this chapter is to review and discuss the preclinical safety evaluation strategy for vaccine approaches to the prophylaxis and treatment of viral diseases. This chapter will discuss the newer approaches to vaccination and will include recombinant proteins, peptides, polysaccharides, DNA plasmids, and viral vectors with and without adjuvants. It is outside the scope of this chapter to discuss whole cells expressing immunogens, live attenuated viruses, bacteria, or parasites.

31.2 BACKGROUND

Billions of doses of vaccines were safely administered over the last century to millions of infants, children, and adults [1,4]. Vaccine-associated adverse events were nevertheless identified in a minority of patients. Many of the adverse events were directly related to the vaccine; others as in the case of MMR have not been substantiated with data but still cause considerable public unease [1]. One documented case is that of vaccination with a formalin-inactivated respiratory syncytial virus (RSV) that, when given prophylactically, caused enhanced disease after exposure to the virus and resulted in the death of some children [1,4,5]. An increased incidence of Guillain–Barré syndrome appeared to be associated with a swine flu vaccine that was tested in humans in the late 1970s [1,6]. Guillain-Barré syndrome has also been associated with other vaccines including those for polio, measles, and hepatitis B [6].

Successful vaccination requires both aspects of adaptive (or acquired) immunity: specificity and memory. The primary purpose of a vaccine is to prime the host's immune system with an infectious agent that has been modified so that it is no longer infectious but still immunogenic enough that the host can mount an immune response before the agent produces its adverse effects [7]. Prior to advances in molecular technology that allowed for genetic manipulation of the virus and/or toxoids, the main types of vaccines developed were live attenuated vaccines, inactivated vaccines, and chemically altered exotoxins [7]. The virulence of live attenuated vaccines (e.g., oral polio virus and cholera) was eliminated by various methods, including treatment with heat and chemicals or enzymes, or through multiple passages of the virus in culture [1,7]. Although effective and safe in most individuals, these vaccines were not recommended for people with impaired immune systems, and in rare cases reversion to virulence was noted. For example, after the introduction of oral polio virus sporadic cases of vaccine-associated paralytic polio were observed. It was thought that the few attenuating mutations present in one vaccine strain caused the live polio virus to revert to virulence [1]. However, it was a rare occurrence, and given the risk of polio and the perceived benefit, the vaccine continued to be used until it was replaced by an inactivated or killed vaccine. Although the killed vaccines were associated with fewer adverse effects, they were less effective [7]. The third major type of vaccine at that time was for-malin-inactivated toxoids (e.g., pertussis, diphtheria, and tetanus). Since these vaccines, such as those against whooping cough, developed in the 1940s dem-onstrated good efficacy and safety, they were combined with diphtheria and tetanus toxoids. Similar to the single vaccines, these vaccines exhibited a good safety profile. However, some adverse reactions such as seizures and infantile spasms, observed in the 1970s, caused sufficient public concern that the use of these vaccines declined dramatically [1,8,9]. Not surprisingly, their decline in use was associated with an increased incidence in those diseases [1].

The development of recombinant DNA, large-scale cell culture technolo-gies, and advances in synthetic DNA and protein chemistry introduced a wide range of potential pharmaceutical products including cytokines, receptor ago-nists/antagonists, hormones, growth factors, monoclonal antibodies, and gene therapy products. These advances enabled the development of the next gen-eration of vaccines: recombinant protein, DNA plasmid, and recombinant viral vectors.

31.3   CURRENT TECHNOLOGIES

31.3.1   Recombinant Protein Vaccines

Improvements in genetic engineering facilitated the identification, construc-tion, and production of novel recombinant antigens [1]. This approach was particularly successful for HBV as it reduced the risk that the formulation could be contaminated with residual viral particles [6,10]. Instead of purifying HBV from urine of infected individuals, the segments of the HBV that encode for hepatitis B surface antigen (HBsAg) were inserted into a yeast plasmid using DNA recombinant technology. At first the administration of HBV vaccine was restricted to individuals at high risk of exposure to HBV, but as the vaccine proved to be efficacious and safe, its use increased to the point that it became common practice in some countries to vaccinate all infants. Although reactions were infrequent in adults and rare in infants and children, some reactions were considered significant. A review of all the safety reports with HBV vaccine found that the vaccine-associated reactions included immediate (anaphylaxis and urticaria), delayed (e.g., systemic lupus erythematosus, glomerulonephritis), hematologic, ophthalmic, and neurologic toxicities [11]. Given the temporal relationship to vaccination, the similarity between the serious reactions to the vaccine and the extrahepatic effects of infection with HBV and the potential induction of soluble antigen–antibody complexes indicated that although rare, these reactions were related to vaccination. As the benefit of HBV vaccine far outweighs the potential risks, this vaccine continues to be used [11].

While recombinant protein technology eliminated some of the potential risks associated with vaccine therapy (i.e., reversion to virulence), these vaccines still require adjuvants that can produce adverse local reactions and hypersensitivity on occasion. These newer vaccines will share some of the other potential risks of vaccines such as enhancement of disease or infection, antigenic competition, and cross-reactive antibodies [6]. Toxicity due to molecular mimicry in which antibodies to the viral antigen cross-react with other tissues in the body has been a regulatory concern for many years [4,6,11,12]. Cross-reactive antibodies were a particular issue for the development of vaccines against groups A and B Streptococcus (GAS, GBS), Lyme disease and group B meningococcus [4,13–15]. In one example, rheumatic heart disease developed after vaccination to GAS. It was found that the antigen presented by GAS was similar enough to a host's cardiac antigen that the antibodies attacked the cardiac valve [12].

31.3.2   Virus-like Particles

Structural proteins derived from viruses such as HBV have the ability to spontaneously assemble into particles called virus-like particles (VLPs). These VLPs are similar to virions and consist of highly repetitive and ordered structures, but unlike recombinant protein vaccines, VLPs can elicit both humoral and cellular responses [16]. In addition these particles are easily purified and can be produced in large quantities [16]. Several VLPs are in clinical trials and have shown to be effective. This strategy has been particularly successful for HPV, and one product has been recently approved by the FDA for prophylactic use [17].

31.3.3   DNA Vaccines

Interest in the potential for DNA vaccines was increased after a number of publications reported that bacterial plasmids could produce immune responses following administration to vertebrates [18]. DNA vaccines consist of a bacterial DNA plasmid that contains a gene encoding the antigen of interest, a strong viral promoter, and a terminator sequence to ensure that the gene will be expressed in mammalian cells [18–20]. When injected by various routes of administration (e.g., intramuscularly and intradermally), DNA vaccines are transcribed, translated, and the encoded protein is presented by an antigen-presenting cell (APC) in the context of a self major histocompatibility complex (MHC) [21,22]. DNA vaccines have been found to generate all types of immunity including cytotoxic T cell (CTL) responses, T helper cells, and antibodies [20]. It is thought that DNA vaccines can elicit a CTL response while recombinant proteins cannot because the antigen can be delivered into the cell, allowing the antigen to enter the intracellular processing pathway and resulting in the presentation of its relevant peptides on MHC class I molecules to stimulate a CTL response. Recombinant protein vaccines on the other hand, tend to be taken up by the endolysosomal system where it degrades into peptides and associates with MHC class II molecules that stimulate T helper cells rather then cytolytic T cells [20].

There are potential safety issues with DNA vaccines, some similar to other vaccine strategies and some unique to DNA vaccines. These concerns include induction of autoimmunity, potential integration of plasmid DNA into the host genome, induction of immunological tolerance, immunotoxicity, and altered immune responsiveness to other vaccines and infection [21,23,24].

Induction of Autoimmunity   The bacterial elements of a DNA plasmid can contribute to its immunogenic potency. It is well known that oligonucleotides having the sequence purine-purine-CG-pyrimidine, in which the CpG sequence is unmethylated, can activate antigen-presenting cells in vitro and exert immune stimulating effects in vivo [25–27]. It has also been shown that these CpG motifs can stimulate polyclonal T, B, and NK cells that can release immunomodulatory cytokines such as IL-2, TNFα, γ-interferon, and IL-6 [21,26,28,29]. The safety concern is that the promotion of immune activation could lead to anti-DNA antibodies, which may then contribute to and/or accelerate the development of autoimmunity [21, 23]. Additionally bacterial, but not mammalian, DNA can stimulate production of IgG anti-DNA autoantibodies that can lead to glomerulonephritis in mice [21,30,31]. To assess this risk, the effect of vaccination of several DNA vaccines was investigated in normal Balb/c mice and mice prone to lupus (NZB/W). A threefold increase in the number of B cells secreting IgG antibodies against mammalian DNA was induced when Balb/c mice were repeatedly vaccinated whereas the serum anti-DNA antibody titers only rose 35% to 60% [21]. No effect on the onset or severity of autoimmune disease was observed in either the normal or lupus-prone mice, and therefore these findings indicated that this modest level of autoantibody production was not sufficient to induce autoimmunity [21]. These findings are consistent with other reports where no autoimmune-mediated pathology or development of systemic autoimmune response was observed in normal animals after DNA vaccination [22,23,32,33]. Furthermore other studies performed in a number of species, including rodents, rabbits, and nonhuman primates, have not reported any anti-DNA antibodies [22,23,33,34,35,36].

Integration into Host Genome   DNA plasmid needs to enter the cell to produce an immune response. Therefore a safety concern is whether integration of the plasmid DNA into the host genome occurs, and if so, will the risk of genetic instability or cell growth dysregulation, mutagenesis, and carcinogenicity increase [23,24]. Results from biodistribution and persistence studies have typically shown that although plasmid DNA can be detected in many organs shortly after injection, DNA plasmid could only be detected at the injection site several weeks after injection. [23]. Long-term persistence may facilitate the integration, and in one study, when DNA plasmid was injected intramuscularly in mice, it was still present in the muscle 19 months later [23,37]. However, in this and other studies, no integration was observed; the plasmids were predominantly extrachromosomal [23,37,38,39]. Nevertheless, in one study investigators using a newly developed PCR assay to assess integration identified four independent integration events upon plasmid injection followed by electroporation of the injected muscle in vivo. Electroporation of the injection site was considered to have increased plasmid DNA delivery into cells and increased plasmid integration frequency [23,40]. Biodistribution studies are also useful for assessing for distribution to the gonads, but again studies have found that although plasmid can be detected in the gonads shortly after injection, they do not persist [23].

Immunological Tolerance   Most preclinical studies (for both efficacy and safety) utilize healthy adult animals. However, there is a concern that the risk for certain clinical populations with reduced immune function, including infants, children, and elderly, is not adequately assessed [21]. Evidence suggests that recognition of foreign determinants is acquired at distinct stages of maturation ranging from early gestation until days or weeks after birth. Since the protein encoded by a DNA vaccine is produced endogenously and expressed in the context of self MHC, the potential exists for the neonatal immune system to recognize the vaccine antigen not as foreign but as "self," resulting in tolerance [21]. Experiments with DNA plasmids in neonatal mice showed long-lasting neonatal tolerance (persisting for more than nine months) when newborn Balb/c mice were injected with a DNA plasmid [21]. However, in other experiments treatment with DNA plasmids did not induce tolerance in neonatal mice [23]. Experiments in aged mice demonstrated a diminished immune-response relative to younger animals but cytokine and antibody production increased following repeated administrations suggesting that age-related changes could be overcome with additional dosing [21,23].

A number of DNA vaccines have progressed into clinical trials for the prevention and/or treatment of HIV, malaria, cytomegalovirus (CMV) and hepatitis B and C [23,24]. So far the DNA vaccines have been well tolerated in clinical trials [23] and have produced both humoral and cellular responses in some trials [41], but overall the potency has been disappointing [20]. Although DNA is typically injected intramuscularly, alternative delivery systems have been evaluated. One such system that has been tested clinically for hepatitis B involves coating plasmid DNA onto gold beads, which are then propelled into the epidermis using a needle-free delivery system [20,42,43].

One such delivery system known as PMED (particle-mediated epidermis delivery) was the first to show that DNA vaccines could produce a humoral response in human trials [44,45]. Also this method was associated with an increased response in patients that had not responded to the HBV protein vaccine [20,45,46].

31.3.4 Virus-Based Vectors

In gene therapy where the goal is to replace a malfunctioning gene with a normal gene viral vectors were initially considered to be an efficient method of ensuring integration into the genome. However, early clinical trials proved to be largely unsuccessful, primarily due to immune reactions to the vector [47,48], and in one case an immune reaction is believed to be the cause of the death of a volunteer in a clinical trial for ornithine transcarbamylase (OTC). The high dose of the vector, which was administered by direct infusion into an hepatic artery, apparently produced a cytokine cascade that led to disseminated intravascular coagulation, acute respiratory distress, and multi-organ failure [49]. Second, it has been shown that the production of neutralizing antibodies, even at moderate doses of vector, decrease the uptake of adenoviral vectors by cells, including antigen-producing cells [47,50]. Therefore formation of neutralizing antibodies can clearly restrict the number of repeat doses given in a clinical trial. However, what is considered to be a negative for gene therapy may be seen as a positive for vaccine therapy, since viral vectors can produce both innate and adaptive immune responses [47,48]. A number of vectors are based on viruses, including variola, vaccinia, avipoxivirus, adenovirus, and alphaviruses [51].

Initially adenoviruses were chosen for several reasons: (1) they cause mild disease in humans, (2) their genome has been well characterized (3) they are relatively easy to manipulate genetically, and (4) they exhibit a broad tropism transducing different cell types [47]. Adenovirus are double-stranded DNA viruses with a genome of approximately 34 to 43 kb; they are species specific, and they include a number of distinct serotypes. There are about 51 known human serotypes and 27 simian serotypes including 7 from chimpanzees [47]. Adenoviruses are made replication defective by removing the E1 gene, but there are vectors with other genes such as E3 and E4 that can also be removed [47].

A number of experiments in mice, rabbits, and nonhuman primates have demonstrated the potential utility of adenoviral vectors in producing immune responses against various viral pathogens, as reviewed by Tastis [47]. While a number of preclinical models have demonstrated the potential utility of these vectors, preexisting immunity against human adenoviruses will still likely curtail the number of clinical administrations of the vector. Moreover neutralizing antibodies against the vector can reduce the potential efficacy upon repeated dose [47]. Investigators have started to evaluate other species, and there are several examples of chimpanzee-derived adenoviruses that have been evaluated in preclinical models. A vector produced from the chimpanzee AdC68 virus shares almost 90% homology with the human adenovirus 4 [52] and, similar to the HuAd5 virus, enters the cell via the coxsackie adenovirus receptor (CAR), so this vector should exhibit similar tropism to humans [47]. Although greater than 80% of chimpanzee sera will be positive for neutralizing antibodies, humans tested so far do not have neutralizing antibodies for AdC68 [52,53].

As with any vaccine technology the adenoviral vectors share some of the same potential safety issues already discussed. Like DNA vaccines, adenoviral vectors may integrate into the genome and may produce unacceptable immunotoxicity. In addition there is a risk that a viral vector could combine with an endogenous virus to form a chimera. Administration of a viral vector could produce both an innate immune reaction (at high doses) and an antigen-specific response (at lower doses). However, for vaccine treatment, the vector will typically be administered intramuscularly or intradermally so that the systemic exposure is less than for intravenous administration, which is a common route of administration for gene therapy. Figure 31.1 illustrates these two responses.

Immune-based toxicities of Adenoviral vectors

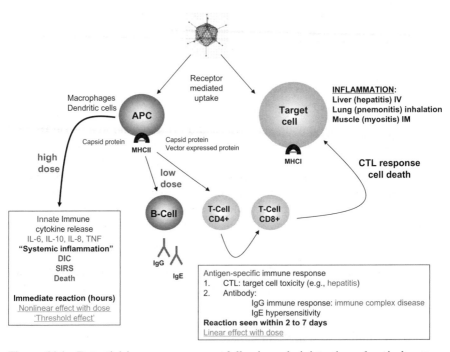

Figure 31.1 Potential immune-responses following administration of a viral vector. DIC: disseminated intravascular coagulation; SIRS: systemic inflammatory response syndrome. Image courtesy of Sarah Taplin.

The risk of adenoviral vector-induced oncogenicity is another potential safety concern as human adenoviruses are known to be oncogenic in rats. However, in humans it is considered to be a low risk, for extensive analysis has failed to find human adenovirus DNA associated with human tumors [54]. Therefore the use of in vivo carcinogenicity assays for adenoviruses may be uninformative given the lack of any association of adenoviruses with human malignancy. Also the known oncogenic component (E1 region) of the nonhuman primate (NHP) adenoviral vectors has been deleted from the product. However, other potential oncogenes may be present, and therefore it may be necessary to assess the oncogenicity of the vector.

31.3.5 Mixed Modality Paradigms

Most of the technologies discussed above have been used as single entities. However, because the potency of DNA vaccines in clinical trials has been disappointing and because neutralizing antibodies to adenoviral vectors may restrict the number of administrations in the clinic, investigators have developed a regimen in which a priming dose of a DNA vaccine is followed by a boost using a different modality such as recombinant protein or recombinant viral vector. This prime/boost regimen is currently being evaluated in a number of animal models [18,20]. In one study rhesus macaques were immunized using a heterologous prime/boost regimen of different adenoviral vectors using a combination of human group C Ad6 or Ad5 vectors with a rare human serotype belonging to subgroup D AD24, or two chimpanzee adenoviruses, C32 and C33. These data showed that the prime/boost regimen increased the HCV T cell responses two- to threefold and that boosting could be delayed for over two years after priming, and thus indicating that there is long-term maintenance of resting memory cells [55]. Another study assessed DNA prime followed by a protein boost. In this study mice were immunized with HIV1084 *env*-coding DNA and then boosted with homologous 1084i gp160. Results showed that although immunization with gp160 produced high-titer antibodies, it required two inoculations, whereas in mice primed with DNA, antibodies were produced after a single boost [56].

31.4 ADJUVANTS AND IMMUNOMODULATORS

Advances in immunology have delivered more specific targeted types of vaccine, such as subunit, peptide, and DNA plasmids rather than inactivated whole organisms. These new types of vaccine represent the result of intensive research into epitope mapping, T and B cell receptor binding, and antigen selection. Unfortunately, the refinement has resulted in a reduction in immunogenicity [57]. Nonliving vaccines generally have proved ineffective at inducing potent cell-mediated immune (CMI) responses, particularly of the Th1 type. Although live vaccines can induce an effective CTL response, they also risk causing disease in immunosuppressed patients who in chronic diseases, for example, HIV and HCV, often form the target patient population. In addition some viruses fail to grow in culture (e.g., HCV) making the development of attenuated viruses difficult. Achieving effective cellular immune-responses while using rationally designed recombinant, peptide, or DNA vaccines is the holy grail of modern vaccine development.

To supplement immunogenicity, adjuvants are required. Adjuvants can be defined as "agents that act nonspecifically to increase the specific immune-response or responses to an antigen." Therefore a particular adjuvant should work with a wide range of antigens. While a great deal of effort is paid to antigen design and mechanism of action, traditionally there has been less effort spent on discovering new adjuvants and understanding their mechanisms of action.

A wide range of unrelated substances can act as adjuvants, including surfactants, oil emulsions, mineral gels, and bacteria-derived substances. Aluminium adjuvants have been in widespread use for over 70 years [58]. Although the exact mechanism of action is still not understood, it is clear that physical association of the antigen with aluminium is required. Usually aluminium hydroxide or aluminium phosphate gels are used. These adjuvants have historically been used as part of bacterial or viral vaccines to help stimulate neutralizing antibodies. However, alum is a weak adjuvant for antibody induction to recombinant protein vaccines, and it induces a Th2 rather than a Th1 response. Alum is also not effective at producing mucosal IgA antibody responses, but it does upregulate costimulatory signals on monocytes and produces a release of IL-4. These adjuvants are not effective at stimulating CMI responses, which are now understood as being important in clearing persistent infections, such as hepatitis C, tuberculosis, and HIV. In these cases a Th1 response consisting of IFNγ production and B cell IgG2a secretion is considered more effective than a Th2 response consisting of IL-4 and IL-5 production and B cell production of IgG1 and IgE. In the laboratory this problem can be overcome by using Freunds complete antigen (FCA), which induces Th1 responses. However, this adjuvant produces injection site necrosis and disseminated granulomatous inflammation that precludes its use in the clinic. Inflammation at the site of vaccination results in the release of cytokines (e.g., TNFα) that induce dendritic cell activation and stimulate the CMI response. Despite the recognized link between local tissue reaction and adjuvant efficacy, there is a need for novel adjuvants that have the efficacy of FCA but the safety profile of aluminium adjuvants. A list of different types of adjuvant which have been tested for use in infectious disease vaccines is provided in Table 31.2.

Adjuvants can be classified into two main groups based on their mechanism of action. The first group are particulate materials that act as vaccine delivery systems and target associated antigens into APC. These include emulsions, microparticles, iscoms, and liposomes. The second group are immunostimulatory and are derived mainly from pathogens. These include lipopolysaccharide

TABLE 31.1 Selection of regulatory guidelines addressing preclinical safety testing

Vaccine Class	Guideline	Date
All vaccines	European Medicines Evaluation Agency (EMEA) notes for guidance of preclinical pharmacological and toxicological testing of vaccines	1997
Combination vaccines	EMEA notes for guidance on pharmaceutical and biological aspects of combined vaccines	1998
Viral vector and DNA vaccines	EMEA note for guidance on the quality, preclinical, and clinical aspects of gene transfer medicinal products	2001
Cell-based vaccines	EMEA points to consider on the manufacture and quality control of human somatic cell therapy medicinal products	2001
Smallpox vaccines	EMEA note for guidance on the development of vaccinia virus-based vaccines against smallpox	2002
Influenza vaccines	EMEA points to consider on the development of live attenuated influenza vaccines	2003
Adjuvanted vaccines	EMEA guideline on adjuvants in vaccines for human use	2005
Recombinant protein/ peptide vaccines	US Food and Drug Administration (FDA) points to consider in the production and testing of new drugs and biologics produced by recombinant DNA technology	1985
Viral vector and cell-based vaccines	FDA guidance for industry: guidance for human somatic cell therapy and gene therapy	1998
Vaccines for pregnant women and women of child-bearing potential	FDA guidance for industry, considerations for reproductive toxicity studies for preventative vaccines for infectious disease indications	2000
DNA vaccines	FDA guidance for industry, considerations for plasmid DNA vaccines for infectious disease indications	2007
All vaccines	World Health Organisation (WHO) guidelines on nonclinical evaluation of vaccines	2003
Includes vaccines but more relevant to other biologics	International Conference on Harmonization (ICH) S6: preclinical safety evaluation of biotechnology-derived pharmaceuticals	1997
All vaccines	ICH S7A: Safety pharmacology studies for human pharmaceuticals	2000

Source: Adapted from LeBron et al. 2005 [62].

(LPS), monophosphoryl lipid A, and CpG DNA. These substances contain pathogen-associated molecular patterns (PAMPs) that are recognized by and stimulate cells of the immune system. Many of these substances, for example, LPS, have been discovered to act as ligands for Toll-like receptors (TLR). These receptors are expressed on APC, recognize highly conserved motifs on bacteria and viruses, and mediate APC activation. Vaccine developers are now focusing

TABLE 31.2 Adjuvants that have been tested for stimulating the immune response to vaccines

Class of Adjuvant	Examples
Mineral Salts	Aluminium hydroxide,* aluminium phosphate,* calcium phosphate*
Immunostimulatory adjuvants	Saponins (e.g., QS21), MDP derivatives, bacterial DNA (CpG oligos), LPS, MPL and synthetic derivatives, lipopeptides, cytokines (e.g., GM-CSF, IL-2, IL-12)
Lipid particles	Liposomes, virosomes,* iscoms, cochleates, emulsions (e.g., Freunds adjuvant, SAF, MF59*)
Particulate adjuvants	Poloxamer particles, virus-like particles, PLG microparticles
Mucosal adjuvants	Cholera toxin (CT), mutant toxin (e.g., LTK63, LTR72), heat labile enterotoxin (LT), microparticles, polymerized liposomes, chitosan

Source: Adapted from Singh and O'Hagan. [57].

Note: All of these adjuvants have been evaluated in clinical trials with the exception of cochleates and polymerized liposomes. Only those adjuvants marked * are currently licensed as adjuvants in approved vaccine products.

on the rational design and selection of adjuvants that act on TLR. A useful way to consider the role of adjuvants in recombinant vaccines is that because the final product resembles infection closely enough to initiate an effective immune-response, they ensure the biological consequences of the vaccine.

The acceptable level of toxicity for an adjuvant will depend on its application. For adjuvants intended for use in therapeutic vaccines the level will be higher than for those intended for prophylactic vaccines in healthy individuals. This is particularly true of therapeutic vaccines intended for treatment of cancer patients or life-threatening infectious disease.

Preclinical evaluation of vaccine adjuvants is normally carried out within toxicity studies that also evaluate the whole vaccine. The injection site is evaluated macroscopically and scored for local reaction (e.g., erythema, edema, skin sloughing) at intervals following dosing (e.g., 1, 2, 3 and 14 days). Photographs of the skin sites may be useful for internal use within companies but are not required by regulatory authorities. In addition all of the other traditional endpoints (e.g., haematology, pathology) are assessed. Novel adjuvants need to be evaluated for toxicity in the absence of other vaccine components. In most cases for biotechnology-derived adjuvants, such as DNA plasmid encoding a human cytokine, this can be achieved by adding an additional group of animals to the toxicity studies evaluating the final product. However, a novel chemical-based adjuvant should be treated as a new chemical entity and therefore requires a classical toxicological programme as outlined in the EMEA guideline on adjuvants (Table 31.1). This will consist of acute and repeat-dose toxicity studies in two species, pharmacokinetic (PK) and tissue distribution studies, genotoxicity testing and testing for hypersensitivity, anaphylaxis and pyrogenicity. Immunological assays are often included as part of the toxicity assessment and are helpful to demonstrate the benefit of the adjuvant. In some studies different potential adjuvant–antigen combinations can be compared for both immunogenicity and toxicity [59].

No adjuvant is licensed as a medicinal product in its own right, but only as a component of a particular vaccine. Therefore preclinical and toxicology studies need to be designed on a case-by-case basis to evaluate the safety profile of the adjuvant and adjuvant/ vaccine combination [60]. Evaluation in preclinical studies is important for identifying the optimum composition and formulation process and also for allowing development of tests for quality control [61]. Data from these studies also helps plan protocols for subsequent clinical trials from which safety and efficacy in humans can be evaluated.

31.5 CONSIDERATIONS FOR PRECLINICAL SAFETY EVALUATION

The wide range of different types of biotechnology-derived vaccines has resulted in the publication of a diverse range of regulatory guidelines. These take the form of a guidance note or points to consider. Rapid changes in technology have required a similarly rapid response from regulators on new requirements for assessing safety (Table 31.1). The relationship between vaccine companies and regulators has been constructive, and input into guidance from all sources has been solicited. The expectation is that toxicity studies will be conducted in animal species on all new vaccines prior to first administration to humans. Exceptions to this rule include combined vaccines containing known antigens. A conservative approach is merited because most vaccines are intended for prophylactic use in healthy humans. The risk–benefit evaluation requires that new vaccines have minimal risk of toxicity. Therapeutic vaccines that are intended for use in patients, frequently with life-threatening diseases such as HIV or hepatitis C infection, have a different risk–benefit evaluation. Thus an effective new vaccine for these diseases might be approved even with a low level of acceptable adverse effects.

Reading the published guidelines represents an important first step in designing a suitable package of toxicity studies. However, early communication with the regulatory authorities is encouraged, and this represents a valuable opportunity for companies to receive feedback on preclinical and clinical plans. The benefit of this dynamic regulatory environment is that it permits companies to design a preclinical development program that does not rely wholly on the published guidelines but rather on scientific justification for each study and endpoint measured. Preclinical safety studies should be performed in compliance with good laboratory practice (GLP) regulations.

31.5.1 Quality Control Testing of Material Intended for GLP Studies

There is a requirement that the test material used in GLP preclinical studies should resemble the same quality of product that will be tested in the clinic.

Therefore quality control (QC) testing of vaccines normally includes the following assays, which must be passed prior to material being released for use in preclinical toxicology studies: sterility, endotoxin, general safety, identity, mass, potency, purity, and stability [62]. These assays should be performed on the final product using the clinical formulation.

Ideally the test material used in the toxicology studies should come from the vaccine lot, produced according to cGMP, that is intended for the FIH clinical trial. However, frequently this is not possible, and non-GMP material may be used subject to demonstrating the comparability of this vaccine lot to the intended clinical lot. For those vaccines that incorporate antigens or adjuvants that are biologically active in limited species, it may be necessary to perform some or all of the testing using homologues. For example, a plasmid expressed cytokine may form part of the adjuvant for a novel vaccine. This expressed cytokine may only be biologically active in humans and chimpanzees. In this situation there will be an ethical case or biological case (e.g., similarity to human skin for dermally applied vaccine) for selecting a lower species and using a homologue form of the cytokine. So suitable QA testing must also be applied to the plasmid encoding the homologue protein prior to its use in preclinical studies. However, there is a regulatory expectation that the final clinical product will also be tested. The formulation should be identical to the intended clinical formulation. Stability of the vaccine is determined before and after the GLP study to ensure adequate stability during storage prior to dosing.

31.5.2 Testing for Viral Contamination

Vaccines produced using eukaryotic cells have the potential to be contaminated with either endogenous or exogenous viruses resulting from accidental introduction at some stage of the process. A battery of analytical and safety tests is applied to the cell banks (master and working), virus seeds (master and working), and vaccine batches to address this concern. These tests are performed in vitro, in vivo, and by laboratory analysis. The range of tests required will depend on species and tissue source of the cells, history of the cells and original virus isolate, and the culture media ingredients.

31.5.3 Immunogenicity Evaluation within Toxicity Studies

Evaluating the immune response to the vaccine at the same time as evaluating toxicity is recommended in a 2003 WHO guideline (Table 31.1). This makes good sense because any toxicity observed with vaccines is frequently related to the immune response, and correlation of these two endpoints provides a fuller explanation of the test results. Assays to measure the immune response include those which measure antigen-specific antibody responses (e.g., ELISA) and cell-mediated responses (e.g., γ-interferon—ELISPOT). Developing these assays can be a challenge for certain species. Therefore the choice of relevant animal model for toxicity testing ideally should be the same as the animal model selected for immunogenicity or efficacy testing. Recent FDA guidance state that preclinical studies to specifically assess if DNA vaccination causes autoimmune disease are no longer required (Table 31.1). This follows experience that any anti-DNA antibodies produced following vaccination are usually at such a low level as to be insufficient to cause disease in normal animals or accelerate disease in autoimmune-prone mice. Similarly the absence of an immune-response against cells expressing the vaccine-encoded antigen (including muscle cells and dendritic cells) suggests that an autoimmune response directed against tissues in which such cells reside is unlikely. It is also recommended that prior to use of a DNA vaccine in children or newborns, the vaccine be first tested for safety and immunogenicity in adults and appropriate animal models be used to evaluate the potential of the vaccine to induce neonatal tolerance. Preclinical testing to evaluate the risk of hypersensitivity is problematic because this type of response is rare and idiosyncratic in the clinic. Conventional endpoints evaluated in the repeat-dose toxicity study provide a screen for the development of hypersensitivity in the animal studies. However, the low number of animals used and the important genetic variability inherent in the human population are important factors in weakening the predictive power of current preclinical studies.

31.5.4 Species Selection

Immunologists will have selected the most appropriate species for establishing immunogenicity of the vaccine. Frequently they will have used animal models of, for example, tolerance or in the case of cancer targets, xenograft models. Usually naive animals that respond to all constituents of the vaccine will also have been used and assays developed for use in this species. For a live viral vaccine, infection and protection studies might have been performed in a species susceptible to infection with the wild-type virus. Regulatory guidelines allow for a single species to be used for the toxicology assessment. The key requirement is that the species chosen should develop a similar immune response to that expected for humans postvaccination [63]. In practice, either rodents or rabbits are often used. However, if elements of the vaccine are inactive in these species, such as plasmid encoding human cytokines, then either an alternative sensitive species, such as a nonhuman primate or a nonhuman homologue of the cytokine, should be used. Which is the correct approach? This is an ambiguous regulatory area for those developing vaccines. On the one hand, there are sound ethical reasons for avoiding the use of nonhuman primates in safety testing, and their use must be justified in each case. On the other hand, there is an expectation by the regulatory authorities that the clinical product should be evaluated in a sensitive species. In the case of a plasmid encoded human cytokine that is only active in nonhuman primates this presents a dilemma. Animal use ethical committees will scrutinize a preclinical study and ask why a homologue of the cytokine cannot be used enabling the use of, for example, rodents instead. However, there remains uncertainty as to whether a safety package developed using a nonhuman homologue would be currently acceptable to regulators for use in risk assessment prior to human studies. This is an area where improved regulatory guidance is clearly required. An example where a murine homologue was used in preclinical toxicity studies is provided by Vical Inc., which tested murine GM-CSF in a repeat-dose toxicity study in mice [32]. However, it is not known if this safety package was acceptable in the absence of testing the clinical product, plasmid DNA encoding multivalent malaria antigens and human GM-CSF, in a nonhuman primate. With increasing species specificity of vaccines incorporating human cytokines, it seems likely that under the current regulatory environment there will be increasing use of nonhuman primates in safety assessment. In any case, studies should be carefully designed to optimize the information obtained with as few animals as possible, especially if nonhuman primates are used.

Phylogenetically, macaques are closely related to humans and, as such, are often used to evaluate vaccine safety and immunogenicity [64]. Vaccine responses in rhesus macaques, as opposed to rodents, have been found to be better predictors of human responses to several malaria vaccine candidates [59]. The rhesus macaque has substantial class II and to a lesser extent class I MHC homology with humans [65], and it has proved useful in selecting malaria vaccine formulations with improved clinical immunogenicity and efficacy [66]. In addition the nonhuman primate allows cutaneous immunologic endpoints, such as delayed-type hypersensitivity (DTH) responsiveness to vaccine-related antigens to be measured. This is an important consideration because for vaccines the possible adverse effects "immunotoxicity" are generally related to the immunological response rather than to any inherent toxicity of the components within the final product.

31.5.5 Design of Safety Assessment Studies

For each vaccine candidate a tailored package of safety assessment studies should be performed. The package will reflect the type of vaccine. As a minimum these should include repeat-dose toxicity, local tolerance, and reproductive and development toxicity. Local tolerance is evaluated by visual assessment of the dosing sites, and the skin reaction is scored according to the Draize method for erythema and oedema formation [67]. Epithelial sloughing can also be scored. Plasmid DNA or adenoviral vectors require studies of biodistribution and integration (Table 31.1), whereas live viral vaccines require virulence and potentially neurovirulence testing. Additional separate studies might include single-dose toxicity and safety pharmacology. In many cases these endpoints can be obtained from the repeat-dose study. This represents an efficient use of animals and enables comparisons among different endpoints for the same animal.

Carcinogenicity and Genotoxicity Tests Carcinogenicity studies and genotoxicity assays are generally not considered appropriate for testing vaccines and are therefore not required. Exceptions to this arise if a new chemical-type adjuvant is included in the formulation, if the vaccine includes components that may be considered a risk for mutagenicity and/or tumorigenicity by virtue of their novel nature (e.g., new adenovirus-derived vectors) or if the production process for the vaccine has used a cell line with a potential risk. Since adjuvants are intended for infrequent use at low dose, the EMEA considers the direct risk of tumor induction by these as negligible and does not require long-term carcinogenicity tests (Table 31.1). Viral vectors may also have the potential to recombine with wild-type viruses, revert to virulence, and cause oncogenic mutations or suppress immune function [68]. Biodistribution studies should be conducted to establish disposition of viral DNA, and separate assays should evaluate if the viral vector is itself pathogenic. If a DNA vaccine contains a vector with extensive homology to the human genome or known oncogenic potential, then close attention must be paid to the results of the biodistribution study, and if positive results are obtained, an integration assay may be needed.

Single-Dose Study Although single-dose studies are advised in the EMEA guideline, they are generally not particularly useful for products intended for repeat dosing in the clinic. Many of the endpoints, such as clinical signs, body weight, and macroscopic observations of the dosing site can be obtained following the first dose during a repeat-dose study. However, if they are needed, for example, for a vaccine designed for single dosing in the clinic, a 14-day period following dosing to study termination is a normal period that enables development of the primary immune response.

Repeat-Dose Study The route of administration, dose, and dosing intervals used in the preclinical safety assessment studies should reflect the intended clinical study as closely as possible. If a particular dosing device is to be used in the clinic, then this device should also be used in preclinical studies. In contrast to the development of small molecules, administering the full clinical dose is acceptable for vaccine candidates, generally in a nonrodent species, rather than large multiples of the clinical dose. In some cases, for example, in small species, it may not be possible to administer the entire clinical dose or use the clinical dosing device. In these situations agreement prior to study start should be reached with regulators.

If immunogenicity studies demonstrate that a similar immune response is obtained at intervals shorter than the proposed clinical dosing interval (e.g., 4–6 weeks), then a truncated dosing interval (2–3 weeks) can be used in the repeat dose safety studies. The FDA recommends that one more dose than the clinical dosing regimen (N) be used in animal studies. This is termed the $N + 1$ rule [61]. The number of animals used per group should be sufficient to detect a treatment-related change. In practice, the number of animals used depends on the species selected for practical and ethical reasons. For example, a rat study might have 10 animals per sex per group. In contrast, a nonhuman primate study might have 3 per sex per group. There are no fixed guidelines for this and group sizes should be justified.

Repeat-dose toxicity studies include a wide range of antemortem and postmortem evaluations. Antemortem evaluations usually include mortality, clinical signs, body weights, food consumption, ophthalmology, urinalysis, serum biochemistry, haematology, coagulation, and blood for immunogenicity assays. Necropsies typically take place at two time points following the final vaccine dose. The first time point at 2 to 7 days evaluates acute changes, both at the final dosing site and systemically. An advantage of waiting until 7 days is that it enables development of an immune response to the final dose which can be assayed. In addition any pathology related to the peak immune response is more likely to be detected at this time point. In contrast, a necropsy at 2 days enables histological evaluation of the acute response at the injection site and systemically. In most cases a judgment can be made on the relative importance of these different aspects to the safety assessment. The second time point at 2 to 4 weeks evaluates delayed toxicity and recovery of any treatment-related effects observed at the earlier time point. At necropsy, gross examination of all major tissues, organ weights, and a complete list of tissues is collected. Selection of tissues for microscopic examination depends to some extent on the type and route of vaccination. However, in all cases major organs and the site of vaccination should be evaluated.

Treatment-related effects are generally related to the development of an immune response and consist of local skin or muscle inflammation, enlarged draining lymph nodes, and potentially increased spleen weight. Effects are also frequently seen in haematology parameters. Since they relate to the expected immune response, these changes are generally not considered adverse. In certain cases additional endpoints to these studies should be added. For example, when testing certain vectors that target the liver such as recombinant adenovirus serotype 5, it may be of use to evaluate effects on hepatic enzymes, because P450 enzymes have been demonstrated to be reduced following dosing and this could affect drug interactions [69].

Safety Pharmacology Studies Safety pharmacology studies test for treatment-related changes in key physiological functions, such as respiratory, central nervous, and cardiovascular systems. WHO guidance suggests that if there are components of the vaccine (e.g., toxoids) that may influence these body systems, then safety pharmacology studies should be performed. However, in those cases where the pharmacology is well characterized and the systemic exposure is low, there may not be a requirement to perform these tests (Table 31.1; ICH S7A). A case-by-case approach is usually followed, and if it is considered that these evaluations are required, then frequently the endpoints can be incorporated into the repeat-dose study. This approach is particularly valuable when a large animal model is being used.

Reproductive Toxicology Studies   Most vaccines are destined to be used in a population that includes women of child-bearing potential. Therefore most vaccines need to be tested for adverse effects on reproduction and development [70]. The general approach taken is that the benefit of vaccination among pregnant women usually outweighs the risk for potential adverse effects on the mother or developing offspring when the risk for disease exposure is high, infection poses a special risk to mother or fetus, and the vaccine is unlikely to cause harm [71]. For example, live virus vaccines are not recommended for use in pregnant women because of the risk of viral transmission to the fetus. There is a continuing medical need for maternal immunization with vaccines that could prevent serious disease in the newborn, for example, group B streptococcal disease.

Currently, unless the vaccine is specifically indicated for maternal immunization, no data are collected regarding the vaccine's safety in pregnant women prior to licensing. Pregnant women are normally excluded from clinical trials, and therefore risk assessment for adverse effects on development is based on developmental toxicity studies in animals. The potential for adverse effects on fertility can also be assessed by careful examination of the reproductive tract tissues in the repeat-dose toxicity studies. Such preclinical data are used to inform the vaccine labeling regarding its use during pregnancy. FDA draft guidance on reproductive toxicity studies for prophylactic vaccines requires that the following be assessed: antibody production in the pregnant animal, antibody transfer from the pregnant female to the fetus, and the persistence and effects of the antibody response in the newborn. The FDA has issued guidance on study design and recommends an embryofetal development protocol that tests effects on the pregnant/lactating female, embryonic and fetal development, and pre- and postnatal development up to weaning (Table 31.1). For embryofetal toxicity studies it is recommended to include a group with immunizations prior to mating in order to achieve antibody exposure during the entire embryofetal period [63]. Vaccination should also take place during pregnancy. Postmating immunization is recommended for females that are not submitted to caesarean for fetal examination. Pups from these immunized dams are necropsied at the end of the lactation period.

The FDA is proposing to amend its labeling regulations and require that a summary assessment of the risks of using a product during pregnancy and lactation be included. This summary would enable a wider discussion of the animal and any human data available.

Biodistribution and Integration Assays   An additional specialized GLP study is normally required to evaluate the dissemination and persistence of DNA plasmid and viral vector-based vaccines. These are termed biodistribution studies, and they track the levels of vector in a panel of tissues at varying times following dosing of vaccine on a single occasion by the clinical route. Mouse, rabbit, and minipig have been used for this purpose [72]. Necropsies are performed at staggered timepoints (e.g., 1 day, 14 day, 28 day, 56 day, and 140 day) and need to be carefully carried out following special precautions to avoid cross-contamination of residual plasmid between tissues [73]. A recommended panel of tissues to be collected as frozen specimens is now provided in the recent FDA guidelines for DNA vaccines and includes blood, heart, brain, liver, kidney, bone marrow, ovaries, testes, lung, draining lymph nodes, spleen, and muscle or skin at the site of administration and subcutis at the injections site (Table 31.1).

Briefly, DNA is extracted from these tissues, and the copy number of vector per microgram of genomic DNA is determined by a sensitive assay, for example, quantitive PCR (Q-PCR). For many of these types of products, wide dissemination to many organs is expected via the blood. This results in low levels of vector being detected at early time points (e.g., days 1–2) in many tissues, including blood, heart, liver, and reproductive organs [74]. However, at later time points (e.g., day 30) these tissues are generally negative as judged by a particular threshold of vector concentration (e.g., 100 copies/μg genomic DNA). In this case there is not considered to be any safety concern. However, persistence above this threshold level at the last time point of the study (e.g., day 140) in any tissue including administration site raises the possibility that the vector will have integrated into genomic DNA at significant levels and thus caused insertional mutagenesis. An alternative explanation is that the vector is persisting episomally and does not represent a risk of mutagenesis. To distinguish between these two explanations, companies are requested to test for integration if plasmid persists in any tissue at levels exceeding 30,000 copies/μg genomic DNA by study termination. Developing a robust and sensitive assay has proved difficult, and there are a number of imperfect options from which to select. In principle, the simplest assay consists of gel purification of genomic DNA using size exclusion in an effort to remove low molecular weight DNA, which contains nonintegrated vector [39]. To confirm a positive result in this assay that is due to integrated vector and not contamination with free vector, an additional assay, the repeat-anchored integration-capture (RAIC) PCR, can be used to confirm genomic insertion sites [40]. To enable risk assessment, the copy number of plasmid persistence should be compared to the spontaneous mutation rate. Literature and regulatory agency experience is developing in this area, and there is now an improved understanding of the biological significance of persistent plasmid DNA.

Virulence and Potency Testing Live attenuated viral vaccines are considered to have a theoretical risk of reversion to virulence that needs to be tested. This is done by monitoring genetic or phenotypic markers of attenuation or virulence and can include in vitro and in vivo potency tests [62].

31.6 CASE STUDIES FOR POTENTIAL HIV THERAPIES

While many infectious diseases are controlled by vaccination, there are other diseases where novel and safe vaccines are urgently required. The obvious example is HIV where no proven vaccination exists. Vaccination for HIV is a difficult prospect for several reasons: (1) it was never considered to be safe enough to trial a live-attenuated virus, (2) effective vaccination requires other approaches than envelope-only constructs, (3) because of the genetic drift of the virus it is unlikely that single variants will be effective, (4) transmission of infection tends to occur from cell to cell contact rather than by free virus particles, and finally (5) there are no relevant animal models [75]. A number of potential vaccine strategies have been evaluated both preclinically and clinically and are discussed below.

31.6.1 Synthetic Peptide

An HIV-1 p17-based synthetic peptide (HGB-30) coupled to a carrier protein (KLH, keyhole limpet hemocyanin) has been administered with alum as an adjuvant [75]. The potential toxicity of HGB30-KLH/alum (HGB-30) was assessed in a number of species. In mice, guinea pigs, and goats the safety evaluation was limited to clinical observations. In chimpanzees, in addition to clinical observations, clinical pathology was also assessed, and in rabbits, dogs and cynomolgus monkeys, autopsies were conducted in addition to the other parameters mentioned above. In general, animals were immunized subcutaneously at doses ranging from 20 to 1000 μg/kg HGB-30 at 2- to 8-week intervals for a total of 2 immunizations. No toxicity or mortality was observed in any of the species. In some cases when the vaccine was administered in Freund's adjuvant, abscesses and/or hypersensitivity reactions occurred and were considered to be related to this adjuvant, particularly as no skin reactions were observed when alum was substituted for Freund's adjuvant. A longer term study (up to 1 year) was carried out in cynomolgus monkeys and chimpanzees. No toxicity was seen following a total of 6 to 8 immunizations. The immune response to the vaccine was also evaluated, and antibodies to HGB-30 were observed in all species by 4 weeks after a booster immunization. T cell proliferative responses to HGB-30 in mice were variable but did reach statistical significance in at least one experiment and CTL responses were inconsistent.

The phase 1 clinical trial for HGB-30 consisted of 18 seronegative healthy volunteers (6/group) who were administered 10, 20, or 50 μg of the vaccine at 0, 6, and 14 weeks. Physical examinations and blood analyses were performed, and all subjects were followed for 1 year. Initial results indicated that the vaccine was not associated with any adverse effects. Similarly to that observed in mice and chimpanzees, antibodies to HGP-30 were observed in volunteers. Since T cell proliferative responses are considered to be optimal with fresh cells, extensive studies were carried out on one volunteer's peripheral blood lymphocytes. Increased T cell proliferation was observed. The T cell proliferation was maximal 6 weeks after the third immunization but then declined at 6 months after the third immunization.

31.6.2 DNA Plasmid

Another strategy for HIV vaccination is the use of DNA plasmid encoding various HIV-1 genes. Different plasmids ranging from the simplest encoding for the Clade B gag gene only, to a combination of six plasmids including Clade B env gene, Clade B gag-pol-nef genes, Clade C gag-pol-nef fusion protein, env protein for Clade C, gag-pol-nef fusion protein for Clade A, and env protein for Clade A were evaluated in repeat-dose toxicity and biodistribution studies [12,76]. These clades represent different HIV subtypes and are prevalent in different areas. For example, Clade C is the most prevalent subtype and predominates in sub-Saharan Africa and Asia [56]. One of the HIV DNA plasmids also contained a cytokine adjuvant (IL-2). In addition plasmids for Ebola, the severe acute respiratory syndrome (SARS) virus, and the West Nile virus were also evaluated in this report.

The repeat-dose toxicity and biodistribution studies were designed to support a phase 1 clinical trial in human subjects. The DNA plasmid was intramuscularly injected using a device called the Biojector 2000 at doses of up to 8 mg/dose DNA plasmid at 3 intervals (0, 1, and 2 months). The Biojector is a needle-free injection system for intramuscular (IM) and subcutaneous (SC) injections of liquid medications including vaccines. In general, rabbits were injected (using the Biojector) with either 3 (to mimic the clinical plan) or 4 immunizations ($N + 1$ in line with current FDA regulatory standards). The dose levels were either 4 or 8 mg, and the rabbits were dosed with one of the different HIV DNA plasmids every 4 weeks. The standards parameters (clinical observations, body weight and food consumption determination, ophthalmoscopy, clinical pathology, organ weight measurements, and gross and microscopic pathologic evaluations) were included in the repeat-dose toxicity study. Animals were necropsied approximately 2 weeks after the final immunization. Treatment-related findings were limited to the injection site and consisted of mild to moderate irritation or inflammation and were recoverable. All other changes were considered to be incidental and not related to treatment.

The biodistribution study evaluated the same DNA plasmids. In one series of studies, 6- to 7-week-old Hsd:ICR (CD-1) mice were administered 100 μg DNA plasmid vaccine by either the IM or intravenous (IV) route. Animals were dosed once and then necropsied (5/sex/group for treated and 1/sex/group for control) on study days 8 and 50. A number of organs including gonads, liver, heart, brain, kidney, lymph nodes, injection site (muscle), lung, bone marrow, and heart were collected for Q-PCR analysis. In a second series of studies, 12- to 13-week old New Zealand white rabbits (same number/group as with the mouse study) were dosed with 2 mg of DNA plasmid delivered IM by the Biojector device. Animals were terminated approximately 1 week and 1 and 2 months after a single injection. A number of organs (similar to the mouse study but including adrenal glands and thymus) were collected for Q-PCR analysis. In a third study, 6- to 7-week-old CD-1 mice were inoculated with 100 µg DNA plasmid intramuscularly, and 28 days later injected muscles were harvested and assessed for possible integration of the DNA plasmid. Results showed that for the most part, plasmids remained at or near the injection site and did not distribute widely throughout the body. Sporadic low-level signals (hundreds to at most thousands of copies) were detected in other tissues in some rabbits, whereas tens of thousands to millions of copies/µg DNA were seen at the injection site. The signal at the injection site steadily decreased 1 and 2 months postdose to a few hundred copies/µg DNA at the 2-month time point. This distribution pattern was observed for all of the different DNA plasmids (including Ebola, SARs, and West Nile virus) tested regardless of backbone, promoters, or gene inserts. Finally no integration was noted in the integration study. These findings show that DNA plasmids are well tolerated, do not distribute widely, and do not appear to integrate into the genome.

31.6.3 Mixed Modality

Investigators are currently assessing the potential safety and efficacy of a mixed modality treatment regimen (i.e., combining a DNA vaccine with a viral vector). In this example preclinical toxicity and biodistribution studies were conducted in mice using a DNA vaccine in combination with a modified vaccinia virus Ankara based HIV vaccine to support a phase 1 trial in healthy HIV-1-uninfected volunteers [77,78].

In this example the DNA vaccine (pTHr·HIVA) is based on a novel direct gene transfer vector pTH [77], and the second component, MVA-HIVA, is based on a modified vaccinia virus Ankara. Both of these components contain most of the HIV-1 clade A *gag* protein coupled to conserved HIV-1 clade A CTL epitopes arranged in a polypeptide string that served as the immunogen [77].

Balb/c mice about 6 to 7 weeks old were selected. Because the CTL epitope is recognized by this strain, Balb/c mice are considered a biologically relevant strain and species. A CTL response was confirmed in all mice following administration. Four groups of mice were assessed for toxicity (10/sex/group) and persistence (10/sex/group for treated mice and 3/sex/group for vehicle group). Mice were administered the vehicle, 2 doses (50 µg/dose) of DNA plasmid intramuscularly on days 29 and 43, 2 doses (10^6 pfu/dose) MVA intradermally on days 29 and 43, or a combination of DNA (on days 1 and 14, same dose) followed by 2 doses of MVA on days 29 and 43 at the same dose. The dose levels selected represented a safety margin of 1750-fold and 70-fold over the proposed clinical dose for DNA and MVA, respectively, based on body mass. All mice for the toxicity evaluation were necropsied on day 49/50. Parameters tested included mortality, clinical observations, local tolerance, ophthalmoscopy, body weight and food consumption, clinical pathology, organ weights, and gross and microscopic evaluation. In the persistence study, one vehicle-treated/sex and three vaccine-treated/sex were evaluated on days 46 and 78.

Remaining animals in the persistence study were retained for possible further assessment.

Treatment with DNA alone, MVA alone, and in combination was well tolerated in mice. Some of the local reactions observed were considered to be related to the injection procedure rather than to the vaccine components. Other findings were considered to be incidental in nature and not related to the vaccine treatment. Persistence was assessed by PCR, and results showed that positive signals were observed at the injection sites on both days 46 and 78. Equivocal positive results were observed in some mice (including vehicle controls) in a few other tissues, and these were most likely due to contamination and the high sensitivity of the PCR method. Since there was no persistence in any other tissue except for the injection site, no integration assays were carried out.

In summary, administration of DNA plasmid alone, MVA alone, and in combination revealed no adverse findings, and furthermore, with the exception of the injection sites, no persistence was noted in any organ including the gonads. For safety testing in the clinic, healthy HIV-1-uninfected volunteers (male and female) were recruited into one of three trials [78]. Women of childbearing potential were included in the trial if they were not pregnant (confirmed by urine test), were not lactating, and were willing to use an approved method of contraception from screening until four months after final vaccination. The contraceptive regimen was required for male volunteers as well.

Twenty-six volunteers were recruited. In the first trial, 18 volunteers received either a 100 µg or 500 µg dose of plasmid THr.HIVA DNA intramuscularly on two occasions (days 0 and 21). In the second trial, 8 volunteers were administered two intradermal injections on days 0 and 21 with 5×10^7 pfu MVA-HIVA, and then in the third trial, 9 volunteers from the first trial were boosted with two doses of MVA-HIVA (21 days apart) 9 to 14 months after their last vaccination with DNA. All volunteers were followed for up to six months to two years after the last vaccination.

In all three trials, the candidate vaccines were well tolerated alone and in combination. Clinical signs were limited to reactions (soreness, redness, etc.) at the intradermal injection site, and no adverse events were considered to be related to vaccine treatment.

REFERENCES

1. O'Hagan DT, Rappuoli R. The safety of vaccines. *Drug Discov Today* 2004;9: 846–54.

2. Anonymous. United Nations Programme on HIV/AIDS. 2004 Report on the Global AIDS Epidemic, 2006. http://www.unaids.org

3. Gomez-Roman VR, Florese RH, Peng B, Montefiori DC, Kalyanaraman VS, Venzon D, Srivastava I, Barnett SW, Robert-Guroff M. An adenovirus-based HIV subtype B prime/boost vaccine regimen elicits antibodies mediating broad antibody-

dependent cellular cytotoxicity against non-subtype B HIV strains. *J Acquir Immune Defic Syndr* 2006;43:270–7.

4. Brennan FR, Dougan G. Non-clinical safety evaluation of novel vaccines and adjuvants: new products, new strategies. *Vaccine* 2005;23:3210–22.

5. Piedra PA. Clinical experience with respiratory syncytial virus vaccines. *Pediatr Infect Dis J* 2003;22:S94–9.

6. Bussiere JL, McCormick GC, Green JD. Preclinical safety assessment considerations in vaccine development. *Pharm Biotechnol* 1995;6: 61–79.

7. Perrie Y. Vaccines: an overview and update. *Pharmaceut* 2006;276:209–12.

8. Strom J. Further experience of reactions, especially of a cerebral nature, in conjunction with triple vaccination: a study based on vaccinations in Sweden 1959–65. *Br Med J* 1967;4:320–3.

9. Stewart GT. Toxicity of pertussis vaccine. *Lancet* 1977;310:1130.

10. Dreesman GR, Hollinger FB, Sanchez Y, Oefinger P, Melnick JL. Immunization of chimpanzees with hepatitis B virus-derived polypeptides, *Infect Immun* 1981;32: 62–7.

11. Grotto I, Mandel Y, Ephros M, Ashkenazi I, Shemer J. Major adverse reactions to yeast-derived hepatitis B vaccines—a review. *Vaccine* 1998;16:329–34.

12. Sheets RL, Stein J, Manetz TS, Andrews C, Bailer R, Rathmann J, Gomez PL. Toxicological safety evaluation of DNA plasmid vaccines against HIV-1, ebola, severe acute respiratory syndrome, or West Nile virus is similar despite differing plasmid backbones or gene-inserts. *Toxicol Scis* 2006;91:620–30.

13. Hayrinen J, Pelkonen S, Finne J. Structural similarity of the type-specific group B streptococcal polysaccharides and the carbohydrate units of tissue glycoproteins: evaluation of possible cross-reactivity. *Vaccine* 1989;7:217–24.

14. Hemmer B, Gran B, Zhao Y, Marques A, Pascal J, Tzou A, Kondo T, Cortese I, Bielekova B, Straus SE, McFarland HF, Houghten R, Simon R, Pinilla C, Martin R. Identification of candidate T-cell epitopes and molecular mimics in chronic Lyme disease. *Nat Med* 1999;5:1375–82.

15. Coquillat D, Bruge J, Danve B, Latour M, Hurpin C, Schulz D, Durbec P, Rougon G. Activity and cross-reactivity of antibodies induced in mice by immunization with a group B meningococcal conjugate. *Infect Immun* 2001;69:7130–9.

16. Boisgerault F, Moron G, Leclerc C. Virus-like particles: a new family of delivery systems. *Expert Rev Vaccines* 2002;1:101–9.

17. Anonymous. Gardasil product description, 2006. http://www.fda.gov/cber/products/hpvmer060806.htm

18. Donnelly JJ, Ulmer JB, Shiver JW, Liu MA. DNA vaccines. *Annu Rev Immunol* 1997;15:617–48.

19. Snodin DJ, Ryle PR. Understanding and applying regulatory guidance on the nonclinical development of biotechnology-derived pharmaceuticals. *Bio Drugs* 2006;20:25–52.

20. Liu MA. DNA vaccines: a review. *J Intern Med* 2003;253:402–10.

21. Klinman DM, Takeno M, Ichino M, Gu M, Yamshchikov G, Mor G, Conover J. DNA vaccines: safety and efficacy issues. *Springer Semin Immunopathol* 1997;19: 245–56.

22. Parker SE, Borellini F, Wenk ML, Hobart P, Hoffman SL, Hedstrom R, Le T, Norman JA. Plasmid DNA malaria vaccine: tissue distribution and safety studies in mice and rabbits, *Hum Gene Ther* 1999;10:741–58.

23. Schalk JA, Mooi FR, Berbers GA, van Aerts LA, Ovelgonne H, Kimman TG. Pre-clinical and clinical safety studies on DNA vaccines. *Hum Vaccines* 2006;2:45–53.

24. Smith HA, Klinman DM. The regulation of DNA vaccines. *Curr Opin Biotechnol* 2001;12:299–303.

25. Donnelly J, Berry K, Ulmer JB. Technical and regulatory hurdles for DNA vaccines. *Int J Parasitol* 2003;33:457–67.

26. Krieg AM, Yi AK, Matson S, Waldschmidt TJ, Bishop GA, Teasdale R, Koretzky GA, Klinman DM. CpG motifs in bacterial DNA trigger direct B-cell activation. *Nature* 1995;374:546–9.

27. Davis HL, Weeratna R, Waldschmidt TJ, Tygrett L, Schorr J, Krieg AM. CpG DNA is a potent enhancer of specific immunity in mice immunized with recombinant hepatitis B surface antigen. *J Immunol* 1998;160:870–6.

28. Halpern MD, Kurlander RJ, Pisetsky DS. Bacterial DNA induces murine inter-feron-gamma production by stimulation of interleukin-12 and tumor necrosis factor-alpha. *Cell Immunol* 1996;167:72–8.

29. Klinman DM, Yi AK, Beaucage SL, Conover J, Krieg AM. CpG motifs present in bacteria DNA rapidly induce lymphocytes to secrete interleukin 6, interleukin 12, and interferon gamma, *Proc Natl Acad Sci USA* 1996;93:2879–83.

30. Gilkeson GS, Ruiz P, Howell D, Lefkowith JB, Pisetsky DS. Induction of immune-mediated glomerulonephritis in normal mice immunized with bacterial DNA. *Clin Immunol Immunopathol* 1993;68: 283–92.

31. Gilkeson GS, Pippen AM, Pisetsky DS. Induction of cross-reactive anti-dsDNA antibodies in preautoimmune NZB/NZW mice by immunization with bacterial DNA. *J Clin Invest* 1995;95:1398–1402.

32. Parker SE, Monteith D, Horton H, Hof R, Hernandez P, Vilalta A, Hartikka J, Hobart P, Bentley CE, Chang A, Hedstrom R, Rogers WO, Kumar S, Hoffman SL, Norman JA. Safety of a GM-CSF adjuvant-plasmid DNA malaria vaccine. *Gene Ther* 2001;8:1011–23.

33. Choi SM, Lee DS, Son MK, Sohn YS, Kang KK, Kim CY, Kim BM, Kim WB. Safety evaluation of GX-12: A new DNA vaccine for HIV infection in rodents. *Drug Chem Toxicol* 2003;26:271–84.

34. Xiang ZQ, Spitalnik SL, Cheng J, Erikson J, Wojczyk B, Ertl HC. Immune responses to nucleic acid vaccines to rabies virus. *Virology* 1995;209:569–79.

35. Tuomela M, Malm M, Wallen M, Stanescu I, Krohn K, Peterson P. Biodistribution and general safety of a naked DNA plasmid, GTU-MultiHIV, in a rat, using a quantitative PCR method. *Vaccine* 2005;23:890–6.

36. Liu MA, McClements W, Ulmer JB, Shiver J, Donnelly J. Immunization of non-human primates with DNA vaccines. *Vaccine* 1997;15:909–12.

37. Wolff JA, Ludtke JJ, Acsadi G, Williams P, Jani A. Long-term persistence of plasmid DNA and foreign gene expression in mouse muscle. *Hum Mol Genet* 1992;1: 363–9.

38. Ledwith BJ, Manam S, Troilo PJ, Barnum AB, Pauley CJ, Griffiths TG, Harper LB, Schock HB, Zhang H, Faris JE, Way PA, Beare CM, Bagdon WJ, Nichols WW.

Plasmid DNA vaccines: assay for integration into host genomic DNA. *Dev Biol* 2000;104:33–43.

39. Ledwith BJ, Manam S, Troilo PJ, Barnum AB, Pauley CJ, Griffiths TG, Harper LB, Beare CM, Bagdon WJ, Nichols WW. Plasmid DNA vaccines: investigation of integration into host cellular DNA following intramuscular injection in mice. *Intervirology* 2000;43:258–72.

40. Wang Z, Troilo PJ, Wang X, Griffiths TG, Pacchione SJ, Barnum AB, Harper LB, Pauley CJ, Niu Z, Denisova L, Follmer TT, Rizzuto G, Ciliberto G, Fattori E, Monica NL, Manam S, Ledwith BJ. Detection of integration of plasmid DNA into host genomic DNA following intramuscular injection and electroporation. *Gene Ther* 2004;11:711–21.

41. Liu MA, Ulmer JB. Human clinical trials of plasmid DNA vaccines. *Adv Genet* 2005;55:25–40.

42. Dean HJ. Epidermal delivery of protein and DNA vaccines. *Expert Opin Drug Deliv* 2005;2:227–36.

43. Montgomery DL, Ulmer JB, Donnelly JJ, Liu MA. DNA vaccines. *Pharmacol Therapeut* 1997;74:195–205.

44. Fuller DH, Loudon P, Schmaljohn C. Preclinical and clinical progress of particle-mediated DNA vaccines for infectious diseases. *Methods* 2006;40: 86–97.

45. Roy MJ, Wu MS, Barr LJ, Fuller JT, Tussey LG, Speller S, Culp J, Burkholder JK, Swain WF, Dixon RM, Widera G, Vessey R, King A, Ogg G, Gallimore A, Haynes JR, Heydenburg FD. Induction of antigen-specific CD8+ T cells, T helper cells, and protective levels of antibody in humans by particle-mediated administration of a hepatitis B virus DNA vaccine. *Vaccine* 2000;19:764–78.

46. Swain WE, Heydenburg FD, Wu MS, Barr LJ, Fuller JT, Culp J, Burkholder J, Dixon RM, Widera G, Vessey R, Roy MJ. Tolerability and immune responses in humans to a PowderJect DNA vaccine for hepatitis B. *Dev Biol* 2000;104:115–9.

47. Tatsis N, Ertl HC. Adenoviruses as vaccine vectors. *Mol Ther* 2004;10:616–29.

48. Basak SK, Kiertscher SM, Harui A, Roth MD. Modifying adenoviral vectors for use as gene-based cancer vaccines. *Viral Immunol* 2004;17:182–96.

49. Anonymous. Assessment of adenoviral vector safety and toxicity: report of the National Institutes of Health Recombinant DNA Advisory Committee. *Hum Gene Ther* 2002;13:3–13.

50. Fitzgerald JC, Gao GP, Reyes-Sandoval A, Pavlakis GN, Xiang ZQ, Wlazlo AP, Giles-Davis W, Wilson JM, Ertl HC. A simian replication-defective adenoviral recombinant vaccine to HIV-1 gag. *J Immunol* 2003;170:1416–22.

51. Polo JM, Dubensky TW, Jr. Virus-based vectors for human vaccine applications. *Drug Discov Today* 2002;7:719–27.

52. Zhou D, Cun A, Li Y, Xiang Z, Ertl HC. A chimpanzee-origin adenovirus vector expressing the rabies virus glycoprotein as an oral vaccine against inhalation infection with rabies virus. *Mol Ther* 2006;14:662–72.

53. Farina SF, Gao GP, Xiang ZQ, Rux JJ, Burnett RM, Alvira MR, Marsh J, Ertl HC, Wilson JM. Replication-defective vector based on a chimpanzee adenovirus. *J Virol* 2001;75:11603–13.

54. Berk AJ. *Adenoviruses In Encyclopaedia of Genetics*. San Diego: Academic Press, 2006;15–9.

55. Fattori E, Zampaglione I, Arcuri M, Meola A, Ercole BB, Cirillo A, Folgori A, Bett A, Cappelletti M, Sporeno E, Cortese R, Nicosia A, Colloca S. Efficient immunization of rhesus macaques with an HCV candidate vaccine by heterologous priming-boosting with novel adenoviral vectors based on different serotypes. *Gene Ther* 2006;13:1088–96.

56. Rasmussen RA, Ong H, Kittel C, Ruprecht CR, Ferrantelli F, Hu SL, Polacino P, McKenna J, Moon J, Travis B, Ruprecht RM. DNA prime/protein boost immunization against HIV clade C: safety and immunogenicity in mice. *Vaccine* 2006;24: 2324–32.

57. Singh M, O'Hagan DT. Recent advances in vaccine adjuvants. *Pharmaceut Res* 2002;19:715–28.

58. Brewer JM. (How) do aluminium adjuvants work? *Immunology Let* 2006;102: 10–15.

59. Pichyangkul S, Gettayacamin M, Miller RS, Lyon JA, Angov E, Tongtawe P, Ruble DL, Heppner DG, Jr., Kester KE, Ballou WR, Diggs CL, Voss G, Cohen JD, Walsh DS. Pre-clinical evaluation of the malaria vaccine candidate P. falciparum MSP1(42) formulated with novel adjuvants or with alum. *Vaccine* 2004;22: 3831–40.

60. Sesardic D. Regulatory considerations on new adjuvants and delivery systems. *Vaccine* 2006;24(Suppl 2):S2–S7.

61. Goldenthal KL, Cavagnaro JA, Alving CR, Vogel FR. Safety evaluation of vaccine adjuvants. National Cooperative Vaccine Development Working Group. *AIDS Res Hum Retroviruses* 1993;9:S45–S49.

62. Lebron JA, Wolf JJ, Kaplanski CV, Ledwith BJ. Ensuring the quality, potency and safety of vaccines during preclinical development. *Expert Rev Vaccines* 2005;4: 855–66.

63. Verdier F, Morgan L. Predictive value of pre-clinical work for vaccine safety assessment. *Vaccine* 2001;20:S21–S23.

64. Kennedy RC, Shearer MH, Hildebrand W. Nonhuman primate models to evaluate vaccine safety and immunogenicity. *Vaccine* 1997;15:903–8.

65. Boyson JE, Shufflebotham C, Cadavid LF, Urvater JA, Knapp LA, Hughes AL, Watkins DI. The MHC class I genes of the rhesus monkey: different evolutionary histories of MHC class I and II genes in primates. *J Immunol* 1996;156:4656–65.

66. Garcon N, Heppner DG, Cohen J. Development of RTS,S/AS02: a purified subunit-based malaria vaccine candidate formulated with a novel adjuvant. *Expert Rev Vaccines* 2003;2:231–8.

67. Anonymous. OECD guideline for testing of chemicals No. 404, 2006. http://www. oecd.org/

68. Chabicovsky M, Ryle P. Non-clinical development of cancer vaccines: regulatory considerations, *Regul Toxicol Pharmacol* 2006;44:226–37.

69. Callahan SM, Ming X, Lu SK, Brunner LJ, Croyle MA. Considerations for use of recombinant adenoviral vectors: Dose effect on hepatic cytochromes P450. *J Pharmacol Exp Therapeut* 2005;312:492–501.

70. Verdier F, Barrow PC, Burge J. Reproductive toxicity testing of vaccines. *Toxicology* 2003;185:213–9.

71. Gruber MF. Maternal immunization: US FDA regulatory considerations. *Vaccine* 2003;21:3487–91.

72. Leamy VL, Martin T, Mahajan R, Vilalta A, Rusalov D, Hartikka J, Bozoukova V, Hall KD, Morrow J, Rolland AP, Kaslow DC, Lalor PA. Comparison of rabbit and mouse models for persistence analysis of plasmid-based vaccines. *Hum Vaccines* 2006;2:113–8.

73. Haworth R, Pilling AM. The PCR assay in the preclinical safety evaluation of nucleic acid medicines. *Hum Exp Toxicol* 2000;19:267–76.

74. Vilalta A, Mahajan RK, Hartikka J, Rusalov D, Martin T, Bozoukova V, Leamy V, Hall K, Lalor P, Rolland A, Kaslow DC. I. Poloxamer-formulated plasmid DNA-based human cytomegalovirus vaccine: evaluation of plasmid DNA biodistribution/persistence and integration. *Hum Gene Ther* 2005;16:1143–50.

75. Naylor PH, Sztein MB, Wada S, Maurer S, Holterman D, Kirkley JE, Naylor CW, Zook BC, Hitzelberg RA, Gibbs CJ, Jr. Preclinical and clinical studies on immunogenicity and safety of the HIV-1 p17-based synthetic peptide AIDS vaccine—HGP-30-KLH. *Int J Immunopharmacol* 1991;13(Suppl 1):117–27.

76. Sheets RL, Stein J, Manetz TS, Duffy C, Nason M, Andrews C, Kong WP, Nabel GJ, Gomez PL. Biodistribution of DNA plasmid vaccines against HIV-1, ebola, severe acute respiratory syndrome, or West Nile virus is similar, without integration, despite differing plasmid backbones or gene inserts. *Toxicol Scis* 2006;91:610–9.

77. Hanke T, McMichael AJ, Samuel RV, Powell LA, McLoughlin L, Crome SJ, Edlin A. Lack of toxicity and persistence in the mouse associated with administration of candidate DNA- and modified vaccinia virus Ankara (MVA)-based HIV vaccines for Kenya. *Vaccine* 2002;21:108–14.

78. Cebere I, Dorrell L, McShane H, Simmons A, McCormack S, Schmidt C, Smith C, Brooks M, Roberts JE, Darwin SC, Fast PE, Conlon C, Rowland-Jones S, McMichael AJ, Hanke T. Phase I clinical trial safety of DNA- and modified virus Ankara-vectored human immunodeficiency virus type 1 (HIV-1) vaccines administered alone and in a prime-boost regime to healthy HIV-1-uninfected volunteers. *Vaccine* 2006;24:417–25.

Preclinical Safety Evaluation of Biopharmaceuticals

MERCEDES A. SERABIAN, MS, DABT, and YING HUANG, PhD

Contents

Preclinical Safety Evaluation of Biopharmaceuticals: A Science-Based Approach to Facilitating Clinical Trials, edited by Joy A. Cavagnaro
Copyright © 2008 by John Wiley & Sons, Inc.

32.1 INTRODUCTION

New discoveries in the field of gene therapy are occurring at a rapid pace, resulting in the identification of genes that contribute in some way to a particular disease or abnormal medical condition. Although marketed therapies may exist for many of these diseases, such as hemophilia or some forms of cancer, these pharmaceuticals can only treat the symptoms of the disease but cannot cure it. The hope of those working in the field of gene therapy is that the products that result from these discoveries will ultimately result in effective treatments, even cures, for many diseases or conditions that arise due to defective genes. The goal is the development of novel vectors engineered to express the "good" genes and delivered to the appropriate targets in the human body, where they will hopefully correct the medical condition for the person's lifetime or for a short period of time, as needed.

There is a scientific process by which to achieve this goal. This pathway involves the application of in vitro and in vivo preclinical studies (Figure 32.1) to generate data to support use of these novel therapeutic agents in humans. Preclinical studies for any experimental pharmaceutical agent, including gene therapy products, are conducted to provide better scientific insight into the potential pharmacologic and toxiologic effects that may result from the administration of the agent in humans. These studies are critical for helping to define the risk–benefit ratio of the experimental agent of interest in the desired clinical population, both prior to initiation of a clinical trial and throughout the development program for the pharmaceutical agent. Early-phase clinical trial design

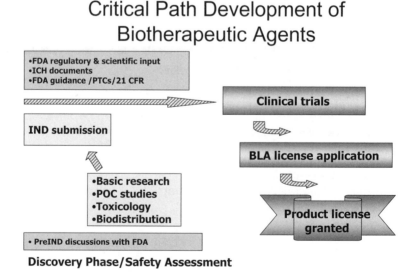

Figure 32.1 Critical path development of gene therapy products in the United States.

can be constrained by inadequate preclinical testing of the investigational product. This chapter provides a perspective of the preclinical assessment of gene therapy products intended for clinical use in therapeutic indications.

32.2   DEFINITION OF GENE THERAPY

Gene therapy is a medical intervention based on the modification of the genetic material (DNA or RNA) of living cells. This intervention can involve the ex vivo modification of autologous, allogeneic, or xenogeneic cells, using replication-deficient viral vectors or nonviral vectors (e.g., plasmid DNA) for subsequent administration into humans, or the intervention may involve the direct in vivo administration of the gene therapy product into humans [1]. According to the scientific literature, experimental human gene therapy is currently being tested for the treatment of various genetic disorders, among these (1) diseases due to inborn errors in a single defective gene, such as severe combined immunodeficiency (SCID), hemophilia, or muscular dystrophy; (2) polygenic diseases, such as diabetes mellitus or coronary heart disease; and (3) acquired genetic diseases, such as cancer or rheumatoid arthritis. Theoretical approaches to correcting faulty genes include (1) insertion of a normal gene into a nonspecific location on the genome to replace a nonfunctional gene, (2) exchanging an abnormal gene for a normal gene through homologous recombination, (3) repair of the abnormal gene through selective reverse mutation that returns the gene to its normal function, or (4) the regulation of a particular gene (i.e., turning "on" or "off").

Only oncolytic viruses that carry a heterologous transgene are defined as gene therapy products. Other oncolytic viruses, such as the naturally attenuated and genetically modified viruses, are classified as viral therapy; these viruses will be briefly discussed in this chapter. The desired property for all oncolytic viruses is the potential to lyse the target tumor cells, although some oncolytic viruses may display other biological effects due to the expressed transgene. All oncolytic viruses are designed or modified to selectively replicate in tumor cells, but with an attenuated viral life cycle in normal cells. This mechanism is usually achieved through the mutation of the viral coding genes that are critical for viral replication in normal cells, but spared in tumor cells, or through the control of viral early gene expression by using tumor-specific promoters. The cellular targets for oncolytic viruses can be cell surface molecules and antigens that are recognized by these viruses for viral entry as well as intracellular components that are responsible for the host interaction with the viral components involved in the viral life cycle [2].

32.3   MODE OF GENE TRANSFER

Two basic modes of gene transfer currently exist for gene therapy products, namely ex vivo or in vivo gene transfer. Ex vivo gene transfer is achieved by administering cells that are transduced with vectors that express the desired transgenes or tumor-associated antigens. A wide variety of somatic cells and hematopoietic cells can be transduced with viral vectors such as adenoviral and retroviral vectors. Certain types of somatic cells can be pulsed with naked DNA plasmid or transduced via a lipid/ligand DNA complex. Somatic cells can also be transduced with microorganism-based vectors, such as bacterial or yeast vectors. The transduced cells can then be administered via a route designed to deliver the gene therapy to the anatomic location where gene expression and the related biological activity are desired. In vivo gene transfer is the direct delivery of biological vectors and vector-based vaccines to the animal or patient. Direct injection can be in situ, which constitutes local delivery such as intratumoral injection, subcutanous injection, and others, or in vivo, which is direct systemic delivery (usually intravenous administration) into the individual.

32.4 DISTINCTIONS BETWEEN PREVENTIVE (PROPHYLACTIC) VIRAL AND PLASMID DNA VACCINES AND THERAPEUTIC GENE THERAPY PRODUCTS

Gene transfer products are used as therapeutic agents and as preventive vaccines. A preventive vaccine, consisting of a live-attenuated microorganism or virus, or plasmid DNA-based, is administered to elicit an immune response(s) that results in the prevention of infectious diseases in humans. On the other hand, a therapeutic vaccination with a gene therapy product is the transfer of a molecule with the intent to generate or intensify a host immune response to an antigen that is related to a disease already present in the patient. For therapeutic vaccines the immune response to the viral particles (i.e., neutralizing antibodies) should be avoided in order to achieve the desired effect in humans that is also safe. Although many of the scientific principles in this chapter can also be applied to viral or plasmid DNA vaccines used to prevent infectious diseases, the focus of this chapter is on the therapeutic gene therapy products that are being developed to treat established diseases (infectious or malignant).

32.5 HISTORICAL BACKGROUND OF GENE THERAPY PRODUCTS

The first gene therapy clinical trials in the United States began in the late 1980s with the ex vivo transduction of tumor-infiltrating lymphocytes (TIL) with a retroviral vector that carried the marker gene NeoR, administered to melanoma patients [3,4]. Another trial quickly followed in 1990, with the injection of autologous lymphocytes that were ex vivo transduced with a retroviral vector expressing the ADA gene into a child with ADA-deficient SCID [5]. The first trial involving the direct injection of a DNA plasmid occurred in 1992 with administration of plasmid expressing HLA-B7 into HLA-B7 positive

Gene Therapy INDs/IDEs

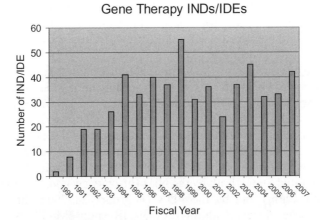

Figure 32.2 Number of applications submitted to the FDA for the conduct of clinical trials using gene therapy products for therapeutic indications (fiscal year encompasses October of the previous year to October of the next year).

tumors [6]. The first clinical trial using adenovirus vector occurred in cystic fibrosis patients in 1993 [7], and was extended to the use of adeno-associated vectors (AAV) in this patient population in 1995 [8]. This was followed by accelerated numbers of clinical trials with a variety of vectors, peaking in 1999. However, with the death of Jesse Gelsinger, a teenager with a mild ornithine transcarbamylase (OTC) deficiency, in September 1999 following the intrahepatic infusion of an adenoviral vector expressing a normal OTC gene and the subsequent regulatory and public scrutiny, the number of new gene therapy clinical trials initiated in the United States was notably reduced (Figure 32.2).

Following this incident, numerous public meetings were held in the United States to discuss inadequacies in the scientific, ethical, and regulatory oversight of clinical trials involving gene therapy. As a result in the United States these study protocols now have more regulatory oversight by FDA/CBER, as well as wider assurance of public exposure and scientific and ethical discussions regarding this area of medical research through the Office of Biotechnology Activities (OBA) at NIH. Many of these research protocols are discussed in a public forum by the NIH Recombinant DNA Advisory Committee (RAC; http://www4.od.nih.gov/oba/RAC/RAC_FAQS.htm). The gene therapy field began to recover when reports of some of the early clinical trials, such as the use of an AAV vector expressing factor IX for hemophilia [9] and an adenoviral oncolytic vector for the treatment of head and neck cancer [10] showed some preliminary evidence of activity. However, many gene therapy trials have ended at an early stage, primarily due to the lack of a lasting biological effect with few products reaching phase 3 clinical trials in the United States. With the exception of one gene therapy product, an adenoviral vector expressing the p53 gene (rAd-*p53*; Gendicine) that was approved in China in 2003 for the treatment of head and neck cancer [11] and a recombinant oncolytic adeno-virus (H101; Oncorine) that was approved in China in 2005 also for the treatment of head and neck cancer [12], there are currently no marketed products in the world.

Elsewhere the success of the administration of autologous hematopoietic cells transduced ex vivo with retrovirus expressing the γc gene for the treatment of children with SCID-X1 disease was reported in 2000 in a clinical trial in France [13]. Unfortunately, several years after administration of the gene therapy product, several children developed a leukemia-like syndrome that was attributed to the combination of the integrating retrovirus and the γc gene itself [14]. As in the aftermath of the Gelsinger death, many public discussionswere held in the United States, both by the NIH (http://www4.od.nih.gov/oba/RAC/SSMar05/index.htm) and by the FDA (February 28, 2003—http://www.fda.gov/ohrms/dockets/ac/cber03.html#BiologicalResponseModifiers; and March 4,2005—http://www.fda.gov/ohrms/dockets/ac//05/transcripts/2005-4093T2_02.htm). Although these events conclusively demonstrated the biological complexity of the gene therapies and the real potential for adverse effects in the clinical population, it did not halt the progression of other clinical trials that used other gene therapy approaches, and in fact catalyzed a move forward with the engineering and testing of potentially safer vectors based on the knowledge that was gained from analysis of these adverse events.

32.6 WORLDWIDE REGULATION OF GENE THERAPY PRODUCTS

As evidenced by the marketing approval of the gene therapy product Gendicine in China, clinical trials of gene therapy products is extending worldwide. Many regulatory bodies are now responsible for evaluating the safety and effectiveness of gene therapy products. In Europe, the European Medicines Agency (EMEA) plays a vital role in the marketing procedure for medicines in the European Union through the Committee for Medicinal Products for Human Use (CHMP). The EMEA/CHMP coordinates the evaluation and supervision of medicinal products via both "centralized (community)" and "decentralized (mutual-recognition)" mechanisms. One of the CHMP working parties, the Gene Therapy Working Party (GTWP), is responsible for providing recommendations to the CHMP on all matters that relate to gene therapy, including the development of regulatory guidance (http://www.emea.europa.eu/htms/human/genetherapy/genetherapy.htm).

Other European agencies that play a role in the regulation of gene therapy products in member states include the French Agency for the Sanitary Safety of Health Products (AFSSAPS; http://agmed.sante.gouv.fr/), the Gene Therapy Advisory Committee (GTAC) in the United Kingdom (www.doh.gov.uk/genetics/gtac/index.htm), and the Paul Erlich Institute in Germany (www.pei.de/themen/gentherapie/gene_therapy_reg.htm).

Regulatory bodies in Asia that evaluate gene therapy products include the Ministry of Health, Labour and Welfare (MHLW) (www.mhlw.go.jp/english) and the Pharmaceuticals and Medical Devices Agency (www.pmda.go.jp/index-e.html) in Japan, the Korean Food and Drug Administration (KFDA) in South Korea (www.kfda.go.kr), and the State Food and Drug Administration (SFDA) in China (www.sfda.gov.cn/eng).

The International Conference on Harmonisation (ICH) has officially recognized the rapidly progressing area of gene therapy through the creation of the Gene Therapy Discussion Group (GTDG), which is made up of regulatory and industry representatives from the United States, European Union, and Japan, as well as experts from Health Canada, WHO, and the European Free Trade Association (EFTA). This group is charged with the monitoring of emerging scientific issues related to gene therapy and communicating principles that may benefit the harmonization of the regulation of gene therapy products through public ICH workshops, and a publicly accessible ICH gene therapy web page containing ICH press statements, GTDG meeting minutes, ICH documents related to gene therapy and links to other major gene therapy public workshops. (http://www.ich.org/cache/html/1386-272-1.htm). In addition the World Health Organization (WHO) has also published guidelines for the nonclinical safety of DNA vaccines (http://www.who.int/).

32.7 COMPLIMENTARY ROLES OF THE FOOD AND DRUG ADMINISTRATION (FDA) AND RECOMBINANT DNA ADVISORY COMMITTEE (RAC) IN GENE THERAPY

The FDA and the National Institutes of Health (NIH) in the United States have complimentary responsibilities with respect to the regulation of human gene therapy. The NIH, through the Office of Biotechnology Activities (OBA), is mandated by Congress to review all clinical trials conducted using gene therapy (1) if the sponsor of the research or the institution where the trial will be conducted receives any money from NIH for DNA research and/or (2) if the institution that develops the product receives funding from NIH for recombinant DNA research. The DNA Recombinant Advisory Committee (RAC), under the purview of OBA, consists of a review panel of up to 21 experts and serves an advisory role to the NIH director and to OBA. The RAC holds regular public meetings to discuss proposed gene therapy trials and issues, focusing on the scientific, safety, and ethical issues involved. Material submitted to the RAC are available for public view [15]. The RAC has no regulatory oversight; this function is held exclusively by the FDA.

The FDA is mandated by US statue as the regulatory body that is responsible for the oversight of pharmaceuticals (including biologics) [16,17]. FDA's primary role is to ensure that manufacturers produce high-quality, safe, and efficacious biologics, drugs, and devices that are properly studied in human subjects prior to approval for commercial marketing. The FDA Center for

Biologics Evaluation and Research (CBER) is responsible for the regulatory review of gene therapy products. All clinical trials conducted in the United States that involve the administration of investigative gene therapy products must be reviewed by CBER. Sponsors of experimental gene therapy products must file a "Notice of Claimed Investigational Exemption for a New Drug" (IND) with the FDA. This regulatory body is responsible for determining whether a particular gene therapy product may be administered to humans as defined by the proposed clinical trial protocol [18]. FDA requires the submission of preclinical data to support the planned clinical trial (21 CFR 312.23), which allow the FDA reviewers to conduct independent reviews to assess the safety of each respective gene therapy product. Unlike the RAC review, the FDA's review is not conducted in a public forum and all information submitted to FDA is confidential (http://www.fda.gov/cber/gene.htm).

32.8 VECTORS USED IN GENE THERAPY PRODUCTS

Gene therapy is one of the most rapidly evolving areas of clinical research. There are a large and increasing number of different vector types that are currently being studied in animals and/or in humans. Many of these vectors are engineered to carry specific genetic material into the cells or tissues of individuals with a myriad of diseases, while others are designed to kill cancer cells by their pathogenic nature alone. The fundamental challenges to generating an effective gene therapy vector for treating diseases are accomplishing efficient gene delivery, obtaining biologically relevant levels of transgene expression in the desired target cell(s), and maintaining expression of the transgene without interfering with host gene expression.

Presented below are summary descriptions of gene therapy vector types that are most representative of the products administered in clinical trials.

32.8.1 Nonviral Vectors

A nonviral vector consists of "naked" plasmid (plasmid DNA alone) or plasmid DNA formulated with other entities designed to assist cell entry of the DNA complex via various mechanisms such as endocytosis; frequently these formulations include an artificial lipid sphere with an aqueous core (liposomes), basic proteins, receptor ligands, or polymers. Generally, nonviral vectors have shown safety advantages over viral vectors because of the reduced cytotoxicity, pathogenicity, and potential for insertional mutagenesis. Potential safety concerns for nonviral vectors include (1) DNA tissue biodistribution and any subsequent adverse biological effects, (2) the potential for insertional mutagenesis mediated by the elements incorporated in the plasmid backbone sequence, (3) clinical toxicities from the formulated plasmid DNA product, (4) toxicities due to the delivery procedure of the plasmid DNA, and (5) toxicities

Nonviral Vectors—Plasmid DNA

Advantages

- Cells do not have to be dividing for transduction
- Episomal replication; low risk of insertional mutagenesis
- Can be directly transferred to host
- Can accommodate large genes

Disadvantages

- Transduction efficiency usually low—need lipid or other transfer technique (i.e., electroporation)
- Duration of expression is low (degradation of gene in cytoplasm)
- Potential interaction with normal cells
- Expression of foreign proteins—concern for autoimmunity

Figure 32.3   Characteristics of plasmid DNA nonviral vectors.

resulting from the expressed protein, such as autoimmunity. While the potential for insertional mutagenesis for plasmid vectors is a safety concern, it remains theoretical as there have been no reports of the occurrence of such an event as a result of the administration of nonviral gene therapy products in animals or humans. This is likely due to the mechanism of episomal replication mediated by the plasmid vector backbone, which contains elements that confer the two essential requirements for extrachromosomal stability: replication of the DNA during the cell cycle and segregation to daughter cells during mitosis [19]. Some characteristics of plasmid DNA as vectors are presented in Figure 32.3.

Plasmid DNA vectors are delivered mainly via direct injection, as the injected DNA can be taken up by a variety of targeted somatic cells, such as skeletal muscle and cardiac muscle. Despite direct injection the injected plasmid DNA retains the ability to distribute via hematogenous spread to nontarget tissues. This DNA biodistribution profile is usually assessed in preclinical studies. Persistence of the injected plasmid DNA at the injection site in rodents for greater than one year following intramuscular injection without chromosome integration has been reported [20]. Several physical methods have been developed to enhance the transfection of plasmid DNA delivered to local tissue. For example, electroporation, which is commonly used, involves the application of controlled electric pulses via a medical device delivered to the DNA injection site following plasmid administration in order to enhance the transfection of plasmid DNA and to contain the DNA at the injection site. The electroporation procedure itself can cause local toxicity such as muscle degeneration, thus the safety of the complete delivery procedure (i.e., device settings) should be assessed in animals.

The plasmid DNA is provided in a vehicle formulation to enable direct injection of the product in vivo. This vehicle may be as simple as phosphate-buffered saline, or it can be more complex; for example, cationic lipid–DNA complexes have been widely used in clinical trials. The potential toxicities of these formulations depend on the physical and chemical properties of the liposome(s) and on the potential interaction of these lipids with the plasmid DNA. Yew and Scheule reported that the body's response to cationic lipid–DNA complexes is highly dependent on both the dose level and the route of administration. High-dose levels of a cationic lipid–DNA complex administered intravenously in mice can activate the innate immune response, resulting in the induction of proinflammatory cytokines and immune cell activation, with lethality as the worst-case outcome. These investigators found that some of these reactions appeared to be related to the structure of the plasmid DNA that was formulated with the lipid [21]. Safety assessment is dependent on the type of lipid(s) that constitute the final DNA complex, the stability of the complex, the route of administration of the complex, and the dose levels administered.

32.8.2   Replication-Deficient Viral Vectors

Adenoviral Vectors   Adenoviral vectors (Ad) are one of the most extensively used viral vectors for ex vivo and in vivo gene transfer that have been studied for use in a diversity of diseases, including cancer. This is mainly due to the advantages these double-stranded DNA viruses have over other viral vectors, such as their high infectivity in certain species including humans, lack of direct virally mediated pathogenesis in their natural hosts including humans, and transduction of a wide spectrum of both proliferating and quiescent cell types. In addition the adenoviral genome remains episomal in the transduced cell, and thus does not have a propensity to integrate, greatly reducing the concerns of insertional mutagenesis. The replication-deficient state of frequently used Ad vectors is established by the deletion of critical viral regulatory genes such as E1 and E3. The deletion of these viral early genes also allows the vectors to accommodate significant lengths of heterologous transgene and promoter sequences to achieve the desired transgene expression. Several generations of replication-deficient Ad vectors have been developed, and the manufacturing process for some of them has been successfully scaled up for clinical use. The "first-generation" Ad vectors have the deletion of the early genes: E1-deleted or E1 and E3-deleted. The "second-generation" Ad vectors have the deletion of E2 and/or E4 genes, in addition to the deletion of E1 or E1 and E3. Helper-dependent Ad vectors have most of the Ad coding sequences deleted. These gutless vectors can be classified as "third-generation" Ad vectors.

Potential safety concerns for Ad vectors include (1) DNA tissue biodistribution and any subsequent adverse biological effects and (2) significant immune response and inflammatory response to the vector. Some characteristics of Ad vectors are presented in Figure 32.4. The use of nonhuman Ad vectors to circumvent the drawbacks of using human Ad vectors, such as an immune

Adenoviral Vectors

<u>Advantages</u>

- Cells do not have to be dividing for transduction
- Able to target cells bearing capsid receptors
- Wide range of tissue and host infectivity
- Episomal replication; low risk of insertional mutagenesis

<u>Disadvantages</u>

- Inflammatory immune response: capsid proteins, viral genes expressed by target cells
- Potential for recombination/complementation

Figure 32.4   Characteristics of adenoviral vectors.

response and an inflammatory response to the protein capsid that coats the virus and/or to the viral genes that are expressed by target cells, is emerging [22]. The safety and viral biodistribution for each type of Ad vector should be established prior to use in humans.

Adeno-associated Viral Vectors (AAV)   Wild-type AAV is a member of the *dependovirus* genus of the family *Parvoviridae*, and is a nonpathogenic human DNA virus. Multiple serotypes of these single-stranded DNA viruses have been identified, and neutralizing antibodies against the AAV capsid proteins are frequently detected in human serum. Recombinant AAV vectors (rAAV) contain no viral-coding sequence. In particular, they do not express Rep proteins that play a key role in the DNA replication, site-specific integration, and cellular growth inhibitory effects of AAV. Thus the transgene and the virus capsid are the only source of foreign antigens. The documented spread of rAAV to the gonadal tissues of various animal species and the presence of rAAV DNA in semen, peripheral blood, and sputum of human subjects injected with rAAV2 vectors raises the concern regarding the risk of rAAV dissemination to various human tissues, especially the reproductive organs [23].

Although AAV remains episomal in the transduced cell, thus reducing the concerns of insertional mutagenesis, the potential to randomly integrate into host DNA exists. There have been no reports of insertional mutagenesis and resulting tumorigenicity from human trials using rAAV-based gene therapy. Although tumors reported in a murine disease model were attributed to rAAV-based gene transfer, tumors in humans attributable to injected AAV vectors have not occurred [24]. The observed persistence of rAAV DNA sequences in human biological samples also raises concerns regarding the potential for horizontal transmission from the subjects injected with the vector and their family members and health care providers.

AAV Vectors

Advantages
- Cells do not have to be dividing for transduction
- No known pathology of wild-type AAV
- Able to target multiple cell types
- Episomal replication; low risk of insertional mutagenesis
- Long-term gene expression

Disadvantages
- Limitations in accommodating the size of heterogeneous sequence
- Potential for recombination and/or complementation
- Potential for immune response to capsid protein
- Unable to halt gene expression if toxicity occurs
- Potential for dissemination and germline transfer

Figure 32.5   Characteristics of adenoviral-associated viral (AAV) vectors.

Potential safety concerns for AAV vectors include (1) DNA tissue biodistribution and any subsequent adverse biological effects, (2) the potential for insertional mutagenesis and any subsequent adverse biological effects, and (3) the immune response to the vector. Some characteristics of AAV vectors are presented in Figure 32.5.

Retroviral and Lentiviral Vectors Recombinant retroviral vectors (*gammretrovirus* genus, *Retroviridae* family) can only transduce actively dividing cells such as hematopoietic cells and stem cells. Although engineered to be replication deficient, retroviral vectors can provide long-term expression because they efficiently and stably integrate into the host genome after the infection of host cells. However, safety concerns regarding the pathogenic potential of retroviral vectors exist: (1) the production of a replication competent retrovirus (RCR) and (2) the potential for insertional mutagenesis, resulting in oncogene activation. An instance where vector contaminated with RCR was injected into monkeys resulted in the development of a T cell lymphoma, presumably due to oncogene activation [25]. The recent findings in the clinical trial using ex vivo retrovirus transduced hematopoietic cells for the treatment of X-linked SCID, have provided the proof that (1) retroviral vector-derived DNA integrated into the cellular DNA of several subjects and (2) this integration resulted in several oncogenic events [26; NIH Recombinant DNA Advisory Committee Meeting, March 11, 2008]. Much scientific discussion on vector engineering to decrease the probability of recombination and insertional mutagenesis is ongoing. Considerations include (1) the use of self-inactivating (SIN) vectors that delete most of the U3 region of the 3′LTR (long terminal repeat) because this site harbors the major transcriptional functions of the retroviral genome, (2) development of vectors from non-oncogenic

Retroviral Vectors

Advantages
- Able to transduce dividing cells
- Stable, long-term gene integration into host genome
- High levels of gene expression

Disadvantages
- Target cells have to be actively dividing; low percentage of cells transduced
- Potential for contamination by RCR
- Potential for insertional mutagenesis
- Potential for germline transfer

Figure 32.6   Characteristics of retroviral vectors.

retroviruses (e.g., lentivirus), and (3) the incorporation of insulator sequences [27]. Additional potential safety concerns for retroviral vectors include (1) DNA tissue biodistribution and any subsequent adverse biological effects and (2) the potential for germline integration following in vivo gene transfer. Some characteristics of retroviral vectors are presented in Figure 32.6.

Lentiviruses (*lentivirus* genus, *Retroviridae* family) can originate from five serogroups: primates, sheep and goats, horses, cats, and cattle. The replication-defective, attenuated lentiviral vectors that have been administered to humans thus far are HIV based. The use of HIV as a basis for lentiviral vectors is attractive because it infects dividing, nondividing, and terminally differentiated cells; it can accommodate long sequences that are stably expressed due to integration into the cell chromosome; and it appears to be less immunogenic. With retroviral vectors, the product used to "treat" many diseases (e.g., severe combined immunodeficiency) is the ex vivo manipulation of stem cells because actively dividing cells are a prerequisite for successful retroviral vector transduction. However, this process is not necessary for lentiviral vectors; they can be administered by direct in vivo injection into humans. Lentiviral vectors carrying a specific transgene have been associated in the scientific literature with possible use in many diseases, such as metabolic diseases, cancer, and neurological diseases, among many others. For example, injection of a lentiviral vector expressing glial cell-derived neurotrophic factor (GDNF) into the striatum and substantia nigra of a rhesus monkey Parkinson disease model resulted in improvement of neurological function and prevention of nigrostriatal degeneration [28].

The lentiviral vectors have safety concerns similar to the retroviral vector-based gene therapy products: (1) the production of a replication competent lentivirus (RCL) during manufacturing and (2) the potential for insertional mutagenesis, resulting in oncogene activation. One concern unique to the lentiviral vectors is the possibility that the vector can be mobilized in vivo,

Lentiviral (HIV-based) Vectors

Advantages
- Infects dividing, nondividing, terminally differentiated cells
- Highly attenuated, SIN constructs
- Inserts into host genome like HIV; stable integration and long-term gene expression
- Less immunogenic

Disadvantages
- Generation of replication-competent virus (RCL)
- Viral mobilization in vivo; infection of human subject
- Unable to halt gene expression if toxicity occurs
- Potential for insertional mutagenesis (Lentiviruses have similar, site-specific integration to HIV)
- Potential for germline transfer

Figure 32.7   Characteristics of lentiviral vectors.

resulting in infection of the injected subject with newly recombinant or wild-type HIV. Various safety modifications are being considered by researchers, including (1) production of the vector using a packaging plasmid that does not contain HIV genes with the potential for facilitating viral recombination and replication, (2) vectors that are self-inactivating (SIN), and (3) testing for specific internal promoters that regulate gene expression but do not introduce the potential for mediating undesired gene expression such as oncogenes. In addition the use of other lentiviruses, such as equine infectious anemia virus (EIAV), is being considered as a strategy to circumvent the issue of host infection. Additional potential safety concerns for these vectors include (1) DNA tissue biodistribution and any subsequent adverse biological effects and (2) the potential for germline integration. Some characteristics of lentiviral vectors are presented in Figure 32.7.

32.8.3   Other Viral Vectors

Other types of replication-deficient viral vectors that have been used in the gene therapy field include *Herpes simplex* viral (HSV) vectors that (1) are able to transduce nondividing cells and (2) are highly infective for neurologic tissue and vaccinia vectors. Vaccinia vectors in turn (1) are able to transduce nondividing cells and (2) have the ability to efficiently infect many types of cells. The primary safety concerns for HSV vectors are the potential for tropism to the CNS and the potential for latency and reactivation. Vaccinia vectors contain the same backbone as the smallpox vaccine, thus the available safety databases for vaccinia administration in humans consist primarily of preventive vaccination in a healthy population. Principal safety concerns with the use of vaccinia vectors include (1) their ability to replicate in humans and possibly the production of a replication competent vaccinia (RCV), (2) the potential for germline integration, and (3) the potential for toxicity in immune-compromised populations such as cancer patients. Any safety concerns regarding the route of administration and dosing regimens for therapeutic vaccinia vectors should be addressed before the vector is used in humans.

32.8.4 Replication-Competent Oncolytic Vectors

The oncolytic viruses include adenovirus, measles, reovirus, vesicular stomatitis virus (VSV), HSV, poxvirus, and vaccinia. Specific examples include (1) ONYX-015, which is an adenoviral oncolytic virus, administered to patients with liver metastases of colorectal cancer and pancreatic cancer [29], (2) Reolysin, which is an oncolytic reovirus administered to patients with glioma [30], and (3) MV-CEA, which is an oncolytic measles virus expressing carcinoembryonic antigen, administered to patients with ovarian cancer [31]. Some oncolytic viruses are wild type and are apparently not pathogenic in humans, such as the Newcastle disease virus (NDV), which is an RNA avian paramyxovirus. PV701, a naturally attenuated, replication-competent strain of NDV, has been administered to patients with advanced solid tumors [32]. The applicability of oncolytic viruses as a therapy for clinical oncology trials is due to their potential selectivity: the ability to kill tumor cells but not normal cells. However, the level of attenuation of viral replication in normal cells is limited for most oncolytic vectors.

The desired properties of these viruses include (1) stable and efficient viral replication in tumor cells in vivo, (2) lateral spread of virus to surrounding tumor cells (i.e., "bystander effect"), (3) tumor-selective killing, also called "controlled" tropism, and (4) avoidance of early detection/"neutralization" by the immune system. Potential safety concerns for this vector class include (1) the potential for viral tropism to normal human cells, (2) increased viral spread and replication in nontarget tissues in immunosuppressed individuals, (3) synergistic potential for viral replication in nontarget tissues when administered in combination with radiation, chemotherapy, prodrugs, and other agents, and (4) any toxicities due to an added transgene. One major challenge for safety assessment of these products is the selection of an animal species that reflects the biology of the respective oncolytic virus in humans (e.g., the use of transgenic mice expressing one of the receptors, CD46, for measles virus) and the availability of adequate tumor-bearing models that can be used to assess antitumor activity.

32.9 USE OF ADJUVANTS WITH THERAPEUTIC GENE THERAPY PRODUCTS

Similar to prophylactic vaccines, many of the therapeutic gene therapy products are administered in conjunction with adjuvants in order to enhance the immune system to respond in a vigorous manner to the injected antigen. The adjuvants can include aluminum salts (aluminum hydroxide, aluminum phosphate, and potassium aluminum sulfate), QS-21 (a saponin extract from the *Quillaja saponaria* [soapbark] tree), bacterial adjuvants, liposomes, and the newer MF59 (an oil-in-water emulsion manufactured by Chiron) and ISCOMATRIX(r) (a saponin-based adjuvant manufactured by CSL Limited). Recombinant proteins such as granulocyte-monocyte colony stimulating factor (GM-CSF), interleukin-2 (IL-2) and interleukin-12 (IL-12), which also serve to stimulate the immune system, have been administered in combination with many therapeutic gene therapy products. The adjuvant list is continually growing as a result of the development of new therapeutic and preventive vaccines that may require novel adjuvants.

The use of an adjuvant concurrent with a gene therapy product could result in toxicity due to the molecular mimicry between a vaccine antigen and a self antigen [33]. By their intended action of increasing the immune response, adjuvants administered with a gene therapy product can potentially exacerbate some toxicities because of an inappropriate immune response. In addition the adjuvants can be toxic, depending on their intrinsic chemical properties. Safety concerns regarding the adjuvant alone can include (1) the potential for proinflammatory effects of immunomodulatory adjuvants like cytokines, (2) the induction of hypersensitivity and autoimmunity, and (3) the intrinsic toxicity of these compounds [34]. General strategies to assess the safety of therapeutic gene therapy vaccines administered with adjuvants should include evaluation of the intended clinical formulation (gene therapy product plus adjuvant) when administered via the intended clinical immunization regimen using a relevant animal species. A major challenge for gene therapy vaccine–adjuvant combination is safety assessment using animal species that display a response similar to the human host response to both the vaccine and the adjuvant. This consideration is more complex in diseased individuals, who may be more vulnerable to any potential risks of therapeutic vaccination compared to normal human populations. For a general scientific discussion and toxicology testing principles for adjuvants, the reader is referred to the adjuvant guideline published by the EMEA [35].

32.10 PRECLINICAL STUDIES FOR GENE THERAPY PRODUCTS

Preclinical studies for any experimental pharmaceutical agent are conducted to provide better scientific insight into the potential pharmacologic and toxicologic effects that may result from the administration of the agent in humans. These studies are critical as they help define the risk–benefit ratio of the experimental agent of interest in the desired clinical population, both prior to initiation of a clinical trial and throughout the development program for the pharmaceutical agent.

32.10.1 Demonstrating Proof of Concept

The initial definitive first step in the movement from the "bench" to the "bedside" is the supportive scientific justification of the use of a particular agent to substantiate an appropriate rationale for use in a specific disease indication (Figure 32.1). This rationale, termed proof-of-concept (POC) studies, focuses on assessing the bioactivity and pharmacology profile of a particular gene therapy product to understand the ability of that product to induce the desired biologic effect via both in vitro (e.g., the trophic effect of an expressed transgene on a specific receptor or cell population) and in vivo (e.g., the use of an animal disease model) systems in order to enable advancement to first use of the product in humans. These POC studies are the initial translation step, as they help establish the basis for conducting the desired clinical trial through the generation of data to show (1) the biological feasibility of the use of the gene therapy product in the target disease, (2) the level of gene expression resulting from administration of the product (the "pharmacokinetic" effect), and (3) the extent of the morphological and functional correction (the "pharmacodynamic" effect) that results from administration of the product. In addition these POC studies help define a pharmacologically active dose range, with establishment of an optimal biological dose (OBD) and a minimally effective dose (MED), determine a potentially optimal route for product administration, and provide guidance regarding a possible dosing regimen/ schedule for the first clinical trial. This pharmacological effect may translate to correction of a genetic defect, such as with an inborn error of metabolism; the amelioration or slowed progression of a disease, such as cancer; or lessened severity/frequency of some of the symptoms of a particular disease, such as Parkinson's disease.

For gene therapy products, the selection of the vector system is put to the test initially in the POC studies. These studies provide the first in vitro assessment of the choice of the viral or nonviral vector, the cell population to be used (if applicable), as well as the selection of a therapeutic transgene (if applicable) to treat a specific disease.

Consideration of Relevant Animal Species One very important goal of the POC studies for a gene therapy product is to establish at least one biologically relevant animal species (if one exists). This selection process can entail assessment of the permissiveness/susceptibility of various animal species to replication by viral vectors, the pharmacological responsiveness to the transgene, the sensitivity of the species to the actions of the administered population of cells, and the comparative physiology of the animal species to humans. Relevancy determination may not stop at the species level as, for example, the responsiveness of particular strains of mice to the gene therapy product of interest may also need to be evaluated. For instance, Mazzolini et al. showed that following systemic injection of AdCMVmIL-12, heterogeneous toxicity was evident in different strains of mice depending on the levels of gene transduction achieved in the livers of these various strains [36]. For some gene therapy products, the relevant species may not be considered a "standard" laboratory animal species for preclinical testing, such as the applicability of cotton rats in the evaluation of the activity and safety of adenovirus [37] or the use of Syrian hamsters to assess oncolytic adenovirus [38]. The expressed transgene also needs to be considered when determining a relevant animal species, as many of the recombinant human protein products have been shown to be biologically active in a restricted number of species, such as human interferon activity in nonhuman primates. For some POC studies that are conducted in rodents the analogous animal transgene (i.e., murine interferon) is used. In these instances additional characterization of the human product and the animal product would be conducted to determine the similarities and differences between the human and animal investigational materials. There are many other examples in the scientific literature, both for the vectors and for the expressed transgenes.

The injection of cells ex vivo transduced to express a specific transgene, such as autologous CD8$^+$ cells transduced with lentiviral vector to express an anti-sense HIV envelope (env) gene [39] or hematopoietic stem cells transduced with retrovirus to express the FAA gene [40], highlights another aspect of the biological relevancy of animals. The injection of human cells into immune competent animals cannot be accomplished due to the immune response of the animal to the foreign cells that will occur. Therefore, for the conduct of POC studies using human transduced cells, the use of immune-incompetent animals, such as genetically immunodeficient rodents (SCID mice, nude rats) or chemically immunosuppressed rodents and large animals (e.g., using cyclosporine), is necessary in order to prevent or slow the rejection of the cells. Another approach that has been used is the administration of the animal cellular analogue, which has been transduced with the clinical vector to express the human transgene into immune competent animals. POC studies have also been conducted using the animal cellular analogue, transduced with the clinical vector encoding the animal transgene, notably in instances where a rodent species has been used in which the human protein was not biologically active. One such example is human autologous bone marrow derived stromal cells (hBMSCs) transduced with plasmid expressing human IL-12 (hIL-12) for peritumoral injection into patients with glioblastoma. Some POC studies were performed using tumor-bearing immune-competent rodents injected with rBMSCs transduced with plasmid expressing mIL-12 [41]. In this situation characterization of the human product—cells and transgene—and the animal product would be conducted to determine significant differences. The degree of understanding of the relationship between an animal cell and its human correlate is an important factor in determining the strength of the extrapolations from findings in animals to human risk assessment.

Another factor that may enter into the selection paradigm for the most appropriate species for evaluation of a specific gene therapy product is the route/method of product administration. For example, if the delivery of the gene therapy product incorporates a system that is more complicated than a needle and syringe (i.e., catheter-pump device delivery system or intracoronary infusion by a cardiac catheter), then the use of a pharmacologically responsive large animal species (if one exists) can also be considered in order to adequately evaluate the activity of the gene therapy product when dispensed according to the anticipated delivery procedure for humans. At times, however, a large animal species may be necessary if an untested delivery device is contemplated for clinical use, in order to evaluate the resulting activity, such as vector spread and resulting transduction pattern in the targeted tissue due to the administration procedure itself.

Knowledge of a product's mechanism of action that is acquired in preclinical trials can be beneficial in the design and conduct of the clinical trials. Ideally the pharmacological response of the species to the gene therapy product will mimic the response seen in humans—which will only be verified following initiation of a clinical trial.

Animal Models of Disease For many of the diseases that are under consideration for treatment with a gene therapy product, a corresponding animal model of disease exists, which to some extent, may reflect the pathophysiology of the disorder. Figure 32.8 depicts some examples of animal models of disease that have been used to study the pharmacological activity of various gene therapy products intended for treatment of a specific human disorder. Existing models include spontaneous disease models such as hemophilic dogs,

Animal Models of Disease to Study Potential Gene Therapies

Animal Model	Disease
CLAD dogs	Leukocyte adhesion deficiency
Gusb mice	MPS VII; Sly disease
mdx mice	Muscular dystrophy
Canine X-linked MD (GRMD)	Duchennes MD
db/db mice	Diabetes
Factor IX-deficient dog	Hemophilia B
PDAPP Tg mice	Alzheimers disease
Aged marmosets	Alzheimers disease
rcd1 dogs	Retinitis pigmentosa
W/W^v mice	Fanconi's anemia
Hbb$^{th3/+}$ mice	ß-thalassemia
Murine tumor xenografts	Cancer
Spontaneous tumors in companion animals	Cancer

Figure 32.8 Examples of animal models of disease that have been used to study potential gene therapy agents.

nonspontaneous disease models (chemically, surgically, immunologically induced) such as the MPTP nonhuman primate model of Parkinson's disease, and genetically modified disease models (transgenics, knockouts, knock-ins) such as the transgenic murine HER-2 model for breast cancer [42].

POC studies using an animal model of disease can then be designed in a manner that reasonably mimics the planned clinical protocol, including the gene therapy product administration schedule and the parameters (both activity and safety) monitored. For example, in a porcine myocardial infarct model, product administration considerations could include the timing of product delivery (using the clinical delivery system) relative to the appearance of the infarct, the number and location of the injections of product into the heart and the product concentration, volume, and rate of administration. The parameters monitored could include functional assessments such as ECGs, echocardiography, and/or SPECT and morphological endpoints such as hematology, serum biochemistry, and cardiac markers (i.e., troponin, LDH, and CPK/CPK-MB) and a comprehensive microscopic examination of the heart. A preclinical study designed in such a manner, using several vector dose levels, would provide insight into the determination of an optimal biological dose level, as well as a no-effect dose level, which would then help to guide the rationale for selection of the dose levels for the subsequent toxicology studies, as well as for the human trial.

While the use of preclinical disease models offers many advantages, such as the potential for identification of biomarkers for clinical trials and a direct estimation of the therapeutic index, there are also disadvantages to this approach. The disadvantages can include a paucity of historical/baseline data and inherent variability of the model, the technical feasibility of using a particular disease model, the onset/severity of the injury in the animals as this may be different from humans, and the fact that the model may only emulate select aspects of the human pathophysiology of the disease [43]. It is important to use behavioral models that have adequate sensitivity and specificity to allow for correlation with morphological and biochemical findings, as in the area of spinal cord injury.

32.10.2 Toxicology Assessment

According to the paradigm depicted in Figure 32.1, the next step on the critical pathway to use of a gene therapy product in a human disease population is the evaluation of the safety of the product of interest through the conduct of toxicology studies. These studies are intended to provide an acceptable risk–benefit ratio to the patients that will receive a particular gene therapy product. While the preclinical studies focus on goals that are similar for small-molecule agents or for traditional biotechnology-derived products (e.g., monoclonal antibodies, cytokines, growth factors), gene therapy products are complex and preclude a standard design of preclinical studies, which is consistent with the "case-by-case" approach to the safety assessment of biotechnology-derived pharmaceuticals.

Relevant Animal Species/Models   The evaluation of the potential toxicity of each gene therapy product should build on the previously conducted POC studies. Important factors for continued product development such as the animal species, the route and procedure for product administration, the potentially effective dose range, and the dosing regimen will have been established from the POC results, providing the rationale for proceeding into preclinical toxicology studies. The collection of toxicity endpoints in the disease models that are used to assess pharmacologic activity is scientifically justified because, if a relevant disease model exists and is readily accessible, the contribution of the disease-related changes in physiology and/or the underlying pathology to any toxicities observed with the use of a particular vector and/or the expressed transgene can be determined. It is important to determine whether administration of the gene therapy product results in exacerbation of the existing disease/disease symptoms or even the induction of a new disease. Caution should be extended, however, in the interpretation of the toxicities that are observed in animal models of disease for the reasons previously stated regarding the POC evaluation in these models. A preclinical study designed to evaluate both activity and toxicology endpoints in a biologically responsive animal model of disease has also been called a "hybrid" study.

Normal, pharmacologically relevant animal species are also often used in toxicology studies to evaluate the safety of gene therapy products. As discussed for the POC studies, many factors of the gene therapy product of interest are considered in the selection of the most appropriate animal species, including vector class, cell population (if applicable), and expressed transgene. The species used should ideally be sensitive not just to infection of the vector but also to the pathological consequences of infection that may be induced by the replication competent virus related to the vector. In some cases lower animal species may be transformed into "humanized" models that express the human target receptor(s) that may not be present or be only partially present in the animals. For example, the use of CD155 transgenic mice, which are engineered to express the CD155 receptor—which is the target for poliovirus [44] or Ifnar (KO) × CD46 transgenic mice that express human CD46 with human-like tissue specificity for the measles virus infection [45]—could be considered biologically applicable animal models for use in evaluation of the potential toxicity of the respective gene therapy product.

The utilization of relevant animal species/models that can mimic the human physiology as closely as possible is critical in order to provide an activity and a safety profile for the gene therapy product of interest. This way measurable boundaries can be obtained for an acceptable risk–benefit ratio that will allow for the administration of the gene therapy product into the desired human population (i.e., bench to bedside translation; Figure 32.9). There should be a justifiable use of the animal resources employed to assess the pharmacology and safety of the gene therapy product.

32.10.3 Overall Toxicology Study Designs

The toxicology assessment of a gene therapy product should be comprehensive enough to identify, characterize, and quantify the potential local and systemic toxicities (Figure 32.10). Outcomes measured are acute/chronic toxicities, reversibility of toxicities, delayed toxicities, and any dose–response effects on these various outcomes. The approach used to ascertain a safety profile for a gene therapy product is novel; therefore the preclinical studies that are designed and conducted for these products are unique. For example, broad safety concerns for both the ex vivo and the in vivo administration of a gene therapy product originate from multiple factors, including (1) the potential for adverse reactions such as immunogenicity, to the ex vivo transduced cells, (2) vector and transgene toxicities, and (3) the potential risks of the delivery procedure. Direct injection of transduced cells or vector to vital organs such as the brain and heart generate questions regarding not only the potential toxicity of the gene therapy product but also the risks associated with the delivery procedure and the delivery device. While certain aspects of the overall scientific principles of internationally recognized guidelines such as those sponsored by the International Conference on Harmonisation (ICH), notably the S6 document, "Preclinical Safety Evaluation of Biotechnology-Derived Pharmaceuticals" [46], can be used, traditional toxicology programs are of minimal value in the determination of safety for gene therapy products. Many times the preclinical testing methodology is developed specifically for the gene therapy product of interest with the incorporation of novel technologies. Guidances for various gene therapy products released by different scientific and regulatory bodies can be utilized, as appropriate, for evaluation of a particular gene therapy product.

Ex vivo Transduced Cells The toxicological assessment of the cellular component of ex vivo transduced cells may include endpoints that are similar to those evaluated for somatic cellular therapies. Depending on the cell population that is transduced, the following considerations should be incorporated for safety assessment: local environmental influence on cell survival, differentiation/phenotype expression, cell migration, host immune response, local and systemic reactions, and tumorigenicity. In addition the potential for induction of an immune response to the transduced cells can result in unwanted toxicities. For example, the expression of surface antigens on the transduced cells may be altered, potentially leading to an autoimmune response. Design of the preclinical studies should include assessment of the induction of autoimmunity or other immune responses. The considerations for the preclinical toxicology assessment of ex vivo transduced cells follow the same pathway as for gene therapy products that are administered directly into the recipient.

Assessment of Safety/Activity

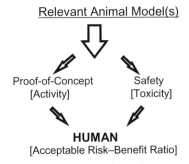

Figure 32.9   Translational studies from preclinical to clinical trials.

Toxicology Assessment for Gene Therapy Products

Evaluate single/repeat exposure to the vector product (V)
- Toxicities related to the vector
- Biodistribution of the vector in blood and tissues

Evaluate the safety of gene expression (T)
- Persistence, level of expression in vivo
- Identify target tissues/functional endpoints
- Delayed toxicities/reversibility of toxicities

Evaluate V + T
- Characterize general toxicities
- Identify specific toxicities
- Characterize dose/exposure

Figure 32.10   Overall paradigm for the assessment of the safety of a gene therapy product.

The development of clonal T cell proliferation in several children with X-SCID postadministration of autologous hematopoietic cells transduced ex vivo with retrovirus expressing the γc gene raised the awareness of the gene therapy scientific community regarding the potential safety concerns of an integrating vector from theoretical to actual [26,47]. The FDA has issued a draft guidance document that discusses the potential risks of delayed adverse events following exposure to gene therapy products as a consequence of persistent biological activity of the genetic material or other components of the products used to carry the genetic material, which could result in adverse effects on normal cell function. As listed in the guidance, factors that are likely to increase the risk of delayed adverse events in humans include persistence of the viral vector, integration of genetic material into the host genome, prolonged expression of the transgene, and altered expression of the host's genes [48].

In vivo Administration of a Gene Therapy Product

Vector Considerations For the design of the most clinically applicable toxicology studies the route of administration, and the dosing schedule, knowledge of the planned clinical use of the gene therapy product regarding the dose level range, is important. Most gene therapy products are given either as a single administration or as a minimal number of repeat administrations over a relatively limited time interval. The route of administration and the dosing schedule for each gene therapy product in animals should mimic the intended clinical scenario as closely as possible. The presence and persistence of the vector in target and nontarget tissues, termed biodistribution, can help to provide insight toward extrapolation of the safety and rationale for the timing of multiple injections in humans. This evaluation, discussed in more detail later in this chapter, is analogous to the determination of a pharmacokinetic profile for a biological pharmaceutical in the instance of a recombinant human protein.

In parallel with an understanding of the injected vector's biodistribution profile should come an understanding of its potential toxicities. Adverse effects in animals can be dependent on the vector class and the route of administration. For example, the inflammatory reactions in response to adenovirus capsid proteins are well documented in the scientific literature. Intravenous administration of adenovirus in normal C57Bl/6 mice resulted in an acute inflammatory response in the liver [49], and direct instillation into the lungs of cotton rats resulted in a dose-related inflammatory reaction in the bronchioles [50]. In addition the toxicities observed in an animal model of disease given the same vector type can be potentially different. For example, the altered biodistribution of adenoviral vectors following intravascular administration in cirrhotic rats resulted in pulmonary hemorrhagic edema due to the presence of pulmonary intravascular macrophages resulting in notable vector biodistribution to the lungs [51].

It is well documented that humans generate neutralizing antibodies to select adenoviral and AAV vector serotypes (e.g., Ad5 and AAV2) following administration. These neutralising antibodies can prevent vector distribution to target tissue, accelerate clearance of the virus, and decrease transgene expression/persistence of expression [52]. In addition to reducing the kinetic and activity profile of the gene therapy product, induction of autoimmunity or other adverse immune effects may occur. The potential for stimulating an immune response (humoral and/or cellular) to the nucleic acid, the viral protein, or other parts of the vector construct is always a possibility and thus should be appropriately assessed.

The nature of the vector under investigation should be considered in the design of preclinical studies. For example, for preclinical evaluations of vectors that have a documented potential to integrate, such as gammaretrovirus and lentivirus, or possess the potential for latency and reactivation, such as the

Herpes virus, there could be used instead a tiered approach consisting of an assessment of the vector persistence followed by vector integration, latency, and/or reactivation, depending on the vector type.

Transgene Considerations   The safety of the expressed transgene should be evaluated in appropriately designed preclinical studies as well. In most cases, the same animal species that is biologically sensitive to the vector of interest is also responsive to the translated protein. However, in some instances, the transgene product, such as human interleukin-12 or interferon, is biologically active only in humans and nonhuman primates, potentially necessitating the use of monkeys in toxicology studies. In other instances where published toxicology data exist for a transgene product that is active only in humans or nonhuman primates, another species analogue, such as murine IL-12, may suffice for the transgene product [53].

Similar to the recombinant human proteins, the potential for an immune response (cellular or humoral) to the expressed transgene exists. For example, delivery of transgenes that encode various endogenous enzymes, receptors, and structural proteins may elicit antibodies against both the transgene and the endogenous components expressed in normal cells and tissues, resulting in an autoimmune response. Similarly clinical delivery of transgenes that express fusion or chimera proteins can theoretically be immunogenic because of to their foreign nature. Thus the potential development of an immune response (humoral or cell mediated) for each gene therapy product should be investigated, as appropriate.

While persistent transgene expression may be a desired endpoint for some gene therapy products, toxicity can be an undesired outcome of transgene overexpression and/or a delayed abnormal immune response. Prolonged expression of transgenes such as growth factors, growth factor receptors, or immunomodulating agents may be associated with long-term risks due to from unregulated cell growth and malignant transformation, autoimmune reactions to self-antigens, or other unanticipated adverse effects. Long-term preclinical studies should be considered to evaluate these concerns.

The relationship between the dose level of the gene therapy product administered and the level and persistence of transgene expression in specific tissues and any toxicities that are observed should be determined. These data are important to ascertain, as they will affect the clinical monitoring and planned dose escalation in the clinical trials.

32.10.4   General Considerations

The design of the preclinical toxicology studies incorporates the basic tenets used in toxicology study designs for biological and small-molecule pharmaceuticals. The design should allow for the inclusion of appropriate control groups (may be more than one group, e.g., untreated controls, sham controls, null vector controls, vehicle controls), several dose groups, adequate numbers of animals per gender in each group for each sacrifice time point, and a clinically relevant route of administration. The controls could consist of the vehicle formulation, a sham control if the administration procedure is unique or an unknown delivery device is used, or an empty vector if a novel vector system is used. Several groups of animals that will be given the gene therapy product at dose levels that bracket and exceed the intended dose level range in humans, if possible, should be included. The multiples of the human dose required to determine an adequate safety margin can vary with the vector class, the "equivalency" of the injection route used in animals to the clinical route (i.e., intratumoral in human vs. subcutaneous or intramuscular in animals), and the relevance of the animal species/model to humans. The duration of each study conducted is dependent on the product, the dosing scheme, and the subject population of interest. The biodistribution and persistence profile of the vector and the expression profile of the transgene often guide the duration of the toxicology studies and the time intervals selected for sacrifice of animals.

The inclusion of safety endpoints such as clinical signs, physical exams, body weights, food consumption/appetite, serum chemistry, hematology, coagulation, urinalysis, organ weights, gross pathology, histopathology, and anti-vector/anti-transgene antibody measurements are considered routine for preclinical toxicology studies for gene therapy products. Other endpoints specific for the assessment of potential adverse effects due to the class of vector (e.g., neuropathology for Herpes virus), due to the transgene product (e.g., undesired cell proliferation due to a growth factor), or due to the proposed clinical population (e.g., diabetes or cancer) can include ECGs and other cardiac parameters, ophthalmology exams, immunotoxicity assessment, behavioral assessment, neurotoxicity evaluation, specialized histopathology (i.e., immunohistochemistry, special stains), as well as other parameters.

The traditional carcinogenicity study as described in the ICH S1B guideline and the standard battery of genotoxicity studies as described in the ICH S2 guidelines are generally not applicable to gene therapy products [54–56]. As previously discussed, the concern for insertional mutagenesis of the vector is an important potential safety issue that should be addressed, and the tumorigenic potential of an expressed transgene of concern should be evaluated in adequately designed preclinical studies.

32.10.5 Good Laboratory Practice (GLP)

In the United States preclinical toxicology studies performed in support of the use of gene therapy products in clinical trials should be conducted in compliance with good laboratory practice (GLP) as per the US regulation, 21 CFR part 58. Preclinical in vivo pharmacology studies (i.e., proof of concept) and in vitro pharmacology studies are not expected to be conducted under GLP. In the early stages of the development program for a gene therapy product the preclinical studies are not always conducted in full compliance with GLP. The

FDA has agreed that these preclinical studies can be conducted at a facility that is capable of complying with a prospectively designed study protocol. Non-GLP studies are acceptable as long as they are performed in accordance with a prospectively designed protocol and the data are of sufficient quality and integrity to support the proposed clinical trial. The study report that is submitted to FDA should identify any areas that deviate from the prospectively designed protocol and the potential impact of these deviations on study integrity. Many times initial preclinical toxicology data for these products are collected in proof-of-concept studies conducted using an animal model of disease, which may require unique animal care issues; thus complete compliance with GLP may be difficult. The expectation is that pivotal toxicology studies submitted to support a marketing application will be conducted under GLP.

32.10.6 Non-GLP Studies

In addition to the GLP toxicology studies and well-controlled non-GLP studies conducted for various gene therapy products, published information in peer-reviewed scientific journals, as well as from public presentations and discussions, can be consulted to support the safety of the gene therapy product of interest. For example, all information regarding a specific gene therapy product that is submitted to the NIH Recombinant DNA Advisory Committee (RAC), located in the Office of Biotechnology Activities (OBA), is considered to be in the public domain. Thus the toxicology information for one vector serotype in a class (e.g., adeno-associated viruses) may help in the safety evaluation of another serotype in the same vector class. If extensive preclinical or clinical safety data for the same or similar vector type exist, toxicity assessment of the gene therapy product of interest may be less extensive, depending on such factors as the dose levels, dosing regimen, route of administration, and expression cassette that were previously used. Depending on the extent of the change to a particular vector that has been administered to humans, in vitro or small in vivo bridging studies may suffice.

The data generated from the toxicology studies should allow a determination of a no-observable-adverse-effect-level, or NOAEL, and should characterize the relationship of the documented toxicities to the dose of the gene therapy product that is given. The extrapolation of this NOAEL to the clinical arena is accomplished in several ways, including body weight, body surface area, and organ weight/volume. An understanding of the association of the dose levels employed in the toxicology studies to the resulting toxicities, as well as the effect of administration route and dosing schedule on any toxicities observed in the animals, is the desired goal.

32.10.7 Biodistribution Considerations

While the determination of the overall safety of an experimental agent is a desired common objective for all pharmaceutical agents, the approach used to achieve this goal for a gene therapy product is distinct from the approach used for small-molecule products, as well as for the traditional biologic therapies (e.g., monoclonal antibodies and recombinant cytokines). A specific difference is reflected in the determination of the pharmacokinetic profile of a gene therapy product. While standard absorption, disposition, metabolism, and excretion (ADME) studies are conducted for small-molecule products and pharmacokinetic assessment is applied for biologics, the localization or biodistribution of the vector is assessed in animals. Following administration via (ideally) the planned clinical route, the determination of the dissemination of the vector to the intended therapeutic site(s), as well as to nontarget tissues, provides an important part of the overall safety profile of each gene therapy product (Figure 32.11). Such data should guide the toxicology further study designs, with respect to dose levels, dosing schedule, and route of administration. The biodistribution study should include appropriate control animals and groups of animals given dose levels of the gene therapy product that overlap the dose levels used in the toxicology studies. Multiple sacrifice intervals are also included in order to capture a comprehensive kinetic profile to show peak vector levels and to characterize the persistence of vector signal in certain tissues and biological fluids (i.e., blood, semen) over time.

Biodistribution analysis is conducted at the molecular level. The current gold standard is a quantitative polymerase chain reaction (Q-PCR) assay that detects the number of vector copies per microgram of genomic DNA. Biological fluids and tissue samples are carefully harvested (to avoid cross-contamination) from control and gene therapy product-injected animals at

Vector Biodistribution to Intended
Therapeutic Site/Unintended Site(S)

Presence of vector sequence via Q-PCR analysis
•Dissemination of vector to nontarget tissues
•Dissemination of vector to the germline
•Vector persistence and clearance profile

Study conducted prior to phase 1 trials when:
• New class of vector, with no/little experience (e.g., capsid modification)
• Change in formulation (e.g., lipid carrier)
• Change in ROA with an established vector
• Change in dosing schedule
• New transgene; potential toxicities unknown
• Potential for the transgene to induce toxicity if aberrantly expressed in nontarget tissue

Figure 32.11 Considerations for the assessment of vector biodistribution.

several time points postadministration. Usually a default panel of tissues is collected and analyzed, including blood, injection site(s), gonads, brain, liver, kidneys, lung, heart, and spleen. Depending on the vector type and the transgene expressed, as well as the route of administration, other tissues should be analyzed (i.e., draining lymph nodes and contralateral sites of injection, bone marrow, and eyes) [48].

Another very important outcome of this analysis is the determination of vector presence in the germline (Figure 32.5). For every biodistribution study conducted, samples of gonadal tissue (testes or ovaries) from each animal should be harvested and analyzed. If a significant, persistent positive signal is detected using the state-of-the-art methodology, then a more extensive testing paradigm may be necessary. Further studies to determine the cell type that is positive for vector presence (i.e., germ cells, stromal cells, leukocytes) should be the next step. If the outcome continues to implicate inadvertent germline transfer, then the conduct of reproductive and developmental toxicology studies may be needed in order to assess the potential for vertical transmission of the gene sequences. The ICH S5(R2) guideline should be consulted for the overall design of these studies [57]. The risk of inadvertent germline transmission and the subsequent potential for integration are currently the major focus of the ICH GTDG. This group has released a consideration paper on this issue entitled "General Principles to Address the Risk of Inadvertent Germline Integration of Gene Therapy Vectors" (for more information, refer to the ICH Web site for details, http://www.ich.org/cache/html/1386-272-1.htm).

The presence of a vector sequence in nontarget tissues at significant levels should suggest the need for further analysis of the tissue to determine the levels of transgene expressed. These data, coupled with results of other safety endpoints, such as clinical pathology and histopathology evaluation, will determine whether vector presence or gene expression is correlated with any detrimental effects on the tissue.

Instances in which the biodistribution studies are conducted prior to use in humans can include the following: when the gene therapy product belongs to a new vector class, when there is little or no published data on the vector or the transgene of interest, if there is a change in the vector backbone for an established vector, if there is a change in formulation, if there is a change in the route of vector administration, or if there is a known or suspected potential for the transgene to induce toxicity that may be aberrantly expressed in nontarget tissues. For example, Cearly and Wolfe showed that injection of AAV 7, 8, 9, and rh10 vectors containing the same genome into the same area of rodent brains resulted in distinctly different transduction patterns due to the different capsid proteins. These differences translate into potential effects on (1) product activity if each vector displays unique capabilities at transducing different substructures of the brain and on (2) product toxicity if overexpression occurs in unwanted areas of the CNS to which the vector has disseminated [58].

If biodistribution studies are not performed prior to initiation of clinical trials, these studies should be incorporated in the development program of the gene therapy product so that data are generated prior to beginning any large pivotal studies in humans.

32.10.8 Later Stage Product Development

As the gene therapy product development program continues into the later phase clinical trials and toward the ultimate goal of a marketed product (Figure 32.1), additional consideration has to be given to the components of a product label (i.e., the package insert) that require data from preclinical studies, on mutagenicity, carcinogenicity, and reproductive toxicity. The intent of the label is to convey information on the safety and effectiveness of the approved product to the patient population receiving the respective product and to communicate any associated or perceived risk to both the physician and to the patient. Sponsors of gene therapy products should consult with the applicable regulatory agencies early in the product development program to ensure that the timing and design of the necessary preclinical studies are in place in accordance with the regulators' expectations.

32.11 CONCLUSION

Included on the Web site of the American Society of Gene Therapy (ASGT) is a section entitled "Brief History of Gene Therapy." This synopsis is a snapshot of the notable advances and setbacks in this field since 1966. Although these biologics are complex, rapid advances have been made with the discovery of new and novel viruses, as well as with the re-engineering of existing viruses. Without preclinical studies that are appropriately designed to provide insight on dose/activity and dose/toxicity relationships for the gene therapy products that are to be used in predetermined disease settings, early phase clinical trial designs are limited. Careful and thorough evaluation of the biological plausibility and safety of a gene therapy product is an essential first step on the critical pathway to a successful clinical product development program [59,60]. Unique and comprehensive preclinical testing approaches using biologically relevant animal species/models are critical elements in risk assessment of such novel products. The preclinical study designs will need to consider the vector system, the expressed transgene, the transduced cell type (as applicable), and the clinical indication to adequately assess the potential risks of each gene therapy product. Since risk assessment leads to risk communication, the preclinical data provide an effective means of risk communication to the physicians that manage the clinical trials, as well as to the individuals consenting to receive these experimental therapies. Ultimately any such risk communication will transfer to the marketed label for the approved gene therapy product.

ACKNOWLEDGMENTS

The authors wish to acknowledge the helpful contributions of many colleagues in the Office of Cellular, Tissue, and Gene Therapies. We are especially grateful to Drs. Richard McFarland, Stephanie Simek, and Daniel Takefman for their thorough and helpful review of the manuscript during its preparation.

REFERENCES

1. *FDA Guidance for Industry: Guidance for Human Somatic Cell Therapy and Gene Therapy*, March 1998. http://www.fda.gov/cber/gdlns/somgene.pdf

2. Bell J, Lichty B, Stojdl D. Getting oncolytic virus therapies off the ground. *Cancer Cell* 2003;4:7–11.

3. GeMCRIS, Gene Transfer Protocol Reports. www.gemcris.od.nih.gov

4. Rosenberg SA, Anderson WF, Blaese M, Hwu P, Yannelli JR, Yang JC, Topalian SL, Schwatzentruber DJ, Weber JS, Ettinghausen SE, Parkinson DN, White DE. The development of gene therapy for the treatment of cancer. *Ann Surg* 1993;218:455–63.

5. Blaese RM, Culver KW, Miller AD, Carter CS, Fleisher T, Clerici, M, Shearer G, Chang L, Chiang Y, Tolstoshev. P, Greenblatt JJ, Rosenberg SA, Klein H, Berger M, Mullen CA, Ramsey WJ, Muul L, Morgan RA, Anderson WF. T-lymphocyte-directed gene therapy for ADA-SCID: initial trial results after 4 years. *Science* 1995; 270:475–80.

6. Nabel GJ, Nabel EG, Yang ZY, Fox BA, Plautz GE, Gao X, Huang L, Shu S, Gordon D, Chang AE. Direct gene transfer with DNA-liposome complexes in melanoma: expression, biologic activity, and lack of toxicity in humans. *Proc Na Acad Sci USA* 1993;23:11307–11.

7. Crystal RG, Jaffe A, Brody S, Mastrangeli A, McElvaney NG, Rosenfeld M, Chu CS, Danel C, Hay J, Eissa T. A phase 1 study in cystic fibrosis patients of the safety, toxicity, and biological efficacy of a single administration of a replication deficient recombinant adenovirus carrying the cDNA of the normal cystic fibrosis transmembrane conductance regulator gene in the lung. *Hum Gene Ther* 1995;6:643–66.

8. Flotte T, Carter B, Conrad C, Guggino W, Reynolds T, Rosenstein B, Taylor G, Walden S, Wetzel R. A phase I study of an adeno-associated virus-CFTR gene vector in adult CF patients with mild lung disease. *Hum Gene Ther* 1996;7: 1145–59.

9. Kay MA, Manno CS, Ragni MV, Larson PJ, Couto LB, McClelland A, Glader B, Chew AJ, Tai SJ, Herzog RW, Arruda V, Johnson F, Scallan C, Skarsgard E, Flake AW, High KA. Evidence for gene transfer and expression of factor IX in hemophilia patients treated with an AAV vector. *Nat Genets* 2000;24:257–61.

10. Khuri FR, Nemunaitis J, Ganly I, Arseneau J, Tannock IF, Romel L, Gore M, Ironside J, MacDougall RH, Heise C, Randlev B, Gillenwater AM, Bruso P, Kaye SB, Hong WK, Kirn DH. A controlled trial of intratumoral ONYX-015, a selectively-replicating adenovirus, in combination with cisplatin and 5-fluorouracil in patients with recurrent head and neck cancer. *Nat Med* 2000;8:879–85.

11. Peng Z. Current status of Gendicine in China: recombinant human Ad-p53 agent for treatment of cancers. *Hum Gene Ther* 2005;16:1016–27.

12. Guo J, Xin H. Chinese gene therapy: splicing out the west? *Science* 2006;314: 1232–5.

13. Cavazzana-Calvo M, Hacein-Bey S, de Saint Basile G, Gross F, Yvon E, Nusbaum P, Selz F, Hue C, Certain S, Casanova JL, Bousso P, Deist FL, Fischer, A. Gene therapy of severe combined immunodeficiency (SCID)-X1 disease. *Science* 2000;288:669–72.

14. Thrasher AJ, Hacein-Bey-Abina S, Gaspar HB, Blanche S, Davies EG, Parsley K, Gilmour K, King D, Howe S, Sinclair J, Hue C, Carlier F, von KalLe C, de Saint BasiLe G, Le Deist F, Fischer A, Cavazzana-Calvo M. Failure of SCID-X1 gene therapy in older patients. *Blood* 2005;105:4255–7.

15. National Institutes of Health. Amended Charter: Recombinant DNA Advisory Committee. Updated April 13, 2005. http://www4.od.nih.gov/oba/rac/RACCharter2005.pdf

16. The Public Health Service Act. Title 42. Approved on July 1, 1944. http://www.fda.gov/opacom/laws/phsvcact/phsvcact.htm

17. Federal Food, Drug, and Cosmetic Act, as amended through December 31, 2004. http://www.fda.gov/opacom/laws/fdcact/fdctoc.htm

18. Kessler DA, Siegel JP, Noguchi PD, Zoon KC, Feiden KL, Woodcock J. Regulation of somatic cell-therapy and gene therapy by the Food and Drug Administration. *N Engl J Med*, 1993;329:1169–73.

19. Glover DJ, Lipps HJ, Jans DA. Towards safe, non-viral therapeutic gene expression in humans. *Nat Rev Genet* 2005;6:299–310.

20. Wolff JA, Budker V. The mechanism of naked DNA uptake and expression. *Adv Genet* 2005;54:3–20.

21. Yew NS, Scheule RK. Toxicity of cationic lipid-DNA complexes. *Adv Gene* 2005; 53:189–214.

22. Bangari DS, Mittal SK. Current strategies and future directions for eluding adeno-viral vector immunity. *Curr Gene Ther* 2006;6:215–26.

23. Tenenbaum L, Lehtonen E, Monahan PE. Evaluation of risks related to the use of adeno-associated virus-based vectors. *Curr Gene Ther* 2003;3:545–65.

24. Donsante A, Vogler C, Muzyczka N, Crawford JM, Barker J, Flotte T, Campbell-Thompson M, Daly T, Sands MS. Observed incidence of tumorigenesis in long-term rodent studies of rAAV vectors. *Gene Ther* 2001;8:1343–6.

25. Donahue RE, Kessler SW, Bodine D, McDonagh K, Dunbar C, Goodman S, Agri-cola B, Byrne E, Raffeld M, Moen R, Bacher J, Zsebo KM, Nienhuis AW. Helper virus induced T cell lymphoma in nonhuman primates after retroviral mediated gene transfer. *J Exp Med* 1992;176:1125–35.

26. Hacein-Bey-Abina S, Von Kalle C, Schmidt M, McCormack MP, Wulffraat N, Lebouch P, Lim A, Osborne CS, Pawliuk R, Morillon E, Sorensen R, Forster A, Fraser P, Cohen JI, de Saint Basile D, Alexander I, Wintergerst U, Frebourg T, Aurias A, Stoppa-Lyonnet D, Romana S, Radford-Weiss I, Gross F, Valensi F, Delabesse E, Macintyre E, Sigaux F, Soulier J, Leiva LE, Wissler M, Prinz C, Rabbitts TH, Le Deist F, Fischer A, Cavazzana-Calvo, M. LMO2-associated clonal

T-cell proliferation in two patients after gene therapy for SCID-XI. *Science* 2003;302:415–9.

27. Anson D. The use of retroviral vectors for gene therapy—What are the risks? A review of retroviral pathogenesis and its relevance to retroviral vector-mediated gene delivery. *Genet Vaccines Ther* 2004;2:9–22.

28. Loewen N, Poeschla EM. Lentiviral vectors. *Adv Biochem Eng/Biotech* 2005;99: 169–91.

29. Biederer C, Ries S, Brandts CH, McCormick F. Replication-selective viruses for cancer therapy. *J Mol Med* 2002;80:163–75.

30. Stoeckel J, Hay JG. Drug evaluation: Reolysin-wild type reovirus as a cancer thera-peutic. *Curr Opin Mol Therapeu* 2006;3:249–60.

31. Hasegawa K, Pham L, O'Connor MK, Federspiel MJ, Russell SJ, Peng KW. Dual therapy of ovarian cancer using measles viruses expressing carcinoembryonic antigen and sodium iodide symporter. *Clin Cancer Res* 2006;6:1868–75.

32. Pecora AL, Rizvi N, Cohen GI, Meropol NJ, Sterman D, Marshall JL, Goldberg S, Gross P, O'Neil JD, Groene WS, Roberts MS, Rabin H, Bamat MK, Lorence RM. Phase I trial of intravenous administration of PV701, an oncolytic virus, in patients with advanced solid cancers. *J Clin Oncol* 2002;20:2251–66.

33. Schijns VE, Tangrås A. Vaccine adjuvant technology: from theoretical mechanisms to practical approaches. *Dev Biol* 2005;121:127–34.

34. Brennan FR, Dougan G. Non-clinical safety evaluation of novel vaccines and adju-vants: new products, new strategies. *Vaccine* 2005;23:3210–22.

35. EMEA Guideline on Adjuvants In Vaccines for Human Use, January 2005. www. emea.eu.int/pdfs/human/vwp/13471604en.pdf

36. Mazzolini G, Narvaiza I, Perez-Diez A, Rodriguez-Calvillo M, Qian C, Sangro B, Ruiz J, Prieto J, Melero I. Genetic heterogeneity in the toxicity fo systemic adeno-viral gene transfer of interleukin-12. *Gene Ther* 2001;8:259–67.

37. Prince GA, Porter DD, Jenson AB, Horswood RL, Chanock RM, Ginsberg HS. Pathogenesis of adenovirus type 5 pneumonia in cotton rats (Sigmodon hispidus). *J Virol* 1993;67:101–11.

38. Thomas MA, Spencer JF, La Regina MC, Dhar D, Tollefson AE, Toth K, Wold WS. Syrian hamster as a permissive immunocompetent animal model for the study of oncolytic adenovirus vectors. *Cancer Res* 2006;3:1270–6.

39. Manilla P, Rebello T, Afable C, Lu X, Slepushkin V, Humeau LM, Schonely K, Ni Y, Binder GK, Levine BL, MacGregor RR, June CH, Dropulic, B. Regulatory considerations for novel gene therapy products: a review of the process leading to the first clinical lentiviral vector. *Hum Gene Ther* 2005;1:17–25.

40. Williams DA, Croop J, Kelly P. Gene therapy in the treatment of Fanconi anemia, a progressive bone marrow failure syndrome. *Curr Opin Mol Therapeut* 2005;5: 461–6.

41. December 3–4, 2003, Recombinant DNA Advisory Committee (RAC) meeting. http://www4.od.nih.gov/oba/rac/meeting.htm

42. Disis ML, Scholler N, Dahlin A, Pullman J, Knutson KL, Hellstrom KE, Hellstrom, I. Plasmid-based vaccines encoding rat neu and immune stimulatory molecules can elicit rat neu-specific immunity. *Mol Cancer Ther* 2003;10:995–1002.

43. Cavagnaro JA. Preclinical safety evaluation of biotechnology-derived pharmaceuticals. *Nat Rev* 2002;1:469–75.

44. Dragunsky EM, Ivanov AP, Abe S, Potapova SG, Enterline JC, Hashizume S, Chumakov KM. Further development of a new transgenic mouse test for the evaluation of the immunogenicity and protective properties of inactivated poliovirus vaccine. *J Infect Dis* 2006;194:804–60.

45. Peng KW, Frenzke M, Myers R, Soeffker D, Harvey M, Greiner S, Galanis E, Cattaneo R, Federspiel MJ, Russell SJ. Biodistribution of oncolytic measles virus after intraperitoneal administration into Ifnar(tm)-CD46Ge transgenic mice. *Hum Gene Ther* 2003;16:1565–77.

46. International Conference on Harmonisation (July 1997). *S6: Preclinical Safety Evaluation of Biotechnology-Derived Pharmaceuticals.* http://www.ich.org/cache/compo/502-272-1.htm

47. Couzin J, Kaiser J. As Gelsinger case ends, gene therapy suffers another blow. *Science* 2005;307:1028.

48. [Draft] *FDA Guidance for Industry: Gene Therapy Clinical Trials—Observing Participants for Delayed Adverse Events*, August 2005. http://www.fda.gov/cber/gdlns/gtclin.pdf

49. Zhang Y, Chirmule N, Gao GP, Qian R, Croyle M, Joshi B, Tazelaar J, Wilson JM. Acute cytokine response to systemic adenoviral vectors is mediated by dendritic cells and macrophages. *Mol Ther* 2001;5:697–707.

50. Bauer SR, Pilaro AM, Weiss KD, Testing of adenoviral vector gene transfer products: FDA expectations. In *Adenoviral Vectors for Gene Therapy*. Curiel DT, Douglas JT. eds. San Diego: Academic Press, 2002; 615–53.

51. Smith JS, Tian J, Lozier JN, Byrnes AP. Severe pulmonary pathology after intravenous administration of vectors in cirrhotic rats. *Mol Ther* 2004;6:932–41.

52. Jiang H, Couto LB, Patarroyo-White S, Liu T, Nagy D, Vargas JA, Zhou S, Scallan CD, Sommer J, Vijay S, Warren D, Mingozzi F, High KA, Pierce GF. Effects of transient immunosuppression on adeno associated virus-mediated liver-directed gene transfer in rhesus macaques and implications for human gene therapy. *Blood*, prepublished online, July 25, 2006; DOI 10.1182.

53. Sung MW, Chen SH, Thung SN, Zhang DY, Huang TG, Mandeli JP, Woo SL. Intratumoral delivery of adenovirus-mediated interleukin-12 gene in mice with metastatic cancer in the liver. *Hum Gene Ther* 2002;6:731–43.

54. International Conference on Harmonisation (July 1997). *S1B: Testing for Carcinogenicity of Pharmaceuticals.* http://www.ich.org/cache/compo/276-254-1.htm

55. International Conference on Harmonisation (July 1995). *S2A: Guidance on Specific Aspects of Regulatory Genotoxicity Tests for Pharmaceuticals.* http://www.ich.org/cache/compo/276-254-1.htm

56. International Conference on Harmonisation (July 1997). *S2B: Genotoxicity: A Standard Battery for Genotoxicity Testing of Pharmaceuticals.* http://www.ich.org/cache/compo/276-254-1.htm

57. International Conference on Harmonisation (Nov, 1995; amended Nov, 2000). *S5(R2): Detection of Toxicity to Reproduction for Medicinal Products and Toxicity to Male Fertility.* http://www.ich.org/cache/compo/276-254-1.htm.

58. Cearley CN, Wolfe JH. Transduction characteristics of adeno-associated virus vectors expressing cap serotypes 7, 8, 9, and rh10 in the mouse brain. *Mol Ther* 2006;13:528–37.

59. Leiden JM. Human gene therapy: the good, the bad, and the ugly. *Circul Res* 2000;86:923–5.

60. Borellini F, Ostrove J. The transfer of technology from the laboratory to the clinic: In process controls and final product testing. In Meager A, ed. *Gene Therapy Technologies, Applications and Regulations*. New York: Wiley, 1999;359–73.

CHAPTER 33

Considerations in Design of Preclinical Safety Evaluation Programs to Support Human Cell-Based Therapies

JOY A. CAVAGNARO, PhD, DABT, RAC

Contents

Preclinical Safety Evaluation of Biopharmaceuticals: A Science-Based Approach to Facilitating Clinical Trials, edited by Joy A. Cavagnaro
Copyright © 2008 by John Wiley & Sons, Inc.

33.1   INTRODUCTION

The sixteenth-century German-Swiss physician, Philippus Aureolus Theophrastus Bombastus von Hohenheim ("aka Paracelsus") may be credited with the earliest references to cell therapy. Although Paracelsus is probably best recognized as the "father of toxicology" for his pioneering work in systematizing the study of effects of chemicals and drugs, he spoke of healing of the heart with heart, lung with lung, spleen with spleen—indeed as "like heals like" in his 1536 book *Der grossen Wundartzney* [1]. Four centuries later, the Swiss physician. Paul Niehans would, by chance, become known as "the father of cell therapy" after treating a patient, whose parathyroid was accidentally removed by a fellow physician, with a homogenate of the parathyroid gland of an ox. Niehans claimed that he could cure illnesses through injection of live cells extracted from healthy organs. He believed that adding new tissue stimulated rejuvenation and recovery (see Table 33.1). In the 1960s the use of cells and tissue extracts from young or fetal animals, "fresh cell therapy," was still popular in Germany, and this practice lasted until the late 1990s when it was finally banned following increases in severe immune-mediated allergic diseases resulting from repeated injections of heterologous antigenic materials.

Today, with the exception of bone marrow for hematopoietic reconstitution, therapeutic cellular transplantation is an emerging technology. In recent years novel approaches in the potential restoration of function through cellular transplantation have included the use of fetal human or xenogeneic neural tissue for Parkinson's disease, ectopically implanted pancreatic islets for diabetes, Schwann cells and olfactory ensheathing glia for spinal cord injury, encapsulated chromaffin cells for pain, and various types of stem cells for the treatment of diabetes, cardiac disease, and central nervous system injuries or disease [2]. There have also been trials of encapsulated cells to provide enzymes that either remove "toxic" products or provide activation of prodrugs to therapeutics, usually anticancer derivatives.

Today the field of "regenerative medicine" refers to the broad range of disciplines adopted by groups working toward a common goal of replacing or regenerating damaged or diseased cell populations or tissues. There are approximately 270 cell types in the human body [3]. Understanding the biology as well therapeutic potentials of the many cell types is an important reason for pursing research on embryonic stem cells. Theoretically embryonic stem cells represent a source of cells capable of development into normal

TABLE 33.1   Selected milestones in the field of cell-based therapies

1931	First injection of living cells (parathyroid cells from an ox)
1937	Implantation of cerebral cells
1949	First injection of lyophilized cells
1956	Successful engraftment of bone marrow cells in mice following irradiation
1963	Self-renewing cells discovered in mouse bone marrow
1964	Single cell in teratocarcinoma isolated and remained undifferentiated in culture
1968	First successful bone marrow transplantation between two siblings
1978	Hematopoietic stem cells discovered in human cord blood
1981	Murine embryonic stem cells derived from mouse inner cell mass
1983	Fetal cells reported to repair spinal cord injury
1988	Isolation of murine hematopoietic stem cells
1988	Fetal pancreatic cells used in diabetic patients
1991	Fetus-to-fetus cell therapy
1992	Neural stem cells cultured in vitro as neurospheres
1995	Law to prohibit federal funds for research where human embryos are created or destroyed
1997	Cloning of Dolly the sheep by somatic cell nuclear transfer (SCNT)
1997	Isolation of putative progenitor endothelial cells
1997	Fresh cell therapy banned in Germany
1998	First human embryonic stem cell line derived (hESC)
1998	First established culture of human embryonic germ cells (hEGC)
1998	Bone marrow derived dendritic cells first described
1999	Cardiac tissue formation after bone marrow transplantation
2000	Development of neurons from bone marrow
2001	Cloning of first early (4 to 6 cell) human embryos for purpose of generating hESCs
2001	hESCs differentiated into early-stage neuronal cells
2001	Muscle tissue formation after bone marrow transplantation
2001	Stem cells from adipose tissue produce cartilage, bone, muscle
2001	Restriction of US federal funding for hESC research (use of approved cells only)
2003	Children's primary teeth as new source of stem cells
2005	Cord blood derived embryonic-like stem cell derived from umbilical cord blood
2006	hESC lines derived from single blastomeres
2007	Discovery of new type of stem cell in amniotic fluid
2007	hESC-based progenitor cells produce multiple nerve growth factors

differentiated cells that, when properly engineered can replace diseased tissues and restore normal function. In addition to selection of the most appropriate cell type, several different modes of transfer may be used to deliver cells to optimize therapeutic benefit. Cells may be directly infused, surgically implanted, or contained within an encapsulating membrane. Cells can be delivered through catheters, implanted in devices, or delivered through extracorporeal devices. In some cases genes can also be introduced into the cells to improve the efficacy and/or safety of the various types of cell-based therapies. The combination of cell and gene therapy using both nonviral and viral gene transfer vectors is beyond the scope of this chapter (see Chapter 32).

Over 500 companies are currently involved in cell therapy technology, and of these 121 are involved in stem cell therapies [4]. Clinical proof of principle has been demonstrated across several diseases for transplanted cells including multipotent fully differentiated cells in culture, cells for in vivo terminal differentiation, mixtures of multipotent and differentiated cells, and pluripotent cells for restoring function. No single source of cells is best or even suitable for all disease indications. In addition more than one source of cells may be used for the same indication; for example, adult bone marrow derived cells, endothelial progenitor cells, resident cardiac cells, and embryonic stem cells are all being studied for cardiac repair [3,6–8]. In diabetes sources of new β islet cells have included fetal pancreas, ex vivo expansion of endogenous progenitors β cell from adult pancreas, xenotransplants, umbilical cord blood, adult bone marrow, and embryonic stem cell lines [9,10] (see Table 33.2).

Most applications for cell-based therapies are still in the experimental research and clinical trial stages. As novel cell-based therapies move from discovery research to the clinic, developers and regulators will face new and continually evolving issues and uncertainties involving long-term efficacy and safety. The success of cell-based therapy will depend on optimal selection, manufacture, and survival of the implanted cells. However, because of the heterogeneity in cell types and scope of indications, the preclinical development, strategies, clinical development, and evaluation requirements are expected to be optimized according to product attributes and clinical indica-

TABLE 33.2   No single source of cells is suitable for all indications

Intervention	Indication	Types of Cells
Hematopoietic, immune replacement	Cancer Autoimmune disorders Immunodeficiencies	Lymphocyte-based therapies, autologous tumor cell vaccines, blood, bone marrow, UCB stem cells, HSCs, hMSCs, etc.
Metabolic replacement. support	Ophthalmic disorders Diabetes Lysosomal storage diseases Renal/liver failure	Human retinal stem cells, tissue-derived stem cells, islet cells, bioartificial kidney, bioartificial liver, hepatocytes, etc.
Tissue repair, regeneration	Cardiovascular disorders Neurological/ neurodegenerative Disorders Bone and joint disorders Wound healing[a]	hMSCs, cardiomyocytes, tissue-derived stem cells including olfactory cells neural cells, osteoblasts, chondrocytes, keratinocytes, dermal fibroblasts, hESCs, etc.

[a]The FDA has approved several cell therapy products as devices for skin replacements; for the treatment of acute (e.g., burns) and chronic (e.g., diabetic ulcers) inflammatory skin disorders.

tion. As is true for other novel biopharmaceuticals, the diversity of potential products coupled with uncertainties about unique product specific attributes creates a challenge for toxicologists responsible for predicting and characterizing their safety and estimating potential risks. However, knowledge gained from traditional biopharmaceuticals developed and approved throughout the 1980s and 1990s can be applied to novel cellular therapies. The challenges in moving cell therapy to the clinic is to understand what aspects of the results obtained with animal models can be easily translated to therapy and where caution must be exercised in extrapolating animal studies to ultimate human treatment [5].

33.2   REGULATION OF CELL-BASED THERAPIES IN THE UNITED STATES AND EUROPE

The FDA regulates cellular products as biological products. The Center for Biologics Evaluation and Research (CBER) is designated as the agency with primary jurisdiction for the pre-market review and regulation. Cellular products intended for use as somatic cell therapy are subject to regulation pursuant to the PHS Act (42 USC 251) and also fall within the definition of drugs (21 USC 312 (g)). Somatic cell therapy products are defined as autologous (i.e., self), allogeneic (i.e., intraspecies), or xenogeneic (i.e., interspecies) cells that have been propagated, expanded, selected, pharmacologically treated, or otherwise altered in biological characteristics ex vivo to be administered to humans and applicable to the prevention, treatment, cure, diagnosis, or mitigation of disease or injuries [11]. Specific examples of cellular products regulated by FDA as biological cellular products include (1) autologous or allogeneic lymphocytes activated and expanded ex vivo including lymphokine-activated killer cells (LAK) and tumor infiltrating lymphocytes (TIL cells); (2) encapsulated autologous, allogeneic, or xenogeneic cells or cultured cell lines intended to secrete a bioactive factor or factors (e.g., insulin, growth hormone, neurotransmitters); (3) autologous or allogeneic somatic cells including genetically modified cells (e.g., hepatocytes, myocytes, fibroblasts, bone marrow- or blood-derived hematopoietic stem cells, lymphocytes that have been genetically modified; (4) cultured cell lines; and (5) autologous or allogeneic bone marrow transplants using expanded or activated bone marrow cells [12]. Transplantation of minimally manipulated bone marrow and vascularized whole organs is regulated by the Health Resource Services Administration (HRSA), and allogeneic unrelated bone marrow transfer falls under the authority of the National Bone Marrow Donor Program standards under HRSA.

In accordance with the statutory provisions, cellular products must be in compliance with CFR part 312 regardless of whether the finished product is shipped across state lines; this is due to the use of ancillary products used in manufacture. Ancillary products (e.g., bioreactors and cell culturing systems; components of culture media; agents used to purge, select, or stimulate specific cell populations) are not intended to be present in final products, but they may have an impact on the safety, purity, or potency of the products. At the investigational stage these products must be in compliance with part 312. Therefore clinical trials are to be conducted under INDs. Although products regulated by FDA as biological products must also meet drug or device requirements, the agency does not require duplicate pre-market approvals.

Prior to 1993 the FDA did not require pre-marketing approval for many types of transplantation, including bone marrow transplants. To the extent that some bone marrow transplantation products are subject to extensive manipulation prior to transplantation, they are treated the same as somatic cell therapy and gene therapy products. FDA defined "manipulation" as the ex vivo propagation, expansion, selection, or pharmacological treatment of cells, or other alteration of their biological characteristics (11). Over the past two decades the FDA has published a number of guidance documents outlining various expectations for ensuring the safety of cellular therapies (13) (see Table 33.3).

The first guidance document relating to regulatory expectations for a cellular therapy product was entitled Points to Consider in the Collection, Processing, and Testing of Ex vivo Activated Mononuclear Leukocytes for Administration to Humans, and published in August 1989. In February 1996, FDA published a guidance for manipulated autologous structural (MAS) cells, which are autologous cells manipulated and then returned to the body for structural repair or reconstruction. Manipulation required for MAS cell products is more than that required for autologous bone marrow, where the source of material is harvested but otherwise undergoes minimal manipulation. Therefore MAS cell products were considered to fall within the definition of cellular therapy products. One year later the FDA published A Proposed Approach to the Regulation of Cellular and Tissue-Based Products.

The regulatory framework of the Proposed Approach document is a tiered risk-based approach: Products thought to present greater risk receive more regulatory oversight, and require more extensive control in manufacturing and clinical studies as well as more product characterization. The approach focuses on three general areas: (1) prevention of use of contaminated tissues or cells with the potential for transmitting infectious disease; (2) prevention of improper handling or processing that might contaminate or damage tissue or cells, and (3) assurance that clinical safety and effectiveness is demonstrated for tissue or cells that are highly processed, are used for other than their normal function, are combined with nontissue components, or are used for metabolic purposes. The manufacturing issues for cells lie in the preparation of the cell cultures and the assurance that cells are free of microbial contamination, such as mycoplasma (if cultured), or otherwise sterile. Appropriate screening/testing of donor tissue for communicable disease is essential as such criteria are necessary for accepting donor source materials to initiate production.

Consistency in lot-to-lot preparation of cells is paramount in the demonstration of manufacturing control. Critical manufacturing controls include

REGULATION OF CELL-BASED THERAPIES

TABLE 33.3   Key FDA regulatory guidance documents relating to cell-based therapies

Points to Consider in the Collection, Processing, and Testing of Ex vivo Activated
   Mononuclear Leukocytes for Administration to Humans (August 1989)
Guidance on Applications fro Products Comprised of Living Autologous Cells
   Manipulated Ex vivo and Intended for Structural Repair and Reconstruction
   (May 1996).
FDA Proposed Approach to Regulation of Cellular and Tissue-Based Products
   (February 1997)
Guidance for Industry: Guidance for Human Somatic Cell Therapy and Gene
   Therapy (March 1998)
PHS Guideline on Infectious Disease Issues in Xenotransplantation. OMB Control
   No.0910-0456 (January 2001)
Guidance for Industry: Source Animal, Product, Preclinical, and Clinical Issues
   Concerning the Use of Xenotransplantation Products in Humans (final guidance)
   (April 2003)
Guidance for Reviewers: Instructions and Template for Chemistry, Manufacturing,
   and Control (CMC) Reviewers of Human Somatic Cell Therapy Investigational
   New Drug Applications (INDs) (draft guidance) (August 2003)
Guidance for FDA Review Staff and Sponsors: Content and Review of Chemistry,
   Manufacturing, and Control (CMC) Information for Human Gene Therapy
   Investigational New Drug Applications (INDs) (draft guidance) (November 2004)
Current Good Tissue Practices for Human Cell, Tissue, and Cellular Tissue-Based
   Product Establishments; Inspection and Enforcement (November 2004)
Guidance for Industry: Minimally Manipulated, Unrelated, Allogeneic Placental/
   Umbilical Cord Blood Intended for Hematopoietic Reconstitution in Patients
   with Hematologic Malignancies. (draft guidance) (December 2006)
Guidance for Industry: Cell Selection Devices for Point of Care Production of
   Minimally Manipulated Autologous Peripheral Blood Stem Cells (PBSCs)
   (July 2007)
Guidance for Industry: Preparation of IDEs and INDs for Products Intended to
   Repair or Replace Knee Cartilage (draft guidance) (July 2007)
Guidance for Industry: Eligibility Determination for Donors of Human Cells,
   Tissues, and Cellular and Tissue-Based Products (HCT/Ps) (August 2007)
Guidance for FDA Reviewers and Sponsors: Content and Review of Chemistry,
   Manufacturing, and Control (CMC) Information for Human Somatic Cell Therapy
   Investigational New Drug Applications (INDs) (April 2008)

Note: See http://www.fda.gov/cber/guidelines.htm.

standardization and optimization of reagents and processing criteria. Product
characterization and development of acceptance criteria is also important,
including (1) establishing specific characteristics to ensure product integrity,
(2) identifying product parameters that anticipate adverse events, (3) developing analytical approaches for evaluating proposed acceptance criteria for in-
process intermediates and final cellular product, and (4) controlling purity and
impurity profiles of the final cellular product. Impurities arising from the scale-
up of manufacturing such as host-cell contaminants, endotoxin contamination,
and residual DNA levels are all potential safety concerns. Stability of the

protein sequence and posttranslational modifications are additional concerns for cell-based gene therapy products. Use of bovine serum is acceptable in the United States provided on that the source of the serum is demonstrated to be from herds reared for the entirety of their lives in certified BSE-free countries, although concerns have been expressed for use of bovine materials. Karyotypic analysis for determining genetic stability is also important for cells cultured for a long time.

In 2001 FDA put in place a comprehensive system consolidating the regulation of human cells, tissues, and cellular and tissue-based products (HCT/Ps) into one regulatory program. The definition of human cells, tissues, and cellular and tissue-based products (HCT/Ps) includes a broad range of cell- and tissue-based therapies and is intended to cover HCT/Ps at all stages of their manufacture, from recovery through distribution. The final new part 1271 regulation of chapter 21 is made up of six subparts. Subpart part A includes general provisions pertaining to the scope and applicability of part 1271, definitions and subpart B includes registration and listing procedures. The donor-suitability proposed rule contains subpart C of part 1271, and the GTP proposed rule contains subparts D, E, and F (see Table 33.3).

In Europe, the Council of Ministers approved the EC Regulation on Advance Therapy Medicinal Products in May 2007. Directive 2001/83/EC covers genetic medicinal products and somatic cell therapy medicinal products. Additional requirements are laid down in Regulations (EC)No726/2004 and a series of other European Commission Directives. The Advanced Therapy Medicinal Product (ATMP) regulations are amendments to Directive 2004/23/EC that provide quality and safety rules for the donation, testing, processing, preservation, storage, and distribution of human cells and tissues. All member states support the Regulation, which was implemented across the European Union at the end of 2007. The regulation governs production, distribution, and use of advanced therapies, including stem cell therapies for treating or preventing disease in humans. The Regulation also brings all innovative therapies into a single legislative framework and sets up a centralized marketing authorization procedure for such treatments.

The United Kingdom was first in Europe to introduce legislation covering human embryo research in 1990 following passage of the Human Fertilisation and Embryology (HFE) Act. The HFE Act included provisions in connection with human embryos and any subsequent development of such embryos prohibiting certain practices with embryos and gametes and the establishment of a Human Fertilisation and Embryology Authority. Currently in the United Kingdom the regulatory framework for human stem cell research is split into two, governing storage and use of human embryos and storage and use of human tissues and somatic cells. In July 2007 new regulations further implementing the EU Tissues and Cells Directive came into force in the United Kingdom. The Human Tissue (Quality and Safety) Regulations 2007 and the Human Fertilisation and Embryology (Quality and Safety) Regulations 2007 amend the current regulations governing the licensing of facilities in carrying out work in relation to human tissues and cells intended to be used in human applications. The Regulations 2007 set out requirements for obtaining a license from the relevant authority, either the Human Fertilisation and Embryology Authority (HEFA) or the Human Tissue Authority (HTA) in order to carry out the various acts covered by the Directive in relation to human derived tissue and cells that are intended for use in human applications. In September 2007, following considerable debate that will likely continue among experts over the next few years, the HFEA decided to permit the creation of hybrid or chimera embryos (human–animal) for research purposes.

33.3   TYPES OF CELL-BASED THERAPIES

33.3.1   Ex vivo Activated Mononuclear Leukocytes

Adoptive immunotherapy is a general term describing the transfer of immunocompetent cells to a tumor-bearing host. The major research challenge in advancing adoptive immunotherapies has been to develop immune cells with specific antitumor reactivity that can be generated in large enough quantities for transfer to tumor-bearing patients. Examples of passive nonspecific immunotherapy include transfer of lymphokine-activated killer (LAK) cells or tumor-infiltrating lymphocytes (TIL), activated in vitro by interleukin 2 (IL 2) or other lymphokines. Examples of passive specific immunotherapy include transfer of specific immune cells, such as NK cells, draining lymph node cells or "antigen-loaded" pulsed dendritic cells. The pulsed dendritic cells function as potent immunostimulators of native T cells. A key safety issue for these various cellular therapies is related to potential contamination with autologous malignant cells and the selection of immunoresistant malignant cells by the ex vivo activation procedure. The potential for cells cultured through many passages to transform to an exogenous growth factor-independent phenotype should also be addressed.

Initial studies of systemic administration of autologous LAK cells and rIL2 in patients with advanced cancer were reported by Rosenberg and others in the early to mid-1980s [14–16]. The regimen was based on animal models in which the systemic administration of LAK cells plus rIL2 mediated the regression of established pulmonary and hepatic metastases from a variety of murine tumors in several strains of mice. Patients showed some benefit; however, LAK cells had to be generated form lymphocytes obtained through multiple leukaphereses [17,18]. Methods have subsequently been developed to shorten the culture period and increase the proliferation of cells to improve the cell yield.

Infusion of tumor-infiltrating lymphocytes (TIL) isolated from tumor samples and expanded in vitro with rIL2 resulted in a more efficient tumor reduction in animal models [19] and showed activity in clinical studies [20]. A significant impediment to generating therapeutic TILs resides in the inherent limitations of the immunogenicity of the tumor from which the TILs are derived. In animal models using poorly immunogenic tumors, the therapeutic efficacy of TILs is limited. Tumors genetically engineered to produce certain cytokines have been found to contain TILs with enhanced in vitro and in vivo antitumor activity. Studies have shown that efficacy has been improved with TILs that are characterized by less time in tissue culture, longer telomeres, and a less differentiated phenotype.

In 1996 Celluzi et al. reported that active immunization strategies using antigen-pulsed dendritic cells were useful for inducing tumor-specific immune responses [21]. The authors showed that the major histocompatability complex class I–presented peptide antigen pulsed onto dendritic antigen-presenting cells (APCs) induced protective immunity in mice to lethal challenge by a tumor transfected with the antigen gene. The immunity was antigen specific, requiring expression of the antigen gene by the tumor target, and its elimination by in vivo depletion of CD8-T lymphocytes [21]. The first therapeutic tumor antigen vaccine evaluated by the FDA was Sipuleucel-T (Provenge(r)), a peptide-pulsed dendritic tumor cell vaccine manufactured by Dendreon for treatment of men with asymptomatic metastatic androgen independent prostate cancer (AIPC). Dosing is based on a minimal number of total nucleated cells in the starting material, which contains T, B, and NK cells and monocyte populations and a minimum number of CD45+ cells in the final product. The proposed mechanism of action of Sipuleucel-T is presentation of prostatic acid phosphatase (PAP) antigen by activated APCs to stimulate tumor-specific T cells in the patient [22]. Following a favorable advisory committee review in March 2007, the FDA issued an "approvable letter" in May requesting additional data from the sponsor in order to support a final approval.

In July 2007, a US biotech firm, Northwest Biotherapeutics, received approval form the Swiss Institute of Public Health to market to selected centers in Switzerland the first brain cancer vaccine, DCVax-Brain®, an autologous patient-specific dendritic cell based vaccine.

33.3.2 Living Autologous Cells Manipulated Ex vivo Intended for Structural Repair or Reconstruction (MAS Cells)

MAS cells are derived from a patient's tissues. The cells are manipulated ex vivo and then implanted into the same patient with the intent of providing repair or reconstruction of a structure rather than via systemic action of the cells. The manipulation of MAS cells involves dissociation of the selected tissue into individual cells, which are then propagated and expanded into large numbers of cells using tissue culture methods. Since MAS cells are implanted within an enclosed space, they are considered to be more similar to tissue and device products. Examples of MAS cells include chondrocytes for repair of focal cartilage defects, autologous fat cells for cosmetic augmentation, and autologous keratinocytes for dermal wound healing. In 1997 FDA approved the first MAS cellular therapy product under an accelerated approval procedure, Carticel® manufactured by Genzyme Tissue Repair, which involves the autologous transfer of healthy chondrocytes into damaged knee joints following ex vivo cell culture and proliferation.

33.3.3 Adult Stem Cells (Somatic Stem Cells)

Adult stem cells are cells found in a number of differentiated tissues that can self-renew and differentiate (with certain limitations) to give rise to the specialized cell types of the tissue. Adult stem cells may also be able to give rise to specialized cell types of a completely different tissue, a phenomenon known as transdifferentiation or plasticity. However, the presence of pluripotent adult stem cells remains a subject of scientific debate.

Identification of stem cells from different sources has broadened the prospects for clinical applications. The types of stem cells that can be isolated from adult bone marrow include hematopoietic stem cells, endothelial progenitors, and mesenchymal stem cells. The adult brain contains neural stem cells that can generate the brains three major cell types of the brain, namely nerve cells (neurons) and nonneural cells, astrocytes, and oligodendrocytes. Epithelial stem cells in the lining of the digestive tract can give rise to a number of cell types, including absorptive cells, goblet cells, and enteroendocrine cells. Skin stem cells in the basal layer of the epidermis can give rise to keratinocytes, and follicular stem cells at the base of the hair follicle can give rise to both the hair follicle and the epidermis.

There are two characteristics that distinguish stem cells from other types of cells: stem cells can self renew, and they can differentiate into other types of cells. Stem cells renew themselves for long periods through cell division, and given certain conditions, they can be induced to become cells with special functions.

33.3.4 Hemapotopoietic Stem Cells

Hematopoietic stem cells (HSCs) can be derived from bone marrow, umbilical cord blood, placenta, or mobilized peripheral blood. The hemapoietic tissues may have cells with long- and short-term regeneration capacities and committed multipotent, oligopotent, and unipotent progenitors. HSCs give rise to all the blood cell types including myeloid and lymphoid lineages as wells as some dendritic cells. There is a growing body of evidence suggesting that HSCs are plastic and that, at least under certain circumstances, HSCs may participate in the generation of tissues other than those of the blood system. HSCs are phenotypically identified by their small size and certain surface markers. Murine HSCs have been demonstrated to be negative for lineage markers (Lin-), including myeloid and B and T cell lineages, and positive for c-kit, Sca-1, and CD34 [17]. The cell markers used to characterize the commonly accepted type of human HSCs include $CD34^+$, $CD59^+$, Thy/$CD90^+$, $CD38^{lo/-}$, C-kit$^{-/lo}$, and lin- [23]. However, not all HSCs are covered by these combinations; for example, some cells lack CD34 [24,25].

33.3.5   Endothelial Progenitor Cells (EPCs)

Adult endothelial progenitor cells were first described by Asahara and colleagues showing that a purified subpopulation of CD34-expressing cells isolated from the blood of adult mice could differentiate into endothelial like cells in vitro [26]. Endothelial progenitor cells derived from bone marrow have the ability to differentiate into endothelial cells (cells that line blood vessels). These progenitor cells have been reported to express CD34, CD133, CD31, VE-cadherin, VEGFR2, and c-Kit. CD133 and CD34 are often used as markers for selection and purification because CD133 is not found on mature endothelial cells, and CD34 is not found on the undifferentiated stem cells from which endothelial progenitor cells derive [27,28].

Endothelial progenitor cells have been shown to participate in a number of regenerative activities. They contribute to pathologic angiogenesis such as that found in retinopathy and tumor growth. There is evidence that circulating EPCs play a role in the repair of damaged blood vessels after a myocardial infarction. Higher levels of circulating endothelial progenitor cells detected in the bloodstream predict better outcomes and fewer repeat heart attacks [29]. Recently tissue-resident stem cells have been isolated from the heart, and they are capable of differentiating to the endothelial lineage [30]. There is also increasing evidence suggesting that there are additional bone marrow derived cell populations (e.g., myeloid cells and mesenchymal cells) and non–bone marrow derived cells that can give rise to endothelial cells [28]. Although the role of EPCs in neovascularization has been convincingly shown by several groups, their precise function in neovascularization remains undefined.

33.3.6   Mesenchymal Stem Cells (MSCs)

Mesenchymal stem cells represent a rare population of bone marrow derived cells that do not express CD34 or CD133. Under defined in vitro and in vivo conditions mesenchymal cells can differentiate into a variety of cell types, including osteoblasts, chondrocytes, adipocytes, myocytes, and stromal fibroblasts [31,32,33]. Human MSCs have high expansion potential, genetic stability, and reproducible characteristics as has been proved in many laboratories. They have the ability to migrate to sites of tissue injury and to modify the response of immune cells. The later characteristic may support the development of allogeneic stem cell approaches when autologous stem cells are not readily available [34]. Because MSCs can produce important growth factors and cytokines, they may also be able to exert their effect without direct participation in long-term tissue repair. MSCs have not been shown to be capable of regenerating or maintaining a whole tissue compartment as has been shown for hematopoietic stem cells (HSCs). Although MSCs can engraft and differentiate to some extent in host tissue, they do not have an ability comparable with the de novo tissue-forming ability of embryonic stem cells in embryoid bodies.

33.3.7 Human Embryonic Stem Cells (hESC)

Human embryonic stem cells (hESCs) were first derived from the inner cell mass (ICM) from the blastocyst stage (~100–200 cells) of embryos generated by in vitro fertilization [35,36]. In humans the blastocyst is an early-stage embryo, approximately 4 to 5 days old. The blastocyst can be formed by means of either in vitro fertilization or somatic cell nuclear transfer, in which the nucleus of a somatic cell is combined with an enucleated oocyte. Methods have been developed to derive hESCs from the late morula stage (30–40 cells) and from arrested embryos (16–24 cells incapable of further development), and more recently from single blastomeres isolated from 8-cell embryos (37).

Human embryonic stem cells are defined by the presence of several transcription factors and cell surface proteins. The transcription factors oct-4, nanog, and sox2 ensure the suppression of genes that lead to differentiation and the maintenance of pluripotency [38]. The cell surface proteins most commonly used to identify hESCs are the glycolipids SSEA3 and SSEA4 and the keratin sulfate antigens Tra-1-60 and Tra-1-81 [39]. The characteristic features of hESCs include their proliferative and self-renewing properties and their ability to differentiate into derivatives of all three primary germ cell layers: ectoderm, endoderm, and mesoderm. hESCs maintain pluripotency through multiple cell divisions. Although hESCs can form all somatic tissues, they cannot form all of the other "extraembryonic" tissues necessary for complete development, such as the placenta and membranes, so they cannot give rise to a complete new individual [40]. The only other cells with proven pluripotency similar to that of hESCs are embryonic germ cells (hEGCs) derived from primordial germ cells [40]. Biologically hEGCs have many properties in common with hESCs [41]. In humans, hEGCs were first established in culture in 1998 from tissue derived from an aborted fetus [42].

As of October 2006, 500 hESC lines had been reported in the literature (including posters and meeting abstracts). Of these, 455 were normal, no-disease-related cell lines and 45 were disease related [43]. In response to concerns regarding the ethics of deriving hESCs from early-stage embryos, the US federal government initiated a moratorium on the use of federal funds to derive and/or work on hESCs after August 9, 2001 [44]. At this time, a total of 71 hESC lines were identified as being acceptable for study using US government funds. Only 15 of the 27 hESCs lines that are eligible are fully characterized and available for research to scientists around the world [43]. All hESCs derived after August 9, 2001, are considered by the US government to be ineligible for NIH funding. As of October 2006, 384 of these lines were derived from normal embryos. Of these, 73 have been fully characterized, karyotyped, shown to express hESC "stemness" markers, demonstrated to differentiate into derivatives of all three germ cell layers both in vitro and in vivo, and fully described with respect to derivation and propagation methods [43].

As long as embryonic stem cells in culture are grown under certain conditions, they can remain undifferentiated (unspecialized). But if cells are allowed to clump together to form embryoid bodies they begin to differentiate spontaneously into specific cell types (muscle cells, nerve cells, etc.). To generate cultures of specific types of differentiated cells, various growth factors are used in the culture media [45].

The scope of current stem cells research is larger than providing cells for transplantation. Cultured pluripotent stem cells are also being used in toxicity testing, identifying drug targets, studying cell differentiation, and understanding the prevention and treatment of birth defects.

33.3.8 Xenogeneic Cells

Xenogeneic cell therapy refers to live cells or tissues from a nonhuman animal source administered to a human recipient in vivo or ex-vivo. The main interest for using xenogeneic cells and tissues is the insufficient supply of human cells or organs. While attempts have been made to implant xenogeneic cells or tissues into patients, these attempts have often failed due to immunological incompatibility. From the public health point of view, the risk of cross-species transmission of infectious agents remains the most serious obstacle for using xenogeneic cells in humans.

33.4 CASE-BY-CASE APPROACH BASED ON PRODUCT ATTRIBUTES AND INDICATION

Ideally cell-based therapy products should (1) proliferate sufficiently to generate desired quantity of cells, (2) differentiate into desired cell type(s), (3) retain normal chromosomal complement, (4) survive in recipient after transplantation, (5) integrate into the surrounding tissue after transplantation, (6) exhibit controlled proliferation, (7) function appropriately for the duration of the recipient's life, and (8) avoid harm to the recipient. The source of cells in addition to the clinical indication influence the type and level of concern regarding safety [46] (see Table 33.4). While some concerns can be generalized across various cell types—such as about the migratory potential of transplanted cells in vivo and the possibility of infectious contamination—concerns regarding genetic instability, inherent or culture-induced tumorigenic potential, and the potential immunogenicity of host versus graft and graft versus host are more specific to the particular cell types. The remainder of this chapter will focus on the preclinical development considerations related to adult and embryonic stem cell based therapies to enable clinical trials.

TABLE 33.4 Product attributes based on source of cell-based therapies

Product Attributes	Primary Cells (Allogeneic)	Adult Stem Cells (Autologous)	Adult Stem Cells (Allogeneic)	Embryonic Stem Cells (Allogeneic)
• Accessibility • Proliferative capacity	• Easy • None	• Easy • Limited (multipotent); reprogram to become more "stem-like"?	• Easy • Limited (multipotent); reprogram to become more "stem-like"?	• Difficult • Unlimited (pluripotent)
• Differentiation capacity	• None	• Restricted (decreases with age of donor as well as time in culture; may not differentiate into cells that are needed)	• Restricted (decreases with age of donor as well as time in culture; may not differentiate into cells that are needed)	• Unlimited (reliable selection procedures needed to produce homologous cell populations)
• Genetic manipulation	• None	• None	• More difficult than ESCs	• Can be manipulated to incorporate foreign nucleic acid sequences in a stable manner
• Quality (reproducibility)	• No	• Yes	• Yes, not derived as single clones	• Yes, single clone
• Immunologic risk (transplant rejection)	• Possible	• Low (culturing ex vivo could lead to allogeneic epitopes)	• Possible	• Possible
• Safety (transmission of infectious agent(s))	• High risk	• Low risk	• Moderate risk	• Moderate risk
• Safety (tumorigenicity)	• No concern	• No concern	• Increased concern based upon length of culture period	• Moderate to high concern
• Economic feasibility/advantage	• High cost	• High cost	• Moderate cost	• Potentially lower cost
• Ethical/legal concerns	• None	• None	• Fewer	• Many

33.5 PRINCIPLES OF PRECLINICAL SAFETY EVALUATION FOR STEM CELL BASED THERAPIES

Stem cells are a dynamic biological entity and are intended to persist in the transplant environment for prolonged periods. They respond to their environment and undergo changes that are dependent on extrinsic signals as well as their intrinsic cellular properties and are thus more complex than defined metabolic pathways of drugs. However, the principles of preclinical safety evaluation for stem cell based therapies are similar to those of small-molecule drugs and closely parallel biopharmaceutical products. Studies are expected to define a safe starting dose and dose escalation scheme for clinical trials, to provide information to support the route of administration and the application schedule, to identify target organs of toxicity and parameters to use in monitoring clinical trials and the extent of follow up, and to determine populations that may be at greater risk for toxicity [47–52].

Study designs should take into consideration the type of cells that will be evaluated, selection of a relevant animal model, including a model that mimics the intended clinical population or disease state, and the treatment regimen, including route of administration. In most cases animal models of disease will be the most relevant model to assess not only proof of concept but also safety.

Two approaches have been used for predicting how stem cells will behave after transplantation into humans. Either human cells are transplanted into animals (generally rodents) with or without immune suppression or labeled, or unlabeled analogous cells are transplanted into the respective animal species. Both approaches have their limitations since transplantation is regulated by a species-specific network of biologically active molecules such as growth factors, cytokines, cell adhesion molecules and receptors, and extracellular matrices that may differ among species and thus influence engraftment [5].

Cells derived from humans at the same stage of development with the same overall characteristics may also differ significantly, as humans show a high frequency of allelic variability, which may be greater than the transplant models that frequently use inbred strains. In addition human cells tested in animal models may behave differently than human cells transplanted into humans because of provoked immune responses and/or intrinsic differences in cell properties or host environments for which limited information is available [5]. Although the overall properties may seem similar when analogous products are compared, there may be significant biological differences in cells isolated at similar stages of development in terms of developmental patterns, environmental cues, and growth factor dependence in culture as well as expression of specific markers for more restricted precursors that makes isolation and purification of subsets of progenitors more difficult [5].

When the data from analogous cell products are used to guide clinical trials, in-depth comparison between the animal and human cells is needed. The concerns with determining product comparability are not unlike those raised when using homologous or analogous proteins [49]. Potential processing, formulation, and storage may be different; cellular morphology, phenotype, and the level of engraftment and persistence may differ; and the cells may have different function or regulation (e.g., species-specific signaling may be present). Limited characterization of the animal product may also introduce uncertainty for extrapolation (e.g., potentially different impurities/contaminants). Ensuring comparability is even more important when assessing toxicity, as extrapolation of an initial safe starting dose is generally based on safety rather than activity in animals.

33.6 PHARMACOLOGY

Before initiating clinical studies, it is essential to demonstrate that cell preparations possess well-defined biological activity. Studies should be adequate to demonstrate the intended pharmacological activity in relevant in vitro and in vivo models. Initially in vitro studies, addressing cell and tissue morphology, proliferation, phenotype, heterogeneity, and the level of differentiation may be used to support pharmacological activity [52]. Relevant animal model selection is based on the biological and structural goal of the study, the disease under study, the animal's anatomy and physiology and size, availability, housing requirements, cost and technical feasibility, as well as historical experience with the model.

Animal transplant models of human disease support a rationale for conducting the initial clinical trials in patients. These studies provide information concerning the feasibility of the treatment and explore the establishment of a dose–response relationship between the cellular product and activity outcomes. The studies are also designed to understand the basic mechanisms of structure and function, host–implant interface, and systemic effects after transplantation. Such observations are particularly important for products that contain cells that are not terminally differentiated at the time of transplantation. Since most human diseases do not occur spontaneously in animals, animal models of human disease that are generally created by chemical, surgical, or immunological methods are often imperfect [5]. In all cases the abilities and limitations of each animal model including level of characterization of the model should be considered for extrapolating findings to humans.

Ideally biomarkers of activity should be identified at various times over the course of the study to support the pharmacodynamic activity (e.g., normalization of insulin, improvement in beta cell function as measured by C-peptide level, or control of glucose following transplantation of β pancreatic islet cells); improvement of motor coordination in mice with spinal cord damage following transplant of neurons; or repair of heart function (e.g., functional measures such as LV ejection fraction, pressure volume loops, ventricular pressure and heart wall thickness). Such markers may also be useful in subsequent clinical

TABLE 33.5 In vivo preclinical demonstration of POC: Stem-cell based cellular therapies

- Identify which cell(s) will be used.
- Characterize cell population(s) using multiparametric analytical testing.
- Establish comparability of cellular products if an analogous product is being evaluated.
- Perform studies in animal transplant model of human disease (consider cell biology, anatomy, pathophysiology, biomechanics, etc; immunosuppression regimen, identify limitations).
- Consider reasonable group size such as 10/group or 5/sex/group for rodents; total of 3 to 5/group for large animals (consider attrition based on surgical procedures, concomitant treatments, historical information on the model, etc.; consider incorporation of various controls including placebo, sham, and positive controls).
- Explore dose–response relationship (determine minimal or optimal cell number, maximum feasible dose).
- Assess feasibility of intervention (timing of lesion by chemical or surgical insult, location of cell transplant, route of administration, biocompatibility of delivery device, etc.).
- Determine biomarkers of activity.
- Define functional activity (desired effect), and justify timing and frequency of assessments (assessors should be blinded to treatment groups).
- Assess early response and durability of response (justify timing).
- Identify possible incorporate safety endpoints.
- Establish comparability of clinical material over the course of clinical development.
- Consider more than one species to enhance knowledge of cell placement and dose extrapolation.

trials. If the intended use is to restore function of deficient cells (tissue regeneration) functional tests should be implemented to demonstrate that function is restored. If the intended use is adoptive immunotherapy or vaccination in cancer patients, immune assays to assess immunological effects should be used [52]. Studies should also be designed to determine the optimal amount of cells needed to achieve the desired effects and the extent that immunosuppressive agents act synergistically in promotion of graft survival. (see Table 33.5)

33.7 SAFETY PHARMACOLOGY

Cells by themselves or by secreting pharmacologically active substances may have effects on the CNS, cardiac, respiratory, renal, or GI systems. Safety pharmacology should therefore be considered on a case-by-case basis depending on the specific characteristics of the cell-based product [52]. In general, specific assessments are made as part of the toxicology assessments rather than as stand-alone studies consistent with the assessments made with protein-based biopharmaceuticals [50]. The fundamental physiological differences (e.g., total blood volume, pulmonary capillary surface area, and volume) should be considered when extrapolating across species as well as specific attributes of the cells including viability and potential cell aggregates. Flow rate is particularly important when administering cells by the intravenous route. Assessment of CNS effects will be more relevant to therapeutic interventions to the nervous system.

33.8 EXPOSURE ASSESSMENT

Although the practices for conventional PK/ADME studies are not relevant for cell-based therapies, the principles of understanding exposure are relevant to determining optimal dose and understanding cell localization and migration. Various noninvasive (nonterminal) imaging modalities including positron emission tomography (PET), single-photon emission tomography (SPECT), or magnetic resonance imaging (MRI), fluorescence, and bioluminescence imaging provide visualization of grafted cells, evaluation of targeting of transplants to specific areas, and monitoring the regenerative process changes after cell therapy. Ensuring accurate cell delivery to the correct physiological site is fundamental to determining the activity and safety of cell-based products. Therefore studies are conducted to determine spatiotemporal information about cellular trafficking patterns, tissue distribution (biodistribution), and persistence. It is also important to characterize the dynamics of cell proliferation, growth, alterations in phenotype, and the kinetics of cell death. If there is no effect after cell transplantation, it is important to determine if that is due to incorrect cell function or to improper cellular targeting. In addition the unintended migration of the cells including release of bioactive products to "ectopic sites" may result in adverse effects.

Various strategies are used for cell labeling and tissue visualization. Ideally labeling techniques should not perturb the target cell, be able to quantify the cell number, have minimum transfer to nontarget cells, and be compatible with histochemical methods used for morphological analysis. Examples of labeling strategies include radioisotopes, fluorescent dyes, and 5-bromo-2-deoxyuridine (BrdU). BrdU binds to DNA during its synthesis and labels the nucleus. It can be identified in both frozen and paraffin-embedded sections by either immunostaining as brown staining (peroxidase) or red staining (alkaline phosphatase) after treatment with an appropriate anti-BrdU antibody [53]. Chloromethylbenzamido-DiI-derived (cm-DiI), a red autofluorescent dye that binds to the cell membrane, can be identified in frozen sections [54].

While these techniques are sensitive, they can be hampered by cytotoxic side effects of the labeling procedures and can be limited by dilution and loss of the marker over time as a result of cell division [55]. Thus, while useful for measuring the efficiency of acute delivery, these techniques may offer minimal long-term information regarding cell survival, proliferation, and differentiation [56].

Use of viral transduction methods allows stable integration of reporter genes—such as green (GFP) or yellow (YFP) fluorescent proteins, lacZ, alkaline phosphatase, or firefly luciferase—permitting the evaluation of viable cells by fluorescence microscopy and flow cytometry. Reporter gene imaging can be used to track long-term cell survival, migration, division, and differentiations, and this method provides information on location and numbers of cells [57,58]. Cells can also be labeled via in situ hybridization for Y chromosome showing survival of male donor cells into female recipients [59]. Human cells can further be tracked in animal tissue by qPCR for human specific sequences. The disadvantages of reporter gene, Y chromosome, and qPCR methods is the requirement of a biopsy or animal sacrifice for the performance of the cell tracking in tissues [60].

Magnetic resonance imaging (MRI) can be used to track cells labeled with contrast materials. The two classes of contrast material that are generally used as MRI imaging labels are gadolinium chelates and iron oxide nanoparticles [61]. Iron oxide particles are a class of superparamagnetic MRI contrast agents. The particles range from tens of nanometers in diameter, termed ultrasmall superparamagnetic iron oxide (USPIO), to 100 nm (superparamanetic iron oxide [SPIO]), to some larger than 1 μM, known as micrometer-sized iron oxide particles (MPIOs). These compounds consist of magnetite (iron oxide) cores that are coated with dextran or siloxanes encapsulated by a polymer or further modified to facilitate internalization. They can confirm cell delivery and monitor short-term migration into surrounding tissues and can also be used in larger animals and humans [61–64]. MRI methods are, however, unable to distinguish between viable and nonviable cells. Nuclear labeling techniques, such as ^{18}F, can theoretically be used in combination with tracking methods to evaluate the anatomy of the transplant in relation to its function [60,65].

Ultimately multiple imaging modalities as well as newer more sensitive approaches to track live cells may be needed for complete functional monitoring of the various cellular repair processes.

33.9 GENERAL TOXICITY

Although guidance documents have been issued by regulatory agencies to provide assistance in the preclinical safety of cellular products [51,52], toxicologists should recognize that the ultimate study designs including appropriate animal models may be product specific (see Table 33.6). Ideally toxicology studies designed to support product safety are fully GLP compliant.

However evaluation of safety in animal models of disease may be difficult to conduct with strict adhere to current good laboratory practices (cGLPs) due to novel routes of administration, limited animal numbers, uniqueness of the animal model of disease, and/or novel surgical procedures. In such cases the principles of the regulation can still be followed, and where deviations occur, they should be evaluated for their impact on the expected clinical application and discussed. An in-depth discussion should be provided to support a regulatory submission.

TABLE 33.6 In vivo preclinical safety evaluation: Stem-cell based cellular therapies

Exposure assessment

- Determine cellular fate/ biodistribution and persistence (cell migration/trafficking, engraftment, differentiation, cell phenotype, fusion, tissue integration, proliferation, survival). Use of noninvasive (nonterminal) imaging modalities and special histological stains (terminal). Determine presence of ectopic foci. Justify multiple time points (e.g., 1 week, 1 month, 3 months, 6 months or 12 months).

General toxicity assessment

- Select one or more available relevant models (e.g., age of animal, relevance to human disease).
- Select test article (human cells or comparable analogous cells).
- Determine whether immunosuppressive agents are needed and their affect on activity.
- Justify number of animals/sex/group (e.g., 10/group or 5/sex/group for rodents; total of 3 to 5/group for large animals per time point).
- Justify dose levels (include minimum effective dose, multiples of proposed human dose; consider negative and positive controls).
- Justify route and timing of administration (if device is used, assess biocompatibility with cells).
- Determine general health status.
- Assess daily food consumption.
- Assess weekly body weights.
- Assess clinical laboratory parameters (hematology, coagulation, serum chemistry).
- Assess local tolerance (infusion toxicity, implant site reaction, local microenvironment, release of paracrine factors).
- Assess host immune response (inflammatory response in target/nontarget tissue, auto-antibodies, sensitized cells against normal tissues/organs).
- Assess morphologic response in target/nontarget tissue.
- Identify functional and other laboratory endpoints (assessors should be blinded to treatment groups).
- Identify target tissues.
- Characterize toxicities (delayed toxicity/ reversibility of toxicity).
- Assess macroscopic pathology (gross observations) at justified sacrifice intervals.
- Assess microscopic pathology (histopathology) at justified sacrifice intervals; analyze multiple sections from site of transplantation. Consider specific IHC staining in addition to standard staining.

Tumorigenicity assessment

Established cell lines, embryonic pluripotent stem cells, adult tissue derived multipotent stem cells-extended culture
- Determine one relevant animal model (chemically immunosuppressed rodent, genetically immunocompromised/immunodeficient rodent species).
- Confirm cellular engraftment in animal model via intended clinical route of administration.
- Justify number of animals/sex/group (e.g., minimum of 20/group; 10/sex/group).
- Justify dose level(s) (consider maximum feasible dose, positive and negative controls).
- Justify study duration (minimum of 6 months up to 12 months).
- Assess microscopic pathology (interpretation of findings—frequency of tumor formation, inappropriate proliferation without malignant formation, etc.).

When preclinical studies are conducted "in house" or are reported in peer-reviewed journals and intended to support clinical trials, they should be well-controlled and designed to answer specific toxicological questions. The data should also be available in sufficient detail to allow an independent review of the studies. Ideally study designs include not only efficacy but toxicological endpoints such as defined clinical laboratory parameters, macroscopic, and microscopic evaluation of tissues.

As is true for all biopharmaceuticals, toxicity studies should be performed in relevant animal models. For cellular therapies these models are often in animal models intended to mimic the human disease. When possible the intended human cells are utilized for assessments with or without low-dose immunosuppressants (e.g., 10 mg/kg, i.p. dose of cyclosporine A in rats). The immunosuppressive drug is generally administered prior to the cell dose and extended for a specified period after the transplant. In cases where it is not feasible to use the intended clinical material, largely due to the inability of the cells to engraft sufficiently into the host, analogous cells can be used to assess preclinical safety and activity. In such cases it is important to understand the potential impact of any differences between the analogous product and the clinical product in order to improve extrapolation of safe and active cell doses to humans.

In many cases, only one relevant animal model of disease may be available to assess activity and/or safety; in other cases, more than one model may be available and sufficiently characterized to allow for meaningful extrapolation. Two species, including larger animal species, can be used to assist extrapolation of dose to humans and/or to test the safety of cell-based product with the intended clinical delivery device. In the latter case, it is important to assess not only biocompatibility of the cells with the delivery device but the delivery reproducibility, namely the quantitative recovery of cells after injection based on the formulation and concentration to be used.

Usually three dose levels are assessed, including the minimal effective dose and a maximum feasible dose. It is also good to look at previous preclinical and clinical experience with similar products for estimating clinical dose. Doses are extrapolated based on body weight, body surface area, or target organ volume, depending on the route of administration. The rate of delivery is especially important for cells administered intravenously. Other considerations include cell concentration and delivery volume, the number of injections, and cell viability. Cell viability is generally equal or greater than 70%.

Multiple time points are included in study designs to assess acute and late effects as well as the reversibility of any adverse effects. The route of administration should reflect the intended clinical use. Repeated-dose toxicity studies are only relevant if the clinical use includes multiple dosing. For example, in the case of β pancreatic islet cells, toxicity studies should mimic the clinical scenario of retransplantation assessment of acute toxicities and cumulative effects that would preclude retransplantation.

The potential for autoimmunity should be considered when cells are used for immunotherapy purposes [52]. The basic local alignment search tool

(BLAST) is generally used to identify the potential cross-reactivity with endogenous molecules which could signal an autoimmune concern [66].

33.10 REPRODUCTIVE AND DEVELOPMENTAL TOXICITY

The need for reproductive and developmental toxicity studies is dependent on the product, the clinical indication, and the intended patient population [50,52]. Consideration is based on the nature of any expressed products and/or inappropriate biodistribution. Effects to the reproductive system that were identified in exposure and general toxicity assessments that suggest a cause for concern must be addressed in these more specific studies. If studies are necessary, study designs will likely need to be altered to accommodate selection of relevant animal model, dose selection, and dosing frequency.

33.11 GENOTOXICITY

Similar to protein-based biopharmaceuticals, the standard battery of genotoxicity studies is not considered to be relevant for cell-based therapies unless there is a specific cause for concern regarding the nature of any expressed products that would indicate a potential interaction directly with DNA or other chromosomal material [50,52]. The conduct of genotoxicity studies for assessing the genotoxic potential of process related contaminants is also not considered to be appropriate [50].

33.12 TUMORIGENICITY

One of the greatest concerns about using undifferentiated stem cells is their potential to develop tumors [67,68]. The investigation of immortalization, malignant transformation, and tumorigenicity, however, are unlikely to be addressed by conventional rodent bioassays for carcinogenicity or the alternative short-term transgenic mouse assays (see Table 33.7).

Human stem cell lines are actually defined by their formation of benign tumors (teratomas) following injection of cells into an ectopic site in immunocompromised mice. The teratomas are comprised of differentiated tissue originating from all three embryonic germ layers, thus confirming the ability of the cell lines to give rise to all cell types in the body [45]. To date, tumor formation has not been reported in animal or human studies with stem cell therapies when passaged for standard periods such as 6 to 8 weeks. However, there has been at least one report of late-passaged mesenchymal stem cells (16–20 weeks) developing chromosomal abnormalities and spontaneous cancerous transformation in vitro [69].

TABLE 33.7 Dose extrapolation for FIH dose: Stem-cell based cellular therapies

Points to consider

- Comparability to clinical product if analogous product is used (processing, cellular morphology, phenotype, species-specific signaling, impurities, contaminants, formulation and storage)
- Response to cytokines, chemokines, growth factors, adhesion molecules, and their receptors

- Inherent limitation of animal model compared to human disease (e.g., etiology, progression, phenotype, pathology; acute vs. chronic disease)
- Influence of host environment of human recipient (age, disease, medical history)
- Allelic variability in humans (compared to inbred animal strains)
- Transplant and surgical technique impacting diffusion and growth of cells
- Timing of transplantation
- Physiological and biological in the response of the transplanted cells to the local environment
- Immune response
- Dose administration (concentration, volume, rate of delivery, location of injection, number of injections, cell stability, delivery device)
- Scaling factor (e.g., body weight, body surface area, volume of target organ)
- Cross species validation (if more than one animal model is available)

The need for assessment of tumorigenic risk should therefore be considered based on the cell type (including cell source and "stemness" of the cells) as well as the degree of post collection ex vivo manipulation. Analysis may include assessments of proliferative capacity, dependence on exogenous stimuli, and response to apoptosis stimuli or genomic modification.

When needed, a tumorigenicity study should be performed with cells that are at the limit or beyond routine cell culturing. Generally, tumorigenicity is evaluated in genetically immunodeficient or chemically immunosuppressed rodents (mice or rats), 20 animals per group, via the intended clinical route of administration for at least 6 months duration. Although in some cases, based on specific product attributes, cells may be minimally detectable at 6 or 12 months even in the presence of immunosuppressive regimes. Ideally the study should be designed to include both negative and positive control groups. A pilot study is often performed to confirm cell engraftment. One dose group may be sufficient, if it is the maximum feasible dose. Tissues found to contain cells or expressed products during the biodistribution studies should also be analyzed with special emphasis during the tumorigenicity study [52].

33.13 LOCAL TOLERANCE

One of the goals of preclinical evaluation is to improve efficacy and safety by optimizing both the method of cell delivery and the site of cell delivery (transplantation site). Thus many novel routes of delivery have been employed based on specific product attributes and intended clinical indication. For example, various sites have been successful for transplantation of β islet cell-based therapies in experimental animal models, including intraportal, kidney subcapsule, intrasplenic, intrathymic, intraperitoneal, anterior chamber of the eye, subcutaneous, intra-abdominal, and omental pouch. Other unique routes of dosing include autologous adult olfactory neuroepithelial-derived neuronal progenitor cells for spinal cord repair delivered via the intralesional route, allogeneic adult bone marrow derived MSC for acute myocardial infarction via the intravenous route, and human fetal-derived progenitor cells for treatment of myelodegenerative CNS disease via the intracerebral route.

As a result of these unique delivery routes, there is an increased potential for toxicity to tissues at or near the injection site. Assessment of local tolerance and tissue compatibility of the clinical formulation is usually evaluated as part of the animal model of efficacy and/or general toxicity study, thus obviating the need for separate local tolerance studies. There may be additional concerns in cases where analogous products are used including potential differences in formulation, stability, and so forth.

33.14 EXPECTATIONS FOR PRE-PREIND FILING IN THE UNITED STATES

The Office of Cell Tissue and Gene Therapy (CBER/FDA) has historically encouraged sponsors that are developing products in an emerging field to engage in early dialogue to better understand the current regulatory concerns and expectations. The information necessary to engage in early discussions with the agency includes (1) a summary description of the intended clinical product; (2) a summary outline (e.g., one page) of the proposed clinical trial, to include the subject population, possible dose levels, dosing regimen, route of administration, dosing procedure (devices, if intended for delivery of the product), and parameters that will be assessed; (3) a comprehensive summary of all preclinical (in vitro and in vivo) activity/proof-of-concept and toxicity studies conducted and the results obtained, including relevant publications; (4) a detailed discussion, with protocol outlines, regarding what additional preclinical studies (toxicity/safety and proof of concept) are planned to adequately address the safety of the product; and (5) specific questions relating to pharmacology and toxicology issues/assessments. While the comments made during these early discussions with FDA are nonbonding, they are intended to help in preparing the subsequent pre-IND submission. The agency, however, discourages the conduct of pivotal preclinical studies if there are significant questions related to the proposed approach. The general issues and specific considerations are provided in the Appendix. In the EU, the scientific advice procedures in various countries and at the EMEA level are also useful in guiding sponsors developing novel therapies.

33.15 THE TRANSITION INTO CLINICAL TRIALS

As novel cell-based therapies move from preclinical studies into the clinic, researchers and regulators face new and evolving issues and uncertainties involving long-term safety and efficacy. Justification for proceeding with clinical trials is based on establishment of a rational scientific basis, demonstrated proof of concept, and an adequate demonstration of safety in relevant animal model(s). In comparison to pharmaceuticals, cell therapies require an increased coordination and logistical consideration to implement the clinical trial. It is obviously important to be vigilant against ex vivo contamination of the cell-based products.

The first in human trial (FIH) for cell-based therapies is in patients often with no available alternative therapies rather than in normal volunteers. These are also populations where clinical effects are less easy to manifest themselves and where adverse events may be difficult to distinguish from disease-associated events. The surgical procedures and use of immunosuppressants may also contribute to the adverse event profile. Therefore it is even more important to understand the nature and extent of the pathological process underlying the disease symptoms of the patients enrolled in the early clinical trials.

The timing of the transplant as well as location of the transplant are important considerations in the trial design. Dose extrapolation algorhythms differ from conventional pharmaceuticals [52]. In many cases the highest dose in animals may be limited to a maximum feasible dose. Extrapolations need to take into consideration the cell concentration and number of cell injections and expected cell migration due to potential differences in anatomy and physiology. Fewer dose groups are generally employed (e.g., 3 to 4) to define an optimal biological dose rather than a maximum tolerated dose. A review of published clinical trials with similar products and indications is therefore useful to support initial dose and dose escalation schemes. If an analogous product has been used to support preclinical evaluations, comparability assessment is needed to reduce the uncertainty of extrapolations.

Although it may be difficult to definitively assess location and function at a cellular level, a variety of nonivasive technologies are currently being explored to track cells and to observe changes in metabolic activity in specific tissue areas, such as monitoring glucose metabolism using PET in stroke patients. The potential for immune reactions against implanted cells is also closely monitored and may depend not only on the source of cells but on the extent of tissue damage or bleeding at the implantation site(s).

Other aspects of trial design including randomization, acceptability of sham operation in a placebo arm, appropriate statistical approaches, as well as stopping rules and duration of follow-up. The duration of follow-up to monitor for complications and any delayed effects including, in some cases, detection of possible malignant change or chromosomal abnormalities will differ based on the specific product or product class and indication.

33.16 CONCLUSIONS

During the past two decades there have been rapid and exciting advancements in cell therapy research. Today stem cell-based therapy is a therapeutic possibility. A number of cell-based therapy products have transitioned into clinical development for a range of applications including genetic diseases, cancer, cardiac disorders, diabetes, diseases of the nervous system, bone and joints, and wounds of the skin and soft tissues. While a single source of cells may not best or even suitable for all indications, some cells may have the potential to be definitive therapies for replacement, restoration of function, or reconstruction of various tissues. Current manufacturing technologies also have the potential to provide an unlimited number of defined and standardized cells for transplantation, but rigorous characterization is needed to address biological heterogeneity, variability, and incomplete cellular definition.

Cell-based products present similarities as well as complex issues not encountered with "traditional biologicals." Innovative uses of animal models have contributed to advances toward clinically applicable treatment options based on studies designed to answer specific questions. Novel models and experimental paradigms are best considered as a case-by-case approach applied to each specific product. Noninvasive imaging methods play a critical role in cell therapy by identifying how many cells reach the desired target and, if they survive, divide and differentiate to fulfill their intended function.

Successful translation of cell-based therapies into clinical benefit, however, still faces many challenge, including developing more efficient methods for differentiation into the desired cell type(s), maintaining genetic stability during long-term culture, ensuring the absence of potentially tumorigenic cells, optimizing the implantation medium to reduce infusion toxicity, and optimizing the surgical delivery procedures (see Table 33.8). Process and analytical methods as well as definition of the final product will likely evolve throughout the clinical trials, and therefore assessing safety will be an ongoing iterative process during clinical development.

Regulatory and ethical issues are often inextricably linked with novel therapies. Since cell-based therapy is a rapidly evolving field for both researchers and regulators, it is essential that each potential new cellular therapy be considered individually and that researchers maintain frequent and personal contact with regulatory agencies. Developers and regulators need to identify the issues that must be considered in order to best evaluate the risks and the benefits.

TABLE 33.8   Current challenges of stem-cell based cellular therapies

- Understanding cell specialization (biological signals to differentiate cells into specific cell types required for normal organ function)
- Understanding cell cycle control (regulation/control of cell division/differentiation)
- Establishing specific cell characteristics to ensure product integrity
- Ensuring availability of clinical grade ancillary products (cytokines, growth factors, transcription factors)
- Improving cell scalability
- Optimizing cell preservation techniques
- Ensuring long term genetic stability of cells
- Optimizing cell delivery
- Improving evaluation and understanding of cell–host interactions for improving graft retention and survival
- Understanding potential risks if undifferentiated or partially differentiated stem cells are needed to show benefit
- Identifying exogenous controls if inappropriate function of cells or unregulated cell growth (malignant cells)
- Minimizing ethical and political constraints while encouraging proper control of the sources and procedures

APPENDIX   PHARMACOLOGY/TOXICOLOGY CONSIDERATIONS REGARDING SOMATIC CELL PRODUCTS

General Questions to Ask Regarding the Completed and Planned Preclinical Studies

- Do toxicological data derived from preclinical models provide information for the clinical management of potential toxicities?
- How predictive will be the preclinical activity/toxicity data for the human response?
- What will be the impact of the preclinical data on clinical development?

Product Used in Preclinical Studies:

Data should be provided to show the comparability of the product lot used in the POC studies, the toxicology studies, and the cell trafficking studies to the intended clinical lot. When possible, the intended clinical product should be used to conduct the pivotal preclinical toxicology studies. Immune tolerance to human cells (genetically or chemically immunosuppressed animals) allows use of the intended clinical product. In cases where analogous animal cells are used, comparability to the human product should be provided.

Product Delivery Issues

Ideally preclinical safety evaluation studies should be designed based on the intended clinical route of administration using the intended clinical delivery device (if applicable).

Animal Species/Models

Studies should be designed in a relevant model. Consideration should be given to the usefulness/ability of existing models to (1) mimic the disease/human population (activity/efficacy) and (2) predict safety (toxicity) in the context of the similarity in anatomy and pathophysiology. A discussion of whether the disease status of the animal has an impact on pharmacologic/toxicologic activity and whether the investigative therapy has an impact on the disease status of the animal should be provided.

While toxicology studies can be conducted in healthy animals, considerations should be given to hybrid pharmacology-toxicology study designs when possible for incorporation of both activity and toxicity endpoints. In any case, adequate numbers dose groups should be used, and time points should be justified. In most cases both genders should be used.

Cellular Fate Post Transplantation

The fate of the cells should be determined, including comprehensive histopathological evaluation of cell trafficking/migration, engraftment/survival posttranslation (e.g., differentiation, plasticity, transdifferentiation and/or fusion), as well as unwanted expression or alteration of phenotypes.

Tumorigenicity Potential

Tumorigenicity should be considered based on product attributes and intended clinical indication. If performed, the clinically relevant route of administered should be used, and the appropriate animal species, including the appropriate study design and duration, should be justified.

ACKNOWLEDGMENTS

The author would like to thank Mercedes Serabian, MS, Dr. Richard Lewis and Professor Anthony Dayan for their critical reading of this chapter and their thoughtful comments.

REFERENCES

1. Kuettner H. Verimpfung an stelle der transplantation hochwertiger organe. *Zentralblatt fuür Chirugie* 1912;1:390–7.
2. Sagen J. Cellular therapies for spinal cord injury: What will the FDA need to approve moving from the laboratory to the human? *J Rehab Res Dev* 2003;40:71–80.
3. LeBlanc K, Pittenger MH. Mesenchymal stem cells: progress toward promise. *Cytotherapy* 2005;7:36–45.
4. Cell Therapy—Technologies, Markets and Companies. Strategic Report Cell Therapy Technologies, Markets and Companies. Jain PharmaBiotech, 2007;1–690

(http://pharmabiotech.ch/reports/celltherapy/) http://www.piribo.com/publications/drug_delivery/cell_therapy.html

5. Ginis I, Rao MS. Toward cell replacement therapy: promises and caveats. *Exp Neurol* 2003;184:61–77.

6. Honold J, Addmus B, Lehman R, Zeiher AM, Dimmeler S. Stem cell therapy of cardiac disease: An update. *Nephrol Dial Transplant* 2004;19:1673–7.

7. Lewis RM, Gordon DJ, Poole-Wilson PA, Borer JS, Zannad F. Similarities and differences in design considerations for cell therapy and pharmacologic cardiovascular trials. *Cardiology* 2008;110:73–80.

8. Boyle AJ, Schulman SP, Hare JM. Is stem cell therapy ready for patients? Stem cell therapy for cardiac repair ready for the next step. *Circulation* 2006;114:339–52.

9. Skyler JS. Cellular therapy for type 1 diabetes. Has the time come? *JAMA* 2007; 297:1599–600.

10. Burns CJ, Persaud SJ, Jones PM. Stem cell therapy for diabetes: So we need to make beta calls? *J Endocrinol* 2004;183:437–43.

11. Application of Current Statutory Authority to Human Somatic Cell Therapy Products and Gene Therapy Products. Federal Register 1993;58(197):53248–51.

12. Brady RP, Newberry MS, Girard VW. The Food and Drug Administration's Statutory and Regulatory Authority to Regulate Human Pluripotent Stem Cells. In Ethical Issues in Human Stem Cell Research, vol. 1. Report and Recommendations of the National Bioethics Advisory Commission, Appendix D, pp. 93–8.

13. Halme DG, Kessler DA. FDA regulation of stem-cell-based therapies. *N Engl J Med* 2006;355:1730–5.

14. Grimm EA, Mazumder A, Zhang HZ, Rosenberg SA. Lymphokine-activated killer cell phenomenon: lysis of natural killer resistant fresh solid tumor cells by interleukin-2 activated autologous human peripheral blood lymphocytes. *J Exp Med* 1982;155:1823–41.

15. Rosenberg S. Lymphokine activated killer cells: a new approach to the immunotherapy of cancer. *J Cancer Inst* 1985;75:595–603.

16. Lafreniere R, Rosenberg SA. Successful immunotherapy of murine experimental hepatic metastases with lymphokine-activated killer ceils and recombinant interleukin-2. *Cancer Res* 1985;45:3735–41.

17. Rosenberg SA, Lotze MT, Muul LM, Leitman S, Chang AE, Ettinghausen SE, Matory YL, Skibber JM, Shiloni E, Vetto JT, et al. Observations on the systemic administration of autologous lymphokine-activated killer cells and recombinant interleukin-2 to patients with metastatic cancer. *N Engl J Med* 1985;313:1485–92.

18. Bar MH, Snzol M, Atkins MB, et al. Metastatic malignant melanoma treated with combined bolus and continuous infusion interleukin-2 and lymphokine activated killer cells. *J Clin Oncol* 1990;8:1138–47.

19. Rosenberg SA, Spiess P, Lafreniere R. A new approach to the adoptive immunotherapy of cancer with tumor infiltrating lymphocytes. *Science* 1986;233:1318–21.

20. Kradin FL, Lazarus DS, Dubinett SM, et al. Tumor infiltrating lymphocytes and interleukin-2 in treatment of advanced cancer. *Lancet* 1989;2:577–80.

21. Celluzzi CM, Mayordomo JI, Storkus WJ, Lotze MT, Faolo LD, Jr. Peptide-pulsed dendritic cells induce antigen-specific CTL-mediated protective tumor immunity. *J Exp Med* 1996;183:283–7.

22. Sipuleucel-T, Dendreon (BLA-STN 125197) Indicated for the Treatment of Men with Asymptomatic Metatatic Hormone Refractory Prostate Cancer. Cellular, Tissue and Gene Therapies Advisory Committee Meeting March 29, 2007. http://www.fda.gov/ohrms/dockets/ac/cber07.htm#CellularTissueGeneTherapies

23. Berger JA, Spoo A, Dwenger A, Burger M, Behringer D. CSCR4 chemokine receptors (CD184) and alpha4beta1 integrins mediate spontaneous migration of human CD34+ progenitors and acute myeloid leukaemia cells beneath marrow stromal cells (pseudoemperipolesis). *Br J Haemat* 2003;122:579–89.

24. Bhatia M, Bonnet D, Murdoch B, Gan OI, Dick JE. A newly discovered class of hematopoitic cells with SCID-repopulating activity. *Nat Med* 1998;4:1038–45.

25. Gou Y, Lubbert M, Engelhardt M. CD34-Hematopoietic stem cells: current concepts and controversies. *Stem Cells* 2003;21:15–20.

26. Asahara T, Murohara T, Sullivan A, Silver M, Van der Zec R, Li T, Witzenbichler B, Schatteman G, Isner JM. Isolation of putative progenitor endothelial cells for angiogenesis. *Science* 1997;275:964–7.

27. Hristov M, Erl W, Weber PC. Endothelial progenitor cells: isolation and characterization. *Trends Cardiovas Med* 2003;13:201–6.

28. Urbich C, Dimmeler S. Endothelial progenitor cells. Characterization and role in vascular biology. Circulation *Res* 2004;95:343–53.

29. Werner N, Kosiol S, Schiegl T, Ahlers P, Walenta K, Link A, Bohm M, Nickenig G. Circulating endothelial progenitor cells and cardiovascular outcomes. *N Engl J Med* 2005;353:999–1007.

30. Beltrami AP, Barlucchi L, Torella D, Baker M, Limana F, Chimenti S, Kassahra H, Rota M, Musso E, Urbanek K, Leri A, Kajstura J, Nadal-Ginard B, Anversa P. Adult cardiac stem cells are multipotent and support myocardial regeneration. *Cell* 2003; 114:763–76.

31. Caplan AI. Mesenchymal stem cells. *J Orthopedic Res* 9:641–50.

32. Prockop DJ. Marrow stromal cells as stem cells for nonhematopoietic tissues. *Science* 1997;276:71–4.

33. Pittenger MF, Mackay AM, Beck SC, et al. Multilineaege potential of human mesenchymal stem cells for nonhematopoietic tissues. *Science* 1999;284:143–7.

34. Le Blanc K, Pittenger MF. Mesenchymal stem cells: progress toward promise. *Cytotherapy* 2005;7:36–45.

35. Thomson JA, Itskovitz-Eldor J, Shapiro SS, Waknitz MA, Swiergiel JJ, Marshall VS, Jones JM. Embryonic stem cell lines derived from human blastocysts. *Science* 1998; 282:1145–7.

36. Reubinoff BE, Pera MF, Fong CY, Trounson A, Bongso A. Embryonic stem cell lines from human blastocysts: somatic differentiation in vitro. *Nat Biotech* 2000; 18:399–404.

37. Klimanskaya I, Chung Y, Becker S, Lu S-J, Lanza R. Human embryonic stem cell lines derived from single blastomeres. *Nature* 2006;444:481–4.

38. Boyer LA, Lee TI, Cole MF, et al. Core transcriptional regulatory circuitry in human embryonic stem cells. *Cell* 2005;122:947–56.

39. Adewumi O, Aflatoonian B, Ahrlund-Richter L, et al. Characterization of human embryonic stem cells by the International Stem Cell Initiative. *Nat Biotech* 2007; 25:803–16.

40. de Wert G, Mummery C. Human embryonic stem cells: research, ethics and policy. *Hum Reprod* 2003;18:672–82.

41. Schamblott MJ, Axelman J, Littlefield JW, Blumenthal PK, Huggins GR, Cui Y, Cheng L, Gearhart JD. Human embryonic germ cell derivatives express a broad range of developmentally distinct markers and proliferate extensively in vitro. *Proc Nat Acad Sci USA* 2001;98:113–8.

42. Shamblott MJ, Axelman J, Wang S, Bugg EM, Littlefield JW, Donovan PJ, Blumenthal PK, Huggins GR, Gearhart JD. Derivation of pluripotent stem cells form cultured human primordial germ cells. *Proc Nat Acad Sci USA* 1998;95:13726–31.

43. Strulovici Y, Leopold PL, O'Connor TP, Pergolizzi RG, Crystal RG. Human embryonic stem cells and gene therapy. *Mol Ther* 2007;15:850–66.

44. National Institutes of Health. Information on eligibility criteria for federal funding of research on human embryonic stem cells. Stem Cell Information, 2001. http://stemcells.nih.gov/policy

45. Hentze H, Graichen R, Colman A. Cell therapy and the safety of embryonic stem cell-derived grafts. Elsevier (www.sciencedirect.com), 2006. http://www.aseanbiotechnology.info/Abstract/21020806.pdf

46. Schletter J. Regulatory requirements for stem cell-based therapies. *Regul Affairs J* 2003;14.

47. Vogel G. Read or not? Human ES cells head toward the clinic. *Science* 2005; 308:1534–8.

48. Parson A. The long journey from stem cells to medical product. *Cell* 2006; 125:9–11.

49. Cavagnaro JA. Preclinical safety evaluation of biotechnology-derived pharmaceuticals. *Nat Rev Drug Discov* 2002;1:469–75.

50. ICH S6 Preclinical Safety Evaluation of Biotechnology-derived Pharmaceuticals. http://www.fda.gov/cder/guidance/index.htm

51. Guidance for Industry. Guidance for Human Somatic Cell Therapy and Gene Therapy, March 1998. http://www.fda.gov/cber/guidelines.htm

52. CHMP Guideline on Human Cell-Based Medicinal Products EMEA/CHMP/410869/206, January 2007. http://www.emea.eu.int

53. Horan PK, Melnicoff MJ, Jensen BD, Slezak SE. Fluorescent cell labeling for in vivo and in vitro cell tracking. Methods in *Cell Biol* 1990;33:469–90.

54. Fukuhara S, Tomita S, Nakatani T, et al. Comparison of cell labeling procedures for bone marrow cell transplantation to treat heart failure: long-term quantitative analysis. *Transplant Proc* 2002;34:2718–21.

55. Lyons AB. Analyzing cell division in vivo and in vitro using flow cytometric measurement of CFSE dye dilution. *J Immunol Meth* 2000;243:147–54.

56. Edinger M, Cao Y-A, Verneris MR, Bachman MH, Contag CH, Negrin RS. Revealing lymphoma growth and the efficacy of immune cell therapies using in vivo bioluminescence imaging. *Blood* 2003;1010:640–8.

57. Tohill MP, Mann DJ, Mantovani CM, Wiberg M, Terenghi G. Green fluorescent protein is a stable morphological marker for Schwann cell transplants in bioengineered nerve conduits. *Tissue Eng* 2004;10:1359–67.

58. Brazelton TR, Blau HM. Optimizing techniques for tracking transplanted stem cells in vivo. *Stem Cells* 2005;23:1251–65.

59. Shen LH, Li Y, Chen J, Cui Y, Zhang C, Kapke A, Lu M, Savant-Bhonsale S, Chopp M. One-year follow-up after bone marrow stromal cell treatment in middle-aged female rats with stroke. *Stroke* 2007;38:2150–6.

60. Boersma HH, Tromp SC, Hofstra L. Stem cell tracking: reversing the silence of the lamb. *J Nucl Med* 2005;46:200–3.

61. Rogers WJ, Meyer CH, Kramer CM. Technology insight: in vivo cell tracking by use of MRI. *Nat Clin Pract Cardiovas Med* 2006;3:554–62.

62. Jendelova P, Herynek V, Urdzikova L, et al. Magnetic resonance tracking of transplanted bone marrow and embryonic stem cells labeled by iron oxide nanoparitcles in rat brain and spinal cord. *J Neurosci Res* 2004;76:232–43.

63. Bulte JWM, Zhang S-C, van Gelderen P, Herynek V, Jordan EK, Duncan ID, Frank JA. Neurotransplantation of magnetically labeled oligodendrocyte progenitors: magnetic resonance tracking of cell migration and myelination. *Proc Nat Acad Sci USA* 1999;96:15256–61.

64. Barnett BP, Arepally A, Karmarkar PV, Qian D, Gilson WD, Walcak P, Howland V, Lawler L, Lauzon C, Stuber M, Kraitchman DL, Bulte JWM. Magnetic resonance-guided, real-time targeted delivery and imaging of magnetocapsules immunoprotecting pancreatic islet cells. *Nat Med* 2007;13:986–91.

65. Ma B, Hankenson K, Dennis J, Caplan A, Goldstein S, Kilbourn M. A simple method for stem cell labeling with fluorine 18. *Nucl Med Biol* 2005;32:701–5.

66. NIH BLAST. http://0-www.ncbi.nlm.nih.gov.catalog.llu.edu/BLAST/

67. Vogel G. Ready or not? Human ES cells head toward the clinic. *Science* 2005;308:1534–8.

68. Brickman JM, Burdon TG. Pluripotency and tumorigenicity. *Nat Genet* 2002;32:557–8.

69. Rubio D, G-C J, Martin MC, de la Fuente R, Cigudosa JC, Lloyd AC, Bernad A. Spontaneous human adult stem cell transformation. *Cancer Res* 2005;65:3035–9.

Preclinical Safety Evaluation of Biopharmaceuticals: Combination Products (Biologic/Device)

BRUCE BABBITT, PhD, and BARRY SALL

Contents

Preclinical Safety Evaluation of Biopharmaceuticals: A Science-Based Approach to Facilitating Clinical Trials, edited by Joy A. Cavagnaro
Copyright © 2008 by John Wiley & Sons, Inc.

34.1 INTRODUCTION

Combination products include a wide variety of products that merge medical devices, pharmaceuticals, and/or biologics. Combinations can be physical, such as a drug-coated coronary stent [1,2] where a drug is applied to the implantable device, or they can involve specialized delivery devices for either pharmaceuticals or biologics where contact between the device and biologic is brief. Such delivery devices can include intravascular catheters, pen injectors, or even nebulizers and inhalers. In some of these cases the linkage between the biologic and the device may be through labeling, rather than physical contact. As these examples indicate, the range of combination products is very wide, involving a nearly limitless number of technical, clinical, and regulatory challenges. New technologies such as tissue-engineering (see Chapter 35) and nanotechnology are already in development, and they will add to this complexity as they move closer to the clinic.

The preclinical testing program for a biologic-device combination product should adequately address safety issues associated with device components and those that involve the biologic. However, these two topics can not be considered in isolation. The device component and associated manufacturing processes have the potential to affect the biologic, and vice versa. This interaction forces those responsible for developing the preclinical testing program to utilize a multidisciplinary approach [3]. One of the many challenges involved in this effort is the fact that the technical people are usually familiar with either device or biologic testing, but not both. Combining ICH mandated testing requirements with ISO 10993 testing requirements and adding other specialized testing in a cost-effective and timely manner is the challenge that this chapter will examine.

This chapter discusses the key issues that should be considered when preparing a preclinical development plan for a combination product that includes components generally regulated as medical devices and biologics. It is intended to provide the reader with examples of major elements of a preclinical development plan along with a discussion of the rationale for selecting particular options. Key issues that should be addressed for any biologic-device combination product are discussed in general terms. Then a strategy for a specific hypothetical product is explored in detail.

34.2 DEFINITION OF COMBINATION PRODUCTS

The FDA defines combination products in 21 CFR 3. Four types of combination products are described:

TYPES OF COMBINATION PRODUCTS	BIOLOGIC/DEVICE EXAMPLE
A product comprised of two or more regulated components; i.e., drug/device, biologic/device, drug/biologic, or drug/device/biologic, that are physically, chemically, or otherwise combined or mixed and produced as a single entity	Antibody coated coronary artery stent
Two or more separate products packaged together in a single package or as a unit and comprised of drug and device products, device and biological products, or biological and drug products	BMP putty and spinal cage
A drug, device, or biological product packaged separately that according to its investigational plan or proposed labeling is intended for use only with an approved individually specified drug, device, or biological product where both are required to achieve the intended use, indication, or effect and where upon approval of the proposed product the labeling of the approved product would need to be changed; e.g., to reflect a change in intended use, dosage form, strength, route of administration, or significant change in dose	A novel biologic administered using a 510(k) cleared pen injector
Any investigational drug, device, or biological product packaged separately that according to its proposed labeling is for use only with another individually specified investigational drug, device, or biological product where both are required to achieve the intended use, indication, or effect	Gene therapy agent and delivery catheter

Combinations of two biologics or two devices are not considered combination products in this context.

Once a Sponsor determines that their product fits one of the definitions of a combination product, the sponsor then must determine the lead Center within the FDA that will assume regulatory responsibility for the product. This determination is made by considering the primary mode of action (PMOA) [4] of the product. In simple terms, if the main function of the product is a device function, then it is likely that the Center for Devices and Radiological Health (CDRH) will have primary responsibility for the product. On the other hand, either the Center for Biologics Evaluation (CBER) or the Center for Drug Evaluation and Research (CDER) will be assigned primary review responsibility based on whether the PMOA of the product is dependent on the pharmacological effects of a synthetic drug or a well-characterized biologic (CDER) versus other more complex biologics (CBER). Responsibility means that the Center managing the regulatory review uses its regulatory mechanisms to authorize the clinical trial and, ultimately, commercialization of the product. If CDRH is responsible for the product, it would follow the Investigational Device Exemption (IDE) and PreMarket Approval (PMA) pathways. If CBER is the lead Center, an Investigational New Drug Application (IND) and Biologic License Application (BLA) would be necessary, whereas if CDER has primary responsibility, then an IND and New Drug Application (NDA) would be the regulatory pathway. In many cases, precedents created with other similar products will provide clear direction as to the responsible Center. In other cases, jurisdiction is less clear such that the Sponsor may choose to submit a Request for Designation (RFD) [5] to the Office of Combination Products (OCP). The RFD contains a description of the product, available data on its use and mechanism of action, as well as a suggested product designation. OCP will review the RFD and inform the Sponsor of their decision. Some redacted decision letters are available at the OCP Web site (http://www.fda.gov/oc/combination/rfd.html). Once the responsible Center is identified, the Sponsor can then begin to assess preclinical data requirements and determine the scheduling for the necessary studies.

34.3 GENERAL POINTS APPLICABLE TO ALL DEVICE-BIOLOGIC COMBINATION PRODUCTS

Developers of combination products should rigorously evaluate their product in order to construct a preclinical testing plan that is scientifically and medically sound and take into account business objectives. Often biologic-device combination product development efforts involve collaborations between a biotech company and a more traditional device company. Each organization brings its own technical and business expertise and expectations to the project. Biologic developers are accustomed to designing comprehensive, multi-species preclinical testing programs that by themselves may take two or more years to complete. This is in large contrast to many device companies whose entire product life cycle, from development through end-of-commercial sales, typically takes little more than two years. Furthermore, preclinical testing for biologic products follows CBER/CDER and ICH guidances that are quite different from the medical device ISO 10993 standard. Therefore, the preclinical development team for a biologic-device combination product needs to address "cultural" as well as technical issues. The following sections describe in general terms the broad issues that should be considered when designing the preclinical development program for a biologic-device combination product.

34.3.1 Functionality of the Biologic

Whether a biologic is directly physically associated with the surface of a device (via some type of chemical cross-linking or simple adsorption), or alternatively, embedded in some type of matrix that is used to coat the device, it is very likely that the pharmacology/toxicology profile of the biologic will be altered when compared to administration of the biologic as a single agent.

If the physical association of the biologic with the device causes even small changes in the structure of the molecule (either while bound to the device or upon release into the local environment), then it is possible to decrease or even eliminate its intrinsic receptor binding activity and downstream physiological effects. Alternatively, the possibility exists to increase the overall binding affinity and resultant pharmacological and/or toxicological effects of the biologic, in vivo, if multivalent binding (e.g., of an antibody to its cognate antigen) results from the presence of high-density clusters of the molecule on the surface of the device.

A major challenge for both developers and regulators of biologic/device combination products is the potential need to re-define certain key parameters, for example, "dose"/exposure, distribution, and persistence, that have historically formed the basis for a comprehensive preclinical characterization of the pharmacology/toxicology profile of stand-alone biologics. As is the case with most biological drug products, while the basic principles of toxicological assessment are much the same, actual practices may vary from the traditional drug approach. It is likely in certain cases that new animal models or analytical methods will be needed in order to adequately define potential human toxicities and/or safe starting doses and an appropriate dose escalation scheme.

34.3.2 Functionality of the Device

If the device component of the biologic/device combination product has already been cleared or approved as a stand-alone product, some aspects of device functionality will be known. However, the effect of the biologic will need to be investigated. In the case where the device and biologic are physically associated with each other, the process used to join the two components can affect device performance in a variety of ways. Easily determined parameters such as dimensions and clearances must be confirmed. More subtle issues arise when physical performance and durability are assessed. Additional manufacturing procedures associated with the antibody coating could, at least in theory, alter the properties of the entire device. In some cases, test methods that have been successfully employed for stand-alone devices may need to be modified to accurately assess all relevant parameters that must be considered for the combination product.

34.3.3 Properties of the Combined Product

While it is important to evaluate the component parts of the combination product, the fully integrated finished product(s) must be evaluated as well.

Devices that have long histories of reliability as stand-alone products may behave differently when associated with a biologic. Conversely, when a biologic is associated with a device, a variety of chemical, physical, or conformational modifications could occur and alter its biologic activity in some manner. In the preclinical development phase, proof-of-concept (POC) testing is used to make a preliminary efficacy determination and is often designed to generate safety data.

Combining the device and biologic will almost certainly affect stability. Packaging systems may frequently be altered in significant ways. The form of the biologic may also change from, for example, a lyophilized powder to a form bound to a solid surface or entrapped in a matrix. Furthermore, the manufacturing methods used to combine the two components may significantly affect the biologic's stability. In any case, stability studies should be conducted with product that has undergone the full manufacturing, packaging, and sterilization processes.

Sterilization methods should be carefully considered. Many medical devices undergo terminal ethylene oxide (EtO) or radiation sterilization. Both of these processes can alter a biologic component, either through chemical modification or radiolysis. Whatever sterilization method or bioburden limit is selected, it must balance the competing needs of product safety and product integrity. Preclinical testing will need to utilize a product that has undergone all processing steps, including sterilization and packaging, to ensure that preclinical testing uses test articles that have been exposed to all the product stresses encountered in the commercial manufacturing process.

34.3.4 Regulatory Issues

The overall regulatory approach for a combination product is governed by several considerations. First, one must consider which Center has primary jurisdiction for the product and if the other Center will participate in a collaborative or consultative role. Once these parameters are defined, the Sponsor will know the type of submissions necessary to gain approval for the clinical trial(s), and ultimately, for the marketing application. Second, if either or both of the components (biologic and device) are already approved in the case of the biologic or cleared in the case of the device, the Sponsor should obtain authorization to cross-reference data in those submissions and determine which data are relevant to the combination product. As discussed in the following specific example (see below), not all data from component parts are relevant to the combination product. Several FDA guidance documents [6,7] should be reviewed when preparing the initial regulatory evaluation. Last, regulatory staff should contact the FDA, either the responsible Center or OCP, early in the process and confirm that their plans are consistent with FDA expectations. Such contacts, while important, are not a substitute for a formal pre-IDE or a type B pre-IND meeting [8,9] (CDRH types of meetings), but they do address key questions early in the development process.

34.4   MODEL COMBINATION PRODUCT: ANTIBODY-COATED STENT

In order to present clearly and specifically the unique preclinical testing challenges associated with the early-stage development of biologic/device combination products, an antibody-coated stent will be used as a model. For this particular case study the antibody chosen for manufacturing has either not yet been approved for use in humans or, if it has, not for the newly targeted indications. In addition, the combination product utilizes a previously approved stent and delivery system.

The rationale for selection of a monoclonal antibody (mAb) as the biologic component of our model biologic-device combination product is based primarily on the following two major factors: (1) there seems to be a high degree of interest in these next-generation type of products due to the potential for very high affinity interactions with specific targets (antigens), in vivo, with the potential for a much more favorable risk–benefit ratio of the therapy as compared to the use of more conventional "nonspecific"drugs, and (2) antibodies represent a very well-characterized class of biologics from a manufacturing, preclinical, clinical, and regulatory standpoint.

Another reason for focusing on antibody-coated stents throughout the remainder of this chapter is that discussion of preclinical strategy covering the very broad range of biologic-device combination products currently under development would, by definition, require both the writers and readers to have a solid working knowledge of the basic science aspects of a broad array of biologics (living cells, genes, etc.). (See Chapters 32 and 33 for a discussion of specific considerations for developing gene and cellular therapies, respectively.)

34.5   PRECLINICAL TESTING CONSIDERATIONS

One of the first decisions to be made in order to formulate an adequate preclinical testing strategy for biologic-device combination products is to determine a relevant form(s) of the product to test in selected animal species for assessment of potential pharmacological and toxicological effects in humans. In general, one can approach an analysis of the potential in vivo effects of a device-biologic combination product from the following two mechanistically distinct standpoints: (1) local effects arising from the direct interaction of living cells and/or soluble factors with the device or the antibodies bound to the surface of the device, and (2) local or systemic effects arising from the interaction of living cells or soluble factors with any of a variety of antibody-containing species capable of eluting off of the surface of the implanted device. In addition, it may be necessary to consider evaluation of the mAb alone in addition to assessing the combination product, based on intrinsic attributes of the mAb as well as the availability of relevant preclinical and clinical safety and efficacy data.

Finally, a major challenge for both developers and regulators of biologic-device combination products is the potential need to reconsider the way that certain key parameters typically associated with preclinical assessment, such as dose in the case of the biologic and durability in the case of the device, are defined, measured, and analyzed.

34.5.1   Biologic Orientation on the Device

In antibody-coated stents it is possible for the heterogeneity in the overall orientation of the antibody molecule on the surface of the device to lead to different pharmacological and/or toxicological effects, in vivo. The degree of heterogeneity is likely to be strongly influenced both by the intrinsic nature of the antibody (primary, secondary, and tertiary structure) and by the particular method (adsorption, chemical cross-linking, etc.) selected for binding the selected antibody to the device.

For example, if a high percentage of the device-associated antibody molecules are attached "backward" to the surface of the device—that is, with their antigen binding domains (Fab) facing inward and their F_c domains facing outward—then there is a relatively high likelihood of local interactions of the immobilized antibodies with circulating immune cells expressing high levels of F_c receptors (Figure 34.1). It is the responsibility of the manufacturing team

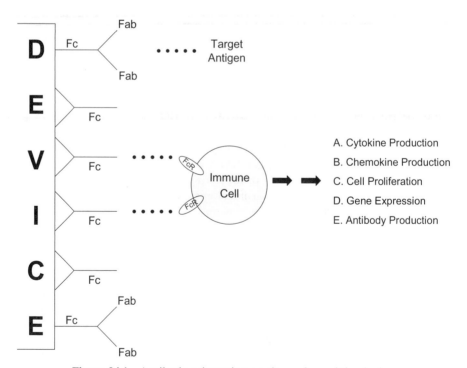

Figure 34.1   Antibody orientation on the surface of the device.

to fully characterize and control (minimize) this potential variability in the orientation of the biologic prior to the start of preclinical testing.

Once immune cells become bound to the surface of the antibody-coated stent via multivalent interactions with exposed F_c domains, there is the potential for a variety of immunomodulatory effects (cytokine release, inhibition of normal F_c receptor mediated events, etc.) that could lead to the generation of adverse events, in vivo.

As a worst-case scenario the possibility exists to break natural tolerance to human F_c and lead to the formation of anti-F_c antibodies, in vivo, due to the "presentation" of such a high local concentration of F_c domain epitopes to various components of the cellular immune system. As a result, the generation and function of endogenous immunoglobulins could be negatively affected by the presence of these circulating antibodies (immunosuppression).

In addition, although the typical antibody-coated device will likely be designed to allow rapid elution of the drug into the local microenvironment over a relatively short period of time (hours to days), the short-term ability of the device to interact with target antigens present in the local milieu will be negatively affected by the presence of improperly oriented antibody molecules on the device surface.

34.5.2 Potential Elution (Biologic) Species

It is straightforward that the final implantable combination product, as a finished product, needs to be assessed for both potential device-related and biologic-related pharmacological effects and potential toxicities in one or more animal species. However, once the biologic component of the combination product starts to elute off of the device (again, focusing on antibody-coated stents as a model, and assuming that the intention of the product is to "deliver" the biologic to the local microenvironment), attention must be paid to the changing nature of the implanted biologic/device and the appearance over time of various antibody-containing species (cells and/or soluble factors) first in the microenvironment around the device, and thereafter in the general circulation.

In terms of antibody-coated stents, the following is a list of potential antibody-containing species that could, in theory, be eluted directly from the surface of the implanted biologic/device combination product, in vivo (Figure 34.2):

- Monomeric antibody molecules (native conformation)
- Monomeric antibody (altered conformation)
- Aggregated antibodies (native or altered conformation)
- Degradation products (antibody derived peptides)
- Antibody–antigen complexes
- Antibody–cell complexes

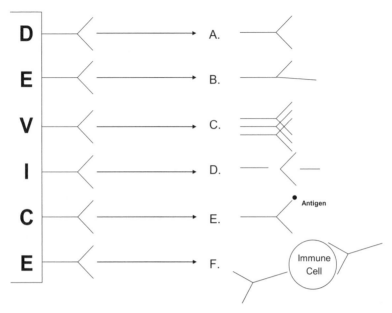

Figure 34.2   Antibody-containing elution species.

Again, the combination device would be optimized during the manufacturing process to ensure a consistent antibody coupling and control for the various species. In order to determine which, if any, of the antibody-containing elution species have the potential to exert either pharmacological or toxic effects in humans, the various species could be generated and tested, ex vivo, via extended exposure of the combination product to various biological fluids (e.g., whole blood, serum, plasma), and then to assess potential effects of the "supernatant" from these experiments in at least one animal species. If any meaningful effects are uncovered, then studies could be designed to determine which molecular entity is responsible for the observed effects.

This experimental approach has limitations in that it ignores the potential critical interactions of immune cells and other living cells, in vivo, with the antibody-coated surface of the device. These cellular "interactions" can occur either via direct binding to the device surface of cells expressing receptors (e.g., cognate antigen) capable of recognizing various antibody domains, or alternatively, via secretion of cellular enzymes capable of directly modifying these antibodies. As such, further in vivo studies would be needed to characterize potential toxicities.

34.6   PHARMACOLOGICAL / TOXICOLOGICAL ASSESSMENT

Based on the inherent complexity of biologic/device combination products, together with the assumption that the potential in vivo adverse effects of the combination is not simply equal to the sum of what is known regarding their component parts, it is clear that the design of an adequate program for the preclinical characterization of a biologic-device combination product will need to be approached on a case-by-case basis. In theory, the potential adverse effects of the combination product can be derived from in vivo interactions with the implanted biologic device, as designed, the biologic device modified by local physiological activities, or any of a broad array of molecular (or cellular) species eluting off of the surface of the device over time capable of exerting either local or systemic effects (see Section 34.5.2 above).

Another key factor in defining an adequate preclinical testing program for these products is whether a biopharmaceutical company chooses to use a biologic (antibody in this case) that has already received FDA approval for use in humans, even though it is likely not for the same indication targeted by the stent manufacturer. Use of an approved biologic with the device may provide information as to what to expect under a worst-case scenario, such as all of the biologic being released immediately into the systemic circulation. However, it is still very important to understand what impact attaching the mAb to the surface of a given medical device and implanting the combination product into a patient (route of administration) has on potential toxicity. For example, release of the mAb directly into the coronary artery might be expected to result in a different PK/PD profile than a direct IV or IM injection of the biologic alone. In addition, if the mAb has not previously been administered to the same patient population that was previously treated with the stand-alone medical device, potential differences between the different patient populations must also be very carefully considered.

34.6.1 Definition of New Terms

A major challenge for both developers and regulators of biologic-device combination products is the potential need to reconsider how to measure certain key parameters typically associated with the preclinical assessment of stand-alone medical devices and biologics with the goal toward extrapolation of the information to humans.

These parameters include, but are not limited to, establishment of a minimal effective dose (MED), a no observable dose (NOEL), a no observable adverse effect dose (NOAEL), and a maximum tolerated dose (MTD). From the standpoint of our antibody-coated stent model, and antibody "dose," it is possible that the product (device) labeling could limit the dose of mAb a patient is allowed to receive to how much protein is able to be coated onto just one stent. Alternatively, since stents are made in various lengths in order to match the length of the lesion, the longer the stent, the more antibodies that can be delivered.

Issues related to PK, distribution, persistence, and stability will also need to be considered. Optimizing methods to assess local effects as well as potential changes in the immunogenicity of the biologic component of the combination product may also be needed. Careful consideration must be given to identification of the most relevant animal models, including use of an animal model of disease to better assess toxicity.

Quantitative assessment of these key parameters could require the development of new analytical methods compared to the relatively well established methods currently in use for characterization of stand alone medical devices and biologics.

34.6.2 Choice of Animal Species/Pharmacology Studies

Given that the various animal species and experimental protocols typically used for preclinical testing of conventional devices versus biologics are quite different, a major challenge for developers of biologic-device combination products is to determine the best way to combine the essential elements of these studies into a manageable number of predictive models for their particular product. A very basic aspect of this challenge is that, in general, animal species used for preclinical testing of implantable devices (especially proof-of-concept (POC) type of studies) tend to consist of larger animals due to their greater compatibility with surgical procedures. For example, porcine models have been used extensively for testing of drug-coated stents [1,2]. For biologics such as mAbs the most important product attribute for defining a relevant preclinical species is whether the target antigen or epitope is present in sufficient amounts in the chosen animals. In some cases a species may be selected for its similarity to humans based on its potential off-target binding to tissues as demonstrated by tissue cross-reactivity studies.

It is likely that manufacturers of devices (e.g., stents) will strongly prefer testing their antibody-coated products in the established porcine models for POC type of studies in order to make critical go or no go decisions regarding choice of antibody besides proceeding into toxicology studies and then human testing. If so, developers will need to screen their antibodies for their ability to bind to porcine tissues in order to perform POC studies without any complications (e.g., immunogenicity due to species-specific effects) that would compromise their ability to evaluate the results of the study. In certain cases companies might be faced with having to use immunosuppressed animals or a porcine homologue of the antibody (surrogate antibody) in order to carry out "gold standard" POC studies, Alternatively, development of a different animal model that will bind the antibody and allow implantation of the stent may be needed as well. A practical challenge in this area might be that contract research organizations experienced in performing the POC type studies with devices may not have experience with biological products and associated assays, and vice versa.

From a pharmacological standpoint, monomeric antibodies in their native conformation (whether free, cell-bound, or still attached to the device) are most likely to maintain their intrinsic ability to bind stably to their target antigens, in vivo, leading to the desired therapeutic effect. However, while device-associated or locally released mAbs would be expected to exert mostly local pharmacological or toxicological effects, cell-bound antibodies have the potential to exert more systemic effects as a result of the trafficking of immune cells to or from the site of the implanted device. In addition, it is possible that target antigens bound to antibodies on the surface of various immune cell subsets would not be cleared via the same pathways typically used to clear more conventional antibody–antigen complexes. These potential concerns would need to be addressed in the preclinical safety evaluation program for the biologic-device combination product.

34.6.3 Toxicology Testing

General Biologic/Device Considerations The following is a list of potential unique considerations for assessing the safety of biologic-device combination products:

1. As mentioned above, the types of animal species typically used to assess the toxicology profile of the mAb may not be the same species typically chosen for ISO 10993 device safety testing.
2. Toxicology testing for devices typically focuses greatly on local effects of the product, while there is always a major focus on potential systemic effects with biologics.
3. The issue of species-specific interactions is unique to biologics and complicates the design, performance, and interpretation of biologic-device pharm/tox study results.
4. Patients have much shorter exposures to most biologics (e.g., months, intermittent) compared to conventional devices (e.g., chronic, lifetime).
5. Compared to the majority of biologics, which are typically fully catabolized in vivo into amino acids over the short-term (hours, days), devices are expected to change very little in vivo even after long-term exposure to most biological fluids.
6. The potential for immune responses against biologics (hypersensitivity, anti-drug antibodies, immune complexes, etc.) is something that most stent (alone or as drug-coated stents) manufacturers have not had to consider in prior development programs.
7. ISO 10993 testing is intended to evaluate materials such as metals and polymers that essentially do not interact directly with the human immune system. However, the presence of an antibody on the device surface introduces the potential for cross-species reactions that may not be indicative of performance in humans. These interactions may affect some or all ISO 10993 in vivo tests. For example, the duration of chronic toxicity testing may be limited based on induction of immune responses or carcinogenicity studies may not be appropriate based on the specific product attributes of the antibody.

8. The biologic could be attached to the surface of the device using a broad array of materials and coupling techniques. Therefore, in addition to the conventional device-based biocompatibility testing for coating materials, close attention must be paid to potential in vivo effects derived from the presence of biologic-device attachment factor complexes or derivatives that could be generated following implantation of the device in humans.

Considerations Unique to Antibody-Coated Stents From a toxicological standpoint, the release of aggregated antibodies (native or altered conformation) from the surface of an antibody-coated stent into the microenvironment or systemic circulation has the potential to induce an array of immunomodulatory effects via direct interaction with several key components of the human cellular immune system (dendritic cells, macrophages, neutrophils, B cells, NK cells, etc.). For example, aggregated antibodies have the potential to bind with high affinity and cross-link F_c receptors on the surface of various immune cells resulting in (1) overproduction of proinflammatory cytokines and chemokines, (2) increase in the level of tyrosine phosphorylation of intracellular proteins, (3) induction of new gene expression, (4) increase in phagocytic activity, (5) increase in antigen presentation, (6) increase in cell cycle progression (cell proliferation), and (7) increase in the production and release of reactive oxygen species. These predominantly immunostimulatory effects can often lead to toxic reactions (adverse events) in humans.

In addition, since it is now well established that aggregated proteins are much more immunogenic in animals and in humans than native monomeric versions of the same proteins, the potential exists for aggregated antibodies released into the circulation from the surface of antibody-coated stents to induce human antihuman antibody (HAHA) responses with the theoretical potential to cross-react against endogenous related immunoglobulins. The local release from the surface of the implanted biologic/device of pre-formed antibody–antigen complexes, or alternatively, much larger immune cell–antibody complexes, followed by deposition of these complexes into the nearby vasculature could lead to inflammation and subsequent damage to blood vessels, tissues, and joints in close proximity to the combination product. It is less likely, but still possible, that these immune complexes could also exert negative effects, in vivo, via systemic access to the kidneys, lungs, skin, and other organs.

Since all of the potential immunotoxicological effects mentioned above related to the use of antibody-coated stents are typically highly concentration dependent, it is possible that the use of only very small amounts of protein on the surface of the device to exert a desired localized therapeutic effect, will mitigate, but certainly not eliminate these potential toxicities. Nevertheless, the purpose of the preclinical toxicological evaluation will be to address the potential impact of these theoretical concerns.

34.7 DEVICE CONSIDERATIONS

Assessment of biologic/device combination product functionality needs to include all of the testing typically performed on bare metal stents (BMS). In the case of our antibody-coated stent model the BMS have been previously approved by CDRH, allowing some of the BMS data to be cross-referenced and not repeated when the effect of the antibody coating on the functionality of the device is considered negligible. These judgments must be made on a case-by-case basis and should be confirmed with the Office for Device Evaluation.

The finished, packaged and sterilized product must be considered as a whole. In accordance with the Design Control provisions of the Quality System Regulation (21 CFR 820.30) medical devices undergo a formal risk analysis throughout product development. Such an analysis identifies potential risks inherent in the design, materials, and method of use of the device ranks the risks and ensures that unacceptable risks are mitigated. The original risk analysis for the BMS must be re-evaluated to consider the addition of the antibody coating. The risk analysis should consider the physical effects of the coating, packaging modifications, or manufacturing process modifications as well as the physiological and immunological effects discussed above. Considerable effort will be directed to the physiological and immunological effects, but developers should not lose sight of some of the more practical concerns, such as deliverability of the stent and the effect of packaging modifications on handling of entire system. Experts with a good understanding of these technical areas must be brought into the risk analysis process. Human factor issues should also be addressed, especially if there have been any modifications to the instructions for use for the delivery system.

34.8 REGULATORY CONSIDERATIONS

As discussed, successful development of a combination product will require a thorough understanding of the requirements for the individual components as well as an understanding of what questions need to be asked based on the specific product attributes when the individual components are combined. It will be important to determine early in development which FDA Center will have primary responsibility for the combination product as that will likely influence the development strategy. As the products will likely be unique with little regulatory precedent, it will be important for Sponsors to communicate with the FDA, again early in the development process, to ensure that the program addresses all the important issues necessary for introducing the product into humans for the first time.

REFERENCES

1. J&J Cypher SSE. http://www.fda.gov/cdrh/PDF2/P020026b.PDF
2. BSC Taxus SSE. http://www.fda.gov/cdrh/pdf3/P030025b.pdf
3. Getting Started with a Combination Product. Part I: Overcoming the Regulatory Challenges in This Ever-Expanding Field Yields Rewards. http://www.devicelink.com/mddi/archive/03/03/018.html
   Getting Started with a Combination Product. Part II: European Regulations. The European Union adds further wrinkles to the combination product market. http://www.devicelink.com/mddi/archive/03/04/019.html
4. Definition of Primary Mode of Action of a Combination Product. http://www.fda.gov/OHRMS/DOCKETS/98fr/05-16527.htm
5. Guidance for Industry and FDA Staff: How to Write a Request for Designation (RFD). http://www.fda.gov/oc/combination/Guidance-How%20to%20Write%20an%20RFD.pdf
6. Guidance for Industry and FDA Staff: Early Development Considerations for Innovative Combination Products. http://www.fda.gov/oc/combination/innovative.pdf
7. Guidance for Industry and FDA Current Good Manufacturing Practice for Combination Products. http://www.fda.gov/oc/combination/OCLove1dft.pdf
8. Early Collaboration Meetings under the FDA Modernization Act (FDAMA); Final Guidance for Industry and for CDRH Staff. http://www.fda.gov/cdrh/ode/guidance/310.pdf
9. Guidance for Industry. Formal Meetings with Sponsors and Applicants for PDUFA Products. http://www.fda.gov/cber/gdlns/mtpdufa.htm

CHAPTER 35

Tissue Engineered Products: Preclinical Development of Neo-Organs

TIMOTHY A. BERTRAM, DVM, PhD, and MANUEL JAYO, DVM, PhD

Contents

35.1 INTRODUCTION

In the early 1930s during his tenure at Rockefeller University, Charles Lindbergh, the aviator, first contemplated preclinical development of manufactured human organs (neo-organs) for implantation into the body [1]. However, it took 50 years of scientific research and technology advancements

Preclinical Safety Evaluation of Biopharmaceuticals: A Science-Based Approach to Facilitating Clinical Trials, edited by Joy A. Cavagnaro
Copyright © 2008 by John Wiley & Sons, Inc.

for the idea of augmenting or replacing diseased organs with laboratory-grown components to emerge into the realm of possibility. Today technologies have matured to the point that a diseased or missing organ can be regenerated de novo with a tissue-engineered neo-organ.

The term *tissue engineering* was coined at a National Science Foundation workshop in 1987 to mean "the application of principles and methods of engineering and life sciences toward fundamental understanding of structure-function relationships in normal and pathological mammalian tissues and the development of biological substitutes to restore, maintain or improve tissue function" [2]. Tissue engineering draws on specialized expertise from two traditional disciplines: engineering and the life sciences. The combination of these technologies forms a foundation upon which the commercial development of neo-organs is possible.

Preclinical development of neo-organs faces complex scientific questions and regulatory hurdles. The term *neo-organ product* will be used to indicate any product composed of synthetic or natural biodegradable materials, with or without living cells and/or cellular products, implanted in the body to incorporate, replace, and/or regenerate a damaged tissue or organ. Today ex vivo development of partial and complete neo-organs by the emerging regenerative medical industry fulfills a significant unmet medical need for patients who have partial or complete organ or tissue loss. In this chapter we will consider development challenges and available solution strategies for bringing these transformational technologies to patients in need.

35.2 MEDICAL NEEDS AND CHALLENGES

Currently a patient's diseased organ replacement requires the transplantation of whole organs (e.g., kidneys, livers, hearts, lungs, and pancreases) donated or taken from another body system or living being (human–autologous/allogeneic or animal–xenogeneic). Regardless of source, organs are in finite supply, and complications such as chronic metabolic alterations, immunologic rejection, and product shelflife have rendered this therapeutic approach both costly and risky. Furthermore patients who receive nonautologous organ transplants require life-long chemical immunosuppression or face partial or complete organ rejection.

Recent scientific advances involving tissue engineering technologies and their use in regenerative medicine have helped us better understand host tissue responses and basic needs during healing, repair, and regeneration. With these advances comes a need to establish product development pathways that fit into existing and emerging regulatory guidelines while remaining commercially viable. Production of a neo-organ requires defined raw materials and a reproducible manufacturing process whereby the appropriate constituents (i.e., cells and biomaterials) can be cultured and combined ex vivo to form an implantable neo-organ product. Following implantation, both partial to complete neo-organs must become vascularized by host tissues, integrate, heal, grow, respond to physiological needs or injury, and otherwise function at a level sufficient to support the patient's life.

As mentioned above, development of regenerative medical products for organ augmentation and/or replacement is dependent on the availability of appropriate raw materials. Important factors to consider include the source, quality, and handling by which the raw materials are processed into an implantable product. The life-sustaining role of the organ being augmented or replaced must also be considered when sourcing raw materials. As a rule, the manufacturing challenges presented by simple organs (e.g., skin) will be fundamentally different than those presented by vital organs (viscous or solid organs, e.g., heart, kidney, liver, pancreas). Nonetheless, there are fundamental aspects shared by regenerative medical products for which generalizations can be made regarding development approaches and potential regulatory pathways.

Tissue engineering has progressed to the point where neo-organ products are ready now for wholesale manufacturing and commercialization. In response to these advances, the United States Food and Drug Administration (FDA) established the Office of Combination Products (OCP) as the entry point into the regulatory review process for companies seeking approval for combination products, as these products are expected to increase as technological advances continue to merge therapeutic products and blur the historical lines of sepapration between FDA's medical product centers. In the case of neo-organ products composed of a device (e.g., scaffold), biological (e.g., cells), and/or biological active (e.g., pharmaceutical), one or two product centers could be involved.

35.3 REGULATORY HISTORY/DEVELOPMENT

The OCP was established in 2002 under the Medical Device User Fee and Modernization Act (MDUFMA) to address the regulatory complexity for combination products. The MDUFMA gave OCP broad responsibilities, covering the regulatory life cycle of drug-device, drug-biologic, and device-biologic combination products—categories that encompass most neo-organ products being developed today. However, the OCP assigns primary regulatory responsibility for, and oversight of, combination products on a case-by-case basis to one of three product centers based on the product's primary mode of action.

The three product centers that can lead the regulatory review of a neo-organ product include Center for Devices and Radiological Health (CDHR), Center for Biologics Evaluation and Research (CBER), and the Center for Drug Evaluation Research (CDER). CDRH is responsible for regulating those products that are primarily medical devices. A medical device is defined as "An instrument, apparatus, implement, machine, contrivance, implant, or other similar or related article, including a component, part, or accessory, which is: (1) recognized in the official National Formulary, or the United States Pharmacopoeia, or any supplement to them; (2) intended for use in the diagnosis of disease or other conditions, or in the cure, mitigation, treatment, or prevention of disease, in man or other animals; or (3) intended to affect the structure or any function of the body of man or other animals, and which does not achieve any of [its] primary intended purposes through chemical action within or on the body of man or other animals and which is not dependent upon being metabolized for the achievement of any of its primary intended purposes" [3]. CDER's primary objective is to ensure that all prescription and over-the-counter (OTC) medications are safe and effective. In contrast, CBER is responsible for regulating human tissue, cells, and/or their products under CFR 21, 1270, and 1271 and biologics under 351 of PHS Act 610 of CFR 21. Because the final product produced by tissue engineering and regenerative medicine technologies frequently involves the combination of two or more FDA-regulated components, one or more of the above-mentioned FDA Centers may be assigned to regulate a neo-organ product.

For example, the scaffold or biomaterial component of a neo-organ would normally fall under CDRH jurisdiction, while biological components (i.e., cells) would normally fall under CBER's authority if these components were being used alone. Similarly a biologically active pharmaceutical product would normally be reviewed by CDER. However, review of a combination product can require expertise from multiple centers and the lead center is assigned based on the component that the FDA decides is delivering the primary mode of action.

35.4 ESTABLISHING A REGULATORY PATHWAY FOR NEO-ORGAN

Certain regenerative products may fit into existing regulatory pathways for drugs, devices, or biologicals. Since these singular pathways are already well established, the focus of this discussion will be on neo-organ products composed of a combination of materials (biologics, drugs, and/or devices). In recent years substantial clarification about appropriate regulatory pathways for evaluating combination product neo-organs has occurred. Presently the United States occupies a lead position in establishing regulatory pathways for combination products. The OCP is providing tissue engineering and regenerative medicine industries with guidance as the regulatory authority (21 CFR 3) [4] for combination product development.

A combination product is composed of any combination of a drug and a device; a biological product and a device; a drug and a biological product; or a drug, device, and a biological product. Under 21 CFR 3.2 [4] a combination product is defined to include the following:

1. A product comprised of two or more regulated components (i.e., drug-device, biologic-device, drug-biologic, or drug-device/biologic) that are

physically, chemically, or otherwise combined or mixed and produced as a single entity.

2. Two or more separate products packaged together in a single package or as a unit and comprised of drug and device products, device and biological products, or biological and drug products.

3. A drug, device, or biological product packaged separately that according to its investigational plan or proposed labeling is intended for use only with an approved individually specified drug, device, or biological product where both are required to achieve the intended use, indication, or effect and where, upon approval of the proposed product, the labeling of the approved product would need to be changed (e.g., to reflect a change in intended use, dosage form, strength, route of administration, or significant change in dose).

4. Any investigational drug, device, or biological product packaged separately that according to its proposed labeling is for use only with another individually specified investigational drug, device, or biological product where both are required to achieve the intended use, indication, or effect. [7]

A neo-organ product represents a combination product that is composed of two or more regulated components, under 21 CFR 3.2, that may be mixed together to form a single entity, or that are separate but cannot achieve their intended use without being used together. A sponsor seeking to obtain regulatory guidance for a combination product prepares a Request for Designation (RFD) document [5], laying out key information requested by the FDA (Table 35.1).

The RFD document presents the sponsor's recommendation and rationale for how the combination product should be regulated. The FDA's decision about regulatory pathway rests on its evaluation of the primary mode of action, a judgment that focuses on the primary therapeutic process whereby the neo-organ activates the therapeutic outcome—usually a choice between scaffold and cellular or constitutive components. If a product is sufficiently related to a product already regulated by a particular center or one that has

TABLE 35.1   Request for designation information needed for the food and drug administration

Name of product
Composition of product
Primary mode of action
Method of manufacture
Related products currently regulated by the FDA
Duration of product use by the patient
Science supporting product development
Primary route of administration

a defined pathway, FDA's requirements for preclinical support of clinical trials may mirror the precedent product's regulatory pathway. The FDA has 60 days from the date of RFD submission to render its decision. Once a pathway is identified, the sponsor can engage the lead reviewing center's personnel for the optimal study plan to support their first clinical trials.

Specific guidance on engaging the OCP and establishing communications with the FDA can be found at the FDA's Web site [6]. Interacting with OCP prior to establishing a preclinical development approach can assist in linking to the proper regulatory authority and necessary regulatory guidelines. For some products the primary mode of action is not readily apparent, and the designation of lead center may be based on the most relevant therapeutic activity, intended therapeutic use, or the most relevant safety and efficacy questions. The guidelines of the designated lead regulatory center will provide the framework for a potential regulatory pathway for entry into the clinic and ultimate product registration. A current assignment algorithm can be obtained at the FDA's Web site [4].

35.5   DEVELOPMENT OF NEO-ORGAN PRODUCTS

The first tissue-engineered and regenerative medical products were device products for skin conditions, regulated by CDRH, and based on culturing skin cells in simple layers. The earliest clinical applications of tissue engineering revolved around the use of essentially flat materials designed to stimulate wound care. The cellular component was considered more as a physical barrier than a biologically active component of the product itself. Dermagraft®, a product originally manufactured by Advanced Tissue Sciences, Inc. that is now manufactured by Smith & Nephew, used skin cells isolated from neonatal foreskins seeded onto a polymeric scaffold. Apligraf®, a product from Organogenesis Inc., used similar technology to seed and culture cells on collagen-based scaffolds. Tissue-engineered skin substitutes dominated the regulatory and development pipeline in the late 1990s. The FDA regulated these products as class III devices. As these products moved from the laboratory to the clinic, development issues such as cell source (allogeneic or autologous), scaffold materials (natural or synthetic), and bioreactor design encountered additional safety challenges, including immunocompatibility responses in patients. As these challenges were solved, further commercial demands for scale-up and cost-of-goods considerations had to be reconciled against the magnitude of incremental medical benefit over existing approaches (i.e., cadaveric skin).

Medtronic, Inc. markets one of the first commercial products that combined a device and a biologically active compound, bone morphogenic protein (BMP). Medtronic's INFUSE® Bone Graft/LT-CAGE® lumbar tapered fusion device contains a collagen sponge infused with the BMP peptide housed within a metal cage. This product was developed as a combination product in which CDRH maintained a leadership role for regulatory guidance and consultation with CBER and CDER occurred for complete regulatory oversight. The combination product was approved for treatment of lower spine disc disease via the FDA's premarket approval (PMA) process. The individual components were each regulated by the appropriate pathway: the recombinant human BMP2 (manufactured in accordance with biologics regulations), the collagen sponge to carry the protein (manufactured under device regulations), the sterile water to resuspend the protein (manufactured by a supplier in compliance with drug regulations), and the metal cage device (manufactured under device guidelines) housing the sponge plus protein that is surgically implanted between the patient's vertebrae. Later CDRH approved INFUSE® Bone Graft, consisting of the collagen, sterile water, and protein components (no metal cage) for use in open fractures of the tibia. The product is used in addition to standard treatment protocols, which may or may not include using an intramedullary nail to stabilize the fracture.

Many of these early successes in the tissue engineering field were gained in relatively simple two-dimensional (2D) skin tissue or 3D bone fracture structures with limited vital organ function required immediately after implantation. Organ regeneration goes beyond traditional tissue engineering, which focuses on using in vitro and ex vivo methods to replace as much of the tissue as possible before implantation. Tissue engineering techniques are applied to regenerative medical products, but these products also focus on utilizing the natural healing processes of the body to recapitulate the organ being augmented or replaced.

One example of a regenerative medicine product in development is Tengion, Inc.'s focus to replace complex organs while developing the basic biological understanding necessary to ensure integration into the patient's own body. Tengion is currently bringing forward advanced neo-organ technology designed to augment or replace failing internal organs. Tengion's product used preclinical and clinical development pathways offered by the OCP. The regulatory lead center was assigned to CBER based on the FDA's assessment of primary mode of action (cells–biologics) with collaboration from CDRH to cover the device (scaffold) components.

Tengion's technology platform brings functionality and vascularization of a complex organ by using autologous and homologous progenitor cells, isolated and cultured ex vivo, which are then seeded onto a degradable biomaterial whose shape and biomechanical properties are optimized to the body organ being augmented or replaced. The cell-seeded neo-organ construct provides the minimal raw materials necessary for tissue regeneration and the target organ's physiologic function at the time of surgical implantation. Following implantation, the product's scaffold is degraded, bioabsorbed, and replaced by organized stroma within the patient. Final and complete parenchymal organ regeneration is patient specific.

Using the neo-organ construct as a template, the body regenerates healthy tissue, restoring function to the patient's failing organ. By providing the patient with an autologous-homologous neo-organ for tissue regeneration, many of the necessary co-therapies used in traditional donor transplantation techniques are avoided, such as immunosupression. Deriving the biologically active cellular component from the patient avoids the traditional issue of limited organ donor supply.

In considering the development pathways traveled by these early transformational products, we can begin to see a framework that combines established technologies with emerging regulatory pathways and defines preclinical and clinical development strategies for products that address previously untreatable diseases. Development of therapeutic modalities to treat and potentially cure such maladies as diabetes, heart disease, renal failure, and other diseases caused by malfunctioning, damaged, or failing tissues is now a reality with regenerative medical therapies envisioned by the US Department of Health and Human Services [7] as "tissues for life" (Executive Summary, para. 2).

35.6 NEO-ORGAN PRODUCTS

Since most neo-organs will be regulated as combination products, a tiered format of analyses allows for each component to be evaluated as well as the final combination product. The neo-organ preclinical development program can be based on a foundation of current risk analysis principles combined with clinically relevant functional endpoints to establish structure–function relationships before entry into human clinical trials. Ultimately the scientific approach employed will include established anatomical, surgical, clinical, cell biological, physiological, and material sciences principles appropriate for the specific neo-organ product under development [8–14].

Neo-organ safety studies will include both acute and chronic studies, since the product will develop into an organ that remains with the patient for a lifetime. Importantly, long-term studies provide evidence for at least two outcomes vital for all products within this category: product durability and the neo-organ's capacity for becoming responsive to each individual patient's need (i.e., capacity or size). Regenerative processes are dynamic and can continue for several months. Therefore short-term studies are focused primarily on characterization of acute host tissue biological responses, biomaterial degradation, neo-tissue integration, and neo-organ functional failure or comorbidity. Longer term studies focus on evaluating the capability of the neo-organ to integrate and mold within the patient's organ systems or body size over time, neo-organ functionality, and the absence of chronic inflammatory or neoplastic processes.

35.6.1 Development Strategies

Planning for clinical testing involves defining the unmet medical need (disease characterization), determining how the intended use of the neo-organ product addresses the need, and defining processes that yield reproducible production of a safe and efficacious product for placement into patients. Developing a scientifically based definition of what constitutes a successful outcome (i.e., primary clinical endpoint) is a prerequisite for entering clinical trials. Applying existing regulatory guidelines for product testing and manufacture will be required during preclinical testing prior to its use in a human subject.

Defining the optimal regulatory pathway is done in partnership with the FDA, most likely through the OCP. With this information in hand, a sponsor can initiate preclinical testing, from which considerations for clinical testing emerge. A scientifically based program produces a foundation for exploratory clinical testing where final product characteristics are defined, production processes are standardized, and justifications that indicate readiness for entering into the clinical testing phase are anticipated. Table 35.2 presents an overview of a prototypical neo-organ product development process.

Transitioning into an initial exploratory clinical evaluation rests upon safety and functional understanding built during preclinical evaluation. The preclinical program establishes assessment objectives related to specific product characteristics and the supporting production processes. Translational medicine study results define the extent to which preclinical information demonstrates

TABLE 35.2   Overview of a potential testing program to support clinical entry of a prototypical neo-organ product

Process manufacturing control

- Define product production and early manufacturing processes
- Establish cell, tissue, and biomaterial sourcing and qualify vendors
- Validate in-process and final release testing schemes
- Characterize adventitious agents and impurities for each raw material
- Define lot-to-lot consistency criteria
- Validate quality control procedures

Preclinical studies

- Complete in vitro and in vivo safety testing
- Define toxicity testing of raw materials
- Evaluate biomaterial biocompatibility
- Establish immunogenic and inflammatory responses to raw materials
- Develop rationale for animal and in vitro models to test product function
- Define endpoints for establishing individual component and/or final product safety
- Define endpoints for establishing organ or tissue functionality
- Define endpoints for establishing organ or tissue durability

Clinical trials

- Develop rationale for safety and clinical benefit (risk–benefit analysis)
- Design exploratory and confirmatory trials
- Select patient population and define inclusion/exclusion criteria
- Identify investigational comparators and control treatments
- Establish primary and secondary study endpoints
- Consider options for data analysis and potential labeling claims

TABLE 35.3 Preclinical data collection prior to clinical study initiation

	In vitro	In vivo
Raw materials supply		
Cells[a]	+	±
Scaffold	+	±
Manufacturing process controls: In-process and potency		
Cellular processing[a]	+	−
Biomaterial processing	+	−
Final combination product[a]	+	+
Preclinical development studies		
Safety and efficacy	+	+
Endpoint selection	+	+
Translation into clinical design	±	+

[a]Products comprised of scaffold material and biologically active substances (e.g., pharmaceutical agents) do not require evaluation of cellular components.

the desired clinical outcome [15,16]. Relevant clinical endpoints need to be incorporated, wherever possible, into the animal studies. As such the endpoints need to be identified before the design of animal studies is finalized. Table 35.3 provides an overview of the preclinical data that can be generated prior to exploratory clinical trial initiation.

Regulatory considerations impact the types of data required and production process technologies that must be in place prior to initiating clinical trials. There are three considerations that have significant impact on the preclinical development plan: the extent of cellular manipulation, relationship between cell source and application, and scaffold characteristics. Table 35.4 summarizes some regulatory considerations for cellular and scaffold components.

35.6.2 Raw Material Testing

Cells Cellular components are living "raw" materials. They can be derived from the patient (autologous), other donors (allogenic), or animals (xenogenic). An additional consideration is the relationship between the cell source and the target tissue of the neo-organ product. Homologous cells are derived from the organ to be augmented or replaced. Heterologous cells are derived from a tissue or organ other than the augmentation or replacement target. Cell quality standards have been extensively reviewed and defined. Major objectives are controlling introduction of infectious agents and preventing contamination during neo-organ manufacturing. Contamination concerns include cross-contamination between patients and environmental contamination from the facility and equipment. Infectious agents may come into production with the cell source or be exogenously introduced via materials that come in contact with neo-organ materials during production (e.g., bovine-derived material).

TABLE 35.4   Regulatory considerations for the development of a neo-organ product

	Description	Impact
Manipulation of cells	For structural and nonstructural tissues, manipulation is minimal if it involves centrifugation, separation, cutting, grinding and shaping, sterilization, lyophilizing, or freezing (e.g., cells are removed and reintroduced in a single procedure). Manipulation is not minimal if cells are expanded during culture or growth factors are used to activate cells to divide or differentiate. Defined in 21 CFR 1271.3(f); see also [27].	More extensive regulatory requirements applied to neo-organ products when cellular manipulation is more than minimal.
Cell source and application	Homologous use is interpreted as the augmentation tissue using cells of the same cellular origin. Examples include applying bone cells to skeletal defects and using acellular dermis as a urethral sling. Nonhomologous use examples include using cartilage to treat bladder incontinence or hematopoietic cells to treat cardiac defects. Defined in 21 CFR 1271.3(c); see also [27].	Nonhomologous use triggers additional requirements for entering clinical trials [28].
Scaffold characterization	Final scaffold composition and design determine whether the neo-organ product is characterized as a device, a biologic, or a combination product. Defined in Quality Systems Regulations (QSRs) in 21 CFR 820 [22]; see also [29].	Devices are held to the QSRs in 21 CFR 820 [22], biologics are required to comply with good manufacturing processes (GMPs) [29] and combination products are often required to comply with both sets of regulations and guidelines.

Neo-organs designed to regenerate an entire organ must contain a sufficient number of viable cells of the proper type(s) at the time of implantation to support and/or promote de novo growth of multiple tissue layers resulting in the development of a functional, persistent organ. Therefore a cell source must exist that can expand to the required numbers in vitro or in vivo. Scientific efforts are focused on establishing cellular sources (e.g., stem cell and progenitor cells) that can be expanded and guided to differentiate into the required cell type. Following implantation, these cells must retain functional and structural consistency with the tissue and organ being replaced. Each manipulation along a differentiation process carries a potential safety risk. The total number of manipulations required to align cell source and tissue target must be determined. Also assessments to determine persistence of differentiated phenotype and function must be defined and tested in preclinical studies.

Many stem cells can be expanded and guided along a differentiation pathway to achieve a terminal functional state. Preclinical development of stem cells for neo-organ products must also demonstrate that the selected cellular raw material can safely restore original tissue structure and function (Table 35.5). Additionally, because stem cells have been manipulated into a new phenotype and incorporated into a neo-organ, preclinical studies must determine that safe maturation of a multilayered tissue occurs ex vivo or in vivo, depending on the product's primary mode of action. Finally, the safety of augmentation or regeneration processes must be assessed along with determining whether the implanted cells persist in their new (or final) phenotype and/or remain localized to the target organ site for the duration of the organ's life expectancy.

Differentiation stability and phenotype/localization persistence must also be determined for cells obtained from heterologous sources such as umbilical cord tissue and blood (UCB) [17] or adipose tissue (AT) [18]. Endothelial progenitor cells are isolated with UCBs from the blood component, adipose tissues and Wharton's jelly-derived myofibroblasts from tissue biopsies [18] contain cells capable of becoming multiple cell lines: adipogenic, osteogenic, chondrogenic, and myogenic [18]. When using these or similar heterologous

TABLE 35.5   Cell source and potential safety risk

Source	Ex vivo Manipulation	Potency	Safety Risks[a]
Embryonic stem cell	Extensive	Pluripotent	+++
Bone marrow	High	Multipotent	++
Umbilical cord	High	Multipotent	++
Adipose tissue	High	Multipotent	++
Adult tissue progenitor	Minimal to moderate	Unipotent	+

Note: + to +++ = progressively increasing levels of risk.
[a]Safety risks estimation is proposed and based on (1) biological controls for cellular stability, immunogenicity, tissue growth differentiation (i.e., risk of dysplasia or neoplasia), and (2) extent of ex vivo manipulation required to produce a neo-organ product.

cell sources, the preclinical program must evaluate purity, homogeneity, and the potentials for dysplasia, metaplasia, and neoplasia. However, one benefit of using adult stem cells from bone marrow (BM) or AT is the cells' ability to express growth factors and drive angiogenesis. This benefit must be weighed against the potential for the emergence of an undefined functional fate and possible cell expansion limits imposed by the need to maintain required phenotype characteristics, lineage compositions, and/or immunological behavior [19].

Within cell lineage differentiation pathways, the inherent potency of the starting material may be restricted based on original source. Bone marrow derived cells have the ability to differentiate into eosinophils, erythrocytes, megakaryocytes, osteoclasts, and lymphoid cells [20]. However, these hematopoietic lineages have limited potential to become a distinct tissue such as liver. Mesenchymal stem cells, on the other hand, can differentiate into a broader array of distinct tissues such osteocytes, chondrocytes, adipocytes, myocytes, and bone marrow stromal cells [20]. This plurality of outcomes requires identification of circumstances under which an aberrant outcome is manifested.

Regardless of cell source, the preclinical program demonstrates that the chosen raw cellular materials are capable of regenerating into a functional new organ. The cellular component must also be shown to function in accordance with the requirements of the native tissues and organ being replaced or augmented. Committed adult progenitor cells obtained from the same tissue being replaced (homologous tissue source) represent the lowest tier of safety concern, especially when they are returned to their original location to recapitulate homologous organ function.

Currently there is scientific interest around manipulating less differentiated cellular material (e.g., embryonic stem cells) to become differentiated and functional cells that may form tissues and, ultimately, functioning organs. The greater the pluripotency of the starting cell population, the higher the potential for becoming a different cell type (dysplasia) and/or exhibiting uncontrolled growth (neoplasia). Neo-organ products using less differentiated cells or cells from an allogenic source carry potential risks of immune response, rejection, and/or altered homestatic controls, including neoplasia. Any of these responses can lead to abnormal cellular and tissue growth. Driving undifferentiated cells to a steady state by ex vivo manipulation during the manufacture of neo-organs can introduce high concentrations of growth factors or involve manipulation techniques whose effects may persist postimplantation. Potential consequences of these ex vivo manipulation techniques include unresponsive or overresponsive cell growth, altered differentiation, and abnormal tissue growth, organic structure, and function.

Preclinical development programs are required to establish modeling systems that adequately evaluate and/or detect potential risks associated with cellular differentiation, tissue growth, and organogenesis—all necessary components of a neo-organ regenerative process. Sufficient control studies are needed to evaluate in vivo proliferation and differentiation of a neo-organ's cellular components. Additionally tests must be designed to distinguish normal differentiation and growth from adverse and uncontrolled tissue growth patterns. Moreover, if a patient receiving a neo-organ product requires medication with immunocompromising drugs, the neo-organ's capacity to integrate with native tissue could be affected. As such, postimplantation studies under a variety of co-therapeutic conditions may need to be incorporated into the preclinical development strategy.

The goal of these studies would be to demonstrate postimplantation neo-organ function and maintenance of the desired cellular differentiation and phenotypic state. Cellular components of neo-organ products may have the potential to undergo excessive proliferation (risk of hyperplasia), altered cellular differentiation (risk of dystrophy), or respond abnormally to homeostatic control of tissue growth (risk of dysplasia). Certain categories of risks that a preclinical program must evaluate can be predicted by the combination of cell source and target location. Table 35.6 illustrates this principle and lists some of the assays that should be incorporated into preclinical evaluation of neo-organ products depending on which combination applies. In all cases preclinical programs should be designed to provide evidence that the implanted neo-organ product produces stable organic function and proper therapeutic outcome by integrating into the body's systems and maintaining life.

For neo-organ product development, simply demonstrating that the cellular constituent is stable is insufficient. Cellular components of neo-organ products are expected to follow normal cell cycle and differentiation pathways. They are also expected to become part of a functioning tissue. Furthermore the neo-organ product is expected to develop into a life-sustaining organ. Achieving this ultimate level of de novo tissue regeneration and organ function generally requires the use of a structural component that forms a scaffold or temporary biocompatible frame upon which cellular components can achieve the desired integration and maturation. Testing of the scaffold or device components used in neo-organ products is well-established from a long history of traditional device product development.

Scaffold   When cells are placed onto a scaffold, scientific and regulatory considerations focus on ensuring that both the raw materials comprising the scaffold and its three-dimensional characteristics are biocompatible [21]. Biocompatibility testing involves evaluation of the scaffold's potential cytotoxicity at several levels. The first level is biocompatibility with cells placed onto the scaffold. The second level is potential toxicity to the recipient's tissues postimplantation. The third level is the consequences of a patient's immune and inflammatory responses to the neo-organ product following implantation. Biocompatibility must continue throughout the in vivo regeneration process; therefore biocompatibility testing should parallel preclinical evaluation of the scaffold's biomechanical properties during new tissue or organ growth.

TABLE 35.6 Risk-based assay selection for the evaluation of cellular constituent in neo-organ products

	Cell Source/Neo-Organ Product				
	Autologous Homologous	Autologous Heterologous	Allogeneic Homologous	Allogeneic Heterologous	Embryonic Homologous/Heterologous
In vitro					
Karylogy	+	+	+	+	++
Phenotype	+	+	+	+	+++
Cell cycle	+	+	+	+	+++
Metabolic	+	+	+	+	++
Cytokine	+	++	+	++	++
Endocrine	+	++	+	++	++
In vivo					
Morphology	+	+	+	+	++
Function	+	++	+	++	+++
Tissue Integration	+	++	++	++	++
Organ Physiology	+	+	+	+	++
Systems biology	+	++	+	++	+++
Special					
Immunotoxicity	–	–	++	++	++
Dystrophy	–	+	–	++	+++
Chorista	+	–	++	–	++
Hamartia	–	+	–	++	+++
Anaplasia	–	+	–	++	+++
Neoplasia	–	+	–	++	+++

Note: Estimated risk is proposed based on considerations outlined in the text. – = limited or no risk; + to +++ = progressively increasing levels of risk and extent of study required for each area to be assayed. Chorista is defined as a focus of tissue that is histologically normal but not normally found in the organ or structure in which it is located. Hamartia is defined as a formation defect characterized by the abnormal arrangement or combination of tissues normally present in a specific area.

Synthetic, natural or semi-synthetic composite materials are readily available from various commercial sources, but the quality control of a material varies substantially between medical and research grades. Many aspects of device testing have been outlined in 21 CFR 820 [22]; however, during the preclinical phase of testing the most relevant of these guidelines are biomaterial composition, process validation, and design controls.

Typically the design input phase is a continuum beginning with feasibility and formal input requirements and ending with early physical design activities. Engineering input on final prototype specifications follows the initial design input phase and establishes the design reviews and qualification. For a combination neo-organ product, defining quality for the chemical polymer (e.g., polyglycolic acid or PGA) or natural material (e.g., collagen), including any residues introduced during machine processing (e.g., mineral oil), can require quality systems regulations (QSR) integration into a product that would otherwise be regulated as a biologic. Since most neo-organ products are combination products, testing of scaffold, cells, and the cell-seeded scaffold (i.e., construct) are required to ensure that in exploratory clinical trials, the product is sterile, potent, fit for use, and composed of the appropriate raw materials to function properly following in vivo placement.

Scaffolds can be made from natural or synthetic materials. Such materials fall under the category of biomaterials. A biomaterial can be considered a single element or compound, which is a composite or mixture of elements, and is synthesized or derived to be used in the body to preserve, restore, or augment the structure or function of the body. Examples of natural materials for scaffold construction are: extracellular matrix, collagen, fibrin, and polysaccharides (e.g., chitosan or glycosaminoglycans). Natural materials, unless they are obtained from the patient who receives the neo-organ implant, will cause an immunogenic response. This is not always the case with synthetic materials.

Commonly used synthetic materials include polylactic acid (PLA), polyglycolic acid (PGA), polycaprolactone (PCL), and poly(lactic-co-glycolic acid) (PLGA). PLGA copolymer has been approved for use by the FDA in a number of surgical products and is commonly used by the biomedical industry. Two benefits of PLGA are its biodegradability and biocompatibity. Biodegradability is important because it allows the scaffold to be absorbed by the surrounding tissues without surgical removal (e.g., PGA undergoes spontaneous hydrolysis in body tissues). Biocompatibility is important as it supports the appropriate cellular activity and facilitates molecular and mechanical signaling systems. These characteristics help optimize tissue regeneration without eliciting undesirable cellular effects or inducing undesirable local or systemic responses in the host tissue following implantation.

For newly developed, as yet unapproved, novel biomaterial scaffolds, the regulatory preclinical guidelines developed for device materials evaluation are particularly useful in guiding the pre-clinical program of a neo-organ product. In general, the following preclinical tests should be included for such scaffold materials: acute, subchronic, and chronic toxicity; irritation to skin, eyes, and mucosal surfaces; sensitization; hemocompatibility; genotoxicity; carcinogenicity; and the materials' effect on reproduction and embryonic development. Last, target organ toxicity evaluations, such as neurotoxicity and/or immunotoxicity assays, may be necessary as part of the preclinical development. For listings of evaluation tests to consider, see Tables 35.7 and 35.8.

Collectively these guidelines serve as points to consider for preclinical development program of any neo-organ composed of a biocompatible biomaterial-based scaffold. The ultimate focus of biomaterial and scaffold testing is to evaluate its in vivo behavior following implantation. Characterizing the degradation profile ensures that the scaffold's supportive properties are maintained long enough to allow the regenerating tissue to acquire functional and structural integrity. Defining scaffold breakdown products identifies biochemical factors that may impact reparative, inflammatory, immunologic, and regenerative processes following product implantation. Measuring biomechanical properties such as stress–strain relationships and other characteristics ensures that the scaffold portion of the combination product will perform properly after implantation into the body.

35.6.3 Final Neo-Organ Product Testing

Model System Selection Safety and function evaluation of a neo-organ product is conducted in animals, and these findings are foundational to the design of the first clinical trial protocol. Translational studies are the basis for safely transitioning a potential neo-organ product into clinical testing. Since the neo-organ and its components can invoke multiple homeostatic (e.g., metabolic), defense (e.g., immune), and healing (e.g., inflammation) pathways, animal studies provide an approach to understand the inherent function of the neo-organ product.

Preclinical studies can be conducted in large (e.g., dog, goat, pig) or small (e.g., rat, mouse) animal models for the purpose of translating safety and function to the clinical trial design. Selection of the correct animal model should be based on clinical endpoint similarities between the animal model's pathophysiological, physiological, and structural characteristics and those observed in the clinical indication. Exploratory clinical trials for most medical products utilize normal human volunteers as the first line of clinical testing. However, some neo-organ products cannot be tested outside of the intended clinical population. As such, the animal model employed in translational medicine should resemble the human condition as closely as possible—immune status, inflammatory response, and healing pathways. Medical treatment approaches used to treat the human condition (e.g., surgical procedure) and monitoring methods to follow a clinical benefit or risk (e.g., imaging) should also be mimicked as closely as possible in the animal model.

Surgical aspects of implanting the neo-organ product may enter into the preclinical development paradigm. If new surgical procedures are required, or the new technology uses approved products in an off-label manner, an assess-

TABLE 35.7 Initial evaluation tests for consideration

Device Categories			Biological Effect							
Body Contact (see 4.1)		Contact Duration A Limited (24h) B Prolonged (24h to 30 days) C Permanent (>30 days)	Cytotoxicity	Sensitization	Irritation or Intracutaneous Reactivity	System Toxicity (Acute)	Subchronic toxicity (Subacute Toxicity)	Genotoxicity	Implantation	Haemocompatibility
Surface devices	Skin	A	×	×	×	—	—	—	—	—
		B	×	×	×	—	—	—	—	—
		C	×	×	×	—	—	—	—	—
	Mucosal membrane	A	×	×	×	—	—	—	—	—
		B	×	×	×	0	0	—	0	—
		C	×	×	×	0	×	×	0	—
	Breached or compromised surfaces	A	×	×	×	0	—	—	—	—
		B	×	×	×	0	0	—	0	—
		C	×	×	×	0	×	×	0	—
External communicating devices	Blood path, indirect	A	×	×	×	×	—	—	—	×
		B	×	×	×	×	0	—	—	×
		C	×	×	0	×	×	×	0	×
	Tissue/bone dentin communicating +	A	×	×	×	0	—	—	—	—
		B	×	×	0	0	0	×	×	—
		C	×	×	0	0	0	×	×	—
	Circulating blood	A	×	×	×	×	—	0	—	×
		B	×	×	×	×	0	×	0	×
		C	×	×	×	×	×	×	0	×
Implant devices	Tissue bone	A	×	×	×	0	—	—	—	—
		B	×	×	0	0	0	×	×	—
		C	×	×	0	0	0	×	×	—
	Blood	A	×	×	×	×	—	—	×	×
		B	×	×	×	×	0	×	×	×
		C	×	×	×	×	×	×	×	×

Source: Reproduced from [22].

Note: X = ISO evaluation tests for consideration; 0 = additional tests which may be applicable; note + tissue includes tissue fluids and subcutaneous spaces; note ∧ for all devices used extracorporeal circuits.

TABLE 35.8 Supplementary evaluation tests for consideration

Device Categories			Biological Effect							
Body Contact (see 4.1)		Contact duration A Limited (–24 h) B Prolonged (24 h to 30 days) C Permanent (>30 days)	Cytotoxicity	Sensitization	Irritation or Intracutaneous Reactivity	System Toxicity (Acute)	Subchronic toxicity (Subacute Toxicity)	Genotoxicity	Implantation	Haemocompatibility
Surface devices	Skin	A	—	—	—	—	—	—	—	—
		B	—	—	—	—	—	—	—	—
		C	—	—	—	—	—	—	—	—
	Mucosal membrane	A	—	—	—	—	—	—	—	—
		B	—	—	—	—	—	—	—	—
		C	0	—	—	—	—	—	—	—
	Breached or compromised surfaces	A	—	—	—	—	—	—	—	—
		B	—	—	—	—	—	—	—	—
		C	0	—	—	—	—	—	—	—
External communicating devices	Blood path, indirect	A	—	—	—	—	—	—	—	—
		B	—	—	—	—	—	—	—	—
		C	×	×	—	—	—	—	—	—
	Tissue/bone dentin communicating	A	—	—	—	—	—	—	—	—
		B	—	—	—	—	—	—	—	—
		C	0	×	—	—	—	—	—	—
	Circulating blood	A	—	—	—	—	—	—	—	—
		B	—	—	—	—	—	—	—	—
		C	×	×	—	—	—	—	—	—
Implant devices	Tissue bone	A	—	—	—	—	—	—	—	—
		B	—	—	—	—	—	—	—	—
		C	×	×	—	—	—	—	—	—
	Blood	A	—	—	—	—	—	—	—	—
		B	—	—	—	—	—	—	—	—
		C	×	×	—	—	—	—	—	—

Source: Reproduced from [22].

ment of new safety risks may be needed that are not directly related to the product itself. The number of possible new approaches or new applications of current surgical products is sufficiently large that each needs to be considered on a case-by-case basis in close collaboration with the FDA or regulatory agency responsible for ensuring safety. Such considerations are beyond the scope of this chapter.

The biological activity of a neo-organ product may preclude the use of commonly used animal models for safety testing (e.g., rats and dogs). Safety evaluation programs should include the use of species relevant to both safety testing and providing proof-of-concept evaluation of the neo-organ's ability to function and sustain homeostasis. A relevant species is one in which the test product is biologically active in regenerating or replacing the native organ.

Safety evaluation programs have historically used two relevant species. However, in certain cases one relevant species may suffice when biological activity (e.g., organ function) or technical feasibility (e.g., surgical implantation) considerations render the use of another species irrelevant. Even under circumstances where two species may be necessary for short-term toxicity studies, it may be possible to justify using only one species to evaluate durability, growth potential, and full regenerative outcome in subsequent long-term toxicity studies. Long-term studies may need to extend for months or even years to demonstrate that the neo-organ can function in a safe and appropriate manner.

For neo-organ products, safety studies in nonrelevant species may actually provide misleading results. Lower order species have a greater potential for regeneration, allowing a product to appear to have more regenerative capacity than would be manifested in humans. New developments in animal models of human diseases may bring these advanced technologies to greater use in studying the replacement and augmentation of diseased organs (e.g., transgenic animal models reflecting human disease pathogenesis). These models may provide further insight, not only in determining the mechanism of regeneration but also in safety evaluation (e.g., evaluation of undesirable promotion of disease progression). Scientific justification for safety evaluations using these animal models of human disease should be provided.

Since a neo-organ must function at the moment of implantation, animal studies provide an understanding of how to evaluate initial body responses as well as longer term outcomes reflecting the desired benefit—an augmented or replaced tissue or organ. Since most neo-organs remain with the patient for a lifetime following surgical implantation, translational study duration should extend to a time when final clinical outcome is achieved. Considerable thought should be given to the duration of preclinical studies. Since the implications of these therapies relates to patient longevity, the duration of these studies may extend from months to years. Nonetheless, the final outcome is frequently achieved in a shorter time period of time, so the potential to conduct shorter duration studies based on final patient outcome may present a rational solution to testing clinical utility in the shortest possible time while ensuring a high outcome benefit–risk ratio.

Endpoint Selection As with other medical products, preclinical development can be conducted using selected toxicological endpoints (e.g., in-life, serum chemistry, hematological, urinalysis, and target and sentinel organ histological evaluation) based on the target organ being replaced or augmented. Final organ function will influence the appropriate endpoints to monitor during in-life and postmortem analysis. Neo-organ safety evaluation would also focus on the mechanism of product function, extent of neo-organ integration into the body, neo-organ structure–function relationships, appropriate cellular, local and target tissue, and systems biology aspects.

In-life observations, serum chemistry, hematology, urinalysis, and body weight gain coupled with imaging and other clinically relevant procedures can be used to monitor the progression of neo-organ incorporation into the body and assumption of a functional role in homeostasis. Abnormal tissues, areas of adhesion, and any macroscopically or functionally abnormal tissues should be collected and evaluated postmortem. Histopathological evaluation of target organ tissues, potential target organs, and peripheral tissues should be evaluated postmortem to evaluate adverse effects and document the neo-organ's function(s). Immunohistochemical evaluation may also be conducted to demonstrate cell phenotype, tissue morphogenesis, and neo-organ characteristics.

Cellular analysis will depend on cell source, with higher risk cell sources requiring more extensive in vitro, in vivo, and ex vivo analysis. Genetic stability and cell phenotypic analysis are also focus areas in preclinical studies, since they provide evidence of appropriate regeneration and function of the cellular component in the neo-organ product.

Understanding which endpoints are available and appropriate for first clinical trials is achieved through translation of preclinical development study results. Standards are provided for the proper safety evaluation of neo-organ products whether they are regulated as a device [23] or a biological product [24,25]. Although the optimal testing strategy will typically be product specific [23], some basic guidelines for testing device-like neo-organ products can be found in the ISO10993-1 guidance document [26]. These guidelines also provide insight into possible testing strategies to evaluate the final product after all components are combined (Table 35.9).

Final neo-organ products that are cell based or neo-organs in which the primary mode of action is mediated through cellular constituents of a scaffold-cell combination product require an assortment of studies. Scaffold and cellular components are evaluated through appropriate endpoint selection. Endpoints selected should have direct translation to the clinical testing phase,

TABLE 35.9 Test categories described in ISO10993-1 (USP 71)

In vitro Assays	In vivo Assays
Cytotoxicity	Irritation
Pyrogenicity	Sensitization
Hemocompatability	Acute systemic toxicity
Genotoxicity/genetic tests	Subchronic toxicity
	Local tolerance

TABLE 35.10   General preclinical development testing paradigms for a cell-based neo-organ product

Cellular Component	Scaffold	Combination
Phenotype characterization	Early stage (acute)	Early stage (acute toxicity)
Genetic stability	Late stage (chronic)	Late stage (chronic toxicity)
	Biocompatability	
	Biomechanical properties	
	Degradation profile	

emphasizing the importance of having matching endpoints for both clinical and laboratory situations.

Experimental Design   Experimental design for both in vitro and in vivo translational studies is influenced by the endpoints that will be evaluated in clinical studies. The experimental design should also recognize that new endpoints may need to be evaluated in clinical trials. An example of a preclinical development program for a combined cell-based neo-organ product is presented in Table 35.10.

Specific testing approaches are not absolutely defined. However, testing approaches and their scope for a specific neo-organ product can often be predicted by comparison with development strategies used for related component technology platforms. As more combination products are approved for clinical use, the choice of related technology platforms for comparison will broaden.

Transitioning a neo-organ product from preclinical development to a scientifically based clinical evaluation involves several steps. First to be demonstrated is the ability of the neo-organ to invoke a bodily response that has therapeutic benefit. Second, a controlled and reproducible manufacturing process must be in place. Finally, the safety of each component and the final product (a safe and functioning neo-organ) must be demonstrated. This transition to clinical evaluation is typically the first point of regulatory authority and governance body interactions, and an area where there are established procedural approaches and controls to review and clarify the experimental design of preclinical studies.

35.7   TRANSITION TO CLINICAL TESTING

35.7.1   Defining and Testing a Prototype

Prior to initiating a clinical testing program, a neo-organ product's specific characteristics must be defined to the point that the product can be repeatedly and reproducibly manufactured for in vitro and in vivo testing as defined above. Product characteristics should be sufficiently stable to allow for data-driven demonstration of their clinical utility. Once a prototype is defined, its characteristics can be evaluated in a series of tests to define the limits of the initial design criteria. Durability testing establishes failure points, limits of neo-organ application, and evaluates the achievement of design criteria.

Anticipating the clinical conditions, complications, and untoward events that may arise during clinical testing also establishes a prototype product's potential for clinical utility. A neo-organ product is seldom introduced as a final functioning organ, since even highly engineered neo-organ products require scaffold degradation, neo-vascularization, tissue integration, and functional maturation stages to be complete prior to healing. Therefore characterization of pharmacological responsiveness and electrophysiological parameters, along with determining phenotypic and structural features of the emerging neo-tissue and/or neo-organ following implantation, are key data for supporting claims about the product's ultimate clinical benefit.

Human testing of specific design elements of a final neo-organ prototype is the culmination of a series of biological, physical, and chemical evaluations obtained during the preclinical prototyping phase. As defined above, these evaluations span sourcing and control of raw materials, assembly processes (i.e., in-process testing), and release criteria. Additionally the product's shelf life, shipping conditions (temperature, humidity, nutrients, etc.), stability, sterility, and method of use are established in the preclinical testing phase. Translational studies provide anticipated protocols for unique surgical procedures, recovery times, and clinical management practices during and after implantation once a final prototype product with the fully embodied characteristics is available.

Using previously tested technology platforms can accelerate neo-organ product entry into clinical testing. Leveraging prior approval of scaffold materials, cell processing methods, culture media components, or transport containers can greatly reduce the number of variables that need to be tested in product prototyping and preclinical testing phases. Additionally availability of historical data for employed technologies can assist in the development of final prototype testing strategies and early clinical trial designs.

35.7.2 Production of Neo-Organs for Preclinical Testing

Production process definition for neo-organ products in the preclinical testing stage of development takes on increasing importance relative to traditional noncombination devices, drugs, and biologics. Clearly, established product characteristics, standard operating procedures, and the use of clinical-grade production in late-stage preclinical testing can accelerate the deployment of a facility to manufacture final preclinical prototype products and extend to the manufacture of GMP-grade products for initial human trials. Neo-organ technologies can vary substantially, but small GMP facilities can meet neo-organ production needs for both late-stage preclinical testing and early clinical trials

TABLE 35.11 Regulated practices for consideration when taking a neo-organ to clinical testing

	Regulation
Good tissue practices	21 CFR 1271
Good manufacturing practices	21 CFR 210 and 211
Good laboratory practices	21 CFR 58
Good clinical practices	21 CFR 50
Quality systems regulations	21 CFR 820[a]

[a]Replaced cGMPs for neo-organ products regulated as devices.

for some products. Facility design considerations are outside of the scope of this chapter, but a GMP-qualified facility that can provide the required clean room processing, shipping and receiving procedures, and HVAC systems for airflow maintenance should be identified as part of the preclinical development phase of neo-organ product-development strategies.

Production of a neo-organ product for preclinical testing can be regulated by a number of different guidelines depending on the combination product composition (Table 35.11). Good tissue practices and good manufacturing practices established in the preclinical testing phase may go through an IND/BLA under 21 CFR 312/601 or IDE/PMA 21 CFR 812/814. Preclinical testing programs using the final neo-organ product or process may require that the test product be manufactured in a manner consistent with the conditions required for making the human neo-organ.

When designing the preclinical testing program for a neo-organ product, consideration is given to not only the clinical testing phase but also the bioprocessing activities required to manufacture a neo-organ product. Testing of any neo-organ product requires defining the bioprocess approach that will be used in early clinical testing. Without this planning, bioprocesses used in the preclinical testing may be dissimilar to those used in the clinical trials. Differences in the process may impact final neo-organ product characteristics to such a degree that release and in-process testing results established in the preclinical stage of development no longer apply to the product being tested in the clinical trials. Such an outcome may render the preclinical test results invalid or inappropriate for the product intended for clinical testing.

35.8 BRINGING NEO-ORGAN PLATFORMS TO CLINICAL TESTING

As discussed above, technology platforms that intend to recapitulate a tissue (e.g., skeletal muscle, bone, cardiac muscle) or an organ may address a range of unmet medical needs from simple cosmetic defects (tissue-focused technologies) to life-threatening maladies (organ and organ system replacement). Bringing a neo-organ technology to clinical testing may rest on the scope of unmet medical need and availability of alternative therapies. The array of available alternative therapies influences the early testing strategy of a particular product by determining comparable products to be evaluated, selection of animal models, appropriate endpoints, and amount of preclinical information needed to enter into clinical testing. Ultimately the risk–benefit analysis between safety and functionality of the prototype product and other available products has a direct influence on the ability to test the product in human trials.

Tissue-focused technologies, such as bone and tendon repair, may move through preclinical development into clinical trials via routes that have been established by previous successes (e.g., Depuy's Restore®). If animal models and alternative therapeutic approaches are established, comparing the benefit of a proposed product to an existing therapy may be an one approach to potential clinical testing. Ultimately comparing the benefit of a complex tissue or neo-organ versus the "gold standard" commercial product or surgical therapy is the foundational rationale for evaluating potential human use.

Neo-organ technologies offer the promise of offsetting the worldwide organ shortage. Despite this great promise the pathway to clinical testing for a product that replaces an entire organ is the least clearly defined. Although definitive clinical benefit, discernable endpoints, established animal models, and delivery mechanisms may exist, the procedures for "connecting" the neo-organ product to other parts of the body pose substantial development hurdles and require extensive preclinical testing programs.

The complexity of whole organ replacement by neo-organ products spans defining what is actually being replaced through defining what ancillary products may be needed if all organ functions are not recapitulated by the neo-organ product. Traditional therapeutic approaches have generally focused on one pathway or target (e.g., pharmaceutical) or possibly two therapeutic benefits such as structural and functional restoration (e.g., cartilage repair products). However, products that replace an entire organ (e.g., kidney) or body part (e.g., limbs) will need to consider broad functional testing of both exocrine/excretory, metabolic, structural, and endocrine functions before clinical testing can be considered.

The transition to clinical testing of more complex neo-organ products will have commensurate preclinical testing requirements to demonstrate not only the functionality of each component being replaced or augmented but also the biological responsiveness of the integrated organ to native homeostatic mechanisms (e.g., integration with blood pressure or glucose control). Matters such as building percutaneous conduits and controlling skin infections and/or biofilms may be substantial development hurdles for the use of products outside the body. For products intended for use inside the body, clinical testing may hinge on finding solutions for vascular connections, waste product release pathways (e.g., urinary tract and GI), and clinical monitoring of neo-organ development. Similarly the length of time it takes to achieve clinical outcome may need to be determined before clinical testing can be considered.

Biosensors and integration of biosensors with neo-organ products are becoming a reality. Moving into clinical testing with these products requires definition of "recovery pathways" in the event of product failure. Adjunct therapies to be applied concurrently with neo-product use if all organ functions are not replaced with the neo-organ itself need to be defined. An understanding of neo-organ durability/longevity and replacement methods in the event that the neo-organ "wears out" needs to be developed. Finally, developing an understanding of product failure frequency and rate is important for proper clinical management.

Despite these hurdles, the lure of replacing an entire organ is considerable. The benefit to society of replacing a kidney or pancreas would be unimaginable. As technologies for in vitro organ growth advance and regenerative templates for entire organs are pioneered (e.g., through such technologies as organ printing), the potential to replace, regenerate, repair, and restore entire organ systems is being considered. Regenerative medical approaches may yield solutions for devastating human conditions including congenital agenesis, cancer, degenerative disorders, and infectious diseases. However, entry into clinical testing with such products has not yet been defined.

35.9 CONCLUSIONS

It is inevitable that, in the future, neo-organ products will represent an important class of treatments for patients needing neo-organ and tissue replacements, especially for many diseases in which available therapeutic options offer suboptimal outcomes. These products have the potential to satisfy significant unmet medical needs with an almost unimaginable benefit—a cure, not just a treatment. Currently regenerative medical products hold out the hope that downside risk is limited, since they reduce or even eliminate the potential for rejection without the onerous cost and difficulties associated with immunosuppressive therapy. Autologous-homologous products represent the best example. These products may offer unmatched risk–benefit profiles with the potential for rapid approval and introduction into the appropriate patient populations. Anticipated results include reductions in health care costs and substantial patient benefits, particularly when there are no medically acceptable alternatives.

The path to clinical entry has been partially paved for some of these breakthroughs, especially those that can emerge from application of established development strategies. It is conceivable that neo-organ products can be brought to market more rapidly and efficiently than traditional medical products (e.g., pharmaceuticals) and offer unknown advantages by their customized and individually tailored nature. Furthermore logistical advantages occur with patient-specific neo-organs, so well-defined studies (rather than time-consuming and costly large-scale preclinical studies to define unknown risks), smaller trial sizes (due to the customized nature of the products), and postregistration follow-up (these products, once implanted, become part of the patient) can all be considered in the development of this transformational technology.

ACKNOWLEDGMENTS

The authors thank Belinda Wagner for her guidance and assistance in helping us to present this new material in a clear and concise fashion. We would also like to thank David Watson for gathering information needed to compile this chapter.

REFERENCES

1. Nelson JW. The lone eagle as medical researcher. *Navy Med* 2003;94:18–22.
2. Viola J, Bhavya L, Grad O. Emergence and evolution of a shared concept. In *The Emergence of Tissue Engineering as a Research Field*. Washington, DC: National Science Foundation, 2003. from, http://www.nsf.gov/pubs/2004/nsf0450/emergence.htm
3. FDA. Is the product a medical device? *Device Advice*, 1998. http://www.fda.gov/cdrh/devadvice/312.html#contents
4. FDA. 21 CFR Part 3: Product Jurisdiction, 2006. http://www.fda.gov/oc/ombudsman/part3&5.htm
5. FDA. Guidance for Industry and FDA Staff: How to Write a Request for Designation, 2005. http://www.fda.gov/oc/combination/howtowrite.html
6. FDA. Office of Combination Products, 2006. http://www.fda.gov/oc/combination/
7. US Department of Health and Human Services. 2020: A New Vision—A Future for Regenerative Medicine, 2006. http://www.hhs.gov/reference/newfuture.shtml
8. Anderson JM. Biological responses to materials. *Ann Rev Mater Res* 2001;31: 81–110.
9. ASTM F981-99. Standard Practice for Assessment of Compatibility of Biomaterials for Surgical Implants with Respect to Effect of Materials on Muscle and Bone. 1999.
10. Cotran RS, Kumar V, Collins T. *Robbin's Pathologic Basis of Disease*, 6th ed. Philadelphia: WB Saunders, 1999.
11. Lewis RW, et al. Recognition of adverse and nonadverse effects in toxicity studies. *Toxicol Pathol* 2002;30:66–74.
12. Long G. Recommendations to guide determining cause of death in toxicity studies. *Toxicol Pathol* 2004;32:269–70.
13. Ratner BD, et al. *Biomaterials Science: An Introduction to Materials in Medicine*. San Diego: Elsevier Science/Academic Press, 1996.
14. Rubin E, et al. *Rubin's Pathology*. 4th ed. Philadelphia: Lippincott/Williams Wilkins, 2005.
15. Preti RA. Bringing safe and effective cell therapies to the bedside. *Nat Biotechnol* 2005;23:801–4.

16. Weber DJ. Navigating FDA regulations for human cells and tissues. *BioProcess Int* 2004;2:22–7.

17. Schmidt D. et al. Engineering of biologically active living heart valve leaflets using human umbilical cord-derived progenitor cells. *Tissue Eng* 2006;12:3209–21.

18. Zuk PA, et al. Multilineage cells from human adipose tissue: implications for cell-based therapies. *Tissue Eng* 2001;7:211–28.

19. Haider H. Bone marrow cells for cardiac regeneration and repair: current status and issues. *Expert Rev Cardiovasc Ther* 2006;4:557–68.

20. Ikada Y. Challenges in tissue engineering. *J R Soc Interface* 2006;3:589–601.

21. FDA. Required Biocompatibility Training and Toxicology Profiles for Evaluation of Medical Devices: May 1, 1995 (G95-1). http://www.fda.gov/cdrh/g951.html

22. FDA. 21 CFR part 820: Quality System Regulation, 2006, http://www.accessdata.fda.gov/scripts/cdrh/cfdocs/cfcfr/CFRSearch.cfm?CFRPart=1271

23. FDA. Proposed Approach to Regulation of Cellular and Tissue-Based Products, 1997. http://www.fda.gov/cber/gdlns/celltissue.txt

24. FDA. Biological Products Regulated under Section 351 of the Public Health Service Act; Implementation of Biologics License; Elimination of Establishment License and Product License, 1999. http://www.fda.gov/cber/rules/elapla.pdf

25. FDA. Guidance for Industry FDA Staff: Minimal Manipulation of Structural Tissue Jurisdictional Update, 2006. http://www.fda.gov/oc/combination/manipulation.html

26. ISO 10993-5. Biological Evaluation of Medical Devices. Part 5: Tests for In vitro Cytotoxicity. 1999.

27. FDA. 21 CFR part 1271: Human Cells, Tissues, and Cellular and Tissue-Based Products, 2006. http://www.accessdata.fda.gov/scripts/cdrh/cfdocs/cfcfr/CFRSearch.cfm?CFRPart=1271

28. Halme DG, Kessler DA. FDA regulation of stem-cell-based therapies. *N Engl J Med* 2006;355:1730–5.

29. FDA. Medical Device Quality Systems Manual: A Small Entitiy Compliance Guide, 1997. http://www.fda.gov/cdrh/dsma/gmpman.html

PART VII

PRECLINICAL STUDY DESIGN, IMPLEMENTATION, AND ANALYSIS

CHAPTER 36

GLP Requirements and Current Practices

TANYA SCHARTON-KERSTEN

Contents

36.1 BACKGROUND FOR GLP REGULATIONS

Regulations and guidelines for the conduct of preclinical testing of drugs and biologics were introduced by US and other governments to ensure the quality and integrity of preclinical data submitted in support of clinical trial applications (IND, CTA, etc.) and/or marketing approvals (BLA, NDA, MAA, etc.). The good laboratory practices (GLP) regulations and guidelines foster mutual acceptance of test data in the international community, serve to minimize redundant testing, minimize animal use, and maximize protection of human health. The purpose of this chapter is to provide guidance on compliance with GLP provisions in the conduct of preclinical (nonclinical) laboratory studies of biopharmaceuticals. Application of the US promulgated GLP provisions

Preclinical Safety Evaluation of Biopharmaceuticals: A Science-Based Approach to Facilitating Clinical Trials, edited by Joy A. Cavagnaro
Copyright © 2008 by John Wiley & Sons, Inc.

(21 CFR 58) is the primary focus, with more limited reference to global GLP regulations and compliance.

Within the United States, the Food and Drug Administration (FDA) regulates the conduct of preclinical laboratory studies under part 58, Good Laboratory Practice for Nonclinical Laboratory Studies, of title 21 of the Code of Federal Regulations (21 CFR 58). The most current version of the GLP regulations may be accessed through the US National Archives and Records Administration Web site [1]. A similar but distinct set of GLP regulations is used by the US Environmental Protection Agency (EPA) to govern laboratory studies of pesticides [2] and other toxic chemical substances [3].

The GLP provisions promulgated by the FDA specifically apply to preclinical safety data generated in test systems both in vitro and in vivo. In section 58.3(d) of the GLP regulations, the FDA defines the term nonclinical laboratory study as "in vivo or in vitro experiments in which test articles are studied prospectively in test systems under laboratory conditions to determine their safety." Examples include, but are not limited to, physical-chemical testing, toxicity studies, mutagenicity studies, tissue residue depletion studies, and analytical and clinical chemistry testing. Basic exploratory or proof-of-principle studies carried out to determine whether a test article has any potential utility or to determine physical or chemical characteristics of a test article are excluded from the US GLP regulations. However, complete exclusion of many elements of GLP preclinical animal studies has become relatively unusual as both industry and the regulatory community recognize the ethical, scientific and long-term cost saving benefits associated with application of GLP provisions. Animal use is reduced when study designs are rigorously reviewed. Careful execution of studies also minimizes the need to repeat testing, thereby further reducing animal use and costs associated with test redundancy. Rigorous documentation during study conduct data collection facilitates communication of study results in both scientific publication and to regulatory agencies.

From the FDA perspective it is expected that all preclinical safety studies supporting the safety of research or marketing application (IND, CTD, BLA, NDA, etc.) will be performed in a manner consistent with GLP provisions and that Sponsors justify any nonconformance (21 CFR 312.23(a)(8)(iii)). Nonetheless, it is neither a regulatory requirement nor often feasible to conduct all preclinical studies within a drug (biologic) development program in 100% GLP compliance. The lack (or perceived lack) of an independent quality unit in small companies or academic organizations can prohibit 100% GLP compliance for internally conducted studies. Alternatively, technical resources for specialized studies, particularly those where both pharmacological and safety testing are combined; limited capacity, particularly for biologics testing; and prohibitive costs can impact outsourcing of studies to GLP knowledgeable contractors.

There are many misconceptions surrounding GLP principles. For example, sponsors often believe that the GLP provisions may be applied to the testing of samples from clinical studies. However, the introductions to the FDA GLPs in 21 CFR part 58 and to the Organization for Economic Cooperation and Development (OECD) Principles of GLP state that applicable studies do not include studies utilizing human subjects or clinical studies or field trials in animals. The FDA and other regulatory authorities do require a demonstration of the quality of test data from clinical studies. However, this is by means of compliance with good clinical practice (GCP) and International Conference for Harmonization (ICH) provisions as well as conformance with CLIA (Clinical Laboratories Improvement Act). There is also a common but inappropriate use of the term GLP to refer to the quality of test material used in preclinical studies. Test material that is not fully GMP compliant should be stated as such. The term GLP cannot be used to indicate less than GMP material. Other common terminologies used to designate non-GMP material include, "research grade" or "pre-GMP" material.[1]

Application of GLP principles to testing of biopharmaceuticals, including cell therapies and infectious agent vaccines and therapies, can be difficult. Biological test materials often require special handling and/or less conventional animal models for preclinical safety testing. For example, development of vaccines and therapies for counterterrorism applications and for infectious diseases such as human immunodeficiency virus associated with the acquired immune deficiency syndrome (AIDS) is fostering novel vaccines approaches and therapies. Handling of the related test materials, and even the test systems, can require adherence to defined biosafety level (BSL) containment provisions [4]. Similarly the toxicity testing may require conduct in species other than rodents and dogs, which have been the conventional models for pharmaceuticals. As a consequence test facility options for biological materials are relatively limited when compared to that available for drug compounds. To accommodate the required studies, sponsors are often faced with either long wait times at test facilities, building GLP compliance capacity within their own organizations, bringing necessary scientific, permitting, and general biologic expertise to conventional test facilities, and/or educating university and smaller private laboratories on GLP provisions. In all cases it has become increasingly important for the sponsor to have a pragmatic understanding of domestic and global GLP provisions in order to select the test laboratory (qualification) and to ensure that study performance and reported data meet acceptable standards (monitoring) for both scientific validity and regulatory compliance.

The chapter aims to (1) provide an overview of US and global GLP regulations and (2) discuss pragmatic application of GLP elements to preclinical studies, particularly those where conventional 100% GLP compliance may not be feasible.

---

[1]While one may insert such terms in a study report, and CROs may accept such descriptions, it should be noted that the FDA and other regulatory agencies expect that the definitive safety studies be conducted with test article that is comparable to the product proposed for the initial clinical studies. Any differences, compliance (GMP/nonGMP) or other (manufacturing methods, product attributes), must be justified within the relevant regulatory submissions (e.g., IND or BLA/CTD).

36.2   HISTORY AND SCOPE OF GOOD LABORATORY PRACTICE (GLP) REGULATIONS

The Federal Food Drug and Cosmetics Act (FD&C) Act and Public Health Service (PHS) Act (biologics only) require that sponsors of FDA-regulated products submit evidence of their product's safety and efficacy in research (IND, IDE) and/or marketing applications (BLA, NDA, PMA). These products include human drugs and biological products, and human medical devices. FDA uses these data to answer questions regarding the toxicity profile of the test article, the observed no adverse effect dose level (NOAEL) in the test system, the risks associated with clinical studies involving humans or animals, the potential teratogenic/reproductive, genotoxic, carcinogenic, or other adverse effects of the article, and the level of use that can be approved.

The GLP regulations (21 CFR 58) were promulgated in the mid-1970s based on inspections of animal laboratories revealing unsuitable industry practices within studies submitted to the FDA [5–8]. The quality and integrity from such studies were not considered adequate to ensure product safety in accord with the FD&C Act, PHS Act, and other applicable laws. As a result of these findings the FDA promulgated the good laboratory practice (GLP) regulations. The proposed GLP regulations were published in the Federal Register of November 1976 [9]. The regulations establish standards for the conduct and reporting of animal laboratory studies and are intended to ensure the quality and integrity of safety data submitted to FDA.

The final rule for GLP regulations was published in the Federal Register of December 22, 1978 (43 FR 59986), and it became effective on July 20, 1979 [10]. Revisions to the cGLP regulations, to reduce regulatory and paperwork burdens, were proposed in the Federal Register of October 29, 1984 (49 FR 43530), with the final amendment published in the Federal Register of September 4, 1987 (52 FR 33768) [11,12]. Two ancillary documents published by the FDA—Guidance for Industry: Good Laboratory Regulations Management Briefings [13] and Good Laboratory Practices: Questions and Answers [14]—provide pragmatic information on application of the GLP regulations and the FDA's interpretations thereof. Answers to many common questions and conceptions, may be found within these documents. The FDA/ORA Bioresearch Monitoring Information Web page contains numerous US based GLP resources [15].

In May 1981 the member countries for the Organization for Economic Cooperation and Development (OECD) approved the OECD Principles of Good Laboratory Practice. The GLP Web site of the OECD contains detailed reference information and links for global GLP compliance [16]. Revised OECD GLP principles were adopted by the Council on November 26, 1997. The complete OECD GLP regulations are comprised of a series of guidance documents with the first document, No. 1 OECD Principles of Good Laboratory Practice, providing the overarching guidance for GLP compliance among the member countries [17–30].[2] The OECD GLP provisions are the most commonly referenced global standards for GLP compliance.

Within the European Union, the European Commission (EC) has codified the GLP requirements for medicinal products in the Introduction and General Principles chapter of Directive 2003/63/EC [31]. Within this document it is stated that nonclinical (pharmacotoxicological) studies must be carried out in conformity with the provisions related to GLP laid down in Council Directives 87/18/EEC[3] on the harmonization of regulations and administrative provisions relating to the application of the principles of GLP and the verification of their application for tests in chemical substances; and 88/320/EEC[4] (corrigenda 1, 2, and 3) on the inspection and verification of GLP [32,33]. The OECD principles have been adopted by the European Union and published, in their revised form, in the appendix to Directive 2004/10/EC [32]. The GLP Web site of the EC contains detailed reference information and links for member state GLP compliance [34].

Establishment of global GLP standards as well as mutual recognition agreements permit sharing of data among regulatory authorities and reduces the need for redundant testing by product sponsors. Data generated in an OECD member country, in accordance with OECD test guidelines and the Principles of Good Laboratory Practice, are accepted by regulatory agencies of other OECD member countries. The US FDA has also established specific Memorandum of Understanding (MOU) for GLP compliance with several European and non-European countries. The European Union has concluded Mutual Recognition Agreements for GLP provisions within its member states and with Israel, Japan, and Switzerland. By means of the Treaty of the European Economic Area (EEA) of December 13, 1993, the European Regulations and Directives also apply to Iceland, Liechtenstein, and Norway. The Web sites of the various national GLP compliance and monitoring bodies may be consulted to verify mutual data recognition [35].

36.3 COMMON ELEMENTS OF GLP REGULATIONS

Both the OECD and US FDA GLP regulations are intended to establish minimal standards for conducting and reporting preclinical laboratory studies. Study organization, personnel, control of test and reference materials, the test system, data collection, reporting, communication, and storage are all covered within the domestic and global GLPs. The required period(s) of storage for raw data, documentation, protocols, specimens, and interim and

---

[2]The OECD member countries are Australia, Austria, Belgium, Canada, the Czech Republic, Denmark, Finland, France, Germany, Greece, Hungary, Iceland, Ireland, Italy, Japan, Korea, Luxembourg, Mexico, the Netherlands, New Zealand, Norway, Poland, Portugal, the Slovak Republic, Spain, Sweden, Switzerland, Turkey, the United Kingdom, and the United States.
[3]Directive 2004/10/EC replaces Directive 87/18/EEC.
[4]Directive 2004/9/EC has replaced Directive 88/320/EEC as of March 11, 2004.

final reports is defined within the GLP regulations (e.g., 21 CFR 58.190 and 195).

The US FDA GLP regulations (21 CFR 58) are comprised of 11 subparts (A–K), beginning with a definition of the scope and terminology (subpart A, General Provisions), followed by minimal requirements for the following:

- Organization and personnel (subpart B)
- Facilities (subpart C)
- Equipment (subpart D)
- Test facilities operation (subpart E)
- Test and control articles (subpart F)
- Protocol for conduct of a nonclinical laboratory study (subpart G)
- Records and reports (subpart J)

The FDA regulations end with a discussion of procedures for Disqualification of Test Facilities (subpart K).

A critical feature of the GLP regulation is the integral role of an independent quality assurance unit (QAU). Per 21 CFR 58.35 the quality assurance unit, an entity that is entirely separate and independent of the personnel engaged in the direction and conduct of the study, is responsible for monitoring each study to ensure management that the facilities, equipment, personnel, methods, practices records, and controls are in conformance with the GLP provisions. Specific responsibilities include maintenance of a master schedule, maintenance of copies of all protocols, inspection of each laboratory study with documented communication of any problems to management and the study director, submission of periodic status reports on each study to management and the study director, determination that no deviations from approved protocols or SOPs were made without proper authorization and documentation, review of the final report to ensure accuracy of the methods and reported data, preparation and signature of a statement to be included in the final report with the date of inspections and findings reported to management, and maintenance of records for review by authorized FDA employees during inspections. In many cases it is either the lack of internal resources to perform these activities or a lack of understanding of the nature of the QAU responsibilities that preclude a sponsor from performing GLP regulated studies in-house. Moreover the need for integrated quality assurance within *all* GLP studies primarily precludes even the best planned and documented studies from claiming full GLP adherence if the responsibilities are not considered and implemented prior to study initiation.

Similarly the OECD GLP regulations (GLP Principles No. 1 in the series) begin with the definition of scope and terminology (section I, Scope and Definition of Terms), followed by 10 subparts (section II) providing minimal requirements for the following:

- Test facility organization and personnel (subpart 1)
- Quality assurance programme (subpart 2)
- Facilities (subpart 3)
- Apparatus, material, and reagents (subpart 4)
- Test systems (subpart 5)
- Test and reference items (subpart 6)
- Standard operating procedures (subpart 7)
- Performance of the study (subpart 8)
- Reporting of study results (subpart 9)
- Storage and retention of records and materials (subpart 10)

Additional guidance is found in the remaining series of documents (Nos. 2–14) of the OECD GLP series, which covers aspects such as management of multisite studies [29] and responsibilities of the study director [25] and the sponsor [27].

36.4 GLP REGULATIONS AND COMPLIANCE IN THE UNITED STATES

The FDA relies on documented adherence to GLP requirements by preclinical laboratories in judging the acceptability of safety data submitted in support of research and/or marketing permits. The FDA monitors compliance with the GLP requirements through a program of regular facility inspections and targeted data audits at private, government, and public laboratories. A precedent for the current inspection program was established in December 1976 when the FDA began a pilot inspection program of representative testing programs to ascertain how well toxicology laboratories (sponsor, contract, and university facilities) were adhering to the proposed GLP regulations. The results of the inspection program were published in OPE Study 42, Results of the Nonclinical Toxicology Laboratory Good Laboratory Practices Pilot Compliance Program [36].

Laboratory compliance with GLP requirements is still monitored by the FDA through a facility inspection and data audit program according to criteria described in chapter 48 of its Compliance Program Guidance Manual [6]. The FDA conducts surveillance and directed inspections. Surveillance inspections are periodic, routine determinations of a laboratory's compliance with GLP regulations. These inspections include a facility inspection and audits of on-going and/or recently completed studies. Directed inspections are conducted to achieve a specific purpose, such as verifying the reliability, integrity, and compliance of critical safety studies being reviewed in support of pending applications or investigating issues involving potentially unreliable safety data and/or violative conditions brought to the FDA's attention. At the end of each inspection the facility is issued an Establishment Inspection Report (EIR). Inspectional observations may also be listed on a form FDA-483. Findings listed on the 483 represent inspectional observations that have not been detected and corrected by the firm through its internal procedures and are either not considered minor in nature or are more than one-time occurrences that may impact on the firm's operations, study conduct, or data integrity. All findings, regardless of reporting on the 483, are listed on the EIR and are discussed with the firm's management [6]. Depending on the nature of the findings a warning letter may or may not follow the issuance of the 483. A warning letter differs from a 483 in that the warning is issued from the FDA's district office after higher level FDA officials have concluded that the 483 and EIR findings warrant further formal notification to the firm where, the FDA believes, serious violations exist. In most cases a firm will prepare a formal reply to FDA within one to two weeks of receiving either a 483 or warning letter. The warning letter serves to prompt voluntary corrective action at the test facility or firm and to establish a history of warning(s) should further regulatory action be required at a later date (i.e., injunction or prosecution). For reviews of the history and present use of the FDA-483 as well as the procedures for firms responding to form 483 and warning letters, the reader is referred to articles by two former compliance officials [37,38]. Receipt of warning letters by GLP laboratories is relatively uncommon, whereas many larger and longstanding test laboratories have received a 483s at one time in their tenure.

The FDA Web site contains a list of the testing facilities that have been inspected since October 1, 1989 [39]. The list provides the current name and former (if known) names of the testing facility, the dates the facility has been inspected, and the classification of the inspection results. Active toxicology laboratories, university laboratories, foreign laboratories, and inactive laboratories are listed. The list is updated quarterly. The most common outcome of inspections include NAI (no action indicated), VAI (voluntary action indicated), and OAI (official action indicated). For inspections with an OAI classification, regulatory and administrative actions will be recommended. Warning letters may or may not be issued with an OAI classification.

Results of FDA inspections are available through a variety of sources. The official classification of a facility's inspection is reported on the FDA's compliance Web site [39], which contains the results from current and all previous inspections. Alternatively, many contract laboratories are quite willing to provide a regulatory inspection history for the past five years and/or the actual EIRs or 483s with their response letters to FDA upon request. Finally, the EIRs may be requested through the Freedom of Information Act (FOIA) [40]. The latter option, while a formal possibility, can be a very lengthy process. Unlike the European GLP monitoring programmes, the US FDA does not issue certificates or other documents of compliance. Warning letters are immediately available, upon issuance, on the FDA Web site [41].

36.5 GLOBAL GLP REGULATIONS AND COMPLIANCE

From a compliance perspective, Directive 2004/9/EC [33] lays down the obligation of the member states to designate the authorities responsible for GLP inspections in their territory. The Directive requires that the OECD Revised Guides for Compliance Monitoring Procedures for GLP and the OECD Guidance for the Conduct of Test Facility Inspections and Study Audits must be followed during laboratory inspections and study audits. Directive 2004/10/EC [32] requires member states to take all measures necessary to ensure that laboratories carrying out safety studies on chemical products (cosmetics, industrial chemicals, medicinal products, food additives, animal feed additives, pesticides) comply with the OECD Principles of Good Laboratory Practice.

Test facilities within the European Union are required to notify their national GLP monitoring authority as soon as they claim to conduct studies in accordance with the OECD GLP principles. All laboratories claiming GLP compliance are entered into a periodic national compliance program to monitor GLP adherence. The core of the compliance-monitoring program is a periodical inspection scheme, with an intended frequency of one inspection every two years. As circumstances require, the inspection schedule may be intensified. If a test facility is considered to operate in compliance with the OECD GLP principles, an Endorsement of Compliance will be issued, as indicated in Directive 2004/9/EC. This endorsement only states that the facility was operating in compliance at the time of the inspection. It may be used for inclusion in study reports to indicate that the test facility has been inspected for GLP compliance with good results. The endorsement of compliance also states which areas of expertise are operating in compliance with GLP provisions.

Foreign laboratories may apply for inspection by various European monitoring programs. The monitoring authorities are generally willing to accommodate such requests if (1) the facilities submit evidence that data produced by them are or will soon be submitted to the regulatory (receiving) authorities, (2) there is no recognized monitoring authority in the country, and (3) the requesting facility is willing to bear the full costs of the inspection. The GLP Web site for the European Union [34] contains information on the application of GLP Directives in the European Union by the member states including the legislative adoption or "transposition" of the GLP directives, contact information for the national authorities on GLP, and public lists of inspected test facilities.

The Japanese drug regulatory body is the Ministry of Health, Labor and Welfare (MHLW). The standards concerning the nonclinical safety testing of pharmaceuticals (good laboratory practices) have been in place since 1982 in the form of administrative instruction. Such standards have been enforced since April 1997 as ministerial ordinances. One of the Ministry's 11 bureaus, the Organization for Pharmaceutical Safety and Research (OPSR/KIKO or Drug Organization) is responsible for GLP compliance monitoring. Thus, as in the United States and Europe, pivotal safety studies must comply with good laboratory practice (GLP) standards. For those studies to which GLP applies, the preclinical testing facilities will be subject to GLP compliance inspections that occur after an application is submitted. Based on the findings of the KIKO, a facility will receive one of three ratings: (1) class A for compliance with GLP, (2) class B indicating some improvements are possible, but the effects of non-compliance on the data's reliability are not considered significant (improvements are encouraged), or (3) class C where there is noncompliance with GLP. The MHLW will accept the test results from facilities receiving a class A or B rating. Mutual acceptance of GLP inspection results and data from several countries is provided through the bilateral agreements. Japan is one of the three (tripartite) members of the International Conference on Harmonization (ICH) and a member state of the OECD. An overview of the competent authorities for GLP compliance and regulations within Japan, as well as the applicable laws, regulations, and administrative provisions stipulating the principles of GLP verification and confirmation, may be found in Sectoral Annex A of the January 1, 2002, Japan-EC Mutual Recognition Agreement [42].

36.6 COMPARISON OF FDA AND OECD GLP REGULATIONS

The FDA has published a reference table with a side-by-side comparison of OECD, 21 CFR 58 (FDA) and US EPA GLP provisions [43]. As stated throughout the chapter, the objectives of the GLP principles are similar, but the methods of implementing GLP provisions, the programs for ensuring GLP compliance, and the scope of the provisions vary considerably between regions. With respect to scope, the GLP provisions of the OECD are generally applicable to all nonclinical testing of chemicals, whereas the 21 CFR 58 regulations pertain to food and color additives, animal food additives, human and animal drugs, medical devices for human use, and biological products and electronic products (21 CFR 58.1).

Another important difference between the US FDA and OECD regulations is that the former is, in a formal sense, limited to collection of toxicological data, whereas the OECD regulations are applied to both toxicological and pharmacological data. Sponsors considering submission to non-US agencies should strongly consider collection of both data sets in compliance with relevant GLP regulations. In practice, current industry practice even in the United States is to collect both toxicological and pharmacological data in compliance with applicable aspects of the GLP regulations, such as under a protocol, with a final report, with a study director, and with some QA oversight, whenever possible.

The programs for assuring GLP compliance have already been described above in Sections 36.4 and 36.5. In summary, the European Union guided by OECD requires registration of all facilities claiming conduct of studies under GLP in a program for GLP compliance. The identified laboratories are inspected by regional authorities on a periodic basis, and they are issued certificates of endorsement that support GLP compliance in technical disciplines within the European Union. In contrast, the US FDA relies on documentation of GLP compliance by the sponsor. The FDA periodically inspects some but not all facilities claiming GLP compliance and study data thereof. The FDA does not issue certificates or other documents of compliance. Establishment inspection reports and/or FDA 483s are often available from the laboratories and are always available by request through the Freedom of Information Act.

36.7 PRAGMATIC APPROACH TO GLP COMPLIANCE

As noted earlier in the chapter, it is not always possible or feasible to conduct studies in 100% compliance with GLPs. From a regulatory perspective the sponsor is responsible for describing and justifying areas of noncompliance. Section 21 CFR 312.23(a)(8)(iii), which pertains to IND content and format states: "For each nonclinical laboratory study subject to the good laboratory practice regulation under part 58, a statement that the study was conducted in compliance with the good laboratory practice in part 58, or if the study was not conducted in compliance with the regulation, a brief statement of the reason for non-compliance." In the case of novel biopharmaceuticals or pharmaceuticals, it may not always be possible to begin the clinical development program with preclinical testing run under full GLP compliant conditions. For example, the sponsor may lack a quality assurance unit internally, or external laboratories may not have animal models suitable for conducting the primary study. Ultimately the decision on site selection for preclinical studies is based on a matrix of considerations, and rational departures from full GLP compliance may be necessary.

The lack of full GLP compliance, particularly for preclinical studies collected early in a development program, does not inhibit data from being submitted and reviewed by regulatory agencies, provided that the sponsor adequately describes and justifies areas of noncompliance. The FDA in its 1981 Question and Answer Document [14] clearly indicates that even safety supporting preclinical studies with areas of noncompliance may be acceptable provided that the quality and integrity of the study has not been impacted [14]:

Q: Does FDA reject nonclinical laboratory studies that have not been conducted in full compliance with GLPs?

A: Not necessarily. The GLP compliance program provides guidance on this issue. For FDA to reject a study it is necessary to find that there were deviations from the GLPs and that these deviations were of such a nature as to compromise the quality and integrity of the study covered by the agency inspection.

TABLE 36.1 Examples of GLP (non)compliance statements that may be included in preclinical study reports or within FDA submissions

This study will not be/was not conducted in full compliance with part 58 of 21 CFR. However, the study will be/was conducted according to the study protocol and standard operating procedures of _____. There is no formal involvement of a quality assurance unit

Currently acceptable practices of good animal husbandry will be followed, e.g., Guide for the Care and Use of Laboratory Animals: DHHS Publication No. (NRC) 86-23, revised 1996.

This study will not be conducted in full compliance with part 58 of 21 CFR. However, the study will be conducted according to the study protocol and standard operating procedures of _____. There is no formal involvement of a quality assurance unit.

Currently acceptable practices of good animal husbandry will be followed, e.g., Guide for the Care and Use of Laboratory Animals: DHHS Publication No. (NRC) 86-23, revised 1996.

This study was not performed in strict compliance with the US FDA good practice regulations (GLPs) as amended (21 CFR, part 58). GLPs were followed, except that no in-life critical phase audits were conducted. Efforts were made to operate with documented procedures, standard operating procedures, and the study protocol. No circumstances occurred during the study that might have affected the quality or integrity of the data. The raw data contained in this report were subjected to a final audit.

Source: Adapted Cavagnaro [44].

Nonetheless, a movement toward full compliance is expected during the evolution of the development program. During the interim, reports from such studies should state the reasons for noncompliance and the sponsor must justify the noncompliance within submissions to the FDA. Recently a framework for the staged application GLP provisions to preclinical testing of novel biologics has been presented in the context of gene therapy product development [44]. Sections of the presentation have been adapted to provide detailed examples of compliance statements that might be used to describe studies not conducted in full compliance with GLP provisions (Table 36.1) and to describe regulatory expectations for GLP compliance of pharmacology, biodistribution, and toxicology studies (Table 36.2). The latter table also indicates elements of the GLP provisions that can be applied such as use of a study plan, documented test methods, assignment of a single point of control, and inclusion of quality assurance oversight.

36.8 SITE SELECTION FOR PRECLINICAL STUDIES

Preclinical studies may either be conducted in house (within a sponsor's own laboratories) or outsourced to a contract laboratory or grantee. When a

TABLE 36.2 Framework for application of GLP provisions to novel biologics: Example for gene transfer research

Type of Study	Level of Compliance	Example Language or Comments
Pharmacology—in vitro or in vivo activity and/or mechanism	By convention non GLP	• Use of laboratory procedures • Novel in vitro test systems/animal models • Use of research grade vector preparation and possibly more than one lot • Limited information on product characteristics
Proof of concept—in vivo assessment of efficacy and safety in the same model	In accordance with the principles of GLP ...	• Study protocol • Animal model of disease (unvalidated) • Research grade or early GMP preparation • Limited or no quality assurance oversight
Biodistribution studies—PCR testing, etc.	In compliance with GLPs with the exception of ...	• Study protocol may be a part of the toxicology study • Methodology/standardization of assays evolving (level of sensitivity improving) • Pre-GMP test material • Laboratory procedures; draft SOPs • QA review of the final report only
Pilot toxicology studies—selection of relevant species	In compliance with GLPs with the exception of ...	• Study protocol/outline • Limited numbers; not statistically relevant • Research/representative test material not GMP/clinical • Limited stability data for test article
Pivotal toxicology studies—support route of administration, dose, regimen, patient population selection, etc.	In full compliance with GLP provisions	• Study protocol and amendments • SOPs • Test material clinical GMP or pre-validation lot • Stability and product characterization data • QA audit all phases

Source: Adapted Cavagnaro [44].

decision is made to outsource, it is critical for the sponsor to remember that GLP compliance and scientific integrity are ultimately the sponsor's responsibility. When the service of a consulting laboratory, contractor, or grantee is used, the final responsibility for the quality of the study still resides with the sponsor. It is the sponsor's obligation to notify the other party that the service is part of a preclinical laboratory study that must be conducted in compliance with GLP provisions.

Once the a decision has been taken to outsource a preclinical study, contractor selection based on quality and technical standards is a key element of successful study conduct. Generally, one begins with identification of laboratories that are capable of conducting the proposed scope of work, followed by quality audits to ensure that the test facility has can conduct the study(ies) in a GLP compliant manner. The FDA inspection Web site is often a good resource for identifying potential contractors, particularly when used in combination with referrals from industry representatives conducting similar studies. Whenever possible, the screening of contract research organizations (CROs) should go beyond business development representatives to potential study directors or operational heads to ensure that technical needs, containment requirements (BSL1-4), and/or desired animal models are accessible. To this end it is advisable to communicate as many details as possible regarding the type of test article, animal species/test system, duration of study, and so forth, to ensure that the information provided is accurate. When the list of potential contractors has been narrowed down to two or three, a more formal qualification process should be initiated. Generally, this begins with a confidentiality agreement (CDA) followed by a qualification exercise, consisting of both an offsite and onsite review of the facility's quality and technical expertise.

An example of a contractor selection plan for a preclinical study requiring GLP compliance is provided in the tables below. Tabular (checklist) type of examples are provided for:

- Activities to conduct prior to scheduling the audit (Table 36.3),
- Scheduling the audit (Table 36.4),

TABLE 36.3   Example checklist of test facility selection and inspection tools prior to scheduling audit

Activity	Complete
• Execute confidentiality agreement	
• Communicate a detailed scope of work	
• Identify one or more potential study directors	
• Identify the primary test facility and all offsite (secondary or subcontract) facilities that could be utilized[a]	
• Collect physical addresses of all potential facility areas for study	

[a]Subcontract and offsite areas must be identified at this stage.

TABLE 36.4   Example checklist of scheduling audit one to four weeks prior to visit

Activity	Complete
• Set audit schedule based on scope of work and physical sites proposed for study conduct[a]	
• Provide proposed agenda and previsit document request (below)	
• Schedule travel and communicate travel schedule to contract laboratory	

[a]Six to 8 hours for primary facility and additional time, including transportation, for offsite or satellite facilities.

TABLE 36.5   Example checklist of previsit document request two weeks prior to visit

Activity	Received
• Company prospectus; if available	
• Regulatory inspection history[a]	
• Index of Standard Operating Procedures for relevant functional areas	
• Organizational Diagram for relevant functional areas	
• CV of proposed study director(s) and principle investigator(s)	
• Test item receipt instructions and example intake form	
• SOP(s) for protocol deviation and amendments	
• SOP(s) for in-phase study inspections	

[a]EU GLP compliance certificate or US inspection history with most recent Establishment Inspection Report.

- Previsit document requests (Table 36.5),
- Audit agenda (Table 36.6)
- Structure of an audit report (Table 36.7)

Issues that are of particular relevance for biopharmaceuticals include the following:

- Time constraints imposed by transport of test material to the test site that may involve permits from either the CDC or USDA, or other national requirements when test material or the contract laboratory is located outside of the United States.
- Identification of appropriate test article receipt and storage conditions at the test facility with consideration of any required facility departures from conventional procedures for test material receipt, handling, and storage.
- Review of standard facility procedures for test material preparation for dosing and/or delivery. Test materials for biopharmaceuticals tend to be very limited in quantity and handled in much smaller quantities than that used for pharmaceuticals. Many test facilities are not used to handling

TABLE 36.6 Example checklist of audit agenda one week prior to visit

Activity	Time Frame
Opening meeting/introductions	5–10 minutes
Suggested attendees: proposed study director, QA representative, client services representative, management representative	
Sponsor overview and proposed scope of work	15 minutes
Brief contractor overview of company and services	15 minutes
	15 minutes
Discussion of GLP inspection history; compliance issues	2–4 hours
Facility tour and document request during tour	
• Test and control article receipt/storage/archival/distribution • Test article formulation • Test article analysis • Animal husbandry support areas • Animal husbandry and treatment areas • Necropsy • Clinical pathology • Histopathology • Other relevant laboratory areas • Computer systems/backup • Document archival • Tissue and slide archival	
	1–1.5 hour
Record review	
Training records, environmental records, AAALAC or equivalent certification, feed and water monitoring data, animal health records, etc.	
Review assay validation(s) or qualifications, as needed.	
Review procedures for project management within the contract facility	
SOPs	1–1.5 hour
Close out	15–30 minutes

small volumes and do not routinely use the disposable and small quantity equipment (e.g., micropipets, plasticware) that are second nature in cell and molecular biology laboratories.

• Availability of stability data to support the operational conditions that will need to be used by the contract test facility to execute the sponsor's proposed activities. The test facility may require several hours or days to dose a series of treatment groups. Often times vaccines may only be stable

TABLE 36.7   Example of the structure of an audit report

- Logistical details
Date of visit, sponsor and contractor participants with contact information, addresses of all facilities visited
- Overview of findings (critical, major, minor)
- Facilit(ies) description
- GLP inspection information
- Detailed narrative of functional areas reviewed and all findings (critical, major, minor) with classification rationale within relevant narrative
- List of SOPs reviewed with comments as needed
- List of non-SOP documents with comments as needed
- Signature page for auditor(s) and date of finalization of report

Optional

- Recommendations for corrective and preventative actions
- Space for contractor responses to be included in body of report

at room temperature for several hours. This information needs to be communicated early to the test facility such that appropriate adjustments to test material handling can be considered and incorporated into the protocol or supporting study specific documents.

The purpose of the qualification/audit is for the sponsor to investigate the standard practices of the contractor. Quality as well as technical capabilities should be evaluated. One should determine where the test article will actually be stored, the department that will conduct the in-life portion, make an assessment of procedures (SOPs) for dosing, identify differences between the sponsor's general practices and the facilities operating procedures (protocol/study-specific procedures (SSPs), and assess the process of interim data exchange and the method of reporting of SOP and protocol deviations to the study director and the sponsor.

Protocol development begins the formal process of establishing study details. Study-specific procedures may be used to append important technical details specified by the sponsor. Most contractors will hold a prestudy initiation meeting, which is an opportunity for the sponsor to meet study staff via teleconference and to provide to critical study staff an overview of the study objectives, last minute details on special handling, and so forth. Study monitoring, particularly of the first day of dosing and at critical necropsy time points, can be very valuable for ensuring appropriate study conduct and in establishing a sponsor's quality and technical expectations. As the data become available, technical and quality review of raw data, including querying any delays in reporting and/or any discrepancies with data in real time, often saves considerable time during the reporting stage.

36.9   CONCLUSIONS

Conduct of preclinical testing in compliance with GLP regulations has become an established part of clinical development. US and global regulatory agencies require that sponsors describe and justify all areas of noncompliance for safety (United States/Europe/Japan) and pharmacological (Europe) supporting studies. For novel biopharmaceuticals and pharmaceuticals it is not always possible to achieve 100% GLP compliance due to the technical requirements and/or unique animal models that may be used to assess safety. Limited resources early in product development particularly impact adherence to GLP compliance. As a product progresses in development, the regulatory expectation is that the GLP knowledge of the sponsor and full compliance of the studies will also evolve. The chapter provides a starting point for US and global GLP compliance and a pragmatic approach to contractor selection for studies intended for full or partial GLP compliance.

In conclusion, the GLP provisions are a regulatory tool to ensure the integrity and quality of the preclinical study data submitted in support of a product's safety for use in humans. GLP regulations pertain to preclinical safety testing within the United States (21 CFR 58) and to both safety and efficacy (pharmacological) testing globally (OECD GLP provisions). Compliance with GLP principles is ultimately the responsibility of the sponsor of the research or marketing application, regardless of the laboratory (in house, contractor, or grantee) that performs the studies for a given product. GLP compliance itself should not be interpreted as inferring scientific competency or a facility's compliance with other regulatory standards. From this perspective the GLP provisions are only one facet of the regulatory expectation for preclinical testing. Other standards include, but are not limited to, 9 CFR test parameters: virus safety testing [45], ICH guidances for analytical methods and safety testing [46], relevant FDA guidance for Industry [47], standards for animal care and use [48], and import/export permits for the test materials from CDC [49] and USDA [50]. Finally, guidance from the World Health Organization on GLP regulations may also be considered, particularly for global development of novel biopharmaceuticals [51].

REFERENCES

1. United States National Archives and Records Administration1. www.gpoaccess. gov/cfr/index.html

2. US EPA. Toxic Substances Control, Good Laboratory Practice standards, Code of Federal Regulations, Title 40, Part 792, effective December 29, 1983. http://www. epa.gov/compliance/monitoring/programs/fifra/glp.html

3. US EPA. Pesticide Programs, Good Laboratory Practice Standards, Code of Federal Regulations, Title 40, Part 160, effective May 2, 1984. http://www.epa.gov/ compliance/monitoring/programs/fifra/glp.html

4. US Department of Health and Human Services, Centers for Disease Control and Prevention, and National Institutes of Health. *Biosafety in Microbiological and Biomedical Laboratories (BMBL)*, 4th ed. Washington: US Government Printing Office, 1999. http://www.cdc.gov/OD/OHS/biosfty/bmbl4/bmbl4toc.htm

5. Marshall E. The murky world of toxicity testing. *Science* 1983;220:1130–2.

6. US FDA. Compliance Program Guidance Manual, Program 7348.808, Chapter 48, Bioresearch Monitoring, Good Laboratory Practice, Completion Date 09/03/93. http://www.fda.gov/ora/compliance_ref/bimo/7348_808/48-808.pdf

7. Anderson MA. *GLP Quality Audit Manual*, 3rd ed, Boca Raton: CRC Press, 2000.

8. RAPS. Chapter 18. Good Laboratory Practices and Good Clinical Practices. In *2005 Fundamentals of US Regulatory Affairs*. Rockville: Regulatory Affairs Professional Society, 2005.

9. US FDA. Good Laboratory Practice (GLP) Regulations, Proposed Rule. Federal Register, November 19, 1976. Vol. 41:51206–51230. http://www.fda.gov/ora/compliance_ref/bimo/GLP/76proposedrule.pdf

10. US FDA. Good Laboratory Practice (GLP) Regulations, Final Rule. Federal Register, December 22, 1978. Vol. 43:59985–60025. http://www.fda.gov/ora/compliance_ref/bimo/GLP/78fr-glpfinalrule.pdf

11. US FDA. Good Laboratory Practice (GLP) Regulations, Proposed Rule. Federal Register. October 29, 1984. Vol. 49:43530–43537. http://www.fda.gov/ora/compliance_ref/bimo/GLP/84proposedrule.pdf

12. US FDA. Good Laboratory Practice (GLP) Regulations (Amendment), Final Rule. Federal Register. September 4, 1987. Vol. 52:33768–33782. http://www.fda.gov/ora/compliance_ref/bimo/GLP/87fr-glpamendment.pdf

13. US FDA. Guidance for Industry. Good Laboratory Practice Regulations Management Briefings. Post Conference Report. August 1979 (Minor editorial and formatting changes made November 1998). http://www.fda.gov/ora/compliance_ref/bimo/q_as.htm

14. US FDA. Good Laboratory Practice Regulations, Questions and Answers. June 1981 (Minor editorial and formatting changes made December 1999, September 2000). http://www.fda.gov/ora/compliance_ref/bimo/GLP/qna.htm

15. US FDA ORA/FDA/ORA Bioresearch Monitoring Information Page (general) http://www.fda.gov/ora/compliance_ref/bimo/default.htm.

16. GLP Web site of the OECD. http://www.oecd.org/department/0,2688,en_2649_34381_1_1_1_1,00.html

17. OECD. No. 1: Principles on Good Laboratory Practice, revised 1997. http://www.olis.oecd.org/olis/1998doc.nsf/LinkTo/env-mc-chem(98)17

18. OECD. No. 2: Revised Guides for Compliance Monitoring Procedures for Good Laboratory Practice. http://www.olis.oecd.org/olis/1995doc.nsf/LinkTo/ocde-gd(95)66

19. OECD. No. 3: Revised Guidance for the Conduct of Laboratory Inspections and Study Audit. http://www.olis.oecd.org/olis/1995doc.nsf/LinkTo/ocde-gd(95)67

20. OECD. No. 9: Guidance for the Preparation of GLP Inspection Reports. http://www.olis.oecd.org/olis/1995doc.nsf/LinkTo/ocde-gd(95)114

21. OECD. No. 4: Quality Assurance and GLP, revised 1999. http://www.olis.oecd.org/olis/1999doc.nsf/LinkTo/env-jm-mono(99)20

22. OECD. No. 5: Compliance of Laboratory Suppliers with GLP Principles, revised 1999. http://www.olis.oecd.org/olis/1999doc.nsf/LinkTo/env-jm-mono(99)21

23. OECD. No. 6: The Application of the GLP Principles to Field Studies, revised 1999. http://www.olis.oecd.org/olis/1999doc.nsf/LinkTo/env-jm-mono(99)23

24. OECD. No. 7: The Application of the GLP Principles to Short&Term Studies, revised 1999. http://www.olis.oecd.org/olis/1999doc.nsf/LinkTo/env-jm-mono(99)24

25. OECD. No. 8: The Role and Responsibilties of the Study Director in GLP Studies, revised 1999. http://www.olis.oecd.org/olis/1995doc.nsf/LinkTo/ocde-gd(95)115

26. OECD. No. 10: The Application of the Principles of GLP to Computerised Systems, 1995. http://www.olis.oecd.org/olis/1995doc.nsf/LinkTo/ocde-gd(95)115

27. OECD. No. 11: The Role and Responsibility of the Sponsor in the Application of the Principles of GLP. http://www.olis.oecd.org/olis/1998doc.nsf/LinkTo/env-mc-chem(98)16

28. OECD. No. 12: Requesting and Carrying Out Inspections and Study Audits in Another Country. http://www.olis.oecd.org/olis/2000doc.nsf/LinkTo/env-jm-mono(2000)3

29. OECD. No. 13: The Application of the OECD Principles of GLP to the Organisation and Management of Multi-site Studies. http://www.olis.oecd.org/olis/2002doc.nsf/LinkTo/env-jm-mono(2002)9

30. OECD. No. 14: The Application of the Principles of GLP to In vitro Studies. http://appli1.oecd.org/olis/2004doc.nsf/linkto/env-jm-mono(2004)26

31. Directive 2003/63/EC. Commission Directive 2003/63/EC of 25 June 2003 Amending Directive 2001/83/EC of the European Parliament and of the Council on the Community Code Relating to Medicinal Products for Human Use. http://europa.eu.int/eur-lex/lex/LexUriServ/LexUriServ.do?uri=CELEX:32003L0063:EN:HTML

32. Directive 2004/10/EC of the European Parliament and of the Council of 11 February 2004 on the Harmonization of Laws, Regulations and Administrative Provisions Relating to the Application of the Principles of Good Laboratory Practice and the Verification of Their Applications for Tests on Chemical Substances. http://ec.europa.eu/enterprise/chemicals/legislation/glp/directives_en.htm

33. Directive 2004/9/EC of the European Parliament and of the Council of 11 February 2004 on the Inspection and Verification of Good Laboratory Practice (GLP). http://ec.europa.eu/enterprise/chemicals/legislation/glp/directives_en.htm

34. GLP Web site of the European Commission. http://ec.europa.eu/enterprise/chemicals/legislation/glp/index_en.htm

35. US FDA. International cooperative agreements. http://www.fda.gov/oia/

36. US FDA. OPE Study 42. Results of the Nonclinical Toxicology Laboratory Good Laboratory Practices Pilot Compliance Program. September 1977.

37. Chesney DL. The FDA-483: its history and present use. *BioPharm* 1996;9(4):30–2.

38. Chesney DL, Kelly AE. Responding to FDA-483's and warning letters. *BioPharm* 1998;11(10):26–9. http://www.ispe.org/page.ww?section=Technical+Articles&name=Responding+to+483's+and+Warning+Letters

39. US FDA. ORA/FDA/ORA Bioresearch Monitoring Information Page (GLP specific). http://www.fda.gov/ora/compliance_ref/bimo/glp/default.htm

40. US FDA. Freedom of Information Requests. http://www.fda.gov/opacom/backgrounders/foiahand.html

41. US FDA. Warning Letters. http://www.fda.gov/foi/warning.htm

42. Japan. EU–Japan Mutual Recognition Agreement, 1 January 2002. Sectoral Annex on Good Laboratory Practice (GLP) for Chemicals. http://www.mofa.go.jp/region/europe/eu/agreement-glp.pdf

43. US FDA. Comparison Chart of FDA, Environmental Protection Agency (EPA) and Organization for Economic Co-Operation and Development (OECD) Good Laboratory Practices, June 2004. http://www.fda.gov/ora/compliance_ref/bimo/comparison_chart/

44. Cavagnaro J. Regulatory oversight of gene transfer products: good science and good sense. Session II: Preclinical Development of Gene Therapy Vectors from Petri Dish to Patient. Presentation 5th Annual American Society of Gene Therapy Meeting, Boston, MA.

45. 9 CFR 113 APHIS regulations. http://www.access.gpo.gov/nara/cfr/waisidx_04/9cfr113_04.html

46. International Conference for Harmonization (ICH) Quality and Safety Guidelines. http://www.ich.org/cache/compo/276-254-1.html

47. CBER Guidances/Guidelines/Points to Consider. http://www.fda.gov/cber/guidelines.htm

48. Institute of Laboratory Animal Research, Commission on Life Sciences, National Research Council. Guide for Care and Use of Laboratory Animals, NIH Publication No. 85-23, revised 1985.

49. Centers for Disease Control and Prevention. Etiologic Agent Import Program. http://www.cdc.gov/od/eaipp/

50. USDA Animal and Plant Health Inspection Service. Import and Export regulations and instructions. http://permanent.access.gpo.gov/lps3025/index-33.htm

51. WHO Handbook for Good Laboratory Practice (GLP): Quality Practices for Regulated Non-clinical Research and Development. http://www.who.int/tdr/publications/publications/pdf/glp-handbook.pdf

CHAPTER 37

Preclinical Safety Study Design Templates and Estimated Costs

GARY W. WOLFE, PhD, DABT

Contents

Preclinical Safety Evaluation of Biopharmaceuticals: A Science-Based Approach to Facilitating Clinical Trials, edited by Joy A. Cavagnaro
Copyright © 2008 by John Wiley & Sons, Inc.

37.1   INTRODUCTION

Preclinical studies are conducted to support the use of the test article in humans in the clinic. The preclinical studies are designed to identify target organs, and biomarkers and to set starting dose levels, recommend dose-escalation schemes and target organs of toxicity. In designing the preclinical study it is important to design the study to answer specific questions concerning the test article while maximizing the use of the animals. An example would be in the dose range studies to design studies using a minimum number of animals to answer the question "What is the toxicity following a single dose in that species and what doses should be used in acute and repeat dose studies in the rodent?" Studies to support safety should comply with GLPs possibly except for some of the initial single dose studies. It is also important to have the pre-clinical plan with preclinical study designs reviewed by the regulatory agencies as part of a pre-IND of IND process.

One important aspect in the conduct of the preclinical studies is the iden-tification of a qualified contract research organization (CRO) when studies are not performed internally. These CROs may be identified via the internet websites, literature from national and local toxicology meetings, and regula-tory documents such as 483's. In addition to checking references with col-leagues, the CRO should be visited and procedures, facilities, staff, and previous experience should be evaluated before entrusting your preclinical program with the CRO (see Chapter 39).

Study designs are provided for the following study types:

Dose escalation studies in rodent and nonrodent   These studies are gener-ally the first time the test article is administered to a living system. They provide an initial indication of toxicity, organs involved, and doses that can be used in longer term studies. Many times these studies are not conducted in full compliance with GLPs.

Acute toxicology studies in rodent and nonrodent   These studies are used to identify doses causing no adverse effects and doses causing significant life-threatening effects. In addition to toxicity these studies frequently include toxicokinetics to identify the disposition of the test article in the rodent and nonrodent. These studies also provide additional support for the dose levels to be used in longer term studies.

Four-week toxicology studies in rodent and nonrodent   The four-week studies are designed for subchronic exposure of rodents and nonrodents to the test article. These studies also look at reversibility of any toxicity observed. Many times these are the pivotal studies used to support the first in human dosing. Toxicokinetic assessments are generally included in repeat-dose toxicity studies. When testing biopharmaceuticals, stud-ies also include assessment and characterization of immune response (immunogenicity).

Three-month toxicology studies in rodent and nonrodent   These studies have a similar design to the four-week studies but support repeated human dosing up to three months.

Six or nine-month toxicology study in rodent and nonrodent   These studies have a similar design to the 4- and 13-week studies but support chronic repeated human dosing beyond 6 months.

Carcinogenicity study in mice and rats   These studies are designed to iden-tify a tumorigenic potential and to assess the relevant risk in humans. These studies are conducted for pharmaceuticals that are generally administered over the life of a human and are generally not conducted for biopharmaceuticals (see Chapters 19 and 27).

Immunotoxicity studies in rats and nonhuman primates   Immunotoxicity of pharmaceuticals and biopharmaceuticals includes hematology, organ weights, and pathology of immune-sensitive organs from the repeat-dose studies (4- and 13-week studies). For biopharmaceuticals these tests may need to be extended to T cell dependent antibody responses, imunophenotyping, natural killer cell assays, host resistance studies, and macrophage/neutrophil function. A potential design for a natural killer cell assay is presented in these designs.

Vaccine study in rabbits   Vaccines are evaluated in rabbits following the dosage regimen that is intended for humans. In many cases these studies include the same dose as is used in humans. In cases where achieving a full human dose cannot be assessed in rodents, nonrodents are needed in particular to determine the local reactogenicity of a full human dose (Draize Score).

Biodistribution study in rats for plasmids, cellular and gene therapies   Biodistribution and in many cases integration, depending on the type of vaccine, are evaluated in rats following single or multiple doses using qPCR. In many cases these studies can be combined with repeat-dose studies.

Reproduction studies in rats and rabbits   Reproductive effects are evaluated on the gametes, in the developing organism (teratology), and in the progeny. These studies are generally conducted for all pharmaceuticals, but on a case-by-case basis for biopharmaceuticals.

Safety pharmacology studies in rodent and nonrodent   These studies are designed to identify undesirable pharmacological effects in several systems primarily the cardiovascular, respiratory, and CNS systems. Other studies may be included based on the pharmacological activity of the test article. In many cases these studies are not required for biopharmaceuticals and/or may be included in the 4- and 13-week studies and 6- and 9-month studies.

Genetic toxicology studies   These studies designed to identify potential point mutations, and/or clastogenic damage/chromosomal alterations are required for pharmaceuticals but generally not required for biopharmaceuticals, since they are not applicable for proteins.

Tissue cross-reactivity (TCR) studies   Tissue cross-reactivity studies with human tissues (or cells if applicable) are conducted prior to Phase 1 to search for cross-reactions with the intended target and/or nontarget tissue. In special cases of bispecific antibodies, each parent antibody is evaluated individually in addition to testing the bispecific product. Human cells or tissues are surveyed immunocytochemically or immunohistochemically with appropriate controls. Animal species are also surveyed to determine relevant species for toxicology studies.

Cost estimates Cost estimates are provided for planning and budgetary purposes, and they vary widely based on a number of factors with each individual CRO. The estimates are based generally on average prices for the study designs presented; but the final price may vary for specific circumstances:

- Final design. Numbers of animals, blood collection intervals and time points, clinical pathology intervals, and tissues examined.
- Special study requests. CTD tables, additional QA inspections, peer review, or accelerated report submission.
- Percentage of each study conducted in house. Cost increases due to specialty sections (e.g., pathology, clinical pathology) being subcontracted by the CRO.
- Discounted individual studies. A program having a large number of studies.
- Unutilized capacity of CRO. Price decreases to fill CRO's available space.
- Flexibility in initiation and reporting. Proper planning tends to decrease the CRO's costs.

In summary, a well-designed preclinical program that addresses questions of toxicity conducted internally or at a well-qualified CRO is necessary for a satisfactory preclinical safety evaluation program to support successful clinical development.

37.2 STUDY OUTLINES AND COST ESTIMATES

37.2.1 Dose Escalation Study in Rodents

Purpose	What is the toxicity following a single dose to the nonrodent?
	What doses should be used in acute and repeat dose studies in the rodent?
Timeline initiation report	4 to 6 weeks following authorization
	4 to 8 weeks following termination
Estimated cost	$15,000 to $35,000
Regulatory guidelines and compliance	No specific guidelines and FDA GLP optional
Total animals	36 (18/sex) rats (or mice)
Number/sex/group	2 rats/sex/group with 4 groups in dose escalation phase
	5 rats/sex/group with 2 groups in MTD phase

Dosing route	Generally a parenteral route (IV, IM, or sc) for biopharmaceuticals
	Oral route usually for pharmaceuticals
Dosing frequency	Day 1 and every 72 hours thereafter 2 animals/sex dosed for a total of 4 escalating doses to determine MTD
	5 rats/sex/group dosed with the vehicle and at the MTD either as a single dose or multiple doses up to 14 days
Formulations	Usually biopharmaceuticals dosed as received if clinical formulation is available
	Pharmaceuticals formulated by the CRO and require formulation analysis for concentration, homogeneity, and stability
Clinical signs	Twice daily
Clinical observations	0.5, 1, and 2 hours after each dose and daily in the MTD phase
Body weights	Before and after each dose in the dose escalation phase and prior to initiation, weekly, and at termination in the MTD phase
Food consumption	Weekly in the MTD phase
Clinical pathology (optional)	Not required
Terminal necropsy	2–3 days after dosing in the dose escalation phase
	14 days after dosing in the MTD phase
Organ weights (optional)	See Appendix C
Tissue preservation (optional)	See Appendix D
Histopathology (optional)	MTD groups gross lesions only or all tissues
Report	One copy of the draft final report
	One bound and unbound copy of the final and an electronic copy in Word and PDF
Archive	Yes for at least 1 year at CRO

37.2.2 Dose Escalation Study in Nonrodents

Purpose	What is the toxicity following a single dose to the nonrodent?
	What doses should be used in acute and repeat-dose studies in the nonrodent?

Timeline	
initiation	4 to 8 weeks following authorization
report	4 to 8 weeks following termination
Estimated cost	$50,000 to $75,000
Regulatory guidelines and compliance:	No specific guidelines and FDA GLP optional
Total Animals	12 monkeys or dogs (6/sex)
Number/sex/group	2 monkeys or dogs/dose with up to 4 doses/animal
	2 monkeys or dogs/group with 2 groups in MTD phase
Dosing route	Generally a parenteral route (IV, IM, or sc) for biopharmaceuticals
	Oral route usually for pharmaceuticals
Dosing frequency	Day 1 and every 72 hours thereafter the same 2 animals/sex dosed for up to 3 escalating doses to determine MTD
	2 animals/sex/group dosed with vehicle and at the MTD either as a single dose or multiple doses up to 14 days
Formulations	Usually biopharmaceuticals dosed as received if clinical formulation is available
	Pharmaceuticals are formulated by the CRO and require formulation analysis for concentration, homogeneity, and stability
Clinical signs	Twice daily
Clinical observations	0.5, 1, and 2 hours after each dose each dose and daily in the MTD phase
Body weights	Before and after each dose in the dose escalation phase and prior to initiation, weekly, and at termination in the MTD phase
Food consumption	Weekly in the MTD phase
Clinical pathology (optional)	Not required
Terminal necropsy	2 to 3 days after dosing in the dose escalation phase
	14 days after dosing in the MTD phase
Organ weights (optional)	See Appendix C
Tissue preservation (optional)	See Appendix D
Histopathology (optional)	MTD groups gross lesions only or all tissues
Report	One copy of the draft final report
	One bound and unbound copy of the final and an electronic copy in Word and PDF
Archive	Yes for at least 1 year at CRO

37.2.3   Acute Toxicology Study in Rodents

Purpose	What are the toxicities and toxicokinetics of a test article after a single dose?
	What doses should be used in acute and repeat dose studies in the rodent?
Timeline	
initiation	4 to 6 weeks following authorization
report	6 to 10 weeks following termination
Estimated cost	$20,000 to $40,000
Regulatory guidance and compliance	Single–dose acute toxicity testing for pharmaceuticals (August 1996) and FDA GLP
Total Animals	40 without toxicokinetics
	76 with toxicokinetics
Number/sex/group—Main	5/sex/group in groups 1–4 rats (or mice)
Number/sex/group—TK (optional)	6/sex/group in groups 2–4 (assumes <1 ml of blood/rat/time point and <0.1 ml of blood/mouse/time pont)
	Additional volumes will require additional animals
Dosing route frequency	Generally a parenteral route (IV, IM, or sc) for biopharmaceuticals
	Oral route for pharmaceuticals
Dosing frequency	Single dose at 4 dose levels (control, low, mid, and high dose)
Formulations	Usually biopharmaceuticals dosed as received if clinical formulation is available
	Pharmaceuticals are formulated by the CRO and require formulation analysis for concentration, homogeneity, and stability
Clinical signs	Twice daily
Clinical observations	Weekly
Body weights	Weekly and prior to necropsy
Food consumption	Weekly
Toxicokinetics	Day 1 TK animals are bled at 6 time points (3/sex/group) after dosing
Antibodies (for biopharmaceuticals only)	Prior to study initiation and at termination
Clinical pathology (optional)	Day 14
Hematology	See Appendix B
Clinical chemistry	See Appendix B
Coagulation	See Appendix B
Urinalysis	See Appendix B
Terminal necropsy	Day 14—full necropsy

Organ weights (optional)	See Appendix C
Bone marrow smears	Yes from sternum
Tissue preservation	See Appendix D
Histopathology (optional)	Groups 1 and 4 all tissues
	Groups 2 and 3—target tissues and gross lesions
Report	One copy of the draft final report
	One bound and unbound copy of the final and an electronic copy in Word and PDF
Archive	Yes for at least 1 year at CRO

37.2.4 Acute Toxicology Study in Nonrodents

Purpose	What are the toxicities and toxicokinetics of a test article after a single dose when administered to monkeys or dogs?
	What doses should be used in acute and repeat-dose studies in the nonrodent?
Timeline	
initiation	4 to 8 weeks following authorization
report	6 to 10 weeks following termination
Estimated cost	$100,000 to $120,000 (dogs)
	$150,000 to $200,000 (monkeys, IV bolus)
	$175,000 to $225,000 (monkey 4-hour infusion)
Regulatory guidelines and compliance	Single–dose acute toxicity testing for pharmaceuticals (August 1996) FDA GLP
Total animals	16 monkeys or dogs
Number/sex/group	2 monkeys or dogs/sex/group
Dosing route	Generally a parenteral route (IV, IM, or sc) for biopharmaceuticals
	Oral route for pharmaceuticals
Dosing frequency	Single dose at 4 dose levels (control, low, mid, and highdose)
Formulations	Usually biopharmaceuticals dosed as received if clinical formulation is available
	Pharmaceuticals are formulated by the CRO and require formulation analysis for concentration, homogeneity, and stability
Clinical signs	Twice daily
Clinical observations	Twice daily
Body weights	Weekly and prior to necropsy
Food consumption	Daily
Toxicokinetics	Day 1 TK animals are bled at 6 time points after dosing

Antibodies (for biopharmaceuticals only)	Prior to study initiation, and on day 14
Clinical pathology (optional)	Day 14
Hematology	See Appendix B
Clinical chemistry	See Appendix B
Coagulation	See Appendix B
Urinalysis	See Appendix B
Terminal necropsy	Day 14—full necropsy
Organ weights (optional)	See Appendix C
Tissue preservation (optional)	See Appendix D
Histopathology (optional)	Groups 1 and 4 all tissues
	Groups 2 and 3—target tissues and gross lesions
	Recommended—All tissues in all groups
Report	One copy of the draft final report
	One bound and unbound copy of the final and an electronic copy in Word and PDF
Archive	Yes for at least 1 year at CRO

37.2.5 Four-Week Toxicology Study in Rodents

Purpose	What are the subchronic toxicities and toxicokinetics of a test article when administered for 4 weeks?
	What is the reversibility, persistence, or delayed occurrence of any effect after a 4-week treatment-free period?
Timeline	
initiation	4 to 8 weeks following authorization
report	10 to 12 weeks following termination
Estimated price	$200,000 to $250,000
Regulatory compliance	FDA GLP
Total animals	88 male and 88 female rats (or mice)
Number/sex/group—Main	15/sex/group in groups 1–4
Number/sex/group—Recovery	5/sex/group in groups 1 and 4
Number/sex/group—TK	6/sex/group in groups 2–4 (assumes <1 ml of blood/rat/timepoint and <0.1 ml of blood/ mouse/time pont)
	Additional volumes will require additional animals
Dosing route	Generally a parenteral route (IV, IM, or sc) for biopharmaceuticals
	Oral route for pharmaceuticals

Dosing frequency	Dosed daily for 4 weeks for pharmaceuticals, but for biopharmaceuticals frequency based on TK data or proposed clinical regimen
Formulations	Usually biopharmaceuticals dosed as received if clinical formulation is available
	Pharmaceuticals are formulated by the CRO and require formulation analysis for concentration, homogeneity, and stability
Clinical signs	Twice daily
Clinical observations	Weekly
Body weights	Weekly and prior to necropsy
Food consumption	Weekly
Ophthalmology	Prior to initiation and during weeks 4, and 8
Toxicokinetics—optional if conducted in an earlier study	Days 1 and 28 TK animals (3/sex/group) are bled at 6 time points after dosing
Antibodies (for biopharmaceuticals only)	Prior to study initiation, and weeks 4 and 8
Neutralizing antibodies (for biopharmaceuticals only)	Prior to study initiation, and weeks 4 and 8
Clinical pathology	During weeks 4 ad 8
Hematology	See Appendix B
Clinical chemistry	See Appendix B
Coagulation	See Appendix B
Urinalysis	See Appendix B
Terminal necropsy	Week 4—full necropsy in 15/sex/group in groups 1–4
Recovery necropsy	Week 8—full necropsy in 5/sex/group in groups 1 and 4
Organ weights	See Appendix C
Bone marrow smears	Yes from sternum
Tissue preservation	See Appendix D
Histopathology	Groups 1 and 4 all tissues (terminal and recovery)
	Groups 2 and 3, and recovery—target tissues and gross lesions
Report	One copy of the draft final report
	One bound and unbound copy of the final and an electronic copy in Word and PDF
Archive	Yes for at least 1 year at CRO

37.2.6 Four-Week Toxicology Study in Nonrodents

Purpose	What are the subchronic toxicities and toxicokinetics of a test article when administered to monkeys/dogs for 4 weeks?
	What is the reversibility, persistence, or delayed occurrence of any effect after a 4-week treatment-free period?
Timeline	
initiation	6 to 8 weeks following authorization
report	10 to 12 weeks following termination
Estimated cost	$400,000 to $450,000 (dogs)
	$500,00 to $550,000 (monkey IV bolus)
	$550,00 to $650,000 (monkey 4-hour infusion)
Regulatory guidelines	FDA GLP
Total animals	32 monkeys or 40 dogs
Number/sex/group—main	3 monkeys or 4 dogs/sex/group in groups 1–4
Number/sex/group—recovery	2/sex/group in groups 1–4
Dosing route	Generally a parenteral route (IV, IM, or sc) for biopharmaceuticals
	Oral route for pharmaceuticals
Dosing frequency	Dosed daily for pharmaceuticals but for biopharmaceuticals frequency based on TK data or proposed clinical regimen
Formulations	Usually biopharmaceuticals dosed as received if clinical formulation is available.
	Pharmaceuticals are formulated by the CRO and require formulation analysis for concentration, homogeneity, and stability
Clinical signs	Twice daily
Clinical observations	Weekly
Body weights	Weekly and prior to necropsy
Food consumption	Weekly
Ophthalmology	Prior to initiation and during weeks 4 and 8
Toxicokinetics—optional if conducted in earlier studies	Day 1, and at termination, animals are bled at least at 6 time points after dosing
Antibodies (for biopharmaceuticals only)	Prior to study initiation, and weeks 4 and 8
Neutralizing antibodies (for biopharmaceuticals only)	Prior to study initiation, and weeks 4, and 8

Clinical pathology	Prior to study initiation
	During weeks 4 and 8 in all surviving animals
Hematology	See Appendix B
Clinical chemistry	See Appendix B
Coagulation	See Appendix B
Urinalysis	See Appendix B
Terminal necropsy	Week 4—full necropsy in all main study animals
Recovery necropsy	Week 8—full necropsy in recovery animals
Organ weights	See Appendix C
Bone marrow smears	Yes from sternum
Tissue preservation	See Appendix D
Histopathology	Groups 1 and 4 all tissues Groups 2 and 3—target tissues and gross lesions
	Recommended—all tissues in all groups
Report	One copy of the draft final report
	One bound and unbound copy of the final and an electronic copy in Word and PDF
Archive	Yes for at least 1 year at CRO

37.2.7 Three-Month Toxicology Study in Rodents

Purpose	What are the subchronic toxicities and toxicokinetics of a test article when administered to rats for 3 months?
	What is the reversibility, persistence, or delayed occurrence of any effect after the 3-month period?
Timeline	
initiation	6 to 8 weeks following authorization
report	10 to 12 weeks following termination
Estimated cost	$250,000 to $300,000
Regulatory compliance	FDA GLP
Total animals	176
Number/sex/group—main	15/sex/group in groups 1–4 rats (or mice)
Number/sex/group—recovery	5/sex/group in groups 1 and 4
Number/sex/group—TK	6/sex/group in groups 2–4 (assumes <1 ml of blood/rat/timepoint and <0.1 ml of blood/mouse/time point)
	Additional volumes will require additional animals
Dosing route	Generally a parenteral route (IV, IM, or sc) for biopharmaceuticals
	Oral route for pharmaceuticals

Dosing frequency	Dosed daily for 13 weeks for pharmaceuticals but for biopharmaceuticals frequency based on TK data or proposed clinical regimen
Formulations	Usually biopharmaceuticals dosed as received if clinical formulation is available
	Pharmaceuticals are formulated by the CRO and require formulation analysis for concentration, homogeneity, and stability.
Clinical signs	Twice daily
Clinical observations	Weekly
Body weights	Weekly and prior to necropsy
Food consumption	Weekly
Ophthalmology	Prior to initiation, and during weeks 13 and 17
Toxicokinetics—optional if conducted in a previous study	Days 1 and 90 TK animals (3/sex/group) bled at 6 time points after dosing
Antibodies (for biopharmaceuticals only)	Prior to study initiation, and weeks 4, 13, and 17
Neutralizing antibodies (for biopharmaceuticals only)	Prior to study initiation, and weeks 4, 13, and 17
Clinical pathology	During weeks 13 and 17 in all main study animals
Hematology	See Appendix B
Clinical chemistry	See Appendix B
Coagulation	See Appendix B
Urinalysis	See Appendix B
Terminal necropsy	Week 13—full necropsy in 15/sex/group in groups 1–4
Recovery necropsy	Week 17—full necropsy in 5/sex/group in groups 1 and 4
Organ weights	See Appendix C
Bone marrow smears	Yes from sternum
Tissue preservation	See Appendix D
Histopathology	Groups 1 and 4 all tissues (main and recovery)
	Groups 2 and 3, and recovery—target tissues and gross lesions
Report	One copy of the draft final report
	One bound and unbound copy of the final and an electronic copy in Word and PDF
Archive	Yes for at least 1 year at CRO

37.2.8 Three-Month Toxicology Study in Nonrodents

Purpose	What are the subchronic toxicities and toxicokinetics of a test article when administered to monkeys or dogs for 3 months?
	What is the reversibility, persistence, or delayed occurrence of any effect after the 3-month period?
Timeline	
initiation	4 to 8 weeks following authorization
report	10 to 12 weeks following termination
Estimated cost	$450,000 to $500,000
Regulatory compliance	FDA GLP
Total animals	32 monkeys or 40 dogs
Number/sex/group—main	3 monkeys or 4 dogs/sex/group in groups 1–4
Number/sex/group—recovery	2/sex/group in groups 1–4
Dosing route	Generally a parenteral route (IV, IM, or sc) for biopharmaceuticals
	Oral route for pharmaceuticals
Dosing frequency	Dosed daily for 13 weeks for pharmaceuticals but for biopharmaceuticals frequency based on TK data or proposed clinical regimen
Formulations	Usually biopharmaceuticals dosed as received if clinical formulation is available
	Pharmaceuticals are formulated by the CRO and require formulation analysis for concentration, homogeneity, and stability
Clinical signs	Twice daily
Clinical observations	Weekly
Body weights	Weekly and prior to necropsy
Food consumption	Weekly
Ophthalmology	Prior to initiation, and during weeks 13 and 17
Toxicokinetics—optional if conducted in earlier studies	Days 1 and 90 all animals bled at least at 6 time points after dosing
Antibodies (for biopharmaceuticals only)	Prior to study initiation, and weeks 4, 13, and 20
Neutralizing antibodies (for biopharmaceuticals only)	Prior to study initiation, and weeks 4, 13, and 20 (for biopharmaceuticals only)

Clinical pathology	Prior to study initiation
	During weeks 13 and 17 in all surviving animals
Hematology	See Appendix B
Clinical chemistry	See Appendix B
Coagulation	See Appendix B
Urinalysis	See Appendix B
Terminal necropsy	Week 13—full necropsy in all main study animals
Recovery necropsy	Week 17—full necropsy in recovery animals
Organ weights	See Appendix C
Bone marrow smears	Yes from sternum
Tissue preservation	See Appendix D
Histopathology	Groups 1 and 4 all tissues (main and recovery)
	Groups 2 and 3—target tissues and gross lesions
	Recommended—all tissues in all groups
Report	One copy of the draft final report
	One bound and unbound copy of the final and an electronic copy in Word and PDF
Archive	Yes for at least 1 year at CRO

37.2.9 Six-Month Toxicology Study in Rodents

Purpose	What are the toxicities and toxicokinetics of a test article when administered for 6 months?
Timeline	
initiation	6 to 10 weeks following authorization
report	10 to 12 weeks following termination
Estimated cost	$350,000 to $550,000
Regulatory guidelines and compliance	S4A duration of chronic toxicity testing in animals (rodent and nonrodent testing) and FDA GLP
Total animals	156 Sprague–Dawley rats (or mice)
Number/sex/group—main	15/sex/group in groups 1–4
Number/sex/group—TK	6/sex/group in groups 2–4 (assumes <1 ml of blood/rat/time point and <0.1 ml of blood/mouse/time point)
	Additional volumes will require additional animals
Dosing route	Generally a parenteral route (IV, IM, or sc) for biopharmaceuticals
	Oral route for pharmaceuticals

Dosing frequency	Dosed daily for 26 weeks for pharmaceuticals but for biopharmaceuticals frequency based on TK data or proposed clinical regimen
Formulations	Usually biopharmaceuticals dosed as received if clinical formulation is available
	Pharmaceuticals are formulated by the CRO and require formulation analysis for concentration, homogeneity, and stability
Clinical signs	Twice daily
Clinical observations	Weekly
Body weights	Weekly and prior to necropsy
Food consumption	Weekly
Ophthalmology	Prior to initiation, and during week 26
Toxicokinetics—optional if conducted in earlier studies	Day 1, and at termination, animals (3/sex/ time point) bled at least at 6 time points after dosing
Antibodies (for biopharmaceuticals only)	Prior to study initiation, and weeks 4, 13, and 26
Neutralizing antibodies (for biopharmaceuticals only)	Prior to study initiation, and weeks 4, 13, 26, 39, and 43
Clinical pathology	At termination
Hematology	See Appendix B
Clinical chemistry	See Appendix B
Coagulation	See Appendix B
Urinalysis	See Appendix B
Terminal necropsy	Week 26—full necropsy
Organ weights	See Appendix C
Bone marrow smears	Yes from sternum
Tissue preservation	See Appendix D
Histopathology	Groups 1 and 4 all tissues
	Groups 2 and 3—target tissues and gross lesions
Report	One copy of the draft final report
	One bound and unbound copy of the final and an electronic copy in Word and PDF
Archive	Yes for at least 1 year at CRO

37.2.10 Nine-Month Toxicology Study in Nonrodents

Purpose	What are the chronic toxicities and toxicokinetics of a test article when administered to monkeys or dogs for 9 months?

Timeline	
initiation	8 to 12 weeks following authorization
report	10 to 12 weeks following termination
Estimated cost	$450,000 to $650,000
Regulatory guidelines and compliance	S4A duration of chronic toxicity testing in animals (rodent and nonrodent testing) and FDA GLP
Total animals	32 beagle dogs
	24 cynomolgus monkeys
Number/sex/group—main	4 dogs/sex/group in groups 1–4
	3 monkeys/sex/group in groups 1–4
Dosing route	Generally a parenteral route (IV, IM, or sc) for biopharmaceuticals
	Oral route for pharmaceuticals
Dosing frequency	Dosed daily for 39 weeks for pharmaceuticals but for biopharmaceuticals frequency based on TK data or proposed clinical regimen
	For biopharmaceuticals 6-month duration generally appropriate
Formulations	Usually biopharmaceuticals dosed as received if clinical formulation is available
	Pharmaceuticals are formulated by the CRO and require formulation analysis for concentration, homogeneity, and stability
Clinical signs	Twice daily
Clinical observations	Weekly
Body weights	Weekly and prior to necropsy
Food consumption	Weekly
Ophthalmology	Prior to initiation, and during Weeks 39
Electrocardiograms	Prior to initiation, and at termination
Toxicokinetics—optional if conducted in earlier studies	Day 1, and at termination, animals are bled at least at 6 time points after dosing
Antibodies (for biopharmaceuticals only)	Prior to study initiation, and weeks 4, 13, 26, and 39
Neutralizing antibodies (for biopharmaceuticals only)	Prior to study initiation, and weeks 4, 13, 26, and 39 (for biopharmaceuticals only)
Clinical pathology	Prior to study initiation
	During weeks 4, 13, 26, and 39 in all surviving animals
Hematology	See Appendix B
Clinical chemistry	See Appendix B
Coagulation	See Appendix B
Urinalysis	See Appendix B

Terminal necropsy	Week 39—full necropsy in all surviving animals
Organ weights	See appendix C
Bone marrow smears	Yes from sternum
Tissue preservation	See Appendix D
Histopathology	Groups 1 and 4 all tissues
	Groups 2 and 3—target tissues and gross lesions
	Recommended—all tissues in all groups
Report	One copy of the draft final report
	One bound and unbound copy of the final and an electronic copy in Word and PDF
Archive	Yes for at least 1 year at CRO

37.2.11   Carcinogenicity Study in Sprague–Dawley Rats

Purpose	What is the carcinogenic potential of a test article when administered to Sprague–Dawley Rats for at least 104 weeks?
Timeline	
initiation	8 to 10 weeks following authorization
report	26 to 30 weeks following termination
Estimated cost	$1.0 to 1.5 M
Regulatory guidance and compliance	S1A need for long-term rodent carcinogenicity studies of pharmaceuticals and S1B testing for carcinogenicity of pharmaceuticals and FDA GLP
Total animals	480 Sprague–Dawley rats
Number/sex/group—Main	60/sex/group in groups 1–4
Dosing route	Generally a parenteral route (IV, IM, or sc) for biopharmaceuticals
	Oral route for pharmaceuticals
Dosing frequency	Dosed daily for 104 weeks for pharmaceuticals but for biopharmaceuticals frequency based on TK data or proposed clinical regimen
Formulations	Usually biopharmaceuticals dosed as received if clinical formulation is available
	Pharmaceuticals are formulated by the CRO and require formulation analysis for concentration, homogeneity, and stability
Clinical signs	Twice daily
Clinical observations	Weekly with special attention to tumor development

Body weights	Weekly for the first 13 weeks, and every 4 weeks thereafter
Food consumption	Weekly for the first 13 weeks, and every 4 weeks thereafter
Blood smears	At 12 and 18 months and prior to necropsy a blood smears obtained from all animals
	Smears are read in the high-dose and control only unless indicated by toxic effects
Terminal necropsy	Week 104—full necropsy in all surviving animals
Organ weights	See Appendix C
Bone marrow smears	Sternum at termination
Tissue preservation	See Appendix D
Histopathology	Minimum—all tissues in groups 1 and 4 and target tissues, tumors, and gross lesions from groups 2 and 3
	Recommended—all tissues in all groups
Report	One copy of the draft final report
	One bound and unbound copy of the final and an electronic copy in Word and PDF
Archive	Yes at least 1 year at the CRO

37.2.12 Carcinogenicity Study in Mice

Purpose	What is the carcinogenic potential of a test article when administered to mice for at least 104 weeks?
Timeline	
initiation	8 to 10 weeks following authorization
report	26 to 30 weeks following termination
Estimated cost	$1.0 to 1.5 M
Regulatory guidelines and compliance	S1A need for long-term rodent carcinogenicity studies of pharmaceuticals and S1B testing for carcinogenicity of pharmaceuticals and FDA GLP
Total animals	480 mice
Number/sex/group	60/sex/group in groups 1–4
Dosing route	Generally a parenteral route (IV, IM, or sc) for biopharmaceuticals
	Oral route for pharmaceuticals
Dosing frequency	Dosed daily for 104 weeks for pharmaceuticals but for biopharmaceuticals frequency based on TK data or proposed clinical regimen

Formulations	Usually biopharmaceuticals dosed as received if clinical formulation is available
	Pharmaceuticals are formulated by the CRO and require formulation analysis for concentration, homogeneity, and stability
Clinical signs	Twice daily
Clinical observations	Weekly
Body weights	Weekly for the first 13 weeks, and every 4 weeks thereafter
Food consumption	Weekly for the first 13 weeks, and every 4 weeks thereafter
Blood smears	At 12 and 18 months and prior to necropsy a blood smear obtained from all animals
	Smears are read in the high-dose and control only unless indicated by toxic effects
Terminal necropsy	Week 104—full necropsy in all surviving animals
Organ weights	See Appendix B
Bone marrow smears	Sternum at termination
Tissue preservation	See Appendix D
Histopathology	Minimum—all tissues in groups 1 and 4 and target tissues, tumors, and gross lesions from groups 2 and 3
	Recommended—all tissues in all groups
Report	One copy of the draft final report
	One bound and unbound copy of the final and an electronic copy in Word and PDF
Archive	Yes at least 1 year at CRO

37.2.13 Carcinogenicity Testing using the Transgenic Mouse (p53+/−, rasH2, or Tg.AC)

Purpose	What is the carcinogenic potential of a test article when administered to a transgenic mouse for 26 weeks?
Timeline	
initiation	12 to 16 weeks following authorization
report	13 to 17 weeks following termination
Estimated cost	
Pilot	$250,000 to $350,000
Main	$650,000 to $750,000

Regulatory guidelines and compliance	S1A need for long-term rodent carcinogenicity studies of pharmaceuticals and S1B testing for carcinogenicity of pharmaceuticals and FDA GLP
Total animals	
Pilot	80 mice
Main	200 mice
Animal model strain	p53+/− mice for genotoxic drugs, rasH2 for nongenotoxic drugs, or Tg.AC mice for dermal administration
Number/sex/group	Pilot 10/sex/group in groups 1–4
	Main 25/sex/group in groups 1–4
Dosing route	Generally a parenteral route (IV, IM, or sc) for biopharmaceuticals
	Parenteral or oral route for pharmaceuticals
	Dermal route for Tg.AC mice
Dosing frequency	Generally dosed daily for 4 (pilot) or 26 weeks (main) for pharmaceuticals and biopharmaceuticals
Formulations	Usually biopharmaceuticals dosed as received if clinical formulation is available
	Pharmaceuticals are formulated by the CRO and require formulation analysis for concentration, homogeneity, and stability
Clinical signs	Twice daily
Clinical observations	Weekly
Body weights	Weekly
Food consumption	Weekly
Clinical pathology (optional)	Hematology, coagulation, and clinical chemistry at termination
Terminal necropsy	Pilot study (week 4) or main study (week 26)—full necropsy in all surviving animals
Organ weights	See Appendix B
Tissue preservation	See Appendix D
Histopathology	Minimum—all tissues in groups 1 and 4 and target tissues, tumors, and gross lesions from groups 2 and 3
	Recommended—all tissues in all groups
Report	One copy of the draft final report
	One bound and unbound copy of the final and an electronic copy in Word and PDF
Archive	Yes at least 1 year at CRO

37.2.14 Immunogenicity Study in Sprague–Dawley Rats

Purpose	What is the T cell dependent antibody response to KLH (keyhole limpet hemocyanin) in the rat?
	(Note: this design may be incorporated with other short-term rat studies)
Timeline	
initiation	4 to 8 weeks following authorization
report	10 to 12 weeks following termination
Estimated price	$200,000 to $250,000
Regulatory compliance	FDA GLP
Total animals	24 male and 24 female Sprague–Dawley rats
Number/sex/group—main	6/sex/group in groups 1–4
Dosing route	Generally a parenteral route (IV, IM, or sc) for biopharmaceuticals
	Oral route for pharmaceuticals
Dosing frequency	Dosed daily for 2 to 4 weeks for pharmaceuticals but for biopharmaceuticals frequency based on TK data or proposed clinical regimen
Formulations	Usually biopharmaceuticals dosed as received if clinical formulation is available
	Pharmaceuticals are formulated by the CRO and require formulation analysis for concentration, homogeneity, and stability
Clinical signs	Twice daily
Clinical observations	Weekly
Body weights	Weekly and prior to necropsy
Food consumption	Weekly
KLH administration	1 and 2 weeks prior to termination, KLH is administered
Blood collection	Serial collections at one or more time points
Terminal necropsy	Spleen collected on ice
Organ weights	Spleen
Assay	Titers for anti-KLH antibodies
Report	One copy of the draft final report
	One bound and unbound copy of the final and an electronic copy in Word and PDF
Archive	Yes for at least 1 year at CRO

37.2.15 Immunotoxicity Study in Monkeys

Purpose	What is the T cell dependent antibody response to KLH (keyhole limpet hemocyanin) in the monkey?
	(Note: this design may be incorporated with other short-term monkey studies)
Timeline	
initiation	6 to 8 weeks following authorization
report	10 to 12 weeks following termination
Estimated cost	$200,000 to $300,000
Regulatory guidelines	FDA GLP
Total animals	16 monkeys
Number/sex/group	2 monkeys /sex/group in groups 1–4
Dosing route	Generally a parenteral route (IV, IM, or sc) for biopharmaceuticals
	Oral route for pharmaceuticals
Dosing frequency	Dosed daily for pharmaceuticals but for biopharmaceuticals frequency based on TK data or proposed clinical regimen
Formulations	Usually biopharmaceuticals dosed as received if clinical formulation is available
	Pharmaceuticals are formulated by the CRO and require formulation analysis for concentration, homogeneity, and stability
Clinical signs	Twice daily
Clinical observations	Weekly
Body weights	Weekly and prior to necropsy
Food consumption	Weekly
KLH administration	1 and 2 weeks prior to termination, KLH is administered
Blood collection	Serial collections at one or more time points
Terminal necropsy	Spleen collected on ice
Organ weights	Spleen
Assay	Titers for anti-KLH antibodies
Report	One copy of the draft final report
	One bound and unbound copy of the final and an electronic copy in Word and PDF
Archive	Yes for at least 1 year at CRO

37.2.16 Vaccine Study in Rabbits

Purpose	What are the subchronic toxicities and toxicokinetics of a vaccine when administered to rabbits?
Timeline	
initiation	6 to 8 weeks following authorization
report	10 to 12 weeks following termination
Estimated cost	$400,000 to $450,000
Regulatory guidelines	FDA GLP
Total animals	72 rabbits
Number/sex/group	9 rabbits/sex/group in groups 1–4
Dosing route	Generally intramuscular or subcutaneous
Dosing frequency	Dosed based on clinical regimen, generally at 2 to 3 week intervals for 2 to 3 doses
Formulations	Usually vaccines are dosed as received if clinical formulation is available
Clinical signs	Twice daily
Clinical observations	Weekly
Body weights	Weekly and prior to necropsy
Food consumption	Weekly
Draize scoring	0, 24, 48, 72, 96, and 120 hours after each dose
	See Appendix E for scoring
Clinical pathology	Prior to study initiation
	2 to 3 days after each dose
Hematology	See Appendix B
Clinical chemistry	See Appendix B
Coagulation	See Appendix B
Urinalysis	See Appendix B
Terminal necropsy	3 days after final dose
Recovery necropsy	15 days after final dose
Organ weights	See Appendix C
Bone marrow smears	Yes from sternum
Tissue preservation	See Appendix D
Histopathology	Groups 1 and 4 all tissues
	Groups 2 and 3—target tissues and gross lesions
Report	One copy of the draft final report
	One bound and unbound copy of the final and an electronic copy in Word and PDF
Archive	Yes for at least 1 year at CRO

37.2.17 Phototoxicity Study in Rodents

Purpose	What is the potential phototoxic effect on the eyes and skin of rodents after a single dose followed by exposure to radiation from a xenon lamp (simulate sunlight)?
Timeline	
initiation	4 to 6 weeks following authorization
report	6 to 10 weeks following termination
Estimated cost	$40,000 to $50,000
Regulatory guidance and compliance	Photosafety testing (May 2003) and FDA GLP
Total animals	50 Long–Evans rats
Number/sex/group	5/sex/group in groups 1–5
Dosing route	Generally a parenteral route (IV, IM, or sc) for biopharmaceuticals
	Oral route for pharmaceuticals
Dosing frequency	Single dose at 4 dose levels (control, low, mid, and highdose) plus positive control
Formulations	Usually biopharmaceuticals dosed as received if clinical formulation is available
	Pharmaceuticals are formulated by the CRO and require formulation analysis for concentration, homogeneity, and stability
Clinical signs	Twice daily
Body weights	Daily and prior to necropsy
Exposure procedure	At appropriate intervals after dosing (e.g, 24 and 120 hours for eyes, and 4, 24, and 120 hours for skin) rats are anesthetized, restrained, and placed approximately one meter from the UVR source at the time of UVR exposure
	An instrumental UVR response dose equivalent to approximately 0.5 minimal erythema dose (MED) is delivered to each rat
Clinical observations	Prior to exposure and 1 and 4 hours after dosing, continuously during anesthesia and exposure, and daily for 3 days

Skin observations	Prior to exposure, 30 minutes after completion of each UVR exposure, and on days 2, and 3 after exposure
Ophthalmological observations	Prior to exposure and at termination
Terminal necropsy	Three days after the final UVR exposure
Tissue preservation	Eyes and skin from all animals
Histopathology	Eyes and skin from control and high-dose animals
Report	One copy of the draft final report
	One bound and unbound copy of the final and an electronic copy in Word and PDF
Archive	Yes for at least 1 year at CRO

37.2.18   Biodistribution Study in Sprague–Dawley Rats

Purpose	What is the biodistribution of a gene therapy product when administered to Sprague–Dawley rats after a single dose or after repeated dosing?
Timeline	
initiation	4 to 8 weeks following authorization
report	10 to 12 weeks following termination
Estimated price	$200,000 to $250,000
Regulatory compliance	FDA GLP
Total animals	24 male and 24 female Sprague–Dawley rats
Number/sex/group	6/sex/group in groups 1–4
Dosing route	Generally a parenteral route (IV, IM, or sc) for biopharmaceuticals
Dosing frequency	Either a single dose or dosing daily for 2 to 4 weeks for gene therapy products or based proposed clinical regimen
Formulations	Usually gene therapy products are dosed as received if clinical formulation is available.
Clinical signs	Twice daily
Clinical observations	Weekly
Body weights	Weekly and prior to necropsy
Food consumption	Weekly
Terminal necropsy	Week 4

PCR analysis	The following tissues are removed in the order listed below with a fresh set of clean instruments for each organ. The tissues (at least 0.5 g sample for each tissue-weight not required for protocol fulfillment) are snap frozen in liquid nitrogen and stored at or below $-70\,°C$:

1. Blood ($X \geq 0.6$ ml of blood is collected into an EDTA tube and then transferred to a cryovial and snap frozen)
2. Ovaries/testes (paired)
3. Liver (left lateral lobe)
4. Thymus
5. Heart (apex)
6. Lung (right
7. Small intestine (representative sample as site it not specified
8. Kidney
9. Spleen (median)
10. Mesenteric lymph nodes
11. Representative skin and subcutis (at exposure site)
12. Representative thigh muscle (at exposure site)
13. Bone marrow
14. Brain

	All tissues are processed for the presence of the gene therapy agent in the tissues using a GLP validated method for biodistribution. Skin and subcutis and thigh muscle are processed for the incorporation of gene therapy agent using a GLP validated method. Tissues are not be pooled for analysis. Analysis includes qPCR (quantitative polymerase chain reaction) for the presence of the gene therapy agent in the tissue.
Report	One copy of the draft final report
	One bound and unbound copy of the final and an electronic copy in Word and PDF
Archive	Yes for at least 1 year at CRO

37.2.19 Study of Fertility and Early Embryonic Development to Implantation in Sprague–Dawley Rats (Segment 1)

Purpose	What are the potential effects of a test article on gonad function, mating behavior, implantation, and general fertility in male and female rats when administered through mating and implantation?
Timeline	
initiation	4 to 6 weeks following authorization
report	6 to 8 weeks following termination
Estimated cost	$125,000 to $175,000
Regulatory guidance and compliance	ICH-S5A detection of toxicity to reproduction for medicinal products and FDA GLP
Total animals	100 males and 100 females
Number/sex/group	25/sex/group in groups 1–4, control, low dose, mid dose, and high dose, respectively
Dosing route	Generally a parenteral route (IV, IM, or sc) for biopharmaceuticals
	Oral route for pharmaceuticals
Dosing frequency	Males dosed for 4 weeks prior to mating (up to 10 may be required), throughout the mating period, and through the day prior to termination
	Females dosed 2 weeks prior to mating, throughout the mating period, and through GD 7
	Frequency may differ for biopharmaceuticals based on TK data or proposed clinical regimen
Formulations	Usually biopharmaceuticals dosed as received if clinical formulation available
	Pharmaceuticals are formulated by the CRO and require formulation analysis for concentration, homogeneity, and stability
Clinical signs	Twice daily
Clinical observations	Weekly

Body weights	Males weighed on the first day of treatment prior to dosing, twice weekly during treatment, and at termination
	Females weighed on the first day of treatment prior to dosing, twice weekly during premating treatment phase, and twice weekly during mating
	Confirmed-mated females are also weighed on days 0, 3, 7, 10, and 13 of presumed gestation
Estrous cycle determination	During the 2-week dosing premating phase, daily vaginal smears assessed for stage of estrus
	Estrous cycle determination continued until confirmation of mating occurred or the mating phase ended
Mating	1:1 with identification of both parents of a litter
Uterine examinations	Performed at any point after midpregnancy but generally on GD 13
	Uterine contents are examined for corpora lutea, implantation sites, and live and dead conceptuses
Necropsy	Necropsy of males and unconfirmed females include an examination of the external features of the carcass; external body orifices; and cervical, abdominal, and thoracic viscera
	Special attention given to the organs of the reproductive tract
Antibodies (for biopharmaceuticals only)	Prior to initiation and at termination
Sperm evaluation	Sperm count and motility in the males surviving to termination.
Tissue preservation	Testes, epididymides, ovaries, and uteri from all animals
Histopathology	Not conducted unless indicated by treatment-related effects
Report	One copy of the draft final report
	One bound and unbound copy of the final and an electronic copy in Word and PDF
Archive	At the CRO for at least one year

37.2.20   Study for Effects on Embryofetal Development and Toxicokinetics in Rats (Segment 2)

Purpose	What is the maternal and embryofetal toxicity and teratogenic potential and toxicokinetics of a test article when administered daily to pregnant rats from implantation to closure of the hard palate?
Timeline	
initiation	4 to 6 weeks following authorization
report	8 to 12 weeks following termination
Estimated cost	$100,000 to $125,000
Regulatory guidance and compliance	ICH-S5A detection of toxicity to reproduction for medicinal products and FDA GLP
Total females	118 time-mated ($\leq$GD3) females received
Number/group	25/sex/group in groups 1–4, control, low dose, mid dose, and high dose, respectively
Number/group for TK	6/sex/group in groups 1–4
Dosing route and frequency	Generally a parenteral route (IV, IM, or sc) for biopharmaceuticals
	Oral route for pharmaceuticals
	Dose GD 6 to 17 for pharmaceuticals, but frequency for a biologic based on TK data or proposed clinical regimen
Formulations	Usually biopharmaceuticals dosed as received if clinical formulation available
	Pharmaceuticals are formulated by the CRO and require formulation analysis for concentration, homogeneity, and stability
Clinical signs	Twice daily
Body weights	Main study animals weighed on GD 0, 4, 6, 8, 10, 12, 14, 16, 18, and 20
	Toxicokinetic animals weighed on GD 0, 4, 6, 8, 10, 12, 14, 16, and 18
Food consumption	Beginning on GD 4, food consumption measured at body weight intervals
Toxicokinetics	Blood samples obtained from 3 animals/ time point on GD 6 and 17 of the treatment phase at approximately 0.5, 1, 2, 4, 8, and 24 hours postdose ($\pm$2 min)

Uterine examinations	Performed on GD 20
	Uterine contents are examined for corpora lutea, number of live and dead fetuses, and gross lesions
Antibodies (for biopharmaceuticals only)	Prior to study initiation, and at termination
Fetal examinations	Each fetus (live or dead) sexed, weighed, and examined for external abnormalities
	Approximately half of all fetuses from each litter processed for visceral examination
	Heads preserved in Bouin's fixative, and evaluated by Wilson's technique
	Internal organs of the thoracic and abdominal cavities of the fetuses examined in the fresh state using Staples's technique
	Remaining fetuses eviscerated, processed for skeletal examination using the Alizarin Red S staining method, and evaluated
	Findings are judged to be variations or malformations:
	Malformations are developmental deviations that (1) are gross structural changes, (2) are incompatible with life, or (3) may affect the quality of life. Variations are structural deviations that are thought to have no effect on body conformity or the well-being of the animal.
Tissue preservation	All fetuses retained in Bouin's fixative or glycerin
Report	One copy of the draft final report
	One bound and unbound copy of the final and an electronic copy in Word and PDF
Archive	At the CRO for at lest one year

37.2.21 Study for Effects on Embryofetal Development and Toxicokinetics in New Zealand White Rabbits (Segment 2)

Purpose	What are the maternal and embryofetal toxicity, teratogenic potential, and toxicokinetics of a test article when administered to pregnant rabbits from implantation to closure of the hard plate?

Timeline	
initiation	4 to 6 weeks following authorization
report	8 to 12 weeks following termination
Estimated cost	$125,000 to $150,000
Regulatory guidance and compliance	ICH-S5A detection of toxicity to reproduction for medicinal products and FDA GLP
Total females	92 Time-mated female Hra:(NZW)SPF rabbits
Number group	20/group in groups 1–4
Number/group for TK	3/group in groups 1–4
Dosing route	Generally a parenteral route (IV, IM, or sc) for biopharmaceuticals
	Oral route for pharmaceuticals
Dosing frequency	Dose GD 7 to 20 for pharmaceuticals, but frequency for a biologic may differ based on TK data or proposed clinical regimen
Formulations	Usually biopharmaceuticals dosed as received if clinical formulation available
	Pharmaceuticals are formulated by the CRO and require formulation analysis for concentration, homogeneity, and stability
Clinical signs	Twice daily
Body weights	Main study rabbits are weighed on GD 0, 4, 7, 9, 11, 13, 15, 18, 21, 24, 27, and 29
	TK rabbits are weighed on GD 0, 4, 7, 9, 11, 13, 15, and 18
Food consumption	Food consumption is measured for the main study rabbits at GD 4 to 5, 5 to 7, 7 to 9, 9 to 11, 11 to 13, 13 to 15, 15 to 17, 17 to 18, 18 to 20, 20 to 21, 21 to 22, 22 to 24, 24 to 26, 26 to 27, and 27 to 29
Toxicokinetics	Blood samples obtained from 3 animals/time point on GD 7 and 20 of the treatment phase at approximately 0.5, 1, 2, 4, 8, and 24 hours postdose (±2 min)
Uterine examinations	Performed on GD 29
	Uterine contents examined for corpora lutea, number of live and dead fetuses, and gross lesions
Antibodies (for biopharmaceuticals only)	Prior to study initiation, and at termination

Fetal examinations	Each live fetus weighed and examined for external abnormalities
	Live fetuses killed and a midcoronal slice made in the head of each fetus to evaluate the contents of the cranium
	Internal organs of the thoracic and abdominal cavities of all fetuses examined in the fresh state using Staples's technique, and the sex of each fetus determined
	Viscera removed and discarded
	Carcasses processed for skeletal examination using the Alizarin Red S staining method and evaluated
	Findings judged to be variations or malformations
	Malformations are developmental deviations that (1) are gross structural changes, (2) are incompatible with life, or (3) may affect the quality of life. Variations are structural deviations that are thought to have no effect on body conformity or the well-being of the animal.
Tissue preservation	All fetuses are retained in Bouin's fixative or glycerin
Report	One copy of the draft final report
	One bound and unbound copy of the final and an electronic copy in Word and PDF
Archive	At the CRO for at last one year

37.2.22   Study for Effects on Pre- and Postnatal Development, Including Maternal Function in Sprague–Dawley Rats (Segment 3)

Purpose	What are the effects of the test article on pregnant and lactating dams and on the development of the conceptus and offspring following exposure of the dams from implantation through weaning?
Timeline	
initiation	4 to 6 weeks following authorization
report	8 to 10 weeks following termination
Estimated cost	$200,000 to $250,000
Regulatory guidance and compliance	ICH-S5A detection of toxicity to reproduction for medicinal products and FDA GLP

Total animals	100 F_0 time mated (≤GD 4) females received
Number/sex/group	25/sex/group in groups 1–4
Dosing route	Generally a parenteral route (IV, IM, or sc) for biopharmaceuticals
	Oral route for pharmaceuticals
Dosing frequency	Implantation through the end of lactation, generally daily from GD 6 through PND 20
	Frequency may differ for biological, based on TK data or proposed clinical regimen
	F_1 generation not dosed
Formulations	Usually biopharmaceuticals dosed as received if clinical formulation available
	Pharmaceuticals are formulated by the CRO and require formulation analysis for concentration, homogeneity, and stability
Clinical signs	Twice daily
Clinical observations	Weekly
F_0 Body weights	GD 0, 4, 6, 8, 10, 12, 14, 16, 18, and 20 and on PND 0, 4, 7, 10, 14, 17, and 21
F_0 Food consumption	GD 4–6, 6–8, 8–10, 10–12, 12–14, 14–16, 16–18, and 18–20
	Food consumption will not be measured during lactation
F_1 Litter observations	At birth—litter size (number alive and dead), and the sex, weight, and clinical observations of individual pups
	At PND 4—litter size and sex, weight, and observations of individual pups prior to culling; litters with more than 8 pups culled to 4 males and 4 females
	At PND 7, 14, 21—litter size and sex, weight, and observations of individual pups
	General development—pinna unfolding (PND 1), surface righting (PND 4), hair growth (PND 7), incisor eruption (PND 7), eye opening (PND 11), and auditory startle (PND 21)
Weaning	1 pup/sex/litter randomly selected for F_1 generation

Postweaning	Pup observation may include the following:
	Vaginal opening—starting on PND 30
	Cleavage of the balanopreputial gland—starting on PND 35
	Locomotor activity—PND 22 ± 1 day
	Water maze—PND 30 ± 2
F_1 breeding	Following 7 weeks of postweaning one female and one male from the same groups are selected to cohabit; sibling mating avoided
	Mating confirmed by presence of vaginal plug or sperm
F_1 body weights	GD 0, 7, 14, and 20 and on PND 0.
F_2 litter observations	At birth—litter size (number alive and dead), and the sex, weight, and clinical observations of individual pups
	PND 0—all pups killed and preserved in 10% NBF
Necropsy	F_0 females
	F_1 males and females
Antibodies (for biopharmaceuticals only)	Prior to study initiation, and at termination
Tissue preservation	Gross lesions
Histopathology	Not conducted unless indicated by treatment-related effects
Report	One copy of the draft final report
	One bound and unbound copy of the final and an electronic copy in Word and PDF
Archive	At the CRO for at least one year

37.2.23 Evaluation of Cardiovascular (Hemodynamic) Function in the Conscious Telemetered Nonrodent

Purpose	What is the effect of the test article on the hemodynamic function in the conscious telemetered nonrodent?
Timeline	
initiation	2 to 4 weeks following authorization
report	6 to 8 weeks following termination
Estimated cost	$100,000 to $150,000
Regulatory guidelines and compliance	ICH S7A safety pharmacology studies for human pharmaceuticals and FDA GLP
Total animals	8 cynomolgus monkeys or beagle dogs
Number/sex	4/sex/dose

Dosing route	Expected clinical route of administration when feasible
	Generally a parenteral route (IV, IM, or sc) for biopharmaceuticals and oral route for pharmaceuticals
Dosing frequency	4 animals/sex treated with 4 doses (control, low, mid, and high dose) with at least 7 days between doses
Formulations	Usually biopharmaceuticals dosed as received when clinical formulation available
	Pharmaceuticals are formulated by the CRO and require formulation analysis for concentration, homogeneity, and stability
Clinical signs	Twice daily
Clinical observations	Prior to and following each dose
Body weights	Prior to each dose
Cardiovascular analysis	In instrumented dogs, blood pressure (diastolic, mean, and systolic) recorded every 15 minutes for the first 4 hours with hourly measurements thereafter for 24 hours and ECGs to include P duration, PR interval, QRS interval, R amplitude, and QT/QTc interval recorded every 15 to 30 minutes for the first 4 hours and hourly thereafter for 8 hours
	Times may vary based on toxicokinetic parameters
Report	One copy of the draft final report
	One bound and unbound copy of the final and an electronic copy in Word and PDF
Archive	At least one year at CRO

37.2.24 Neuropharmacology Study in Sprague–Dawley Rats

Purpose	What are the neuropharmacology effects (functional observational battery, spontaneous motor activity, and motor coordination) in Sprague–Dawley rats following a single dose?
Timeline	
initiation	2 to 4 weeks following authorization
report	6 to 8 weeks after termination
Estimated cost	$20,000 to $40,000

Regulatory guidelines and compliance	ICH S7A safety pharmacology studies for human pharmaceuticals and FDA GLP
Total animals	120 Sprague–Dawley rats
Number/sex/group	10 males/group in groups 1–4 for each test (functional observational battery, spontaneous motor activity, and rotarod)
	Tests may be conducted in 5 rats/sex/ group
Dosing route	Expected clinical route of administration when feasible
	Generally a parenteral route (IV, IM, or sc) for biopharmaceuticals and oral route for pharmaceuticals
	Oral route usually for pharmaceuticals
Dosing frequency	Prior to each test
Formulations	Usually biopharmaceuticals dosed as received when clinical formulation available
	Pharmaceuticals are formulated by the CRO and require formulation analysis for concentration, homogeneity, and stability
Functional observational battery	Rats dosed and placed in open field and observed for signs of pharmacological or toxicological activity at 15, 30, and 45 minutes, 1, 2, 3, 4, and 24 hours following treatment
	Observation times may vary based on the toxicokinetics of the test article
	Observances for the following will include:
	Seizures/convulsions, awareness reaction, startle response, vocalization, irritability, decreased abdominal tone, increased secretion, body tremors, decreased grip strength, immobility, motor activity, ataxia, abnormal posture, stereotypy, excretion, decreased respiration, piloerection, loss of righting, pupil size, nociceptive (pain) response, corneal reflex, and pinnal reflex
	Body temperatures taken on all animals at 60 minutes (± 5 min) following dose administration

Rotarod	Rats are pre-trained and act as their own control to maintain themselves on the rotarod for one minute
	Rats are tested on the rotarod at 30 and 60 minutes (±2 minutes) postdose
	Observation times may vary based on the pharmacokinetics of the test article
Spontaneous motor activity	Rats are orally dosed, and individually placed in a photobeam activity system for 60 minutes postadministration of the test article/vehicle, to count spontaneous motor activity over a 20 minute period
	Spontaneous motor activity is counted at the following time intervals (minutes): 0–5, 5–10, 10–15, 15–20
	Observation times may vary based on the pharmacokinetics of the test article
Report	One copy of the draft final report
	One bound and unbound copy of the final and an electronic copy in Word and PDF
Archive	At least one year at the CRO.

37.2.25 Pulmonary Assessment in the Conscious Rat

Purpose	What are the potential effects on pulmonary function in the conscious rat?
Timeline	
initiation	2 to 4 weeks following authorization
report	4 to 6 weeks after termination
Estimated cost	$25,000 to $45,000
Regulatory guidelines and compliance	ICH S7A safety pharmacology studies for human pharmaceuticals and FDA GLP
Total animals	16 male Sprague–Dawley rats
Number sex/group	4 males/group in groups 1–4
Dosing route and frequency	Generally a parenteral route (IV, IM, or sc) for biopharmaceuticals
	Oral route usually for pharmaceuticals prior to each test

Methods	Pleural pressure transmitters surgically implanted using aseptic surgical techniquein each rat
	Rats trained initially for two days in the head-out plethysmographic chamber for 15 minutes each
	On day of dosing, each rat placed in its plethysmographic chamber and allowed to stabilize for 5 minutes
	Following stabilization, the following respiratory parameters are measured for five minute for baseline levels:
	Airway Resistance $(cmH_2O/ml/s)$, Tidal Volume (ml/breath), minute volume (ml/min), and respiratory rate (breaths/min)
	Rats then removed from the chambers and dosed with the test article or vehicle
	30 minutes following the dosing, rats returned to the plethysmographic chamber and respiratory parameters measured continuously for 5 minutes
	After 1, 2, and 4 hours, each animal returned to its designated plethysmographic chamber and respiratory parameters are measured continuously for 5 minutes following a 5-min stabilization period
Report	One copy of the draft final report
	One bound and unbound copy of the final and an electronic copy in Word and PDF
Archive	At least one year at the CRO

37.2.26 Evaluation of Cardiovascular Function Using Cloned hERG Channels Expressed in Human Embryonic Kidney (HEK293) Cells

Purpose	What is the potential of the test article to prolong the human QT interval in vivo by assessing the rapidly inward rectifying potassium current (Kr) conducted by hERG (human ether-a-go-go related gene) channels stably expressed in a HEK293 cell line?
Timeline	
initiation	2 to 4 weeks following authorization
report	4 to 6 weeks following termination
Estimated cost	$15,000 to $20,000

Regulatory guidelines and compliance	ICH S7A safety pharmacology studies for human pharmaceuticals and FDA GLP
Cells	HEK293 cells from *Homo sapien* embryonic kidney epithelial cell line transformed with adenovirus 5 DNA and maintained in cell culture incubators
Dosing route	In vitro
Formulations	Biopharmaceuticals or pharmaceuticals dissolved in physiological saline containing 0.1% DMSO to obtain at least 5 different concentrations
	Biopharmaceuticals and pharmaceuticals formulated by the CRO and require formulation analysis for concentration, homogeneity, and stability
Positive control	Cisapride, a potent blocker of hERG channels, expressed in HEK293 cells and clinically shown to result in QT prolongation and ventricular arrythmias
Study design	Cells harvested using trypsin/EDTA and plated onto glass cover slips prior to evaluation
	Following whole-cell patch clamp with demonstration of stable hERG current, control values taken followed by exposure of the cells to the vehicle, then each concentration of the test article from lowest to highest concentration and finally the positive control
Parameters	Peak tail currents from the last 30s of the baseline period averaged and compared to 30s of data recorded in the presence of each test article solution
	Current inhibition calculated as percent according to Inhibition (%) = $100 \times (I_{test}/I_{baseline})$, where I_{test} is the peak tail current measured in the presence of the test solution and $I_{baseline}$ is the peak tail current measured prior to exposure to the test solution
Report	One copy of the draft final report
	One bound and unbound copy of the final and an electronic copy in Word and PDF
Archive	At least one year at CRO

37.2.27 Evaluation of Cardiovascular Function Using Action Potential Parameters in Isolated Dog Purkinje Fibers

Purpose	What is the potential of the test article to prolong the human QT interval in vivo by assessing the action potential parameters in the Beagle dog Purkinje fibers?
Timeline	
initiation	2 to 4 weeks following authorization
report	4 to 6 weeks following termination
Estimated cost	$20,000 to $25,000
Regulatory guidelines and compliance	ICH S7A safety pharmacology studies for human pharmaceuticals and FDA GLP
Total animals	4 beagle dogs
Dosing route	In vitro
Formulations	Biopharmaceuticals or pharmaceuticals dissolved in Tyrodes's solution to obtain at least 5 different concentrations
	Biopharmaceuticals and pharmaceuticals formulated by the CRO and require formulation analysis for concentration, homogeneity, and stability
Positive control	dl-soltalol, a β-adrenergic antagonist that prolongs cardiac action potential by selectively blocking the rapidly activating delayed rectifier potassium current (IKr)
Study design	4 Purkinje fibers obtained from 4 different dogs isolated from dog hearts and placed in a recording chamber and perfused with Tyrode's solution at 35–38 °C
	Fibers electrically paced via bipolar silver electrodes and impaled with 3M KCl-filled glass microelectrodes
	Action potentials continuously monitored
	Control values taken, followed by exposure of fibers to vehicle, then each concentration of the test article from lowest to highest concentration and finally the positive control

Action potential parameters	Resting membrane potential (RMP)
	Maximum rate of depolarization of the action potential upstroke (V_{max})
	Action potential amplitude (APA)
	Overshoot (OS)
	Action potential duration at 30%, 50%, and 90% (APD_{30}, APD_{50}, and APD_{90}) repolarization
Report	One copy of the draft final report
	One bound and unbound copy of the final and an electronic copy in Word and PDF
Archive	At least one year at CRO

37.2.28 *Salmonella typhimurium/Escherichia coli* Plate Incorporation Mutation Assay in the Presence and Absence of Induced Rat Liver S-9

Purpose	What is the potential of a test article with and without metabolic activation to produce point mutations in bacteria strains with base substitutions and frameshift mutations in operons coding for synthesis of specific amino acids?
Timeline	
initiation	2 to 4 weeks following authorization
report	4 to 6 weeks following termination
Estimated cost	$10,000 to $15,000
Regulatory guidelines/compliance	ICH S2A specific aspects of regulatory genotoxicity tests for pharmaceuticals, S2Bgenotoxicity: a standard battery for genotoxicity testing of pharmaceuticals and FDA GLPs
Metabolic activation	Standard rat liver S-9 prepared by inducing male Sprague–Dawley rats with Aroclor-1254 or Phenobarbital and/or β-naphthoflavone
Test system identification	*Salmonella typhimurium* strains—TA98, TA100, TA1535, TA1537
	Escherichia coli strain—WP2 uvrA
Positive controls	2-AA, 2-NF, 9-AA, NaAz, and MMS
Determination of solubility/miscibility	Conducted to determine the maximum achievable concentration of ANS 201 in the selected solvent (water, DMSO, acetone, or ethanol).

Dose selection	Performed with and without S-9 activation using tester strains TA100 and WP2 uvrA only to identify test article concentrations that produce 0–100% toxicity.
Mutation assay	Performed using the four *Salmonella typhimurium* strains (TA98, TA100, TA1535, TA1537) and the *Escherichia coli* strain WP2 uvrA strain bu plate incorporation method of treatment Plates incubated at 37 °C for 36 to 72 hours and then scored for number of revertants per plate
Confirmatory assay	If mutation assay negative, the same strains and test article concentrations is tested using the preincubation method of treatment
Criteria of response	Negative, if all stains treated with test article had mean reversion frequencies that are less than twice those observed in the corresponding solvent control plates in TA98 and TA100 and less than three times in TA 1535, TA1537, and WP2 uvrA, and there is no evidence of a concentration–response Positive, if either TA98 or TA 100 exhibit a mean reversion frequency that is at least double those observed in the corresponding control in at least one concentration, or if TA1535, TA1537, or WP2 uvrA exhibit a threefold increase in mean reversion frequency compared to the solvent control in at least one concentration and the response must be concentration-dependent
Report	One copy of the draft final report One bound and unbound copy of the final and an electronic copy in Word and PDF
Archive	At least one year at the CRO

37.2.29 Chemical Induction of Micronucleated Polychromatic Erythrocytes in Mouse Bone Marrow Cells

Purpose	What is the potential of a test article to produce clastogenic genetic damage as measured by induced micronucleated polychromatic erythrocytes (MPCE) in bone marrow cells?
Timeline	
initiation	2 to 4 weeks following authorization
report	4 to 8 weeks following termination
Estimated cost	$15,000 to $25,000
Regulatory guidelines/ compliance	ICH S2A specific aspects of regulatory genotoxicity tests for pharmaceuticals, S2Bgenotoxicity: a standard battery for genotoxicity testing of pharmaceuticals and FDA GLPs
Abbreviations	PCE—polychromatic erythrocytes
	NCE—normochromatic erythrocytes
	MPC—micronucleated polychromatic erythrocytes
Total mice	90 CD-1 mice (or rats)
Number/sex/group	10/sex/group in groups 1–4 (control, low, mid, and high dose) and 5/sex in the positive control group
Positive control	Cyclophosphamide (CP) at 80 mg/kg or trimethylenemelamine (TEM) at 1.0 mg/kg
Dosing route	Generally a parenteral route (IV, IM, or sc) for biopharmaceuticals
	Oral route for CP or intraperitoneal for TEM
Range finding	Performed only if sufficient information is not available on the toxicity of the test article in mice.
Assay	Approximately 24, 48, or 72 hours after dosing, mice killed and bone marrow obtained from both femurs
	Slide of a bone marrow suspension prepared, stained with Wright-Giemsa stain, dried, and scored blind
	Number of PCE among the total erythrocytes (PCE + NCE) determined for each animal by counting at least 200 erythrocytes
	Number of MPCE scored for 1000 or 2000 PCE per animal

Criteria of response	Positive, if there is a positive dose–response trend or statistically significant increase in the number of MPCE at one or more dose levels compared to control
Report	One copy of the draft final report
	One bound and unbound copy of the final and an electronic copy in Word and PDF
Archive	At least one year at the CRO

37.2.30 Lymphoma Mutagenesis in the L5178Y TK+/– Mouse with Colony Size Evaluation in the Presence and Absences of Induced Rat Liver S-9 with a Confirmatory Study

Purpose	What is the potential of a test article with and without metabolic activation to induce forward mutations at the thymidine kinase locus of L5178Y TK+/– mouse lymphoma cells?
Timeline	
initiation	2 to 4 weeks following authorization
report	4 to 8 weeks following termination
Estimated cost	$15,000 to $25,000
Regulatory guidelines/compliance	ICH S2A specific aspects of regulatory genotoxicity tests for pharmaceuticals, S2B genotoxicity: a standard battery for genotoxicity testing of pharmaceuticals and FDA GLPs
Metabolic activation	Standard rat liver S-9 prepared by inducing male Sprague–Dawley rats with Aroclor-1254 or Phenobarbital and/or β-naphthoflavone
Positive control	Hycanthone methanesulfonate (HYC)—induces mutations at the TK locus without metabolic activation
	7,12-Dimethylbenz[α]anthracene (DMBA)—induces mutations at the TK locus with metabolic activation
Dose selection	Performed to identify the concentrations that produce 0–100% toxicity.

Mutation assay	Positive controls (HYC and DMBA) and five concentrations of the test article used with and with metabolic activation
	Cells exposed to each dose, and the supernatant obtained, and incubated for 20 and 44 hours
	After a 2-day expression period, the cultures cloned with the restrictive agent trifluorothymidine (allows the growth of TK–/– cells only) or vehicle control
Results	Mutation frequency (MF) calculated as mean of all mutants per plate ÷ mean of all colonies in corresponding plates
	Induced MF also calculated
Criteria	Positive response is if at least one culture had an MF that is two times or greater than the average MF of the corresponding solvent control cultures, and the response is concentration dependent
Confirmatory assay	Performed without S-9 activation and exposure period extended to 24 hours to confirm mutation assay results
Report	One copy of the draft final report
	One bound and unbound copy of the final and an electronic copy in Word and PDF
Archive	At least one year at the CRO

37.2.31   In vitro Chromosomal Aberration

Purpose	What is the potential of a test article with and without metabolic activation to induce structural chromosome alterations in Chinese hamster ovary (CHO) cells?
Timeline	
initiation	2 to 4 weeks following authorization
report	4 to 8 weeks following termination
Estimated cost	$15,000 to $25,000
Regulatory guidelines/compliance	ICH S2A specific aspects of regulatory genotoxicity tests for pharmaceuticals, S2B genotoxicity: a standard battery for genotoxicity testing of pharmaceuticals and FDA GLPs

Metabolic activation	Standard rat liver S-9 prepared by inducing male Sprague–Dawley rats with Aroclor-1254 or Phenobarbital and/or β-naphthoflavone
Positive control	Methyl methanesulphonate, ethyl methanesulfonate, ethylnitrosurea, mitomycin, or 4-nitroquinone-N-oxide for the nonmetabolic activation and benzo(a)pyrene or cyclophosphamide for the metabolic activation
Dose selection	Performed as the loss of growth potential of cells induced by a 4-hour expression in growth medium
Assay	Approximately 10^6 cells treated with at least three doses of the test article with and without the S9 fraction for two hours at $37\,°C$ in growth medium
	Exposure period stopped by two washing the cells twice with saline
	Following the addition of fresh growth medium and BrdU (5-bromo-2'-deoxyuridine), cells incubated for 20 hours.
	Colcemid included in the medium the last three hours
	Slides are then prepared with 10% Giemsa for scoring of chromosomal aberrations
Results	Standard forms are used to score 100 to 200 cells for gaps, breaks, fragments, reunion figures, and numerical aberrations such as polyploidy cells
Criteria	Type of aberration, frequency, and dose–response considered when evaluating the potential of a test article to induce chromosomal aberrations
Report	One copy of the draft final report
	One bound and unbound copy of the final and an electronic copy in Word and PDF
Archive	At least one year at the CRO

37.2.32 Tissue Cross-Reactivity

Purpose	What is the potential for expected or unexpected tissue binding (or cross-reactivity) of antibodies (test articles) in human and animal tissues?
	What is the relevance of a given species for use in toxicity studies with that antibody?
Timeline	
initiation	2 to 4 weeks following authorization
report	4 to 6 weeks following termination
Estimated cost	Human tissue cross-reactivity (3 donors) $45,000 to $50,000
	Animal tissue cross-reactivity (2 donors) $65,000 to 70,000
Regulatory guidelines/ compliance	No specific guidelines and FDA GLP optional
Staining methods	Avidin-biotin (ABC) for biotinylated test articles or
	Tertiary antibody detection for FITC labeled test article or
	Precomplexing with a labeled anti-human IgG for an unlabeled test article
Negative control	Tissue element or cell line that does not express the target antigen or
	Beads coated with an irrelevant antigen or
	Irrelevant antigen spotted and cross-linked to UV-resin slides
Assay control	Used to define background
Positive control	Tissue element or cell line known to express the target antigen or
	Sepharose or agarose beads coated with target antigen target antigen spotted and cross-linked on UV-resin slides
Results	Specific reactions of the antibody with the positive control material and lack of specific reactivity with the negative control material demonstrate the sensitivity, specificity, and reproducibility of the assay
	In a typical cross-reactivity assay, a staining method most appropriate for the antibody is developed
	In a typical tissue cross-reactivity study (see Appendix J, cryosections of normal human (3 unrelated donors) and/or animal (2 unrelated donors) tissues are stained

Criteria	Slides initially evaluated to determine if the tissue is adequate and normal
	Staining judged specific (CDR mediated) or nonspecific (non-CDR mediated) by comparison with control slides
	Any specific staining judged to be an expected or unexpected reactivity based on the known expression of the target antigen
	Any staining judged to be specific scored for intensity, frequency, and staining affinity
Report	One copy of the draft final report
	One bound and unbound copy of the final and an electronic copy in Word and PDF
Archive	At least one year at the CRO

APPENDIX A   NORMAL HUMAN TISSUES USED IN TISSUE CROSS-REACTIVITY TESTING

Adrenal

Bladder

Blood cells

Bone marrow

Breast

Cerebellum

Cerebral cortex

Colon

Endothelium

Eye

Fallopian tube

Gastrointestinal tract

Heart

Kidney (glomerulus, tubule)

Liver

Lung

Lymph node

Ovary

Pancreas

Parathyroid

Pituitary

Placenta

Prostate

Skin

Spinal cord

Spleen

Striated muscle

Testis

Thymus

Thyroid

Ureter

Uterus (cervix, endometrium)

APPENDIX B CLINICAL PATHOLOGY PARAMETERS

Hematology

Red blood cell (erythrocyte) count	Platelet count
Hemoglobin	White blood cell (leukocyte) count
Hematocrit	Differential blood cell count
Mean corpuscular volume	Blood smear
Mean corpuscular hemoglobin	Reticulocyte count
Mean corpuscular hemoglobin concentration	

Coagulation

Prothrombin time	Activated partial thromboplastin time
Fibrogen (optional)	

Clinical Chemistry

Glucose	Alanine aminotransferase
Urea nitrogen	Alkaline phosphatase
Creatinine	Gamma glutamyltransferase
Total protein	Aspartate aminotransferase
Albumin	Calcium
Globulin	Inorganic phosphorus
Albumin/globulin ratio	Sodium
Cholesterol	Potassium
Total bilirubin	Chloride

Urinalysis

Bilirubin	Blood
Glucose	Ketones
Microscopic examination of sediment	pH
Protein	Specific gravity
Volume	Urobilinogen
Appearance/color	

APPENDIX C   ORGAN WEIGHTS

At scheduled sacrifices, the following organs (when present) are weighed; paired organs are weighed together:

Adrenal (2)	Prostate
Brain	Salivary gland (mandibular) (2)
Epididymis (2)	Seminal vesicle
Heart	Spleen
Kidney (2)	Testis (2)
Liver	Thymus
Lung	Thyroid (2 lobes) with parathyroid
Ovary (2)	Uterus
Pituitary gland	

Organ-to-body weight and organ-to-brain weight ratios are generally reported as percentages

APPENDIX D   TISSUE PRESERVATION

The following tissues (when present) from each animal are preserved in 10% neutral-buffered formalin, unless otherwise indicated below:

Adrenal (2)	Pancreas
Aorta	Pituitary gland
Brain	Prostate
Cecum	Rectum
Colon	Salivary gland [mandibular (2)]
Duodenum	Sciatic nerve
Epididymis (2)[a]	Seminal vesicle (except dogs)
Esophagus	Skeletal muscle (biceps femoris)
Eye (2 with optic nerve)[a]	Skin
Femur with bone marrow (articular surface of the distal end)	Spinal cord (cervical, thoracic and lumbar)
	Spleen
Gallbladder (except rats)	Sternum with bone marrow
Harderian gland[a]	Stomach

Heart
Ileum
Injection site(s) if applicable
Jejunum
Kidney (2)
Lesions
Liver
Lung with large bronchi
Lymph node (mesenteric and/or mesenteric)
Mammary gland (females)
Ovary (2)

Testis (2)[a]
Thymus
Thyroid (2 lobes) with parathyroid
Tongue
Trachea
Urinary bladder
Uterus
Vagina

[a]Preserved in modified Davidson's fixative.

APPENDIX E   DRAIZE SCORES

The following scores are based on the Draize scale for scoring skin irritation:

ERYTHEMA AND ESCHAR FORMATION

0   No erythema
1   Very slight erythema (barely perceptible)
2   Well-defined erythema
3   Moderate to severe erythema
4   Severe erythema (beet redness) to slight eschar formation (injuries in depth)

Maximum possible = 4

EDEMA FORMATION

0   No edema
1   Very slight edema (barely perceptible)
2   Slight edema (edges of area well defined by definite raising)
3   Moderate edema (raised approximately 1 mm)
4   Severe edema (raised more than 1 mm and extending beyond area of exposure)

Maximum possible = 4

J. H. Draize, G. Woodard, and H. O. Calvery (1944). Methods for the study of irritation and toxicity of substances applied topically to the skin and mucous membranes. *J. Pharmacol. Exp. Ther.* 82: 377–390.

APPENDIX F ANALYTICAL/BIOANALYTICAL COSTS

Dose Analysis

Method validation	$10,000 to $20,000

- Method transferred or developed using an aqueous vehicle
- Validation includes the proposed concentrations and storage periods to be used in the toxicology studies
- Stability determined for 24 hours and up to 8 days
- Report is included in the study report
- Analyses conducted following GLPs

Study analysis	$5000 to $7500

Bioanalytical Method Validation and Sample Analysis

Method validation for a pharmaceutical (generally LS/MS/MS) or biopharmaceutical (ELISA)	$15,000 to $30,000

- Method transferred or developed using an serum or plasma
- Validation includes the proposed concentrations anticipated in the toxicology studies
- Long-term stability included
- Report is included in the study report
- Analyses conducted following GLPs
- Method validation for additional species is generally about 75% to 80% of initial species

Individual sample analysis	$60 to $100

Toxicokineic Blood Collection Cost per Time Interval

Rodent	$10,000 to $20,000
Nonrodent	$15,000 to $25,000

APPENDIX G SPECIAL STAINS

STAIN	AFFINITY
Alcian Blue	Mucopolysaccharides
Acid Fuchsin	Connective tissue
Dunn-Thompson	Hemoglobin
Hematoxylin and Eosin	Nuclei (hematoxylin) and cytoplasm (eosin)

STAIN	AFFINITY
Immunoperoxidase (Horseradish peroxidase)	Antibody–antigen interactions
Immunofluorescence (FITC, Rhodamine, or Texas Red)	Antibody–antigen interactions
Oil Red O (ORO)	Fat
PAS (Periodic Acid-Schiff)	Glycogen, mucin, mucoprotein, glycoprotein, fungi
Perl's Iron Stain	Iron
Silver Stain (Gomori Methenamine Silver Stain)	Fungi and *Pneumocystis carinii*
Trichrome	Collagen
Verhoeff'Elastic Stain	Elastic fibers
Wright-Giemsa	Peripheral blood smears
Wright Stain	Differentiation of blood cells

APPENDIX H   REFERENCES

For additional details see ICH Guidance Documents at:
http://www.fda.gov/cder/guidance/index.htm

Single Dose Acute Toxicity Testing for Pharmaceuticals (1996)

M3 Nonclinical Safety Studies for the Conduct of Human Clinical Trials for Pharmaceuticals	11/1997
S1C Dose Selection for Carcinogenicity Studies of Pharmaceuticals	3/1995
S1C(R) Guidance on Dose Selection for Carcinogenicity Studies of Pharmaceuticals: Addendum on a Limit Dose and Related Notes	12/4/1997
S2A Specific Aspects of Regulatory Genotoxicity Tests for Pharmaceuticals	4/1996
S2B Genotoxicity: A Standard Battery for Genotoxicity Testing of Pharmaceuticals	11/21/1997
S3A Toxicokinetics: The Assessment of Systemic Exposure in Toxicity Studies	3/1995
S3B Pharmacokinetics: Guidance for Repeated Dose Tissue Distribution Studies	3/1995
S4A Duration of Chronic Toxicity Testing in Animals (Rodent and Nonrodent Toxicity Testing)	Posted 6/25/99
S5A Detection of Toxicity to Reproduction for Medicinal Products	9/1994
S5B Detection of Toxicity to Reproduction for Medicinal Products: Addendum on Toxicity to Male Fertility	4/1996

S6 Preclinical Safety Evaluation of Biotechnology-Derived   11/1997
   Pharmaceuticals
S7A Safety Pharmacology Studies for Human   7/2001
   Pharmaceuticals
S7B Nonclinical Evaluation of the Potential for Delayed   10/19/2005
   Ventricular Repolarization (QT Interval Prolongation)
   by Human Pharmaceuticals
S8 Immunotoxicity Studies for Human Pharmaceuticals   4/12/2006

Points to Consider in the Manufacture and Testing of Monoclonal Antibody
Products for Human Use (1997)

APPENDIX I ESTIMATED COSTS FOR GLP COMPLIANT PRECLINICAL STUDY DESIGNS TO SUPPORT CLINICAL DEVELOPMENT

Study Title	Guidelines	Timelines		Estimated cost (USD)
		Weeks to Initiation after Authorization	Weeks for Report after Termination	
Safety Pharmacology				
Evaluation of Cardiovascular Function Using Cloned hERG Channels Expressed in Human Embryonic (HEK293) Cells	ICH S7B The Nonclinical Evaluation of the Potential for Delayed Repolarization (QT Interval Prolongation) by Human Pharmaceuticals	2–4	4–6	15,000–20,000
Evaluation of Cardiovascular Function Using Action Potential Parameters in Isolated Purkinje Fibers	ICH S7B The Nonclinical Evaluation of the Potential for Delayed Repolarization (QT Interval Prolongation) by Human Pharmaceuticals	2–4	4–6	20,000–25,000
Evaluation of Cardiovascular (Hemodynamic) Function in the Conscious Telemetered—Nonrodent	ICH S7A Safety Pharmacology Studies for Human Pharmaceuticals and ICH S7B The Nonclinical Evaluation of the Potential for Delayed Repolarization (QT Interval Prolongation) by Human Pharmaceuticals	2–4	6–8	100,000–150,000
Neuropharmacology study in Sprague-Dawley Rats	ICH S7A Safety Pharmacology Studies for Human Pharmaceuticals	2–4	6–8	20,000–40,000
Pulmonary Assessment in the Conscious Rat	ICH S7A Safety Pharmacology Studies for Human Pharmaceuticals	2–4	4–8	25,000–45,000
Tissue Cross-Reactivity (TCR)				
Human tissue cross-reactivity (3 donors)	NA	2–4	4–6	45,000–50,000
Animal tissue cross-reactivity (2 donors)	NA	2–4	4–6	65,000–70,000

APPENDIX I *Continued*

Study Title	Guidelines	Timelines		Estimated cost (USD)
		Weeks to Initiation after Authorization	Weeks for Report after Termination	
General Toxicity				
Dose Escalation Study in Rodents[a]	NA	4–6	4–8	15,000–35,000
Dose Escalation Study in Nonrodents[b]	NA	4–8	4–8	50,000–75,000
Acute Toxicology Study in Rodents[a]	Single Dose Acute Toxicity Testing for Pharmaceuticals (August 1996)	4–6	6–10	20,000–40,000
Acute Toxicology Study in Nonrodents[b]	Single Dose Acute Toxicity Testing for Pharmaceuticals (August 1996)	4–8	6–10	100,000–250,000
Four-Week Toxicology Study in Rodents[a]	ICH M3 Timing of Nonclinical Studies for the Conduct of Human Clinical Trials for Pharmaceuticals	4–8	10–12	200,000–250,000
Four-Week Toxicology Study in Nonrodents[b]	ICH M3 Timing of Nonclinical Studies for the Conduct of Human Clinical Trials for Pharmaceuticals	6–8	10–12	400,000–650,000
Three-Month Toxicology Study in Rodents[a]	ICH M3 Timing of Nonclinical Studies for the Conduct of Human Clinical Trials for Pharmaceuticals	6–8	10–12	250,000–300,000
Three-Month Toxicology Study in Nonrodents[b]	ICH M3 Timing of Nonclinical Studies for the Conduct of Human Clinical Trials for Pharmaceuticals	4–8	10–12	450,000–500,000

Six-Month Toxicology Study in Rodents[a]	ICH S4A Duration of Chronic Toxicity Testing in Animals (Rodent and Non-rodent Testing)	6–10	10–12	350,000–550,000
Nine-Month Toxicology Study in Nonrodents[a]	ICH S4A Duration of Chronic Toxicity Testing in Animals (Rodent and Non-rodent Testing)	8–12	10–12	450,000–650,000
Genotoxicity				
Salmonella typhimurium/ Escherichia coli Plate Incorporation Mutation Assay in the Presence and Absence of Induced Rat Liver S-9	ICH S2A Specific Aspects of Regulatory Genotoxicity Tests for Pharmaceuticals, ICH S2B Genotoxicity: A Standard Battery of Genotoxicity Testing of Pharmaceuticals	2–4	4–6	10,000–15,000
In vitro Chromosomal Aberration	ICH S2A Specific Aspects of Regulatory Genotoxicity Tests for Pharmaceuticals and ICH S2B Genotoxicity: A Standard Battery of Genotoxicity Testing of Pharmaceuticals	2–4	4–8	15,000–25,000
Lymphoma Mutagenesis in the L5178YTK +/– Mouse with Colony Size Evaluation in the Presence and Absence of Induced Rat Liver S-9 with a Confirmatory Study	ICH S2A Specific Aspects of Regulatory Genotoxicity Tests for Pharmaceuticals and ICH S2B Genotoxicity: A Standard Battery of Genotoxicity Testing of Pharmaceuticals and	2–4	4–8	15,000–25,000
Chemical Induction of Micronucleated Polychromatic Erythrocytes in Mouse Bone Marrow Cells	ICH S2A Specific Aspects of Regulatory Genotoxicity Tests for Pharmaceuticals and ICH S2B Genotoxicity: A Standard Battery of Genotoxicity Testing of Pharmaceuticals	2–4	4–8	15,000–25,000
Carcinogenicity Assessment				
Carcinogenicity Study in Sprague-Dawley Rats	ICH S1A The Need for Long-term Rodent Carcinogenicity Studies of Pharmaceuticals and ICH S1B Testing for Carcinogenicity of Pharmaceuticals (2yr)	8–10	26–30	1–1.5M

APPENDIX I *Continued*

Study Title	Guidelines	Weeks to Initiation after Authorization	Weeks for Report after Termination	Estimated cost (USD)
			Timelines	
Carcinogenicity Study in Mice	ICH S1A The Need for Long-term Rodent Carcinogenicity Studies of Pharmaceuticals and ICH S1B Testing for Carcinogenicity of Pharmaceuticals (2 yr)	8–10	26–30	1–1.5 M
Carcinogenicity Testing Using the Transgenic Mouse (p53+/−, ras H2, or Tg.AC)	ICH S1A The Need for Long-term Rodent Carcinogenicity Studies of Pharmaceuticals and ICH S1B Testing for Carcinogenicity of Pharmaceuticals (6 months)	12–16	13–17	650,000–750,000
Reproductive/Developmental Toxicity Studies				
Study of Fertility and Early Embryonic Development to Implantation in Sprague-Dawley Rats (Segment 1)	ICH S5A Detection of Toxicity to Reproduction for Medicinal Products and FDA	4–6	6–8	125,000–175,000
Study for Effects on Embryofetal Development and Toxicokinetics in Rats (Segment 2)	ICH S5A Detection of Toxicity to Reproduction for Medicinal Products	4–6	8–12	100,000–125,000
Study for Effects on Embryofetal Development and Toxicokinetics in New Zealand White Rabbits (Segment 2)	ICH S5A Detection of Toxicity to Reproduction for Medicinal Products	4–6	8–12	125,000–150,000

Study for Effects on Embryofetal Development and Toxicokinetics in the Monkey (Segment 2)	ICH S5A Detection of Toxicity to Reproduction for Medicinal Products	39–52	13–26	750,000–1,250,000
Study for Effects on Pre- and Postnatal Development, Including Maternal Function in Sprague-Dawley Rates (Segment 3)	ICH S5A Detection of Toxicity to Reproduction for Medicinal Products	4–6	8–10	200,000–250,000
Study for Effects on Pre- and Postnatal Development, Including Maternal Function in the Monkey (Segment 3)	ICH S5A Detection of Toxicity to Reproduction for Medicinal Products	39–52	21–34	1,000,000–1,500,000
Local Tolerance				
Rabbit Ear Vein		2–4	4–6	1000–5000
Other Toxicity Studies				
Irritation and sensitization—rabbit, guinea pig	NA	2–4	4–6	9000–15,000
Hemolytic Potential	NA	2–4	4–6	6000–10,000
Photoxicity Study in Rodents[a]	NA	4–6	6–10	40,000–50,000

[a] Rodent (mouse or rat).
[b] Nonrodent (dog or monkey).
[c] ICH Guidance Documents (www.ich.org).
[d] Single Dose Acute Toxicity Testing for Pharmaceuticals (August 1996).

CHAPTER 38

Practical Considerations in the Design of Preclinical Safety Assessments for Biopharmaceuticals

DAMON R. DEMADY, PhD

Contents

38.1 INTRODUCTION

While good scientific principles should always be applied to preclinical assessments of biopharmaceuticals, practical considerations for the implementation of said methods should be given equal consideration when designing and conducting these studies. Some of these considerations are the subject of this chapter and will be discussed briefly mainly through tabular illustration.

A number of recent FDA developments and initiatives have addressed novel approaches to biopharmaceutical product development and regulatory review, ranging from reorganization that has led to a fundamental shift of primary regulatory authority for therapeutic biologics from the Center for

Preclinical Safety Evaluation of Biopharmaceuticals: A Science-Based Approach to Facilitating Clinical Trials, edited by Joy A. Cavagnaro
Copyright © 2008 by John Wiley & Sons, Inc.

Biologics Evaluation and Research (CBER) to the Center for Drug Evaluation and Research (CDER) through guidance documents and concept papers on key initiatives issued or under way. The result of the transfer of the biopharmaceuticals from CBER to CDER has resulted in a partial adaptation of CDER guidelines and preferences superimposed on prior CBER and ICH precedents as they relate to the contrasts between biologics and small-molecule drug development. More and more, regulatory agencies are requiring assessments for biologics that have increasingly similar features to what one would undertake in a small-molecule development program, although it is not clear in all cases that the additional studies that may be required provide important additional information to support clinical trials.

The primary goals of preclinical safety evaluation articulated in ICH S6 are namely (1) to identify an initial safe dose and subsequent dose escalation schemes in humans, (2) to identify potential target organs for toxicity and for the study of whether such toxicity is reversible, and (3) to identify safety parameters for clinical monitoring. These goals are generally accepted across all product classes.

Small-molecule pharmaceuticals typically require two species for general toxicology evaluation that have large historical databases within a CRO and/or the public literature. In contrast, biologics should be evaluated in at least one, preferably two, species in which the test article is biologically active, namely a receptor or other entity that specifically recognizes the test article and elicits a specific pharmacological response.

38.2 SPECIES SELECTION

The evaluations to determine relevant species for toxicity evaluation include various receptor binding assays and tissue cross-reactivity assessments, the later being routinely performed for monoclonal antibody based products (see Chapters 10 and 26). Species specificity can be determined using properly controlled in vitro cell-based response assays, cloning of receptors and ligands to determine compatibility, receptor-based response assays, immunoassays, genomic-based assays, and traditional biochemical-based assays as well as in vivo assessments with validated endpoints and markers for specificity.

The ICH S6 guidance states that toxicity studies in nonrelevant species may be misleading and so are discouraged. When no relevant species exists, the use of relevant transgenic animals expressing the human receptor or the use of homologous proteins should be considered.

A pragmatic consideration for long-term toxicology studies of biopharmaceuticals is the development of antibodies against the test article in question. If these antibodies are neutralizing, then exposure to active drug over the long term (roughly longer than 3–4 weeks) is unlikely, negating the utility of the study to qualify the safety and characterize exposure in the species in question. It is not uncommon for biopharmaceuticals not to be pharmacologically active in the standard toxicology species of rats, dogs, or pigs. While surrogate molecules active in rodent species can be acceptable, typically a nonhuman primate (NHP) is the relevant species to assess safety and characterize exaggerated pharmacology, but properly controlled studies should be conducted to determine responsive species in particular to justify the use of NHPs.

38.3 ANIMAL USE, NUMBERS, AND GENDER

Once a species is selected, the number of animals per group must be decided. The interrelationship between the probability of a given toxic effect in humans and the numbers of animals required in a toxicology study to ensure the same toxic effect can be observed in Table 38.1. Clearly, to pick up low probability events would be prohibitive in terms of animal usage. In efforts to maximize the chances of seeing an effect, it is generally accepted that toxicology studies use a lower number of animals per group number, and use a higher dose multiple or dose frequency (within reason, ethical guidelines, and test article-driven feasibility) to compensate for commonly underpowered studies especially NHP studies. This approach maximizes the chances of observing relevant test article-related toxicity. Particularly in the case of NHPs, higher dose multiples, more frequent monitoring, and sample collections incorporating noninvasive pharmacodynamic or toxicity evaluations and longer duration studies, are factors that can help compensate for smaller sample size.

On average, 10 to 15 rodents and 3 to 5 nonrodents per sex per group are used for repeat-dose toxicity studies. If possible, 5 rodents and 2 to 3 nonrodents per sex per group should be used for recovery arms. The reuse of nonrodent species is a common practice, particularly for pharmacokinetic studies and in studies in which telemetry is used. Early pilot non-GLP studies for dose selection purposes may also involve the reuse of animals. However, it may not be appropriate in all instances to reuse animals based on the level of

TABLE 38.1   Relationship between animal numbers and observing human toxicity

Probability of Toxic Effects in Human	Animals in Experiments ($p = 0.95$)
100	1
80	2
60	4
50	5
40	8
20	14
10	29
5	59
2	149
1	299
0.1	2,995
0.01	29,956

invasiveness of the procedure, the degree of pain and distress, or the potential for underlying toxicity from a previous compound. When testing is performed on a novel compound or an innovative family class, or when a rare effect is expected, minimization of animal numbers per study group could be risky or counterproductive [1].

To investigate a possible gender effect, regulatory testing should be performed on both genders. One gender can be used for investigative and exploratory studies (e.g., mechanistic studies). Such an approach may also be possible in pilot studies when the absence of a gender effect has been confirmed previously or if the intended clinical indication is for use in a single gender. In safety and toxicity studies, the use of a control group is scientifically justified. Current guidelines recommend the use of control groups in some cases, and this may mean both positive and negative controls. In most toxicity studies, control groups are necessary to evaluate test article related effects. Individual animal variation among nonrodent animals remains an important consideration. The control group is critical when evaluating subtle clinical effects or histological lesions because such findings can be hidden by spontaneous anomalies and individual animal variability. In most toxicity studies a control group is required. However, in some cases, a control group may not be required (e.g., in pilot, exploratory, or dose-finding studies, or when there are adequate in-house historical data of the vehicle used in the formulation) [1].

38.4   QUALITY OF THE TEST ARTICLE

"Safety concerns may arise from the presence of impurities or contaminants. It is preferable to rely on purification processes to remove impurities and contaminants rather than to establish a preclinical testing program for their qualification. In all cases, the product should be sufficiently characterized to allow an appropriate design of preclinical safety studies. In general, the product that is used in the definitive pharmacology and toxicology studies should be comparable to the product proposed for the initial clinical studies." (ICH S6)

One of the primary issues repeatedly arising from the guideline and from the very nature of the complexities of process development, scale up, and eventual large-scale manufacture of biologics is what material is appropriate to use during the various stages of nonclinical development. As stated above, the material should be representative of the anticipated clinical material. This needs to be supported by data, namely identity, purity, stability, and potency. See Table 38.2 for suggested analytical tests for test article used in preclinical studies.

The material need not be made under fully GMP compliant conditions to be comparable or representative of the clinical lots. As with all material used for pivotal IND enabling studies, the characterization described in the certificate of analysis should be conducted under GLP conditions. Lots used for

TABLE 38.2   Suggested analytical tests for test articles used in preclinical studies

Analytical Test Performed	Sterile Injectable	Pellet Implant	Solution or Ointment for Ophthalmic Administration	Inhalation Products	Oral Dosage Forms
Sterility	X	X		X	
Identity	X	X	X	X	X
Assay (potency)	X	X	X	X	X
Purity	X	X	X	X	X
Endotoxin (LAL)	X				
Particulates/aggregates	X				
Release rate		X			
pH	X		X	X	X
Microbial limits	X	X	X	X	X
Contaminants (product related, process related)	X	X	X	X	X
Dissolution					X
Homogeneity				X	X

(Column header spanning "Sterile Injectable", "Pellet Implant", "Solution or Ointment for Ophthalmic Administration", "Inhalation Products", "Oral Dosage Forms": **Dosage Form Sampled**)

toxicology, pharmacology, and safety assessments should be less pure than clinical material if they are to be different than the clinical lot.

Bioburden testing is required for biologics used in pivotal preclinical studies to support clinical development and registration. Endotoxin levels are the primary concern in this regard. There are several major regulatory documents listed below (taken from Associates of Cape Cod Inc. Web site: *http://www.acciusa.com/*) that describe how drugs, devices, dialysate, water, and other substances are to be tested for endotoxin.

- Guideline on Validation of the Limulus Amebocyte Lysate Test as an End-Product
- Endotoxin Test for Human and Animal Parenteral Drugs, Biological Products, and Medical Devices, FDA, December, 1987.
- Interim Guidance for Human and Veterinary Drug Products and Biologicals, Kinetic LAL Techniques, FDA, July 1991.
- Bacterial Endotoxins Test, United States Pharmacopoeia
- Transfusion and Infusion Assemblies and Similar Medical Devices, United States Pharmacopoeia (USP)
- Bacterial Endotoxins Test, European Pharmacopoeia
- Bacterial Endotoxins Test, Japanese Pharmacopoeia XIV

The USP now recognizes two tests—the pyrogen test conducted with rabbits and the bacterial endotoxins test, also termed the limulus amebocyte lysate

(LAL) test. Additionally the agency has approved the use of the bacterial endotoxins test for many drug and device products.

The endotoxin limits (measured by endotoxin units, or EU) apply for drugs and devices administered to humans or animals are listed below:

- Limit for parenteral drugs: 5.0 EU/kg. Assume a 70 kg human adult, unless administering drugs to children.
- Limit for drugs being injected intrathecally: 0.2 EU/kg.

Vehicle selection is an important consideration in all animal investigations. The vehicles should offer optimal absorption and exposure of test article. Consideration should be given for time of absorption before exposure but should not influence the results obtained for the test article under investigation, and as such they should ideally be biologically inert, have no effect on the biophysical properties of the compound, and have no toxic effects on the animals. If a component of the vehicle has biological effects, the dose should be limited such that these effects are minimized or not produced. Simple vehicles used to administer test articles include aqueous isotonic solutions, buffered solutions, co-solvent systems, suspensions, and oils. When administering suspensions, the viscosity, pH, and osmolality of the material need to be considered. The use of co-solvent systems needs careful attention because the vehicles themselves have dose-limiting toxicity. Laboratories are encouraged to develop a strategy to facilitate selection of the most appropriate vehicle based on the animal study being performed and the properties of the substance under investigation. Table 38.3 lists some of the common vehicles used for test article administration that are generally considered to be nontoxic and nonirritating.

38.5 DOSE SELECTION AND ADMINISTRATION

Body weights and surface area are considered in dose selection (see Table 38.4). A variety of physiological parameters are also considered in dose considerations. (see Table 38.5 through 38.8)

Toxicology studies are designed to establish a no observable adverse effect level (NOAEL) and a maximum tolerated dose (MTD) or a maximum feasible dose (MFD). The later is determined in part by the dosage form and maximum volumes that can be administered in an animal via the intended route of administration. (see Tables 38.9 through 38.11)

38.5.1 Determination of No Observed Adverse Effect Level (NOAEL)

The common definition of NOAEL is "the highest experimental point that is without adverse effect" or "the highest dose used that produces no evidence of adverse effects using the most susceptible but appropriate species and the

TABLE 38.3   Common vehicles for test article administration

Oral	Water
	Methyl cellulose (0.5–5% aqueous suspension)
	Carboxymethyl cellulose
	Hydroxypropylmethyl cellulose
Dermal	Physiological saline
	Water
	Ethanol
	Acetone
	Mineral oil
Parenteral	Physiological saline (sterile)
	Water (sterile)

TABLE 38.4   Equivalent surface area dosage conversion factors

	Mouse (20 g)	Rat (150 g)	Monkey (3 kg)	Dog (8 kg)	Minipig (15 kg)	Human (60 kg)
Mouse	1	1/2	1/4	1/6	1/11	1/12
Rat	2	1	1/2	1/3	1/6.4	1/6
Monkey	4	2	1	3/5	1/2.7	1/3
Dog	6	4	3/2	1	1/1.8	1/2
Minipig	11	6.4	2.7	1.8	1	0.9
Human	12	7	3	2	1/1.1	1

Example: 50 mg/kg in the mouse to equivalent in monkeys assuming equal mg/m^2: 50 mg/kg * 1/4 = 13 mg/kg.

TABLE 38.5   Comparative physiological reference values

Species	Average Life Span (years)	Body Weight (kg)	Food Consumption Factor (g/day)	Food Consumption Factor[a]	Water Consumption (ml/day)	Inhalation Rate (m^3/day)
Human	70	70	2000	0.028	1400	20
Mouse	1.5–2	0.03	4	0.13	6	0.052
Rat	2	0.35	18	0.05	50	0.29
Hamster	2.4	0.14	12	0.083	27	0.13
Guinea pig	4.5	0.84	34	0.040	200	0.40
Rabbit	7.8	3.8	186	0.049	410	2
Cat	17	3	90	0.030	220	1.2
Dog	12	12.7	318	0.025	610	4.3
Monkey (rhesus)	18	8	320	0.040	530	5.4

Source: Modified from US EPA, Development of Statistical Distributions or Ranges of Standard Factors Used in Exposure Assessments, Office of Health and Environmental Assessments, EPA No. 600/8-85/010, NTIS, PB85-242667, 1985.

[a]Fraction of body weight consumed per day as food.

TABLE 38.6 Comparative physiological parameters

	Mouse (0.02 kg)	Rat (0.25 kg)	Rabbit (2.5 kg)	Monkey (5 kg)	Dog (10 kg)	Human (70 kg)
Surface area (m2)	0.008	0.023	0.17	0.32	0.51	1.85
Mean life span potential (yr)	2.7	4.7	8.0	22	20	93
Total plasma protein (g/100 ml)	6.2	6.7	5.7	8.8	9.0	7.4
Plasma albumin (g/100 ml)	3.3	3.2	3.9	4.9	2.6	4.2
Hematocrit (%)	45	46	36	41	42	44
Total ventilation (L/min)	0.03	0.12	0.80	1.7	1.50	8.0
Respiratory rate (L/min)	163	85	51	38	2	12
Heart rate (beats/min)	624	362	213	192	96	65
Oxygen consumption (ml/hr/g body wt)	1.6	0.85	0.5	0.4	0.34	0.20

Source: Adapted from B. Davies and T. Morris (1993). Physiological parameters in laboratory animals and humans. *Pharmaceutical Research* 10(7):1093–1095.

TABLE 38.7 Comparative volumes of various organs and body fluids

	Mouse (0.02 kg)	Rat (0.25 kg)	Rabbit (2.5 kg)	Monkey (5 kg)	Dog (10 kg)	Human (70 kg)
Organ volumes (ml)						
Brain	—	1.2	—	—	72	1,450
Liver	1.3	19.6	100	135	500	1,700
Kidneys	0.35	3.7	15	30	60	300
Heart	0.095	1.2	6	17	120	300
Spleen	0.1	1.3	1	—	36	200
Lungs	0.1	2.1	17	—	120	1,200
Gut	1.5	11.3	120	230	500	1,700
Muscle	10.0	245	1,400	2,500	5,500	35,000
Adipose	—	10.0	120	—	—	10,000
Skin	3.0	40.0	110	500	—	7,800
Blood	1.7	13.5	165	375	900	5,200
Total body water (ml)	15.0	167	1,800	3,500	6,000	42,000
Intracellular fluid (ml)	—	93.0	1,200	2,400	3,300	24,000
Extracellular fluid (ml)	—	75.0	625	1,000	2,800	18,000
Plasma volume (ml)	1.0	7.8	110	225	500	3,000

Source: Adapted from B. Davies and T. Morris (1993). Physiological parameters in laboratory animals and humans. *Pharmaceutical Research* 10(7):1093–1095.

TABLE 38.8 Comparative cardiovascular characteristics

| Species | Energy Metabolism | | Cardiac Function | | | | | Arterial Blood Pressure (mm Hg) | |
	cal/kg/day	Cal/m²/day	Heart Wt. (g/100 g)	Heart Rate (beats/min)	Stroke Vol (ml/beat)	Cardiac Output (L/min)	Cardiac Index (L/m²/min)	Systolic	Diastolic
Rat	120–140	760–905	0.24–0.58	250–400	1.3–2.0	0.015–0.079	1.6	88–184	58–145
Rabbit	47	810	0.19–0.36	123–330	1.3–3.8	0.25–0.75	1.7	95–130	60–90
Monkey	49	675	0.34–0.39	165–240	8.8	1.06	—	137–188	112–152
Dog	34–39	770–800	0.65–0.96	72–130	14–22	0.65–1.57	2.9	95–136	43–66
Human	23–26	790–910	0.45–0.65	41–108	62.8	5.6	3.3	92–150	53–90
Pig	14–17	1100–1360	0.25–0.40	55–86	39–43	5.4	4.8	144–185	98–120

Source: Adapted from M. A. Hollinger and M. J. Derelanko (2002). *Handbook of Toxicology*, 2nd ed. New York: CRC Press LLC, pp. 1275.

TABLE 38.9 Suggested ranges of needle sizes for test article administration

Species	Gavage	IV		IP		SC		IM	
	Recommended	Ideal	Range	Ideal	Range	Ideal	Range	Ideal	Range
Mouse	Premature infant feeding tube cut to 70 mm, marked at 38 mm.	25 or 27	25–30	25 or 27	22–30	25 or 27	22–30	25 or 27	22–30
Rat	3-inch ball-tipped intubation needle	25	25–30	25	22–30	25	25–30	25	22–30
Rabbit	Number 18 French catheter, cut to 15 inches, marked at 12 inches	21	21–22	21	18–23	25	22–25	25	22–30
Dog	Kaslow stomach tube 12Fr> 24 inches: Davol 32Fr>intubation tube	21	21–22	—	—	22	20–23	21 or 25	20–25
Monkey	Number 8 French tube (nasogastric gavage)	25	25–30	—	—	22	22–25	25	22–25

Source: Adapted from C. S. Auletta (2002), *Handbook of Toxicology*, 2nd ed. New York: CRC Press LLC, pp. 98.

TABLE 38.10   Recommended test article administration volumes (considered maximal)

Species	Route and Volumes (ml/kg)					
	Oral	SC[a]	IP	IM[b]	IV (bolus)	IV (slow)
Mouse	10 (50)	10 (40)	20 (80)	0.05[c] (0.1)	5	(25)
Rat	10 (40)	5 (10)	10 (20)	0.1[c] (0.2)	5	(20)
Rabbit	10 (15)	1 (2)	5 (20)	0.25 (0.5)	2	(10)
Dog	5 (15)	1 (2)	1 (20)	0.25 (0.5)	2.5	(5)
Macaque	5 (15)	2 (5)	(10)	0.25 (0.5)	15	(4)
Marmoset	10 (15)	2 (5)	(10)	0.25 (0.5)	2.5	(10)
Minipig	10 (15)	1 (2)	1 (20)	0.25 (0.5)	2.5	(5)

Source: Adapted from K. Diehl, R. Hull, D. Morton, R. Pfister, Y. Rabemampianina, D. Smith, J. M. Vidal, and C. van de Vorstenbosch (2001). A good practice guide to the administration of substances and removal of blood, including routes and volumes. *Journal of Applied Toxicology* 21: 15–23.

[a]Maximum of 2–3 SC sites per day.
[b]Maximum of two IM sites per day.
[c]Values in ml/site.

TABLE 38.11   Repeated intravenous infusion: dose volumes/rates (and possible maximal volumes/rates)

Daily infusion period (hours)	Mouse	Rat	Rabbit	Dog	Macaque	Minipig
	Total daily volume (ml/kg)					
4	20	20	[a]	20	15	[a]
24	96 (192)	60 (96)	24 (72)	24 (96)	60	24
	*Rate (ml/kg * h)*					
4	[a]	5	[a]	5	10	[a]
24	4 (8)	2.5 (4)	1 (3)	1 (4)	4	1

Source: Adapted from K. Diehl, R. Hull, D. Morton, R. Pfister, Y. Rabemampianina, D. Smith, J. M. Vidal, and C. van de Vorstenbosch (2001). A good practice guide to the administration of substances and removal of blood, including routes and volumes. *Journal of Applied Toxicology* 21: 15–23.

Note: In some cases two sets of values are shown. Those in parentheses are the possible maximal values.
[a]Wide variability of values, nonstandardized.

most sensitive indicator." The NOAEL must, by definition, be one of the experimental doses tested.

The NOAEL is used by regulatory agencies to establish acceptable doses. Safety factors are often used to adjust from the NOAEL to a dose that is deemed safe for initial human trials, typically 10 to 100-fold. While there are some inherent weaknesses in the concept of the NOAEL (minimizing the dose–response, in general, in favor of a single point and the probabilistic concept that exposures that test fewer animals tend to produce larger NOAELs), it is still widely used in toxicological evaluations. Dorato et al. [2] discuss the working definitions of the NOAEL, factors to be taken into account when determining the NOAEL, as well as the shortcomings inherent in the methods employed for determining the NOAEL.

When planning nonclinical studies that are focused on establishing a NOAEL to support the next phase of clinical development, a few major considerations should be kept in mind:

1. Number of animals per dose group. The larger the n, the higher is the probability of identifying toxicity.
2. Number and range of doses administered. The more dose groups and the wider the range of doses, the more likely toxicity will be observed.
3. Endpoints. The more numerous the evaluations (organ weights, tissue histology, clinical pathology, etc.) the more likely toxicity will be observed.

38.5.2   Determination of the Maximum Tolerated Dose (MTD)

The MTD is defined generally as the highest dose of the test agent that is predicted not to alter the animals' longevity or growth because of noncancer effects. The MTD thus varies inversely with the toxicity of a chemical. The major endpoints factoring into the determination of a MTD are as follows:

1. *Mortality*. Generally a mortality rate of 10% to 15% of a dose group due to test article administration indicates that a MTD has been achieved at that dose.
2. *Body weight changes*. Generally, a 10% to 15% decrease in percent body weight gain (not absolute body weight) compared to control groups indicates that a MTD has been achieved at that dose.
3. *Histology*. The identification of target organs with effects clearly attributable to test article indicates that a MTD has been achieved at that dose.

The three parameters above are not the sole set of criteria for determining a MTD, but rather, they are the more significant indicators of toxicity to guide the investigator in characterizing the toxicity of a test article and implementing subsequent studies. The MTD thus determined applies only to that particular study type for the duration of the in-life portion. When planning a preclinical study with preexisting relevant data from a previous study, it is generally applicable to use the previously established MTD to set doses for the subsequent study by selecting a high dose lower than that of the MTD, and then decreasing doses from there to round out mid and lower doses. This will maximize the probability of dose groups surviving the duration of the study in adequate numbers.

38.6   PHARMACOKINETICS (PK) AND TOXICOKINETICS (TK)

The S6 guidelines mention the difficulty of standard guidances for PK and TK studies for biologics. However, single- and repeat-dose PK studies along with tissue distribution studies can be useful. It should be noted as in the discussion concerning immunogenicity that the formation of neutralizing antibodies against the biologic can affect exposure by clearing the drug, thus significantly reducing or eliminating exposure as well as quenching the pharmacodynamic responses to drug action (e.g., ablation of neopterin response after neutralizing antibody formation against human interferon beta treatment in rhesus monkeys). Some cases, as is the case with interferons exposure, are best assessed through the measurement of pharmacodynamic biomarkers of activity.

Biologics are mostly administered parenterally: subcutaneously (SC), intramuscularly (IM), and intravenously (IV). Intravenous administration is the most pharmocokinetically reliable mode of administration, but IM or SC is preferred for biopharmaceuticals that will be administered chronically. Absorption of biopharmaceutical products is influenced by molecular weight but also by non-compound dependent factors like co-administration of albumin, depth of injection, blood flow at injection site, exercise, rubbing, and temperature [3].

The site of administration also influences their pharmacokinetic behavior. Following SC or IM administration, the bioavailability of biopharmaceuticals is often lower than with small molecules due to proteolysis during interstitial and lymphatic transit. Oral delivery of biopharmaceuticals is limited by barriers such as enzymatic and pH-dependent degradation in the gastrointestinal tract, low epithelial permeability, and instability under formulation conditions. Therefore biopharmaceuticals have an extremely low (<1%) and erratic bioavailability after oral administration [3].

Immunogenicity assays for investigating the frequency and consequences of antibody development against a protein therapeutic agent are typically based on an immunoassay technique (mostly ELISAs of various types). However, other assay formats are available such as radioimmunoprecipitation assay, surface plasmon resonance, and electrochemiluminescence [3]. Assays for measuring antibody response should be established in the early preclinical stage of development to estimate the value of the applied animal models (see Chapters 16 and 20).

Because of the catabolism of proteins to (mostly) endogenous amino acids, classical biotransformation studies as performed for small molecules are not needed. Additionally, limitations of current analytical methods to detect and distinguish metabolites and the putative lack of pharmacological or toxicological activity of the metabolites, remain obstacles. Similarly mass balance studies usually used to determine the excretion pathways of small molecules (and their metabolites) are not useful for biologics [3].

For radiolabeled proteins, placement of the radiolabel is critical to the success of the study in regards to tissue distribution and other parameters related to "absorption-distribution-metabolism-excretion" or ADME characterization.

38.7 BLOOD SAMPLING AND MAXIMUM BLOOD VOLUME

An important parameter to consider in the design of toxicology studies is the amount of blood that can be obtained for use, not only in pharmacokinetic/toxicokinetic assessments but for the monitoring of routine clinical pathology parameters (hematology, coagulation, clinical chemistry) as well as other pharmacodynamic markers and other endpoints that may be included specific to the product class. Tables 38.12 through 38.14 provide guidance with respect to the method of blood draw as well as maximal volumes and recoveries for various species.

TABLE 38.12 Advantages and disadvantages of various methods of blood sampling

Route/Vein	General Anaesthesia	Tissue Damage[a]	Repeat Bleeds	Volume	Species
Jugular	No	Low	Yes	+++	Rat, dog, rabbit
Cephalic	No	Low	Yes	+++	Macaque, dog
Saphenous/lateral tarsal	No	Low	Yes	++(+)	Mouse/rat, marmoset/ macaque, dog
Marginal ear	No (local)	Low	Yes	+++	Rabbit, minipig
Femoral	No	Low	Yes	+++	Marmoset/macaque
Sublingual	Yes	Low	Yes	+++	Rat
Lateral tail	No	Low	Yes	++(+)+	Rat, mouse/ marmoset
Central ear artery	No (local)	Low	Yes	+++	Rabbit
Cranial vena cava	No	Low	Yes	+++	Minipig
Tail tip amputation (<1–3 mm)	Yes	Mod	Limited	+	Mouse/rat
Retrobulbar plexus	Yes	Moderate/ high	Yes	+++	Mouse/rat
Cardiac[b]	Yes	Moderate	No	+++	Mouse/rat/rabbit

Source: Adapted from K. Diehl, R. Hull, D. Morton, R. Pfister, Y. Rabemampianina, D. Smith, J. M. Vidal, and C. van de Vorstenbosch (2001). A good practice guide to the administration of substances and removal of blood, including routes and volumes. *Journal of Applied Toxicology* 21: 15–23.

[a]The potential for tissue damage is based on the likely incidence of it occurring and the severity of any sequelae, (e.g., inflammatory reaction or histological damage).

[b]Only carried out as a terminal procedure under general anaesthesia.

TABLE 38.13 Comparative total blood volumes and recommended maximum blood sample volumes per body weight

Species (weight)	Blood Volume (ml)	7.5% (ml)	10% (ml)	15% (ml)	20% (ml)
Mouse (25 g)	1.8	0.1	0.2	0.3	0.4
Rat (250 g)	16	1.2	1.6	2.4	3.2
Rabbit (4 kg)	224	17	22	34	45
Dog (10 kg)	850	64	85	127	170
Macaque (rhesus) (4 kg)	280	21	28	42	56
Macaque (cynomolgus) (5 kg)	325	24	32	49	65
Minipig (15 kg)	975	73	98	146	195

Source: Adapted from K. Diehl, R. Hull, D. Morton, R. Pfister, Y. Rabemampianina, D. Smith, J. M. Vidal, and C. van de Vorstenbosch (2001). A good practice guide to the administration of substances and removal of blood, including routes and volumes. *Journal of Applied Toxicology* 21: 15–23.

TABLE 38.14 Limit volumes for blood sampling and recovery periods

Single Sampling		Multiple sampling	
Circulatory Blood Volume Removed (%)	Approximate Recovery Period	Circulatory Blood Volume Removed in 24 h (%)	Approximate Recovery Period
7.5	1 week	7.5	1 week
10	2 weeks	10–15	2 weeks
15	4 weeks	20	3 weeks

Source: Adapted from K. Diehl, R. Hull, D. Morton, R. Pfister, Y. Rabemampianina, D. Smith, J. M. Vidal, and C. van de Vorstenbosch (2001). A good practice guide to the administration of substances and removal of blood, including routes and volumes. *Journal of Applied Toxicology* 21: 15–23.

38.8 ASSESSMENT OF TOXICITY

In addition to measuring various "in-life" parameters, postmortem assessments provide useful information with respect to understanding potential toxicities as well as insight as to potential mechanisms of toxicity. A summary of comparable weights of various target organs is provided in Table 38.15. This table is also useful when considering dose for specific targeted deliveries (e.g., via intercranial, intercardiac, or inhalation routes). An understanding of both incidence and severity of a histopathological finding is important to the understanding of toxicity (see Tables 38.16 and 38.17). For example a low incidence of a finding graded as severe could be predictive of a response in a subset of patients in a clinical population. Likewise a dose-related increase in a finding of lower severity may be a predictor of a potential adverse clinical response. The recommendations of a safe starting dose and dose escalation scheme and

TABLE 38.15   Comparative weights of various organs

	Mouse (0.025 kg)	Rat (0.25 kg)	Rabbit (2.5 kg)	Rhesus monkey (4 kg)	Dog (10 kg)	Human (70 kg)
Organ weights (g)						
Brain	0.4	2.0	14	90	80	1400
Liver	1.9	10.0	80	150	320	1800
Kidneys	0.3	2.0	15	25	50	300
Heart	0.08	1.0	5	19.0	80	340
Spleen	0.1	0.9	1	8	25	180
Adrenals	0.004	0.05	0.5	1.4	1	14
Lung	0.14	1.5	20	33	100	1000

TABLE 38.16   Common abbreviations and codes used in histopathology assessments

Code	Finding or Observation
+ (1)	Minimal grade lesion
++(2)	Mild or slight grade lesion
+++(3)	Moderate grade lesion
++++(4)	Marked or severe grade lesion
+++++(5)	Very severe or massive grade lesion
(No entry)	Lesion not present or organ/tissue not examined
+	Tissue examined microscopically
–	Organ/tissue present, no lesion in section
A	Autolysis precludes examination
B	Primary benign tumor
I	Incomplete section of organ/tissue or insufficient tissue for evaluation
M	Primary malignant tumor
M	Organ/tissue missing, not present in section
N	No section of organ/tissue
N	Normal, organ/tissue within normal limits
NCL	No corresponding lesion for gross finding
NE	Organ/tissue not examined
NSL	No significant lesion, organ/tissue within normal limits
P	Lesion present, not graded (e.g., cyst, anomaly)
U	Unremarkable organ/tissue, within normal limits
WNL	Organ/tissue within normal limits
X	Not remarkable organ/tissue, normal
X	Incidence of listed morphology, lesion present

Source: Adapted from J. C. Peckham (2002). *Handbook of Toxicology*, 2nd ed. New York: CRC Press LLC, pp. 655.

TABLE 38.17 Frequently used grading schemes (severity scores) for histopathology findings

Severity Degree	Proportion of Organ Affected	(A) Grade	Percentage of Organ Affected	(B) Grade	Percentage of Organ Affected	(C) Grade	Percentage of Organ Affected	(D) Grade	Percentage of Organ Affected	(E) Grade	Quantifiable Finding
Minimal	Very small amount	1	(A1) < 1–25% (A2) < 1–15%	1	<1%			1	<1%	1	<1%
Slight	Very small to small amount			2	1–25%	1	1–25%			1	1–4 foci
Mild	Small amount	2	(A1) 26–50% (A2) 16–35%			2	26–50%	2	1–30%	2	5–8 foci
Moderate	Middle or median amount	3	(A1) 51–75%	3	26–50%	3	51–76%	3	31–60%	3	9–12 foci
Marked	Large amount	4	(A1) 76–100% (A2) 61–100%							4	>12 foci
Moderately severe	Large amount			4	51–75%						
Severe	Very large amount			5	76–100%	4	76–100%	4	61–90%		
Very severe or massive	Very large amount							5	91–100%		

Source: Adapted from J. C. Peckham (2002). *Handbook of Toxicology*, 2nd ed. New York: CRC Press LLC, pp. 656.

clinical monitoring parameters are based on the totality of the toxicology and exposure data.

ACKNOWLEDGMENTS

The author thanks Joshua Bender of the Pittsburgh Technology Council for his assistance in compiling the tables presented in this chapter.

REFERENCES

International Symposium on Regulatory Testing and Animal Welfare. Recommendations on best scientific practices for safety evaluation using nonrodent species. *ILAR J* 2002;43(Suppl).

Dorato MA, Engelhardt JA. The no observed adverse effect level in drug safety evaluations: use, issues, and definitions. *J Appl Toxicol* 2005;21:15–23.

Baumann A. Early development of therapeutic biologics—pharmacokinetics. *Curr Drug Metab* 2006;7:15–21.

■■■■■■ CHAPTER 39

Survey of Preclinical Toxicology Programs for Approved Biopharmaceuticals

ANITA MARIE O'CONNOR, PhD

Contents

39.1 INTRODUCTION

This chapter provides a survey of US marketed biopharmaceuticals approved over the past 20 years. It is a simply a profile of the species and types of toxicology studies done for each drug for marketing approval. For a complete list of all preclinical studies for a biopharmaceutical, the reader is directed to the Web sites of the Food and Drug Administration (FDA) and the European Medicines Agency (EMEA).

The information found in Table 39.1 was obtained from a variety of sources: personal communications with the toxicologists who designed the programs, the FDA Web site, the EMEA Web site, and the package insert for the product

Preclinical Safety Evaluation of Biopharmaceuticals: A Science-Based Approach to Facilitating Clinical Trials, edited by Joy A. Cavagnaro
Copyright © 2008 by John Wiley & Sons, Inc.

TABLE 39.1 Toxicology studies to support biopharmaceutical approvals

Biopharmaceutical	Description ↔ Target	Indication	Toxicology Studies[a]
Abraxane™ (paclitaxel formulated in human serum albumin in a 1 : 9 ratio) (US) Approval: 2005	Albumin bound form of paclitaxel ↔ causes apoptosis in cancer cells	Metastatic breast cancer	<u>Single dose</u>: rats, dogs, swine[b] <u>Repeat dose</u>: athymic nude mice implanted with MX-1 tumors; other studies were complicated by immune reactions to human serum albumin <u>Fertility and early embryonic development</u>: rats <u>Developmental</u>: rats <u>Prenatal and postnatal development</u>: none <u>Genetic toxicology</u>[c]: Ames test, human lymphocyte chromosomal aberration assay, CHO/HGPRT gene mutation assay, mouse micronucleus assay <u>Carcinogenicity</u>: none
Actimune® (interferon gamma-1b) (US) Approval: 1999	Human recombinant interferon gamma-1b ↔ multiple targets within the lymphokine regulatory network	Infections associated with chronic granulomatous disease; malignant osteopetrosis	<u>Fertility and early embryonic development</u>: cynomolgus monkeys (male and female), mice (surrogate, male and female) <u>Developmental</u>: primate[d] <u>Prenatal and postnatal development</u>: primate <u>Genetic toxicology</u>: Ames test, micronucleus assay in mice <u>Carcinogenicity</u>: none
Activase® (alteplase) (US) Approval: 1996	Recombinant human tissue plasminogen activator ↔ plasminogen with fibrin present	Restoration of function of central venous access devices as assessed by the ability to draw blood	<u>Developmental</u>: rats, rabbits <u>Genetic toxicology</u>: Ames test, human lymphocyte chromosomal aberration assay <u>Carcinogenicity</u>: short-term experiments in rodents (i.e., not standard 2-year study)

Product (Approval)	Mechanism	Indication	Toxicology studies
Adlurazyme® (laronidase) (US) Approval: 2003	Laronidase ↔ enzyme replacement therapy	Mucopolysaccharidosis-1	Single dose: rats, dogs Repeat dose: dogs, cynomolgus monkeys Fertility and early embryonic development: rats Developmental: rats Prenatal and postnatal development: none Genetic toxicology: none Carcinogenicity: none
Alferon (interferon alpha-N3) (US) Approval: 1989	Interferon alpha-N3 derived from leukocytes ↔ multiple targets within the lymphokine regulatory network	Refractory or recurring external condylomata acuminata	Fertility and early embryonic development: none Developmental: none Prenatal and postnatal development: none Genetic toxicology: none Carcinogenicity: none
Amevive® (Alefacept) (US) Approval: 2003	Dimeric glycosylated fusion protein ↔ binds to CD2 on T lymphocytes	Chronic plaque psoriasis	Single dose: rats (not relevant), baboons Repeat dose: baboons, cynomolgus monkeys Fertility and early embryonic development: none Developmental: cynomolgus monkeys Prenatal and postnatal development: cynomolgus monkeys Genetic toxicology: in vitro and in vivo Carcinogenicity: evaluated in a chronic cynomolgus monkey study Other: flow cytometry and immunhistochemical analysis of lymphoid tissues for peripheral lymphocyte subsets; humoral immunity

TABLE 39.1 *Continued*

Biopharmaceutical	Description ↔ Target	Indication	Toxicology Studies[a]
Apidra® (insulin glulisine) (US) Approval: 2004	Recombinant human insulin analogue (rapid-acting insulin) ↔ glucose metabolism	Diabetes	Single dose: mice, rats, dogs Repeat dose: rats, dogs Fertility and early embryonic development: rat (male and female) Developmental: rats, rabbits Prenatal and postnatal development: none Genetic toxicology: Ames test, in vitro mammalian chromosome aberration test in V79 Chinese hamster cells, and in vivo mammalian erythrocyte micronucleus test in rats Carcinogenicity: used the 12-month repeat dose study instead of a standard 2-year bioassay Other: cardiovascular study in dogs; drug interaction study with NPH insulin; immunogenicity in rabbits
Apligraf® (living human skin substitute) [US(CDRH)] Approval: 2000	Living, bi-layered skin substitute containing type 1 bovine collagen Extracted and purified from bovine tendons and viable allogeneic human fibroblast and keratinocytes cells isolated from human infant foreskin	Leg and diabetic foot ulcers	In vitro immunology, and Athymic nude mice proof of concept studies

Aranesp™ (darbepoetin alpha) (US) Approval: 2001	Hyperglycosylated recombinant human erythropoietin ↔ stimulation of erythropoiesis	Anemia associated with chronic renal failure; anemia due to nonmyeloid malignancies in patients treated with chemotherapy	Single dose: rats, dogs Repeat dose: rats, dogs Fertility and early embryonic development: rats Developmental: rats, rabbits Prenatal and postnatal development: rats Genetic toxicology: in vitro bacterial and CHO cell assays, mouse micronucleus assay Carcinogenicity: proliferation in vitro and in vivo Tissue cross-reactivity: human tissues Other: safety studies in a variety of species
Avastin™ (bevacizumab) (US) Approval: 2004	Recombinant human monoclonal antibody ↔ binds to vascular endothelial growth factor	Metastatic colorectal cancer in combination with 5-fluorouracil based chemotherapy	Single dose: none Repeat dose: cynomolgus monkeys Fertility and early embryonic development: rabbits Developmental: rabbits Prenatal and postnatal development: none Genetic toxicology: none Carcinogenicity: none Tissue cross-reactivity: rabbit, cynomolgus tissues Other: wound healing, hemolytic potential, blood compatability, Cisplatin renal injury induced in rabbits, rabbit thrombosis model
Avonex® (interferon beta-1a) (US) Approval: 1996	Recombinant human interferon beta-1a ↔ binds to multiple receptors	Multiple sclerosis	Single dose: rhesus monkeys Repeat dose: rhesus monkeys Fertility and early embryonic development: none Developmental: none Prenatal and postnatal development: none Genetic toxicology: Ames test Carcinogenicity: none

TABLE 39.1 *Continued*

Biopharmaceutical	Description ↔ Target	Indication	Toxicology Studies[a]
Betaseron® (interferon beta-1b) (US) Approval: 2003	Human recombinant interferon beta-1b ↔ multiple targets within the lymphokine regulatory network	Multiple sclerosis	Single dose: African green monkeys (subacute) Repeat dose: none (due to antibody development) Fertility and early embryonic development: rhesus monkeys Developmental: rhesus monkeys Prenatal and postnatal development: none Genetic toxicology: Ames test, in vitro transformation assay, human peripheral blood lymphocyte assay Carcinogenicity: none
Bexxar® (tositumomab and I[131] tositumomab) (US) Approval: 2003	Tositumomab is a murine IgG lambda monoclonal antibody ↔ targets the CD20 antigen on normal and malignant B cells I[131] tositumomab is tositumomab covalently linked to I[131]	CD20 positive follicular non-Hodgkin's lymphoma	Fertility and early embryonic development: none Developmental: none Prenatal and postnatal development: none Genetic toxicology: none Carcinogenicity: none

Campath® (alemtuzumab) (US) Approval: 2001	Recombinant humanized monoclonal antibody ↔ directed against CD52, which is expressed on the surface of normal and malignant B and T lymphocytes, NK cells, monocytes, macrophages, and tissues of the male reproductive system	B cell chronic lymphocytic leukemia	Single dose: cynomolgus monkeys Repeat dose: cynomolgus monkeys Fertility and early embryonic development: none Developmental: none Prenatal and postnatal development: none Genetic toxicology: none Carcinogenicity: none Tissue cross-reactivity: human tissues Other: cardiovascular and respiratory safety studies in anesthetized cynomolgus monkeys
Carticel® (autologous cultured chondrocytes) (US) Approval: 1997	Autologous cultured chondrocytes	Repair of clinically significant, symptomatic, cartilaginous defects of the femoral condyle (medial, lateral or trochlear) caused by acute or repetitive trauma	Other: proof of concept/safety studies in dogs and rabbits
CEA-Scan® (arcitumomab; technetium-99 labeled) (US) Approval: 1996	Acritumomab labeled with technetium-99 ↔ radiodiagnostic agent	Imaging agent for colorectal cancer	Fertility and early embryonic development: none Developmental: none Prenatal and postnatal development: none Genetic toxicology: none Carcinogenicity: none

TABLE 39.1 *Continued*

Biopharmaceutical	Description ↔ Target	Indication	Toxicology Studies[a]
Cerezyme® (imiglucerase) (US) Approval: 1994	Recombinant beta-glucocerebrosidase ↔ enzyme replacement therapy	Type I Gaucher's disease	Single dose: rats Repeat dose: rats, cynomolgus monkeys Fertility and early embryonic development: none Developmental: none Prenatal and postnatal development: none Genetic toxicology: Ames test Carcinogenicity: none
Elaprase (idursulfase) (US) Approval: 2006	Recombinant human idursulfase ↔ enzyme replacement therapy	Hunter syndrome (Mucopolysaccharidosis II)	Single dose: rats, cynomolgus monkeys Repeat dose: cynomolgus monkeys Fertility and early embryonic development: male rats Developmental: none Prenatal and postnatal development: none Genetic toxicology: none Carcinogenicity: none
Elitek® (rasburicase) (US) Approval: 2002	Recombinant urate oxidase ↔ catalyzes enzymatic oxidation of uric acid	Malignancy-associated or chemotherapy-induced hyperuricemia	Fertility and early embryonic development: rats (male and female) Developmental: none Prenatal and postnatal development: none Genetic toxicology: Ames test, unscheduled DNA synthesis, chromosome analysis, mouse lymphoma and micronucleus tests Carcinogenicity: none

Elspar (asparaginase) (US) Approval: 1994	Recombinant L-asparaginase ↔ depletion of aspargine: a metabolic defect of asparagine synthesis in malignant cells which are dependent on an exogenous source of asparagine	Acute lymphocytic leukemia in combination with chemotherapy	Single dose: rabbits Repeat dose: dogs, monkeys Fertility and early embryonic development: none Developmental: mice, rats, rabbits Prenatal and postnatal development: none Genetic toxicology: Ames test Carcinogenicity: none
Enbrel® (etanercept) (US) Approval: 1998	Fusion protein (TNFR:Fc) ↔ competitive inhibitor of TNF	Rheumatoid arthritis; Psoriatic arthritis; Ankylosing spondylitis; Psoriasis	Single dose: none Repeat dose: cynomolgus monkeys, rats, mice, rabbits Fertility and early embryonic development: none Developmental: rats, rabbit Prenatal and postnatal development: rats (abbreviated) Genetic toxicology: battery of in vitro and in vivo tests Carcinogenicity: none
Epicel® (cultured epidermal autografts) (US) Approval: unclear if ever formally approved by FDA marketed since 1987	Autologous keratinocytes are co-cultured with irradiated murine cells to form cultured epidermal autografts	Permanent skin replacement product for patients with life-threatening burns	This product was on the market in 1987, before a regulatory framework was put in place by FDA.

TABLE 39.1 *Continued*

Biopharmaceutical	Description ↔ Target	Indication	Toxicology Studies[a]
Epogen®/Procrit® (epoetin alfa) (US) Approval: 1993	Recombinant human erythropoietin ↔ committed erythroid progenitors in bone marrow by replacing or increasing erythropoietin	Anemia of chronic renal failure patients, zidovudine-treated HIV-infected patients and cancer patients on chemotherapy; reduction of allogeneic blood transfusion in surgery patients	Fertility and early embryonic development: rats Developmental: rats Prenatal and postnatal development: rats Genetic toxicology: Ames test, chromosomal aberrations in mammalian cells, micronuclei in mice, gene mutation at the HGPRT locus Carcinogenicity: none
Erbitux™ (cetuximab) (US) Approval: 2004	Chimeric monoclonal antibody ↔ inhibits the EGF receptor	Metastatic colorectal cancer (in combination with irinotecan based chemotherapy)	Single dose: mice (not relevant), rats (not relevant) Repeat dose: rats, cynomolgus monkeys Fertility and early embryonic development: none Developmental: none Prenatal and postnatal development: none Genetic toxicology: Ames test, micronucleus test in rats (not relevant) Carcinogenicity: none Tissue Cross-Reactivity: monkey, goat, rat, rabbit, and human tissues, hepatic tissues of numerous species

Product	Description	Indication	Toxicology
Exubera® (insulin) (US) Approval: 2006	Human insulin inhalation powder ↔ glucose metabolism	Type 1 or type 2 diabetes	Single dose: rats, monkeys (nonpivotal exploration studies) Repeat dose: rats, cynomolgus monkeys Fertility and early embryonic development: none Developmental: none Prenatal and postnatal development: none Genetic toxicology: Ames test Carcinogenicity: none Other: cardiovascular study in dogs
Fabrazyme® (agalsidase beta) (US) Approval: 2003	Recombinant human alpha galactosidase ↔ enzyme replacement therapy	Fabry's disease	Single dose: rats Repeat dose: rats Fertility and early embryonic development: none Developmental: none Prenatal and postnatal development: none Genetic toxicology: none Carcinogenicity: none Other: cardiovascular function in dogs
Gem 21S® (Growth factor enhanced matrix) [US(CDRH)] Approval: 2005	Tissue growth factor, recombinant human platelet-derived growth factor, and a synthetic bone matrix	Periodontal bone defects	Single dose: mice Repeat dose: none Fertility and early embryonic development: none Developmental: none Prenatal and postnatal development: none Genetic toxicology: Ames test Carcinogenicity: none Other: dermal sensitization in guinea pigs, in vitro cytotoxicity, intracutaneous reactivity in rabbits, muscle implantation in rabbits

TABLE 39.1 *Continued*

Biopharmaceutical	Description ↔ Target	Indication	Toxicology Studies[a]
Genotropin (somatropin) (US) Approval: 1995	Recombinant human growth hormone ↔ hormone replacement therapy	Growth hormone deficiency; growth failure in children and adults	Fertility and early embryonic development: rats Developmental: rats, rabbits Prenatal and postnatal development: rats Genetic toxicology: Ames test, gene mutations in mammalian cells grown in vitro (mouse L5178Y cells), and chromosomal damage in intact animals (bone marrow cells in rats) Carcinogenicity: none
Glucagen® (glucagon) (US) Approval: 1998	Recombinant human glucagon ↔ hormone replacement therapy	Hypoglycemic reactions in diabetic patients and as a diagnostic aid to reduce organ motility during radiologic examination of the gastrointestinal tract	Single dose: rats, mice Repeat dose: rats, dogs Fertility and early embryonic development: none Developmental: rats, rabbit Prenatal and postnatal development: none Genetic toxicology: Ames test, human lymphocyte, micronucleus assay in mice Carcinogenicity: none Other: cardiovascular and respiratory function in dogs
Glucagon (glucagon) (US) Approval: 1998	Recombinant human glucagon ↔ hormone replacement therapy	Hypoglycemic reactions in diabetic patients and as a diagnostic aid to reduce organ motility during radiologic examination of the gastrointestinal tract	Fertility and early embryonic development: rats Genetic toxicology: Ames test Other: approval was based mainly on a bioequivalence study comparing the recombinant product to the sponsor's animal sourced product

Drug (Approval)	Description	Indication	Toxicology
Herceptin® (trastuzumab) (US) Approval: 1998	Recombinant humanized monoclonal antibody ↔ HER2	Breast cancer	Single dose: mice, rhesus monkeys; Repeat dose: rhesus monkeys, cynomolgus monkeys; Fertility and early embryonic development: cynomolgus monkeys; Developmental: cynomolgus monkeys; Prenatal and postnatal development: cynomolgus monkeys; Genetic toxicology: Ames test, chromosome aberration assay in human peripheral lymphocytes, in vivo mouse micronucleus; Carcinogenicity: none; Tissue cross-reactivity: human and monkey tissues
Humatrope (somatropin) (US) Approval: 1987	Recombinant human growth hormone ↔ hormone replacement therapy	Growth hormone deficiency; growth failure in children and adults	Fertility and early embryonic development: none; Developmental: none; Prenatal and postnatal development: none; Genetic toxicology: unclear; Carcinogenicity: none
Humira™ (adalimumab) (US) Approval: 2002	Antitumor necrosis factor human monoclonal antibody ↔ binds to TNF-α	Rheumatoid arthritis; psoriatic arthritis; ankylosing spondylitis	Single dose: mice, rats; Repeat dose: mice, cynomolgus monkeys; Fertility and early embryonic development: none; Developmental: cynomolgus monkeys; Prenatal and postnatal development: none; Genetic toxicology: Ames test, in vivo mouse micronucleus; Carcinogenicity: none; Tissue cross-reactivity: human tissues

TABLE 39.1 *Continued*

Biopharmaceutical	Description ↔ Target	Indication	Toxicology Studies[a]
Infergen® (Interferon alfacon-1) (US) Approval: 1997	Recombinant nonnaturally occurring type-1 interferon ↔ multiple targets within the lymphokine regulatory network	Hepatitis C	Single dose: golden Syrian hamsters, rhesus monkeys Repeat dose: golden Syrian hamsters, rhesus monkeys Fertility and early embryonic development: golden Syrian hamsters Developmental: golden Syrian hamsters, rhesus monkeys, cynomolgus monkeys Prenatal and postnatal development: none Genetic toxicology: Ames test, cytogenicity assay in human lymphocytes Carcinogenicity: none
Intron A® (interferon alpha-2b) (US) Approval: 1983	Recombinant interferon alpha 2b ↔ multiple targets within the lymphokine regulatory network	Hairy cell leukemia, malignant melanoma, follicular lymphoma, condylomata acuminata, AIDS-related Kaposi's sarcoma hepatitis C, hepatitis B	Single dose: mice, rats, rhesus monkeys Repeat dose: mice, rats, rabbits, cynomolgus monkeys Fertility and early embryonic development: rats, rabbits Developmental: rats, rabbits, rhesus monkeys Prenatal and postnatal development: rats, rabbits Genetic toxicology: mutagenicity studies Carcinogenicity: none

Kepivance® (Palifermin) (US) Approval: 2004	Human recombinant keratinocytes growth factor ↔ KGF receptor	Oral mucositis in cancer patients	Single dose: rats, rhesus monkeys Repeat dose: athymic nude mice, rats, rhesus monkeys, cynomolgus monkeys Fertility and early embryonic development: rats Developmental: rabbits, rats Prenatal and postnatal development: none Genetic toxicology: Ames test, in vitro mammalian chromosome aberration assay, in vivo mouse micronucleus assay Carcinogenicity: Tg.rasH2 transgenic mouse model Other: antigenicity in guinea pigs, mice, and rats; tumor cell lines (effects of the product on proliferation); human tumor xenografts in athymic nude mice; hemolytic potential studies
Kineret™ (anakinra) (US) Approval: 2001	Human interleukin-1 receptor antagonist ↔ multiple targets within the lymphokine regulatory network	Rheumatoid arthritis	Single dose: rats, cynomolgus monkeys Repeat dose: rats, rhesus monkeys, cynomolgus monkeys Fertility and early embryonic development: rats Developmental: rabbits, rats Prenatal and postnatal development: none Genetic toxicology: none Carcinogenicity: none Other: antigenicity study in rhesus monkeys
Lantus® Insulin glargine (US) Approval: 2000	Recombinant glargine insulin (insulin analogue; long-acting) ↔ glucose metabolism	Diabetes	Single dose: mice, rats, dogs Repeat dose: rats, dogs Fertility and early embryonic development: rats Developmental: rats, rabbits Prenatal and postnatal development: rats Genetic toxicology: Ames test, in vitro mammalian chromosome aberration assay, in vivo cytogenetic test, HGPRT test with V79 cells Carcinogenicity: 2-year study in mice, 2-year study in rats study Other: immunotoxicity studies in rabbits and guinea pigs

TABLE 39.1 *Continued*

Biopharmaceutical	Description ↔ Target	Indication	Toxicology Studies[a]
Leukine® (sargramostim) (US) Approval: 1991	Recombinant human granulocyte macrophage colony-stimulating factor ↔ stimulates the production of neutrophils, monocytes/ macrophages, myeloid-derived dendritic cells	Following induction chemotherapy in older patients with acute myelogenous leukemia, after BMT, and before and/or after PBSCT	No information in the label
Levemir (insulin) (US) Approval: 2005	Recombinant insulin detemir (insulin analogue; long-acting basal) ↔ glucose metabolism	Diabetes type I (adults and pediatrics) and type II (adults)	Single dose: mice, rats Repeat dose: rats, dogs Fertility and early embryonic development: rats Developmental: rats, rabbits Prenatal and postnatal development: rats Genetic toxicology: in vitro reverse mutation study in bacteria, human peripheral blood lymphocyte chromosome aberration test, in vivo mouse micronucleus test. Carcinogenicity: none Other: mitogenicity in CHO-K1 and human B10 osteosarcoma cells, human hepatoma cells and MCF-7 cells to include drug binding study to IGF-1 and insulin receptors; local tolerance in pigs; immunogenicity studies in rabbits

Name	Description	Indication	Nonclinical studies
Lucentis™ (ranibizumab) (US) Approval: 2006	Recombinant humanized monoclonal antibody fragment (Fab) ↔ binds to vascular endothelial growth factor (VEGF)	Neovascular (wet) age-related macular degeneration	Single dose: none Repeat dose: cynomolgus monkeys Fertility and early embryonic development: none Developmental: none Prenatal and postnatal development: none Genetic toxicology: none Carcinogenicity: none Tissue cross-reactivity: human tissues Special toxicology studies: intravitreal in rabbits and cynomolgus monkeys hemolytic potential, blood compatibility and vitreal fluid compatibility, IV verteporfin photodynamic therapy following laser-induced choroidal neovascularization in cynomolgus monkeys
Mylotarg™ (gemtuzumab ozogamicin) (US) Approval: 2000	Recombinant humanized IgG4 kappa monoclonal antibody conjugated with calicheamicin ↔ chemotherapy agent, binds to CD33 on leukemic blasts and immature normal cells of myelomonocytic lineage	CD33 positive acute myeloid leukemia	Single dose: rats, cynomolgus monkeys, chimpanzees, mice, dogs Repeat dose: rats, cynomolgus monkeys Fertility and early embryonic development: rats (male and female) Developmental: rats Prenatal and postnatal development: none Genetic toxicology: mouse in vivo micronucleus test Carcinogenicity: none Tissue cross-reactivity: human, cynomolgus monkey, and rat tissues Other: cardiovascular safety in dogs, in vitro blood compatibility, derivatives of gamma calicheamicin on murine bone marrow hematopoietic colony formation in vitro; in vitro stability of hP67.6 conjugate in human, monkey, and rat plasma

TABLE 39.1 *Continued*

Biopharmaceutical	Description ↔ Target	Indication	Toxicology Studies[a]
Myozyme® (alglucosidase alfa) (US) Approval: 2006	Alglucosidase alfa ↔ enzyme replacement therapy	Pompe disease	Single dose: rats, dogs Repeat dose: rats, mice, monkeys Fertility and early embryonic development: mice Developmental: mice Prenatal and postnatal development: none Genetic toxicology: none Carcinogenicity: none
Naglazyme™ (galsulfase) (US) Approval: 2005	Recombinant human N-acetylgalactosamine 4-sulfase ↔ lysosomal hydrolase that cleaves the sulfate ester at the end of glycosaminglycans	Enzyme replacement therapy for mucopolysacch- aridosis VI	Single dose: rats, dogs Repeat dose: cynomolgus monkeys Fertility and early embryonic development: rats Developmental: rats Prenatal and postnatal development: none Genetic toxicology: none Carcinogenicity: none
Neulasta™ (pegfilgrastim) (US) Approval: 2002	Recombinant human pegylated recombinant methionyl granulocyte colony stimulating factor ↔ hematopoetic cells	Reduction of incidence of infection in non- myeloid cancer patients	Single dose: rats Repeat dose: rats, cynomolgus monkeys Fertility and early embryonic development: rats Developmental: rats, rabbits Prenatal and postnatal development: rats Genetic toxicology: none Carcinogenicity: none Tissue cross-reactivity: none Other: antigenicity in dogs and chimpanzees (these studies were done as pharmacology and PK studies) placental transfer in pregnant rats

Neumega (oprelvekin) (US) Approval: 1997	Recombinant human interleukin-11 ↔ stimulates the proliferation of hematopoietic stem cells, megakaryocyte progenitor cells, lymphoid cells, and induces the differentiation of megakaryocytes into platelets	Prevention of chemotherapy-induced thrombocytopenia and reduction of the need for platelet transfusions in patients with nonmyeloid malignancies	Single dose: rats, cynomolgus monkeys Repeat dose: rats, cynomolgus monkeys Fertility and early embryonic development: rats Developmental: rats Prenatal and postnatal development: none Genetic toxicology: human lymphocyte metaphase analysis, mammalian cell mutation assay, mouse micronucleus test Carcinogenicity: none Other: interaction study in cynomolgus monkeys using Il-11 and G-CSF or GM-CSF
Neupogen® (filgrastim) (US) Approval: 1991	Recombinant human granulocyte colony stimulating factor (G-CSF) ↔ hematopoetic cells	Chemotherapy-induced neutropenia	Single dose: mice, rats, hamsters, cynomolgus monkeys Repeat dose: hamster, rats, dogs, cynomolgus monkeys Fertility and early embryonic development: rats Developmental: rats, rabbits Prenatal and postnatal development: none Genetic toxicology: Ames test Carcinogenicity: none
Norditropin® (somatropin) (US) Approval: 2000	Human recombinant growth hormone ↔ connective tissue, mineral, protein, carbohydrate, and lipid metabolism	Growth failure due to lack of endogenous growth hormone in pediatrics	Single dose: mice Repeat dose: rats Fertility and early embryonic development: none Developmental: none Prenatal and postnatal development: none Genetic toxicology: none Carcinogenicity: none Other: transgenic human somatropin mice tested for immunogenicity

TABLE 39.1 *Continued*

Biopharmaceutical	Description ↔ Target	Indication	Toxicology Studies[a]
Novolog (insulin aspart) (US) Approval: 2000	Rapid-acting insulin analogue ↔ glucose metabolism	Diabetes type I and II	Single dose: mice Repeat dose: rats, dogs Fertility and early embryonic development: rats (males and females) Developmental: rats, rabbits Prenatal and postnatal development: rats Genetic toxicology: Ames tests, mouse lymphoma cell forward gene mutation test, human peripheral blood lymphocyte chromosome aberration test, in vivo micronucleus test in mice and ex vivo UDS test in rat liver hepatocytes Carcinogenicity: 2 one-year studies in rats Other: cardiovascular effects in pigs
Nutropin depot (somatropin) (US) Approval: 1999	Sustained release growth hormone ↔ connective tissue, mineral, protein, carbohydrate, and lipid metabolism	Growth failure due to lack of endogenous growth hormone in pediatrics; replacement of growth hormone in adults; Turner Syndrome; nongrowth hormone deficient short stature; growth failure associated with renal failure	Single dose: none Repeat dose: rhesus monkeys Fertility and early embryonic development: none Developmental: none Prenatal and postnatal development: none Genetic toxicology: none Carcinogenicity: none Other: immunogenicity in transgenic mice expressing rhGH

Drug (Approval)	Description	Indication	Toxicology studies
Ontak (denileukin diftitox) (US) Approval: 1999	Cytotoxic fusion protein composed of diphtheria toxin fragments A and B and Il-2 ↔ cytocidal action of diphtheria toxin to cells that express the IL-2 receptor	Persistent or recurrent cutaneous T cell lymphoma whose malignant cells express the CD25 component of the IL-2 receptor	Fertility and early embryonic development: none Developmental: none Prenatal and postnatal development: none Genetic toxicology: Ames test, chromosomal aberration assay Carcinogenicity: none
Oncaspar® (pegaspargase) (US) Approval: 1994	Pegylated (PEG) recombinant human L-asparaginase ↔ depletion of asparagine for leukemic cells	Acute lymphoblastic leukemia	Fertility and early embryonic development: none Developmental: none Prenatal and postnatal development: none Genetic toxicology: Ames test Carcinogenicity: none
Omnitrope (somatropin) (US) Approval: 2006	Human recombinant growth hormone ↔ connective tissue, mineral, protein, carbohydrate, and lipid metabolism	Growth failure in pediatrics due to lack of endogenous growth hormone; replacement hormone therapy in adults	*(follow-on protein product)* Fertility and early embryonic development: rats (males and females) Developmental: rats, rabbits Prenatal and postnatal development: rats Genetic toxicology: none Carcinogenicity: none

TABLE 39.1 *Continued*

Biopharmaceutical	Description ↔ Target	Indication	Toxicology Studies[a]
Orencia™ (abatacept) (US) Approval: 2005	Soluble fusion protein that consists of the extracellular domain of human cytotoxic T lymphocyte associated antigen 4 (CTLA-4) linked to the modified Fc (hinge, CH2, and CH3 domains) portion of human immunoglobulin IgG ↔ binds to T lymphocyte antigens CD80 and CD86 thus blocking interaction with CD28	Rheumatoid arthritis	Single dose: cynomolgus monkeys Repeat dose: mice, rats, cynomolgus monkeys Fertility and early embryonic development: rats Developmental: rats, mice, rabbits Prenatal and postnatal development: rats Genetic toxicology: Ames reverse mutation, Chinese hamster ovary ↔ hypoxanthine guanine phosphoribosyl-transferase forward point mutation assay, cytogenetics in human lymphocytes Carcinogenicity: 2-year assay (subcutaneous in mice)
Orthoclone OKT3® (muromomab-CD3) (US) Approval: 1992	Murine monoclonal antibody ↔ binds to the CD3 antigen of T lymphocytes	Rejection of transplanted organs	Fertility and early embryonic development: none Developmental: none Prenatal and postnatal development: none Genetic toxicology: unclear Carcinogenicity: none
Osteocel® (bone matrix) (US) Approval: 2005	Allogeneic bone matrix ↔ repair, replacement, and/or reconstruction of bone defects	Regeneration of bones in orthopedic indications	Does not require pre-market approval by the FDA because it meets the regulatory definition of human cells, tissue, and cellular and tissue-based products, or HCT/Ps.

Product	Structure/Mechanism	Indication	Toxicology
Pegasys® (peginterferon alfa-2a) (US) Approval: 2002	Covalent conjugate of interferon alfa-2a with a single branched bis-monomethoxy polyethylene glycol (PEG) chain ↔ multiple targets within the lymphokine regulatory network	Hepatitis C, hepatitis B	Single dose: cynomolgus monkeys Repeat dose: cynomolgus monkeys Fertility and early embryonic development: male rhesus monkeys, female cynomolgus monkeys Developmental: rhesus monkeys Prenatal and postnatal development: none Genetic toxicology: Ames test, in vitro chromosomal aberration assay in human lymphocytes Carcinogenicity: none
Peg-Intron™ (pegylated interferon alfa-2b) (US) Approval: 2001	Covalent conjugate of recombinant interferon alfa-2b with monomethoxy polyethylene glycol (PEG) ↔ multiple targets within the lymphokine regulatory network	Hepatitis C	Single dose: mice, rats, cynomolgus monkeys, rhesus monkeys Repeat dose: rats, cynomolgus monkeys Fertility and early embryonic development: cynomolgus monkeys Developmental: rhesus monkeys Prenatal and postnatal development: none Genetic toxicology: Ames test, chromosomal aberrations in human lymphocyte assay, mouse micronucleus test Carcinogenicity: none
Proleukin, IL-2® (aldesleukin) (US) Approval: 1992	Recombinant human interleukin-2 ↔ receptors on T cells and NK (natural killer) cells	Metastatic renal cell carcinoma, metastatic melanoma	Single dose: none Repeat dose: rats Fertility and early embryonic development: none Developmental: rats Prenatal and postnatal development: unclear Genetic toxicology: none Carcinogenicity: none

TABLE 39.1 *Continued*

Biopharmaceutical	Description ↔ Target	Indication	Toxicology Studies[a]
Pulmozyme® (dornase alfa) (US) Approval: 1993	Recombinant human DNAase ↔ cleaves DNA in sputum of lungs of cystic fibrosis patients to reduce sputum viscosity	Respiratory complications in cystic fibrosis	Single dose: rats, monkeys (inhalation) Repeat dose: rats, monkeys (inhalation) Fertility and early embryonic development: rats Developmental: rats, rabbits Prenatal and postnatal development: rats, cynomolgus monkeys Genetic toxicology: Ames tests, chromosomal aberrations in cultured human peripheral blood lymphocytes, in vivo mutagenicity test (mouse bone marrow) Carcinogenicity: 2-year rat inhalation study Other: intravenous and intratracheal studies in rats and monkeys; blood and serum compatability (human and monkey), ocular toxicity
RAPTIVA™ (efalizumab) (US) Approval: 2003	Recombinant humanized monoclonal antibody ↔ binds to CD 11a on leukocytes	Moderate to severe plaque psoriasis	Single dose: chimpanzees, mice (surrogate antibody) Repeat dose: mice (surrogate antibody), chimpanzees Fertility and early embryonic development: mice (surrogate antibody Developmental: mice (surrogate antibody) Prenatal and postnatal development: mice (surrogate antibody) Genetic toxicology: none Carcinogenicity: none Tissue cross-reactivity: human, chimpanzee tissues, mouse tissue (surrogate antibody) Other: immunotoxicity in mice (surrogate antibody)

Drug (Approval)	Description	Indication	Preclinical studies
Remicade® (infliximab) (US) Approval: 1998	Chimeric monoclonal antibody ↔ binds with high affinity to the soluble and transmembrane forms of TNFα and inhibits binding of TNFα with its receptors	Crohn's disease, rheumatoid arthritis, ankylosing spondylitis, psoriatic arthritis, ulcerative colitis	Single dose: rats (not relevant), chimpanzees; Repeat dose: rats (not relevant), chimpanzees, mice (surrogate); Fertility and early embryonic development: mice (surrogate); Developmental: mice (surrogate); Genetic toxicology: Ames, mouse micronucleus, human lymphocyte; Prenatal and postnatal development:; Genetic toxicology: Ames test, mouse micronucleus, human lymphocyte; Carcinogenicity: TNFα knockout mice, anti-murine TNFα antibodies on tumor development, 6-month mouse (surrogate antibody)
Reopro® (abciximab) (US) Approval: 1997	Fab fragment of chimeric monoclonal antibody 7E3 ↔ glycoprotein IIb/IIIa and vitronectin receptors	Reduction of acute blood clot related complications; treatment of unstable angina	Tissue cross-reactivity: human tissues; Fertility and early embryonic development: none; Developmental: none; Prenatal and postnatal development: none; Genetic toxicology: in vitro and in vivo tests; Carcinogenicity: none

TABLE 39.1 *Continued*

Biopharmaceutical	Description ↔ Target	Indication	Toxicology Studies[a]
Rebif® (interferon beta 1-a) (US) Approval: 2002	Recombinant interferon beta 1-a ↔ multiple targets within the lymphokine regulatory network	Multiple sclerosis	Single dose: rats, mice, cynomolgus monkeys Repeat dose: rats, cynomolgus monkeys Fertility and early embryonic development: built into repeat-dose study in cynomolgus monkeys Developmental: cynomolgus monkeys Prenatal and postnatal development: none Genetic toxicology: Ames test, "unscheduled DNA synthesis" in cultured HeLa cells, chromosome aberrations in human lymphocytes, micronucleus induction in bone marrow cells of mice, chromosome aberration in the Chinese hamster bone marrow Carcinogenicity: none
Retavase® (reteplase) (US) Approval: 1996	Nonglycosylated deletion mutation of tissue plasminogen activator (tPA) containing the kringle 2 and the protease domains of human tPA ↔ catalyzes the cleavage of endogenous plasminogen to generate plasmin	Acute myocardial infarction	Other: peripheral blood leukocytes derived from humans, mice, rats, rabbits, dogs, and cynomolgus monkeys in vitro Single dose: rats, rabbits, cynomolgus monkeys Repeat dose: rats, dogs, cynomolgus monkeys Fertility and early embryonic development: rats Developmental: rats, rabbits Prenatal and postnatal development: unclear Genetic toxicology: Ames test, chromosome aberration test, micronucleus tests in mice and rats Carcinogenicity: none

Product (Approval)	Description	Indication	Preclinical studies
Rituxan™ (rituximab) (US) Approval: 1997	Chimeric murine monoclonal antibody ↔ binds to the CD20 antigen	CD20 positive B cell non-Hodgkin's lymphoma, arthritis	Single dose: mice, guinea pigs (both not relevant species), cynomolgus monkeys; Repeat dose: cynomolgus monkeys; Fertility and early embryonic development: none; Developmental: cynomolgus monkeys; Prenatal and postnatal development: cynomolgus monkeys; Genetic toxicology: none; Carcinogenicity: none; Tissue cross-reactivity: various human tissues
Roferon-A® (interferon alfa-2a) (US) Approval: 1984	Interferon alfa-2a ↔ multiple targets within the lymphokine regulatory network	Hepatitis C, chronic myelogenous leukemia, hairy cell leukemia	Fertility and early embryonic development: rhesus monkeys; Developmental: rhesus monkeys; Prenatal and postnatal development: rhesus monkeys (late fetal development); Genetic toxicology: Ames tests, chromosome damage in human lymphocytes; Carcinogenicity: none
Simulect® (basiliximab) (US) Approval: 1998	Chimeric murine monoclonal antibody ↔ reacts with the CD25 antigen on T cells, inhibiting the binding of interleukin-2 (IL-2) to its receptor (IL-2R)–appears to bind only to activated T lymphocytes and to monocytes ↔ macrophages	Prevention of rejection episodes in kidney transplant recipients	Single dose: none; Repeat dose: rhesus monkeys; Fertility and early embryonic development: none; Developmental: cynomolgus monkeys; Prenatal and postnatal development: none; Genetic toxicology: Ames test, chromosomal aberration tests with V79 Chinese hamster cells; Carcinogenicity: none; Tissue cross-reactivity: human tissues

TABLE 39.1 Continued

Biopharmaceutical	Description ↔ Target	Indication	Toxicology Studies[a]
Synagis™ (palivizumab) (US) Approval: 1998	Recombinant humanized monoclonal antibody ↔ epitope in the A antigenic site of the F protein of respiratory syncytial virus (RSV)	Prevention of respiratory tract disease caused by syncytial virus in pediatric patients	Single dose: cynomolgus monkeys, rabbits Repeat dose: rats Fertility and early embryonic development: none Developmental: none Prenatal and postnatal development: none Genetic toxicology: none Carcinogenicity: none Tissue cross-reactivity: human tissues, cynomolgus monkeys tissues
Synvisc® (hylan G-F 20) [US(CDRH)] Approval: 1997	Mixture of Hylan A and Hylan B polymers derived from chicken combs ↔ lubrication of knee joint	Lubrication of the knee joint and reduction of pain in an osteoarthritic knee	Single dose: mice, rabbits Other: immunogenicity in owl monkeys, in vitro cytotoxicity in mouse fibroblast cell lines, hemocompatibility, pyrogenicity, tissue implantation in rabbits
Thyrogen® (thyrotropin alfa for injection) (US) Approval: 1998	Recombinant human thyroid stimulating hormone ↔ TSH receptors	Adjunctive diagnostic used in screening of cancer patients with thyroid cancer without thyroid glands	Single dose: rats Repeat dose: rats Fertility and early embryonic development: none Developmental: none Prenatal and postnatal development: none Genetic toxicology: Ames test Carcinogenicity: none
Thymoglobulin® [anti-thymocyte globulin (rabbit)] (US) Approval: 1999	Anti-thymocyte globulin (rabbit) ↔ selective depletion of T cells	Immunosuppressive polyclonal antibody used in conjunction with other immune suppression treatments to treat acute rejection in renal transplant	Fertility and early embryonic development: none Developmental: none Prenatal and postnatal development: none Genetic toxicology: none Carcinogenicity: none

Drug	Mechanism	Indication	Studies
Tnkase™ (tenecteplase) (US) Approval: 2000	Tissue plasminogen activator ↔ binds to fibrin and converts plasminogen to plasmin	Decrease in mortality associated with myocardial infarction	Single dose: rats, rabbits, dogs Repeat dose: rats, rabbits, dogs Fertility and early embryonic development: none Developmental: rabbit Prenatal and postnatal development: none Genetic toxicology: none Carcinogenicity: none Other: local intra-arterial tolerance in the rabbit, local paravenous tolerance in the rats; in vitro hemolytic potential and blood compatibility testing Special toxicology studies: renal safety in dogs, cardiovascular safety in cynomolgus monkeys, cardiovascular and respiratory safety in rabbits
Tysabri® (natalizumab) (US) Approval: 2004	Recombinant humanized IgG4 antibody ↔ binds to the α4β1 subunit of integrin	Multiple sclerosis	Single dose: guinea pigs, mice Repeat dose: cynomolgus monkeys, albino mice, rhesus monkeys (drug interaction study with Avonex and Tysabri) Fertility and early embryonic development: guinea pigs Developmental: guinea pigs, cynomolgus monkeys Prenatal and postnatal development: cynomolgus monkeys Genetic toxicology: mouse lymphoma, human lymphocytes Carcinogenicity: (see Other) Tissue cross-reactivity: yes Other: xenograft SCID mice, xenograft athymic nude mice, proliferative in vitro studies with tumor cells

TABLE 39.1 *Continued*

Biopharmaceutical	Description ↔ Target	Indication	Toxicology Studies[a]
V Ectibix™ (panitumumab) (US) Approval: 2006	Fully human monoclonal antibody ↔ targets human epithelial growth factor receptor	Metastatic colorectal cancer	Single dose: none Repeat dose: cynomolgus monkeys Fertility and early embryonic development: cynomolgus monkeys Developmental: cynomolgus monkeys Prenatal and postnatal development: none Genetic toxicology: none Carcinogenicity: none Tissue cross-reactivity: human, cynomolgus monkey, rodent, rabbit tissues Other: safety pharmacology study in cynomolgus monkeys
Xigris™ (drotrecogin alfa) (US) Approval: 2001	Recombinant activated protein C ↔ hydrolyzes coagulation factors Va and XIIa	Sepsis	Single dose: cynomolgus monkeys, rhesus monkeys (continuous infusion), mice Repeat dose: cynomolgus monkeys Fertility and early embryonic development: rabbits Developmental: rats Prenatal and postnatal development: none Genetic toxicology: none Carcinogenicity: none Tissue cross-reactivity: none

Xolair® (omalizumab) (US) Approval: 2003	Recombinant humanized monoclonal antibody ↔ targets IgE	Asthma	Single dose: mice (not relevant), monkeys Repeat dose: cynomolgus monkeys Fertility and early embryonic development: cynomolgus monkeys Developmental: cynomolgus monkeys Prenatal and postnatal development: cynomolgus monkeys Genetic toxicology: Ames test Carcinogenicity: none
Zenapax® (daclizumab) (US) Approval: 1997	Recombinant humanized monoclonal antibody ↔ directed against the high-affinity interleukin-2 receptor	Prophylaxis of acute organ rejection in de novo allogeneic renal transplantation; used concomitantly with an immunosuppressive regimen, including cyclosporine and corticosteroids in patients who are not highly immunized	Tissue cross-reactivity: human, cynomolgus tissues Single dose: mice, rabbit, cynomolgus monkeys Repeat dose: cynomolgus monkeys Fertility and early embryonic development: none Developmental: none Prenatal and postnatal development: none Genetic toxicology: Ames test Carcinogenicity: none Other: renal and cardio allograft studies in cynomolgus monkeys
Zevalin™ (ibritumomab tiuxetan) (US) Approval: 2002	Immunoconjugate murine anti-CD20 monoclonal antibody + Y⁹⁰ + In¹¹¹ ↔ reacts with normal and malignant B lymphocytes	B cell non-Hodgkin lymphomas	Single dose: cynomolgus monkeys Repeat dose: cynomolgus monkeys Fertility and early embryonic development: none Developmental: none Prenatal and postnatal development: none Genetic toxicology: none Carcinogenicity: none Tissue cross-reactivity: B cell cross-reactivity (only)

TABLE 39.1 *Continued*

Biopharmaceutical	Description ↔ Target	Indication	Toxicology Studies[a]
Zorbtive (somatotropin) (US) Approval: 2003	Recombinant human somatotropin ↔ receptors on a variety of cell types including myocytes, hepatocytes, adipocytes, lymphocytes, and hematopoietic cells.	Short bowel syndrome	Fertility and early embryonic development: unclear Developmental: rats, rabbits Prenatal and postnatal development: unclear Genetic toxicology: none Carcinogenicity: none

Source: The main source of the information in this table is either the Food and Drug Administration (FDA) Web site or European Medicines Agency (EMEA) Web site. For biopharmaceuticals approved before 1995 limited information is available so the author used the most recent label (package insert) to derive the reproductive, carcinogenticity, and genetic toxicology studies completed for marketing approval.

[a]For brevity, only the pivotal toxicology studies are given. Examples of studies not included are proof-of-concept, comparability, toxicokinetic, pharmacokinetic, pharmacodynamic, local tolerance, and miscellaneous in vitro and in vivo studies. Pharmacokinetic and pharmacodynamic experiments generally used the pivotal toxicology animal model(s) because of the species specificity of the biopharmaceutical.

[b]It should not be inferred from the table that only one toxicology study per species was conducted for each biopharmaceutical. For example, several repeat-dose studies of different durations could have been conducted in the same species.

[c]Genetic toxicology language is from package inserts (most recent label).

[d]The primate species is not clarified in the label (package insert) for Actimune®.

(i.e., the label). There is a dearth of public information for drugs that came on the market before 1995, but sufficient public records exist for biopharmaceuticals approved during the last 10 years. Some of the early drug labels are lacking in descriptions of the genetic, reproductive, and carcinogenicity studies, particularly the radiopharmaceuticals, and in these cases the table is left blank.

39.2 TISSUE CROSS-REACTIVITY

Tissue cross-reactivity studies are required by FDA for monoclonal antibody products to determine if the product binds to target and/or nontarget tissues. They are also performed for nonmonoclonal biopharmaceuticals if warranted. For example, ARANESP™ was tested in a human tissue panel ex vivo to determine if it bound to nontarget tissues or cross-reacted with related cytokine receptors. These studies are also used to explore known or potential clinical adverse safety events (i.e., mechanism of toxicity). For example, one patient in a Raptiva™ study developed unilateral hearing loss. This finding was further evaluated by cross-reactivity studies with human optic chiasm, acoustic nerve, and inner ear tissues.

39.3 SINGLE-DOSE TOXICITY

The classic single-dose study using highly exaggerated doses (10–1000 times the human dose) of drug is not always feasible for large molecular weight biopharmaceutical drugs. Biopharmaceuticals are traditionally not oral drugs. Thus there is a limit to the amount of drug that can be formulated for intravenous or subcutaneous administration. Moreover there is a limit to the volume of drug solution that can be infused into a preclinical animal model without causing toxicities resulting in a rapid expansion of the extra cellular fluid volume and/or infusion of large quantities of a foreign protein.[1] Also one of the goals of the single-dose study for both animal and human drugs is to determine the toxicities that could occur due to an overdose. This is less of a concern with biopharmaceutical drugs, since many must be administered in a clinic setting. For all of these reasons the single-dose toxicology study[2] is not as germane for biopharmaceuticals as for traditional small-molecule drugs. Examples of biopharmaceuticals for which no single dose studies were conducted are Lucentis™, Avastin™, Simulect™, and Vectibix™.

---

[1]Thus safety factors tend to be lower (e.g., 2–10× on average) for biopharmaceuticals compared to small molecules.

[2]The classic single-dose study is actually more useful as a single-dose pharmacokinetic study than a toxicity study.

39.4 REPEAT-DOSE TOXICITY

A more relevant study for biopharmaceuticals is the repeat-dose study where exaggerated clinical doses are given to an animal model using the intended clinical route of administration. For most biopharmaceuticals this is the intravenous route of administration. Interesting exceptions are Lucentis™ and Pulmozyme®, given intraocularly and by inhalation, respectively, in the pivotal repeat-dose studies.

A unique problem encountered in a biopharmaceutical repeat-dose study is the development of antibodies to the drug, specifically neutralizing antibodies that diminish or eliminate its pharmacological activity. For example, the highly species specific Avonex® (interferon beta 1-alpha) causes neutralizing antibody formation within two weeks. Thus the pivotal repeat dose study for this drug was only a 14-day study in rhesus monkeys. Repeat-dose studies for Abraxane™ were complicated by immune reactions to its human serum albumin component. Another example is the pivotal repeat dose study in cynomolgus monkeys for Campath®, whose results were confounded by antibody development. However, there are products for which it is possible to dose through antibody development (i.e., Rituxan).

Determining the species specificity of a biopharmaceutical is an important first step in designing a toxicology program. This is accomplished with in vitro assays and tissue cross-reactivity experiments. For example, in vitro binding studies are done to assess the binding of the product to receptors in various species. By this approach it was determined that only primate IgE receptor binds to Xolair® precluding use of any species lower than primate in the preclinical program. Tissue cross-reactivity studies with rabbit and cynomolgus tissues were done to justify the use of these two species as the pivotal study animal models for Avastin™. However, there are biopharmaceuticals for which there is no relevant species in which to test the drug, except for the chimpanzee. In these cases a surrogate product may be developed. Raptiva™, for example, is only pharmacologically active in chimpanzees, a species for which limited data can be collected in a toxicology study (i.e., no necropsies permitted). A mouse surrogate antibody was thus developed and tested for Raptiva™ in single-dose, repeat-dose, and reproductive toxicity studies. A mouse surrogate antibody was also developed for the early Remicade® studies. There are examples of biopharmaceuticals that are relatively nonspecies specific and multiple animal models can be used for toxicity testing (i.e., ORENCIA™). Since many biopharmaceuticals are not active in lower species, the cynomolgus monkey is frequently used in the safety assessment of biopharmaceuticals.

The safety pharmacology studies in which the respiratory, CNS, and cardiovascular systems are evaluated in a nonrodent model are not de facto for a biopharmaceutical. Quite frequently the safety endpoints are in the protocols for the pivotal repeat-dose studies, such as a cynomolgus study, obviating the need for separate safety pharmacology studies.

39.5   GENETIC TOXICITY

Genetic toxicity testing is not required per ICH guidelines (ICH S6 [1]). The existence of genetic toxicity tests for biopharmaceuticals in the accompanying table is due, in part, to drug development prior to publication of the ICH guideline. There are no instances of positive outcomes for genetic toxicity testing with biopharmaceuticals except for ABRAXANE™, which was (not surprisingly) positive in genetic toxicity tests due to the paclitaxel component of the drug, and MYLOTARG™, positive in a mouse micronucleus test. The positive result for MYLOTARG™ is consistent with the known ability of calicheamicin (a component of the drug) to cause double-stranded breaks in DNA.

39.6   CARCINOGENICITY

The traditional two-year rodent carcinogenicity bioassay is also not required per ICH guidelines (S6 [1]) and is rarely done for biopharmaceuticals. However, because many biopharmaceuticals are immunosuppressive, there are concerns that specific products (e.g., growth factors) may cause inappropriate proliferation leading to neoplasm, especially if the drug is given chronically to patients. In these cases alternative carcinogenicity studies may be considered (i.e., Tg.rasH2 transgenic mouse model for KEPIVANCE®). Carcinogenicity (or tumorigenicity potential) has also been evaluated in chronic repeat-dose toxicology studies in primates (i.e., AMEVIVE®, APIDRA®).

39.7   REPRODUCTIVE/DEVELOPMENTAL TOXICOLOGY

The cynomolgus monkey model has been utilized for species specific biopharmaceuticals (e.g., Herceptin). One advantage of cynomolgus monkeys is that they cycle monthly compared to rhesus monkeys, which only experience an estrus cycle twice a year. The standard model (rat) is also used if the rat is deemed a relevant species, as are surrogate molecules for use in the rat. The segment 1, 2, and 3 studies are sometimes combined into one study, depending on the needs of the development program. Another alternative is to deduce the toxic effects of a biopharmaceutical on the reproductive system from the anatomical pathology results of the pivotal repeat dose study. For example, in the cynomolgus repeat dose studies for AVASTIN™, there were dose-dependent adverse effects on uterine and ovarian weights and follicular development.

39.8   IMMUNOTOXICITY

Immunotoxicity testing in various animal models is common for biologics because of their immunomodulatory nature. Since most biopharmaceuticals are humanized proteins, the minimum requirement is to define the antibody response to the biopharmaceutical. Other aspects of the humoral response can also be evaluated in repeat-dose studies. Immunohistochemical staining of lymphoid organs and lymphocyte phenotyping have also been components of repeat-dose studies. The appearance of product specific antibodies may not be associated with acute or target organ toxicity (i.e., ORENCIA™). More important, immune system responses to a human biopharmaceutical in an animal model are not necessarily predictive of the effects on the human immune system to the biopharmaceutical.

39.9   CONCLUSIONS

It can be deduced from Table 39.1 that most biopharmaceuticals approved to date are monoclonal antibodies and the most common indication is oncology. However, barring oncology, the biopharmaceuticals span an impressive range of indications. In addition to monoclonal antibodies, other prevalent types of biopharmaceuticals are fusion or conjugate proteins, growth factors, replacement enzymes, and peptides. Cellular and tissue therapies are rarer but becoming more prevalent.

Although the preclinical programs for the biopharmaceuticals in Table 39.1 are each unique and were developed with an experimental, case-by-case approach, they do have some practices that distinguish them from small molecule drugs. The most important practice is that the species chosen for the toxicology study generally had the greatest pharmacological activity when pretested in a variety of species by binding assays. It was not automatically assumed that a two-year carcinogenetic study was informative if the biopharmaceutical had proliferative properties; other approaches such as cell assay and short-term rodent models were used. Tissue-binding studies were always conducted for monoclonal antibodies; use of tissue cross-reactivity studies for other types of biopharmaceuticals were found to be informative on a case-by-case basis. It was not assumed that a single-dose toxicology study was required for the preclinical program; in many cases this study was supplanted by a thoughtfully designed repeat-dose study. Genetic toxicology studies were rarely needed for biopharmaceuticals. If conducted, these studies were always negative, except for drugs having a chemical component. The cynomolgus monkey model, developed for biopharmaceuticals, often supplanted the traditional rat reproductive toxicology study. Endpoints of the segment 1 and 3 studies were frequently built into the segment 2 study. Last, immunotoxicity testing in variety of forms is a critical component of the preclinical program for biopharmaceuticals because most biopharmaceuticals are currently believed to either trigger an immune response (humoral or cellular) or suppress the immune system.

ACKNOWLEDGMENTS

The author thanks Theresa Reynolds and Mary Ellen Cosenza for their insightful comments on preclinical strategies for biopharmaceuticals.

REFERENCES

1. ICH Guidance S6. *www.fda.gov/cder/guidance/1859fnl.pdf*

PART VIII

TRANSITIONING FROM PRECLINICAL DEVELOPMENT TO CLINICAL TRIALS

Science and Judgment in Establishing a Safe Starting Dose for First-in-Human Trials of Biopharmaceuticals

JENNIFER VISICH, PhD, and RAFAEL PONCE, PhD, DABT

Contents

40.1 INTRODUCTION

A significant milestone in the development of a new therapeutic is the first administration into humans. Whereas this is generally accompanied by a sense of excitement at the prospect of advancing a promising therapeutic toward treatment of patients, there is also a strong focus on the potential for harm, particularly harm that was not predicted by the available preclinical studies. This

Preclinical Safety Evaluation of Biopharmaceuticals: A Science-Based Approach to Facilitating Clinical Trials, edited by Joy A. Cavagnaro
Copyright © 2008 by John Wiley & Sons, Inc.

central concept of benefit versus risk forms the primary basis for decisions used by the developing institution, the regulatory authorities, and the clinical community in establishing acceptable parameters for the first clinical trial for novel therapeutic agents, and the underlying lynchpins of this assessment are the initial dose and the subsequent dose escalation strategy. This chapter reviews the decision processes surrounding the determination of the initial dose of a novel biopharmaceutical agent to be administered to subjects in clinical trials.

40.1.1 General Considerations for Approaching the First Human Dose

It is not practical to consider development of specific regulatory guidance for each of the diverse biologic therapeutics under development to treat various diseases. Rather, current practice is to rely on a risk-based strategy to protect subject safety. It is within this framework that the regulatory agencies rely on current scientific knowledge, best practices within the industry, and a case-by-case approach that is tailored to each therapeutic agent and specific subject population to evaluate the initial clinical testing of a novel biopharmaceutical. Specific case examples, which are presented later in this chapter, will provide some insight into how these concepts are applied.

A number of regulatory guidance documents touch on various aspects of the transition from preclinical to clinical study of a novel biopharmaceutical. The primary guidance documents describing the conduct and use of preclinical safety evaluation in supporting the initial clinical trials are as follows:

- Preclinical Safety Evaluation of Biotechnology-Derived Pharmaceuticals (ICH S6) [1]
- Non-clinical Safety Studies for the Conduct of Human Clinical Trials for Pharmaceuticals (ICH M3) [2]
- Points to Consider in the Manufacture and Testing of Monoclonal Antibody Products for Human Use [3]
- Estimating the Maximum Safe Starting Dose in Initial Clinical Trials for Therapeutics in Adult Healthy Volunteers [4]
- Guideline on Strategies to Identify and Mitigate Risks for First-in-Human Clinical Trials with Investigational Medicinal Products [5]

In practice, the regulatory framework governing the first dose of a biopharmaceutical in humans is designed around several fundamental tenets: know the safety profile for the test agent, maintain a positive risk–benefit profile in each subject population, and beware of the unknown.

40.1.2 Establishing the Safety Profile for the Biological Therapeutic

As described in ICH S6 guidance, preclinical safety studies for biopharmaceuticals are designed to identify potential toxicities (and their reversibility) associated with treatment under conditions that mimic the intended clinical use (i.e., dose route, duration, and frequency with representative drug product). In so doing, these studies inform the clinicians, ethical review committees and regulators regarding the nature of potential side effects and appropriate subject monitoring, and guide the initial dose selection and dose escalation strategy.

Because biopharmaceuticals are often designed to mimic an endogenous human molecule (i.e., protein, peptide, nucleotide or other derivative), the burden is on the developer to demonstrate that the species used in the safety studies are appropriate surrogate models for humans; see [1]. This requirement recognizes the potential for broad interspecies differences in DNA/protein sequence homology, binding affinity, target distribution, and underlying biological pathways or processes that ultimately affect the value of the animal model to predict the human response. The requirement for such species justification data in the preclinical evaluation of biopharmaceuticals is an important area of divergence from the preclinical assessment of small molecules. Thus it is not meaningful to interpret the lack of toxicity observed for biopharmaceutical in species that have no demonstrated binding, activity, or other data to justify their use as predictive models of potential human response.

As the basis for decisions about the first dosing in humans, the preclinical safety program needs to mimic the intended clinical regimen. Although these studies are commonly conducted in normal healthy animals, they may also require development and use of an animal model that mimics the health status or condition if it is deemed to possibly sensitize the subject to treatment. For example, we have conducted studies evaluating the safety of recombinant human Factor XIII in an animal model of extracorporeal blood circulation [6] and the safety of recombinant human thrombin in an animal model of hepatic resection [7].

Dose selection and administration route are likewise defined by the intended clinical use. Of particular relevance to the selection of the initial clinical starting dose is the dose range used in the preclinical study and the dose–response relationship for identified toxicities. Under current regulatory practice [4], dose selection in the phase 1 enabling regulatory safety study should establish a no adverse effect level (NOAEL) and a maximal tolerated dose (MTD). Thus the design of the phase 1 enabling preclinical safety study often relies on data from prior pilot animal studies that define the tolerated dose range. But tolerability data in the preclinical species alone is generally not sufficient to establish an intended clinical dosing regimen because of potential interspecies differences in receptor/target affinity, distribution, or potency, or pharmacokinetic differences in biodistribution or clearance. Whereas an accurate human pharmacokinetic profile for the biopharmaceutical can only be established upon clinical testing, ex vivo and in vitro testing of human and animal cells can be used to identify differences in receptor/target affinity, distribution, or pharmacological activity. Accounting for such interspecies differences in selecting the final doses of the preclinical study provides a rational strategy that is matched to a target clinical dose range.

40.1.3   Factors That Increase Concern in Transitioning from Preclinical to Clinical Dosing

We have acknowledged that regulatory and clinical practices rely on a risk-based approach to establish the starting dose and dose escalation strategy for the initial clinical evaluation of a novel biopharmaceutical. But what are those factors that raise concern when transitioning from preclinical to clinical dosing? As a rule, agents associated with a threshold dose–response relationship for toxicity that lack premonitory biomarkers of toxicity, or that cause irreversible toxicity will have a markedly more conservative clinical program compared with agents that have a shallow dose–response relationship for toxicity, have clearly established premonitory biomarkers, that undergo complete reversibility of the toxicity. For example, preclinical safety evaluation of recombinant human Factor XIII demonstrated a threshold dose–response relationship for toxicity associated with few premonitory signs [8]. Thus clinical development of this compound was associated with a low starting dose, cautious dose escalation strategy, and intensive monitoring for evidence of toxicity.

In addition first-in-class therapeutics, particularly those with potential for serious adverse reactions, warrant an extra level of caution based on the pharmacological mechanism of action to account for our lack of knowledge. Recent experience with an experimental monoclonal antibody, TGN1412 (produced by TeGenero AG, Germany), against CD28 has galvanized interest in the process surrounding first-in-human trials. In March 2006, six healthy volunteers received a single 0.1 mg/kg body weight intravenous infusion of TGN1412 [9]. Within 1 to 2 hours after infusion, all six patients reported multiple symptoms including headache, myalgia, nausea, vomiting, bowel urgency and diarrhea, fever, erythema, peripheral vasodilation, hypotension, and tachycardia. Between 16 and 20 hours after treatment, the subjects had neurological, pulmonary, and renal impairment; disseminated intravascular coagulation; and lymphopenia and monocytopenia. Treatment with corticosteroids and/or an IL-2R mAb was used to downregulate the cytokine response. It was ultimately surmised that treatment with TGN1412 led to a systemic inflammatory response syndrome attributed to the release of TNF-α, IFN-γ, and IL-2.

Preclinical studies of TGN1412 were conducted in rhesus (*Macaca mulatta*) and cynomolgus (*Macaca fascicularis*) monkeys and demonstrated no evidence of a similar cytokine release response. Dose selection was based on a 500-fold margin of safety against the NOAEL established in cynomolgus monkeys (50 mg/kg). Comparison of the human and cynomolgus monkey CD28 sequence revealed an identical amino acid sequence in the critical region associated with TGN1412 contact, and TGN1412 binds to T cells from various nonhuman primates and humans [10]. Preclinical safety studies demonstrated no clinical toxicity at doses up to 50 mg/kg in cynomolgus monkeys, although increased serum cytokines were observed, including IL-2, IL-5, and IL-6 [11]. Subsequent data from TeGenero AG revealed comparable in vitro cytokine induction and T cell activation and proliferation for human and cynomolgus monkey peripheral blood mononuclear cells [10]. The basis for the marked interspecies difference in response to TGN1412 has not been established but may relate to evolutionary differences in T cell response to stimulation between humans and nonhuman primates [12] or T cell co-stimulation related to F_c-receptor binding [13–15], or could represent faulty assumptions regarding dose extrapolation [16].

The experience with TGN1412 has resulted in an industrywide introspection regarding our uncertainty and lack of knowledge regarding interspecies extrapolation of safety findings, mechanism of action for novel pharmacologic pathways, and conduct of first-in-human (FIH) trials. These have been summarized in a number of reviews and editorials (e.g., [17,18–20]). In addition the European Medicines Agency (EMEA) has recently released guidance on requirements for first-in-human clinical trials for potential high-risk therapeutics [5]. Under this guidance, high-risk therapeutics are defined by the mode of action, including novelty, knowledge of the proposed mode of action and underlying physiology, type of dose–response relationship, and relevance of animal models. Agents that have a pleiotropic mechanism with the potential for systemic effects (e.g., the immune system) or that bypass physiological control mechanisms (e.g., CD3 or CD28 (super-)) agonists are identified as examples. As in our prior example, we would include agents with the potential to directly stimulate plasma coagulation to this list.

The EMEA guidance presents a departure from NOAEL-based methods for establishing the starting dose for FIH trials when the therapeutic is considered to be a high-risk agent. Rather, for high-risk agents, the FIH dose should be based on the anticipated minimal anticipated biological effect level (MABEL) *in humans* with incorporation of appropriate safety factors. The assessment of whether a particular agent is considered to fall under the high-risk category is conducted on a case-by-case basis, as summarized in Table 40.1. The concept of a MABEL is also described in the FDA maximum recommended starting dose (MRSD) guidance by the inclusion of the term PAD (pharmacologically active dose) [4]. According to the FDA guidance, the PAD is to be considered for cases where it may be a more sensitive indicator of potential toxicity than the NOAEL (certain classes of drugs or biologics where toxicity may arise via exaggerated pharmacologic such as vasodilators, anticoagulants, monoclonal antibodies, or growth factors). As such, it is recommended that the PAD would warrant lowering the MRSD. The terms MABEL and PAD will be used interchangeably in the remainder of this chapter. This is a good reflection of how safety margins should be considered for therapeutic proteins.

40.2 CALCULATION OF STARTING DOSES FOR BIOLOGICS

The preceding section describes the kinds of preclinical safety studies performed to enable the characterization of both the pharmacodynamics and the

TABLE 40.1 Characteristics of standard versus high-risk therapeutics

	Standard Therapeutic	High-Risk Therapeutic
Mode of action	• Follow-on agent or therapeutic target • Well-understood mechanisms • Target has limited physiological interactions • Target has linear or sublinear dose–response relationship • Easily monitored pharmacology/toxicity • Toxicity is reversible	• Novel • Poorly understood mechanism • Pleiotropic or systemic activity • Bypasses or overwhelms physiological controls • Potential for amplification, supralinear, or threshold dose–response • Lack of biomarkers of effect/toxicity • Irreversible toxicity
Nature of target	• Good specificity of therapeutic to target or disease • Target is noncritical, has redundancy	• Poor specificity of therapeutic to target or disease • Inherent risk of targeting specific structures, nonredundant systems • Critical biological effect
Relevance of animal models	• Good structural homology, target distribution, and signaling pathways • Comparable pharmacological effects • Animal models established and considered predictive	• Poor structural homology, target distribution, signaling pathways, and pharmacological effects • Animal models are of limited relevance to study pharmacology and toxicology • Disease state alters relevance of studies in normal animals
Basis for first-in-human dose	• NOAEL-based approach • Healthy volunteers possible • Utilize all available in vitro and in vivo data, including receptor binding and occupancy, concentration–response relationships, PK data in relevant species • Apply appropriate safety factor	• MABEL-based approach • Patient population likely • Utilize all available in vitro and in vivo data, including receptor binding and occupancy, concentration–response relationships, PK data in relevant species • Apply appropriate safety factor

toxicities associated with a new biopharmaceutical. At this point the toxicologist must utilize the information gathered to estimate a scientifically justified, safe starting dose in humans. There is no fixed algorithm used to estimate a safe starting dose. The estimation is performed on a case-by-case basis and must be justified both with regard to science and risk–benefit considerations.

The first step in the process is to understand the nature of the toxicity and the dose at which there is no observed adverse effect (NOAEL) and as described in the preceding sections, in the case of high-risk therapeutics, if possible, the minimal anticipated biological effect level (MABEL) or PAD and/or the dose at which there is no effect at all (NOEL). The NOAEL, the MABEL or PAD, and the NOEL are important starting points at which to base safe first doses in humans. However, there are many situations where the mechanism of action of a protein therapeutic is not measurable in healthy animals or where there is measurable pharmacology resulting from every dose tested (no NOEL estimated; MABEL or PAD is estimated), or where a NOAEL is not determined because an MTD has not been reached. In these cases the most relevant dose level should be used for the estimation of the first dose. The decision on which dose level should be based on the population to be included in the phase 1 and the risk–benefit scenario for these subjects. If the first phase 1 is conducted in healthy subjects, the goal may be that the first dose does not elicit a pharmacology of any kind; thus a dose based off the NOEL or the MABEL (or PAD) is desirable. If the first phase 1 is in subjects with disease, there may be a higher tolerance for the first dose to cause some pharmacologic effect but minimal adverse events; thus a dose based on the NOAEL or the MABEL (or PAD) is satisfactory.

In addition to in vivo data, in vitro receptor affinity and density data should be included in the first-in-human estimations when applicable. These data can be used to calculate the predicted receptor occupancy over a range of concentrations of the biopharmaceutical. The concentrations that result in a minimal receptor occupancy (e.g., 5–10%) should be compared to the circulating concentrations that correspond to the in vivo NOAEL, NOEL, and MABEL (or PAD). For example, ReoPro (abciximab) is a F_{ab} fragment designed to bind to the platelet GPIIb/IIIa receptor and inhibit platelet aggregation. Preclinical animal models demonstrated that with more than 80% receptor blockade arterial thrombosis was prevented. Thus dose extrapolation from animals to humans could be used to estimate clinical doses associated with an 80% receptor blockade (and that could be monitored via flow cytometric analyses) and to define a rational dose escalation strategy. Alternatively, Mehrishi et al. have estimated more than 80% CD28 receptor occupancy among the six subjects treated with TGN1412 using equilibrium-binding calculations based on reported affinity data and assumptions of the number of cells and receptors/cell [16].

The final two steps of calculating a starting dose include the conversion of the NOEL, MABEL (or PAD), or the NOAEL to a human equivalent dose (HED) and the application of a safety factor that reduces the estimation of the human starting dose to allow for sensitivity differences in humans that may result in adverse events. The dose conversion can be done either using a pharmacokinetic-based interspecies scaling or a weight or surface area dose normalization. The safety factor applied to the calculated HED can be based on several factors, including nature of the dose–toxicologic response relationship, what is known about the safety of other proteins with similar mechanism of actions, and in vitro sensitivity comparisons of the preclinical species versus human.

40.2.1   Calculation of a Human Equivalent Dose for Protein Therapeutics

Once the appropriate dose levels (NOAEL, NOEL, MABEL, and/or PAD) have been determined using both in vivo and in vitro data, these levels should be scaled for human estimation. In most cases the preclinical species have received repeated doses of the biopharmaceutical, resulting in increased exposure over the intended human exposure of a single dose. While total exposure in preclinical species (e.g., weekly or monthly) can be leveraged to calculate safety margins over expected human exposures in studies following the initial single ascending dose study, the emphasis for first-in-human dose estimations is most commonly on a dose-to-dose comparison, not on total weekly or monthly doses.

Pharmacokinetic-Based Interspecies Scaling   Allometric scaling is commonly used for the prediction of pharmacokinetic parameters of small molecules in humans. Allometric scaling is based on the assumption that there are anatomical, physiological, and biochemical similarities among the species included in the scaling. The power equation $Y = aW^b$ in its logarithmic form, $\log Y = \log a + b \log W$, has been used to describe the relationship of body weight (W) to both physiological properties (Y) such as organ weight or cardiac output to pharmacokinetic properties such as clearance, volume of distribution, and half-life. In the case of pharmacokinetic scaling, the weights of the animals tested and their observed PK parameters of interest (most commonly clearance) are plotted on a log–log plot where the y-intercept (a) and the slope (b) are calculated and then applied to a calculation of the predicted parameter in humans. The resulting estimate for clearance in humans can be used to estimate the first dose by using the following equation [21]:

$$\text{Human dose (mg)} = \frac{\underset{(\text{mg}*\text{h/L})}{\text{AUC in animal}} \times \underset{(\text{L/h})}{\text{Predicted clearance in humans}}}{\text{Safety factor}}.$$

In addition pharmacokinetic modeling can be used to predict human exposures, but these models are also based on parameter estimates that are initially scaled from preclinical species.

In the case of biopharmaceuticals, while two species are recommended, often times there is only one relevant species included in general preclinical safety studies because of species specificity. In either case, one or two species data are not sufficient to estimate the needed allometric terms. Therefore allometric scaling is not commonly used for biopharmaceuticals. There have been a number of publications by Mahmood et al. (e.g., [22,23,24]) on the addition of additional factors (maximum life-span factors, brain weights, etc.) to improve the allometric scaling of protein drugs, but these improved methods still require data from greater than two species for accurate estimations. Last, as stated above, one of the major assumptions is that the drug will be handled similarly from species to species. In the case of biopharmaceuticals it is quite common for the species tested to have different sensitivities to protein drugs due to receptor density, receptor affinities, and interspecies differences in receptor signaling. These species specific differences are overlooked in the basic allometric estimations.

Weight and Body Surface Area Interspecies Scaling   The simplest scaling method is a one-to-one conversion of the animal dose of interest to a human equivalent dose (HED) via weight based (mg/kg) or body surface area normalization (mg/m²). Choice of weight based versus body surface area scaling is usually on a case-by-case basis and requires some knowledge about the NOAEL, NOEL, or MABEL (or PAD) in several preclinical species and that the source of the observed toxicity is based on an exposure parameter that is correlated with doses administered by weight. For biopharmaceuticals, body surface area normalization is more widely used as it leads to a more conservative estimation of the starting dose. The FDA MRSD guidance provides tables that enable the conversion of several species doses to HEDs based on the following calculation:

$$ \text{HED} = \text{Animal dose (mg/kg)} \times \left(\frac{\text{Animal weight (kg)}}{\text{Human weight (kg)}} \right)^{0.33}. $$

The body surface area conversion factors (BSA-CFs) included in the FDA guidance are based on an average species body weight.

Application of a Safety Factor   Following the conversion of the NOAEL, MABEL (or PAD), or NOEL to a human equivalent dose (HED), the resulting dose is usually divided by a safety factor in order to calculate the proposed starting dose in humans. This safety factor provides a safety margin between a safe dose in preclinical species and the first humans receiving the therapeutic. The default safety factor for most first-in-human studies is 10-fold, however, the assignment of this factor should be science-driven.

40.2.2   Examples of Estimations of First-in-Human Doses for Protein Therapeutics

The examples below illustrate strategies that have been implemented successfully in the estimation of safe first-in-human doses of biopharmaceuticals. Each of the molecules is characterized in terms of the type of therapeutic, whether it is a standard or high-risk therapeutic and why, the relevant toxicology specie(s) studied, its mechanism of action (MOA), mechanism of toxicity (MOT), the planned phase 1 study design and population, and the identified NOAEL, NOEL, and MABEL (or PAD), where applicable. The molecule characterization is followed by a summary of the estimation of the first-in-human dose using the algorithm supplied by the FDA MRSD to calculate the HED and applying a safety margin based on case-by-case considerations.

Example 1

Type of molecule	Fusion protein
Classification	Standard (well-understood MOA, easily monitored pharmacology)
Toxicology species	Mouse, monkey
MOA	Known, not novel, dose-responsive biomarkers present in two relevant toxicology species
MOT	Known, exaggerated pharmacology
Phase 1 study	Single, escalating-dose in healthy subjects
NOAEL	No AEs observed at any dose levels
NOEL	No NOEL determined in either species
MABEL/PAD	5 mg/kg in mouse and monkey

The MABEL/PAD in the mouse and the monkey were divided by the BSF-CFs to calculate the corresponding HEDs:

$$\text{HED (mg/kg)} = \frac{\text{MABEL}_{\text{mouse}}}{13} = 0.38 \, \text{mg/kg},$$

$$\text{HED (mg/kg)} = \frac{\text{MABEL}_{\text{monkey}}}{3} = 1.67 \, \text{mg/kg}.$$

The lowest resulting HED was chosen (0.3 mg/kg) and a 10-fold margin was applied to estimate the first-in-human dose of 0.03 mg/kg.

Example 2

Type of molecule	Cytokine
Classification	High-risk (poorly understood MOA and MOT)
Toxicology species	Monkey
MOA	Poorly understood, dose-responsive biomarkers in 1 toxicology species
MOT	Poorly understood, monitorable
Phase 1 study	Repeat, escalating dose in end stage disease population
NOAEL	NOAEL identified; 100 µg/kg

NOEL	No NOEL determined
MABEL/PAD	10 µg/kg in monkey
Other	In vitro studies showed similar receptor affinity for human and monkey

The HED was calculated using the MABEL/PAD observed in monkeys:

$$HED = \frac{MABEL_{monkey}}{3} = 3.3\,\mu g/kg.$$

Because the phase 1 study was planned in end-stage disease patients, the in vitro receptor affinity was similar between monkey and human, and the NOAEL was 10-fold higher than the MABEL/PAD; a 3-fold safety margin was applied to the MABEL/PAD-based HED resulting in a safe first-in-human dose of 1.0 µg/kg.

Example 3

Type of molecule	PEGylated cytokine
Classification	High-risk (toxicity in one species and not the other)
Toxicology species	Mouse, monkey
MOA	Known, not novel, dose-responsive biomarkers measured in monkey
MOT	Unknown, observed in mice only
Phase 1 study	Single escalating dose in healthy subjects
NOAEL	No NOAEL identified in mice, no AEs observed at any dose level in monkeys
NOEL	NOEL identified in monkey; 0.015 mg/kg
MABEL/PAD	Not determined

The mouse data included histologic evidence of mild cardiac injury that increased in incidence with increasing dose (0.3, 3, and 30 mg/kg) but had no functional consequences. The monkey data showed no evidence of these histologic findings. Similar findings were noted in mouse studies performed with a marketed agent in the same class as the tested biopharmaceutical, but likewise not observed in monkeys or humans. The NOEL in monkeys was based on a biomarker thought to be closely linked to the mechanism of action of the biopharmaceutical. The HED was calculated as follows:

$$HED = \frac{NOEL_{monkey}}{3} = 0.005\,mg/kg.$$

A 10-fold safety margin was applied to the HED and the resulting safe starting dose was 0.5 µg/kg. In addition this starting dose resulted in a 46-fold safety margin over the lowest dose tested in the mouse. The phase 1 study was conducted in healthy subjects and included additional cardiac monitoring.

40.3 DOSE ESCALATION AND PROPOSED TOP DOSES

The examples above illustrate the kinds of considerations that should be included in estimations of first-in-human dosing of biopharmaceuticals. In addition to the starting dose, the proposed dose escalation and the margin of safety surrounding the proposed top dose should also be considered carefully. In terms of dose escalation, the nature of the dose–response curve and inadequate knowledge of the mechanism of action and/or toxicity are the most important determinants of the need for caution in designing an ascending dose schema in humans. Many escalations with highly potent biopharmaceuticals begin with a conservative starting dose and proceed with dose doubling for several cohorts before eventually switching to half-log increases once the chance of unexpected toxicities has lessened. The proposed top dose of a single ascending dose escalation is usually designed to be a moderate multiple of the estimated therapeutic dose of the biopharmaceutical in humans. At a minimum, it is important to design preclinical safety studies to include a dose that at least matches the proposed top dose in humans (when appropriately scaled), although some regulatory reviewers have asked for a 10-fold or higher multiple in the preclinical study. The rationale for such a design should depend on the risk–benefit profile and the feasibility of achieving such doses. One should be mindful that for many biopharmaceutical agents that work through specific receptor-mediated processes, one would not expect to see significant novel biological activity with doses that exceed saturation of the receptor other than nonspecific toxicity associated with excessive protein loading.

40.4 BEYOND PHASE 1

Once the phase 1 has been completed, next steps include the comparison of observed human exposure data (maximum concentration, C_{max} and area under the concentration–time curve, AUC) to the exposures observed in the supportive preclinical studies, prediction of the human exposure in future clinical trials (based on dose level and frequency) and the calculation of the "actual" safety margins provided by the repeat-dose preclinical toxicology studies. The need for safety margins (based on preclinical safety and single-dose human data) to support phase 1b or phase 2 dosing is usually considered on a case-by-case basis.

40.5 CONCLUSIONS

Calculation of the starting dose in first-in-human trials with biopharmaceuticals requires a good understanding of the science behind both the mechanism of action and the mechanism of toxicity of the test article. The FDA has provided an algorithm in its MRSD guidance to calculate a human equivalent dose based on the NOAEL in the most sensitive species tested. However, thoughtful design of the supportive preclinical safety studies includes consideration of the estimated therapeutic human dose level and dose ranges that will allow for the estimation of a NOAEL, and ideally a NOEL, and/or a MABEL (or PAD), if possible. Based on the risk classification of the biopharmaceutical, the most appropriate preclinical dose level (NOAEL, NOEL, or MABEL) should be used to calculate the HED, and the application of a safety factor should be based on data gathered during in vitro and in vivo preclinical development.

REFERENCES

1. ICH, Topic S6. Note for Guidance on Preclinical Safety Evaluation of Biotechnology-Derived Pharmaceuticals, 1998 (CPMP/ICH/302/95).

2. ICH, Topic M3 (R1). Note for Guidance on Non-clinical Safety Studies for the Conduct of Human Clinical Trials for Pharmaceuticals, 2000 (CPMP/ICH/286/95).

3. FDA CBER, Points to Consider in the Manufacture and Testing of Monoclonal Antibody Products for Human Use, 1997.

4. FDA CDER, Guidance for Industry: Estimating the Maximum Safe Starting Dose in Initial Clinical Trials for Therapeutics in Adult Healthy Volunteers, 2005.

5. EMEA CPMP, Guideline on Strategies to Identify and Mitigate Risks for First-in-Human Clinical Trials with Investigational Medicinal Products (EMEA/CHMP/SWP/28367), 2007.

6. Ponce R, Armstrong K, Andrews K, Hensler J, Waggie K, Heffernan J, Reynolds T, Rogge M. Safety of recombinant human factor XIII in a cynomolgus monkey model of extracorporeal blood circulation. *Toxicol Pathol* 2005;33(6):702–10.

7. Heffernan JK, Ponce RA, Zuckerman LA, Volpone JP, Visich J, Giste EE, Jenkins N, Boster D, Pederson S, Knitter G, Palmer T, Wills M, Early RJ, Rogge MC. Preclinical safety of recombinant human thrombin. *Regul Toxicol Pharmacol* 2007;47(1):48–58.

8. Ponce RA, Visich JE, Heffernan JK, Lewis KB, Pederson S, Lebel E, Andrews-Jones L, Elliott G, Palmer TE, Rogge MC. Preclinical safety and pharmacokinetics of recombinant human factor XIII. *Toxicol Pathol* 2005;33(4):495–506.

9. Suntharalingam G, Perry MR, Ward S, Brett SJ, Castello-Cortes A, Brunner MD, Panoskaltsis N. Cytokine storm in a phase 1 trial of the anti-CD28 monoclonal antibody TGN1412. *N Engl J Med* 2006;355(10):1018–28.

10. Duff GC. Expert scientific group on phase 1 clinical trials (Interim report). 2006; 356 pages. www.dh.gov.uk/en/consultations/closedconsultations/DH_4139038.

11. Doi F, Kakizaki S, Takagi H, Murakami M, Sohara N, Otsuka T, Abe T, Mori M. Long-term outcome of interferon-alpha-induced autoimmune thyroid disorders in chronic hepatitis C. *Liver Int* 2005;25(2):242–6.

12. Nguyen DH, Hurtado-Ziola N, Gagneux P, Varki A. Loss of Siglec expression on T lymphocytes during human evolution. *Proc Natl Acad Sci USA* 2006;103(20): 7765–70.

13. Wise MP, Gallimore A, Godkin A. T-cell costimulation. *N Engl J Med* 2006; 355(24):2594–2595; author reply 2595.

14. Colaco CA. T-cell costimulation. *N Engl J Med* 2006;355(24):2595; author reply 2595.

15. Sharpe AH, Abbas AK. T-cell costimulation—biology, therapeutic potential, and challenges. *N Engl J Med* 2006;355(10):973–5.

16. Mehrishi JN, Szabo M, Bakacs T. Some aspects of the recombinantly expressed humanised superagonist anti-CD28 mAb, TGN1412 trial catastrophe lessons to safeguard mAbs and vaccine trials. *Vaccine* 2007;25(11):3517–23.

17. Liedert B, Bassus S, Schneider CK, Kalinke U, Lower J. Safety of phase I clinical trials with monoclonal antibodies in Germany—the regulatory requirements viewed in the aftermath of the TGN1412 disaster. *Int J Clin Pharmacol Ther* 2007;45(1):1–9.

18. Schneider CK, Kalinke U, Lower J. TGN1412—a regulator's perspective. *Nat Biotechnol* 2006;24(5):493–6.

19. Kenter MJ, Cohen AF. Establishing risk of human experimentation with drugs: lessons from TGN1412. *Lancet* 2006;368(9544):1387–91.

20. Hanke T. Lessons from TGN1412. *Lancet* 2006;368(9547):1569–70; author reply 1570.

21. Mordenti J. Dosage regimen design for pharmaceutical studies conducted in animals. *J Pharm Sci* 1986;75(9):852–7.

22. Mahmood I. Interspecies scaling of protein drugs: prediction of clearance from animals to humans. *J Pharm Sci* 2004;93(1):177–85.

23. Mahmood I. The correction factors do help in improving the prediction of human clearance from animal data. *J Pharm Sci* 2005;94(5):940–5; author reply 946–7.

24. Mahmood I, Green MD, Fisher JE. Selection of the first-time dose in humans: comparison of different approaches based on interspecies scaling of clearance. *J Clin Pharmacol* 2003;43(7):692–7.

PART IX

AFTERWORD

A Retrospective

ANTHONY D. DAYAN, LLB, MD, FRCP, FRCPath, FFOM, FFPM, FIBiol

If you don't know where you're going you'll end up some place else.
—Yogi Berra

It may seem perverse to end such a comprehensive and critical account of the preclinical testing of biopharmaceuticals with ideas that are directed as much at the "what" and "how" to investigate as at the ultimate evaluation of experimental results. But, as the depth of the opening quotation subtly suggests, it is essential to consider and reconsider the objectives of toxicity experiments before it is possible to decide the value of their results in permitting safe and effective development of these novel and sometimes surprising products.

GENERAL NATURE OF BIOPHARMACEUTICALS AND OBJECTIVES OF PRECLINICAL TESTING

The objectives of preclinical testing to support development of new medicines are to detect and characterize unwanted actions, whether inherently toxic or secondary to pharmacological effects of the substance and its pharmacokinetics, to exclude predicted harmful effects, and as far as possible to reveal other, potentially valuable actions. All this must be done in such a way that the results are both scientifically and administratively useful, as GLP and GMP considerations are essential, and the duration and costs of the of the studies are minimized. In this way the necessary resources of scientists, experimental animals, and laboratory facilities can be minimized in order to make the development of products to treat sick patients as efficient, humane, speedy, and economical as possible.

The full range of biotechnology products nowadays comprises various types of pharmaceuticals derived from living systems, mainly cells, bacteria, and fungi but also including various types of proteins from specially modified animals or plants, engineered or otherwise modified tissues or living cells from humans and other animals, and engineered viruses and other vectors of transgenes. Hurrying a short distance behind are entirely synthetic substances, artificial organisms or cell-like forms, and more complex medical devices that will release biotechnology products in the body under special conditions.

The common features of this wide range of potential medicines are that they have been selected because of their very particular biological properties, they are all complex and so unsuitable for control just by conventional chemical or biochemical analyses, and they have very powerful effects on specific targets and particular biological processes. Their potency in affecting sometimes fundamentally important physiological or pathological processes, which makes them therapeutically valuable, may also entail powerful counterresponses by the body because of the nature and extent of the disturbances they produce in basic body mechanisms and processes. The biological nature of these products may stimulate immune responses or other counteractions by the body, which may limit or enhance their therapeutic activities and may even result in potentially harmful immunological reactions.

The origin of some products of biotechnology from certain types of living systems or cells carries potential risks of diverse types due to the potential transmission of infectious organisms or prions from the producing system. So far at least few of these products have been manufactured by chemical synthesis, because of the chemical and structural complexity, although that route may become more important in the future.

The potential risks that the toxicologist must consider If a living organism itself is employed as the therapeutic agent, for example, a living organism as a vaccine or a viral vector in gene therapy, will include any potential for infection of the staff administering the therapy as well as the inadvertent bystander in the community for as long as the viable agent may be excreted. Manufacture, storage, and transport of these agents will entail possible hazards to the responsible staff. Those aspects of occupational health and environmental protection are so specialized that they require separate consideration.

It will be seen that the scope of preclinical investigation of a product of biotechnology is likely to be much wider than that of a conventional "New Chemical Entity." There must be particularly close coordination of the manufacturing, analytical, and other pharmaceutical procedures that define the exact nature of the product as it is supplied for investigation and would become available subsequently the clinical use, it is then essential to plan the strategy of preclinical testing by reference to the biological nature of the product, to its pharmacological, immunological, and any other biological effects and the body's possible immune or other counterreactions to it and, as appropriate, to consider any environmental or occupational risk that requires investigation.

The breadth of the questions to be asked and answered in the preclinical investigation mean that the conventional procedures of toxicity testing, which are rightly designed to be general so that both expected and unexpected effects can be detected, will almost certainly require extension to include many investigations that are primarily focused on pharmacological and physiological actions of the test material. The range of the studies must be adapted to the product and its uses, including the abnormalities caused by the disease to be treated and the nature of the patients in whom it occurs, but always leaving the investigator alert to any clue, no matter how subtle, to any action, anticipated or unexpected, that might be beneficial or harmful—having first excluded chance effects and artifacts from the complex test procedures that are required.

Pharmacokinetics and "drug metabolism" may initially appear simpler in their application to biopharmaceuticals than when dealing with conventional NCEs. That is rarely correct, however, because of the technical problems of following low concentrations of proteins in complex body fluids and tissues, the difficulty of detecting and characterizing the immune response to a foreign protein or cell, possibly still in the presence of the target antigen, and our still limited knowledge of how signal molecules, such as the cytokines, influence both energy and xenobiotic metabolic processes in the host. Applying the concepts of "pharmacokinetics" to a transplanted, possibly engineered cell or tissue, to a transgene, or to a therapeutic effect induced in utero or in a young baby that might affect subsequent development indicates the broad scope and sometimes considerable depth of the questions that must be asked and answered about the onset and duration of the therapeutic effect and the reasons for any change that may occur over time.

The toxicologist responsible for a biotechnology product must be skilled and knowledgeable in toxicology, pharmacology, physiology, and pathophysiology as much as in immunology. Concerns about detailed cell structure and metabolism, about molecular biology and genetics, are important in planning the overall strategies of these types of preclinical investigations. Scientific understanding, medical knowledge, and astute biological perception are all just as necessary as understanding of regulatory guidance and the complexities of the development process in ensuring appropriate and efficient preclinical development.

Preclinical testing in the present context is not an end in itself. It exists as an essential part of the development of medicines for the treatment of serious diseases, so it must be done with scientific vigor, with due consideration of the patients and diseases to be treated, and with proper attention to the ethical and industrial factors that influence the progress of every new pharmaceutical. There must always be careful attention to the scientific purpose and value of proposed studies and whether a result from an in vitro system or an animal experiment would be most appropriate. Official guidance and published guidelines about the information required to support clinical studies and about product registration and the general nature of experiments to produce those data rightly have a considerable influence on efficient development in the industrial setting. However, conformity to general guidance must never be allowed to obscure devising and answering specific questions related to the unique nature and particular properties of the biotechnology product in question and its proposed clinical use. Toxicologists, clinicians, regulators, lawyers, and lay advisers must realize that conforming to guidelines by performing experiments of types described in detail yesterday is not necessarily the most useful or most appropriate way to deal with the products of today or tomorrow. The sciences advance and the need is to be sure that the best methods have been applied to obtain the most useful information in the most effective manner even if that means omitting some favored procedure of yesteryear that can be shown no longer to be scientifically useful or appropriate for the particular product in question.

The scientific responsibility, if you like the "ownership" of the preclinical testing strategy for a novel product of biotechnology, should lie in the hands of a small group of experts in toxicology, immunology, the appropriate areas of pharmacology, pathophysiology, and other areas of experimental biology and medicine. They must be guided by other specialists in manufacturing, pharmaceutics, regulatory requirements, and industrial effectiveness, but there must not be any compromise of the real objective of understanding the potential adverse and beneficial effects of the new therapy under circumstances that support realistic extrapolation to patients.

HELP FROM HISTORY?

Help in understanding the scope of the investigations required may come from looking back at the history of what were once called "biological" products and are now more accurately termed "products of biotechnology" or "biopharmaceuticals."

In the early days of the development of these medicines, at that time almost solely vaccines and antisera, mostly obtained directly from animals and some from laboratory cultures, and the earliest nonimmunological product—insulin—the primary needs were to determine the potency of the therapeutic activity, to rule out any direct pathogenicity of the product, and to exclude or limit adventitious contamination by infectious organisms and unwanted substances from the source system. Subsequently, as more refined investigative procedures became available, as the biological hazards of products obtained from living systems became better recognized and as knowledge of immunology and cognate sciences developed, there has been increasing refinement of investigative techniques to quantify the nature and activity of the therapeutic material and to exclude or limit contamination by organisms, proteins, and other substances. Concurrent advances in manufacture and purification have created their own needs for techniques to verify purity and potency, to exclude by-products, and to show that changes in production have not created new hazards by subtle changes in the detailed structure of the therapeutic substance or organism.

As an example consider the evolution of insulin from an acid extract of animal pancreas to a semisynthetic peptide comprising peptide chains made in engineered cells and possibly assembled in vitro after partial chemical modification. Insulin was standardized at first by assessment of its physiological action of hypoglycaemia but now by refined HPLC and other biochemical and biophysical analytical procedures. Earlier preclinical testing was focused on the effect on blood sugar and on exclusion of pyrogenic and other impurities, whereas nowadays there is at least as much interest in excluding immunogenicity due to trace contamination by aberrant epitopes and in broadly ruling out potentially harmful DNA or agents derived from the engineered cells. In parallel, as understanding of the complementary roles of insulin and Insulin-like growth factors I and II (IGF) has developed, and as their roles in fetal development has been demonstrated, toxicity and other preclinical studies of insulins have come to include biochemically sophisticated investigations in species selected for susceptibility of the actions of new preparations on intrauterine development in relation to maternal blood glucose levels and other metabolic processes. It is easy to produce a developmental effect by giving a high maternal dose of an insulin or IGF to a pregnant animal, but the important question is whether the potentially harmful action (the "hazard") occurs under circumstances relevant to controlled treatment with that medicine in pregnant humans or animals (the true "risk").

Further examples include the evolution of the preclinical investigation of clotting factors and anti-rhesus D immunoglobulin, at first produced by simple fractionation of human blood donations and now from genetically engineered cells, and standardized by measurement of the specific activity as well as by increasingly sensitive techniques to detect and characterize the desired epitopes and to exclude unwanted immunogens and other variants and impurities. The composition, nature, and therapeutic activity of these products have become more precisely defined, and the investigative methods have also been adapted for sensitive detection of trace immunogenicity that might result in loss of effect or immune complex disorders if neutralizing or other types of antibody were produced. Many of those preclinical studies are done in vitro, but others depend on in vivo investigations and ultimately on experience in the clinic.

Look at the ways in which preclinical studies have had to adapt to changes in vaccines from whole organism or complex extracts, largely defined by presence of the desired antigenicity, the absence of pathogenicity, and a minimum of pyrogenicity and other adverse effects (e.g., as initially used in typhoid, tetanus, and diphtheria immunization), to the complexity of current antibacterial and antitoxin vaccines, and even more to antitumour and antimalarial vaccines combining one or more extracted antigens, possibly immunostimulating cytokines from recombinant cells and other multicomponent immunomodulatory adjuvants. In the latter examples the need is for the toxicologist and immunologist working together to follow the nature and extent of the specific immune response and to detect or exclude other actions on immunity and autoimmunity and other major physiological controls and responses in the body. Because of the depth to which immune response mechanisms can now be affected and the ways in which they can be steered, there must also be just as much toxicological interest in showing whether there has been any broader effect on the immune status of the host than the intended therapeutic response, such as immuno-activation potentially leading to allergy, to autoimmunity due to an epitope shared between the vaccine antigen and a normal body component, or to impairment of the mechanisms that control tolerance.

The need to specify what is present and how well it exhibits the desired therapeutic action as well as to exclude or minimize any potentially harmful components has not changed, but the power of modern manufacturing and analytical techniques makes it necessary to specify in ever greater detail the nature and actions of the therapeutic agent and other substances present in the medicine. It is now important not just to seek conventional impurities and degradation products but also more complex biological variants in aminoacid sequence or peptide structure, glycosylation pattern, lipid conjugates, and so forth. The inherent variability in physiological production of complex molecules must be considered as we have begun to realize that cells are not sites of precise syntheses but rather biochemical factories in which manufacture is always likely to be affected by changing physiological factors both in normal cells in the healthy or diseased body and in manufacturing fermentation vats. In turn, that drives the preclinical testing to look ever more broadly on a case-by-case basis at what can be evaluated, always balanced against the question of what is worth doing because of our knowledge of the therapeutic agent and the manufacturing process. Coordination with pharmacodynamic and pharmacological investigations of the intended therapeutic activity must be close to ensure that the appropriate information is obtained, no matter from which set of experiments, without duplication of effort or resources.

In development the same types of major questions always remain to be answered in appropriate preclinical studies, even if the nature of those experiments has changed as greater understanding and more searching techniques have enabled more precise or more specific questions to be asked. This generalization can be illustrated by the history of the industrial production of interferon and antilymphocyte antibody.

Early manufacture of interferon-α (IFNα-2) was based on its extraction and purification from the supernatant of tissue cultured cells followed by partial biochemical characterization of the protein and particular reliance on assay of antiviral activity. The toxicologist's approach was greatly limited by the species specificity of the therapeutic effects and the immunogenicity of the human-type protein in other species. Preclinical testing was focused on broad changes in leukocyte numbers, certain specific biochemical markers of interferon effects on those cells, and subtle changes in the histological appearances of lymphoid organs. Subsequent advances in knowledge of how that type of interferon acted on certain types of cells has permitted more specific and sensitive examination of particular subtypes of cells, investigation of relevant receptors, assay of the physiological responses of those cells to certain stimuli and of changes in cytokine-mediated and other innate and reactive humoral and cellular defense mechanisms at the cell and whole body levels. Corresponding work at the genomic and metabonomic levels has characterized the extent and time relationships of those types of responses and the body's counterresponses.

Investigation now of a novel interferon of this type prior to its clinical study is likely to include characterization at the molecular and cellular levels of detailed actions and reactions, assessment of the effects on such basic body mechanisms as phagocytosis, cytokine secretion, amplification of cellular responses, and metabolic changes in the liver and perhaps elsewhere and their consequences for the responses to antigens, infections, and tumors, as well as changes in circulating acute phase proteins and immunoglobulins, antibody and immune complex formation and their consequences, and so on. In other words, the effects of treatment on physiological and biochemical mechanisms and cellular and organ systems will be studied at various levels at the same time as various host-response mechanisms and more conventional "toxic" actions, such as fever and changes in liver function. This represents application of the principles now dignified as "systems biology" to preclinical toxicological investigation.

Antilymphocyte globulins present a similar picture of the evolution of preclinical studies from relatively simplistic investigations focused on what was known of the nature and mechanisms of immune responses and graft rejection to more profound exploration of the nature and intensity of effects on immunological mechanisms and their consequences for the host response to grafts, tumors, infectious agents of diverse types, and the normal control of tolerance. The early toxicological studies were based on broad surveillance of haematological and pathological effects in species able to respond to an antihuman antibody, whereas today the depth of investigations would be greatly increased, quantification would be more important, and the range of effects examined would probably be expanded to include more on changes in specific mechanisms and on the likely shorter and longer term consequences of the type of immune suppression produced, as well as any general actions of the antibody formulation.

Both of these instances also exemplify the problem of species selection in any in vivo studies and of the origin of cells used in in vitro work. Initially there might have been relief at finding almost any species that could respond to the agent to be investigated from the small range suitable for toxicological experiments. That pragmatic choice now would need to consider conventional species as well as knockout and knock-in mice expressing human transgenes, other animals bearing grafts of human cells, and spontaneous genetic variants mimicking human diseases as well as human or other cells and tissues in long-term cultures or ex vivo.

As discussed below, the toxicologist's job has always been to ask the same broad questions of any biopharmaceutical product. But both the precision and the breadth of those queries and the ways in which they can be answered have been greatly expanded by the increasing knowledge of biology and pathology.

THE BASIC QUESTIONS IN PRECLINICAL TESTING

A number of primary questions are to be asked and answered by preclinical testing of new products, and sometimes to be applied to existing medicines as new problems are uncovered and novel procedures become available.

1 What Is the Purpose of the Proposed Preclinical Investigations?

This question covers both the main and associated purposes of studies. Does the principal interest lie in acquiring new information for scientific purposes (e.g., generally for learning more about the actions and reactions that might follow clinical administration of the substance to humans or animals), is the goal to study the mechanisms of known or anticipated actions and their consequences, or is it to provide scientifically valid and regulatorily acceptable data are to support formal clinical studies and eventual registration of the product?

Even on their own these are profound issues in the development of any product, but they have very particular implications for the difficult processes of formal pharmaceutical development, clinical trial, and marketing authorization of the full range of biopharmaceuticals. The answers will define major features of how the experimental work is done and the resources required to do it.

2 What Preclinical Studies Should Be Done?

This overlaps with the answer to Question 1, but it goes much further into assessment of the scientific rationale underlying the product, the availability of appropriate background biological, chemical, and pharmaceutical information, consideration of the nature and state of the human or animal patients who will eventually be treated with it, and a definite decision whether the results are needed for product registration or other regulatory purposes. The latter defines the need for and consequences of the application of GLP and GMP requirements.

There must be considerable overlap here between the basic "pharmacodynamic and pharmacological" experimentation, which has shown why the intended product may be of therapeutic value and the mechanisms of that desired activity, and the range of investigations that it is necessary and worthwhile to apply in the types of preclinical studies usually labeled as "toxicology," here including pharmacokinetics.

Available information about the mechanism of the therapeutic action and about the nature of the disease needs to be broadly reviewed. Relevant information from the spontaneous disease in human and animal populations and from analogous genetic disorders and from knockin and knock-out animal models should be taken into account at this stage.

The primary purpose of preclinical investigations is usually to focus on potential toxic or other harmful effects and to understanding their causes in ways that will guide safer use in patients. The opportunity to make more basic observations (e.g., of physiological mechanisms or aspects of immune response processes) should always be exploited provided the primary purpose of the studies is not jeopardized. Although it has been uncommon, observations in toxicity testing have sometimes suggested a new therapeutic use for a product.

The feasibility of informative experiments, whether in vitro or, if necessary, in vivo will depend mainly on the availability of model systems that are sufficiently well understood, and the coverage of the broad types of investigation, as in conventional toxicity experiments where the objective is to try to detect any effect and subsequently to decide whether it is "toxic" or "pharmacological". The need to explore such major features as the concentration–response or dose–response relationship, speed of onset, duration of action and reversibility of effects and their upstream and downstream consequences on other physiological mechanisms, potential interactions with the physiological and pathophysiological status of the patient, and other treatments administered at the same time, will all affect the nature and number of the most relevant experiments.

Two particularly important factors influencing the entire pattern of experimentation at this stage are the availability of in vitro or in vivo systems in which the therapeutic material can exert its specific effect. For example, if the product is directed at a target in human cells, are there other species and other cell types in which it is represented and has a similar activity so that the particular activity can be examined? And, as the majority of biopharmaceuticals are likely to be immunogenic in foreign species if the immune response cannot be avoided, are there means available to follow it and its immediate and later consequences for the administered substance and for any spillover possibly affecting physiological mechanisms dependent on an antigenically related substance (e.g., an endogenous physiological growth factor or cytokine)? If a product has an appropriate target, might it affect the mechanisms that prevent autoimmune disease most of the time?

Answering these questions before planning detailed preclinical investigations is essential because the decisions will define many of the investigations that should be done. It is not a simple task because of the need to collate biological, pharmacological, immunological, and pathological information from a variety of different systems and species.

A further difficulty may arise when the regulatory and other legal needs for the results of the preclinical studies are considered. It may appear simpler just to ask what are the current guidelines for formal studies and to do all those experiments regardless of the nature of the test substance, its properties, and its intended uses. That pathway of naive experimentation is likely to be highly damaging and very expensive because it will probably generate large amounts of uninterpretable information that will confuse the experimenters and obscure the sorts of data the regulators and others need to make the formal and critical evaluation of potential efficacy and safety that should be the sole purpose of "regulatory toxicology." Before planning any preclinical experiment or program of studies intended to support a new product, or in assessing the results obtained, the essential questions that all should answer remain: What scientific questions are being asked at this stage and why? What are the most appropriate methods to answer them? And, how can those experiments be done to provide the largest amount of the most reliable information? It is only when there are satisfactory and clear answer's to those questions that effective and efficient experimental investigations can be designed.

From time to time those considerations will suggest that there is no directly applicable experimental model in vitro or in vivo of the biological or pathological mechanism that should be explored. Perhaps the process is insufficiently well understood or no suitable in vitro or animal model has yet been validated? In such cases, as in trying to avoid the problems caused by an immune response in a heterologous species, in addition to reviewing the evidence from nature's own experiments in disease and genetic disorders, critical consideration should be given to developing and studying the corresponding homologous factor or process in appropriate cell systems or another species. Investigation of analogous factors and processes can be very helpful, but interpretation of the findings and their extrapolation to the target species requires assessment of whether what is being studied has the same role and properties in different biological systems.

There is always the need in preclinical studies, as in any biological experiments, to be aware that many factors may influence the results, not all of which can be controlled. Biological systems are so complex that variation and seemingly chance effects always arise, particularly when the broad endpoints in toxicological investigations are considered, since they have largely been selected because of their responsiveness to a wide range of potential actions. Critical assessment and careful correlation of different types of evidence is as necessary in investigating biopharmaceuticals as in dealing with the NCEs. The former may be designed to have much more specific actions than the latter, but the possibility always exists of chance effects as well as of unanticipated actions. Both such chance effects must be considered and distinguished.

3 How Are the Results to Be Interpreted and Used?

The limiting factors in interpretation and extrapolation from the laboratory to the patient include all those common to preclinical studies of small-molecule products plus some specific to biopharmaceuticals.

Once it is certain that the appropriate studies have been done and that reliance can be placed on the results, the typical considerations comprise species specificity or generalizability of effects seen or not detected, the concentration–response or dose–response relationship, the duration and durability of effects, reversibility of the therapeutic and any adverse actions, whether the findings have been affected by an immune or counterregulatory response in the test system, and the nature and physiological state of the patients to be treated. As biotechnology products become more potent and more intrusive in their actions on fundamental biological mechanisms, it is necessary also to consider the relationship between the effect detected in the experiments, the underlying mechanism, and what its consequences might be in the target species, possibly at a different stage of biological development.

The principles underlying extrapolation from the laboratory system to the human or animal patient for biopharmaceuticals are much the same as those for conventional NCEs, apart from the ever present possibility of an immunological or other biological counterresponse to administration of the product. The preclinical investigator of a product of biotechnology has the difficult but satisfying task, therefore, of deciding whether the most appropriate substance has been studied, whether the experiments done have really been relevant to the intended purpose of the work, and how the effects seen or not detected can be used to predict the probable safety of its use in sick patients under various clinical circumstances. At the same time the value of the studies done or not done will have to be justified in regulatory and other legal procedures, the case for accepting the work as appropriate to support clinical application of the product will have to be argued, and the implications for the resources, cost, and duration of development will have to be justified.

The opening quotation from that great baseball philosopher offers a pithy summary of the problems of the preclinical scientist in this area. It lacks only mention of the excitement and pleasure of solving them.

Preclinical Safety Evaluation of Biopharmaceuticals: A Science-Based Approach to Facilitating Clinical Trials, edited by Joy A. Cavagnaro
Copyright © 2008 by John Wiley & Sons, Inc.

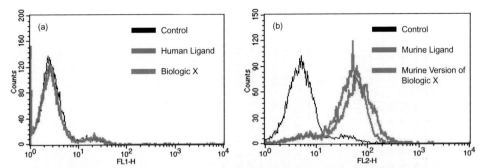

Figure 9.7 Evaluation of biopharmaceutical X binding to mouse bone marrow derived cells. (*a*) Biopharmaceutical X binding to mouse bone marrow-derived cells was evaluated using flow cytometry. Mouse cells were incubated with biopharmaceutical X or the human ligand. Secondary antibodies that cross-reacted with both biopharmaceutical X and the natural human ligand were used to detect binding. Cells were stained with the secondary antibodies only, to detect non-specific binding (control). (*b*) Bone marrow derived mouse cells were stained as described above with a murine version of biopharmaceutical X and the murine ligand for the receptor. Secondary antibodies that cross-reacted with the murine version of biopharmaceutical X and the murine ligand were used to detect binding.

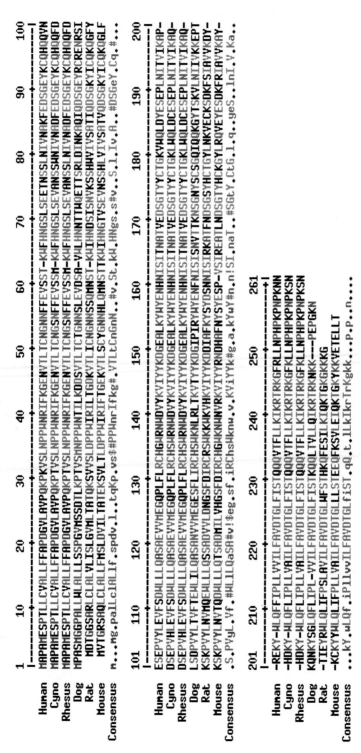

Figure 9.11 Alignment FcεRI-alpha chain protein sequences across species. Human, mouse, rat, dog, cynomolgus macaque, and rhesus macaque protein sequences coding for the alpha chain of the IgE receptor (FcεRI) were aligned and compared. Residues that are identical in all six species are highlighted in red. Residues common to more than half the sequences are listed in blue, and residues found to be identical in half the sequences or less are shown in black.

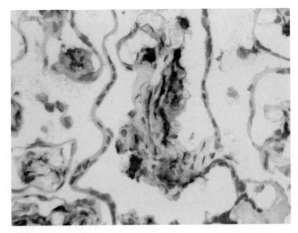

Figure 10.4 FcγR1 in human placenta. CD64 staining of Hofbauer cells and perivascular monocyte/macrophages and dendritic cells. No staining of placental trophoblast epithelium or endothelium.

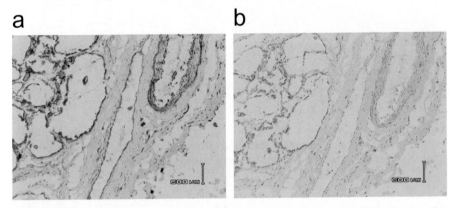

Figure 10.5 (*a*) Unexpected broad-spectrum cross-reactivity with epithelium, endothelium and selected vascular smooth myocytes. No staining of interstitial (stromal) cells, collagen, or nuclei. (*b*) No staining in replicate sections stained by negative control antibody at similar staining concentration.

a

b

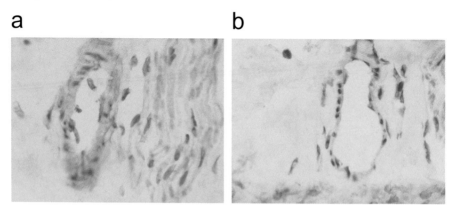

Figure 10.6 (*a*) Unexpected narrow-spectrum cross-reactivity with contractile filaments in vascular smooth myocytes. No staining of interstitial (stromal) cells, collagen,
nuclei, or adjacent peripheral nerve. (*b*) No staining in replicate sections stained by
negative control antibody at similar staining concentration.

a

b

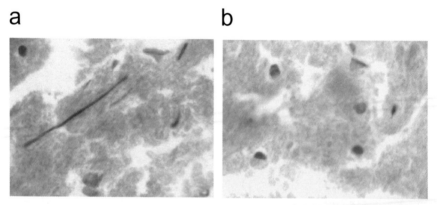

Figure 10.7 (*a*) Unexpected narrow-spectrum cross-reactivity with axons in human
brain. No staining of neural tissue components. (*b*) No staining in replicate sections
stained by negative control antibody at similar staining concentration.

a

b

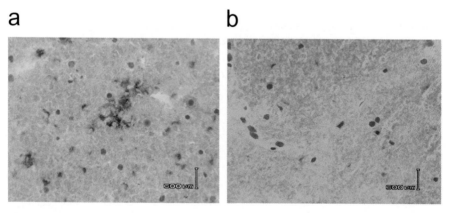

Figure 10.8 (*a*) Unexpected narrow-spectrum cross-reactivity with glial cells in dorsal
tracts of human spinal cord. Clustering of glial cells might indicate a very small glial
scar. No staining of neural tissue components. (*b*) Greatly reduced cross-reactivity with
glial cells in ventral tracts of human spinal cord.

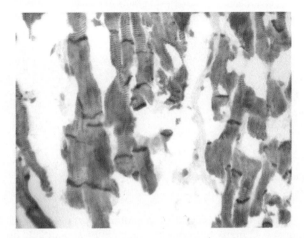

Figure 10.9 Unexpected cross-reactivity with contractile filaments (cross-striations, intercalated discs) in cardiac myocytes. No staining of sarcolemmal cells, interstitial cells or endothelium.

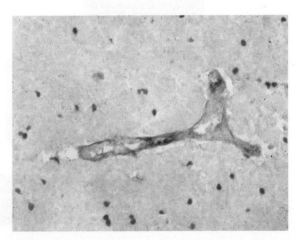

Figure 10.10 Staining of endothelium of human cerebral gray matter with chimeric antibody to a colon carcinoma antigen. The same endothelial staining pattern occurred in cynomolgus monkey cerebral gray matter. ABC Immunoperoxidase.

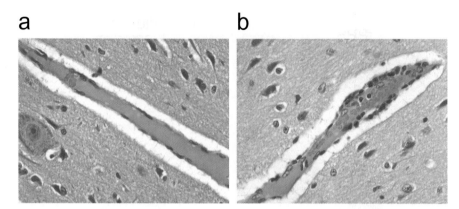

Figure 10.11 Vessels in the cerebral gray matter of control (*a*) and dosed (*b*) of cynomolgus monkey 72 hours following IV injection of an antibody directed against colon carcinoma. Note the leukocytes adherent to the endothelium characteristic of ADCC.

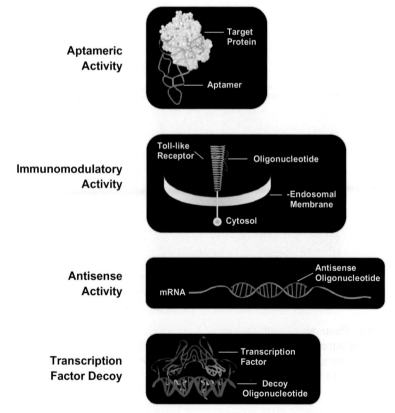

Figure 24.1 Cartoon depicting the mechanism of action of oligonucleotide molecules for aptameric interactions with proteins, interactions with specific receptors of the innate immunity, target mRNAs through hybridization, and transcriptional activators as transcription decoys. Note siRNA works through a hybridization dependent mechanism as depicted for antisense.

PBS

Immunostimulatory
ODN

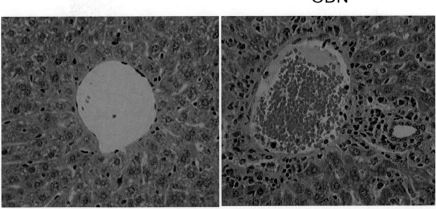

Figure 24.2 Photomicrograph of the renal cortex of a monkey treated with 40 mg/kg/wk for 5 weeks with a typical second generation 20-mer oligonucleotide modified with methoxyethyl groups on the 5 residues at each terminus. Stained with hematoxylin and eosin. The arrows point toward basophilic granules in the cells of the proximal convoluted tubules that are abundant throughout the renal cortex at this dose.

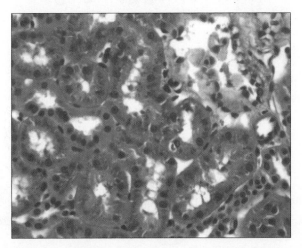

Figure 24.3 Photomicrograph of sections of liver from female CD-1 mice treated by subcutaneous injection with either saline (PBS) or an immunostimulatory oligodeoxynucleoitde at 4 mg/kg ever other day for 1 week. Lymphohystiocytic infiltrates are apparent adjacent to the central vein in the section from the ODN-treated mouse.

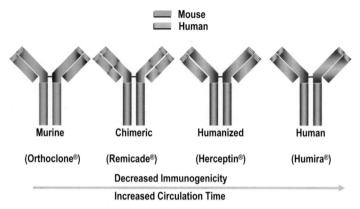

Figure 26.1 Structure of a monoclonal antibody and its interaction with antigen.

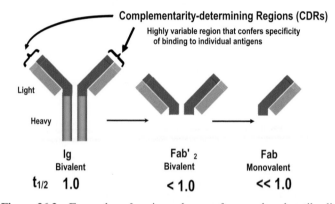

Figure 26.2 Examples of various classes of monoclonal antibodies.

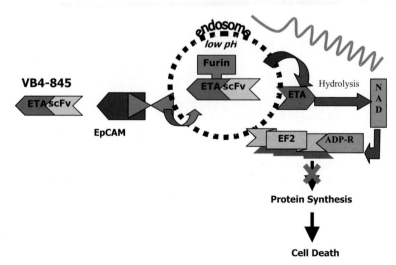

Figure 29.1 Mechanism of action of VB4-845.